James J. Nora M.D

IMMUNOLOGICAL DISEASES

IMMUNOLOGICAL DISEASES

Max Samter, M.D., *Editor*
Harry L. Alexander, M.D., *Associate Editor*

Section Editors: David W. Talmage, M.D., Bram Rose, M.D., William B. Sherman, M.D., John H. Vaughan, M.D.

With 89 Contributing Authors

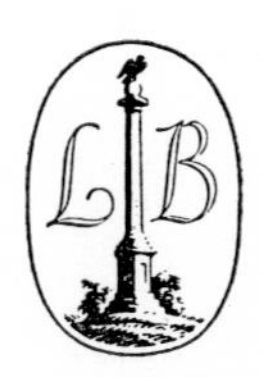

LITTLE, BROWN AND COMPANY
Boston

LIBRARY OF CONGRESS CATALOG CARD NO. 65-22424

Second Printing

Published in Great Britain
by J. & A. Churchill Ltd., London

PRINTED IN THE UNITED STATES OF AMERICA

Preface

It might be suggested that, in time, the amount of knowledge needed before a new discovery could be made would become so great as to absorb all the best years of a scientist's life, so that by the time he reached the frontier of knowledge he would be senile. I suppose this may happen some day, but that day is certainly very distant. In the first place, methods of teaching improve. Plato thought that students in his academy would have to spend ten years learning what was then known of mathematics; nowadays any mathematically minded schoolboy learns much more mathematics in a year.—BERTRAND RUSSELL*

AS THIS BOOK GOES TO PRESS, IT IS comforting to quote a paragraph from Bertrand Russell's essay, which places our intentions into proper perspective. What justifies the effort which goes into a textbook as comprehensive as *Immunological Diseases?* The problem, for all of us, is time. So that it seems only fair to hope that the hours that we have invested are hours saved for those who, "not yet senile," are absorbed in endeavors related to ours and that, to paraphrase Bertrand Russell's sentence, "the immunologically minded scholar will learn much more immunology in a year."

Immunological Diseases, an idea entertained at the Third International Congress of Allergology in Paris, has grown slowly. It took five years and six months to convert a carefree sketch into a formal volume. During periods of discomfort and doubt, Fred Belliveau—friend, counselor, manager of the publisher's medical department—kept assuring us that delays are reasonable and, perhaps, normal for a textbook of this size.

At times we have asked ourselves: "How long will it be before the book is out of date?" We do not feel that obsolescence is imminent, but the answer is as uncertain, of course, as the rate of progress in the investigative efforts reported in the chapters of the book. Approaches to therapy—an obligatory part of a textbook that deals with diseases—occupy only a fraction of the available space but might well prove to be the most vulnerable fraction. After all, no less a philosopher than Francis Bacon concluded that "books must follow sciences, not sciences books."

Some chapters present "pure" science, but the volume has its teleological moments. Authors are bound to inquire whether some of the "factors" and "antibodies" that accompany immunological diseases are misguided responses of cells or serve a purpose that still eludes us. Such inquiries are legitimate and should be encouraged, and we are siding, in this respect, with Kant rather than with Goethe. Questions are simple, but immunology has lost its innocence. Recent advances are sophisticated and complex both in concept and methodology, but the excitement of the search for answers is apparent in many chapters, including some that deal with comparatively common techniques and procedures.

The semantics of allergy and applied immunology have growing pains which have been recognized by the editorial board. The editorial alternatives are obvious; after considering briefly the possible advantages of unified terminology, the editorial board agreed that contributors should be allowed to use their own familiar terms, but should define their meaning clearly so that they could be compared with the terms of other chapters. In order to facilitate comparison, however, of different designations, with the same meanings, of immunoglobulins and their components, we have added (on page xxi) "Notes on Nomenclature" which summarizes the current and proposed usage of terms.

Immunological Diseases has omissions. It would be unrealistic to expect a balanced presentation in a field in which the state of our knowledge is so uneven. The editorial board agreed on basic design, reflected in the allocation of space, but as the book grew, the

* "The Science To Save Us from Science," *The New York Times Magazine,* March 19, 1950.

temperament and skill of our authors accomplished occasional unforeseen shifts in emphasis. Some omissions are deliberate: Air pollution and toxic reactions to chemicals (which might simulate immunological diseases) have not been covered in individual chapters, even though they have attracted considerable attention in recent years. Eosinophilic diseases of the lung are mentioned in various chapters but have not been given a chapter of their own. Some omissions are probably due to lack of editorial judgment. Finally, some omissions, such as twilight areas where the empirical and experimental views on immunological diseases are at odds, simply betray lack of information. Most of these instances have been singled out in editorial introductions and footnotes supplementing the text.

Overlapping—of paragraphs, of parts of chapters, or even of entire chapters—became one of our major editorial headaches. Even so, the editorial board felt that the discussion of the same subject by two different authors is not always undesirable. Strong opinions and occasional differences in interpretation are quite helpful in mapping uncharted territory. The editorial board has welcomed controversy and has tried to present both sides of controversial issues. Since one of the objectives of the textbook is to serve as reference for the many who are attracted to basic and applied immunology, most of the bibliographies are extensive.

It is a privilege to express the thanks of the editorial board to our contributors, who shared our burden, listened patiently to comments and suggestions, revised and rewrote willingly to integrate their specific contributions into the overall design of *Immunological Diseases.* If the correspondence between members of the editorial board and between editors and authors could be made part of the book (which is clearly impractical), it would show how much we have learned from one another. We trust that we have made more friends than enemies.

After the last of our eighty-one chapters had been forwarded to the publishers, we were aware of a feeling of wonder, "how wide the horizons . . . ", and of detached appraisal, "how much remains to be done." And we remembered two lines of Walt Whitman's "Song of Myself" with which we would like to send the book on its way:

> A child said What is the grass? fetching it to me with full hands.
> How could I answer the child? I do not know what it is any more than he.

M. S.

Contents

SECTION I. IMMUNOLOGY OF ATOPIC DISEASES

SECTION II. DIAGNOSTIC PROCEDURES AND FACTORS WHICH COMPLICATE DIAGNOSIS

SECTION III. ALLERGIC RHINITIS

SECTION IV. BRONCHIAL ASTHMA

SECTION V. APPROACHES TO TREATMENT OF ATOPIC DISEASES

SECTION VI. SYMPTOMATIC THERAPY

SECTION VII. ALLERGIC DISEASES OF THE SKIN; REACTIONS TO SERUM, DRUGS, AND INSECTS

SECTION VIII. OTHER DISEASES CAUSED BY ATOPY

SECTION IX. HYPERSENSITIVITY TO PHYSICAL AGENTS

PART FOUR: DISEASES WITH IMMUNOLOGICAL FEATURES

John H. Vaughan, Editor

SECTION I. DISEASES OF THE CONNECTIVE TISSUES

SECTION II. SPECIFIC ORGAN DISEASES

Contributing Authors

Harry L. Alexander, M.D.

EMERITUS PROFESSOR OF CLINICAL MEDICINE, WASHINGTON UNIVERSITY SCHOOL OF MEDICINE, ST. LOUIS

Carl E. Arbesman, M.D.

ASSOCIATE CLINICAL PROFESSOR OF MEDICINE AND ASSISTANT CLINICAL PROFESSOR OF BACTERIOLOGY AND IMMUNOLOGY, STATE UNIVERSITY OF NEW YORK AT BUFFALO, THE SCHOOL OF MEDICINE, BUFFALO

K. Frank Austen, M.D.

ASSOCIATE IN MEDICINE, HARVARD MEDICAL SCHOOL; ASSISTANT PHYSICIAN, MASSACHUSETTS GENERAL HOSPITAL, BOSTON

Domingo M. Aviado, M.D.

ASSOCIATE PROFESSOR OF PHARMACOLOGY, DIVISION OF GRADUATE MEDICINE, SCHOOL OF MEDICINE, UNIVERSITY OF PENNSYLVANIA, PHILADELPHIA

Rudolf L. Baer, M.D.

PROFESSOR AND CHAIRMAN, DEPARTMENT OF DERMATOLOGY, NEW YORK UNIVERSITY SCHOOL OF MEDICINE, NEW YORK

Richard F. Bakemeier, M.D.

ASSISTANT PROFESSOR OF MEDICINE, UNIVERSITY OF ROCHESTER SCHOOL OF MEDICINE AND DENTISTRY, ROCHESTER

Eugene V. Barnett, M.D.

ASSOCIATE PROFESSOR OF MEDICINE, UNIVERSITY OF CALIFORNIA, LOS ANGELES SCHOOL OF MEDICINE, LOS ANGELES

Ray F. Beers, Jr., M.D.

CLINICAL ASSISTANT PROFESSOR OF MEDICINE, UNIVERSITY OF ILLINOIS COLLEGE OF MEDICINE, CHICAGO

William H. Beierwaltes, M.D.

PROFESSOR OF INTERNAL MEDICINE, COORDINATOR, NUCLEAR MEDICINE UNIT, AND DIRECTOR, THYROID RESEARCH LABORATORY, UNIVERSITY OF MICHIGAN MEDICAL SCHOOL, ANN ARBOR

R. E. Billingham, D.Sc., F.R.S.

PROFESSOR AND CHAIRMAN, DEPARTMENT OF MEDICAL GENETICS, UNIVERSITY OF PENNSYLVANIA MEDICAL SCHOOL, PHILADELPHIA

Diana R. Bogdonoff, M.D.
ASSISTANT IN DERMATOLOGY, UNIVERSITY OF ILLINOIS COLLEGE OF MEDICINE, CHICAGO

Dan H. Campbell, Ph.D., Sc.D.
PROFESSOR OF IMMUNOCHEMISTRY, CALIFORNIA INSTITUTE OF TECHNOLOGY, PASADENA

Charles L. Christian, M.D.
ASSOCIATE PROFESSOR OF MEDICINE, COLUMBIA UNIVERSITY COLLEGE OF PHYSICIANS AND SURGEONS, NEW YORK

Henry N. Claman, M.D.
ASSISTANT PROFESSOR OF MEDICINE, UNIVERSITY OF COLORADO SCHOOL OF MEDICINE, DENVER

Leighton E. Cluff, M.D.
PROFESSOR OF MEDICINE, THE JOHN HOPKINS UNIVERSITY SCHOOL OF MEDICINE, BALTIMORE

Edward P. Cohen, M.D.
ASSOCIATE PROFESSOR OF MICROBIOLOGY, INSTITUTE OF MICROBIOLOGY, RUTGERS UNIVERSITY, NEW BRUNSWICK

Sydney Cohen, M.D., Ph.D.
READER IN IMMUNOLOGY, ST. MARY'S HOSPITAL MEDICAL SCHOOL, LONDON, ENGLAND

Frank J. Dixon, M.D.
HEAD, DIVISION OF EXPERIMENTAL PATHOLOGY, SCRIPPS CLINIC AND RESEARCH FOUNDATION, LA JOLLA

William E. Ehrich, M.D.
PROFESSOR AND CHAIRMAN, DEPARTMENT OF PATHOLOGY, DIVISION OF GRADUATE MEDICINE, SCHOOL OF MEDICINE, UNIVERSITY OF PENNSYLVANIA, PHILADELPHIA

Herman N. Eisen, M.D.
PROFESSOR AND CHAIRMAN, DEPARTMENT OF MICROBIOLOGY, WASHINGTON UNIVERSITY SCHOOL OF MEDICINE, ST. LOUIS

Alan R. Feinberg, M.D.
ASSOCIATE IN MEDICINE, NORTHWESTERN UNIVERSITY MEDICAL SCHOOL, CHICAGO; ASSISTANT DIRECTOR, ALLERGY RESEARCH LABORATORY, EVANSTON HOSPITAL, EVANSTON

Samuel M. Feinberg, M.D.
EMERITUS PROFESSOR OF MEDICINE, NORTHWESTERN UNIVERSITY MEDICAL SCHOOL, CHICAGO; DIRECTOR, ALLERGY RESEARCH LABORATORY, EVANSTON HOSPITAL, EVANSTON

Stuart C. Finch, M.D.
ASSOCIATE PROFESSOR OF MEDICINE, YALE UNIVERSITY SCHOOL OF MEDICINE, NEW HAVEN

Charles W. Fishel, Ph.D.

PROFESSOR OF MICROBIOLOGY, UNIVERSITY OF LOUISVILLE SCHOOL OF MEDICINE, LOUISVILLE

Frank W. Fitch, Ph.D., M.D.

ASSOCIATE PROFESSOR OF PATHOLOGY, UNIVERSITY OF CHICAGO, THE SCHOOL OF MEDICINE, CHICAGO

Samuel O. Freedman, M.D.

ASSOCIATE PROFESSOR OF MEDICINE, MCGILL UNIVERSITY FACULTY OF MEDICINE, MONTREAL, CANADA

Arnold P. Friedman, M.D.

ASSOCIATE PROFESSOR OF CLINICAL NEUROLOGY, COLUMBIA UNIVERSITY COLLEGE OF PHYSICIANS AND SURGEONS, NEW YORK

Lorraine Friedman, Ph.D.

PROFESSOR OF MICROBIOLOGY (MYCOLOGY), TULANE UNIVERSITY SCHOOL OF MEDICINE, NEW ORLEANS

Michael L. Furcolow, M.D.

PROFESSOR OF EPIDEMIOLOGY, DEPARTMENT OF COMMUNITY MEDICINE, UNIVERSITY OF KENTUCKY COLLEGE OF MEDICINE, LEXINGTON

Ann E. Gabrielsen, M.A.

RESEARCH FELLOW, PEDIATRICS, UNIVERSITY OF MINNESOTA MEDICAL SCHOOL, MINNEAPOLIS

Frank H. Gardner, M.D.

ASSOCIATE CLINICAL PROFESSOR OF MEDICINE, HARVARD MEDICAL SCHOOL, BOSTON

Justine S. Garvey, Ph.D.

SENIOR RESEARCH FELLOW, DIVISION OF CHEMISTRY AND CHEMICAL ENGINEERING, CALIFORNIA INSTITUTE OF TECHNOLOGY, PASADENA

Robert A. Good, Ph.D., M.D.

AMERICAN LEGION MEMORIAL HEART RESEARCH PROFESSOR OF PEDIATRICS AND MICROBIOLOGY, UNIVERSITY OF MINNESOTA MEDICAL SCHOOL, MINNEAPOLIS

Russell Clark Grove, M.D.

CHIEF OF OTOLARYNGOLOGY AND CHIEF RHINOLOGIST, INSTITUTE OF ALLERGY, ROOSEVELT HOSPITAL, NEW YORK

L. Gyenes, Ph.D.

HELEN HAY WHITNEY RESEARCH FELLOW, DEPARTMENT OF CHEMISTRY, AND LECTURER, DEPARTMENT OF MEDICINE AND CLINICAL MEDICINE, MCGILL UNIVERSITY FACULTY OF MEDICINE, MONTREAL, CANADA

Stanley F. Hampton, M.D.

ASSISTANT PROFESSOR OF CLINICAL MEDICINE, DIRECTOR OF ALLERGY CLINIC, WASHINGTON UNIVERSITY SCHOOL OF MEDICINE, ST. LOUIS

Leonard C. Harber, M.D.

ASSOCIATE PROFESSOR, DEPARTMENT OF DERMATOLOGY, NEW YORK UNIVERSITY SCHOOL OF MEDICINE, NEW YORK

Halsted R. Holman, M.D.

PROFESSOR OF MEDICINE, STANFORD UNIVERSITY SCHOOL OF MEDICINE, PALO ALTO

John H. Humphrey, M.D., F.R.S.

DIVISION OF IMMUNOLOGY, NATIONAL INSTITUTE FOR MEDICAL RESEARCH, LONDON, ENGLAND

Kimishige Ishizaka, M.D.

ASSISTANT PROFESSOR OF MICROBIOLOGY, UNIVERSITY OF COLORADO SCHOOL OF MEDICINE; RESEARCH DIRECTOR, CHILDREN'S ASTHMA RESEARCH INSTITUTE AND HOSPITAL, DENVER

Harold L. Israel, M.D., M.P.H.

CLINICAL PROFESSOR OF MEDICINE, JEFFERSON MEDICAL COLLEGE OF PHILADELPHIA, PHILADELPHIA

Joseph E. Johnson, III, M.D.

ASSISTANT PROFESSOR OF MEDICINE, THE JOHNS HOPKINS UNIVERSITY SCHOOL OF MEDICINE, BALTIMORE

Joseph Barnett Kirsner, M.D., Ph.D.

PROFESSOR OF MEDICINE, UNIVERSITY OF CHICAGO, THE SCHOOL OF MEDICINE, CHICAGO

Henry G. Kunkel, M.D.

PROFESSOR, THE ROCKEFELLER INSTITUTE, NEW YORK

John P. Leddy, M.D.

ASSISTANT PROFESSOR OF MEDICINE, UNIVERSITY OF ROCHESTER SCHOOL OF MEDICINE AND DENTISTRY, ROCHESTER

Irwin H. Lepow, M.D., Ph.D.

ASSOCIATE PROFESSOR OF EXPERIMENTAL PATHOLOGY, INSTITUTE OF PATHOLOGY, WESTERN RESERVE UNIVERSITY, SCHOOL OF MEDICINE, CLEVELAND

Francis C. Lowell, M.D.

ASSISTANT PROFESSOR OF MEDICINE, HARVARD MEDICAL SCHOOL; CHIEF, ALLERGY UNIT, DEPARTMENT OF MEDICINE, MASSACHUSETTS GENERAL HOSPITAL, BOSTON

James A. McLean, M.D.

ASSOCIATE PROFESSOR OF INTERNAL MEDICINE, UNIVERSITY OF MICHIGAN MEDICAL SCHOOL, ANN ARBOR

Mart Mannik, M.D

CLINICAL ASSOCIATE, NATIONAL INSTITUTE OF ARTHRITIS AND METABOLIC DISEASES, NATIONAL INSTITUTES OF HEALTH, BETHESDA

A. S. Markowitz, Ph.D.

HEAD, IMMUNOCHEMISTRY LABORATORY, HEKTOEN INSTITUTE FOR MEDICAL RESEARCH OF COOK COUNTY HOSPITAL, CHICAGO

Kenneth P. Mathews, M.D.

PROFESSOR OF INTERNAL MEDICINE, UNIVERSITY OF MICHIGAN MEDICAL SCHOOL, ANN ARBOR

A. Edward Maumenee, M.D.

PROFESSOR OF OPHTHALMOLOGY, THE JOHNS HOPKINS UNIVERSITY SCHOOL OF MEDICINE, BALTIMORE

John P. Merrill, M.D.

ASSOCIATE CLINICAL PROFESSOR OF MEDICINE, HARVARD UNIVERSITY MEDICAL SCHOOL; DIRECTOR, CARDIORENAL SECTION, PETER BENT BRIGHAM HOSPITAL, BOSTON

Elliott Middleton, Jr., M.D.

ASSOCIATE IN MEDICINE, COLUMBIA UNIVERSITY COLLEGE OF PHYSICIANS AND SURGEONS, NEW YORK

Daniel G. Miller, M.D.

HEAD, LYMPHOMA SECTION, DIVISION OF CLINICAL CHEMOTHERAPY, SLOAN-KETTERING INSTITUTE FOR CANCER RESEARCH, NEW YORK

Harry Louis Mueller, M.D.

CLINICAL ASSOCIATE IN PEDIATRICS, HARVARD MEDICAL SCHOOL; CHIEF, DIVISION OF ALLERGY, CHILDREN'S HOSPITAL MEDICAL CENTER, BOSTON

Philip S. Norman, M.D.

ASSOCIATE PROFESSOR OF MEDICINE, THE JOHNS HOPKINS UNIVERSITY SCHOOL OF MEDICINE, BALTIMORE

Sidney Olansky, M.D.

PROFESSOR OF MEDICINE (DERMATOLOGY), EMORY UNIVERSITY SCHOOL OF MEDICINE, ATLANTA

Elliott F. Osserman, M.D.

ASSOCIATE PROFESSOR OF MEDICINE, COLUMBIA UNIVERSITY, COLLEGE OF PHYSICIANS AND SURGEONS, NEW YORK

Kermit E. Osserman, M.D.

CLINICAL ASSOCIATE IN MEDICINE, COLUMBIA UNIVERSITY COLLEGE OF PHYSICIANS AND SURGEONS; ASSOCIATE ATTENDING PHYSICIAN AND CHIEF, MYASTHENIA GRAVIS UNIT, THE MT. SINAI HOSPITAL, NEW YORK

Charles W. Parker, M.D.

ASSISTANT PROFESSOR OF MEDICINE, WASHINGTON UNIVERSITY SCHOOL OF MEDICINE, ST. LOUIS

Philip Y. Paterson, M.D.

ASSOCIATE PROFESSOR OF MEDICINE, DEPARTMENT OF MEDICINE, NEW YORK UNIVERSITY SCHOOL OF MEDICINE; CAREER SCIENTIST OF THE HEALTH RESEARCH COUNCIL OF THE CITY OF NEW YORK, NEW YORK

Carl M. Pearson, M.D.

ASSOCIATE PROFESSOR OF MEDICINE, UNIVERSITY OF CALIFORNIA SCHOOL OF MEDICINE, LOS ANGELES

Raymond D. A. Peterson, M.D.

ASSISTANT PROFESSOR OF PEDIATRICS, UNIVERSITY OF MINNESOTA MEDICAL SCHOOL; ESTABLISHED INVESTIGATOR, AMERICAN HEART ASSOCIATION, MINNEAPOLIS

David Pressman, Ph.D.

DIRECTOR OF CANCER RESEARCH IN BIOCHEMISTRY, ROSWELL PARK MEMORIAL INSTITUTE, NEW YORK STATE DEPARTMENT OF HEALTH, BUFFALO

Sidney Raffel, M.D.

PROFESSOR OF MEDICAL MICROBIOLOGY, STANFORD UNIVERSITY SCHOOL OF MEDICINE, STANFORD

Ben Z. Rappaport, M.D.

PROFESSOR OF MEDICINE, UNIVERSITY OF ILLINOIS COLLEGE OF MEDICINE, CHICAGO

A. J. Rhodes, M.D., F.R.C.P.E., F.R.S.C.

DIRECTOR, SCHOOL OF HYGIENE, UNIVERSITY OF TORONTO, CANADA

Gerald P. Rodnan, M.D.

ASSOCIATE PROFESSOR OF MEDICINE, UNIVERSITY OF PITTSBURGH SCHOOL OF MEDICINE, PITTSBURGH

Bram Rose, M.D., Ph.D., F.R.S.C.

PROFESSOR OF EXPERIMENTAL MEDICINE, MCGILL UNIVERSITY FACULTY OF MEDICINE; ROYAL VICTORIA HOSPITAL, MONTREAL, CANADA

Geoffrey A. Rose, M.A., D.M., M.R.C.P.

SENIOR LECTURER TO THE MEDICAL UNIT, ST. MARY'S HOSPITAL MEDICAL SCHOOL; SENIOR LECTURER IN EPIDEMIOLOGY, LONDON SCHOOL OF HYGIENE AND TROPICAL MEDICINE, LONDON, ENGLAND

Noel R. Rose, M.D., Ph.D.

ASSOCIATE PROFESSOR OF BACTERIOLOGY AND IMMUNOLOGY AND ASSISTANT PROFESSOR OF MEDICINE, STATE UNIVERSITY OF NEW YORK AT BUFFALO, THE SCHOOL OF MEDICINE, BUFFALO

Adolph Rostenberg, Jr., M.D.

PROFESSOR OF DERMATOLOGY, UNIVERSITY OF ILLINOIS COLLEGE OF MEDICINE, CHICAGO

K. R. Rozee, Ph.D.

ASSOCIATE PROFESSOR, DEPARTMENT OF MICROBIOLOGY, SCHOOL OF HYGIENE, UNIVERSITY OF TORONTO, TORONTO, CANADA

Elvio H. Sadun, Sc.D.

CHIEF, DEPARTMENT OF MEDICAL ZOOLOGY, DIVISION OF COMMUNICABLE DISEASES AND IMMUNOLOGY, WALTER REED ARMY INSTITUTE OF RESEARCH, WALTER REED ARMY MEDICAL CENTER, WASHINGTON, D.C.

Max Samter, M.D.

PROFESSOR OF MEDICINE, UNIVERSITY OF ILLINOIS COLLEGE OF MEDICINE, CHICAGO

Paul M. Seebohm, M.D.

PROFESSOR OF INTERNAL MEDICINE AND DIRECTOR, ALLERGY SECTION, STATE UNIVERSITY OF IOWA COLLEGE OF MEDICINE, IOWA CITY

A. H. Sehon, Ph.D.

PROFESSOR OF CHEMISTRY, MCGILL UNIVERSITY; BIOPHYSICAL CHEMIST, MCGILL UNIVERSITY MEDICAL CLINIC, MONTREAL GENERAL HOSPITAL, MONTREAL, CANADA

John M. Sheldon, M.D.

PROFESSOR OF INTERNAL MEDICINE, UNIVERSITY OF MICHIGAN MEDICAL SCHOOL, ANN ARBOR

William B. Sherman, M.D.

ASSOCIATE CLINICAL PROFESSOR OF MEDICINE, COLUMBIA UNIVERSITY, COLLEGE OF PHYSICIANS AND SURGEONS, NEW YORK

Willys K. Silvers, Ph.D.

ASSOCIATE PROFESSOR OF MEDICAL GENETICS, UNIVERSITY OF PENNSYLVANIA MEDICAL SCHOOL, PHILADELPHIA

Charles E. Smith, M.D., D.P.H.

DEAN, SCHOOL OF PUBLIC HEALTH, UNIVERSITY OF CALIFORNIA, BERKELEY

Wesley William Spink, M.D.

PROFESSOR OF MEDICINE, UNIVERSITY OF MINNESOTA MEDICAL SCHOOL, MINNEAPOLIS

Lisa A. Steiner, M.D.

FELLOW OF THE HELEN HAY WHITNEY FOUNDATION, DEPARTMENT OF MICROBIOLOGY, WASHINGTON UNIVERSITY SCHOOL OF MEDICINE, ST. LOUIS

Arthur J. L. Strauss, M.D.

HEAD, SECTION ON AUTOIMMUNITY, LABORATORY OF IMMUNOLOGY, NATIONAL INSTITUTE OF ALLERGY AND INFECTIOUS DISEASES, NATIONAL INSTITUTES OF HEALTH, BETHESDA

Scott N. Swisher, M.D.

PROFESSOR OF MEDICINE AND HEAD, HEMATOLOGY UNIT, UNIVERSITY OF ROCHESTER SCHOOL OF MEDICINE AND DENTISTRY, ROCHESTER

Andor Szentivanyi, M.D.

ASSISTANT PROFESSOR OF MEDICINE AND MICROBIOLOGY, UNIVERSITY OF COLORADO SCHOOL OF MEDICINE, DENVER

David W. Talmage, M.D.

PROFESSOR OF MICROBIOLOGY, UNIVERSITY OF COLORADO SCHOOL OF MEDICINE, DENVER

Frederick H. Theodore, M.D.

ASSOCIATE CLINICAL PROFESSOR OF OPHTHALMOLOGY, NEW YORK UNIVERSITY SCHOOL OF MEDICINE; ATTENDING OPHTHALMIC SURGEON, THE MT. SINAI HOSPITAL, NEW YORK

Thomas T. B. Tomasi, Jr., M.D.

ASSOCIATE PROFESSOR OF EXPERIMENTAL MEDICINE, UNIVERSITY OF VERMONT COLLEGE OF MEDICINE, BURLINGTON

Jonathan W. Uhr, M.D.

ASSOCIATE PROFESSOR OF MEDICINE, NEW YORK UNIVERSITY SCHOOL OF MEDICINE; DIRECTOR, IRVINGTON HOUSE INSTITUTE FOR RHEUMATIC FEVER AND ALLIED DISEASES, NEW YORK

John H. Vaughan, M.D.

PROFESSOR OF MEDICINE, UNIVERSITY OF ROCHESTER, SCHOOL OF MEDICINE AND DENTISTRY, ROCHESTER

Jan Waldenström, M.D.

PROFESSOR OF INTERNAL MEDICINE, UNIVERSITY OF LUND; HEAD, DEPARTMENT OF MEDICINE, GENERAL HOSPITAL, MALMÖ, SWEDEN

Robert W. Wissler, Ph.D., M.D.

PROFESSOR OF PATHOLOGY, UNIVERSITY OF CHICAGO, THE SCHOOL OF MEDICINE, CHICAGO

Ernest Witebsky, M.D.

DISTINGUISHED PROFESSOR OF BACTERIOLOGY AND IMMUNOLOGY, STATE UNIVERSITY OF NEW YORK AT BUFFALO, THE SCHOOL OF MEDICINE, BUFFALO

Notes on Nomenclature

DURING THE ERA OF RAPID IDENTIfication of new immunoglobulins, their nomenclature (by necessity) was arbitrary; attempts have been made to simplify and to standardize this nomenclature.

The latest proposal of a distinguished ad hoc committee, sponsored by the World Health Organization, is a strong move toward the adoption of uniform terms. This abstract omits the reasons and some detail but lists the essential recommendations.*

The committee recognizes the symbol γ or the abbreviation Ig as appropriate designation for immunoglobulins. These symbols should be accompanied by a capital letter which indicates a specific class of immunoglobulins, but not by arabic numbers which have been used in the past to indicate electrophoretic mobilities.

The following symbols proposed for major classes of immunoglobulin molecules are based on differences in the structure of heavy chains.

Present usage	*Proposed usage*
γ, 7Sγ, 6.6Sγ, γ_2, γss	γG or IgG
β_2A (β_{2A}), γ_1A (γ_{1A})	γA or IgA
γ_1M (γ_{1M}), β_2M (β_{2M}), 19Sγ, γ-macroglobulin	γM or IgM

New immunoglobulins may be indicated by the symbol of the major class followed by a small Roman letter, e.g., IgAa, IgAb, etc.

The polypeptide chains which occur in immunoglobulins were formerly labeled L (or B) for light chains and H (or A) for heavy chains. It is proposed that the heavy chains be designated by small Greek letters corresponding to the Roman capital letters used for the immunoglobulin classes.

Immunoglobulin class	*Heavy chain*
γG or IgG	γ (gamma)†
γA or IgA	α (alpha)
γM or IgM	μ (mu)

* *Bull. WHO* 30:447–450, 1964.

† The choice of the symbol γ for the polypeptide chain is somewhat unfortunate, since γ now appears in two different senses. The committee is hopeful that ambiguity can be avoided (since γ is never used alone), but one wonder if this is a practical proposal.—Ed.

Two forms of light chain (type I and type II) occur in man. The World Health Organization has suggested that the following changes be made:

Present designation

Type I, I, B
Type II, 2, A

Proposed designation

Chain type	*Corresponding immunoglobulin type*
κ (kappa)	Type K
λ (lambda)	Type L

Distinctive proteins related to the immunoglobulins should be classified as "discrete components" or "pathological proteins" but should not be classified precisely in the absence of an appropriate clinical diagnosis. In patients with multiple myeloma or macroglobulinemia they should be termed: (a) G myeloma or A myeloma globulin; (b) M-macroglobulin (Waldenström); (c) light-chain protein or Bence Jones protein depending on the thermosolubility properties associated with them; (d) heavy-chain proteins with the appropriate class designation.

In animal sera the use of γM or IgM is recommended for a class of immunoglobulins with molecular weight of the order of magnitude of 10^6. In addition, other properties of the human γM or IgM—such as high carbohydrate content, dissociation by mercaptoethanol, and antigenic relationship—should be considered.

While it appears logical to extend the proposed terminology to genes and genotypes, identification of individual variants under genetic control has been limited until now to variants detected by serological reagents (Gm groups, allotypes). Progress in this area will require a joint effort of the various disciplines which are involved.

While this abstract does not make any claim to completeness, it illustrates some of the difficulties of classification. In a complex field nomenclature is bound to be complex. It is obvious that the proposal of the committee is only a beginning. It had hardly been published when Rowe and Fahey described, in addition to the γG, γM, and γA globulins, a fourth class, γD.* For a study of the proposed extension of nomenclature to additional classes and chains, to molecular models and to the designation of fragments produced by the cleavage of peptide bonds, readers are advised to consult the World Health Organization's original publication.

* *J. Exp Med.*, 121:185, 1965.

IMMUNOLOGICAL DISEASES

The History of Allergy

HARRY L. ALEXANDER

MOST IMMUNOLOGICAL DISEASES ARE identified with allergy as the term is used in its broadest sense. In this volume allergy has implications which are based on developments in immunology and experimental hypersensitivity as well as in clinical medicine. The history of this broad subject is far too comprehensive to encompass in a brief introductory chapter, and only significant events can be touched upon.

IMMUNOLOGY AND EXPERIMENTAL HYPERSENSITIVITY

Idiosyncrasies in man to foods and medicaments are mentioned in early medical literature. It was not until the last century, however, that several specific instances of experimental hypersensitivity were recorded. Ehrlich [1] cited Morgenroth's statement that it was Magendie who, in 1823, first clearly described the phenomenon. Magendie observed that rabbits tolerated an initial injection of albumin but later reacted to similar doses. Other isolated experiences with hypersensitivity were published subsequently, but with one exception [2] they were not explored extensively until 1890. In that year Robert Koch reported the first experimental studies of allergy to the tubercle bacillus, which came to be known as the Koch phenomenon. Koch [3] observed that although the first injection of tubercle bacilli into the guinea pig caused no immediate response, a similar injection into an infected animal was followed promptly by an inflammatory reaction at the site of the puncture. In some manner the initial exposure had prepared the way for the phenomenon observed on reinjection.

In similar circumstances, with use of other injectable materials, violent reactions began to be recorded. Flexner [4] in 1894 observed that rabbits tolerated the first injection of dog serum but, on reinjection some weeks later, even with smaller doses, they died promptly. In 1895, von Behring [5] pointed out that the guinea pig inoculated with diphtheria toxin became very sensitive to it. He called the phenomenon a "paradoxical reaction" but did not consider it a general response among animals.

In 1898, Charles Richet [6] observed that dogs given injections of eel serum reacted violently on reinjection, but he did not study the response until a few years later. Then, in 1902, with Portier [7] he produced similar effects with Actinaria, marine creatures. Until then, there had been an established principle that the introduction of infectious products (cowpox, rabies vaccine, diphtheria toxin) into man and animal induced immunity—protection from harm—and was prophylactic. Richet and Portier's observations indicated that the initial injections were followed by an effect opposite from prophylaxis, namely, anaphylaxis—without protection.

In 1903, Arthus [8] observed that whereas initial inoculations of horse serum into the rabbit were well tolerated, reinjection after a suitable interval induced immediate shock, as had been known. If, however, the serum were given subcutaneously at intervals of six days, the repeated injections caused increasing local infiltration and only eventually skin necrosis. Arthus interpreted this phenomenon as local anaphylaxis.

In the same year, Hamburger and Moro [9] demonstrated precipitins to horse serum in the blood of individuals some days after they had received the serum. Moreover, the appearance of symptoms coincided with the time that the antibody first could be detected. Two years later, immunological reactions in serum disease were elaborated upon in the classic monograph *Die Serumkrankheit* by Clemens von Pirquet and Bela Schick [10], for this was a period when serum disease became prevalent as antitoxins came into wide clinical use.

Koch's demonstration of the tuberculin-type of hypersensitivity, Richet and Portier's studies of anaphylaxis, the Arthus phenomenon, and the immunological mechanisms that were assumed to mediate the symptoms of serum disease served as foundations upon which much of the concept of hypersensitivity subsequently was built.

Von Pirquet recognized that the introduction of a foreign substance such as an infectious agent into the tissues may alter their capacity to react to subsequent applications of the same material. In 1906, he coined a word for this process, *allergie,* from the Greek terms *allos* (other) and *ergon* (action) [11]. Von Pirquet related such tissue alterations not only to hypersensitivity but also to immunity as it applies to other changes associated with antigenic stimulation. Nevertheless, *allergy* through usage came to be oriented to hypersensitivity, at first in a manner not clearly defined, but later it acquired a specific designation in that it is now the official term for hypersensitivity in standard medical indexes.

By the year 1906 a great interest in hypersensitivity had developed. This was concerned almost entirely with its experimental aspects, and in the following few years a large fund of information about it was published both in this country and abroad. Otto [12] and Friedmann [13] in Germany, Doerr and Russ [14] in Switzerland, Nicolle [15] and Besredka [16] in France, and Theobald Smith, Auer, Wells, and many others in the United States were among the eminent investigators identified with this era. Their observations confirmed earlier ones that in hypersensitivity, antigen-antibody complexes are involved.

Among many areas of research at that time, one that attracted particular attention was related to the underlying mechanisms responsible for anaphylactic shock. Various experiments indicated that the symptoms could be simulated by injections of products of enzymatic digestion of proteins and other substances. Then, Friedberger [17] in 1909 injected into guinea pigs extracts derived from an antigen-antibody complex formed *in vitro* and with them induced typical anaphylactic shock. The product responsible for this phenomenon was referred to as anaphylatoxin. The significance of these early observations is indicated by the continual search through the ensuing years for other substances responsible for the manifestations of hypersensitivity.

Friedberger's humoral theory of circulating toxins soon was challenged by the classic experiments of Schultz [18] in 1910 and of Dale [19] in 1913. These investigators demonstrated that contraction of smooth muscle, a prominent manifestation of anaphylaxis, occurred in sensitized tissue on contact with antigen in the absence of blood. The cellular theory of anaphylaxis thus was introduced. Dale reproduced the muscle contraction by applying histamine, and he suspected that this substance, released from tissues, mediated the reaction of anaphylaxis.

The release of preformed chemical substances in a wide variety of circumstances (transmission of nerve impulses, vagotonia, stress, etc.), at the time called autopharmacology, had a particular orientation to hypersensitivity. The possible role of histamine in this regard became strengthened over the years and was established in 1932 by Bartosch and his associates [20] when they recovered histamine in the perfusate of a sensitized guinea pig lung that had been exposed to specific antigen. Further confirmation, after the introduction of a method for quantitative analysis of histamine by Barsoum and Gaddum [21] in 1935, stimulated research along broad lines [22–25]. Two discoveries of particular note were the identification of the mast cell as the chief repository for preformed histamine [26] and the identification of a number of substances that release histamine from these cells [27, 28].

The pioneer studies of antihistamine substances by Fourneau, Bovet [29], Halpern [30], and Staub [31] were of immense importance, for aside from their therapeutic value they provided more accurate methods for histamine research. Another chemical mediator of hypersensitivity, slow-reacting substance, was discovered by Feldberg and Kellaway [32] in 1938. In time, there followed the identification of other mediators—serotonin, bradykinin, and other plasma kinins. (See Chap. 15.)

Another important area in the developing concepts of allergy has been the passive transfer of hypersensitivity. The earliest relevant record of this phenomenon was the observation by Ehrlich [33] in 1892 that immunity could be transferred by a mother to her fetus as well as during suckling. Then, in 1907, both Otto [12] and Friedmann [13], working independently, transferred anaphylaxis from a sensitized animal to a normal one. The transfer of allergy by blood transfusion [34] in 1919 was soon followed by the classic demonstration by Prausnitz and Küstner [35] that serum from an allergic individual could sensitize skin sites of normal subjects. Landsteiner and Chase [36] demonstrated that hypersensitivity could be transferred by cells by passing peritoneal cells from a sensitized animal to a normal one. A factor thereby was conveyed which permitted the normal animal to react to the sensitizing antigen. The revelation of similar transfer from man to man by leukocytes [37] and the identification of lymphocytes with the transfer of antibody in the experimental animal greatly extended the understanding of hypersensitivity.

A milestone in the history of allergy was the demonstration by Landsteiner [38] that simple chemical compounds (haptens) by conjugating with proteins *in vivo* could become complete antigens and thus induce hypersensitivity. This observation established a new principle in antigen structure and antibody response.

In 1928, Shwartzman [39] described a reaction similar to that of the Arthus phenomenon. Injection of certain bacterial filtrates into the skin of a rabbit caused intense inflammation if the filtrate were reinjected intravenously some 24 hours later. Sanarelli [40] a few years previously had observed profound visceral lesions in rabbits given intravenous injections of sublethal doses of cholera *Vibrios* and later given injections of a small number of colon bacilli. Although these experiments held considerable interest at the time, the discovery that endotoxins are antigenic has focused renewed attention on the so-called Shwartzman-Sanarelli phenomenon which may prove to represent an important immunological development.

In a historical account of experimental allergy, mention should be made of many significant contributions by dermatologists who utilized skin reactions as a means of reflecting both local and systemic sensitization in a wide area of research.

The history of changing concepts of antibody structure, of homografts, and of many other aspects of immunology and experimental hypersensitivity must be deferred for lack of space to the chapters that follow.

CLINICAL ALLERGY

Bronchial asthma was described in the Third Century B.C., and many accounts of it have appeared in subsequent years. Hay fever was recognized as early as the Sixteenth Century, but clinical investigation of allergy dates from the historic publication of Blackley [2] in 1873. Although many years previously hay fever had been found to be due to volatile matter from plants, Blackley reproduced the lesion only in those who had had the disease, by applying specific plant products to the nasal mucosa. Moreover, he induced skin reactions in such patients by rubbing the same material into the scarified epidermis.

The year 1894 marked two historic events. Jadassohn, the founding father of dermatological allergy, described the patch test; and Behring's introduction of diphtheria antitoxin that year was followed shortly by a report of skin eruptions after injection of this material contained in horse serum [41]. In 1895, Johannessen [42] demonstrated that horse serum without antitoxin, when given to nondiphtheritic individuals, produced the same effect. Other manifestations of serum disease then became recognized, and in 1906, Rosenau and Anderson [43] showed that sudden death following the administration of antitoxin was due to the horse serum alone. By that time, hay fever, serum disease, and drug reactions were recognized as the outstanding examples of clinical hypersensitivity.

In 1910, Meltzer [44] noted the similarity of the emphysematous lung of the guinea pig in anaphylactic shock to that of bronchial asthma. He suggested that asthma might be an expression of anaphylaxis. In 1912, Schloss [45] published an account of a child who was intolerant to certain foods. Schloss prepared extracts of various constituents of these foods with which he made superficial skin tests and elicited specific reactions. By this time several investigators sensed the possibility of a broad application of hypersensitivity to clinical medicine.

In these early years, there came a recognition that asthma, hay fever, and urticaria, which long had been known to be somehow associated, were all expressions of hypersensitivity. This was a significant advance in clinical medicine. An important factor that led to the acceptance of this concept was the concurrent demonstration by means of the skin test that the cause of symptoms could be revealed and treatment directed accordingly. It was soon apparent, however, that the clinical practice of allergy is a complex proceeding. Underlying immunological and pathological processes that mediate symptoms were poorly understood, and preparation of allergenic extracts and their testing was tedious. However, numerous physicians were attracted to this aspect of medicine. These were the first allergists, and they were largely self-taught.

In 1911, Noon [46] in England published one of the earliest clinical reports describing the successful treatment of hay fever with pollen extracts. This communication introduced techniques for the preparation of extracts as well as their standardization, testing for sensitivity, and principles of treatment.

Noon believed that the success of therapy was due to the production of an antitoxin, a theory predicated on experiments by Dunbar [47] reported several years previously. Dunbar contended that pollen contained a toxin and that antitoxin developed after its injection into horses. He called the antiserum Pollantin, which at the time became a popular remedy for hay fever. Dunbar's theory was widely held by many physicians who followed Noon's method of injections until 1917, when Cooke *et al.* [48] by animal experimentation demonstrated that the success of therapy was due not to antitoxin but to mechanisms of hypersensitivity.

By 1917, intradermal skin testing, improved methods for preparation and standardization of allergenic extracts, and the fact that asthma and hay fever had a hereditary predisposition had been established [49]. At first, various designations were applied to this new specialty: human hypersensitiveness, protein sensitization, anaphylaxis, and, only later, allergy. In 1929, the usage of that term is indicated in a statement by the editors of the *Journal of Allergy* which appeared on the frontispiece of the first issue. "In view of the differences of opinion of how the word 'Allergy' should be used, we believe it evident that it does not possess an established meaning in scientific usage. However, the term is generally employed by clinicians who apply it to conditions of specific hypersensitiveness exclusive of anaphylaxis in lower animals. Its sense in the title of this Journal corresponds to its current medical usage. . . ." This usage of the word persists, but it has become more inclusive as clinical interest in the wider applications of hypersensitivity has developed. In 1923, the type of allergic individual who has a hereditary background and who demonstrates an immediate type of skin reaction was classified by Coca and Cooke [50] in a particular group for which they coined the word *atopy*. In terms of clinical allergy as well as experimental hypersensitivity, this separation proved to be of great importance. (See Chap. 38.)

By this time, clinical allergy had become recognized as a medical specialty, and it engaged the interest of many investigators who produced important publications concerning both basic and clinical aspects. Between 1920 and 1930, the first allergy clinics were established in the United States, the first national allergy societies were organized, and the *Journal of Allergy* appeared. During the following two decades, clinical allergy expanded to invade many areas of medicine, but attention gradually was given to sorting out clinical experiences in order to separate allergy from other disorders for which, mistakenly, it was alleged to be responsible.

The forerunner of the concept of autoimmune disease dates back many years. Autoantibodies in man long had been identified, and periodic attempts to produce injury in various organs by injections of homologous tissue extracts had been successful occasionally. This was particularly true of brain tissue, and recognition of clinical encephalitis following injection of brain and cord material dates back to the time of Pasteur. A new era of tissue hypersensitivity began, however, with the appearance of Freund's adjuvants in 1942. By adding adjuvants to tissue antigens as described by Freund and McDermott [51], experimental diseases as encephalitis and thyroiditis, which have clinical counterparts, were produced. The coincidental appearance of tissue antibodies remains a subject of current controversy insofar as their role concerns pathogenesis [52].

Development of corticosteroids by Kendall in 1942 and their application to rheumatoid arthritis by Hench *et al.* [53] in 1949 was followed by demonstrations of their effectiveness in a variety of allergic disorders. This discovery was of great importance not only because these steroid drugs possess remarkable therapeutic effectiveness in many expressions of hypersensitivity but because they permit an insight into hormonal mechanisms that underlie allergic reactions.

For the past ten years or more, there has been a decided change in clinical allergy in that it has attracted world-wide interest and there has been a reorientation of attitude toward it. Penetration of interest in this subject is reflected in the representation of forty-one nations from all continents at the International Congress of Allergology held in 1958. At that conference, in a symposium on the status of allergy in many of these lands, accounts varied from a mere foothold to those of highly developed programs. The organization of numerous national allergy societies and regional congresses and appearance of new periodicals testify to the wide interest in allergic disorders.

A broadening of the viewpoint of many allergists appears to have been due in part to their increasing interest in basic immunological principles. The popularity of postgraduate instruction and symposia oriented to fundamental aspects of hypersensitivity, the change in emphasis in this direction in contributions to clinical journals, and the increasing number of research fellowships available and ample funds for their support are examples of this aroused interest.

During this period of reorientation on the part of the allergist, a similar change developed among immunologists. This was due to the recognition that many clinical disorders have immunological implications, and to the constantly increasing number of these that are recognized or suspected. The most common conditions of clinical allergy are bronchial asthma, hay fever, and urticaria, and as these are blended with other disorders of hypersensitivity, they come within the framework of immunological diseases. Thus the interest of the allergist in immunology and the attention of the immunologist to the wide applications of hypersensitivity have arrived on common ground.

Over the years, allergy has become a focal point for the convergence of several disciplines such as immunology, endocrinology, and pharmacology. The current trend to broaden the attitude toward clinical hypersensitivity which embraces a wide variety of clinical disorders corresponds to that which always has been held by microbiologists, immunologists, and physiologists toward its basic aspects. It should be pointed out, however, that such a broad conception of allergy by the medical profession at large, let alone by many allergists, remains far from realized. To promote understanding of it is the purpose of this book.

REFERENCES

1. Ehrlich, P., *et al. Studies in Immunity* (tr. by C. Bolduan) (2nd ed.). New York: John Wiley & Sons, 1910. P. 30.
2. Blackley, C. *Experimental Researches on the Causes and Nature of Catarrhus Aestivus.* London: Ballière, Tindall & Cox, 1873.
3. Koch, R. Weitere Mitteilungen ueber ein Heilmittel gegen Tuberkulose. *Deutsch. Med. Wschr.* 16:1029, 1890.
4. Flexner, S. The pathologic changes caused by certain so-called toxalbumins. *Med. News* 65: 116, 1894.
5. von Behring, E. Leistungen und Ziele der Serumtherapie. *Deutsch. Med. Wschr.* 21:623, 1895.
6. Héricourt, J., and Richet. C. Efféts lointans des injections de sérum de l'anguille. *C. R. Soc. Biol.* (Paris) 50:137, 1898.
7. Portier, P., and Richet, C. De l'action anaphylactique de certaines venins. *C. R. Soc. Biol.* (Paris) 54:170, 1902.
8. Arthus, M. Injections répétées de sérum de cheval chez le lapin. *C. R. Soc. Biol.* (Paris) 55:817, 1903.
9. Hamburger, F., and Moro, E. Ueber die biologisch nachweisbaren Veränderungen des menschlichen Blutes nach der Seruminjektion. *Wien. Klin. Wschr.* 16:445, 1903.
10. von Pirquet, C., and Schick, B. *Die Serumkrankheit.* Leipzig: Franz Deuticke, 1905.
11. von Pirquet, C. Allergie. *München. Med. Wschr.* 53:1457, 1906.
12. Otto, R. Zur Frage der Serum Ueberempfindlichkeit. *München. Med. Wschr.* 54:165, 1907.
13. Friedmann, U. Ueber passive Ueberempfindlichkeit. *München. Med. Wschr.* 54:2414, 1907.
14. Doerr, R., and Russ, V. Studien über Anaphylaxie: II. *Z. Immunitaetsforsch.* 2:109, 1908.
15. Nicolle, M. Contribution à l'étude du phénomène d'Arthus. *Ann. Inst. Pasteur* (Paris) 21:128, 1907.

16. Besredka, A. Du méchanisme de l'anaphylaxie. *Ann. Inst. Pasteur* (Paris) 22:446, 1908.
17. Friedberger, E. Kritik der Theorien über die Anaphylaxie. *Z. Immunitaetsforsch.* 2:208, 1909.
18. Schultz, W. H. Physiological studies in anaphylaxis: 1. *J. Pharmacol. Exp. Ther.* 1:549, 1910.
19. Dale, H. H. An anaphylactic reaction of plain muscle in the guinea pig. *J. Pharmacol. Exp. Ther.* 4:167, 1913.
20. Bartosch, R., Feldberg, W., and Nagel, F. Das Freiwerden eines histaminähnlichen Stoffes bei der Anaphylaxie des Meerschweinchens. *Pflueger. Arch. Ges. Physiol.* 230:129, 1932.
21. Barsoum, G. S., and Gaddum, J. H. Estimation of adenosine and histamine in blood. *J. Physiol.* (London) 85:1, 1935.
22. Dragsted, C. A., and Gebauer-Fuelnegge, E. Studies in anaphylaxis. *Amer. J. Physiol.* 102:512, 1932.
23. Code, C. F. The histamine content of the blood of guinea pigs and dogs during anaphylactic shock. *Amer. J. Physiol.* 127:78, 1939.
24. Rose, B. Blood and tissue histamine during rabbit anaphylaxis. *Amer. J. Physiol.* 129:450, 1940.
25. Roche e Silva, M. Anaphylaxis in the rabbit. *J. Immun.* 38:333, 1940.
26. Riley, J. F., and West, G. B. The presence of histamine in tissue mast cells. *J. Physiol.* (London) 120:528, 1953.
27. Paton, W. D. M. Compound 48/80 a potent histamine liberator. *Brit. J. Pharmacol.* 6:499, 1951.
28. Feldberg, W., and Smith, A. N. Release of histamine by tryptamine and 5-hydroxytryptamine. *J. Physiol.* (London) 122:62, 1953.
29. Bovet, D., Horclois, R., and Walthert, F. Propriétés antihistaminiques de les N-p-méthyloxybenzyl-N-diméthylaminoéthyl-a-amino-pyridine. *C. R. Soc. Biol.* (Paris) 138:99, 1944.
30. Halpern, B. N., and Ducrot, R. Recherches expérimentales sur une nouvelle série chemique de corps doués de propriétés antihistaminiques puissants les dérivés de la thiophénylamine. *C. R. Soc. Biol.* (Paris) 140:361, 1946.
31. Staub, A. M. Récherches sur quelques bases synthétique antagonistes de l'histamine. *Ann. Inst. Pasteur* (Paris) 63:400, 1939.
32. Feldberg, W., and Kellaway, C. H. Liberation of histamine and formation of a lysocithin-like substance by cobra venom. *J. Physiol.* (London) 94:187, 1938.
33. Ehrlich, P. Ueber Immunität durch Vererbung und Säugung. *Z. Hyg. Infektionskr.* 12:183, 1892.
34. Ramirez, M. A. Horse asthma following blood transfusion. *J.A.M.A.* 73:984, 1919.
35. Prausnitz, C., and Küstner, H. Studien ueber die Ueberempfindlichkeit. *Z. Bakt.* 86:160, 1921.
36. Landsteiner, K., and Chase, M. M. Experiments on the transfer of cutaneous hypersensitivity to simple compounds. *Proc. Soc. Exp. Biol. Med.* 49:688, 1942.
37. Lawrence, H. S. The cellular transfer of cutaneous hypersensivity to tuberculin in man. *Proc. Soc. Exp. Biol. Med.* 71:516, 1949.
38. Landsteiner, K. *The Specificity of Serological Reactions* (rev. ed.). Cambridge, Mass.: Harvard University Press, 1947.
39. Shwartzman, G. Studies on *Bacillus typhosus* toxic substances. *J. Exp. Med.* 48:247, 1928.
40. Sanarelli, A. De la pathogénie du choléra. *Ann. Inst. Pasteur.* (Paris) 38:11, 1924.
41. Lublinski, W. Ueber die Nachwirkung der Antitoxins bei Behandlung der Diphtherie. *Deutsch. Med. Wschr.* 20:857, 1894.
42. Johannessen, A. Ueber Injectionen mit antidiphtherischem Serum und reinen Pferdserum bei nicht diphtheriekranken Individuen. *Deutsch. Med. Wschr.* 20:855, 1895.
43. Rosenau, M., and Anderson, J. A study of the cause of sudden death following the injection of horse serum. *U.S. Pub. Health Ser. Lab. Bull.* No. 29, 1906.
44. Meltzer, S. Bronchial asthma as a phenomenon of anaphylaxis. *Trans. Ass. Amer. Physicians.* 25:66, 1910.
45. Schloss, O. A case of allergy to common foods. *Amer. J. Dis. Child.* 3:341, 1912.
46. Noon, L. The prophylactic inoculation against hay fever. *Lancet* 1:1572, 1911.
47. Dunbar, C. P. Zur Frage betreffend die Aetiologie und specifische Therapie des Heufiebers. *Berl. Klin. Wschr.* 40:537 and 569, 1903.
48. Cooke, R. A., Flood, E. F., and Coca, A. Hay fever: The nature of the process and of the mechanism of the alleviating effect of specific treatment. *J. Immun.* 2:217, 1917.
49. Cooke, R. A., and Vander Veer, A. Human sensitization. *J. Immun.* 1:201, 1916.
50. Coca, A., and Cooke, R. A. On the classification of the phenomenon of hypersensitiveness. *J. Immun.* 8:163, 1923.
51. Freund, J., and McDermott, K. Sensitization to horse serum by means of adjuvants. *Proc. Soc. Exp. Biol. Med.* 49:548, 1942.
52. Mackay, I. R., and Burnet, F. M. *Autoimmune Diseases: Pathogenesis, Chemistry and Therapy.* Springfield, Ill.: Charles C Thomas, Publisher, 1963.
53. Hench, P., Kendall, E. C., Slocumb, C. H., and Polley, H. F. Effect of hormone of adrenal cortex (17-hydroxy-11-dehydrocorticosterone) (compound E) and of pituitary adrenocorticotropic hormone on rheumatoid arthritis: Preliminary report. *Ann. Rheum. Dis.* 8:97, 1949.

PART ONE: BASIC IMMUNOLOGY

David W. Talmage, Editor

Rabbit ret. c. ribosomal RNA
↓
E Coli → Hgb

? Immune
Antigen originally foreign

SECTION I. ANTIGENS AND THE IMMUNE RESPONSE

1. The Nature of Antigen and Antibody Combining Regions

DAVID PRESSMAN

ANTIGENICITY

For a substance to be antigenic, it must give rise to circulating antibody or to some other type of immune response when injected into an animal. The term antigenic is relative, since response is frequently a property of the individual animal or species. Thus, although human serum albumin does not cause an antibody response in man, it induces a good response in nearly all other vertebrates. A large variety of substances stimulates the formation of antibodies when injected. Large molecules such as proteins, polysaccharides, polypeptides, and polynucleotides give rise to circulating antibodies which react with the homologous antigen. Also, a host of small molecules also gives rise to antibodies. For example, penicillin and picrylchloride cause sensitization. In such cases it appears that the sensitizing compound combines chemically with protein in order to be antigenic.

A great deal of effort has been devoted to determining whether substances free from protein can be antigenic. It is, perhaps, impossible to solve this problem, since there is always the possibility that injected substances react with protein prior to entering the mechanism for antibody formation. Small molecules which give rise to antibodies, whenever investigated, have been shown to couple to proteins and thus fulfill the protein requirement.

Most proteins, foreign to a species or an individual, are antigenic in that species or individual. Substances do not even have to be foreign to an individual in order to be antigenic. A large body of evidence shows that an animal can produce antibodies against his own constituents. Whether some alteration of the constituent is always induced initially is unknown.

GROUPS AGAINST WHICH ANTIBODIES ARE FORMED

In the case of large molecules such as the proteins, there are apparently many different regions on the molecule against which antibodies are formed. Individual antibody molecules react with the protein, but each reacts with only one type of region. Cross-reactions of an antiserum formed against one protein with a closely related protein are apparently due to the reaction of some of the antibodies with similar regions on both proteins. The same antiserum may contain antibodies which do not react with the second protein. These are apparently formed against groupings present only on the first protein. A classic example of this type of phenomenon is the cross-reaction of antibodies prepared in rabbits against hen egg albumin [1]. Some of the antibodies show extensive reaction with duck egg albumin, but other antibodies react only with hen albumin. The extent of cross-reaction has been particularly well studied in the case of serum albumins from several species [2]. In general, the albumins of phylogenically related species have more groups in common than the albumins of more distant species.

In the case of some protein molecules, for example, bovine serum albumin, it has been possible to split the protein into pieces and show that different fragments react with different groups of antibodies [3]. In the case of polysaccharides, small structural units are repeated many times within the same molecule. Consequently, the number of different antigenic groups against which antibodies are directed may be less than formerly believed [4]. Synthetic polypeptides have been useful in studying the nature of groups that are antigenic [5, 6].

The most precise information about antigenicity of groups and degrees of cross-reaction comes from studies involving antigens composed of proteins combined with small groups of known configuration. These small groups (or haptens) were originally studied by Obermayer and Pick [7] and by Landsteiner and Lampl [8]. When simple substances of known configuration are coupled to protein and injected, antibodies are formed which are directed against the hapten group. The unrelated carrier protein without the hapten does not cross-react with the antibodies being tested. The hapten itself, without being coupled to protein, reacts with these antibodies, as shown by its ability to inhibit precipitation of the antigen-antibody system, or by dialysis equilibrium experiments which show that the simple hapten is bound to antibody. (See Chap. 8.)

Antibodies can be formed against either charged or uncharged haptens. When antibodies are formed against charged haptens, the charge appears to play an important role in the combination. Antibodies have been formed against positively and negatively charged haptens, as for example, against the benzoate group and against the trimethylphenylammonium group. Antibodies have been formed against uncharged groups such as carbohydrate residues, hydrocarbon residues, and halogens. The antibodies formed against naturally occurring products are individually directed against small groupings. If these small groups are isolated, they will combine with the antibody. For example, dextrans are composed of glucose units, and antibodies against the large polysaccharide combine well with the small glucose polymers [9]. In the case of certain proteins, for example, silk fibroin, it has been possible to isolate a sequence of amino acids which combines well with the antibody, indicating that this is a primary sequence against which the antibody is formed [10].

FACTORS OF SPECIFICITY IN COMBINATION OF ANTIBODY WITH ANTIGEN

Closeness of Fit. Antibodies act as though they were formed against the corresponding antigen as a template [11]. The combining region of the antibody fits closely about a part of the surface of the antigenic molecule. A large part of the specificity of interaction is derived from this complementary fit of the antibody about specific groups on the inducing antigen. Only substances containing a group which will fit closely into the combining region of the antibody can combine with it. Other substances cannot, and this selectivity results in a specific reaction. The reason closeness of fit is required for interaction of antigen and antibody is that all of the forces involved are short range. Most of them are also weak and thus require that a fairly large portion of the antigen and antibody molecules come in close apposition.

Forces Involved in Reaction of Antibody with Antigen. Being able to fit together is not sufficient for a specific reaction to take place, since the molecules involved must also stick together strongly enough to avoid dissociation. The arrangement of groups of atoms in the antibody site is complementary to adjacent groups in the antigen, and the various interatomic forces between them provides the energy for holding the antigen and antibody together. The combination takes place not through a strong covalent chemical bond but rather through the weak short-range forces known to exist between various groups [12]. Because these forces are short range, the groups in the antibody site must be properly aligned so that they can interact with those on the antigen. This requirement provides a second factor which determines specificity, i.e., the arrangement of various groups in the antibody combining region.

The effective forces are (1) the electrostatic attraction between negative and positive charges, (2) interaction of permanent dipoles, (3) hydrogen bond formation, (4) van der Waals forces (London dispersion forces), and (5) interaction of nonpolar surfaces.

The charge interaction takes place between a negative or a positive charge on the antigen and the opposite charge on the antibody; similarly, permanent dipoles can contribute to the energy of interaction by proper alignment.

Hydrogen bonding between a proton donor on the antigen and an acceptor on the antibody, or the converse, contributes to the energy of interaction. The magnitude of the energy of interaction due to the formation of the hydrogen bond is tempered somewhat by the fact that the groups forming the bond are hydrated in aqueous solution prior to combination. Unless such groups can form a hydrogen bond during the combination of antibody with antigen, binding will not take place because too much energy would be required to remove the group from the hydrated state. If a hydrogen bond can be formed again in the combination of antigen and antibody, the large expenditure of energy is avoided.

The van der Waals attraction is due to dispersion forces which exist among all atoms owing to the fact that when two atoms approach each other closely, they undergo a mutual polarization with a resultant attractive force. The van der Waals attraction is the type of attraction between molecules which, in the case of a gas, for example, results in a deviation in properties from those predicted by the perfect gas laws.

Finally, when two nonpolar surfaces, one on the antigen and one on the antibody, are brought together, the total water-nonpolar interface is decreased. This results in an overall decrease in energy of the system and an apparent attraction between the nonpolar surfaces. The coalescence of oil drops in water is due to the same phenomenon.

In order for all of these forces to be effective, the interacting groups must be arranged in a complementary manner on the two combining regions so that these groups can come very closely together, essentially in contact. This makes for specificity in the reaction because antibody against one type of antigen will not react equally with another antigen, even though the shapes are identical, if the latter has a different distribution of groups in the combining region. Thus a negative charge on the antigen instead of a positive charge will result in repulsion rather than attraction when there is a negative charge in the combining region of the antibody.

HETEROGENEITY OF ANTIBODIES

Although antibodies act as though they were formed against the antigen as a template, all antibodies directed against a particular antigenic group are not necessarily identical. Antibody activity has been shown to be associated with different types of globulin. (See Chap. 3.) However, even antibodies of one protein type directed against a particular antigen group do not all have an identical combining region. A whole host of different kinds of combining regions can show specificity for the particular antigenic region. Thus, in the case of antibodies to the p-azobenzoate group (Fig. 1-1), the combining regions are formed in a large number of ways complementary to the surface of the benzoate group. All of these will react with this grouping. Antibody can be formed against the whole group or against any part of the surface and be quite strong in its interaction with this particular group.

The fit of the antibody around the hapten cannot be perfect in that the extent of complementariness is limited by the ability of the polypeptide chains of the antibody to orient closely around the antigenic structures. This in turn depends on the flexibility of the backbone and side groups of the polypeptide chain in the antibody molecule. The atoms of the antibody combining region are of the same size as the atoms composing the antigen, occupy space, and are bound to other atoms. Thus the degree to which a close complementary fit can be formed is limited (Fig. 1-2).

These factors of fit and energy of reaction for the combining regions of antigens and antibodies are general factors concerned in any biological interaction, as, for example, between enzyme and substrate.

STRUCTURAL FEATURES OF IMPORTANCE

Much information concerning the complementary nature, closeness of fit, and forces involved has been derived from the studies of antibodies against simple substances of known chemical and steric configuration. The structural features of importance can be evaluated by a study of the interaction of these antibodies with other haptens of known configuration related to the original one.

CLOSENESS OF FIT

As an example, antibodies formed against the p-azobenzoate group appear to fit closely around the van der Waals outline of the group, as shown in Figure 1-3 [13]. Benzoate ion itself combines quite well with this antibody. If a chlorine atom is substituted for a hydrogen atom in the para position, the hapten combines even more strongly than the unsubstituted benzoate. Apparently the chlorine

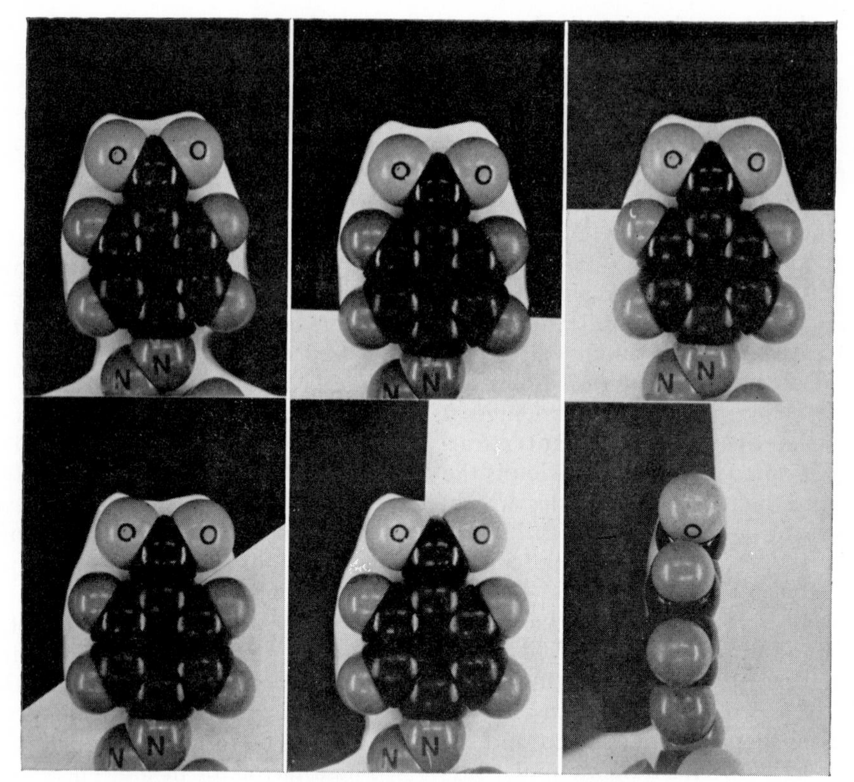

Fig. 1-1. Different degrees of fit of combining regions of anti-p-azobenzoate antibodies.

atom fits into the position occupied by the azo group of the immunizing hapten, is accommodated by this antibody, and provides increased interaction energy relative to the hydrogen atom. When the chlorine atom replaces a hydrogen atom ortho to the benzoate ion, the fit of antibody around the hydrogen group is so close that the larger size of the chlorine atom interferes with the combination. When the chlorine atom is in the meta position, there is

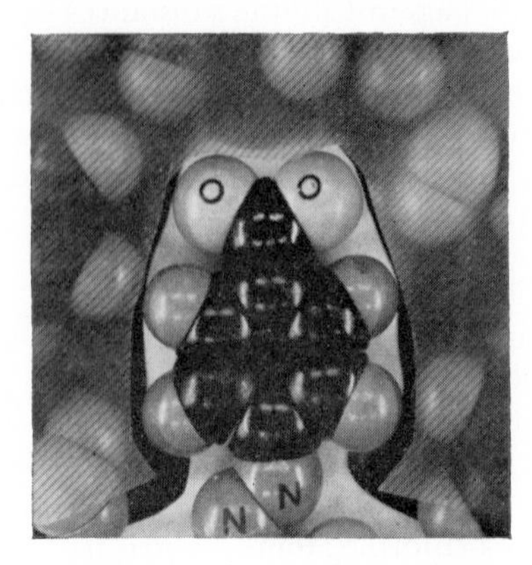

Fig. 1-2. Representation of the combining region of an anti-p-azobenzoate antibody showing atoms of which the antibody is composed.

some interference in the combination. Investigations of this nature show the very close fit of the antibody around the benzoate group.

As for the other structural features [13], the benzene ring plays an important role in the combination with anti-p-azobenzoate antibody. Replacement of a benzene ring by a methyl group to give acetate reduces the binding energy to a very low level. Displacement of the benzene ring by about 1.5 A by inserting a methylene group to give phenylacetate displaces it from its complementary position with respect to the carboxyl and combination does not take place. Similarly, replacement of the benzene ring by cyclohexane, which is somewhat thicker and does not have the polarizability of the benzene ring, causes a large decrease in combination energy. The benzene ring in proper orientation has been found to be very important in many hapten systems.

Antibodies against some haptens appear to fit more closely than do antibodies against other haptens. For example, antibodies against the p-azophenyltrimethylammonium group [14] and the p-(p′-azophenylazo)-phenylarsonate ion [15] seem to fit less closely around the haptens than do antibodies against the p-azo-

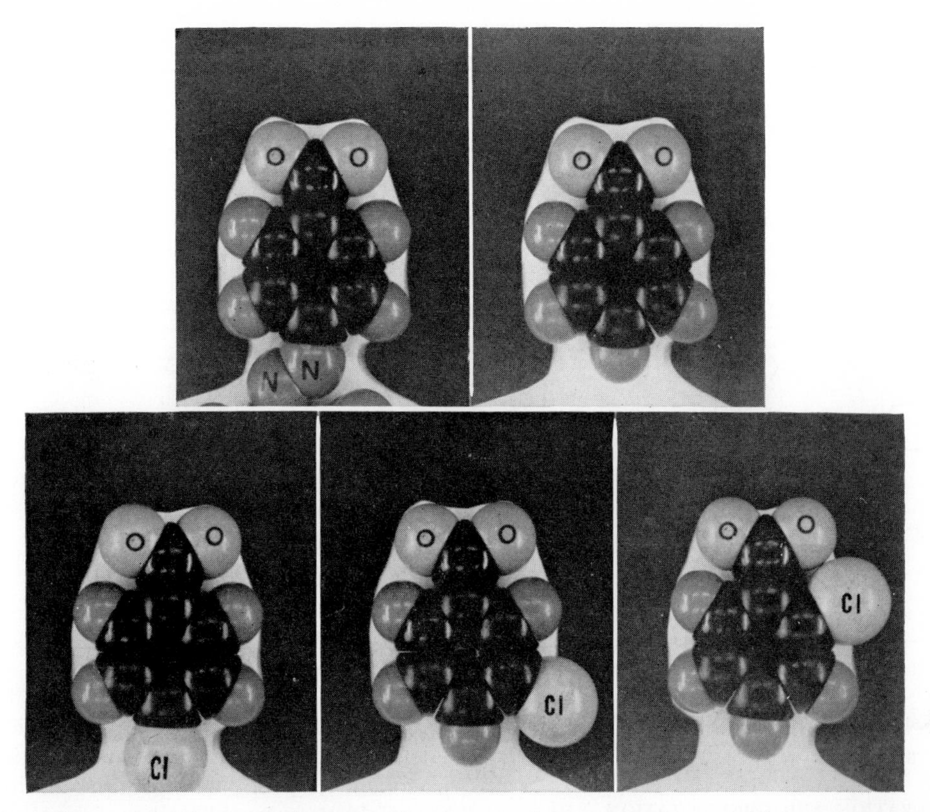

Fig. 1-3. Effect on fit of substitution of azobenzoate and benzoate into combining region of anti-p-benzoate antibody. A chloro group is accommodated in the para position but not in the ortho and meta positions due to steric hindrance.

benzenearsonate [16], the p-azobenzoate [13], or the p-(p-azophenylazo)-benzoate [17] antibodies. This is shown in Table 1-1, where it can be seen that meta- and ortho-methyl substituents do not interfere with the combination with the former antibodies but only with the latter. Indeed, alpha-naphthyl derivatives show increased combination with the former, whereas decreased combination is observed with the latter, indicating that some antibodies can accommodate large substituents on one side, while others cannot. The increase, where observed, is probably due either to increased van der Waals attraction of the naphthalene for the antibody or perhaps to water displacement.

CHARGE

When the antibody is formed against a charged group, the presence of the charge on the hapten is very important for combination. Thus antibody against benzoate shows essentially no combination with the nitrobenzene group in which the charged carboxylate of benzoate is replaced by an uncharged nitro group even though both groups have the same size [13]. Specificity for the nature of the charged group is shown by the fact that if the carboxylate is replaced by the charged groups sulfonate or arsonate, there is essentially no combination, apparently because these charged groups are too large to be accommodated by the antibody directed against the carboxylate grouping.

When there are two charged groups on the hapten and these are very close together, as the two carboxylate groups in the ortho-phthalate group [18], two charges are required on a cross-reacting hapten for strong combination to take place. A single charge as in o-nitrobenzoate is insufficient. In this system, the energy contribution of the charge interaction is so large that the rest of the structure of the hapten is of lesser importance. Thus substituents on the ring are more easily accommodated.

If the haptenic group is not charged, the other types of forces become important and

TABLE 1-1. Closeness of Fit in Various Para-azohapten Systems

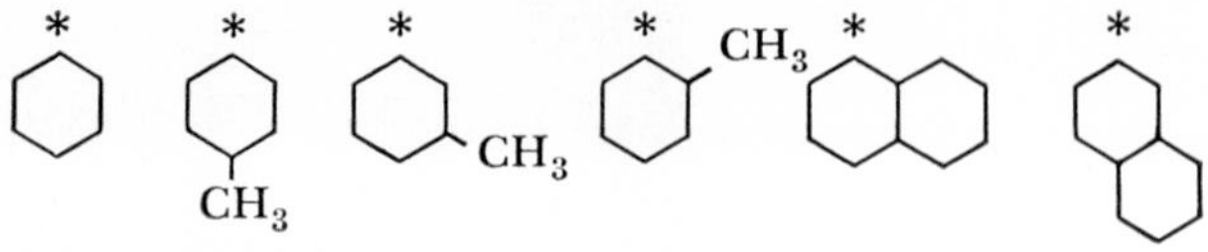

Hapten-specific Antibody	Hapten[a]: * (benzene)	* (benzene), CH_3 para	* (benzene), CH_3 meta	* (benzene), CH_3 ortho	* (naphthalene)	* (naphthalene)
	Relative Binding Constants					
$N=N$ ⬡ $N(CH_3)_3^+$	1.0	1.45	0.86	1.05	2.0	
$N=N$ ⬡ $N=N$ ⬡ AsO_3H-	1.0	2.7	1.1	1.0	2.9	3.9
$N=N$ ⬡ AsO_3H-	1.0	1.9	0.78	0.21	0.52	6.0
$N=N$ ⬡ $N=N$ ⬡ $COO-$	1.0	1.8	0.21	0.03	0.03	1.98
$N=N$ ⬡ $COO-$	1.0	3.0	0.66	0.08	0.18	10.0

[a] The asterisk (*) represents $N(CH_3)_3^+$, AsO_3H^-, or COO^-, depending on the antibody system used.

additively give a comparable amount of energy of interaction.

CONFIGURATION AND CONFORMATION

Antibody formed against one optical isomer usually does not fit the antipode. Since the antibody fits the hapten in a complementary manner as a glove fits a hand, the change from the D to the L configuration interferes much more with combination than a change in the size of the group, just as a right hand will fit into a right-hand glove, even of a different size, much better than into a left-hand glove of correct size.

Another factor which can affect fit is the degree of flexibility of the hapten. If the hapten group is an extended chain, the antibody may be formed against a particular preferred orientation. This appears to be the situation with the azosuccinanilate group, as first pointed out by Landsteiner [8, 19]. This group seems to exist in a coiled configuration in aqueous solution, since antibodies formed against it combine well with succinanilate ion and also with the cis-maleanilate ion but combine only poorly with the trans-fumaranilate ion. Such cyclization of succinanilate could be stabilized by hydrogen bond formation between the carboxylate and the NH group or perhaps through resonance in the carboxyl group (Fig. 1-4). Benzoyl propionate seems to exist in the coiled configuration also. It combines well with antibody against the succinanilate ion, and antibody prepared against the p-azobenzoyl propionate group combines better with the cis-maleanilate ion than with the trans-fumaranilate ion.

Another example of configurational factors is shown by antibody to the 4-azophthalate ion [18]. Although the carboxylate group of benzoate ion is coplanar with the benzene ring, this cannot be the situation for the carboxyl groups of phthalate ion. In the phthalate ion, the carboxylates are titled with respect to each other (Fig. 1-5). This is reflected in the ability of the antibody to combine with

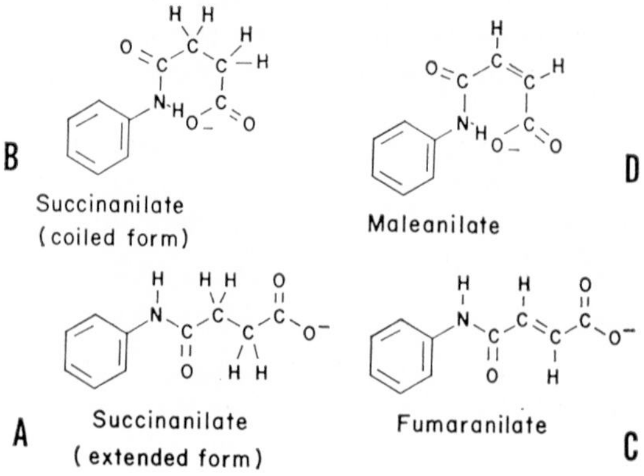

B Succinanilate (coiled form)

D Maleanilate

A Succinanilate (extended form)

C Fumaranilate

Fig. 1-4. Extended (*A*) and coiled (*B*) forms of succinanilate compared with fumaranilate (*C*) and maleanilate (*D*).

the o-sulfobenzoate group although benzene sulfonate does not combine with anti-p-azobenzoate antibodies. The accommodation of a sulfo in place of a carboxylate by antiphthalate antibody may well be due to the fact that the antibody is formed against a much thicker charged region due to the tilting of the groups in the phthalate system, whereas the antibody may be formed against the flat carboxylate group in the benzoate and cannot accommodate the sulfonate group.

HYDRATION

Another factor which affects fit is hydration of the molecule, since water of hydration can act sterically as a substituent on the molecule. The nitrogen of the pyridine ring is hydrated in aqueous solution. This water of hydration is a factor in the reaction with antibody [20]. Antibodies against the o-, m-, and p-azobenzoate ions and p-(p-azobenzeneazo)-benzoate ion react with the pyridine carboxylate ions, picolinate, nicotinate, and isonicotinate, as though there were a large substituent (water) on the ring in the position occupied by the nitrogen atom. The various quinoline carboxylate ions also combine with these antibodies as though there were a large substituent on the ring corresponding to the position of the nitrogen group. These results are consistent with hydration of the ring nitrogen atom. In the combination of antibody formed against the 4-azophthalate ion [18] with pyridine dicarboxylate and with pyrazine dicarboxylate, the relative combining constants are 0.20 and 0.05, indicating a large steric factor due to hydration of one and two ring nitrogen atoms.

Pyridine retains its water of hydration [21] when antibodies are formed against the 3-azopyridine group. This is indicated by a large hole in the antibody site which can accommodate large substituents on haptens in which a benzene ring is substituted for the pyridine group. This hole is very large and will accommodate large groups, e.g., iodo.

Hydration is not limited to the nitrogen atom, but it is probably an important factor with all the various groupings which are either charged or form hydrogen bonds. The energy required to strip water from hydrated small ions is of the order of 50 kcal. per mole or more, and this value is much greater than the free energies of combination or heats of combination of antibody and antigen as determined. It may well be that structures written for many physiologically active substances which neglect the water of hydration are grossly incorrect with respect to their effective steric configurations.

CHEMICAL NATURE OF COMBINING REGION OF ANTIBODY

The combining regions of antibodies directed against different haptens necessarily differ since they have different specificities. Besides differences in complementary configuration, antibody directed against a positively charged group such as a p-azophenyltrimethylammonium group is different from antibody formed against the negatively charged p-azobenzoate group. In this instance, the difference in charge contributes to the specificity, since charge interaction is an important part of antibody-antigen combination. The antibody directed against the positively charged group has a negative charge in the combining region, and the antibody against a negative group has a positive charge in the combining region. The presence of these charges has been shown by the demonstration that the combining region with a negative

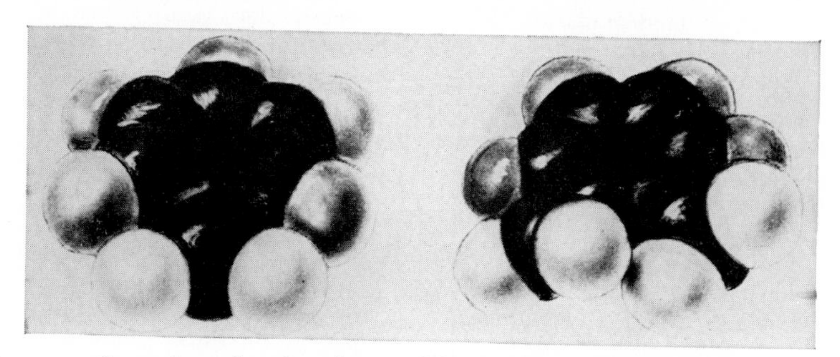

Fig. 1-5. Coplanar configuration of carboxylate and benzene ring in benzoate and tilted orientation in phthalate.

charge attracts inorganic cations nonspecifically [22], while the region with a positive charge attracts anions [23]. Antibodies to an uncharged group do not attract either type of ion preferentially [24].

The negative charge in the combining region of antibody directed to the positive charge on a hapten must necessarily be a carboxylate group. This has been proved to be the case [25]. When such antibodies are treated with diazoacetamide, which is known to esterify carboxylate ions, the ability of the antibody to bind hapten is lost. The greater the degree of reaction, the greater the number of carboxyl groups esterified, the greater the loss of activity. Binding activity can be recovered by exposure of the esterified antibody to alkali which hydrolyzes the ester, liberating the charged carboxylate group. Antibodies against negative charges which presumably contain a positive charge in the combining region are not affected by esterification, indicating that there is no carboxyl group in the combining region. Other evidence of a negative charge in the combining region of the antipositive ion antibody is the fact that the antibody combines ten times as strongly with a hapten containing the trimethylammonium group as with one which contains a tertiary butyl group in its place [26]. The tertiary butyl group has the same size and configuration as the trimethylammonium group but lacks the charge. Calculations based on energy supplied by charge interaction indicate that there must be a negative charge in the combining site close by, within 3 A of closest approach.

The positive charge in the combining region of antibodies against a negative group could be contributed by an amino group such as the ε-amino of lysine or the α-amino at the end of a polypeptide chain, or by the guanidinium group of arginine. In the case of antibodies against benzoate, it appears that the amino group plays a rather limited role, and the positive charge is probably due entirely to a guanidinium residue. On the other hand, amino groups may be important in antibodies against benzenearsonate.

The nonpolar forces are probably contributed through the amino acids with the large hydrocarbon component such as phenylalanine, alanine, leucine, and isoleucine.

The tyrosine residue seems to be particularly important in the antibody combining region. The antibodies of several antihapten antibodies have been found to contain a tyrosine residue, as is shown by various chemical reactions such as iodination and acetylation [27, 28] and by the fact that peptides isolated from the combining region of antibodies have been found to contain tyrosine [29].

REFERENCES

1. Hooker, S. B., and Boyd, W. C. The existence of antigenic determinants of diverse specificity in a single protein: III. Further notes on crystalline hen- and duck-ovalbumins, *J. Immun.* 30:41, 1936.
2. Weigle, W. O. Immunochemical properties of the cross-reactions between anti-BSA and heterologous albumins, *J. Immun.* 87:599, 1961.
3. Lapresle, C. Étude de la dégradation de la sérumalbumine humaine par un extrait de rate de lapin: II. Mise en évidence de trois groupements spécifiques différents dans le motif antigénique de l'albumine humaine et de trois anticorps correspondants dans le sérum de lapin anti-albumine humaine, *Ann. Inst. Pasteur* (Paris) 89:654, 1955.
4. Schiemann, O., and Casper, W. Sind die spezifisch präcipitablen Substanzen der 3 Pneumokokkentypen Haptene? *Z. Hyg. Infektionskr.* 108:220, 1927.
5. Stahmann, M. A., Tsuyuki, H., Weinke, K. F., Lapresle, C., and Grabar, P. Immunochimie-l'antigénicité des polypeptides synthétiques, *C. R. Acad. Sci.* (Paris) 241:1528, 1955.
6. Maurer, P. H., Subrahmanyam, D., Katchalski, E., and Blout, E. R. Antigenicity of polypeptides (poly, alpha amino acids), *J. Immun.* 83:193, 1959.
7. Obermayer, F., and Pick, E. P. Beiträge zur Kenntnis der Präzipitinbildung. Ueber den Begriff der Art-und Zustandspezifizität (originae und konstitutive Gruppierung) und die Beeinflussung der chemischen Eigenart des Tierkörpers, *Wien. Klin. Wschr.* 17:265, 1904.
8. Landsteiner, K., and Lampl, H. Ueber Antigene mit verschiedenartigen Acylgruppen: X. Mitteilung ueber Antigene 3, *Z. Immunitaetsforsch.* 26:258, 1917.
9. Kabat, E. A. Some configurational requirements and dimensions of the combining site on an antibody to a naturally occurring antigen, *J. Amer. Chem. Soc.* 76:3709, 1954.
10. Cebra, J. J. Studies on the combining sites of the protein antigen silk fibroin: III. Inhibition

of the silk fibroin-antifibroin system by peptides derived from the antigen, *J. Immun.* 86:205, 1961.

11. Pauling, L. A theory of the structure and process of formation of antibodies, *J. Amer. Chem. Soc.* 62:2643, 1940.
12. Pauling, L., Campbell, D. H., and Pressman, D. The nature of the forces between antigen and antibody and of the precipitation reaction, *Physiol. Rev.* 23:203, 1943.
13. Pressman, D., Swingle, S. M., Grossberg, A. L., and Pauling, L. The serological properties of simple substances: VIII. The reactions of antiserum homologous to the p-azobenzoic acid group, *J. Amer. Chem. Soc.* 66:1731, 1944.
14. Pressman, D., Grossberg, A. L., Pence, L. H., and Pauling, L. The reactions of antiserum homologous to the p-azophenyltrimethylammonium group, *J. Amer. Chem. Soc.* 68:250, 1946.
15. Pauling, L., Pressman, D., and Grossberg, A. L. The serological properties of simple substances: VII. A quantitative theory of the inhibition by haptens of the precipitation of heterogeneous antisera with antigens, and comparison with experimental results for polyhaptenic simple substances and for azoproteins, *J. Amer. Chem. Soc.* 66:784, 1944.
16. Pressman, D., and Siegel, M. The binding of simple substances to serum proteins and its effect on apparent antibody-hapten combination constants, *J. Amer. Chem. Soc.* 75:686, 1953.
17. Nisonoff, A., and Pressman, D. Closeness of fit and forces involved in the reactions of antibody homologous to the p-(p-azophenylazo)-benzoate ion group, *J. Amer. Chem. Soc.* 79:1616, 1957.
18. Pressman, D., and Pauling, L. The reactions of antiserum homologous to the 4-azophthalate ion, *J. Amer. Chem. Soc.* 71:2893, 1949.
19. Landsteiner, K., and van der Scheer, J. Serological studies on azoproteins: Antigens containing azocomponents with aliphatic side chains, *J. Exp. Med.* 59:751, 1934; and Pressman, D., Bryden, J. H., and Pauling, L. The reactions of antiserum homologous to the p-azosuccinanilate ion group, *J. Amer. Chem. Soc.* 70:1352, 1948.
20. Siegel, M., and Pressman, D. The reactions of antiserum homologous to the p-azohippurate ion, *J. Amer. Chem. Soc.* 75:3436, 1953.
21. Nisonoff, A., and Pressman, D. The annular nitrogen of pyridine as a determinant of immunologic specificity, *J. Amer. Chem. Soc.* 79:5565, 1957.
22. Pressman, D., Nisonoff, A., and Radzimski, G. Specific anion effects with antibenzoate antibody, *J. Immun.* 86:35, 1961.
23. Grossberg, A. L., Chen, C. C., Rendina, L., and Pressman, D. Specific cation effects with antibody to a hapten with a positive charge, *J. Immun.* 88:600, 1962.
24. Grossberg, A. L., Chen, C. C., and Pressman, D. Unpublished data.
25. Grossberg, A. L., and Pressman, D. Nature of the combining site of antibody against a hapten bearing a positive charge, *J. Amer. Chem. Soc.* 82:5478, 1960.
26. Pressman, D., Grossberg, A. L., Pence, L. H., and Pauling, L. The reactions of antiserum homologous to the p-azophenyltrimethylammonium group, *J. Amer. Chem. Soc.* 68:250, 1946.
27. Grossberg, A. L., Radzimski, G., and Pressman, D. Effect of iodination on the active site of several antihapten antibodies, *Biochemistry* (Wash.) 1:391, 1962.
28. Grossberg, A. L., and Pressman, D. Effect of acetylation on the active site of several antihapten antibodies: Further evidence for the presence of tyrosine in each site, *Biochemistry* (Wash.) 2:90, 1963.
29. Pressman, D., and Roholt, O. Isolation of peptides from an antibody site, *Proc. Nat. Acad. Sci. U.S.A.* 47:1606, 1961.

2. *Localization and Fate of Foreign Antigens in Tissues*

DAN H. CAMPBELL AND JUSTINE S. GARVEY

WHEN FOREIGN SUBSTANCES ENTER the parenteral tissue compartments of an animal, they are handled in a variety of ways, depending on the physical and biological properties of the material and the physiological state and homeostatic nature of the animal.* Many foreign materials resist digestion and tattoo tissues for life. For example, the persistence of colloidal dyes injected into the skin is well known; and polysaccharides, such as gum acacia, injected intravenously localize in hepatic tissue and persist for many years in their native form. On the other hand, many substances are immediately excreted intact or rapidly broken down, to be reutilized or excreted. This discussion will be limited to materials (antigens) which persist for varying lengths of time, slowly undergoing degradation after deposition in tissues. During the early period of persistence (perhaps several months), the animal develops a so-called specific immune state which is manifested in one or more ways, such as circulating antibody, hypersensitivity, and enhancement of tissue graft rejection.

Localization of foreign antigenic material has interested immunologists since Metchnikoff first described the phagocytosis of visible particles by phagocytic cells [1]. Subsequent studies clearly showed that localization of various particulate antigens such as bacteria occurred in those organs and tissues which contained the greatest number of phagocytic cells or macrophages (reviewed by Mudd *et al.* [2]). This loosely defined system of cells, termed the RE (reticuloendothelial) system, occurs throughout the body but predominantly in the spleen, lymph nodes, lung, liver, bone marrow, and skin. Subsequent studies with soluble antigens that could be detected by biological activity such as toxicity or by various labels such as fluorescent dyes or radioactive atoms also indicated that the same tissues were primarily involved in removal and localization of soluble antigens. There is some question as to the role of macrophages in antibody formation and immune mechanisms, and the greatest attention is being given to lymphocytes and plasma cells. This suggests that after initial localization in macrophages, antigenic material is modified and transferred to another type of cell and that the initial site of localization of antigen in its native state may not be the actual site of antibody formation.

Little attention was given to the fate of antigen until methodology and tools were developed which permitted tracing of foreign antigenic material† long after the antigen had lost its initial biological and physical properties. However, many of the early immunologists speculated that *in vivo* degradation was one of the important factors for the immunogenicity of any material. Thus Cannon *et al.* [3] felt that degradation of bacteria played an important role in the development of resistance. Wells [4] also believed that ". . . antigenic activity is in some way related to digestive proteolysis." When radioactive isotopes became available, several laboratories utilized them as labels or tracers to study the fate of antigen.

Many current theories of immune mecha-

* The terms physiological state and homeostasis are not entirely synonymous. For example, physiological state applies not only to the normal condition which is based largely on genetic factors but also to conditions which are due to physiological misfunction or stress. Thus, homeostasis may refer to genetic presence of Rh antigen and therefore inability to produce Rh antibodies while physiological state would refer to conditions of stress such that an individual could not produce anti-Rh antibodies.

† With regard to foreign antigenic material, consideration must be given to the material which is still a part of the foreign antigen but partially digested.

nisms relegate antigen and the persistence of antigen fragments to a minor role. For example, some theories of antibody formation are reminiscent of Ehrlich's side chain theory [5],* which postulated that antigen merely stimulated a rather dormant but specific biosynthesis of antibody molecules. However, the degradation and presence of antigenic material deserves serious consideration since it is now known that the number of antigen molecules per cell may be large [6, 7]. Residual antigen may play an important role in immune mechanisms, particularly when the fragment is about the size of an antigenic determinant [8] and associated with some form of ribonucleic acid (RNA) [9, 10], which is intimately involved in the biosynthesis of proteins.

The physical properties and the manner in which a foreign material is handled *in vivo* may well determine the ultimate nature of the host's reaction as to whether antibody will be formed, the heterogeneity of antibody molecules, secondary reaction, delayed hypersensitivity, and so on.

GENERAL EXPERIMENTAL METHODS

Methods used for the study of localization and fate of foreign material have depended to some extent on knowledge of protein chemistry and availability of tools. The first studies were limited to visual examination by the light microscope of cells and tissues following injection of particulate material. Following Metchnikoff's classic studies, use was made of colored tagged proteins by Sabin [11] and by Kruse and McMaster [12] to determine localization as well as rate of disappearance of the native protein antigen after deposition into cells and tissues. An ingenious and extremely valuable technique was initiated by Coons *et al.* [13], who used a specific antibody coupled to a fluorescent dye for the detection of antigen. Thus antigen could be detected by microscopic examination with ultraviolet light of cells or tissue sections after exposure to a solution of antibody (antiserum). Present techniques are basically those described by Coons and Kaplan [14] making use of antibody coupled to fluorescein isothiocyanate. Other special methods based on direct visual observation of antigenic material in tissues involve the use of the electron microscope. For example, Erickson *et al.* [15] followed the localization and morphological changes of tobacco mosaic virus in rabbit tissues. Singer and Schick [16] labeled proteins with ferritin which, because of the high iron content, could be detected with the electron microscope. This technique has many advantages since it can be used to label and detect soluble antigens.

Another method for the detection of antigen by microscopic examination became possible when radioactive isotopes were made available. Thus, due to ionizing radiation similar to that of x-rays, antigens tagged with radioactive elements such as I^{131} and S^{35} produce patterns on photographic emulsions called radioautographs. Figure 2-1 was obtained by placing a photosensitive emulsion on a tissue section from the liver of a rabbit following injection of S^{35}-labeled bovine serum albumin (BSA). In this case, the exposure time was several months. For more details and methodology on radioautography, see Taylor [17].

The use of unique chemical elements other than isotopes for labeling antigens or antibody has received little attention. However, such techniques deserve consideration. Haurowitz *et al.* [18, 19] made some studies on the fate of antigen by using an azoarsanilic acid label on gelatin and then analyzing tissues for arsenic.

Considerable use has been made of classic serological reactions (e.g., specific precipitation, complement fixation, etc.) to follow either antigen or antibody. In general, such techniques have been limited to determinations of the rate of disappearance of either antigen or antibody from the circulation. However, there have been a few broader studies. McMaster *et al.* [20, 21] found that tissue from inoculated mice contained enough antigen after three weeks to actively sensitize normal mice. We [22] followed the serological fate of antigen localized in rabbit liver over a period of weeks and found that specific precipitability with antiserum was soon lost. However, specific hapten inhibition was obtained as long as sufficient antigenic material could be isolated to perform such tests.

In general, the bulk of information regarding localization and persistence of foreign material, particularly soluble antigens, has been

* See also Chapter 6.

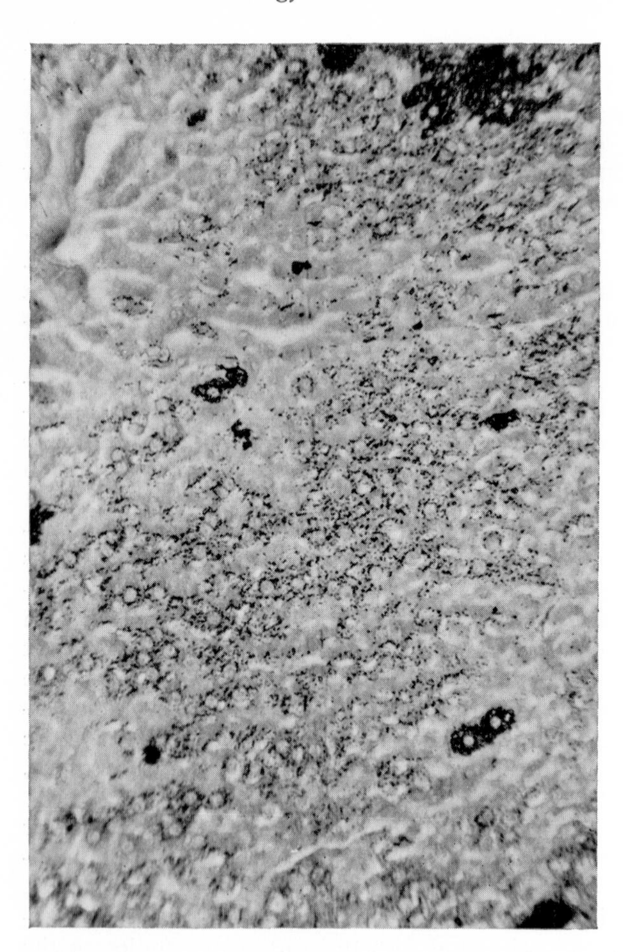

Fig. 2-1. Radioautograph of liver tissue from a rabbit hyperimmune to S^{35}-BSA as a result of seven injections of 10 mg. each over two weeks, followed by a two-week rest, then six injections during two weeks. One week after the last injection, the tissue was obtained, fixed in Carnoy's fluid, embedded in paraffin, sectioned at 10μ, and exposed for about seven months to Kodak stripping film. (× 160 before 30% reduction.) (From Campbell and Garvey [9].)

obtained by use of isotopes. Some of the early studies were carried out with N^{15} or H^2 (deuterium). When radioactive elements became available, attention was directed almost entirely to such tracer elements as C^{14}, I^{131}, S^{35}, and, to a minor extent, H^3 (tritium). Such labels may be used as chemical substituent groups, as, for example, azo-S^{35}-sulfanilic acid or I^{131} coupled to the protein. Proteins or carbohydrates may also be internally labeled by supplying animals with labeled amino acids or sugars obtained by chemical or biological synthesis. Thus internally labeled proteins can be obtained in animals by feeding or injecting yeast which has been grown with $S^{35}O_4$ as a source of sulfur that is incorporated in such sulfur-containing amino acids as methionine and cystine [23]. Other elements, like C^{14} and H^3, can also be incorporated by supplying nutrient supplements which contain amino acids or sugars obtained by chemical or biosynthesis. Although isotopes provide a very sensitive tag, selection must be carefully made according to the nature of the problem. Factors of particular importance are those dealing with the half-life, type of radiation, and *in vivo* behavior, particularly the possibility of transfer from one molecule to another. Recent studies have generally involved S^{35}, C^{14}, and I^{131} because of convenient half-life, ease of addition to protein molecules, and availability. The general problem of the use of radioactive isotopes for biological studies has been reviewed by Kamen [24].

DISTRIBUTION OF ANTIGEN

FACTORS INVOLVED

Since a multiplicity of factors may influence the distribution of antigen, at least the more important of these should be kept in mind in an evaluation of controversial findings and in the planning of future investigations. Varying the route of injection may have a pronounced effect not only on the degree of localization in a particular tissue but also on the number of different tissues involved in localization of antigen and subsequent antibody formation. For example, an injection into the cornea isolates the antigen from the general circulation [25], thereby preventing its distribution to other tissues, whereas intravenous injection usually leads to a widespread distribution of the antigen to various tissues. Some routes of injection may cause a preferential localization of the antigen in certain tissues; e.g., an intra-abdominal injection leads to uptake by mesenteric and sternal nodes, and a foot-pad injection to uptake by popliteal nodes and other regional lymph nodes.

No matter what the route of injection, the concentration of antigen at a particular site changes with time after injection. Following intravenous injection, the maximal concentration occurs in various tissues within a few minutes and thereafter declines. With other routes of injection there may be continuous increase of antigen in certain organs with increasing time as antigen shifts from a localized deposit and becomes more generally distributed. For example, the blood concentration of heterologous diphtheria antitoxin at two hours after subcutaneous injection into a rabbit was one two-hundredth of that in a rabbit given an intravenous injection. The highest blood concentration for the subcutaneous injection occurred after two to three days, when it reached approximately the same value as that for the intravenous injection [26]. The observations of slow dissemination of antigen from a localized site led to useful procedures in applied immunology, e.g., use of subcutaneous and intramuscular routes for injection of immunizing materials and, in some cases, of emulsified soluble antigen to retard further the rate of antigen diffusion.

The type of foreign material studied has varied greatly. In several of the early investigations nonantigenic material, e.g., carbon particles and dyes, both soluble and insoluble, were used. Particulate antigens, e.g., foreign erythrocytes and bacterial cells, and soluble antigens such as foreign serums were also investigated. Regardless of whether such materials were antigenic or nonantigenic, soluble or insoluble, a common factor in distribution early after injection was phagocytosis, and this often led to a limited distribution even if the material was given intravenously. This was particularly so with a small dose of insoluble material, since the RE tissue is widespread and very effective in the initial uptake of foreign material.

Dosage of antigen may have a very noticeable effect on the immune response. A well-known example of this is that pneumococcus polysaccharide at a small dosage level protects the mouse against infection, whereas high dosage levels lead to susceptibility and the phenomenon known as immunological paralysis [27].

Choice of animal species may depend on the technique to be used to detect antibody, since antibody is often correlated with antigen distribution in the first few days to weeks after immunization. The rabbit is often the animal of choice because it produces precipitating antibody that is easily quantitated and, in addition, is of a size suitable for isolation and fractionation of antigen that is retained in the tissues. Mature rabbits produce more antibody than do young rabbits, but among a group of adults there is often a wide variation in precipitin response ranging from none to high, when a soluble antigen such as BSA is used for immunization. A uniform failure of adults to respond to such an antigen as BSA may occur when the initial injection of antigen is close to the time of birth. Animals such as these are known as tolerant or unresponsive [28] and are of considerable interest with regard to their handling of antigen.

DISTRIBUTION IN CIRCULATION

In many of the early investigations of the fate of circulating antigen, living bacteria were used, and the findings had practical application in bacteriology and immunology. If injected directly into the blood stream, the numbers of organisms declined rapidly within a few minutes and the blood became sterile in a few hours. If a previously sensitized animal were used, the rate of clearance was greatly accelerated [29]. Since living materials had obvious disadvantages for handling and in quantitation, these were soon replaced by nonviable antigens. Foreign erythrocytes have been studied for their site of destruction after intravenous injection into rabbits [30]. They are rapidly removed from the circulation and destroyed in the spleen, as are the rabbit's own erythrocytes. As antigens, erythrocytes are particularly useful because of the sensitivity of the assay for hemolysin antibody.

Soluble materials were generally first used in the form of complex mixtures such as whole serum, and the findings were of particular value in practical immunology. Horse serum administered for pneumonia therapy was studied for persistence in human serum by means of specific precipitation [31]; although the foreign serum was detected for several weeks, the level fell severely as antibody formation occurred. Soluble specific substance (SSS) was found to have a long circulatory persistence in the rabbit, a species in which it is not antigenic. The circulatory clearance of heterologous diphtheria antitoxin was described as a three-phase process by Glenny and Hopkins [26]. The first phase, lasting twenty-four hours, consisted in redistribution of antitoxin from the blood into tissues; the next phase, that assigned to metabolic processes, was a period of slow elimination lasting six to seven days. The last phase was marked by a rapidly accelerated loss apparently due to active production of antibody against antitoxin. In animals that had had previous injections, the first phase was unchanged, the second phase was similar to that in a normal animal but shorter, and the last phase was characterized by extremely rapid elimination.

Later work has involved the use of radioactive labels, and I^{131}-labeled protein has been prominent in circulatory clearance studies. A considerable amount of investigation was directed toward determining first the *in vitro* and then the *in vivo* stability of this label. Light labeling, i.e., about 1 iodine atom to 10 protein molecules, was found by Eisen and Keston [32] to produce no significant difference in quantitative precipitation reactions with either tagged or native BSA. When iodide injections were given to prevent thyroid uptake, I^{131} proved to be reliable as a quantitative indicator of labeled BSA in the circulation of rabbits for at least seven days [33], whereas radioactivity and precipitation showed good agreement for fourteen days in the assay of I^{131} human albumin in rabbits [34]. Talmage *et al.* [77] measured the circulatory clearance of I^{131}-labeled bovine γ-globulin injected intravenously into rabbits. The changing rate of clearance practically duplicated the phases of antitoxin clearance previously described by Glenny and Hopkins [26]. In contrast to the rather slow circulatory loss of lightly labeled I^{131} antigen, highly iodinated γ-globulin showed rapid circulatory loss after intravenous injection into rabbits [35]. Dixon's work [36, 37] is an excellent reference for the effect of antibody and other aspects of circulatory clearance of iodoproteins.

Azoproteins such as those used in Landsteiner's studies [38] of serological specificity were studied for their *in vivo* fate by quantitative chemical detection of arsenic [18], by color [39], and later by radioactivity [40]. All azoproteins studied showed faster elimination from the blood than the native proteins from which they were prepared, and the heavier the coupling, the greater the reduction in circulatory time. As with other antigens, sensitization also led to a faster rate of clearance of this group of antigens [41].

URINARY EXCRETION OF ANTIGEN

Information on the excretion of antigen comes from various studies. Among them are those showing excretion in unchanged form of nonantigenic material or material of low antigenicity such as SSS [42] and gelatin [19, 43].

Excretion data were often correlated with circulatory clearance for iodoproteins, and a faster excretion rate was found in sensitized than in normal animals [44]. The slower excretion rate of I^{131} in normal animals was attributed to the intervening influence of cellular degradation, i.e., the iodine-thyroid cycle [45]. Laws [46] showed two breakdown products in urine after injection of I^{131}-labeled protein and presented findings which suggested a difference in proportion of these in sensitized and in normal animals. This work and that of Tong *et al.* [47] on the metabolic fate of diiodotyrosine suggest a need for more work to define better the degradative changes of iodoproteins in tissues, and until this information is obtained, iodoproteins appear to be of questionable value in study of tissue localization.

The deposit of red granules in kidney tubules after injection of azoproteins showed the permeability of renal glomeruli to these antigens [48]. Radioactive labels used on such azoproteins as those listed in Table 2-1 were rapidly excreted, and within one to two days after injection the cumulative excreted radioactivity accounted for all but a small percentage of the injected radioactivity. Comparison of radioactivity data for the two azoproteins S^{35}-BSA and S^{35}-KLH (KLH =

keyhole limpet hemocyanin) indicated characteristic differences in their rates of excretion and also that a sensitized animal excreted antigenic material more rapidly than the normal animal [22]. The detection of radioactivity in urine many months after intravenous injection indicated the slow but continuous loss of antigen from tissues [49].

LOCALIZATION IN EXTRAVASCULAR TISSUES

The cellular fate of antigen and its importance in immunological response was emphasized by some immunologists long before data were available to demonstrate antigen in tissues and to rule out its presence as entrained blood. Thus Wilson and Miles [50] stated the importance of an extravascular fate for antigen in the following way: ". . . it appears that to be an antigen a substance must have certain minimum chemical properties, but it must also be so constructed that it cannot be handled by one of the readily available mechanisms of elimination and thus removed before it has time to exert an antigenic stimulus."

Localization simply means the finding of antigen in tissues, usually very early after injection, but can include an interval of time extending through the rise, as well as decline, in circulating antibody titer. Localization in the sense of antigen remaining in the site of injection into the skin or within draining lymph nodes for long periods of time will not be discussed here. There are fairly recent reports on findings with insoluble material, such as of rickettsiae and virus identified in tissue cells by fluorescent antibody staining [51], tobacco mosaic virus (TMV) rods in the liver by electron microscopy [15], and red cell stromata in various tissues by labeling diazotized sulfanilate with S^{35} [52], but in only the last are quantitative data given. Of the additional investigations to be cited here, most are concerned with the intravenous route of injection and particularly with use of soluble antigen, with quantitative data to support conclusions. The use of soluble antigen permits rapid access to all tissues, and of the quantitative data reported, most have been obtained with radioactive labels. Data from these studies are compiled in Table 2-1; except for the study with P^{32}-TMV, they represent an initial localization.

We [7] performed extensive investigations

TABLE 2-1. Localization of Antigens in Tissues of Normal Animals

Reference No.	Antigen[a]	Animal	Time	% of Dose in Major Sites			
				Liver	Spleen	Lung	Marrow
INSOLUBLE MATERIAL							
52	S^{35}-A stromata	Rabbit, mouse	6-100 min.	73–87	2.0	2–4	1
53	Bacteria[b]	Rabbit	1 hr.				
SOLUBLE MATERIAL							
40	S^{35}-AO	Rabbit	1 hr.	46	1.9	0.5	4.0
35	I^{131}-iodoproteins	Rabbit	1 hr.	27		0.4	
	S^{35}-sulfone proteins	Rabbit	1 hr.	50		1.4	
18	AsA-serum	Rabbit	6 hr.	29	1.5		
41	S^{35}-KLH	Rabbit	6 hr.	20	0.3	0.2	
7	S^{35}-KLH	Rabbit	1 day	17	0.3	0.2	
	S^{35}-BSA	Rabbit	1 day	7			
54	S^{35}-AγG	Mouse	1 day	14	0.4		
55	P^{32}-TMV[c]	Mouse	1 day	63	3.0		

[a] Key to antigens: S^{35}-A stromata, sulfanilate-azo-sheep red cell stromata; S^{35}-AO, sulfanilate azoovalbumin; AsA-serum, arsanilate-azo-serum; S^{35}-KLH, sulfanilate-azo-keyhole limpet hemocyanin; S^{35}-BSA, sulfanilate azo-bovine serum albumin; S^{35}-AγG, sulfanilate-azo-bovine γ-globulin; P^{32}-TMV, P^{32}-labeled tobacco mosaic virus.

[b] Equal average concentrations in spleen and liver; percentages not available.

[c] Prior sensitization as noted in text.

SOURCE: Campbell and Garvey [9].

on the fate of antigens in rabbits given injections of either of two soluble proteins, KLH or BSA. These proteins have been coupled to diazotized S^{35}-labeled sulfanilic acid to prepare antigens that have a high specific radioactivity and are stable *in vivo* with regard to the label (discussed later). The antigen S^{35}-KLH showed a greater degree of localization than did S^{35}-BSA (characteristic differences in urinary excretion of these two antigens were already mentioned), but for the same antigen, the specific radioactivity, i.e., radioactivity per gm. of wet tissue, was not greatly different in liver and in spleen. However, the much greater total weight of liver than of spleen accounts for the percentage variations given in Table 2-1 for these two tissues for the same antigen.

To compare localization in the tissues of normal and immune rabbits, quantitative data were collected both for antigen in tissues and for circulating antibody [41]. Rabbits previously given multiple injections of nonradioactive antigen (SKLH) were bled and the sera used to measure circulating antibody. After bleeding, these same rabbits, as well as normal control rabbits that had never previously received antigen, were given a test injection of S^{35}-KLH. Six hours later, blood and other tissues were sampled and their content of radioactivity was measured. The radioactivity in blood samples was both extremely low (as would be expected with an azoprotein) and not significantly different in normal and immune animals. Of the other tissues, both liver and lung of immune animals showed a greatly increased localization as compared with the same normal tissues. The increase in localization was found to be related to the amount of circulating antibody in the serum just before the test injection. Perfusion with 1 percent saline removed radioactivity from the immune liver tissue to the extent that the remaining radioactivity was essentially that of normal tissue; but perfusion was less effective in reducing the radioactive content of the lung tissue (Fig. 2-2) that control experiments showed to be part of a hypersensitivity reaction. Both antigen and antibody were isolated by dissociation of an insoluble complex recovered from the six-hour perfusate of immune liver tissue. The actual isolation of antigen and antibody from the liver perfusate is probably the first demonstration that antigen-antibody complexes form in the blood stream and are removed as insoluble complexes. Although the relative difference found in normal and immune liver at six hours was observed at seventy-two hours, it was no longer possible to perfuse radioactivity at the later time.

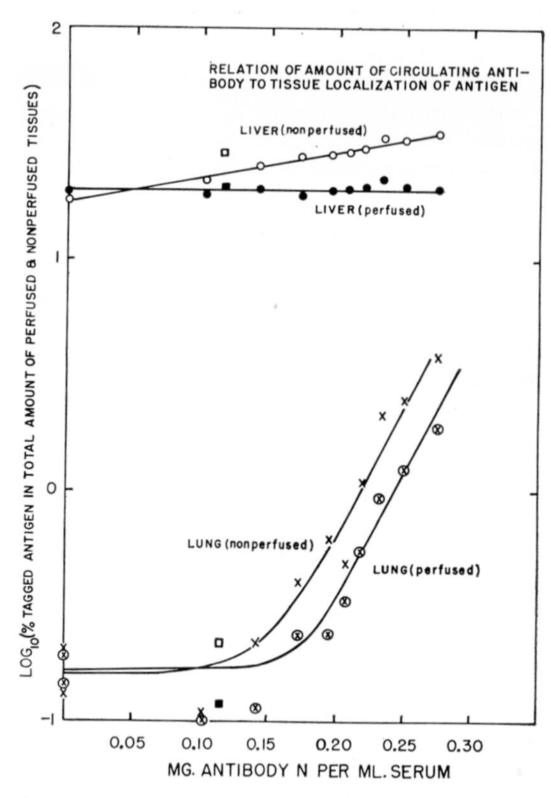

Fig. 2-2. A comparison of total antigen localized in nonperfused and perfused tissue from normal animals (points at zero antibody concentration) and immunized animals (points corresponding to different antibody concentrations). Data for these curves were obtained from actively immunized animals except for passively immunized animal represented by squares. (From Garvey and Campbell [41].)

RETENTION OF ANTIGEN IN TISSUES OF NORMAL AND IMMUNIZED ANIMALS

Ehrlich's side chain theory [5] that specified a normal presence of antibody controlled genetically was challenged after about three decades by a new theory that required antigen as a template for antibody formation [56–59]. As an alternative to the template theory, Burnet and Fenner [60] suggested a complex memory mechanism rather than the continued presence of antigen to account for lasting immunity and gained some acceptance of this theory by emphasizing the absence of direct evidence of persistence of antigen. There had been for many years, however, widely accepted knowledge that such virus infections as smallpox, measles, and yellow fever resulted in long-lasting immunity, but virus had not actually been recovered from tissues. As recounted earlier, numerous investigations, aided particularly by the use of radioactive isotopes, showed significant amounts of antigen localized in tissues, predominantly in liver. Extension of some of these investigations to longer periods of data-collecting showed that persistence (prolonged localization) actually occurred. A notable exception to detection by radioactivity was microscopic observation of blue azoproteins by McMaster and Kruse [20]; this investigation resulted in detection of an azoglobulin for 85 to 120 days after injection and of an azoalbumin for 36 to 44 days after injection.

Although McMaster and Kruse presented direct evidence of long persistence of antigen, Haurowitz and Crampton [6] were the first to emphasize the significance of antigen persistence at the molecular level, i.e., the presence of a large number of molecules per cell. According to their data, 2,000 antigen molecules were found per liver cell 29 days after injection of 86 mg. of iodoovalbumin (as indicated previously, the I^{131} label may not be a good choice for demonstrating antigen in tissues). Ingraham [54] found the greatest concentration of S^{35}-sulfanilic acid-azo-bovine γ-globulin in the liver and spleen of mice where 1 percent and 4 percent respectively of the S^{35} present in the liver 24 hours after injection remained at 200 days.

As described under localization, we [7] labeled two soluble antigens, KLH and BSA, with S^{35}-sulfanilate and used them to follow retention after intravenous injection into rabbits. Since the aim of the research was to isolate and to characterize retained antigen, the tissue of choice was the liver. The choice of liver rather than spleen was based on the fact that at least a 50-fold greater concentration of antigen was available for isolation from the liver even though the specific radioactivities of spleen and liver tissues were often about equal. Thus the choice of studying liver tissue was originally a technical one, but the accumulation of results has shown no evidence that it is not representative of retention occurring elsewhere in the body.

The curves in Figure 2-3 are for single and multiple injections of each of the two antigens, S^{35}-BSA and S^{35}-KLH [7]. When these experimental curves were extrapolated to a three-year interval after injection, the calculated number of molecules per liver cell was about 200 for S^{35}-BSA and 2,000 for S^{35}-KLH. Early data (on circulating antibody) showed for several weeks a rough correlation between the amount of antigen remaining in the liver

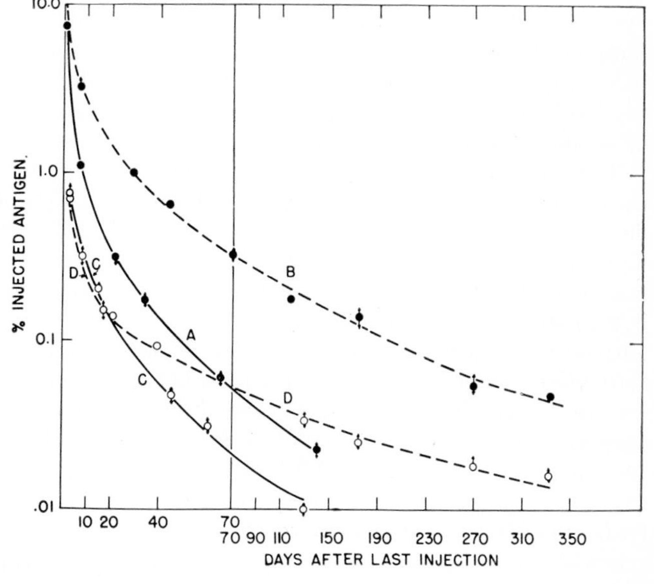

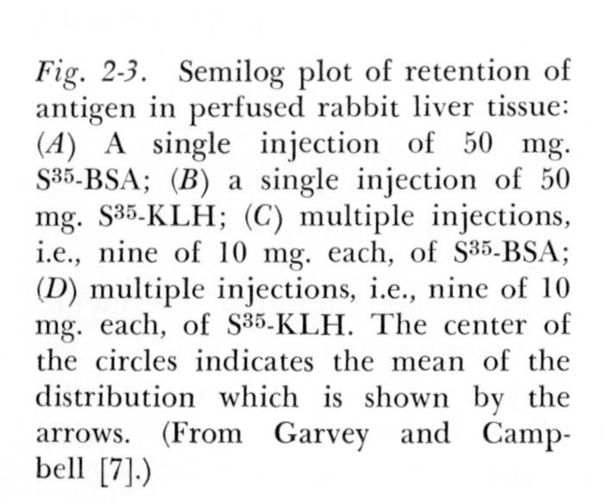
Fig. 2-3. Semilog plot of retention of antigen in perfused rabbit liver tissue: (*A*) A single injection of 50 mg. S^{35}-BSA; (*B*) a single injection of 50 mg. S^{35}-KLH; (*C*) multiple injections, i.e., nine of 10 mg. each, of S^{35}-BSA; (*D*) multiple injections, i.e., nine of 10 mg. each, of S^{35}-KLH. The center of the circles indicates the mean of the distribution which is shown by the arrows. (From Garvey and Campbell [7].)

from multiple injections and the amount of circulating antibody [61]. More recently, persistence of circulating antibody for much longer intervals has been demonstrated by passive hemagglutination [62]. We [63] too have used the passive hemagglutination technique and extended greatly the interval of time during which antibody can be found in the circulation. These findings suggest the possibility that as long as antigen persists, antibody may be circulating, although the concentration may become so low that very sensitive methods are needed for detection.

The curves in Figure 2-3 show that there is less retention from multiple injections than from a single injection. After multiple injections a variable amount of circulating antibody was detectable, but after a single injection comparatively little antibody was present in the circulation, and often none was demonstrable by interfacial ring precipitation technique. An investigation concerning the loss of antigen from multiple injections indicated that loss of the initial injection (the only injection of labeled antigen) was correlated inversely with the quantity of circulating antibody [64] resulting after a series of multiple injections of nonlabeled antigen. Since passively administered antibody proved to be totally ineffective either in causing any loss of antigen from liver or in enhancing the immune response in normal animals, it was obvious that the loss of antigen from liver tissue is at least a consequence of antibody production. It remains to be proved that antigen which is retained, then finally lost by urinary excretion, has a predominant role in antibody production. However, the dynamic state of retained antigen as related to current thinking has been presented in a speculative scheme of antibody production (see Fig. 2-5).

The characterization of retained antigen in the tissues of such animals as have just been described, i.e., those that have produced precipitating antibody, is emphasized in the discussion that follows. Considerable information is available that significant concentrations of antigen are also retained in the tissues of unresponsive animals, e.g., of pneumococcus polysaccharide in tissues of paralyzed mice [27], of S^{35}-BSA in tissues of chickens given injections at hatching [65] and S^{35}-BSA in tissues of rabbits given injections in neonatal life [66]. Quantitative differences in the antigen retained in the tissues of unresponsive animals have failed to account for the lack of a precipitin response. However, qualitative differences in antigen might exist that, if identified, would explain the phenomenon of unresponsiveness and add generally to information concerning the metabolism of antigen.

NATURE OF RETAINED ANTIGENS

The first investigators to study the fate of antigens and their relation to cell constituents were Haurowitz and his collaborators. Thus, using an I^{131}-labeled antigen, Haurowitz and Crampton [6, 67] found that radioactivity 29 days after injection of I^{131}-labeled ovalbumin was associated with the mitochondria and microsomes of liver tissue. Using chromatographic methods, we [7] found that practically all of the radioactivity of S^{35}-sulfanilic azo-labeled bovine serum albumin was associated with soluble ribonucleic acid (SRNA) of liver. The association of antigen with SRNA has been consistently confirmed by using both hemocyanin and bovine serum albumin when mild extraction procedures were used such as freezing and disruption of cells with high pressure and subsequent adsorption of antigen material on a Dowex 2 resin. The original publications gave the antigenic material a molecular weight of about 30,000 [7]. Subsequent studies indicated that this value actually represented the approximate molecular weight of SRNA, while the antigenic fragment weight was only 500 to 1,000, as determined by analytical ultracentrifugation before and after removal of the antigenic material from the SRNA. The physical properties of the antigenic material are still under investigation. Results by Saha *et al.* [68] clearly showed that the antigenic fragment containing the S^{35}-sulfanilic acid group is approximately a pentapeptide and that at least one of the amino acids of the antigen (S^{35}-sulfanilic azo-BSA) is histidine. It appears, therefore, that antigen deposited in the liver is rapidly broken down into fragments consisting of about five amino acids and that these fragments persist in combination with SRNA for many months.

The composition and amino acid sequence of the polypeptide fragment has not been determined. However, it can be assumed that the fragments are heterogeneous and represent various portions of the original native protein molecule, including internal molecular determinants as described by Ishizaka *et al.* [69] and by Lapresle *et al.* [70].

The biological properties of the retained antigen fragments or the complex of antigenic material plus SRNA has received only minor attention. McMaster and his collaborators [21] by using extracts from livers of mice given injections of bovine serum globulin found that enough material was present at 14 weeks to sensitize normal mice. Similar experiments with rabbits failed to detect immunogenic material after 3 weeks following injection. We [7], following the fate of hemocyanin and BSA deposited in rabbit liver, found that immunogenic material could be isolated for as long as 6 weeks after injection and that the fragmented antigen-SRNA complex was more immunogenic than the original native antigen. When isolated and freed from SRNA, the antigenic material lost its ability to precipitate specific antibody after about 10 days, but as long as sufficient material could be obtained for serological testing, it behaved as a simple hapten and inhibited specific precipitation. Also, when the SRNA and antigenic fragment were separated, neither the antigenic fragment nor the SRNA was immunogenic.

CONSEQUENCES OF ANTIGEN RETENTION

It is evident that antigenic material may persist for many months or even years after entering cells. Although the material exists as a degraded fragment of the original protein molecule, this breakdown into a size about that of an antigenic determinant may be quite significant and one of the factors involved in immunogenicity of foreign material. Since the fragment is associated with SRNA, one can speculate that the foreign fragment acts in a specific manner to modify the function of SRNA in the biosynthesis of protein. However, knowledge of the true role of antigen or the products of *in vivo* degradation in the stimulation and production of antibody protein must await information relative to the general problem of the biosynthesis of proteins. A schematic idea of how fragments of partially digested antigenic materials might modify intracellular synthesis of protein is shown in Figure 2-4. The consequence of such a situation is discussed elsewhere by us [9] and

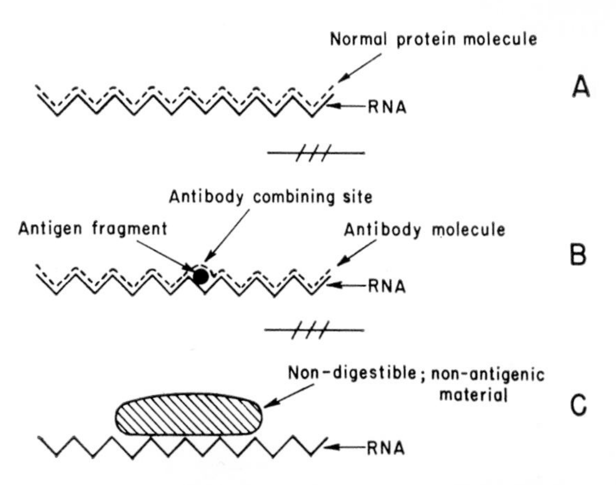

Fig. 2-4. A schematic concept of the role of a fragment of a foreign antigen. (*A*) Normal activity of RNA; (*B*) a molecule of RNA slightly modified by presence of the antigen fragment that results in a slight change in the polypeptide chain; (*C*) the blocking of RNA activity by a large foreign molecule. (From Campbell and Garvey [9].)

in the reviews listed below. Fragmentation and persistence of antigen may also play a role in the formation of clones of antibody-forming cells following secondary exposure to antigen, as described by Coons *et al.* [71, 72]. Thus, as suggested by Campbell and Garvey [73, 10] and Sorkin [74], an initial exposure of a few cells results in antibody formation and sensitization of the few cells which contained antigen. A secondary exposure to antigen results in injury to the sensitized cells and fragments of antigen are released. Some material is taken up by adjacent cells and some is excreted in the urine before it can be taken up by new cells. A schematic representation is shown in Figure 2-5.

Many other possible consequences of intracellular antigen degradation into fragments about the molecular dimension of specific determinants have been given in the reviews already referred to [9, 10, 73] and also in References 75 and 76. If partial degradation is one of the important factors in immunogenicity of foreign material and stimulation of the biosynthesis of specific globulin, the failure of cathepsins to degrade antigen or to do so in a suitable manner may result in a state of unresponsiveness (or immune paralysis), as in neonatal animals [65, 66]. Passive transfer of hypersensitivity by cells may be due to the presence of small amounts of antigen-RNA complexes.

Although the intracellular breakdown of

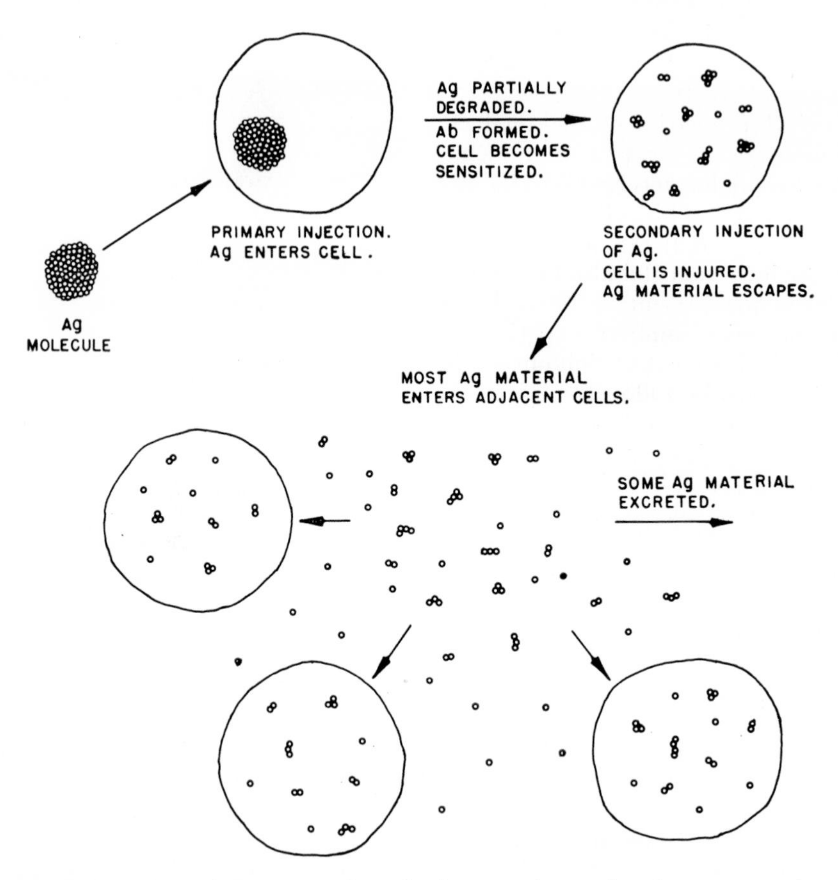

Fig. 2-5. A speculative schematic representation of primary and secondary immune reactions and formation of nonselective clones of antibody-forming cells. *Ag* = immunogenic molecule of antigen consisting of a mosaic of haptenic determinants that become separated on partial intracellular digestion of the antigen molecule. *Ab* = antibody. (From Campbell and Garvey [10].)

antigenic material is well established and provides the basis for much speculation and experimentation related to immune mechanisms, many questions can be answered only after the mechanism of protein synthesis and molecular replication is understood.

REFERENCES

1. Metchnikoff, É. *L'Immunité dans les Maladies Infectieuses.* Paris: 1901. (*Immunity in Infective Diseases* [tr. by F. G. Binnie]. London: Cambridge University Press, 1905.)
2. Mudd, S., McCutcheon, M., and Lucké, B. Phagocytosis. *Physiol. Rev.* 14:210, 1934.
3. Cannon, P. R., Sullivan, F. L., and Neckerman, E. F. Conditions influencing the disappearance of living bacteria from the blood stream. *J. Exp. Med.* 55:121, 1932. (See also Ref. 53.)
4. Wells, H. G. Antigens and Their Specificity. In Jordan, E. O., and Falk, I. S. (Eds.), *The Newer Knowledge of Bacteriology and Immunology.* Chicago: The University of Chicago Press, 1928. P. 704.
5. Ehrlich, P. On immunity with special reference to cell life. *Proc. Roy. Soc.* [Biol.] 66:424, 1900.
6. Haurowitz, F., and Crampton, C. F. The fate in rabbits of intravenously injected I^{131} iodo-ovalbumin. *J. Immun.* 68:73, 1952.
7. Garvey, J. S., and Campbell, D. H. The retention of S^{35}-labeled bovine serum albumin in normal and immunized rabbit liver tissue. *J. Exp. Med.* 105:361, 1957.
8. Kabat, E. A. Heterogeneity in extent of the combining regions of human antidextran. *J. Immun.* 77:377, 1956.
9. Campbell, D. H., and Garvey, J. S. The fate of foreign antigen and speculations as to its

role in immune mechanisms. *Lab. Invest.* 10: 1126, 1961.

10. Campbell, D. H., and Garvey, J. S. Nature of retained antigen and its role in immune mechanisms. *Advances Immun.* 3:261, 1963.
11. Sabin, F. R. Cellular reactions to a dye-protein with a concept of the mechanism of antibody formation. *J. Exp. Med.* 70:67, 1939.
12. Kruse, H., and McMaster, P.D. The distribution and storage of blue antigenic azoproteins in the tissues of mice. *J. Exp. Med.* 90:425, 1949.
13. Coons, A. H., Creech, H. J., and Jones, R. N. The demonstration of pneumococcus antigens in tissues by use of fluorescent antibody. *J. Immun.* 45:159, 1942.
14. Coons, A. H., and Kaplan, M. H. Localization of antigen in tissue cells: II. Improvements in a method for the detection of antigen by means of fluorescent antibody. *J. Exp. Med.* 91:1, 1950.
15. Erickson, J. O., Armen, D. M., and Libby, R. L. The persistence of antigen in the mouse. *J. Immun.* 71:30, 1953.
16. Singer, S. J., and Schick, A. F. The preparation of specific stains for electron microscopy prepared by conjugation of antibody molecules with ferritin. *J. Biophys. and Biochem. Cytol.* 9:519, 1961.
17. Taylor, J. H. Autoradiography at the Cellular Level. In Oster, G., and Pollister, A. W. (Eds.), *Physical Techniques in Biological Research.* New York: Academic Press, Inc., 1956. Vol. III, p. 545.
18. Haurowitz, F., and Breinl, F. Quantitative Untersuchung der Verteilung eines arsenhaltigen Antigens im Organismus. *Z. Physiol. Chem.* 205:259, 1932.
19. Haurowitz, F., Tunca, M., and Schwerin, P. On the failure of azo-gelatin as an antigen. *Biochem. J.* 37:249, 1943.
20. McMaster, P. D., and Kruse, H. The persistence in mice of certain foreign proteins and azoprotein tracer-antigens derived from them. *J. Exp. Med.* 94:323, 1951.
21. McMaster, P. D., Edwards, J. L., and Sturm, E. Active anaphylaxis to a foreign protein induced in mice by the transfer of tissue from animals previously injected with the protein. *J. Exp. Med.* 102:119, 1955.
22. Garvey, J. S., and Campbell, D. H. Studies of the retention and properties of S^{35}-labeled antigen in livers of immunized rabbits. *J. Immun.* 76:36, 1956.
23. Williams, R. B., and Dawson, R. M. C. The biosynthesis of L-cystine and L-methionine labeled with radioactive sulfur (^{35}S). *Biochem. J.* 52:314, 1952.
24. Kamen, M. D. *Isotopic Tracers in Biology.* New York: Academic Press, Inc., 1957.
25. Germuth, F. G., Maumenee, A. E., Pratt-Johnson, J. A., Senterfit, L. B., Van Arnam, C. E., and Pollack, A. D. Observations on the Site and Mechanisms of Antigen-Antibody Interaction. In Shaffer, J. H., LoGrippo, G. A., and Chase, M. W. (Eds.), *Mechanisms of Hypersensitivity.* Boston: Little, Brown, 1959. P. 155.
26. Glenny, A. T., and Hopkins, B. E. Duration of passive immunity. *J. Hyg.* 22:12, 1923.
27. Felton, L. D. The significance of antigen in animal tissues. *J. Immun.* 61:107, 1949.
28. Chase, M. W. Immunologic tolerance. *Ann. Rev. Microbiol.* 13:349, 1959.
29. Wilson, G. S., and Miles, A. A. The Mechanisms Concerned in Specific Antibacterial Immunity. In *Topley and Wilson's Principles of Bacteriology and Immunity* (4th ed.). Baltimore: Williams & Wilkins Company, 1955. Vol. II, Chap. 47.
30. Cary, W. E. The fate of foreign erythrocytes introduced into the blood stream of the rabbit. *J. Infect. Dis.* 17:432, 1915.
31. Longcope, W. T., and Mackenzie, G. M. The relation between the disappearance of foreign proteins from the circulation and the formation of antibodies. *Proc. Soc. Exp. Biol. Med.* 17:133, 1920.
32. Eisen, H. N., and Keston, A. S. The immunologic reactivity of bovine serum albumin labeled with trace amounts of radioactive iodine (I^{131}). *J. Immun.* 63:71, 1949.
33. Knox, W. C., and Endicott, F. C. I^{131} as an antigen label in the circulating serum of nonimmune rabbits. *J. Immun.* 65:523, 1950.
34. Sterling, K. The turnover rate of serum albumin in man as measured by I^{131}-tagged albumin. *J. Clin. Invest.* 30:1228, 1951.
35. Francis, G. E., and Hawkins, J. D. The use of radioactive isotopes in immunological investigations: II. The fate of some chemically modified protein antigens in normal and immune rabbits. *Biochem. J.* 65:570, 1957.
36. Dixon, F. J. The use of I^{131} in immunologic investigation. *J. Allerg.* 24:547, 1953.
37. Dixon, F. J. The metabolism of antigen and antibody. *J. Allerg.* 25:487, 1954.
38. Landsteiner, K. *The Specificity of Serological Reactions.* Springfield, Ill.: Charles C Thomas, Publisher, 1936. Chap. V.
39. Pratt, H. N., and Gregersen, M. I. Studies with colored antigens: I. The rate of disappearance of dye-albumin from the blood. *J. Immun.* 40:163, 1941.
40. Garvey, J. S. An Investigation of the Sites of Antibody Formation by the Use of a Radioactive Antigen. Ohio State University Ph.D. Thesis, 1950.
41. Garvey, J. S., and Campbell, D. H. The relation of circulating antibody concentration to

localization of labeled (S^{35}) antigen. *J. Immun.* 72:131, 1954.
42. Dochez, A. R., and Avery, O. T. The elaboration of specific soluble substance by pneumococcus during growth. *J. Exp. Med.* 26:477, 1917.
43. Oliver, J. New directions in renal morphology: a method, its results and its future. *Harvey Lect.* 40:102, 1944–45.
44. Dixon, F. J., Dammin, G. J., and Bukantz, S. C. Effect of sensitization and irradiation on the fate of I^{131}-labeled bovine gamma globulin in rabbits and mice. *Fed. Proc.* 9:380, 1950.
45. Melcher, L. R., and Masouredis, S. P. The *in vivo* stability of the I^{131} protein label of rabbit antibody in guinea pigs as determined by the quantitative precipitin reaction. *J. Immun.* 67:393, 1951.
46. Laws, J. O. Fate of radioactive protein in the animal body. *Nature* (London) 167:820, 1951.
47. Tong, W., Taurog, A., and Chaikoff, I. L. The metabolism of I^{131}-labeled diiodotyrosine. *J. Biol. Chem.* 207:59, 1954.
48. Smetana, H. The permeability of the renal glomeruli of several mammalian species to labeled protein. *Amer. J. Path.* 23:255, 1947.
49. Garvey, J. S., and Campbell, D. H. Unpublished data, 1958.
50. Wilson, G. S., and Miles, A. A. Ref. 29, Vol. I, p. 303.
51. Coons, A. H., Snyder, J. C., Cheever, F. S., and Murray, E. S. Localization of antigen in tissue cells: IV. Antigens of rickettsiae and mumps virus. *J. Exp. Med.* 91:31, 1950.
52. Ingraham, J. S. Artificial radioactive antigens: III. S^{35}-sulfanil-azo-sheep red cell stromata; preparation and gross distribution in normal rabbits and mice. *J. Infect. Dis.* 96:105, 1955.
53. Sullivan, F. L., Nechermann, E. G., and Cannon, P. R. The localization and fate of bacteria in the tissues. *J. Immun.* 26:49, 1934.
54. Ingraham, J. S. Artificial radioactive antigens: II. The metabolism of S^{35}-sulfanilic acid-azo-bovine γ-globulin in normal and immune mice. *J. Infect. Dis.* 89:117, 1951.
55. Libby, R. L., and Madison, C. R. The distribution of tobacco-mosaic virus in the mouse. *J. Immun.* 55:15, 1947.
56. Breinl, F., and Haurowitz, F. Chemische Untersuchung des Präzipitates aus Hämoglobin und Anti-Hämoglobin-Serum und Bemerkungen über die Natur der Antikorper. *Z. Physiol. Chem.* 192:45, 1930.
57. Alexander, J. Some intracellular aspects of life and disease. *Protoplasma* 14:296, 1932.
58. Mudd, S. A hypothetical mechanism of antibody formation. *J. Immun.* 23:423, 1932.
59. Pauling, L. A theory of the structure and process of formation of antibodies. *J. Amer. Chem. Soc.* 62:2643, 1940.
60. Burnet, F. M., and Fenner, F. *The Production of Antibodies* (2nd ed.). Melbourne: Macmillan & Company, Ltd., 1949.
61. Garvey, J. S., and Campbell, D. H. Studies of the retention and properties of S^{35}-labeled antigen in livers of immunized rabbits. *J. Immun.* 76:36, 1956.
62. Richter, M., and Haurowitz, F. Continuous synthesis of antibody after primary immunization with protein antigens. *J. Immun.* 84:420, 1960.
63. Garvey, J. S., and Campbell, D. H. Unpublished data, 1960.
64. Garvey, J. S., and Campbell, D. H. Effect of secondary injections of antigen upon the retention in liver of a primary injection. *J. Exp. Med.* 107:497, 1958.
65. Hirata, A. A., Garvey, J. S., and Campbell, D. H. Retention of antigen in tissues of serologically suppressed chickens. *J. Immun.* 84:576, 1960.
66. Garvey, J. S., Eitzman, D. V., and Smith, R. T. The distribution of S^{35}-labeled bovine serum albumin in newborn and immunologically tolerant adult rabbits. *J. Exp. Med.* 112:533, 1960.
67. Crampton, C. F., and Haurowitz, F. Deposition of small doses of injected antigen in rabbits. *J. Immun.* 69:457, 1952.
68. Saha, A., Garvey, J. S., and Campbell, D. H. Studies on RNA-antigen complex. *Fed. Proc.* 21:31, 1962.
69. Ishizaka, T., Campbell, D. H., and Ishizaka, K. Internal antigenic determinants in protein molecules. *Proc. Soc. Exp. Biol. Med.* 103:5, 1960.
70. Lapresle, C., Kaminski, M., and Tanner, C. E. Immunochemical study of the enzymatic degradation of human serum albumin: An analysis of the antigenic structure of a protein molecule. *J. Immun.* 82:94, 1959.
71. Coons, A. H. The cytology of antibody formation. *J. Cell. Comp. Physiol.* 52 (supp. 1):55, 1958.
72. Leduc, E. H., Coons, A. H., and Connolly, J. M. Studies on antibody production: II. The primary and secondary responses in the popliteal lymph node of the rabbit. *J. Exp. Med.* 102:61, 1955.
73. Campbell, D. H., and Garvey, J. S. Factors involved in antibody formation. *J. Infect. Dis.* 107:15, 1960.
74. Sorkin, E. Discussion. In *Mechanisms of Antibody Formation,* Holub, M., and Jarošková, L. (Eds.). Prague: Publishing House of the Czechoslovak Academy of Sciences; and New York: Academic Press, Inc., 1960, p. 220.

75. Campbell, D. H., and Garvey, J. S. The fate of labeled foreign antigens in the livers of normal and immunized rabbits. *Int. Arch. Allerg.* 12:70, 1958.
76. Campbell, D. H. Some speculations on the significance of formation and persistence of antigen fragments in tissues of immunized animals. *Blood* 72:589, 1957.
77. Talmage, D. W., Dixon, F. J., Bukantz, S. C., and Dammin, G. J. Antigen elimination from the blood as an early manifestation of the immune response. *J. Immun.* 67:243, 1951.

3. The Structure of Antibody

SYDNEY COHEN

ANTIBODIES IN MAN AND MANY ANImals are associated with a complex group of structurally related proteins, conveniently referred to as the immunoglobulins [1]. This is a heterogeneous family of molecules and it might be anticipated that observed variations in physical and chemical properties would be related to differences in serological specificity. However, much of the structural variability of immunoglobulins appears to be unrelated to combining specificity so that distinct antibodies may be as heterogeneous as the total fraction. Moreover, when different specific antibodies are isolated and analyzed they appear to be indistinguishable in over-all chemical composition. Therefore it is not known whether distinct combining specificities are determined by different amino acid sequences or by variable folding of antibody sites having the same sequences. Particular interest is attached to this fundamental problem because of its relevance to the mechanism of antibody synthesis. The size and complexity of immunoglobulin molecules is such that knowledge of antibody structure has been obtained largely through the study of restricted portions of the molecule which can subsequently be related to the whole. For this reason, this chapter is concerned mainly with properties of the individual polypeptide chains of immunoglobulins and with the characteristics of antibody fragments obtained by enzymatic digestion.

Some immunological reactions, such as delayed hypersensitivity and transplantation immunity, appear to be mediated by specifically modified mononuclear cells of individuals exposed to the antigenic stimulus [2]. This view rests mainly on the observation that these immune states can be passively transferred by lymphoid cells of a sensitized donor, whereas serum is inactive; moreover, these reactions may occur in the absence of a detectable level of circulating antibody of the appropriate specificity. This experimental evidence is inconclusive, and it is possible to account for most of the features of delayed hypersensitivity and transplantation immunity in terms of high affinity antibody present at concentrations too low to be detected by conventional methods [3]. If this hypothesis proves to be correct, it may become possible to account for all immunological reactions in terms of circulating antibody. At present, knowledge of the structural features of antibodies extends only to those known to be associated with the serum immunoglobulins, and the discussion which follows will be confined to these proteins.

HETEROGENEITY OF THE IMMUNOGLOBULINS

Tiselius and Kabat [4] first demonstrated that precipitating antibodies in a strongly immunized rabbit were associated with γ-globulin. This fraction, originally defined as the component which moves most slowly during electrophoresis of serum at alkaline pH, is now known to include three classes of protein. In all species investigated the main component of γ-globulin has a molecular weight of about 150,000 and is usually referred to as 7S γ-globulin; immunoelectrophoresis has shown that protein having the antigenic specificity of 7S γ-globulin extends into the β- and α-globulin regions. About 5 to 10 percent of human γ-globulin consists of protein having a molecular weight of about 1,000,000 and is referred to as 19S γ-globulin; this fraction can be identified by immunoelectrophoresis, when it is usually referred to as β_{2M}- or γ_{1M}-globulin. Immunoelectrophoresis has also led to the identification of a third antigenically distinct type of γ-globulin known as γ_{1A}- or β_{2A}-globulin [5] which is mainly of molecular size similar to that of 7S γ-globulin but, like the 19S fraction, has a relatively high carbohydrate content. Despite their diversity, the three types of γ-globulin have a basically similar structure and all appear to be associated with antibody activity. It is therefore logical, as suggested by Heremans [1], to refer to this family of proteins as the immunoglobulins (IgG). For convenience, the three subfractions will be referred to as IgG (7S γ-globulin), IgM (γ_{1M}-globulin), and IgA (γ_{1A}-globulin). Some properties of these immunoglobulins are summarized below and in Table 3-1.

IgG (7S γ-globulin). This fraction comprises about 85 percent of the total immunoglobulin and contains about 3 percent carbohydrate [6]. IgG can be prepared free from other immunoglobulin fractions by elution of serum from diethylaminoethyl (DEAE) cellulose columns [7, 8]. In all species investigated, molecular weight estimations have fallen within the range 140,000 to 190,000 [9]. Recent studies [10, 11] suggest that this wide scatter arises from differences of technique and that the lower figure, which corresponds to the original estimates of Heidelberger and Pedersen [12], is more probably correct. The heterogeneity of this protein is shown by its wide range of electrophoretic mobility and diffuse spread on ion exchange chromatography [13]. Most of the antibodies which have been studied in detail belong to this subfraction of the immunoglobulins. In the rabbit such antibodies exhibit the same degree of heterogeneity as the whole fraction [14], but human IgG has been separated into a number of chromatographic subfractions in which various antibody activities are unevenly distributed [15].

IgM (19S γ-globulin). This protein fraction has an average molecular weight of about 1,000,000 and constitutes 5 to 10 percent of electrophoretically isolated γ-globulin and ap-

TABLE 3-1. Some Properties of the Subfractions of Human Immunoglobulins

Components	IgG	IgM	IgA
Synonyms	7S γ-globulin	γ_{1M}-globulin	γ_{1A}-globulin
	γ_2-globulin	β_{2M}-globulin	β_{2A}-globulin
	γ_{ss}-globulin	19S globulin	
		γ-macroglobulin	
Serum conc., gm./100 ml.	0.8 to 1.5	0.05 to 0.10	0.05 to 0.20
PHYSICOCHEMICAL PROPERTIES			
% N	15.6	14.5	16.2
% Hexose	1.2	5.2	4.8
% Fucose	0.3	0.6	0.2
% Hexosamine	1.1	2.9	3.8
% Sialic acid	0.2	1.7	1.7
% Total carbohydrate	3.0	10.0	10.0
Electrophoretic mobility	−0.6 to +3.0	About +2	+1.2 to +3.6
pH 8.6 (-10^{-5} cm^{2}V^{-1}sec^{-1})			
Sedimentation coefficient ($S_{20,w}$)	6 to 7	18 to 20	7 (80–85%) 10 to 13 (15–20%)
Range of salting out $(NH_4)_2SO_4$, pH 7	1.2 to 1.8M	1.1 to 1.6M	1.3 to 1.8M
BIOLOGICAL PROPERTIES			
Antibody activity	+	+	+
Allotypic specificity			
Gm	+	−	−
Inv	+	+	+
Complement fixation	+	+	?0

proximately 1 percent of the total protein in human serum [16]. Normal and pathological IgM fractions show a characteristic heterogeneity in the ultracentrifuge; the major component has a sedimentation constant of 19S, and there are two additional components with sedimentation constants of about 29S and 35S to 40S which are thought to be polymers of 19S γ-globulin [16]. The electrophoretic mobility of IgM is intermediate between γ- and β-globulins, and the fraction contains about 10 percent carbohydrate (Table 3-1). Such macroglobulins occur in the serum of many species, including horses [12], rabbits [17], mice [18], and chickens [19]. IgM can be observed by immunoelectrophoresis and can be isolated in relatively pure form by preparative ultracentrifugation [16] or by a combination of chromatography and gel filtration [20]. Heidelberger and Pedersen [12] and Kabat and Pedersen [21] first showed in their classic experiments that horse antipneumococcus antibody has a relatively high molecular weight. Since then, several biologically active proteins have been demonstrated in the human 19S γ-globulin fraction; some of these, including cold agglutinins, antibodies to the O antigen of *Salmonella*, and the rheumatoid factor, are confined to this fraction, while others, such as isohemagglutinins, antithyroglobulin, and the antibodies mediating the Wassermann reaction, are present in both IgG and IgM fractions [16, 22].

IgA (*γ_{1A}-globulin*). This fraction, which comprises about 10 percent of human immunoglobulin, has been isolated from normal serum by a combination of zinc sulfate and ammonium sulfate precipitation and preparative electrophoresis [23]. IgA is usually heterogeneous in the ultracentrifuge; the main component has a sedimentation constant of approximately 7S, but additional components, ranging from 7S to 15S, are usually present [24]. IgA has a relatively high carbohydrate content and an electrophoretic mobility corresponding to γ_1-globulin (Table 3-1). Proteins equivalent to human IgA have been described in the mouse [25] and probably occur also in the horse (T globulin) [26]. Because of the difficulty of isolating IgA in pure, uncontaminated form, some doubt has attached to claims that this fraction is associated with antibacterial [28] and reaginic [29] antibodies. However, the removal of IgA by immune absorption has been shown to eliminate all detectable skin-sensitizing activity from the sera of three ragweed-sensitive individuals, whereas similar absorption of IgG had no detectable effect [30]. In addition, insulin antibodies from two individuals have been shown by immunoelectrophoresis using I^{131}-insulin to be associated with IgA [31], and human antibodies to diphtheria toxoid and to *Brucella abortus suis* have been demonstrated in carefully purified preparations of IgA [32]. It can be accepted, therefore, that the IgA fraction of human immunoglobulin carries antibody activity.

PEPTIDE CHAINS OF ANTIBODY MOLECULES

It is fundamental to the understanding of antibody structure to establish whether immunoglobulin molecules consist of one or more peptide chains. One approach to this problem is to investigate the number and identity of the free terminal amino groups in the molecule. For this purpose, the protein is reacted with fluorodinitrobenzene (FDNB), which combines with the free amino group to give a yellow dinitrophenyl (DNP) amino acid derivative which can be split from the protein by hydrolysis and identified by chromatography [33]. The data obtained by this method for the γ-globulins of different animal species are difficult to reconcile [9]. Human γ-globulin contains one N-terminal aspartic acid residue and up to two glutamic acid residues per mole of protein, which suggests the presence of two or three peptide chains. Rabbit γ-globulin has one terminal alanine residue per molecule together with traces of aspartic acid and serine, and this suggests that the protein may be a single long polypeptide chain. In the γ-globulin of horse and cow some four or five N-terminal amino acids are present, but together add up to less than 1 mole per mole of protein, while pig γ-globulin contains three or four N-terminal amino acid residues per mole. These differences cannot, at present, be attributed to technical factors. Denaturing and reducing agents have failed to reveal unreactive N-terminal amino acids in rabbit γ-globulin [34, 35], while the phenyl isocyanate method of N-terminal amino acid assay gives results for pig and human γ-globulin very similar to those obtained with DNP [36].

These species differences are surprising in view of the over-all similarity of γ-globulin in

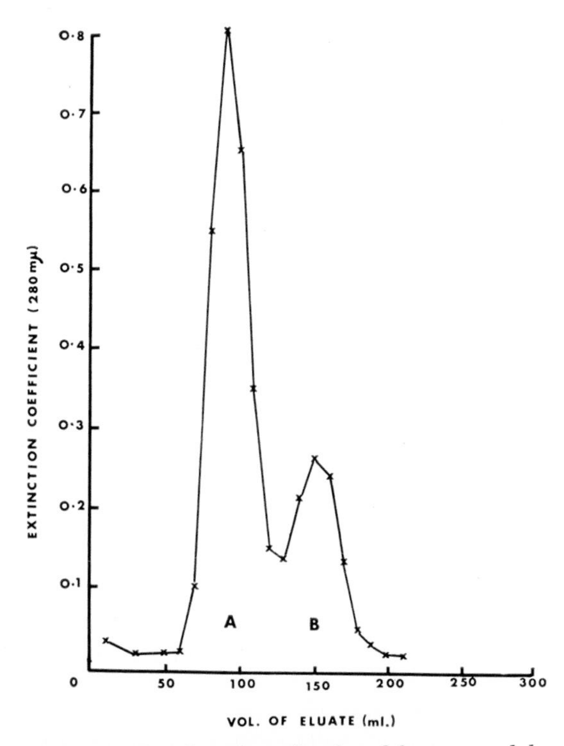

Fig. 3-1. Fractionation of reduced human γ-globulin (IgG) on Sephadex G-75 in N acetic acid showing separation of A and B chains.

various animals. It is therefore of interest that similar discrepancies are not apparent when a different analytical approach is used. In proteins having more than one peptide chain, the units are held together by interaction between adjacent amino acid side chain groups. The disulfide bond of the cystine residues is the only common covalent linkage holding together the constituent chains of a protein molecule. This bond is split by reduction or oxidation, and the consequent fall in molecular weight gives a guide to the approximate number of peptide chains present. Edelman [37] has shown that when human γ-globulin is reduced in the presence of 6 M urea, approximately 15 disulfide bonds are split and the molecular weight falls from about 150,000 to 50,000; the γ-globulins of other species behave similarly [38, 39]. This suggested that all mammalian γ-globulins contain three or possibly four peptide chains. It follows that some of the N-terminal amino acids in human, rabbit, equine, and bovine γ-globulin are blocked or are poorly reactive under the conditions of analysis which have been employed.

The products obtained after reduction of γ-globulin in the presence of urea are separable by chromatography but are biologically inactive and insoluble in aqueous solutions [38]. The chains of γ-globulin can, however, be prepared in soluble form and with several biological activities intact by reduction with mercaptoethanol at pH 8.2 in the absence of urea [40]. These conditions lead to the splitting of 5 of the 20 disulfide bonds present in γ-globulin, but the molecular weight of the protein remains unchanged. However, if the partially reduced alkylated protein is dialyzed against N-acetic or N-propionic acid, it dissociates into two fractions (A and B) which can be separated with 100 percent recovery by gel filtration on Sephadex G-75 columns (Fig. 3-1). On electrophoresis in urea-formic acid starch gels (pH 3.5) the B fraction is diffuse and runs ahead of A, which appears to be relatively homogeneous (Fig. 3-2). It is apparent from their electrophoretic behavior that A and B correspond to the chains referred

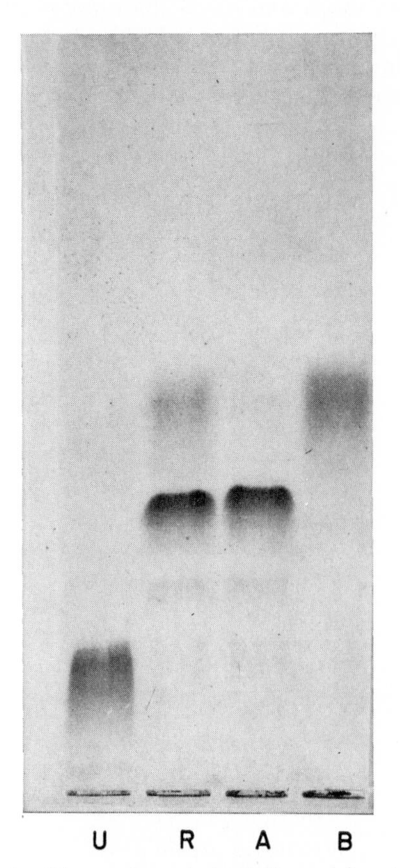

Fig. 3-2. Electrophoresis in 8 M urea-formic acid starch gel (pH 3.5) of human IgG (*U*), reduced IgG (*R*), A chain (*A*), and B chain (*B*).

to as H and L [41], which are obtained after more extensive reduction in the presence of urea.

The A chain of γ-globulin comprises three fourths of the original molecule and has a molecular weight of 50,000; the B chain, which makes up the rest of the molecule, has a molecular weight of 20,000 [11] (Table 3-2). The relative yields and molecular weights suggest that the molecule is made up of two A and two B chains, and this is supported by amino acid analyses. In both rabbit [42] and human γ-globulin [20] the A and B chains have very different amino acid compositions, but the sum of two A plus two B chains gives an amino acid analysis closely similar to that of whole γ-globulin (Table 3-3). The carbohydrate of the molecule appears to be associated almost entirely with the A chain (Table 3-4). The small amounts of carbohydrate present in the B chain may arise from contamination with A, but could be an integral part of some molecules of B.

Both the A and the B chain are chemically heterogeneous, as shown by the fact that the N-terminal aspartic and glutamic acids of human γ-globulin are present on both the separated chains [20]. In addition, both show a broad electrophoretic spread when analyzed in starch or acrylamide gels at alkaline pH. In the case of A, the relative mobility of the chain is related to that of the γ-globulin from which it is derived; this is true of both normal and pathological γ-globulins [43]. The mobility of B, on the other hand, is unrelated to that of its parent γ-globulin. A feature of particular interest is that in all species examined the B chain resolved into about ten distinct components on starch gel electrophoresis in urea-glycine buffer, pH 7 to 8; these subfractions of the human B chain have been numbered B1 to B10 (Fig. 3-3) from the cathodal end of the gel [43, 44]. Control experiments indicate that this complexity is not an artefact resulting from unequal reduction of B chains or from variable hydrolysis of amide groups during fractionation in N-acetic acid; nor can it be attributed to variable reaction of amino groups with cyanate which is in equilibrium with urea at neutral and alkaline pH [45]. The separated fractions of B, on re-electrophoresis, behave as single components with the same mobilities as originally observed. In addition, when myeloma γ-globulins are isolated and

TABLE 3-2. Properties of the Separated Chains of Human 7S γ-Globulin (IgG)

Components	A Chain	B Chain
Synonyms	H	L
Total %	71–76	24–29
Molecular weight	50,000	20,000
Electrophoretic mobility (pH 8)	Related to original γ	Not related to original γ
N-terminal amino acid		
Asp (mole/mole)	0.1	0.2
Glu (mole/mole)	0.4	0.1
Antigenic determinants		
Common to immunoglobulins		
Type I	0	+
Type II	0	+
Specific for IgG	+	0
Genotypic specificity		
Gm	+	0
Inv	0	+
Presence in papain pieces		
S	?	+
F	+	0

TABLE 3-3. Amino Acid Analysis of Human 7S γ-Globulin (IgG) and Its A and B Chains

Amino Acids	A Chain	B Chain	2 A + 2 B	γ-Globulin
	Mole / Mole			
Molecular Wt.	50,000	20,000		140,000
Lys	29	9.7	77	77
His	9.6	2.5	24	25
Arg	12	5.8	36	36
Asp	33	13	92	94
Thr	34	15	98	98
Ser	50	24	148	147
Glu	39	20	118	121
Pro	33	11	88	92
Gly	28	11	78	83
Ala	19	12	62	65
Val	41	13	108	112
Met	3.9	0.6	10	9.9
Ileu	8.2	4.9	25	27
Leu	31	13	88	92
Tyr	17	7.6	49	49
Phe	13	6.0	38	40
Cys	6.9	2.9	20	28
Cys-CH_2COOH	3.6	0.9	9	—
Try	7.5	2.3	20	20

SOURCE: Cohen [20] and Crumpton and Wilkinson [162].

fractionated in exactly the same way, the B chains show only one or two components in urea-glycine starch gels (Fig. 3-4), and this is the strongest evidence that the multiple nature of the normal B chain is not an artefact.

It appears from these data that the B chain of γ-globulin exists in the native molecule in a variety of molecular forms. It is known that these fall into two major antigenic groups referred to as types I and II (see below). B chains isolated from myeloma proteins are of a single antigenic type; these chains show differences in amino acid composition which are most pronounced between type I and type II B chains, even when these are of the same electrophoretic mobility. Thus type I B chains have a significantly higher content of glutamic acid and lower content of proline, glycine, alanine, valine, and tryptophan [43]. These findings are in accordance with the observation that the two antigenic types of Bence Jones protein which appear to be composed of B chains [46] have completely distinct peptide patterns after peptic digestion [47, 90].

Synthesis of the multiple molecular forms of B is presumably controlled by several gene loci. No evidence has been obtained of genetic variation between individuals, and the B chain patterns observed in single subjects belonging to several racial groups and in parents of agammaglobulinemic children are identical [43]. It is, however, of interest that changes in B chain pattern were observed during postnatal development in a calf which had been deprived of colostrum [43]. This suggests that differentiation of the antibody-forming system

TABLE 3-4. Carbohydrate Content of the Peptide Chains of Rabbit 7S γ-Globulin (IgG)

Carbohydrate	γ-Globulin (Mole/Mole 140,000)	A Chain (Mole/Mole 50,000)	B Chain (Mole/Mole 20,000)
Hexose	9.6	4.5	0.27
Hexosamine	8.2	4.0	0.16
Sialic acid	0.9	0.41	0.0

SOURCE: Fleischman *et al.* [42].

following birth may involve a selective activation of the various genes controlling B chain synthesis.

ENZYMATIC CLEAVAGE OF ANTIBODY MOLECULES

The degradation of γ-globulin without loss of antibody activity was demonstrated many years ago in the case of several horse antibodies which can be hydrolyzed to fractions of molecular weight 100,000 without loss of precipitating power. More recently, Porter [48] observed that papain activated by cysteine splits rabbit γ-globulin into three fragments separable by chomatography. The largest of these (piece III) has a molecular weight of about 50,000, is readily crystallized, and contains no antibody activity, although it is associated with other biological activities of the original molecule (Table 3-5). The other fragments (I and II) each have a molecular weight of 45,000, and, although they do not precipitate with the homologous antigen, they specifically inhibit the combination of the whole antibody with the antigen. These results suggested that pieces I and II each contained one unaltered combining site, and direct proof of this has been obtained by equilibrium dialysis studies [49, 50] and by fluorescence quenching [51] employing antihapten antibodies.

The digestion of an IgG subfraction of relatively rapid electrophoretic mobility has been shown to yield fractions I and III, while digestion of more slowly migrating IgG gives fractions II and III [52, 53]. In addition, digestion of purified antibody yields twice as much protein in fraction I as in fraction II, and iodination of the two fractions occurs at significantly different rates [54]. All of these findings indicate that individual γ-globulin molecules contain active fragments of a single chromatographic type. It has now been shown that these univalent fragments have different amino acid compositions consistent with their relative electrophoretic mobilities [55]; whole γ-globulin probably shows corresponding differences, but because of the size of the molecule these have not been detected in analyses of distinct antibodies [56, 57] or electrophoretic subfractions of whole γ-globulin [14].

In Porter's [48] original method for splitting rabbit γ-globulin, cysteine was used to acti-

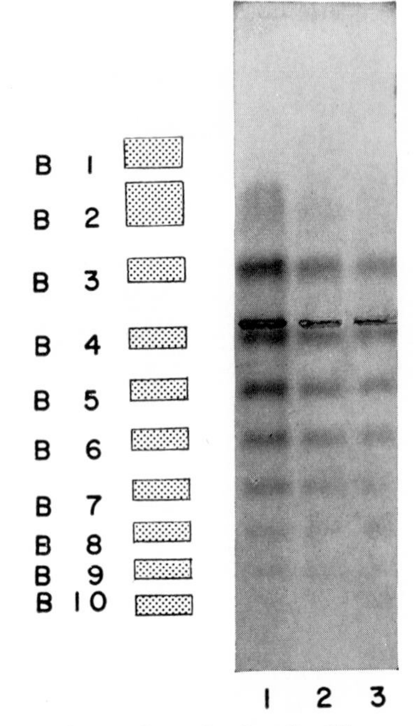

Fig. 3-3. Electrophoresis in 8 M urea-glycine starch gel (pH 7–8) of the B chains from fast (*1*) and slow (*2*) electrophoretic subfractions of normal human IgG and from normal human IgM (*3*). A diagram of the 10 components of the human B chain is shown on the left; designated from the cathodal end as B1 to B10. (See Cohen and Porter [43].)

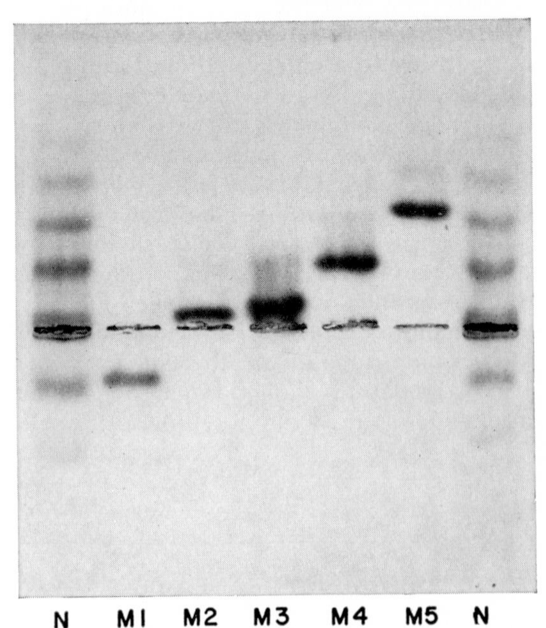

Fig. 3-4. Electrophoresis in 8 M urea-glycine starch gel of the B chains of normal human IgG (*N*) and of five myeloma γ-globulins (*M1* to *M5*). (See Cohen and Porter [43].)

TABLE 3-5. Some Properties of Fragments Obtained by Papain Digestion of Rabbit and Human 7S γ-Globulin (IgG)

Properties	Fragments with Antibody Activity		Fragments with No Antibody Activity	
	Rabbit	Human	Rabbit	Human
Nomenclature	I and II	S or A and C	III	F or B
Molecular weight	45,000	35,000–50,000	50,000	
Proportion of total	⅔	⅔	⅓	⅓
Complement fixation	0	0	+	+
Passage across fetal membranes	0		+	
Skin fixation	0		+	
Combination with rheumatoid factor	0		+	
Antigenic determinants				
Common to immunoglobulins	+	+	0	0
Specific for IgG	0	0	+	+
Allotypic specificity	a and b	Inv	0	Gm

vate the papain. Cebra and co-workers [35] subsequently showed that the resulting fragments are produced by a combination of proteolysis and disulfide cleavage. Thus digestion with insoluble papain ruptures four to five peptide bonds without altering the size of the molecule; subsequent incubation with cysteine leads to a decrease in sedimentation constant to 3.5S and dissociation of the antibody into the three fragments already described.

Papain digestion of γ-globulin from various species gives pieces of molecular size similar to those obtained in the rabbit. Thus human γ-globulin is split by papain and cysteine to yield a component (S) of slow electrophoretic mobility [58] which comprises two thirds of the total and can be separated by chromatography into two fractions called A and C, both of which contain a single antibody combining site [52]. The remaining third of the molecule consists of a more rapidly migrating fragment (referred to as F or B) which is devoid of antibody combining activity; this fraction has been crystallized from digests of concentrated human γ-globulin [59]. It seems likely from these results that fragments obtained by papain digestion of human and rabbit antibodies are basically similar (Table 3-5).

Peptic digestion of rabbit antibody degrades a portion of the molecule which appears to be equivalent to piece III and leaves a 100,000 molecular weight fragment which will precipitate with the antigen. Reduction of a single disulfide bond splits this fragment to give two 50,000 molecular weight pieces which are very similar to the papain pieces I or II [60]; this reaction is partly reversible, so that fragments from different antibodies can be recombined to produce 100,000 molecular weight molecules containing two unrelated combining sites [61].

GENERAL CONFIGURATION OF ANTIBODY MOLECULES

To understand the over-all configuration of antibody molecules it is necessary to relate the fractions obtained by enzymatic digestion to the peptide chains separated by reduction. Fleischman, Pain, and Porter [40] investigated this relationship using rabbit A and B chains and goat antisera specific for piece I and piece III; as shown in Figure 3-5, the B chain reacted only with anti-I sera (or anti-II), while A reacted with antisera to piece I (or II) and piece III. It is evident from this that the A chain must be split during papain digestion, since part of it is present in piece I (or II) and part in piece III.

On the basis of these findings and data sum-

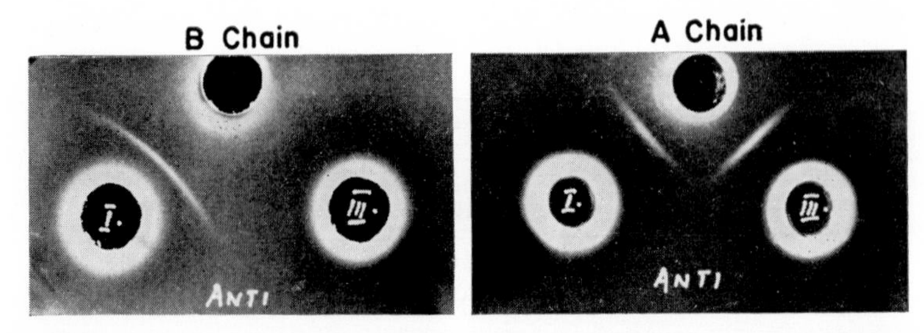

Fig. 3-5. Ouchterlony plate showing the reaction of separate A chains (*right*) and B chains (*left*) from reduced rabbit γ-globulin with goat anti-piece I and anti-piece III; the pieces used for immunization were obtained by papain digestion. (See Fleischman *et al.* [40].)

marized above, Porter [62] proposed that the 7S γ-globulin molecule is made up of two A chains (molecular weight 50,000) and two B chains (molecular weight 20,000) held together by five disulfide bridges (Fig. 3-6). The site of papain cleavage is such that piece III consists only of the A chain; the two fragments (I and II) which carry antibody activity are united by a single disulfide bond and each contains a portion of A and a complete B chain. By reduction of piece I, Fleischman, Porter, and Press [42] isolated this portion of the A chain, which they called A piece, and have shown that it is antigenically distinct from B and contains antigenic sites common to the A chain. Further support for the general con-

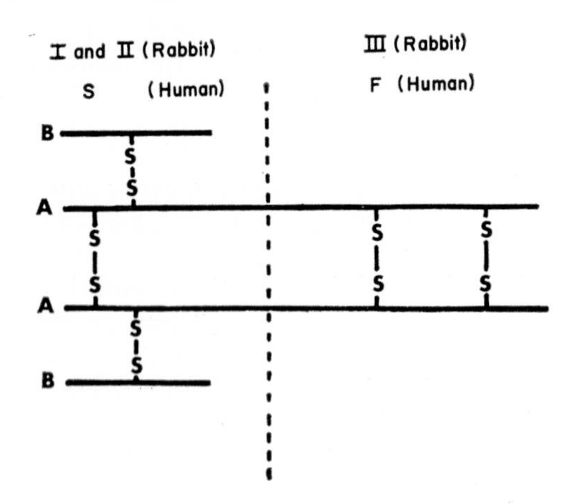

Fig. 3-6. Possible arrangement of the peptide chains of IgG. The molecule is shown made up of two A and two B chains. The dotted line indicates probable site of papain cleavage which separates the molecule into pieces having antibody activity (I and II in the rabbit; S fragments in human) and a piece with no antibody activity (III in rabbit, F in human). (See Porter [62], Fleischman *et al.* [42], Cohen [20].)

figuration shown in Figure 3-6 comes from the fact that tryptic digests of piece I (or II) give the number of peptide spots expected from the content of arginine and lysine residues; piece III, on the other hand, gives only half the number of peptides expected, indicating that it is made up of two identical halves [63].

Porter's proposed four-chain structure was based mainly on studies of rabbit γ-globulin; a closely similar structure for human γ-globulin is suggested by the relative yields of A and B, their amino acid composition and sulfhydryl content (Table 3-3) as well as by the stability of the chains after more complete reduction in the presence of 6 M urea [20] or 6 M guanidine. In the case of human γ-globulin, there is no doubt that the F fragment is made up of A chain since anti-F sera react with A (H) chains [64] and anti-A sera react with F fragment [20]. Similarly, the B chain is present in the S fragment, since B and S give a reaction of identity with anti-B sera [20]. However, serological tests have failed to demonstrate the presence of A chain determinants in the human S fragment [20, 64]. This suggests that the portion of the A chain present in the S fragment may be poorly antigenic or may contain determinants which are common to the B chain.

STRUCTURAL RELATIONSHIPS BETWEEN IMMUNOGLOBULINS

Despite their diversity, all normal and pathological human γ-globulins have a basically similar structure and can be split by reduction and separated by gel filtration into large A and smaller B chains; these chains are present in the same proportions in IgG, IgM, and IgA fractions [20]. The higher molecular weight proteins present in IgM and part of IgA appear to be polymers in which the units of the basic four-chain structure are held together by disulfide bonds. Thus 19S γ-globulin can be dissociated into 7S units by reduction in aqueous solution [65], and reduction of the 9S to 13S components of γ_{1A} myeloma proteins leads to similar dissociation [66, 67]. High molecular weight γ-globulins cannot be regarded as polymers of IgG since the 7S units of human IgM differ from those of IgG in electrophoretic mobility, carbohydrate content, antigenic properties [68], and amino acid composition [69].

The B chains from normal 7S and 19S γ-globulins appear to be identical on electrophoresis at pH 3.5 (Fig. 3-7) and pH 8 (Fig. 3-3) in urea starch gels. In addition, those antigenic and allotypic determinants which are common to all immunoglobulins are associated with the B chain (see below). These findings indicate that all immunoglobulins contain B chains of similar structure. The A chains of normal 7S and 19S γ-globulins (Fig. 3-7) and of pathological γ_{1A}-globulins differ in their electrophoretic behavior; in addition, they are associated with type-specific antigenic and allotypic determinants (discussed later). It appears, therefore, that the three types of immunoglobulins have different A chains. As mentioned earlier, almost all of the carbohydrate of the molecule is present in the A chain, and this may contribute to the observed differences.

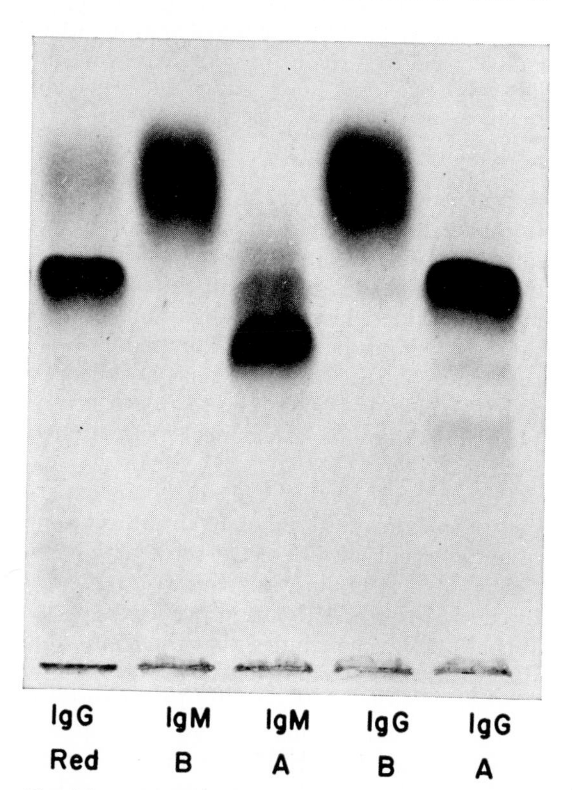

Fig. 3-7. Electrophoresis in 8 M urea-formic acid starch gel of whole reduced human IgG (IgG Red) and the separated A and B chains of IgM and IgG. The B chains of IgG and IgM appear to be identical, but the A chains have different electrophoretic mobilities. (See Cohen [20].)

THE ANTIBODY COMBINING SITE

The combining site is visualized as the surface area of the antibody molecule which is directly involved in combination with the antigen. The size of this active site has been defined in terms of the antigenic groups with which it interacts. Thus Landsteiner and van der Scheer [70] showed that immunization with an azoprotein having arsanilic and succinanilic acid groups attached to the same benzene ring stimulates the production of antibodies specific for only one group; this indicated that the antibody combining site is not sufficiently large to be complementary to both groups. Studies with polyglucose antigens [71] and with large haptenic groups [72] have suggested that the combining site has an area of roughly 700 sq. A, which is equivalent to 1 percent of the surface area of the molecule. There is evidence that antidextran antibodies consist of heterogeneous populations of molecules having combining sites of various sizes [71]; those with smaller and larger combining sites have been separated by specific absorption and elution from insoluble dextran [73]. The upper limit for an antidextran combining site is complementary in size to a hexasaccharide or heptasaccharide, but the lower limit has not been established. The most recent estimate of the size of an antibody combining site suggests that it involves ten to twenty amino acids [74].

The number of combining sites on each 7S antibody molecule is generally agreed to be two; this has been established from equilibrium dialysis measurements and by ultracentrifugation and electrophoresis of antigen-antibody complexes dissolved in excess antigen under conditions in which it can be assumed that all combining sites are saturated [9]. The isolation of two antibody fragments each with a single combining site also indicates very convincingly that antibody molecules are bivalent [48]. Nonprecipitating antibodies found in certain antisera are sometimes regarded as univalent, but there is no proof for this assumption. As already mentioned, it is possible to produce artificially, antibodies with different combining sites [61], but in natural conditions the two sites on a single molecule always appear to have the same specificity [75–77]. Higher molecular weight antibodies probably carry two combining sites per 7S unit. Thus peptic digestion of 19S horse antipneumococcus polysaccharide produces active fragments with molecular weights of about 100,000 which still precipitate with the antigen and are therefore presumably divalent [78].

Rabbit antibodies against different antigens have the same over-all amino acid composition [56, 57], identical N-terminal pentapeptide sequences [34, 79], and closely similar peptide patterns [80]. Since each antibody combining site involves only about 15 of the 1,500 amino acids of the molecule, the apparent identity of different antibodies does not exclude the possibility that specificity is determined by chemical differences at the active sites. Understanding of the structural basis of antibody specificity will require the solution of the complete chemical structure of the combining site; for this reason the location of these sites on the antibody molecule is a matter of particular interest.

The enzymatic cleavage of antibody molecules has led to the isolation of active, univalent fragments having a molecular weight of about 50,000 (Table 3-5). As already shown, these fragments consist of the B chain and a portion of the A chain (Fig. 3-6); the combining site must therefore be present on the B chain or the A piece, or be formed jointly by these chains. Edelman and co-workers [81] have observed reproducible patterns of the B (L) chain characteristic for antibodies of different specificities when fully reduced alkylated guinea pig antibodies were analyzed in urea-formic acid starch gels. On this basis they suggested [81a] that the B chain contained all or part of the antibody combining site. However, B chains from specifically isolated antibodies of horse and rabbit do not show similar evidence of banding when analyzed under the same conditions [62]. In addition, the isolated B chain has never been shown to carry antibody activity, whereas the A chains from horse [42] and rabbit [82] antibodies were found to be active. With a horse antidiphtheria toxoid system the inhibiting activity of the A chain was equivalent on a weight basis to that of the original antibody; this activity was specific, since the A chains from anti-rabbit γ-globulin or inert γ-globulin had no inhibitory power (Fig. 3-8). These experiments indicate that the combining site on horse antibodies is located on the A chain and must be present on that part of the chain which is associated with B in the active fragments obtained by papain digestion. This A piece, which has been isolated by reduction of the active papain fragments, has a molecular weight of about 22,000 [11], so that the complete elucidation of its chemical structure may be feasible.

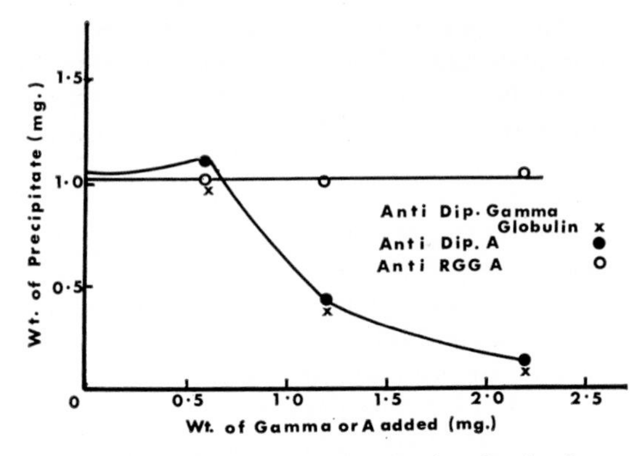

Fig. 3-8. Inhibition of precipitation in the horse anti-(diphtheria toxoid)-diphtheria toxoid system. The degree of inhibition observed with the whole antibody and its A chain are equivalent by weight; the A chain from horse anti-rabbit γ-globulin produces no inhibition. (See Fleischman *et al.* [42].)

Franěk and Nezlin [83], in their experiments on horse antibodies to diphtheria and tetanus toxoid, also detected some activity in the isolated A chains, but this was increased by the addition of either nonspecific or specific B chain. It was concluded that the combining site was on the A chain but that the B chain was necessary for full activity. Edelman *et al.* [84] had similar results with guinea pig antibodies to two bacteriophages and a hapten. Various indirect methods of locating the antibody combining sites have given contradictory and inconclusive results (reviewed by Cohen and Porter [85]). The available data, in which high recoveries of activity have been obtained, indicate that the antibody combining site is on the A chain, but this cannot be accepted without reserve until the role of B chain has been more fully elucidated.

The finding that A chains carry antibody combining sites which may be common to all immunoglobulins is difficult to reconcile with the fact that A chains are also associated with other structural features which are type-specific. This suggests that A, in fact, consists of two separate chains, which would imply that antibody molecules are made up of six chains of approximately equal size. Several other biological observations would be more easily explained on the basis of a six-chain structure [85], but attempts to demonstrate that A consists of two separate chains have been unsuccessful.

ANTIGENIC PROPERTIES OF IMMUNOGLOBULINS

All immunoglobulin molecules carry common antigenic determinants so that antisera to any one of the subfractions will usually cross-react with the other two; in addition, each of the three main types has specific determinants which can be revealed by immunoelectrophoresis and gel diffusion.

Papain digestion splits human γ-globulin into two distinct antigenic fragments which were designated S and F [58]. The common determinant groups responsible for the cross-reactions of human IgG with IgA and IgM as well as with the closely related myeloma proteins, macroglobulins, and Bence Jones proteins are present on the S fragment. On the other hand, the antigenic specificity of 7S γ-globulin is associated with the F fragment [1, 86]; similar findings have been reported for mouse [87] and rabbit γ-globulin [17]. As could be anticipated from these findings and the structural studies described earlier, the common determinants present on the S fragment are actually localized on the B chains, while the type specific determinants are present on A chains [88] (Table 3-2). Thus antisera against purified immunoglobulin fractions can be made specific for the corresponding fraction by absorption with B chain. Similarly, rabbit antisera against the human B chain of IgG give reactions of identity with IgG and IgM, whereas antisera against A chains react only with the corresponding type of immunoglobulin (Fig. 3-9).

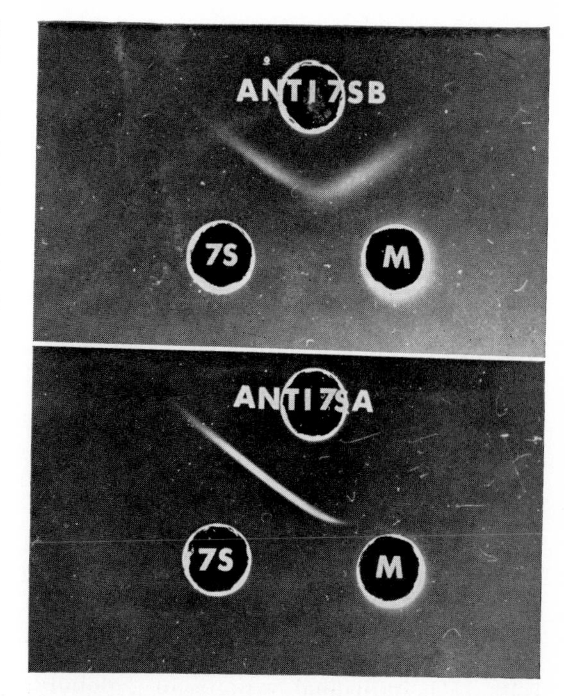

Fig. 3-9. Reaction of normal human IgG (7S) and normal human IgM (M) with rabbit anti-IgG B chain (*above*) and with anti-IgG A chain (*below*). (See Cohen [88].)

The common determinants present on human B chains are of two distinct antigenic types (I and II) [20, 89, 90] which correspond to the variants of Bence Jones proteins originally described by Korngold and Lipari [91]. In both normal [92, 93] and pathological γ-globulins [94–96], these determinants are carried on separate molecules. About 60 percent of normal IgG molecules have B chains of antigenic type I and about 30 percent have B chains of type II; the ratio is similar in preparations of IgA and IgM [93].

Repeated attempts to show that isolated antibodies possess individual antigenic specificity have been unsuccessful. Thus, for example, different antibodies from a single species were found to be antigenically indistinguishable [97], and pneumococcus antibodies from rabbit and chicken do not cross-react when tested as antigens in guinea pigs [98]. In contrast to these findings, however, Kunkel *et al.* [99] have recently demonstrated individual antigenic specificity on several human antibodies which were injected with complete Freund's adjuvant into rabbits. The observed specificity was directed only against the individual antibody used for immunization, and no reactions were observed with antibodies of the same combining specificity obtained from different subjects. Individual specificity has also been demonstrated in myeloma proteins [100], macroglobulins [101, 102], and cold agglutinins [103]. The location of individually specific determinants on immunoglobulin molecules has not been established. It seems likely from the results summarized earlier and from the known heterogeneity of the constituent peptide chains of antibody molecules that the detailed antigenic structure of these chains will prove to be extremely complex.

ALLOTYPES OF IMMUNOGLOBULINS

During recent years it has become apparent that in several species, including rabbit [104–107], guinea pig [108], mouse [109], and man [110, 111], individual variants of γ-globulin occur which can be recognized on the basis of serological differences. These variants, which Oudin named allotypes, were first recognized by injection of specific precipitates of rabbit antibody together with Freund's adjuvant into other rabbits. When the recipients carried a different allotypic specificity from that of the donor, they responded by producing antibodies which precipitated with γ-globulin from the donor rabbit. By use of a gel diffusion technique it has been possible to demonstrate six allotypic specificities in rabbit γ-globulin (A1 to A6). The specificities A1, A2, and A3 appear to be controlled by three allelic genes at one locus (a) and A4, A5, and A6 by three allelic genes at a second locus (b) [112]. Individual sera always contain at least two allotypes, but animals heterozygous at one or both loci may have three or four allotypes. Agar tube analysis of individual sera showed that the nonallelic A1 and A6 were on the same molecules, whereas the allelic forms A1 and A3 were on different molecules [113]. The presence of only one allelic form of allotypic specificity on individual antibody molecules was also suggested by a study of the allotypy of purified antihapten antibodies [114] as well as by quantitative anlyses based on the precipitation of specific allotypes from I^{131}-labeled γ-globulin with antiallotype sera [115, 116]. It therefore appears that, as in the case of hemoglobin [117, 118], nonallelic genes contribute to the formation of a single antibody molecule, whereas allelic genes do not.

Variants of human γ-globulin have been distinguished from one another by differences in their ability to inhibit the agglutination of sensitized cells by sera containing substances serologically related to rheumatoid factors. Since the introduction of this technique by Grubb [110], seven genetically determined types of human γ-globulin have been described. Of these, Gm(a) [119], Gm(b) [120], Gm(x) [121], and Gm(r) [122] are determined by genes at one locus (Gm). In Caucasians, genes controlling the production of Gm(a) and Gm(b) behave as alternate alleles [120], whereas among Negroes these factors appear to be produced by a single allele Gm(ab) [123]. Two alleles at an independent locus (Inv) determine the factors Inv(a) and Inv(b) [124]. The seventh factor, Gm-like [125], is found in Negroes but is extremely rare in other racial groups; this locus is independent of the Inv locus in population studies [126], but its relationship to the Gm locus is uncertain because all Negroes are Gm(a+b+).

The structural differences which exist between allotypic variants of γ-globulin are unknown, but the distribution of specificities on subunits of the molecule has been investigated. The Inv factor, which is found on all types of human immunoglobulins and also on the papain fragment S [127, 128] (Table 3-5), is carried on the B chain, while Gm specificity, which is found only on IgG, is associated with the A chain of that protein [129, 88] and must be localized to that portion of the chain present in the F fragment [127, 128] (Fig. 3-6).

In the case of rabbit γ-globulin, allotypes determined by the two genetic loci are found on both 7S and 19S γ-globulins [130]. The B chain has been shown to be associated only with allotypes determined by the b locus [131]; variants of the a locus would therefore be expected to occur on the A chain. Allotypic specificities determined by the a locus are present in papain fragments I and II [132, 133] and are probably therefore located on the N-terminal portion of the A chain which may be common to IgG and IgM. Experiments reported to date have shown that the A chain contains specificities determined by both a and b loci, and this may indicate that preparations of rabbit A are contaminated by B chain [131].

URINARY EXCRETION OF γ-GLOBULIN FRAGMENTS

The urine of normal subjects contains small amounts of 7S γ-globulin as well as relatively low molecular weight proteins which are antigenically related to serum γ-globulins [134–137]. These low molecular weight proteins are related antigenically to the S fragment of γ-globulin (Fig. 3-6) [138] and to types I and II Bence Jones proteins [138, 139]. These findings suggest that urinary γ-globulin fragments may be composed of B chains. Berggard and Edelman [140] have now demonstrated the close similarity of urinary fragments and B chains in regard to antigenic structure and physical properties. By use of antisera specific for A and B chains, it was found that a normal subject excreted 5 to 10 mg. of free B chain in the urine per twenty-four hours [141]. What appears to be an unrelated antibody fragment has been recovered from the urine of subjects immunized with poliomyelitis virus vaccines and with tetanus toxoid. These fragments have a molecular weight of 13,000 and are able to precipitate with the appropriate antigen, suggesting that each fragment carries two combining sites [142]. However, Rowe [143] was unable to confirm these findings in studies on the urine of a normal subject immunized with typhoid vaccine; in this instance urinary antibody activity was apparently confined to whole γ-globulin and could not be detected in smaller fragments.

The origin of urinary γ-globulin fragments has been studied in radioactive labeling experiments. The results of Franklin [135] and Webb *et al.* [134] indicated that these fragments were derived from the degradation of normal γ-globulin. However, other studies [139] have shown that the urinary proteins which probably correspond to B chains arise as precursors or by-products of γ-globulin synthesis and correspond in this respect to Bence Jones proteins.

COMPLEMENT FIXATION

The term complement* refers to a group of serum factors which, under appropriate conditions, enter into combination with antigen-antibody complexes and play a role in various immunological reactions. Complement fixation can occur with antibodies belonging to both IgG and IgM fractions, but the IgA antibodies which have been studied were inactive in this respect. Thus, Heremans *et al.* [32] identified anti-*Brucella* agglutinins in human IgG, IgM, and IgA and have shown that the first two fractions were able to fix complement but that IgA antibodies lacked this capacity. Similarly, complement-fixing activity has been demonstrated on guinea pig 7S γ_2-globulins but not on 7S γ_1-globulins, which may be analogous to the human IgA fraction [144]. The site for complement fixation is primarily on papain piece III [145, 146] and must be on A; the A chains of IgG and IgM appear to carry the complement-fixing site, but the A chain of IgA may be deficient in this respect. More recent evidence indicates that the enzymatic pieces (I and II) that survive peptic digestion may also be involved in complement fixation [147–149]. Direct evidence that all three enzymatic pieces of the antibody molecule may be involved in complement fixation was provided by Cebra [150]. He showed that rabbit antibody that has been split by insoluble papain, but not dissociated by thiol, precipitates with antigen and binds complement as effectively as the native antibody. When thiol is added to the specific precipitate carrying bound complement, only a partial dissociation occurs, suggesting that the antibody is held together by components of complement bound to all parts of the molecule. The conclusion at present, therefore, seems to be that piece III is predominantly concerned in the binding of complement to antibody reacted with antigen, but that other parts of the molecule are also involved in the process.

TURN-OVER OF IMMUNOGLOBULINS

All plasma protein fractions including γ-globulins are in a state of dynamic equilibrium undergoing constant degradation and replacement by newly synthesized molecules. A homogeneous protein, such as human albumin, when labeled with I^{131}, has a constant rate of breakdown (measured by urinary excretion of label) over a period of several weeks. On the other hand, the fractional catabolic rate of I^{131}-labeled human γ-globulin prepared

* See Chapter 14.

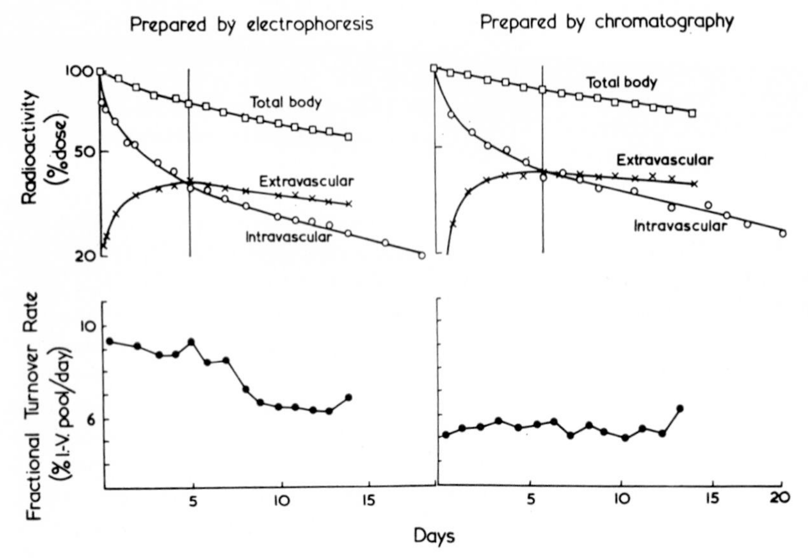

Fig. 3-10. Turn-over of I^{131}-labeled γ-globulin prepared by electrophoresis (IgG and IgM) and by chromatography (IgG only). The daily turn-over rate shown below is calculated from urinary excretion of I^{131} and expressed as a fraction of the total circulating γ-globulin. (See Cohen and Freeman [151].)

by zone electrophoresis falls progressively during the first one or two weeks after injection, suggesting the presence of a mixed population of molecules having different breakdown rates (Fig. 3-10). This metabolic heterogeneity is attributable to differences in the turn-over rates of 19S and 7S fractions. Thus human IgM isolated by ultracentrifugation and zone electrophoresis [151] or by electrophoresis and gel filtration [152] has a relatively high turnover rate, whereas IgG is catabolized at a slower rate; a similar difference in the half-lives of small and large molecular weight antibodies has been reported in rabbits [153]. Little is known about the site and mechanism of immunoglobulin catabolism. On the basis of labeled protein studies it has been suggested that plasma cells which are known to be involved in antibody synthesis may also be responsible for immunoglobulin breakdown [154]. However, perfusion experiments in which biologically screened proteins are used show that the normal rat liver, which is not a site of antibody synthesis, catabolizes IgG at a rate equivalent to 30 percent of the total breakdown *in vivo* [155]. The fractional breakdown rate of IgG can be increased in the mouse by infusing large amounts of either IgG or piece III derived from it, but not by injecting IgA or IgM; the removal of circulating protein by a process such as pinocytosis cannot easily account for such selectivity, and the presence of specific mechanisms controlling immunoglobulin breakdown appears likely [156].

Normal subjects synthesize and break down about 2 gm. of IgG and 0.5 gm. of IgM per day, but in pathological conditions associated with hypergammaglobulinemia the absolute rate of immunoglobulin turn-over may be increased as much as sevenfold [152, 157–160]. Increased rates of immunoglobulin formation presumably result from the replication of antibody-producing cells but are not necessarily associated with an enhanced response to antigenic stimulation [161].

REFERENCES

1. Heremans, J. F. *Les Globulines Sériques du Système Gamma*. Brussells: Arscia, 1960.
2. Gowans, J. L., McGregor, D. D., and Cowen, D. M. Initiation of immune responses by small lymphocytes. *Nature* (London) 196:651, 1962.
3. Karush, F., and Eisen, H. N. A theory of delayed hypersensitivity. *Science* 136:1032, 1962.
4. Tiselius, A., and Kabat, E. A. An electrophoretic study of immune sera and purified antibody preparations. *J. Exp. Med.* 69:119, 1939.
5. Grabar, P., Fauvert, R., Burtin, P., and Hartmann, L. Étude sur les protéines du myélome: L'analyse immuno-électrophorétique des sérums de 30 malades. *Rev. Franc. Etud. Clin. Biol.* 1:175, 1956.
6. Rosevear, J. W., and Smith, E. L. Isolation

and properties of glycopeptides from a fraction of human gamma-globulin. *J. Biol. Chem.* 236:425, 1961.

7. Fahey, J. L., and Horbett, A. P. Human gamma globulin fractionation on anion exchange cellulose columns. *J. Biol. Chem.* 234: 2645, 1959.
8. Vaerman, J. P., Heremans, J. F., and Vaerman, C. Studies of the immune globulins of human serum. *J. Immun.* 91:7P, 1963.
9. Porter, R. R. Gamma-Globulin and Antibodies. In Putnam, F. W. (Ed.). *The Plasma Proteins.* New York: Academic Press, Inc., 1960. Vol. 1, p. 241.
10. Cammack, K. A. Molecular weight of rabbit gamma-globulin. *Nature* (London) 194:745, 1962.
11. Pain, R. H. The molecular weights of the peptide chains of gamma-globulin. *Biochem. J.* 88:234, 1963.
12. Heidelberger, M., and Pedersen, K. O. The molecular weight of antibodies. *J. Exp. Med.* 65:393, 1937.
13. Sober, H. A., Gutter, F. J., Wyckoff, M. M., and Peterson, E. A. Chromatography of proteins: II. Fractionation of serum protein on anion exchange cellulose. *J. Amer. Chem. Soc.* 78:756, 1956.
14. Askonas, B. A., Farthing, C. P., and Humphrey, J. H. The significance of multiple antibody components in serum of immunized rabbits. *Immunology* 3:336, 1960.
15. Sober, H. A., and Peterson, E. A. Protein chromatography on ion exchange cellulose. *Fed. Proc.* 17:1116, 1958.
16. Kunkel, H. G. Macroglobulins and High Molecular Weight Antibodies. Ref. 9, p. 279.
17. Thorbecke, G. J., and Franklin, E. C. Antigenic cross-reactivity between 7S and 19S rabbit gamma-globulin. *J. Immun.* 87:753, 1961.
18. Rask-Nielsen, R., Lontie, R., Clausen, J., Christensen, H. E., Heremans, J. F., and Brauns, G. L'ultracentrifugation des protéines sériques dans trois sortes de leucémies transplantables de la souris. *Rev. Franc. Etud. Clin. Biol.* 5:1000, 1960.
19. Makinodan, T., Gengozian, N., and Canning, R. E. Demonstration of a normal serum macroglobulin co-precipitating with the bovine serum albumin (BSA)-chicken anti-BSA precipitate. *J. Immun.* 85:439, 1960.
20. Cohen, S. Properties of the peptide chains of normal and pathological human gamma-globulins. *Biochem. J.* 89:334, 1963.
21. Kabat, E. A., and Pedersen, K. O. Molecular weights of antibodies. *Science* 87:372, 1938.
22. Fahey, J. L., and Goodman, H. C. Characterization of anti-thyroglobulin factors in human serum. *J. Clin. Invest.* 39:1259, 1960.
23. Heremans, J. F., Heremans, M. T., and Schultze, H. E. Isolation and description of a few properties of the β_2A-globulin of human serum. *Clin. Chim. Acta* 4:96, 1959.
24. Laurell, A. H. F. Sera from patients with myeloma macroglobulinaemia and related conditions as studied by ultracentrifugation. *Acta Med. Scand.*, supp. 367, p. 69, 1961.
25. Fahey, J. L. Immunochemical studies of twenty mouse myeloma proteins: Evidence for two groups of proteins similar to gamma and beta-2 A globulins in man. *J. Exp. Med.* 114: 385, 1961.
26. Pappenheimer, A. M., Lundgren, H. P., and Williams, J. W. Anti-egg albumin antibody in horse. *J. Exp. Med.* 71:247, 1940.
27. Benacerraf, B., Ovary, Z., Bloch, K. J., and Franklin, E. C. Properties of guinea-pig 7S antibodies: I. Electrophoretic separation of two types of guinea-pig 7S antibodies. *J. Exp. Med.* 117:951, 1963.
28. Schultze, H. E. The synthesis of antibodies and proteins. *Clin. Chim. Acta* 4:610, 1959.
29. Heremans, J. F., and Vaerman, J. P. Globulin as a possible carrier of allergic reaginic activity. *Nature* (London) 193:1091, 1962.
30. Fireman, P., Vannier, W. E., and Goodman, H. C. Association of skin sensitizing antibody with the β_2A globulins in sera from ragweed sensitive patients. *J. Exp. Med.* 117:603, 1963.
31. Yagi, Y., Maier, P., Pressman, D., Arbesman, C. E., Reisman, R. E., and Lenzner, A. R. Multiplicity of insulin-binding antibodies in human sera. *J. Immun.* 90:761, 1963.
32. Heremans, J. F., Vaerman, J. P., and Vaerman, C. Studies on the immune globulins of human serum: II. A study of the distribution of anti-brucella and anti-diphtheria antibody activities among γ_{ss}-, γ_1M- and γ_1A-globulin fractions. *J. Immun.* 91:11, 1963.
33. Sanger, F. The free amino groups of insulin. *Biochem. J.* 39:507, 1945.
34. Porter, R. R. A chemical study of rabbit antiovalbumin. *Biochem. J.* 46:473, 1950.
35. Cebra, J. J., Givol, D., Silman, H. I., and Katchalski, E. A two-stage cleavage of rabbit gamma-globulin by a water-insoluble papain preparation followed by cysteine. *J. Biol. Chem.* 236:1720, 1961.
36. Eriksson, S., and Sjoquist, J. Quantitative determination of N-terminal amino acids in some serum proteins. *Biochim. Biophys. Acta* 45:290, 1960.
37. Edelman, G. M. Dissociation of gamma-globulin. *J. Amer. Chem. Soc.* 81:3155, 1959.
38. Edelman, G. M., and Poulik, M. D. Studies on structural units of the gamma-globulins. *J. Exp. Med.* 113:861, 1961.
39. Franěk, F. Dissociation of animal 7S gamma-globulins by cleavage of disulphide bonds. *Biochem. Biophys. Res. Commun.* 4:28, 1961.

40. Fleischman, J. B., Pain, R. H., and Porter, R. R. Reduction of gamma globulins. *Arch. Biochem.*, supp. 1, p. 174, 1962.
41. Edelman, G. M., and Benacerraf, B. On structural and functional relations between antibodies and proteins of the gamma-system. *Proc. Nat. Acad. Sci. U.S.A.* 48:1035, 1962.
42. Fleischman, J. B., Porter, R. R., and Press, E. M. The arrangement of the peptide chains in gamma-globulin. *Biochem. J.* 88:220, 1963.
43. Cohen, S., and Porter, R. R. Heterogeneity of the peptide chains of gamma-globulin. *Biochem. J.* 90:278, 1964.
44. Cohen, S. Structure of gamma-globulin. *Biochem. J.* 88:2P, 1963.
45. Stark, G. R., Stein, W. H., and Moore, S. Reactions of the cyanate present in aqueous urea with amino acids and proteins. *J. Biol. Chem.* 235:3177, 1960.
46. Edelman, G. M., and Gally, J. A. The nature of Bence Jones proteins. *J. Exp. Med.* 116:207 1962.
47. Putnam, F. W., Migita, S., and Easeley, C. W. Structural and Immunochemical Relationships among Bence Jones Proteins. In Peeters, H. (Ed.), *Protides of the Biological Fluids.* Amsterdam: Elsevier Publishing Company, 1962. Vol. 10, p. 93.
48. Porter, R. R. The hydrolysis of rabbit gamma-globulin and antibodies with crystalline papain. *Biochem. J.* 73:119, 1959.
49. Karush, F. Properties of papain-digested purified anti-hapten antibody. *Fed. Proc.* 18:577, 1959.
50. Nisonoff, A., Wissler, F. C., and Woernley, D. L. Properties of univalent fragments of rabbit antibody isolated by specific adsorption. *Arch. Biochem.* 88:241, 1960.
51. Velick, S. F., Parker, C. W., and Eisen, H. N. Excitation energy transfer and the quantitative study of the antibody hapten reaction. *Proc. Nat. Acad. Sci. U.S.A.* 46:1470, 1960.
52. Franklin, E. C. Structural units of human 7S gamma-globulin. *J. Clin. Invest.* 39:1933, 1960.
53. Palmer, J. L., Mandy, W. J., and Nisonoff, A. Heterogeneity of rabbit antibody and its subunits. *Proc. Nat. Acad. Sci. U.S.A.* 48:49, 1962.
54. Stelos, P., Radzimski, G., and Pressman, D. Heterogeneity of rabbit antibody fragments. *J. Immun.* 88:572, 1962.
55. Mandy, W. J., Stambaugh, M. K., and Nisonoff, A. Amino acid composition of univalent fragments of rabbit antibody. *Science* 140:901, 1963.
56. Smith, E. L., McFadden, M. L., Stockell, A., and Buettner-Janusch, V. Amino acid composition of four rabbit antibodies. *J. Biol. Chem.* 214:197, 1955.
57. Fleischer, S., Hardin, R. L., Horowitz, J., Zimmerman, M., Gresham, E., Turner, J. E., Burnett, J. P., Stary, Z., and Haurowitz, F. Composition of antibodies against acidic and basic azo-proteins. *Arch. Biochem.* 92:329, 1961.
58. Edelman, G. M., Heremans, J. F., Heremans, M. T., and Kunkel, H. G. Immunological studies of human gamma-globulin. *J. Exp. Med.* 112:203, 1960.
59. Hershgold, E. J., Cordoba, F., Charache, P., and Gitlin, D. A crystalline fragment from human gamma-globulin. *Nature* (London) 199:284, 1963.
60. Nisonoff, A., Markus, G., and Wissler, F. C. Separation of univalent fragments of rabbit antibody by reduction of a single, labile, disulphide bond. *Nature* (London) 189:293, 1961.
61. Nisonoff, A., and Rivers, M. M. Recombination of a mixture of univalent antibody fragments of different specificity. *Arch. Biochem.* 93:460, 1961.
62. Porter, R. R. The Structure of Gamma-Globulin and Antibodies. In Gellhorn, A., and Hirschberg, E. (Eds.), *Symposium on Basic Problems in Neoplastic Disease.* New York: Columbia University Press, 1962.
63. Seijen, H. G., and Gruber, M. Studies of gamma-globulin structure by peptide mapping of papain-produced fragments. *Biochem. J.* 88: 10P, 1963.
64. Olins, D. E., and Edelman, G. M. The antigenic structure of the polypeptide chains of human gamma-globulin. *J. Exp. Med.* 116:635, 1962.
65. Deutsch, H. F., and Morton, J. I. Human serum macroglobulins and dissociation units: I. Physicochemical properties. *J. Biol. Chem.* 231:1107, 1958.
66. Putnam, F. W. Abnormal Serum Globulins. Ref. 9, Vol. II, p. 345.
67. Fahey, J. L. Physicochemical characterization of mouse myeloma proteins: Demonstration of heterogeneity for each myeloma globulin. *J. Exp. Med.* 114:399, 1961.
68. Reisner, C. A., and Franklin, E. C. Studies of mercaptoethanol dissociated normal human 19S gamma-globulin and pathologic macroglobulins from patients with macroglobulinemia. *J. Immun.* 87:654, 1961.
69. Chaplin, H., Cohen, S., and Press, E. M. Preparation and properties of the peptide chains of normal human 19S gamma-globulin (IgM). *Biochem. J.* (in press).
70. Landsteiner, K., and van der Scheer, J. On cross reactions of immune sera to azoproteins: II. Antigens with azo-components containing two determinant groups. *J. Exp. Med.* 67:709, 1938.
71. Kabat, E. A. Size and heterogeneity of the combining sites on an antibody molecule. *J. Cell. Comp. Physiol.* 50 (supp. 1):79, 1957.
72. Karush, F. The interaction of purified anti-

beta-lactoside antibody with haptens. *J. Amer. Chem. Soc.* 79:3380, 1957.
73. Schlossman, S. F., and Kabat, E. A. Specific fractionation of a population of anti-dextran molecules with combining sites of various sizes. *J. Exp. Med.* 116:535, 1962.
74. Karush, F. Immunologic specificity and molecular structure. *Advances Immun.* 2:1, 1962.
75. Haurowitz, F., and Schwerin, P. The specificity of antibodies to antigens containing two different determinant groups. *J. Immun.* 47:111, 1943.
76. Eisen, H. N., Carsten, M. E., and Belman, S. J. Studies of hypersensitivity to low molecular weight substances. *J. Immun.* 73:296, 1954.
77. Nisonoff, A., Winkler, M. H., and Pressman, D. The similar specificity of the combining sites of an individual antibody molecule. *J. Immun.* 82:201, 1959.
78. Petermann, M. L., and Pappenheimer, A. M. The ultracentrifugal analysis of diphtheria proteins. *J. Phys. Chem.* 45:1, 1941.
79. McFadden, M. L., and Smith, E. L. Free amino groups and N-terminal sequence of rabbit antibodies. *J. Biol. Chem.* 214:185, 1955.
80. Gitlin, D., and Merler, E. A comparison of the peptides released from related rabbit antibodies by enzymatic hydrolysis. *J. Exp. Med.* 114:217, 1961.
81. Edelman, G. W., Benacerraf, B., Ovary, Z., and Poulik, M. D. Structural differences among antibodies of different specificities. *Proc. Nat. Acad. Sci. U.S.A.* 47:1751, 1961. (*a*) Edelman, G. M., Benacerraf, B., and Ovary, Z. Structure and specificity of guinea pig 7S antibodies. *J. Exp. Med.* 118:229, 1963.
82. Utsumi, S., and Karush, F. The separation of purified rabbit antibody into subunits. *Fed. Proc.* 22:496, 1963.
83. Franěk, F., and Nezlin, R. S. Recovery of antibody combining activity by interaction of different peptide chains isolated from purified horse antitoxins. *Folia Microbiol.* (Prague) 8:128, 1963.
84. Edelman, G. M., Olins, D. E., Gally, J. A., and Zinder, N. D. Reconstitution of immunologic activity by interaction of polypeptide chains of antibodies. *Proc. Nat. Acad. Sci. U.S.A.* 50:753, 1963.
85. Cohen, S., and Porter, R. R. Structure and biological activity of immunoglobulins. *Advances Immun.* 4:287, 1964.
86. Franklin, E. C., and Stanworth, D. R. Antigenic relationships between immune globulins and certain related para-proteins in man. *J. Exp. Med.* 114:521, 1961.
87. Askonas, B. A., and Fahey, J. L. Enzymatically produced subunits of proteins formed by plasma cells in mice: II. β_{2A}-myeloma protein and Bence Jones proteins. *J. Exp. Med.* 115: 641, 1962.
88. Cohen, S. Properties of the separated chains of human gamma-globulin. *Nature* (London) 197:253, 1963.
89. Fahey, J. L. Structural basis for the differences between Type I and Type II human gamma-globulin molecules. *J. Immun.,* 91:448, 1963.
90. Schwartz, J. H., and Edelman, G. M. Comparisons of Bence Jones proteins and L polypeptide chains of myeloma globulins after hydrolysis with trypsin. *J. Exp. Med.* 118:41, 1963.
91. Korngold, L., and Lipari, R. Multiple-myeloma proteins, antigenic relationship of Bence Jones proteins to normal gamma-globulin and multiple-myeloma serum proteins. *Cancer* 9: 262, 1956.
92. Mannik, M., and Kunkel, H. G. Two major types of normal 7S gamma-globulin. *J. Exp. Med.* 117:213, 1963.
93. Fahey, J. L. Two types of 6.6S gamma-globulins, β_{2A}-globulins and 18S γ_1-macroglobulins in normal serum and gamma-microglobulins in normal urine. *J. Immun.* 91:438, 1963.
94. Franklin, E. C. Two types of γ_1A-globulin in sera from normals and patients with multiple myeloma. *Nature* (London) 195:393, 1962.
95. Mannik, M., and Kunkel, H. G. Classification of myeloma proteins, Bence Jones proteins and macroglobulins into two groups on the basis of common antigenic characters. *J. Exp. Med.* 116:859, 1962.
96. Fahey, J. L., and Solomon, A. Two types of gamma-myeloma proteins, β_{2A}-myeloma proteins, γ_1-macroglobulins and Bence Jones proteins identified by two groups of common antigenic determinants. *J. Clin. Invest.* 42:811, 1963.
97. Treffers, H. P. Some contributions of immunology to the study of proteins. *Advances Protein Chem.* 1:69, 1944.
98. Cushing, J. F., and Campbell, D. H. *Principles of Immunology.* New York: McGraw-Hill Book Company, Inc., 1957. P. 254.
99. Kunkel, H. G., Mannik, M., and Williams, R. C. Individual antigenic specificity of isolated antibodies. *Science* 140:1218, 1963.
100. Slater, R. J., Ward, S. M., and Kunkel, H. G. Immunological relationships among the myeloma proteins. *J. Exp. Med.* 101:85, 1955.
101. Habich, H., and Hassig, A. Essai d'analyse antigénique des paraprotides dans la macroglobulinémie de Waldenström. *Vox Sang.* 3:99, 1953.
102. Korngold, L., and Van Leeuwen, G. Macroglobulinemia: II. Antisera specific for pathological macroglobulins. *J. Exp. Med.* 106:477, 1957.
103. Mehvotra, T. N. Individual, specific nature of the cold auto-antibodies of acquired haemolytic anaemia. *Nature* (London) 185:323, 1960.

104. Oudin, J. L'allotypie de certains antigènes protéidiques du sérum. *C. R. Acad. Sci.* (Paris) 242:2606, 1956.
105. Oudin, J. Allotypy of rabbit serum proteins: I. Immunochemical analysis leading to the individualization of seven main allotypes. *J. Exp. Med.* 112:107, 1960.
106. Dray, S., and Young, G. O. Differences in the antigenic components of sera of individual rabbits as shown by induced isoprecipitins. *J. Immun.* 81:142, 1958.
107. Dubiski, S., Dubiska, A., Skalba, D., and Kelus, A. Antigenic structure of rabbit gamma-globulin. *Immunology* 4:236, 1961.
108. Benacerraf, B., and Gell, P. G. H. Delayed hypersensitivity to homologous gamma-globulin in the guinea-pig. *Nature* (London) 189: 586, 1961.
109. Kelus, A., and Moor-Jankowski, J. K. An isoantigen ($\gamma\beta^A$) of mouse gamma-globulin present in inbred strains. *Nature* (London) 191:1405, 1961.
110. Grubb, R. Agglutination of erythrocytes coated with "incomplete" anti-RH by certain rheumatoid arthritic sera and some other sera. *Acta Path. Microbiol. Scand.* 39:195, 1956.
111. Dray, S. Three gamma-globulins in normal human serum revealed by monkey precipitins. *Science* 132:1313, 1960.
112. Dray, S., Dubiski, S., Kelus, A., Lennox, E. S., and Oudin, J. A notation for allotypy. *Nature* (London) 195:785, 1962.
113. Oudin, J. On the associated state of rabbit allotypes, the existence of rabbit antibody molecules against two allotypes and the dissociation of human gamma-globulin antigens into smaller molecules. *Biochem. Biophys. Res. Commun.* 5:358, 1961.
114. Gell, P. G. H., and Kelus, A. Deletions of allotypic gamma-globulins in antibodies. *Nature* (London) 195:44, 1962.
115. Dray, S., and Nisonoff, A. Contribution of allelic genes A_b4 and A_b5 to formation of rabbit 7S gamma-globulins. *Proc. Soc. Exp. Biol. Med.* 113:20, 1963.
116. Dray, S., Young, G. O., and Nisonoff, A. Distribution of allotypic specificities among rabbit gamma-globulin molecules genetically defined at two loci. *Nature* (London) 199:52, 1963.
117. Itano, H. A. The human hemoglobins: Their properties and genetic control. *Advances Protein Chem.* 12:215, 1957.
118. Singer, S. J., and Itano, H. A. On the asymmetrical dissociation of human hemoglobin. *Proc. Nat. Acad. Sci. U.S.A.* 45:174, 1959.
119. Grubb, R., and Laurell, A. B. Hereditary serological human serum groups. *Acta Path. Microbiol. Scand.* 39:390, 1956.
120. Harboe, M. A new hemagglutinating substance in the Gm system, anti-Gm^b. *Acta Path. Microbiol. Scand.* 47:191, 1959.
121. Harboe, M., and Lundevall, J. A new type in the Gm system. *Acta Path. Microbiol. Scand.* 45:357, 1959.
122. Brandtzaeg, B., Fudenberg, H., and Mohr, J. The Gm (r) serum group. *Acta Genet.* (Basel) 11:170, 1961.
123. Steinberg, A. G., Stauffer, R., and Boyer, S. H. Evidence for a Gm^{ab} allele in the Gm system of American Negroes. *Nature* (London) 188:169, 1960.
124. Ropartz, G., Lenoir, J., and Rivat, L. A new inheritable property of human sera: The Inv factor. *Nature* (London) 189:586, 1961.
125. Steinberg, A. G., Giles, B. D., and Stauffer, R. A Gm-like factor present in Negroes and rare or absent in Whites: Its relation to Gm^a and Gm^x. *Amer. J. Hum. Genet.* 12:44, 1960.
126. Steinberg, A. G. Progress in the study of genetically determined human gamma-globulin types (the Gm and Inv groups). *Progr. Med. Genet.* 1962, Vol. II.
127. Franklin, E. C., Fudenberg, H., Meltzer, M., and Stanworth, D. R. The structural basis for genetic variations of normal human gamma-globulins. *Proc. Nat. Acad. Sci. U.S.A.* 48:914, 1962.
128. Harboe, M., Osterland, C. K., and Kunkel, H. G. Localisation of two genetic factors to different areas of gamma-globulin molecules. *Science* 136:979, 1962.
129. Lawler, S., and Cohen, S. Distribution of allotypic specificities on the peptide chains of human γ-globulins, *Immunology* (in press).
130. Todd, C. W. Allotypy in rabbit 19S protein. *Biochem. Biophys. Res. Commun.* 11:170, 1963.
131. Kelus, A. S. Gamma-globulin allotypes in the rabbit. *Biochem. J.* 88:4P, 1963.
132. Kelus, A., Marrack, J. R., and Richards, C. B. Specificity of the antigens of rabbit gamma-globulin, hydrolyzed by papain. *Biochem. J.* 76:13P, 1960.
133. Marrack, J. R., Richards, C. B., and Kelus, A. Antigenic Specificity of Hydrolysis Products of Gamma-Globulins. Ref. 47, Vol. 9, p. 200.
134. Webb, T., Rose, B., and Sehon, A. H. Biocolloids in normal human urine: II. Physicochemical and immunochemical characteristics. *Canad. J. Biochem. Physiol.* 36:1167, 1958.
135. Franklin, E. C. Physicochemical and immunologic studies of gamma-globulins of normal human urine. *J. Clin. Invest.* 38:2159, 1959.
136. Stevenson, G. T. Detection in normal urine of protein resembling Bence Jones protein. *J. Clin. Invest.* 39:1192, 1960.

137. Berggard, I. Studies on the plasma proteins in normal human urine. *Clin. Chim. Acta* 6:413, 1961.
138. Hanson, L. A., and Berggard, I. An immunological comparison of immunoglobulins from human blood serum, urine and milk using diffusion-in-gel methods. *Clin. Chim. Acta* 7:828, 1962.
139. Stevenson, G. T. Further studies of the gamma-related proteins of normal urine. *J. Clin. Invest.* 41:1190, 1962.
140. Berggard, I., and Edelman, G. M. Normal counterparts to Bence Jones proteins: Free L polypeptide chains of human gamma-globulin. *Proc. Nat. Acad. Sci. U.S.A.* 49:330, 1963.
141. Cohen, S. Unpublished observations, 1963.
142. Remington, J. S., Merler, E., Lerner, A. M., Gitlin, D., and Finland, M. Antibodies of low molecular weight in normal human urine. *Nature* (London) 194:407, 1962.
143. Rowe, D. S. Human gamma-globulin as antigen and antibody. *Biochem. J.* 88:2P, 1963.
144. Bloch, K. J., Kourilsky, F. M., Ovary, Z., and Benacerraf, B. Properties of guinea-pig 7S antibodies: III. Identification of antibodies involved in complement fixation and haemolysis. *J. Exp. Med.* 117:965, 1963.
145. Taranta, A., and Franklin, E. C. Complement fixation by antibody fragments. *Science* 134:1981, 1961.
146. Amiraian, K., and Leikhim, E. J. Interaction of fragment III of rabbit gamma-globulin and guinea-pig complement. *Proc. Soc. Exp. Biol. Med.* 108:454, 1961.
147. Schur, P. H., and Becker, E. L. Complement-fixing properties of pepsin-treated rabbit and sheep antibodies. *Science* 141:360, 1963.
148. Schur, P. H., and Becker, E. L. Pepsin digestion of rabbit and sheep antibodies. *J. Exp. Med.* 118:891, 1963.
149. Reiss, A. M., and Plescia, O. J. Fixation of complement to fragments of antibody. *Science* 141:812, 1963.
150. Cebra, J. J. In *Conceptual Advances in Immunology and Oncology*. New York: Paul B. Hoeber, Inc., 1963. P. 220.
151. Cohen, S., and Freeman, T. Metabolic heterogeneity of human gamma-globulin. *Biochem. J.* 76:475, 1960.
152. Wochner, R. D., Barth, W. F., Waldmann, T. A., and Fahey, J. L. Metabolism of normal hyman γ-macroglobulin. *Clin. Res.* 11:231, 1963.
153. Taliaferro, W. H., and Talmage, D. W. Antibodies in the rabbit with different rates of metabolic decay. *J. Infect. Dis.* 99:21, 1961.
154. Soons, J. B. J., and Westenbrink, H. G. K. Experiments in the localization of pathological protein synthesis in myelomatosis. *Bull. Soc. Chim. Biol.* 40:1803, 1958.
155. Cohen, S., Gordon, A. H., and Matthews, G. M. E. Catabolism of γ-globulin by the isolated perfused rat liver. *Biochem. J.* 82:197, 1962.
156. Fahey, J. L., and Robinson, A. G. Factors controlling serum γ-globulin concentration. *J. Exp. Med.* 118:845, 1963.
157. Cohen, S. Gamma-globulin metabolism. *Brit. Med. Bull.* 19:202, 1963.
158. Cohen, S., Carrington, S., and McGregor, I. A. Gamma-globulin and acquired immunity to human malaria. *Nature* (London) 192: 733, 1961.
159. Birke, G., Liljedahl, S. O., Olhagen, B., Plantin, L. O., and Ahlinder, S. Catabolism and distribution of γ-globulin. A preliminary study with ^{131}I-labelled γ-globulin. *Acta Med. Scand.* 173:589, 1963.
160. Solomon, A., Waldmann, T. A., and Fahey, J. L. Metabolism of normal 6.6S γ-globulin in normal subjects and in patients with macroglobulinaemia and multiple myeloma. *J. Lab. Clin. Med.* 62:1, 1963.
161. McGregor, I. A., and Barr, M. Antibody response to tetanus toxoid inoculation in malarious and non-malarious Gambian children. *Trans. Roy. Soc. Trop. Med. Hyg.* 56:364, 1962.
162. Crumpton, M. J., and Wilkinson, J. M. Amino acid compositions of human and rabbit gamma-globulins and of the fragments produced by reduction. *Biochem. J.* 88:228, 1963.

4. *The Function of the Thymus**

ROBERT A. GOOD, RAYMOND D. A. PETERSON,
AND ANN E. GABRIELSEN

DURING THE PAST FEW YEARS THERE has been considerable progress in our understanding of the functions of the mammalian thymus, progress stemming largely from the recognition of its profound influence on the ontogenesis of the lymphoid system and adaptive immunity. Two observations served to direct experimental work on the thymus in this direction: the clinical observation of a thymus tumor in an agammaglobulinemic patient in 1953 and, the following year, the discovery of the immunological role of the bursa of Fabricius in birds.

Following the finding of a benign thymoma in a patient with acquired hypogammaglobulinemia (see Chap. 23), MacLean *et al.* [1] removed the thymus from young adult rabbits and studied their antibody response to bovine serum albumin. No differences between thymectomized and control animals were observed, confirming earlier findings in other laboratories [2, 3].

At about this time, Glick and Chang and their associates [4–8] made a key observation in connection with the role of the bursa of Fabricius of the chicken in the development of antibody-producing capabilities. The bursa is an out-pouching of the posterior gut in birds and is similar morphologically and histologically to the thymus. These workers found that chickens subjected to bursectomy in the immediate post-hatching period were deficient in responsiveness to bacterial antigens. Mueller *et al.* [9] confirmed Glick's findings on the effects of surgical bursectomy and also used a method of "hormonal bursectomy" involving the inoculation of the incubating eggs with 19-nortestosterone and similar hormones. The chickens lacking bursas as a result of such hormone treatment were even more deficient immunologically than the surgically bursectomized birds [9], a finding later confirmed by Papermaster *et al.* [10, 11].

In view of the similarities of the thymus to the bursa and the remarkable effect on antibody production of early bursectomy in the chicken, we undertook a series of experiments involving neonatally thymectomized rabbits. Two groups of animals were immunized at 6–8 weeks of age with bovine serum albumin, and a third group with bacteriophage T-2. We found that the thymectomized animals formed less antibody; however, when the results in the three groups of animals were evaluated statistically, only one showed a significant difference [12, 13]. The second was of borderline significance, and the third not significant. Thus, although an effect of neonatal thymectomy on immunological responsiveness had been demonstrated in rabbits, the effect was not great, nor was it consistent. Fichtelius *et al.* [14] made a similar observation in guinea pigs thymectomized early in life.

At about this time, Martinez *et al.* thymectomized newborn inbred mice, using homograft immunity as the means of assessing immunological status of the animals. Complete thymectomy presented a problem at the outset, as did the mortality rate in the thymectomized animals, but it was soon clear that thymectomy on the first day of life depressed homograft immunity sufficiently to permit skin grafts between mouse strains differing at minor (non-H-2) histocompatibility barriers [15, 16]. With improved surgical technique, H-2 histocompatibility barriers were also crossed in inbred mice, first with tumor grafts [17] and later with skin [18]. Miller [19, 20] in independent studies with mice reported similar findings; later, he also demonstrated that thymectomized mice often accepted rat skin as well as skin from genetically distant mouse strains [21]. The antibody response of

* Aided by grants from the U.S. Public Health Service (HE-02085, AI-00798, 5TI-HE-5462), American Heart Association, and the American Cancer Society.

mice thymectomized neonatally is also affected, although this differs with the antigen used [21–24]; recently, Hess *et al.* [24] reported that the effects of thymectomy are more evident in the secondary response to tetanus toxoid than in the primary. Most of the other studies involved a primary response; further delineation of this aspect of the immunological status of the neonatally thymectomized mouse is needed.

It was evident that the immunological depletion of neonatally thymectomized mice was related to a depletion of lymphocytes in the peripheral blood and the peripheral lymphoid tissues (spleen and nodes, in particular), as well as to a probable deficit in plasma cell development [20, 25]. These observations gave substantial support to the thesis, stated in 1900 by Beard [26] and reiterated in recent years by such investigators as Fichtelius [27], Ruth [28], and Auerbach [29], that the thymus is a central source of immunologically effective cells. Morphological and histological studies in baby mice showed that the thymus is the only lymphoid organ at birth [25]. Thus it seemed reasonable that neonatal thymectomy removed this very active lymphoid tissue before its cells had been dispersed to the blood stream, spleen, and lymph nodes of the developing animal, resulting in underdeveloped lymphoid tissues and extreme immunological deficit.

Neonatally thymectomized mice early in life also develop a runting syndrome, which varies in time of onset and severity with the strain of animal [20, 23, 25, 30]. Such growth failure is illustrated in Figure 4-1. Although infectious agents have been suspected, almost all attempts to demonstrate such a factor have failed; recently, East *et al.* [31] demonstrated a hepatotrophic viral agent, but their findings do not suggest that it has a significant role in either the runting process or the early death of the thymectomized mice. The similarity of the post-thymectomy runting syndrome and F_1 hybrid disease (homologous disease, immunological runt disease) has been brought out repeatedly [20, 23, 25, 30]; the course of the animals' condition, their appearance, and the histology of their lymphoid tissues show remarkable parallels. The work of Howard and Woodruff [32] and more recent studies of Blaese *et al.* [33] established another link between the syndromes, since it is clear that mice

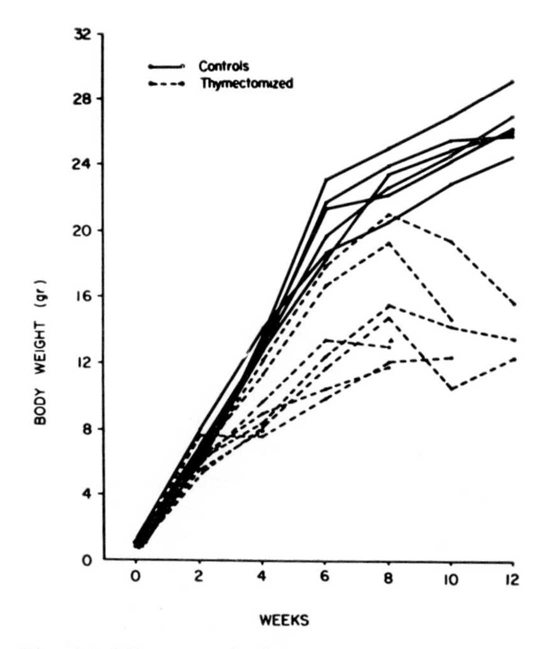

Fig. 4-1. The growth failure of neonatally thymectomized mice, compared to sham-operated controls. Each line represents a single animal.

undergoing immunologically induced runt disease, like neonatally thymectomized mice, have a profound immunological deficiency.

A fruitful approach to the nature of the defect of thymectomized mice has involved efforts to restore the animals both physiologically and immunologically. Miller [20], in the first of these studies, transplanted syngeneic and allogeneic thymus subcutaneously into the neonatally thymectomized animals during the first few days of life. He showed that the grafts prevented the occurrence of the runting syndrome if they were made early and that immunological function was also restored. The thymectomized animals with allogeneic thymuses became chimeric, as indicated by their acceptance of skin from both host and donor strains and as confirmed by chromosome analysis in a system involving a T6 marker. Dalmasso *et al.* [34] made a similar analysis, using the discriminating spleen assay to differentiate host and donor components. The results of the chromosome analyses and the assays of immunological activity showed that the development of the lymphoid tissues of allogeneic-thymus-bearing mice involved both donor and host cells, but host cells for the most part, suggesting that the notion of the thymus as a cell source was perhaps over-simplified. Other means of restoration have also been successful: spleen grafts [34], spleen or lymph node cells [23, 34, 35], and thymocytes [36, 37]; all of these involve population of the peripheral lymphoid tissues of the host with *donor* cells. A high degree of restoration has been attained by these means: the animals have normal life spans, reject allogeneic skin grafts, form antibody, and exercise graft-versus-host activity in appropriate F_1 hybrids. The most notable of the recent results in restoration studies is that of Levey *et al.* [38] and Osoba and Miller [39]. Both groups of investigators have attained significant restoration of neonatally thymectomized mice by intraperitoneal implants of neonatal thymus in Millipore chambers which permit diffusion of humoral products but do not allow egress of cells. Although the degree of immunological restoration possible in these circumstances is still being defined, these simultaneous studies by two different groups have brought the endocrinological role of the thymus to the fore. They suggest that intensive efforts at restoration of thymectomized mice with thymic extracts, heretofore unsuccessful, should be pressed.

Aside from the rabbit and mouse, the most extensive thymectomy experiments have been carried out in rats [40–43] and hamsters [44–46]. Transplantation immunity is affected by neonatal thymectomy in rats: the result was prolonged survival of skin grafts in the random-bred animals studied by Arnason *et al.*, but when inbred rats were thymectomized and grafted with allogeneic skin from donors differing at major histocompatibility loci by Defendi *et al.* [43], rejection of the grafts was not significantly delayed. Antibody production, delayed hypersensitivity, and susceptibility to induction of experimental allergic encephalomyelitis were all significantly affected by neonatal thymectomy of rats studied by the Waksman group [40, 41]. The depression of immunological capability is paralleled by a deficit in circulating lymphoid cells and defects in spleen and lymph node development.

The effects of thymectomy in hamsters have been studied in Philadelphia [43, 46] and in Boston [44, 45]. The influence of neonatal thymectomy on antibody response in the hamster varies with the antigen [43, 45, 46], but both groups of investigators have reported significant depression of transplantation immunity.

ROLE OF THE THYMUS IN THE ADULT ANIMAL

The thymus continues to play a role in the maturing mouse to 40 days and beyond. Martinez *et al.* [15], in some of their earliest studies, showed significant prolongation of graft survival in animals thymectomized as late as 30 days of age, provided the histocompatibility difference between donor and host was slight. Certain parameters, such as susceptibility to runt disease following injection of allogeneic cells, are affected by thymectomy as late as 40 days of age [25].

Dalmasso *et al.* [34] studied the effects of thymectomy at different ages up to 35 days on the graft-versus-host activity of the peripheral lymphoid cells of the animals. They showed that the thymus exercises a significant influence on continuing maturation of these immunological capabilities in mice as late as 35 days of age. Animals thymectomized during this period show an "arrest" of their immunological level; thus the peripheral lymphoid cells of an animal thymectomized at 25 days, assessed 2 months or more later, are very similar in activity to those of an animal killed at 25 days of age (Fig. 4-2).

The thymus apparently continues during adult life to play a role in maintaining integrity of the lymphoid tissues following irradiation and in restoring immunological reactivity following certain kinds of suppression of the immune mechanism. Miller [47] and Globerson *et al.* [48] have shown that the immunological recovery of irradiated mice is greatly hampered by adult thymectomy; they used the response to allogeneic tumor and skin grafts as the criterion of recovery. Auerbach [49], in a similar model, examined the rate of recovery of the lymphoid tissues of mice, thymectomized and not thymectomized, following irradiation, and his findings parallel those of the functional studies. Similarly, Duplan [50] found that the late mortality of lethally irradiated adult mice restored with fetal syngeneic liver suspensions was very different in thymectomized and control animals. The circulating lymphocyte levels of thymectomized mice did not recover, and many of them died between 30 and 60 days after irradiation. In the other groups, the late mortality was negligible, and normal blood lymphocyte levels were observed 50 to 70 days after irradiation.

Archer *et al.* [51] have documented a lag in

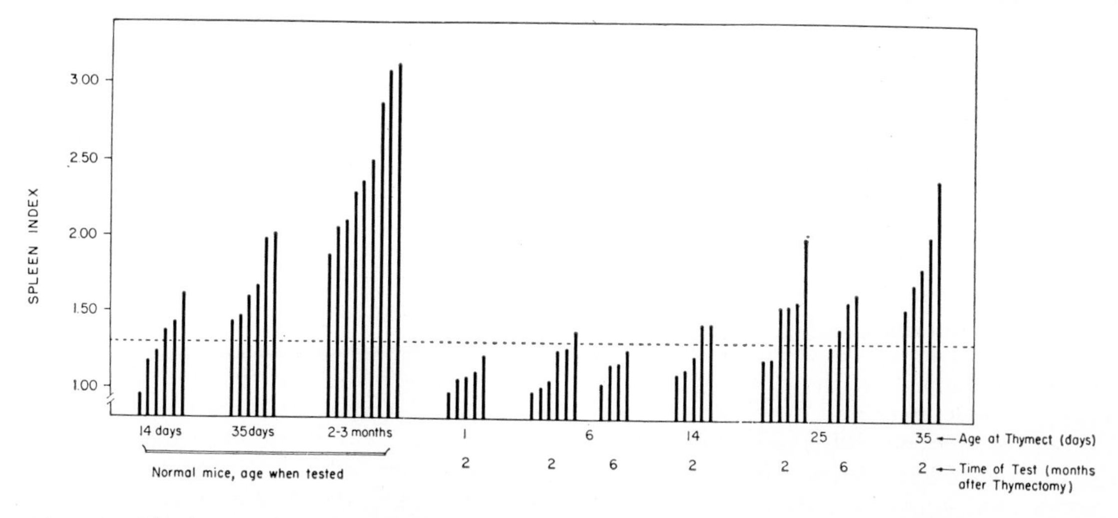

Fig. 4-2. The immunological capability of mice thymectomized at 1, 6, 14, 25, and 35 days of age, as assessed by the capacity of spleen cells from the animals to induce graft-versus-host reactions in appropriate F_1 hybrids. The normal reactivity of cells from unoperated animals killed at 14 and 35 days, and at 2 to 3 months of age is illustrated for comparative purposes. Even when tested as late as six months after thymectomy, the animals showed an "arrest" of immunological reactivity at the level they had presumably attained by the time of thymectomy. (From Dalmasso *et al.* [34], courtesy *J. Exp. Med.*)

immunological recovery of thymectomized adult rabbits, using the level of antibody response to bovine serum albumin as the criterion.

The findings of Claman and Talmage [52] suggest that thymectomy of adult mice also perpetuates another type of immunological failure—tolerance to simple protein antigens. In animals made tolerant in adult life, the effect of thymectomy was reflected in slow recovery of reactivity to the antigen. Mice made tolerant in the newborn period and later thymectomized remained unreactive to the protein antigen for an extended period, far beyond that of controls, apparently reflecting the greater degree of suppression possible in the neonate.

THE THYMUS AND BURSA OF FABRICIUS IN CHICKENS

As noted earlier, the immunological function of the bursa of Fabricius was established several years before the first studies on neonatal thymectomy in rabbits and mice, in the original work of Glick *et al.* [4] and in later work by others [9–11, 53]. These studies involved an assessment of circulating antibody levels after specific antigenic stimulation. The findings of Papermaster and co-workers [10, 11], confirmed by Warner and Szenberg [54], suggested that certain types of homograft immunity are also affected by bursectomy, specifically the development of splenomegaly in chickens following injection of allogeneic cell preparations. Papermaster *et al.* [10] also showed that chemical suppression of bursal development interfered with the development of capacity to reject allogeneic spleen cells. In these experiments the adult allogeneic spleen cells stimulated *in vitro* with *Brucella* antigen showed greater capacity to produce antibody in the hormonally treated chicken than they did in controls, again reflecting the deficiency in capacity of hormonally treated birds to mount a transplantation rejection reaction which would eliminate the foreign spleen cells.

Warner and Szenberg with Burnet [53, 55] have postulated a dissociation of immunological function of the chicken bursa and thymus. Their studies, and those of Aspinall and Wolfe's group [56, 57], suggest that skin homograft survival is prolonged in the absence of a thymus but is not significantly affected by lack of a bursa; and conversely, antibody production is little affected by thymectomy but is greatly affected by bursectomy. Janković *et al.* [58], using susceptibility of chickens to experimental allergic encephalomyelitis and the development of delayed allergy to central nervous system antigens and tuberculin as the criterion of the immunological status of thymectomized and bursectomized chickens, have provided further evidence of a measure of dissociation of function. In our laboratory, Yunis *et al.* [59] have not confirmed the effects of surgical thymectomy of newly hatched White Leghorn chickens on the response to skin homografts. All of the foregoing experiments have involved random-bred White Leghorn chickens. However, Ruth *et al.* [60] assessed the effects of combined bursectomy-thymectomy, on the first post-hatching day, on skin homograft survival in inbred strains of chickens differing at major histocompatibility loci. Despite the fact that the grafts were applied at an early age, these investigators were unable to demonstrate significant prolongation of graft survival following neonatal bursectomy-thymectomy.

Recent work by Cooper *et al.* [60a] involving early thymectomy or bursectomy or both, followed by sublethal irradiation, has provided further evidence of the relative immunological roles of the chicken thymus and bursa. It suggests that the bursa and bursa-dependent lymphoid tissue constitute the production system in antibody production, while the thymus and thymus-dependent lymphoid tissue constitute the recognition system in antibody production, the effector of delayed hypersensitivity, and a major component of homograft rejection.

Another role for the bursa of Fabricius has recently been defined by Peterson *et al.* [61, 62]. The dual role of the mouse thymus in immunogenesis and leukemogenesis suggested that an exploration of the effect of bursectomy and/or thymectomy on the incidence of fowl leukoses warranted investigation. The studies involved a well-characterized model—White Leghorn line 15I, an inbred strain of isolated chickens with a very low incidence of spontaneous lymphocytic malignancy but a well-characterized susceptibility to a range of malignancies following early administration of a virus RPL 12 L31. The experiments showed that bursectomy, at 1 day or 29 days of age, greatly reduces the incidence of visceral lymphomatosis in animals given injections of the virus at 1 or 28 days of age, without affecting the rate of development of the other major malignancies associated with this virus—erythroblastosis and osteopetrosis. Thymectomy alone had little effect.

That there is in the mouse a link of the thymus to leukemia has been known for almost twenty years. Up to the time of the aforementioned studies in the chicken, the only similar observation in another species was that of Gross [63] in rats given Gross passage A virus. He showed that thymectomized rats had a somewhat lower incidence of this virus-induced lymphoma than sham-operated animals.

The experimental evidence of the dual role of the bursa of Fabricius in development of antibody-producing capacity and the manifestation of a viral lymphoma supports the concept of a "central lymphoid tissue" which guarantees the integrity of peripheral lymphoid tissues and the maintenance of certain kinds of cellular proliferation, at least in early life.

THE THYMUS AND MALIGNANT DEVELOPMENT

There is considerable evidence of a thymic role in various types of neoplasia, specifically, an interrelation of defective (or absent) thymus, immunological inadequacy, and certain types of malignant development.

In mice it is clear that the thymus plays different roles with different types of tumor, e.g., mice thymectomized in the newborn period and even as late as age 40 days are unusually susceptible to tumor transplants, whether of mammary adenocarcinoma [17], a mast cell tumor [64], multiple myeloma tumor [65], or a rat leukemia [35]. They are also more prone to tumor development following administration of polyoma virus [43] and treatment with benzopyrene [66]. On the other hand, Martinez [66a] found that mice thymectomized at 6 days of age had a significantly lowered incidence of spontaneous mammary tumors compared to controls.

Many mouse lymphomas will not develop in the absence of the thymus; this is seen with spontaneous tumors [66a] and with lymphomas influenced by radiation, virus administration, hormonal, or carcinogen treatment [67, 67a, 67b]. The nature of the thymic role in leukemogenesis in mice is not known, but clearly it is not as simple as removal of the site of lymphoma development. It was the observation of an anterior mediastinal locus of leukemia development in mice that led to the earliest thymectomy studies; but subsequent studies have shown that the thymic influence extends to nonthymic lymphomas as well [68, 69]. This is demonstrated clearly in the studies of Peterson *et al.* [61, 62]: in chickens, the bursa of Fabricius does not usually show lymphomatous development, but its removal prevents the development of visceral lymphomatosis induced by one of the well-characterized viruses.

With the finding that a role analogous to that of the mouse thymus in leukemogenesis is played by the chicken bursa of Fabricius in a virus-induced lymphoma, it is clear that the problem must be considered in terms of central lymphoid tissue—rather than just thymus, as in the mouse—and in the light of the demonstrated role of this central lymphoid tissue in development of antibody production. Several other recent experimental observations reenforce this linking. Peterson *et al.* [70] have found that mice given Gross passage A virus in the newborn period are defective antibody producers at 3 and 9 weeks of age, a time when they show none of the stigmata of the leukemia. In parallel observations, Linder [71] and Prehn [72] have shown that mice given methylcholanthrene are also immunologically deficient before tumor development actually occurs. Metcalf [73] observed that young mice given repeated injections of the same antigen have a suggestive increase in the occurrence of spontaneous leukemia and especially of reticular tumors. These are animals whose thymus-dependent immunological development is not complete and whose level of immune reactivity is probably depressed by an "antigenic competition" type of mechanism by the repeated exposure to strong antigens [74, 75]. Neither the repeated stimulus to certain types of cellular proliferation in these animals nor their probable immunological depression can be dismissed as factors in the eventual development of uncontrolled proliferation.

It is interesting to reflect on the evidence of the role of various cell types in lymphoma development; the persistence of immature cell types in preleukemic AKR thymuses has been emphasized by Metcalf and Nakamura [76], and Ball [77] and Auerbach [78] have shown, using thymus cell sizes as the criterion, that the thymus of preleukemic mice fails to make a transition from larger to smaller cells as is consistently made in normal mouse thymus.

If some kind of retardation of cellular development in the thymus is basic to leukemogenesis in mice, it is not difficult to see that immunological development might also be stunted in circumstances that interfere with the normal sequence of maturation.

It is obviously not immunological suppression as such that fosters leukemic or lymphomatous development, since the animals with the most extreme deficiency, i.e., the neonatally bursectomized chickens and neonatally thymectomized mice, are protected from lymphoid tumor development. Whatever the thymic (or bursal) contribution to the abnormal proliferation of lymphoid cells, it is essential to this type of malignant development. The thymectomized (bursectomized) animals, however susceptible they are to other agents, will not develop the lymphoid tumors despite the continued presence of virus in the tissues and a very inadequate immune mechanism. On the other hand, when the thymus is present, the immunological depression of mice that have had virus injections or the immunological immaturity of young mice may play a role in the development of the disease process.

ROLE OF THE RABBIT APPENDIX IN IMMUNITY

It has been observed that neonatal appendectomy of the rabbit reduces the antibody-producing capability of the maturing animal and that combined appendectomy-thymectomy produces severe immunological defect. The basis of the experimental exploration of the immunological role of the rabbit appendix has been outlined by Archer *et al.* [79–81]. Briefly, they found that neonatally thymectomized rabbits suffer a temporary delay in lymphoid development of the spleen and lymph nodes and pronounced lymphopenia; the animals recover after a few weeks, however, and by 9 weeks of age the lymph nodes of a neonatally thymectomized rabbit are often very much like those of a sham-operated animal. A certain deficit remains, in the circulating lymphocyte level (10 to 15 percent below normal) (Fig. 4-3) and in antibody-producing capacity. A provocative observation was that the rabbit appendix, which is not a lymphoid organ at birth, develops at about the normal time in thymectomized animals while the lymphoid

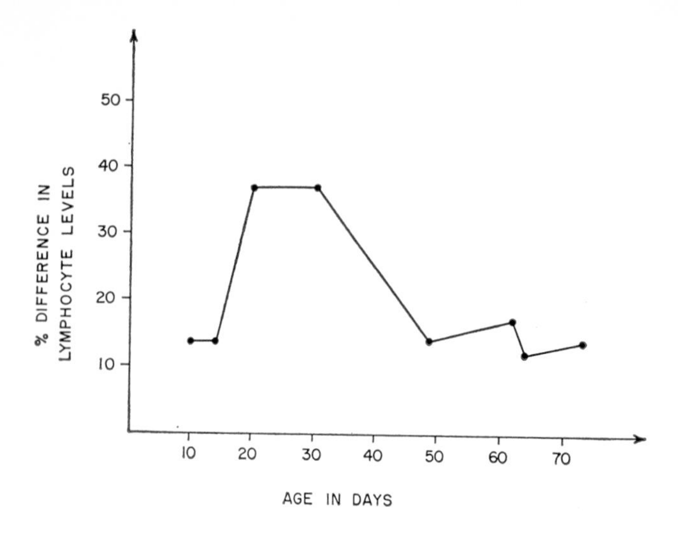

Fig. 4-3. A comparison of the difference between the lymphocyte levels of a normal group of rabbits and a group thymectomized in the newborn period. Depletion of lymphocytes is most marked at 3 to 4 weeks; by about 7 weeks recovery is considerable. This recovery is paralleled by lymphoid development of the spleen and lymph nodes and seems to be attributable, at least in part, to the activity of the appendix. (From Archer *et al.* [80], courtesy *Lab. Invest.*)

development of the spleen and nodes is lagging. The suggestion of an immunological role for the rabbit appendix was further supported by its histological resemblance to the bursa of Fabricius of the chicken [79–81].

As shown in Table 4-1, the thymectomized-appendectomized rabbit has a very low level of responsiveness to primary stimulation with bovine γ-globulin and suffers depletion of circulating lymphocytes. A lack of follicular development in the spleen and lymph nodes is observed well into adult life (12 to 14 weeks at the present writing).

There is some evidence in the rabbit studies that other gut-associated lymphoid tissues, particularly the sacculus rotundus, certain Peyer's patches, and the palatine and pharyngeal tonsils, may also function, to some extent at least, as central lymphoid tissue in immunological development. Much further study is needed to define the central lymphoid tissue of the rabbit and to document the effects of removal of varying portions of it at birth and during the period of immunological maturation.

PHYLOGENIC DEVELOPMENT OF IMMUNOLOGICAL CAPACITY

Interest in the immunological capabilities of invertebrates and lower vertebrates is as old as the concept of adaptive immunity itself. It is well established that birds have immunological capacity comparable to that of mammals and have γ-globulins and plasma cells.

TABLE 4-1. Effects of Neonatal Appendectomy and Thymectomy on Antibody Production in the Rabbit[a]

Group	Antibody to Bovine γ-Globulin, Geometric Mean Titer[b]	Circulating Lymphocytes (%)
I. Sham-operated	3,090 (11)	65
II. Thymectomized	571 (10)	54
III. Appendectomized	1,096 (9)	64
IV. Thymectomized-splenectomized	1,076 (4)	50
V. Appendectomized-thymectomized	121 (10)	41

[a] The animals were stimulated with 10 mg. of bovine γ-globulin in saline at 7–9 weeks and bled nine days later. Antibody determinations were made by the bis-diazotized benzidine hemagglutination method of Gordon *et al.* [94]. The antibody levels in the table are geometric means of the individual titers; the number of animals in the group is given in parentheses.

[b] The differences between antibody levels of group I and those of groups II, III, and V were statistically significant (p less than 0.01). The responses of the appendectomized-thymectomized group (V) were also significantly different from those of groups II and III (p less than 0.01).

The teleost fishes, reptilia, and amphibia have been studied immunologically, and all have adaptive immune responses.

Adaptive immunity, in the sense of specific antibody production, homograft rejection, or immediate and delayed hypersensitivity reactions, has not been demonstrated in invertebrates (reviewed in Ref. 82). Present evidence suggests that phagocytosis, encapsulation by coelomic cells, and nonspecific bactericidal substances provide an adequate defense against invading parasites in these forms. It is by no means certain that adaptive immune responses are totally lacking, however; many of the conclusions reached in studies of the 1920's and 1930's need to be re-examined experimentally with up-to-date methods. More recent work has concentrated on transplantation immunity, an area which is beset with technical problems in many of these organisms. Invertebrates apparently do not have cell systems comparable to the lymphocytic and plasmacytic series of vertebrates (reviewed in Ref. 82). Recent studies by Engle *et al.* [83] failed to disclose evidence of γ-globulins in a number of invertebrate forms; however, Condie [84] has isolated a substance from the hemolymph of a limpet which has the electrophoretic and ultracentrifugation characteristics of a γ-globulin and may have a degree of functional parallel with γ-globulins of vertebrates.

Historically, the least studied portion of the phylogenic scale has been the primitive fishes. Since teleost fishes seemed to have the full range of adaptive immunological responses, which was apparently lacking in invertebrates, the assumption was that study of the lowest vertebrate forms might show the phylogenic origin of this type of reactivity as far as this is possible by study of existing species.

The hagfishes are generally considered the lowest existing vertebrate forms and were the starting point of our investigations. One species, *Eptatretus stoutii,* was studied extensively by Papermaster, Good and Condie [85, 86]. Repeated stimulation with a variety of antigens for as long as seven months failed to induce any discernible antibody response in these animals; certain of the antigens, such as bacteriophage T-2 and hemocyanin, continued to circulate in substantial amounts for periods of 30 days. The hagfish does not develop a delayed hypersensitivity reaction following sensitization with BCG, nor does it show an intense inflammatory response when stimulated repeatedly by Freund's adjuvant. Study of transplantation immunity in the hagfish is subject to some of the technical problems encountered in similar studies in invertebrates. Wound-healing is very limited in this animal, and skin grafts do not regularly heal in place but merely pull away from the sutures as a result of movement of the animal. Similar limitations were encountered in efforts to graft muscle into the myotomes. Syngeneic and allogeneic liver grafts were attempted, in the form of surgical placement of small pieces of liver and the injection of cell suspensions; although a cellular response was noted at the site of such grafts, neither the degree of response nor the cellular components identified the allogeneic as opposed to the syngeneic sites [86].

As shown in Figure 4-4, the hagfish has a

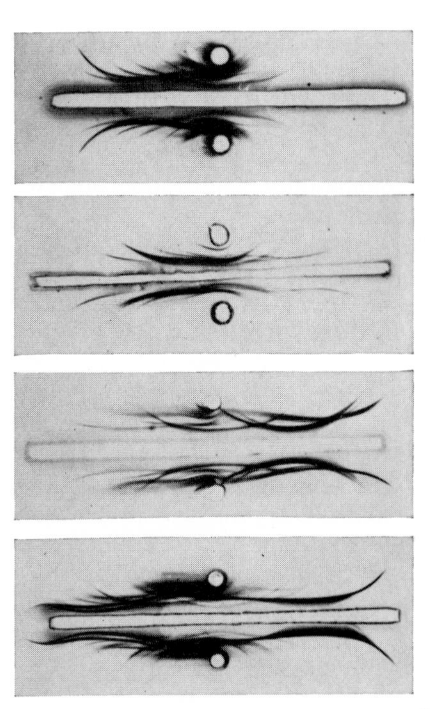

Fig. 4-4. Immunoelectrophoresis of serum of the hagfish (*top*) compared with that of the lamprey, bowfin, and an immunologically normal human being. In each case, the serum was allowed to react with antisera made against itself. The absence of γ-globulin components in the hagfish is associated with complete lack of immunological reactivity by all means tested. The increasing complexity of these proteins in the higher forms parallels a rising level of immunological sensitivity. (From Papermaster *et al.* [91], courtesy *J. Exp. Med.*)

very simple serum protein pattern, lacking in albumin and γ-globulin. It has no plasma cells. It has only one cell which resembles any of the lymphoid cells of higher forms, a small, dark cell, similar to a small lymphocyte; it has no larger lymphocytes. Jordan and Speidel [87], who studied the Atlantic hagfish *Myxine glutinosa* more than thirty years ago, called these small cells lymphocytes. The absence of other lymphocyte cell types and the presence of cell types which seem to be intermediate between these "lymphocytes" and thrombocytes on one hand and red blood cells on the other suggest that these may be a stem cell lymphoid hemoblast. This conclusion is supported by the lack of lymphopoietic tissue in the hagfish; extensive studies have been made of the splenic tissue distributed through the gut tract and sample serial sections have been examined through the entire length of the animal without evidence of any aggregate of these small cells. No thymus tissue has been identified.

Thus, with perhaps a little reservation on the status of transplantation immunity and the functional identity of a small lymphocyte-like cell in the circulating blood, the hagfish seems to be a vertebrate totally lacking in adaptive immunity and its morphological and serological correlates.

The lamprey is a cyclostome, like the hagfish, but is considered to be a higher form phylogenically. Data from recent studies have established unequivocally that the lamprey has a low level of immunological reactivity [88]: it rejects allogeneic grafts, produces a low level of antibody on repeated stimulation with strong bacterial antigens like *Brucella abortus,* develops delayed hypersensitivity lesions following appropriate sensitization and challenge with tuberculin, and shows vigorous mononuclear inflammation at the site of injection of Freund's adjuvant. The serum of the lamprey has a single band in the gamma area on immunoelectrophoresis. On sucrose gradient density and Sephadex column fractionation, the antibody, as measured in diluted whole serum, appears to be contained in a single fraction with sedimentation constant in the neighborhood of 12S [89]. The lamprey has no plasma cells; however, it does have a lymphoid series of cells in the circulation. Salkind [90] in 1914 made extensive studies of the lamprey, focusing particularly on the existence of thymus-like tissue. He concluded that the lamprey had an epithelial-lymphoid thymus. When we examined, at various stages of the lamprey's life cycle, the tissue labeled "epithelial" thymus by Salkind, we, too, often found a few lymphoid cells among the epithelial cells during the larval and newly transformed stages and even extending into late adult life. Further, in the primitive spleens of these animals, located in an invaginated lamina propria of the foregut, small foci of lymphoid cells can be identified. We believe that the thymus and lymphoid cells of these animals are probably the source of the low level of immunity expressed by these animals.

Among the holostean fishes, we have studied *Amia calva* (the dogfish or bowfin) both for antibody production and for sensitivity to *Ascaris lumbricoides* antigen [91]. Both types of responsiveness were present. As with many teleost fishes, the primary response to many antigens is very low; however, this animal had more vigorous immune response to such antigens as T-2 phage following a second injection of antigens and may be able to muster a secondary immune response.

The elasmobranchs, the guitarfish (a ray) and the horned shark, also had a low level of antibody response, not always demonstrable following primary stimulation with certain antigens but usually unmistakable in the secondary response [91]. These animals have thymic tissue, organized lymphoid tissue in the spleen, and circulating lymphoid cells. They seem to be lacking in plasma cell development. Studies of an antibody to hemocyanin formed by the guitarfish by Grey [92] suggest that this is a 19S globulin.

The immunological status of another primitive fish, the paddlefish (*Polyodon spathula*), has been studied extensively [93]. These animals also have the full range of immunological response: a level of antibody response comparable to that of the holostean fish, rejection of allogeneic grafts, and delayed and immediate sensitivity. They have thymic tissue foci, organized lymphoid development in other organs, especially in the spleen, a lymphoid series of cells, and plasma cells. Plasma cells seem to be a relatively late development phylogenically and to some extent dissociated from mere antibody production. Their earliest appearance seems to be associated with more vigorous capacity to produce antibody.

Studies of immunological function in two teleost fishes, the bullhead (*Ameiurus melas*) and the black bass (*Micropterus salmoides*), were made for control purposes [91]. They confirmed the many earlier observations that such fishes produce antibody relatively slowly and in relatively small amounts, particularly on primary stimulation, that temperature is an important variable in the level of reactivity, and that they have thymus tissue, especially early in life, and also have other lymphoid tissue, circulating lymphoid cells, and plasma cells.

Many phases of this work on the phylogeny of immunity need to be filled in; the studies are still in progress, and many of the conclusions must remain tentative. It appears, however, that the phylogenic development of adaptive immunity is paralleled by the development of thymic tissue, circulating cells of the lymphoid series, and foci of lymphoid cells (the first probably a necessary condition for the second and third) and by a simple humoral component with the electrophoretic characteristics of a γ-globulin. Greater organization of lymphoid tissues outside the thymus, increasing complexity of the serum proteins of the γ-globulin type, and, probably around the paddlefish level, the development of plasma cells are all associated with rising levels of immunological reactivity from the lamprey to the elasmobranchs, the dipnoid and holostean fishes, and finally the teleosts. Precipitating antibody to such antigens as hemocyanin is a later phylogenic development than hemagglutinating antibody; this may reflect the greater sensitivity of hemagglutination as a method or a qualitative difference in the antibody produced at the higher phylogenic levels, or both. The data suggest that phylogenically, as well as ontogenically, higher molecular weight antibody is formed first, to be followed later by antibodies of lower molecular weight.

REFERENCES

1. MacLean, L. D., Zak, S. J., Varco, R. L., and Good, R. A. Thymic tumor and acquired agammaglobulinemia—a clinical and experimental study of the immune response. *Surgery* 40:1010, 1956.
2. Hammar, J. A. Experimentelle Untersuchung über die Rolle der Thymus bei der Immunisierung. *Z. Mikr.-Anat. Forsch.* 44:425, 1938.
3. Harris, T. N., Rhoads, J., and Stokes, J., Jr. A study of the role of the thymus and spleen in the formation of antibodies in the rabbit. *J. Immun.* 58:27, 1948.
4. Glick, B., Chang, T. S., and Jaap, R. G. The bursa of Fabricius and antibody production. *Poult. Sci.* 35:224, 1956.
5. Chang, T. S., Rheins, M. S., and Winter, A. R. The significance of the bursa of Fabricius in antibody production in chickens: 1. Age of chickens. *Poult. Sci.* 36:735, 1957.
6. Chang, T. S., Rheins, M. S., and Winter, A. R. The significance of the bursa of Fabricius of chickens in antibody production: 2. Spleen relationship. *Poult. Sci.* 37:1091, 1958.
7. Glick, B. Further evidence for the role of the bursa of Fabricius in antibody production. *Ibid.* P. 240.
8. Glick, B. The Bursa of Fabricius and the Development of Immunologic Competence. In Good, R. A., and Gabrielsen, A. E. (Eds.), *The Thymus in Immunobiology*. New York: Paul B. Hoeber, Inc., 1964.
9. Mueller, A. P., Wolfe, H. R., and Meyer, R. K. Precipitin production in chickens: XXI. Antibody production in bursectomized chickens and in chickens injected with 19-nortestosterone on the fifth day of incubation. *J. Immun.* 85:172, 1960.
10. Papermaster, B. W., Bradley, S. G., Watson, D. W., and Good, R. A. Antibody-producing capacity of adult chicken spleen cells in newly hatched chicks: A study of sources of variation in a homologous cell transfer system. *J. Exp. Med.* 115:1191, 1962.
11. Papermaster, B. W., Friedman, D. I., and Good, R. A. Relationship of the bursa of Fabricius to immunologic responsiveness and homograft immunity in the chicken. *Proc. Soc. Exp. Biol. Med.* 110:62, 1962.
12. Archer, O., and Pierce, J. C. Role of the thymus in development of the immune response. *Fed. Proc.* 20:26, 1961.
13. Archer, O. K., Pierce, J. C., Papermaster, B. W., and Good, R. A. Reduced antibody response in thymectomized rabbits. *Nature* (London) 195:191, 1962.
14. Fichtelius, K. E., Laurell, G., and Philipsson, L. The influence of thymectomy on antibody formation. *Acta Path. Microbiol. Scand.* 51:81, 1961.
15. Martinez, C., Kersey, J., Papermaster, B. W., and Good, R. A. Skin homograft survival in thymectomized mice. *Proc. Soc. Exp. Biol. Med.* 109:193, 1962.
16. Good, R. A. Discussion of Archer and Pierce

[12], at meeting of American Association of Immunologists, Atlantic City, N.J., April, 1961.
17. Martinez, C., Dalmasso, A., and Good, R. A. Acceptance of tumor homografts by thymectomized mice. *Nature* (London) 194:1289, 1962.
18. Dalmasso, A. P., Martinez, C., and Good, R. A. Further studies of suppression of the homograft reaction by thymectomy in the mouse. *Proc. Soc. Exp. Biol. Med.* 111:143, 1962.
19. Miller, J. F. A. P. The immunological function of the thymus. *Lancet* 2:748, 1961.
20. Miller, J. F. A. P. Role of the thymus in transplantation immunity. *Ann. N.Y. Acad. Sci.* 99:340, 1962.
21. Miller, J. F. A. P. Effect of neonatal thymectomy on the immunological responsiveness of the mouse. *Proc. Roy. Soc.* [Biol.] 156:415, 1962.
22. Papermaster, B. W., Dalmasso, A. P., Martinez, C., and Good, R. A. Suppression of antibody-forming capacity with thymectomy in the mouse. *Proc. Soc. Exp. Biol. Med.* 111:41, 1962.
23. Parrott, D. M. V., and East, J. Studies on Fatal Wasting Syndrome of Mice Thymectomized at Birth. Ref. 8.
24. Hess, M. W., Cottier, H., and Stoner, R. D. Primary and secondary antitoxin responses in thymectomized mice. *J. Immun.* 91:425, 1963.
25. Good, R. A., Dalmasso, A. P., Martinez, C., Archer, O. K., Pierce, J. C., and Papermaster, B. W. The role of the thymus in development of immunologic capacity in rabbits and mice. *J. Exp. Med.* 116:773, 1962.
26. Beard, J. The source of leucocytes and the true function of the thymus. *Anat. Anz.* 18:550, 1900.
27. Fichtelius, K. E. On the Destination of Thymus Lymphocytes. In Wolstenholme, G. E. W., and O'Connor, M. (Eds.), *Haemopoiesis*. Boston: Little, Brown, 1960.
28. Ruth, R. F. Ontogeny of the blood cells. *Fed. Proc.* 19:579, 1960.
29. Auerbach, R. Genetic control of thymus lymphoid differentiation. *Proc. Nat. Acad. Sci. U.S.A.* 47:1175, 1961.
30. Parrott, D. M. V. Strain variation in mortality and runt disease in mice thymectomized at birth. *Transplant. Bull.* 29:102, 1962.
31. East, J., Parrott, D. M. V., Chesterman, F. C., and Pomerance, A. The appearance of a hepatotrophic virus in mice thymectomized at birth. *J. Exp. Med.* 118:1069, 1963.
32. Howard, J. G., and Woodruff, M. F. A. Effect of graft-versus-host reaction on the immunological responsiveness of the mouse. *Proc. Roy. Soc.* [Biol.] 154:532, 1961.
33. Blaese, M., Martinez, C., and Good, R. A. Immunologic incompetence of immunologically runted animals. *J. Exp. Med.* 119:211, 1964.
34. Dalmasso, A. P., Martinez, C., Sjodin, K., and Good, R. A. Studies on the role of the thymus in immunobiology: Reconstitution of immunologic capacity in mice thymectomized at birth. *J. Exp. Med.* 118:1089, 1963.
35. Miller, J. F. A. P. Effect of Thymic Ablation and Replacement. Ref. 8.
36. Taylor, R. B. Immunological competence of thymus cells after transfer to thymectomized recipients. *Nature* (London) 199:873, 1963.
37. Yunis, E. J., Hilgard, H., Sjodin, K., Martinez, C., and Good, R. A. Immunological reconstitution of thymectomized mice by injections of isolated thymocytes. *Nature* (London) 201:784, 1964.
38. Levey, R. H., Trainin, N., and Law, L. W. Evidence for function of thymic tissue in diffusion chambers implanted in neonatally thymectomized mice. *J. Nat. Cancer Inst.* 31:199, 1963.
39. Osoba, D., and Miller, J. F. A. P. Evidence for a humoral thymus factor responsible for the maturation of immunological faculty. *Nature* (London) 199:653, 1963.
40. Janković, B. D., Waksman, B. H., and Arnason, B. G. Role of the thymus in immune reactions in rats: I. The immunologic response to bovine serum albumin (antibody formation, Arthus reactivity, and delayed hypersensitivity) in rats thymectomized or splenectomized at various times after birth. *J. Exp. Med.* 116: 159, 1962.
41. Arnason, B. G., Janković, B. D., Waksman, B. H., and Wennersten, C. Role of the thymus in immune reactions in rats: II. Suppressive effect of thymectomy at birth on reactions of delayed (cellular) hypersensitivity and the circulating small lymphocyte. *Ibid.*, p. 177.
42. Waksman, B. H., Arnason, B. G., and Janković, B. D. Role of the thymus in immune reactions in rats: III. Changes in the lymphoid organs of thymectomized rats. *Ibid.*, p. 187.
43. Defendi, V., Roosa, R. A., and Koprowski, H. Effect of thymectomy at birth on response to tissue, cells, and virus antigens. Ref. 8.
44. Sherman, J. D., and Dameshek, W. "Wasting disease" following thymectomy in the hamster. *Nature* (London) 197:469, 1963.
45. Sherman, J. D., Adner, M. M., Costea, N., Schwartz, R., Lewis, F. B., and Dameshek, W. The function of the thymus in the golden hamster. *Fed. Proc.* 22:600, 1963.
46. Roosa, R. A., Wilson, D., and Defendi, V. Effect of neonatal thymectomy in hamsters. *Ibid.*, p. 599.
47. Miller, J. F. A. P. Immunological significance of the thymus of the adult mouse. *Nature* (London) 195:1318, 1962.
48. Globerson, A., Fiore-Donati, L., and Feldman, M. On the role of the thymus in recovery of immunological reactivity following x-irradiation. *Exp. Cell Res.* 28:455, 1962.
49. Auerbach, R. Thymus: Its role in lymphoid

recovery after irradiation. *Science* 139:1061, 1963.
50. Duplan, J. F. Effets de la thymectomie sur la régénération lymphoïde des souris irradiées, restaurées par du foie foetal isologue. *C. R. Acad. Sci.* (Paris) 256:3366, 1963.
51. Archer, O. K., Papermaster, B. W., and Good, R. A. Thymectomy in Rabbit and Mouse: Consideration of Time of Lymphoid Peripheralization. Ref. 8.
52. Claman, H. N., and Talmage, D. W. Thymectomy: Prolongation of immunological tolerance in the adult mouse. *Science* 141:1193, 1963.
53. Warner, N. L., Szenberg, A., and Burnet, F. M. The immunological role of different lymphoid organs in the chicken: I. Dissociation of immunological responsiveness. *Aust. J. Exp. Biol. Med. Sci.* 40:373, 1962.
54. Warner, N. L., and Szenberg, A. Immunological reactivity of bursaless chickens in graft versus host reactions. *Nature* (London) 199:43, 1963.
55. Szenberg, A., and Warner, N. L. Dissociation of immunological responsiveness in fowls with a hormonally arrested development of lymphoid tissues. *Nature* (London) 194:146, 1962.
56. Aspinall, R. L., Meyer, R. K., Graetzer, M. A., and Wolfe, H. R. Effect of thymectomy and bursectomy on the survival of skin homografts in chickens. *J. Immun.* 90:872, 1963.
57. Graetzer, M. A., Wolfe, H. R., Aspinall, R. L., and Meyer, R. K. Effect of thymectomy and bursectomy on precipitin and natural hemagglutinin production in the chicken. *Ibid.*, p. 878.
58. Janković, B. D., and Išvaneski, M. Experimental allergic encephalomyelitis in thymectomized, bursectomized and normal chickens. *Int. Arch. Allerg.* 23:188, 1963.
59. Yunis, E. J., Cooper, M., Peterson, R. D. A., and Good, R. A. Unpublished observations. 1963.
60. Ruth, R. F., Allen, C. P., and Wolfe, H. R. The Effect of Thymus on Lymphoid Tissue. Ref. 8.
60a. Cooper, M. D., Peterson, R. D. A., and Good, R. A. Delineation of the bursal and thymic lymphoid systems in the chicken. Submitted for publication.
61. Peterson, R. D. A., Burmester, B. R., Fredrickson, T. N., and Good, R. A. The prevention of lymphatic leukemia in the chicken by the surgical removal of the bursa of Fabricius. *J. Lab. Clin. Med.* 62:1000, 1963 (abst.).
62. Peterson, R. D. A., Burmester, B. R., Fredrickson, T. N., Purchase, H. G., and Good, R. A. The effect of bursectomy and thymectomy on the development of visceral lymphomatosis in the chicken. *J. Nat. Cancer Inst.* 32:1343, 1964.
63. Gross, L. Serial cell-free passage in rats of the mouse leukemia virus: Effect of thymectomy. *Proc. Soc. Exp. Biol. Med.* 112:939, 1963.
64. McEntegart, M. G., Ross, P. W., and Best, P. V. Growth of the mast cell tumor P.815 in thymectomized mice. *Lancet* 2:611, 1963.
65. Martinez, C., Dalmasso, A. P., and Good, R. A. Homotransplantation of Normal and Neoplastic Tissues in Thymectomized Mice. Ref. 8.
66. Miller, J. F. A. P., Grant, G. A., and Roe, F. J. C. Effect of thymectomy on the induction of skin tumors by 3,4-benzopyrene. *Nature* (London) 199:920, 1963.
66a. Martinez, C. Effect of early thymectomy on development of mammary tumours in mice. *Nature* (London) 203:1188, 1964.
67. Kirschbaum, A., Shapiro, J. R., and Mixer, H. W. The synergistic action of leukemogenic agents. *Cancer Res.* 13:262, 1953.
67a. McEndy, D. P., Boon, M. C., and Furth, J. On the role of the thymus, spleen and gonads in the development of leukemia in a high-leukemia stock of mice. *Cancer Res.* 4:377, 1944.
67b. Kaplan, H. S. Influence of thymectomy, splenectomy and gonadectomy on the incidence of radiation induced lymphoid tumors in strain C57 black mice: *J. Nat. Cancer Inst.* 11:83, 1950.
68. Kaplan, H. S., Brown, M. B., and Paull, J. Influence of post-irradiation thymectomy and of thymic implants on lymphoid tumor incidence in C57Bl mice. *Cancer Res.* 13:677, 1953.
69. Law, L. W., and Miller, J. H. The influence of thymectomy on the incidence of carcinogen-induced leukemia in strain DBA mice. *J. Nat. Cancer Inst.* 11:425, 1950.
70. Peterson, R. D. A., Hendrickson, R., and Good, R. A. Reduced antibody forming capacity during the incubation period of passage A leukemia in C3H mice. *Proc. Soc. Exp. Biol. Med.* 114:517, 1963.
71. Linder, O. E. A. Survival of skin homografts in methylcholanthrene-treated mice and in mice with spontaneous mammary cancers. *Cancer Res.* 22:380, 1962.
72. Prehn, R. Function of depressed immunologic reactivity during carcinogenesis. *J. Nat. Cancer Inst.* 31:791, 1963.
73. Metcalf, D. Induction of reticular tumors in mice by repeated antigenic stimulation. *Acta Un. Int. Cancer* 19:657, 1963.
74. Miller, J., Martinez, C., and Good, R. A. Facilitation of tolerance in weanling mice by enhancing the proliferation of donor lymphoreticular cells. *J. Immun.* 93:331, 1964.
75. Miller, J., Martinez, C., and Good, R. A. Reciprocal competition of a variety of antigens in

the suppression of immunologic reactivity. *J. Immun.* 93:342, 1964.

76. Metcalf, D., and Nakamura, K. Transplantation bioassay of thymuses from preleukaemic AKR mice for the presence of leukaemic cells. *Brit. J Cancer* 15:316, 1961.
77. Ball, W. D. A quantitative assessment of mouse thymus differentiation. *Exp. Cell Res.* 31:82, 1963.
78. Auerbach, R. Experimental Analysis of Mouse Thymus and Spleen Morphogenesis. Ref. 8.
79. Archer, O. K., Sutherland, D. E. R., and Good, R. A. Appendix of the rabbit: A homologue of the bursa in the chicken? *Nature* (London) 200:337, 1963.
80. Archer, O. K., Sutherland, D. E. R., and Good, R. A. The developmental biology of lymphoid tissue in the rabbit: Consideration of the role of thymus and appendix. *Lab. Invest.* 13:259, 1964.
81. Sutherland, D. E. R., Archer, O. K., and Good, R. A. The role of the appendix in development of immunologic capacity. *Proc. Soc. Exp. Biol. Med.* 115:673, 1964.
82. Good, R. A., and Papermaster, B. W. Ontogeny and phylogeny of adaptive immunity. *Advances Immun.* 4:1, 1964.
83. Engle, R. L., Woods, K. R., and Pert, J. H. Studies on the phylogenesis of gamma globulins and plasma cells. *J. Clin. Invest.* 37:892, 1958.
84. Condie, R. M. Unpublished observations, 1962.
85. Good, R. A., and Papermaster, B. W. Phylogeny of the immune response: I. The agnathan, *Polystotrema stouti. Fed. Proc.* 20:261, 1961.
86. Papermaster, B. W., Condie, R. M., and Good, R. A. Immune response in the California hagfish. *Nature* (London) 196:355, 1962.
87. Jordan, H. E., and Speidel, C. C. Blood formation in cyclostomes. *Amer. J. Anat.* 46:355, 1930.
88. Finstad, J., and Good, R. A. Evolution of the immune response III. Immunologic responses in the lamprey. *J. Exp. Med.* 120:1151, 1964.
89. Ashbach, N. E., Finstad, J., Sarnecki, J. C., and Pollara, B. Phylogeny of immunoglobulins: Ultracentrifugal analysis and character of antibody response. *Fed. Proc.* 23:346, 1964.
90. Salkind, J. Contributions histologiques à la biologie comparée du thymus. *Arch. Zool. Exp.* 55:81, 1915.
91. Papermaster, B. W., Condie, R. M., Finstad, J., and Good, R. A. Evolution of the immune response: I. The phylogenetic development of adaptive immunologic responsiveness in vertebrates. *J. Exp. Med.* 119:105, 1964.
92. Grey, H. M. Phylogeny of the immune response: Studies on some physical, chemical and serologic characteristics of antibody produced in the turtle. *J. Immun.* 91:819, 1963.
93. Good, R. A., and Finstad, J. Phylogeny of immune reactions. Immunological capacity of polyodon and other fishes. *Fed. Proc.* 23:285, 1964.
94. Gordon, J., Rose, B., and Sehon, A. H. Detection of "non-precipitating" antibodies in sera of individuals allergic to ragweed pollen by an in vitro method. *J. Exp. Med.* 108:37, 1958.

5. The Histology of Antibody Production

FRANK W. FITCH AND ROBERT W. WISSLER

THE IMMUNOGLOBULINS ARE formed primarily if not exclusively in lymphoid tissue. The histological changes occurring in lymphoid organs after immunization have been studied intensively in relation to the cellular events associated with the immune response [1–10]. In the last two decades, remarkable progress has been made in the understanding of many of the cellular processes involved in the formation of humoral antibody. This chapter is devoted to a consideration of the histological aspects of this phenomenon.

The discussion which follows will not include the immune phenomena of delayed hypersensitivity and the homograft reaction, both of which appear to be mediated largely by sensitized lymphoid cells, although circulating antibody may play a significant role in the homograft reaction. These phenomena are considered in detail in Chapters 11 and 13. The possible role of the eosinophil [11–13] in the immune response is considered in Chapter 17.

HISTORICAL BACKGROUND

The concept of humoral antibody did not develop until nearly a century after clinically induced immunization had been established on a scientific basis by Jenner. By the beginning of the Twentieth Century, however, the role of the spleen and other lymphoid organs in antibody formation had been clearly demonstrated [14]. Many of the early investigators were concerned with immunity to infectious diseases and did not separate the nonspecific factors of host resistance from the specific immune response.

The importance of the reticuloendothelial system in the phagocytosis of bacteria and other antigenic substances was also recognized early [15], and the assumption was made that these phagocytic cells must form antibody. Other data were presented supporting the view that antibodies were formed by macrophages [16, 17]. Investigations with colored antigenic azoproteins in which shedding of cytoplasmic material was associated with appearance of antibody in the blood were interpreted as indicating antibody production by macrophages.

Formation of antibody in individual lymph nodes was unequivocally demonstrated by McMaster and Hudack [18] in 1935. Ehrich and Harris [19] extended these observations and described enlargement of lymph follicles, general lymph node hypertrophy, and outpouring of small lymphocytes into efferent lymph, after immunization with bacterial antigens. Other evidence indicating the role of the small lymphocyte in antibody formation was presented by Dougherty *et al.* [20, 21].

Meanwhile, Bjørneboe and Gormsen [22] showed that intensive immunization of rabbits with polyvalent vaccine resulted in elevation of serum globulin levels and a marked increase in numbers of tissue plasma cells. Fagraeus [23], in a classic study, correlated the splenic histology after multiple antigenic stimulations with the development of humoral antibody. She delineated a series of related cells first evident as rather large cells with pyroninophilic cytoplasm, the transitional cell, which differentiated eventually after several cell divisions into a mature plasma cell. The splenic red pulp, rich in this cell series, formed antibody *in vitro* while the white pulp did not.

Until 1950, only indirect evidence was available to indicate the types of cells which produced humoral antibody. Reiss *et al.* [24] and later Moeschlin and Demiral [25] demonstrated that certain cells from lymph nodes of rabbits immunized with killed *Salmonella* had the capacity of causing bacteria of the immunizing strain to adhere specifically to the cell surface. In almost all cases these cells were plasma cells, although Hayes and Dougherty [26], using a similar technique, found that lymphocytes also gave the specific adherence reaction. Nossal has improved and extended this technique and with Mäkelä [27] applied it to the study of antibody formation by single cells. Other modifications of this method have enabled detection of antibody formed by individual lymphoid cells against bacteria and bacteriophage [27a, 27b]. The adaptation of the fluorescent antibody technique [28] for demonstration of intracellular antibody has furnished direct evidence of the type of cell containing antibody and has made it possible to determine the location of such cells within lymphoid organs. Several of these methods of demonstrating apparent antibody production by cells have been combined with radioactive tracer techniques [29] to determine the kinetics of the cellular populations involved. A technique recently developed by Jerne *et al.* which permits recognition of individual antibody-forming cells promises to be extremely useful since determination of the number of such cells as well as evaluation of their morphology is possible [29a, 117].

Abundant evidence indicates that plasma cells and their precursors contain and presumably produce antibody, but recent histological studies suggest the participation of other cell types as well. For example, proliferation of lymphocytes is frequently prominent following antigenic stimulation, and usually only a few plasma cells are produced after primary immunization. Attardi *et al.* [29b] found antibody production associated with lymphocytes as well as plasma cells. Furthermore, other cells, including primitive reticular cells, macrophages, and eosinophils, may be involved directly or indirectly in the immune response.

INITIATION OF THE HISTOLOGICAL REACTION

It is not known whether activation of the antibody-synthesizing system by antigen involves "instruction" or "selection" of antibody-forming units, nor is it known how or where this essential step occurs (Chap. 6).

Soluble antigens may enter potential antibody-forming cells by pinocytosis (a process similar to phagocytosis) and may be metabolized in the same manner as postulated below for particulate antigens. Recent evidence indicates that relatively few cell types ingest complete protein molecules by pinocytosis although reticular cells, tissue lymphocytes, macrophages [30], as well as very immature plasma cells [31] appear to be active in this process. Immunohistochemical methods have shown antigenically reactive materials in various cells of lymph nodes, spleen, and other organs, including occasional inclusion of antigenic material within cell nuclei [32, 32a]. This technique, however, does not necessarily demonstrate material which has stimulated antibody formation nor does it determine the location of intact protein molecules; it only demonstrates reactive antigenic materials which could be fragments of larger molecules and gives no information about where the antigenic stimulation occurs within the cell.

Studies utilizing horse ferritin as an antigen in the mouse have been interpreted as demonstrating the transformation of "reticular cells" which had ingested the ferritin molecule into mature, presumably antibody-forming, plasma cells [33]. Ferritin, recognizable with the electron microscope by its characteristic molecular configuration, was found in phagosomes of the reticular cells and in dense aggregates within transitional cell forms as well as in mature plasma cells. However, the fact that neoplastic plasma cells from human myelomas may contain hemosiderin [34] and the demonstration that HeLa and other cells are able to synthesize ferritin *in vitro* [35] raise questions concerning the interpretation of these observations.

Although definitive evidence has not been obtained, it seems likely that particulate antigens such as foreign erythrocytes, bacteria, and viruses do not initiate antibody formation before they are ingested by phagocytic cells. If this is so, it is probable that material containing the essential antigenic information is formed during the digestion of the particle by a phagocytic nonantibody-forming cell and that this material then is transferred to nonphagocytic cells having the potential to form antibody. Most evidence indicates that phagocytic cells do not differentiate into antibody-forming cells and that the latter have little if any phagocytic properties.

Presumptive evidence that an active metabolic product is formed from antigen by macrophages has been obtained by Fishman and Adler [36, 37]. Rat peritoneal exudate cells consisting mainly of macrophages were incubated with T-2 bacteriophage *in vitro*. Cell-free extracts prepared from the incubated macrophages stimulated antibody formation by normal rat lymph node cells both *in vitro* [36] and *in vivo* [37]. The active material was of low molecular weight. The presence of antigen fragments was not excluded, but ribonucleic acid (RNA) appeared to play the critical role since stimulatory activity was destroyed by ribonuclease treatment. Friedman [38] has obtained evidence of a similar material in spleen cell homogenates from mice immunized with *Shigella* antigens. Antigenic activity could be demonstrated only after incubation of the ribonucleoprotein fraction of spleen tissue from immunized mice with normal spleen cells *in vitro* followed by transfer of the cells to normal recipients. The material was not active after direct injection into normal animals, suggesting that lymphoid cells probably require a high concentration of the material for activation.

Important information concerning localization of antigen within lymph nodes has been presented by Nossal and co-workers [38a, 38b]. Highly antigenic bacterial flagellar preparations were taken up and retained by macrophages in lymphoid follicles as well as by medullary phagocytes. Nonantigenic proteins were found only in the medullary regions of the node. Thus the phagocytes of lymphoid follicles seemed to exhibit a capacity to recognize "foreignness."

Regardless of the means by which antibody-forming cells are activated, antibody frequently appears in the circulation after an "induction" or "latent" phase lasting only a day or two. The time of appearance of free antibody in the circulation, however, is an inadequate indicator of the onset of antibody synthesis. If antigen remains in the circulation, as is the case after intravenous immunization with serum protein antigens [39] and with some other materials such as foreign erythrocytes from closely related species or some bacteriophage particles [40], the antibody formed early in the response may combine with the circulating antigen. Often, but not always, this results in more rapid elimination of antigen from the circulation. Free antibody may not appear in the circulation in detectable quantities until the antigen has been cleared from the blood. The apparent length of the induction phase also depends on the amount of antigen, route of injection, and species of immunized animal. Of major importance also is the sensitivity of methods used in determining the presence of antibody. The most sensitive measure of antibody formation appears to be the elimination of phage particles from the circulation [40]. This method indicates that antibody formation in the guinea pig may begin as early as 24 hours after immunization.

Although antibody formation may begin very soon after immunization, the *induction* phase is apparently a distinctive process which differs qualitatively from the *production* phase of the immune response. The steps occurring in the period of induction are impaired by x-ray irradiation [41, 42] and by cortisone [43]. Perhaps the most conclusive evidence of distinctive differences between inductive and productive phases comes from *in vitro* studies [44]. Although antibody production which is initiated in the intact animal can be continued *in vitro,* it has not been possible to induce a *primary* response with unaltered antigen in tissue culture. On the other hand, a secondary response has been induced *in vitro* by adding antigen to small bits of lymph nodes from sensitized animals.

The important metabolic processes that occur during the induction period do not have recognized morphological counterparts. The onset of histological changes after immunization varies in different animal species and depends on the type and quantity of antigen injected as well as the route of injection. Proliferation and differentiation of lymphoid cells usually become evident between 12 and 48 hours after immunization.

HISTOLOGICAL CHANGES DURING ANTIBODY FORMATION

The numerous studies of histological alterations during the immune response have been critically reviewed by several authors [1–10]. Multiple antigen injections have often been used to produce maximal cellular response; however, sequential changes are difficult to interpret in such studies. Subcutaneous injection of antigen, especially when given with various adjuvants, results in rather slow and protracted delivery of antigen, as well as migration via lymphatics of locally reacting cells to the regional lymph nodes, thus superimposing cellular reactions of various ages. Adjuvants may also cause cellular reactions unrelated to antibody formation. Evaluation of the

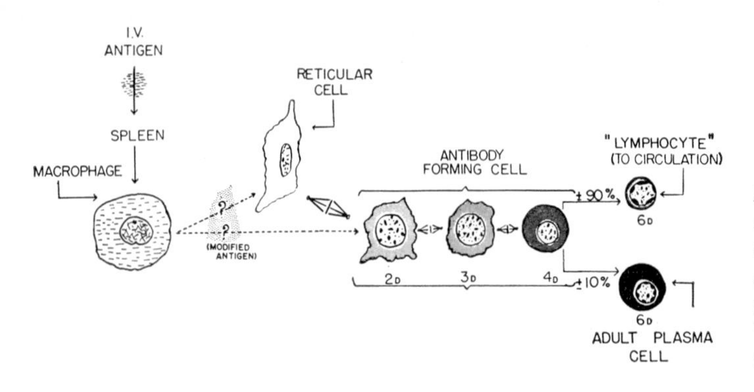

Fig. 5-1. Summary of cellular changes in splenic red pulp during early stages of antibody formation after primary intravenous immunization. (Modified from Fig. 6, R. W. Wissler *et al.* [5], courtesy *J. Cell. Comp. Physiol.*)

splenic histology after a single intravenous injection of particulate antigen appears to offer one of the best opportunities to determine the sequential histological changes. The cells are exposed rapidly and, presumably, in many instances only briefly to the antigen, and under suitable experimental conditions the spleen forms most if not all of the circulating antibody after intravenous immunization.

Although a variety of antigens has been used in several different species, a rather consistent pattern of primary cellular reaction is apparent in the spleen (Fig. 5-1). The essential histological changes in all these situations appear to be the following: One to three days after a single intravenous injection of antigen, large cells with basophilic or pyroninophilic cytoplasm appear in the red pulp, frequently along small trabeculae. These cells have been called plasmablasts, immunoblasts, transitional cells, and antibody-forming cells. There are continuing multiplication and differentiation of these cells for a few days, after which some of them seem to form more mature plasma cells while the majority lose cytoplasm to become cells resembling lymphocytes. These cells persist for only a few hours, then many disappear from the spleen quite suddenly with little evidence of cell rhexis or lysis. As described later, changes are also frequently seen in the lymphatic nodules of the splenic white pulp.

There are conflicting opinions as to the origin of the pyroninophilic cells seen soon after primary immunization. Langevoort [45] has made the most recent, thorough, semiquantitative investigation of the histological changes after a single antigenic stimulation. Rabbits were given injections of horse γ-globulin or H-antigen from paratyphoid-B bacilli. Large pyroninophilic cells which Langevoort called plasmablasts appeared in the periarteriolar lymphoid sheath 24 hours after immunization. It should be noted that in many mammals a continuous lymphoid tissue sheath surrounds the splenic arteries along their course from the trabeculae to their entrance into the red pulp as small penicillar arteries [46]. Lymphatic nodules (Malpighian bodies) are found at irregular intervals adjacent to the artery. Hence Langevoort suggests that the pyroninophilic cells arise within the white pulp lymphatic sheath but not within the lymphatic nodules. Apparent transitional forms between small lymphocytes and plasmablasts were noted, but the possibility that these cells originated from reticular cells in the lymphoid sheath was not definitely excluded. From the second to the fifth day, increasing numbers of "immature plasma cells," presumably derived from plasmablasts by mitosis and differentiation, were observed (Figs. 5-2 and 5-3). These immature plasma cells, characterized by rather abundant pyroninophilic cytoplasm, apparently migrated to the periphery of the periarteriolar lymphocyte sheaths at the border of the red pulp, often appearing to lie within the red pulp but always closely related to arterial capillaries. After the fifth day, there was a striking contrast between the small number of mature plasma cells remaining and the large numbers of immature plasma cells present a few days earlier. Most of the "young plasma cells" were thought to have entered the blood stream directly. This interpretation might appear rather strange since it has been thought that plasma cells are not present in the circulating blood. However, Braunsteiner and Pakesch [47] have described cells in the peripheral blood which are indistinguishable by conventional morphological techniques from medium-sized lymphocytes. Yet these cells have ultrastructural charac-

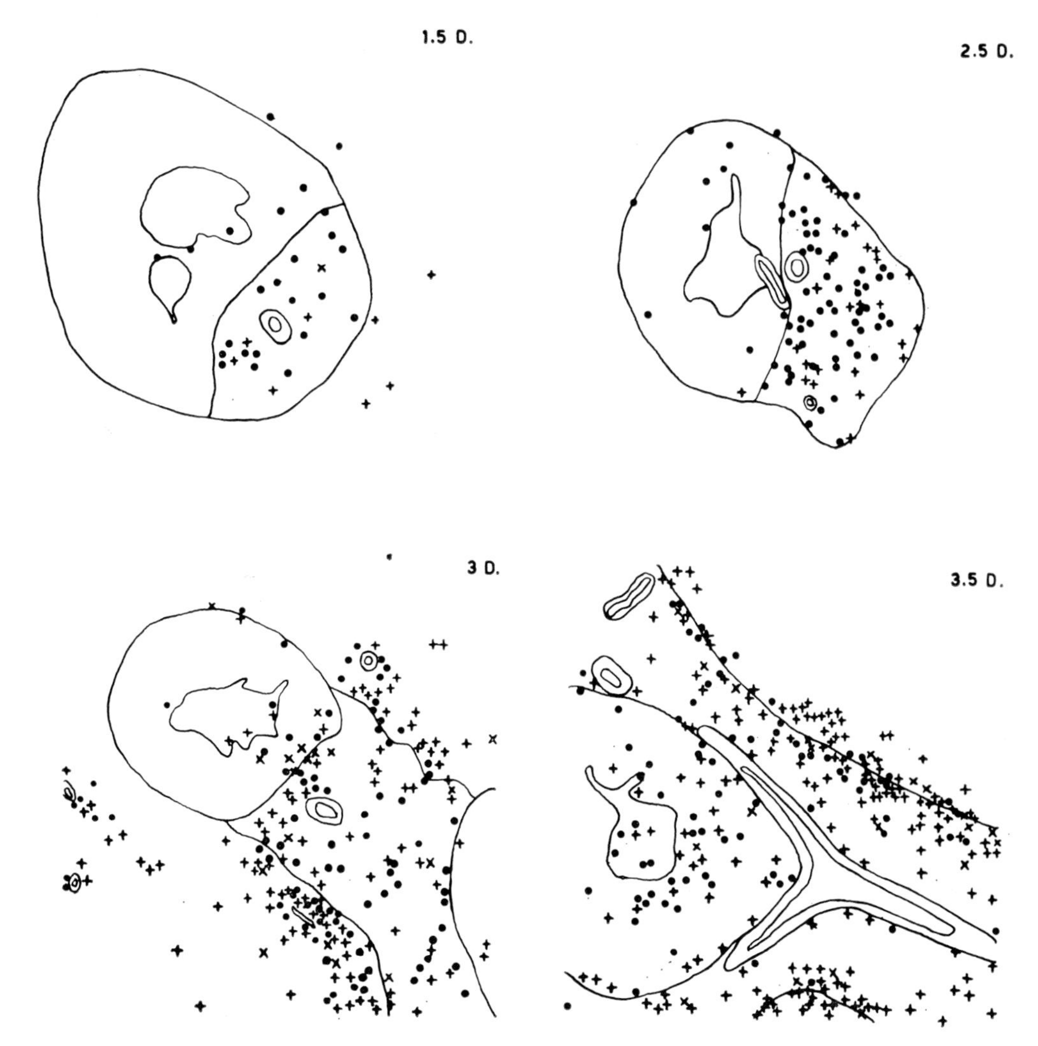

Fig. 5-2. Camera lucida drawings of splenic white pulp after antigenic stimulation. Contours of the periarteriolar sheath (*right*) and a lymphoid follicle (*left*) are shown. "Plasmablasts" (•) first are seen in the periarteriolar lymphoid sheath. "Immature plasma cells" (+) are later seen in here as well as in adjacent red pulp. Mitoses (×) are most numerous the third day after immunization. (From Langevoort [45], courtesy *Lab. Invest.*)

teristics seen under the electron microscope which indicate that they should be considered "plasma cells." It seems that the phenomenon observed by Langevoort is the same as that previously described in our laboratory in the rat [7, 48]. Apparently most of the cells developing in the spleen during the primary response enter the circulation after maturing into a cell which is difficult to distinguish with light microscopy from a lymphocyte.

In Langevoort's studies [45], changes in lymphatic nodules were not evident until the fourth day after immunization and consisted of increased numbers of blast cells and medium-sized lymphocytes. The follicular centers continued to increase in size and by the ninth day were packed with lymphocytes (Fig. 5-4). Four weeks after immunization, the follicle centers were still enlarged but the lymphoid sheaths appeared normal. The antibody titer reached a peak at about 10 days and remained elevated. Thus antibody production continued although cellular change in the splenic red pulp had subsided.

These observations agree in many particulars with the sequential observations made in the rat spleen following intravenous injection of particulate antigen [5, 7, 48–50a]. As discussed in detail later, this evidence is compatible with the concept that circulating

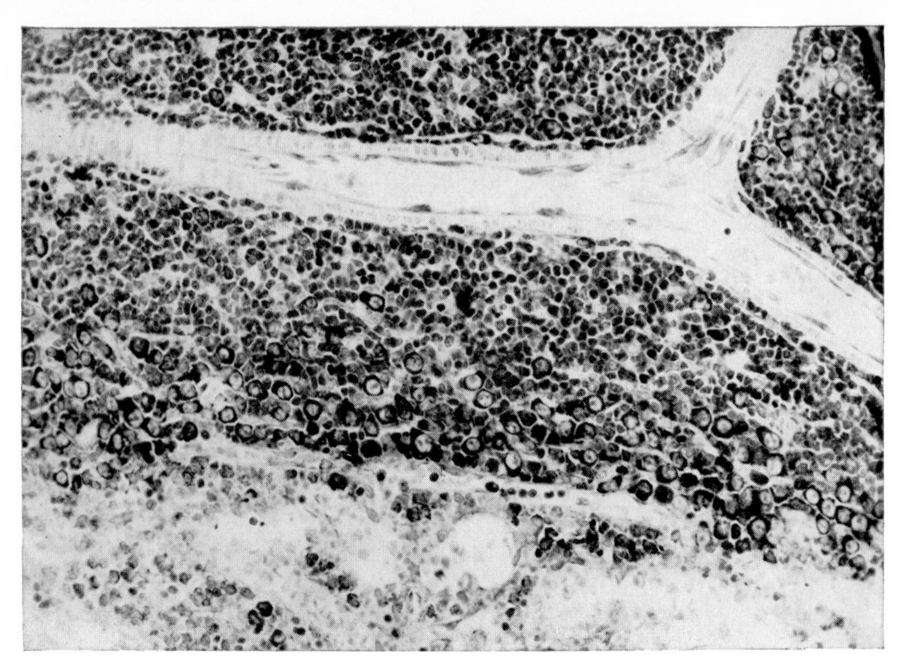

Fig. 5-3. Rabbit spleen three and one-half days after immunization with horse γ-globulin. "Plasmablasts" and "immature plasma cells" are present in peripheral zone of the periarteriolar sheath on the border of red pulp. (×475 before 30% reduction.) (From Langevoort [45], courtesy *Lab. Invest.*)

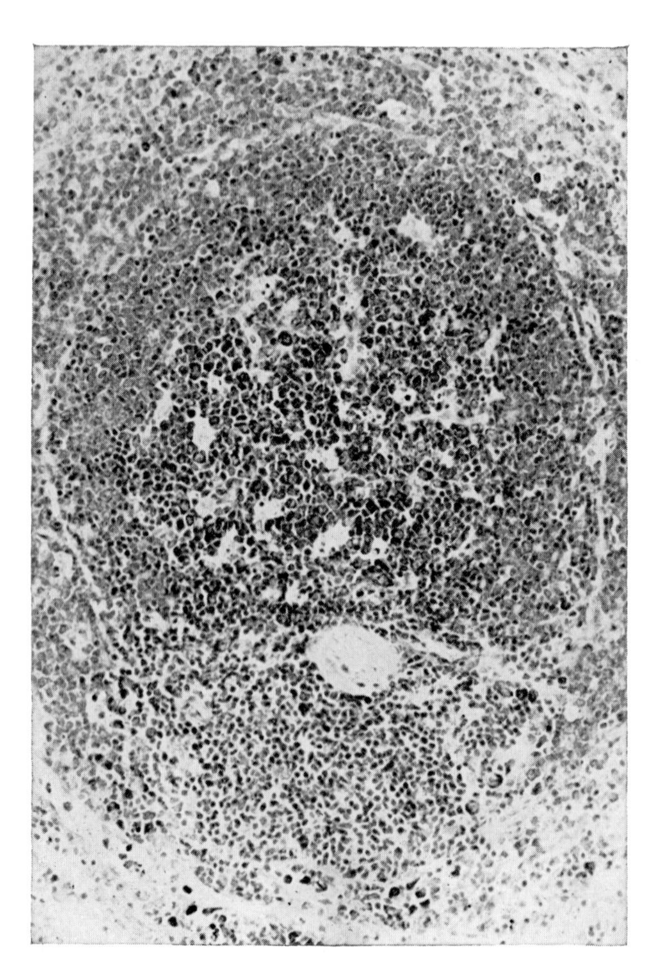

Fig. 5-4. Rabbit spleen seven days after immunization with horse γ-globulin. Follicular center is enlarged and highly active. Numerous medium-sized lymphocytes and *tingibele Körper* are present. (From Langevoort [45], courtesy *Lab. Invest.*)

lymphoid cells released from the splenic red pulp following initial synthesis of antibody may colonize both lymph node follicles and splenic follicles.

Marshall and White [51], using various antigens and schedules of intravenous immunization in the rabbit, noted similar accumulations of basophilic cells located diffusely in the red pulp but particularly in the immediate region of the arterioles of the pulp. These cells were thought to be derived from reticulum cells. Mature plasma cells became prominent only with repeated immunization. Changes in the lymphatic nodules also were noted beginning about four days after immunization. Mitoses of primitive reticular cells and a gradual increase in number of cells with basophilic cytoplasm were seen. With repeated antigen injections, the lymphatic nodules became entirely composed of medium-sized lymphocytes. Qualitatively similar results were obtained by Ward *et al.* [52] after intravenous immunization of rabbits with a single injection of bovine γ-globulin. However, changes in the lymphoid nodules were interpreted as being dominant, and only minimal red pulp change was noted. Bacterial endotoxin, a potent adjuvant, augmented the nodular reaction but did not produce any changes which were qualitatively different.

Histological studies of the spleen in the secondary response indicate a similar sequence of changes [53–55]. However, significant accumulations of "modified reticular cells" in the splenic red pulp and medulla of lymph nodes have been noted. Clusters of mature plasma cells were later observed in these locations, a finding not present in the primary response.

Similar changes have been seen in regional lymph nodes after local injection of antigens [55]. Immunohistochemical methods have demonstrated antibody-containing cells, thought to be plasma cells of varying degrees of maturity, in rather small numbers near the edges of lymphatic nodules and in the medullary cords, but few if any appear within the lymphatic nodules during the primary response [56]. After a second antigen injection, antibody-containing cells were found both within the lymphatic nodules and in the medullary cords [56] (Fig. 5-5). A high proportion of germinal center cells, which appeared to be large and medium-sized lymphocytes, showed faint fluorescence uniformly distributed throughout the cytoplasm. Many clusters of somewhat smaller cells, thought to be members of the plasma cell series in varying degrees of maturity, were found around the medial borders of the follicles and in profusion throughout the medullary cords. White [56] has suggested that the focal lymphopoiesis in regional lymph nodes is an important part of the primary response, perhaps not resulting in much production of antibody but forming the basis for a vigorous secondary response. However, under the conditions of these experiments, one cannot rule out the possibility that many of these lymphoid follicle cells have migrated there from the site of local antigen injection.

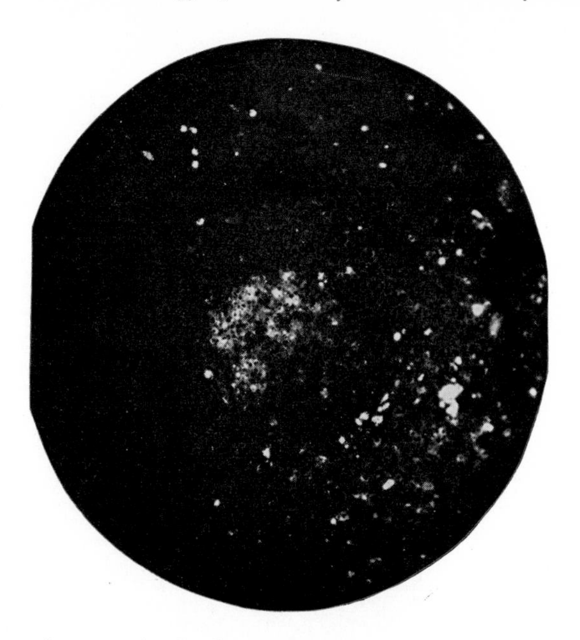

Fig. 5-5. Antibody-containing cells in lymph node. Immunohistochemical method used to demonstrate cells containing antibody in regional lymph node. Four days after second injection of alum-precipitated diphtheria toxoid. Antibody is present in the cytoplasm of a majority of the cells of a germinal center. (From White [56], in Holub and Jarošková [Eds.], *Mechanisms of Antibody Formation,* courtesy (Publishing House of Czechoslovak Academy of Sciences, Prague.)

Histological changes in the spleen of different species after immunization with heterologous erythrocytes as antigens were similar but differed in certain significant respects. We [7] described changes in the red pulp after intravenous immunization of the rat with 1 ml. of 0.25 percent sheep erythrocytes and after immunization with flagellar antigen of *Salmonella typhi* (Fig. 5-6). Large pyronino-

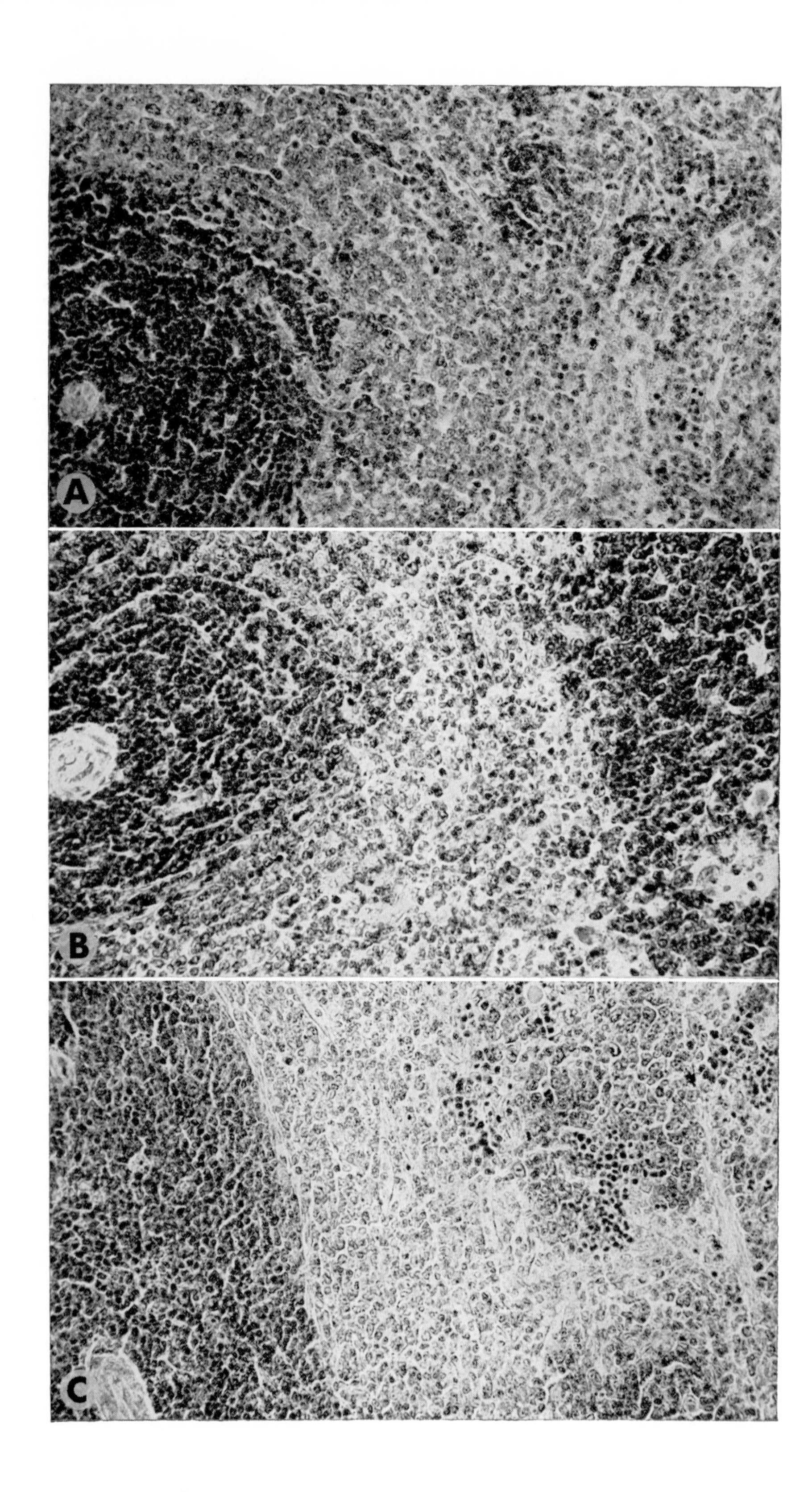
A
B
C

philic cells were first evident in the scattered areas of the red pulp two days after antigen injection. During the next two days, these cells increased in number and became somewhat smaller although the cytoplasm developed more pyroninophilia. Beginning about day 5 and continuing until about day 8, there was a transient appearance of small, dark-staining cells apparently derived from the pyroninophilic cells, which did not seem to break up but rather seemed to leave the spleen. By eight or ten days after immunization, the spleen again appeared to be essentially normal. No appreciable changes were evident in the lymphatic nodules in these circumstances. The level of circulating antibody was correlated with the red pulp changes, reaching a peak about two days after the maximal cellular response and subsiding with regression of the pyroninophilic cells.

Sussdorf [57] measured the relative quantity of splenic red and white pulp after a single intravenous immunization of the rabbit with sheep erythrocytes. There was a significant correlation between mean peak amount of white pulp and the mean hemolysin titers occurring on the days of the white pulp peaks.

Congdon and Makinodan [58] studied the mouse spleen after a single intravenous injection of 1 ml. of 10 percent or 1 percent sheep erythrocytes, both massive antigen doses. Newly formed large cells with basophilic and pyroninophilic cytoplasm were found throughout the white pulp twenty-four hours after immunization, and mitotic figures were numerous. By the fourth day, germinal centers were again evident in the now quite enlarged lymphatic nodules, and large numbers of pyroninophilic cells were seen in the red pulp. From the time these cells appeared in the red pulp there was an increasing amount of serum antibody. It is of interest that although serum antibody levels remained elevated for six weeks, the spleen weight had returned nearly to normal within seven days. White pulp and germinal centers were somewhat hyperplastic, but the large pyroninophilic cells were gone from the red pulp by seven days. Plasma cell collections in the red pulp were somewhat more numerous than in the spleens of normal, nonimmunized mice.

TYPES OF IMMUNOGLOBULINS FORMED DURING THE ANTIBODY RESPONSE

In the past decade there has been increasing awareness of the heterogeneity of antibody molecules found after immunization [59–63]. The time at which the different molecular types of immunoglobulins appear in the serum varies greatly. For example, large molecular weight (19S) antibody appears a few days after immunization, rapidly reaches a peak, and promptly falls (Fig. 5-7). Smaller molecular weight (7S) antibody first appears in the circulation somewhat later, increases more gradually and remains elevated for rather long periods. Formation of this latter kind of antibody apparently "prepares" the animal for an anamnestic response characterized by accelerated and augmented production of this type of antibody; production of 19S antibody apparently does not "prepare" the antibody-forming system for an anamnestic response.

Any attempt to correlate histological changes with formation of humoral antibody must consider the various molecular kinds of antibody formed. This important aspect of the study of cellular changes after antigenic stimulation is almost completely unexplored.

OTHER FACTORS WHICH AFFECT INTERPRETATION OF THE HISTOLOGICAL RESPONSE

A difference between animal species may cause difficulty in interpreting the cellular

Fig. 5-6. Rat spleen (edge of follicle, marginal zone, and red pulp) at different intervals after intravenous immunization with a flagellar preparation of *Salmonella typhi*. With this dose of antigen, most of the changes are in the red pulp, with little apparent alteration in the white pulp. (*A*) Normal rat: note relative emptiness of the red pulp. (*B*) Four days after immunization: numerous large pyroninophilic cells are present in red pulp. The lymphoid follicle is not significantly different from that of a normal rat. (*C*) Six days after immunization: small cells with dark nuclei are present in red pulp areas among larger pyroninophilic cells. The large pyroninophilic cells apparently transform into the smaller cells, which are identical with lymphocytes where conventional morphological techniques are used. (From Wissler *et al.* [7] courtesy *Ann. N.Y. Acad. Sci.*)

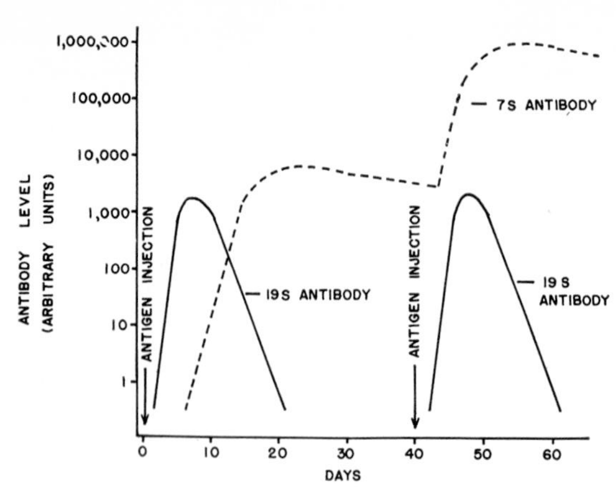

Fig. 5-7. Antibody activity in 19S and 7S immunoglobulins in the primary and secondary immune response. This idealized diagram is based mainly on data of Uhr and Finkelstein [61] and Bauer *et al.* [60]. The general pattern of 19S and 7S antibody response is basically similar after immunization with several antigens. However, with some antigens, such as *Salmonella* O antigen, only 19S antibody is formed in both primary and secondary immune responses.

mechanism of antibody formation. For example, the rat is a rather poor producer of precipitating antibody and develops delayed hypersensitivity less readily than other species [64]. The spleen may in certain circumstances form virtually all the circulating antibody in the rat after intravenous injection of foreign erythrocytes [65], whereas in the rabbit only the early portion of the antibody response to this antigen is the result of splenic production [66]. Such differences make it difficult to compare histological changes in various species after immunization with different antigens.

The ability to relate the cellular reaction to a well-defined time of antigenic stimulation is important in interpreting a cellular response to antigenic stimulation. This is very difficult with living, proliferating agents (bacteria, viruses, tumor cells, etc.). It also may be a serious problem with soluble antigens since such materials may remain in the circulation for long periods and be responsible for antigenic stimulation over a period of days. However, some *in vitro* studies suggest that maximal stimulation with soluble antigens occurs quite rapidly, at least in the secondary response [67].

The varying role played by the spleen after intravenous immunization is another factor which may help to explain the apparent discrepancy between cellular change and antibody level [68]. Intact rats immunized with small doses of *Salmonella* flagella have an early rise in agglutinin levels which reach a peak 6 days after immunization. There is then an abrupt fall lasting several days, followed by a gradual rise in titer to levels frequently exceeding the early peak 4 weeks after antigen injection. Splenectomy immediately after antigen injection prevents antibody formation. Splenectomy up to 8 days after immunization apparently terminates the immune response, indicating that the spleen forms all of the antibody during this early period. However, splenectomy at intervals of 14 days or longer after antigen injection has little effect on the antibody response, and antibody titers remain at presplenectomy levels for several weeks. These findings suggest that immunologically active cells migrate from the spleen during the period of early antibody response and that nonsplenic sites colonized by these cells function in later phases. This interpretation is supported by identification of these cells in the peripheral blood by means of bacterial adherence to specific lymphoid cells [48].

Other investigators have also found immunologically active cells in the circulation. Cells which appear to be medium-sized lymphocytes containing antibody as demonstrated by the immunofluorescent method have been found by Vasquez [69] in the peripheral blood and thoracic duct lymph. Braunsteiner and Pakesch [47] found considerable numbers of cells with prominent ergastoplasm in the thoracic duct, and fewer in the blood of rabbits immunized with typhoid vaccine. Thus it is now clear that antibody-containing (and probably antibody-forming) cells are present in the circulation, at least for brief periods and at specific intervals after antigenic stimulation.

RELATION OF HISTOLOGICAL CHANGES TO HUMORAL ANTIBODY FORMATION

Perhaps the histological changes of the spleen after antigenic stimulation can best be interpreted in the following way: The prominent large cells observed in the red pulp during the first few days after primary immunization and associated with the early appearance of antibody appear to be correlated with the formation of 19S immunoglobulin. These cells lose cytoplasm rapidly as the 19S antibody level increases. Many of them apparently are released directly into the blood stream from the spleen and probably colonize other lymphoid tissues as well as return to the lymphatic nodules of the spleen [50a]. A few may remain in the red pulp as mature plasma cells. Similar cells appear in the medial borders of lymphoid follicles of regional lymph nodes after local antigen injection. These cells migrate into medullary cords and multiply and differentiate. Many are released into efferent lymph.

About the time the splenic red pulp and lymph node medullary reaction is subsiding, changes in the lymphoid follicles become prominent. Indeed, it has been suggested that all "secondary nodules" in lymphoid tissue are the result of antigenic stimulation, since they are not found in neonatal animals [70] and are much less well developed in germ-free animals [71]. Continued division and maturation of these disseminated cells may account for the long-continued production of 7S antibody seen after primary immunization. These numerous, widely disseminated cells probably are able to respond rapidly to a second injection of antigen.

If these interpretations are correct, it may be possible to account for the above-described differences in splenic histological response in various species after immunization with sheep erythrocytes on the basis of types of immunoglobulin molecules formed. Detailed studies of immunoglobulin molecular types after immunization with erythrocytes have not been carried out, but reasonable estimates of the contribution of the different molecular types can be made. The high molecular weight antibody has a short biological half-life ranging from about 1 day in the guinea pig [61] to about 3 days in the rabbit [72]. On the other hand, the smaller, 7S antibody has a half-life of about 5.5 days in several species [61, 72, 73]. Hence the rise to peak titer several days after immunization followed by the rapid decline in total antibody titer is almost certainly due to a brief production of 19S antibody with rather abrupt cessation of antibody formation after a few days. The persisting antibody titer after the early peak is apparently almost all 7S antibody.

It seems likely that the antibody formed by the rat after intravenous immunization with small amounts of sheep erythrocytes is mostly 19S antibody [65]. Certainly the rate of antibody decline after the initial peak is compatible with this hypothesis. In the guinea pig, this pattern of antibody response has been associated with formation of only 19S antibody. In the histological response of the rat spleen after immunization with sheep erythrocytes, proliferation of large pyroninophilic cells in the red pulp predominates, and germinal center changes are minimal.

The mouse probably produces both 19S and 7S immunoglobulins under the immunizing conditions employed by Congdon and Makinodan. The pattern of antibody titer is similar to that seen in other situations where both of these immunoglobulin molecular types are formed [59–61]. Proliferation of large pyroninophilic cells in the red pulp was prominent early, but germinal center changes were rather marked and were quite striking in the secondary response.

It is interesting to speculate about the origin of the proliferating cells seen in the centers of lymphatic nodules during the primary response. These cells may be derived directly from the previously pyroninophilic splenic red pulp cells thought to enter the blood stream directly. Alternatively, they may be derived from cells that have obtained "immunological information" by incorporating nucleoprotein from the previously pyroninophilic splenic red pulp cells broken down and ingested in the germinal centers [74, 75]. In contrast to the lack of nuclear debris in the red pulp areas where the small dark cells are found, abundant fragmented nuclear material is found in the germinal centers at a time the previously pyroninophilic splenic red pulp cells might be expected to find their way to these centers. Future investigations will have to clarify the cellular relationships in this important portion of the cytological response to antigenic stimulation. It is of interest, however, that the lymphocytes (excluding only the large lymphocytes) of thoracic duct lymph appear selectively to colonize the germinal centers of lymphoid tissue and to be able to transform directly into pyroninophilic, immunologically competent cells [76, 77].

A variety of evidence has been presented concerning cell types responsible for formation of the different immunoglobulins. Studies by Burtin [78] were inconclusive. The 19S globulin-containing cells in patients with macroglobulinemia [79–82] and dysgammaglobulinemia [83] and cells containing rheumatoid factor [84] have been described as immature plasma cells, large and medium-sized lymphocytes, lymphocytoid cells, or cells resembling the transitional cells of Fagraeus. It seems likely that cells of this type are also responsible for formation of 19S immunoglobulins. Smith [85] reported that lymph nodes from an infant stimulated with typhoid vaccine contained *neither plasma cells nor plasma cell precursors;* abundant lymphocytes were present, but he observed no secondary follicle formation. This infant formed only 19S antibodies after immunization. Craig [86] described similar transitional cells in rabbits immunized with typhoid vaccine, and undoubtedly he also measured only 19S antibody.

Recently, direct evidence has been presented concerning the type of immunoglobulin contained in or released by lymphoid cells. Mellors and Korngold [86a], using fluorescence immunohistochemistry on human tissues, found all three types of immunoglobulin (γ_2, γ_{1A}, and γ_{1M}) in immature lymphoid cells in germinal centers as well as in plasma cells in medullary cords. Most cells contained only one type of immunoglobulin, although two globulin types were identified occasionally in the same plasma cell or germinal center lymphoid cell. There was no correlation between kind of cell and type of immunoglobulin which it contained. Nossal *et al.* [86b] obtained evidence that rat lymph node cells usually produced either 19S or 7S antibody but that some cells apparently produced both types. There was no correlation between type of immunoglobulin formed and degree of cellular maturity.

Immature and mature plasma cells clearly contain 7S globulin [87]. It is not known whether or not the immature lymphocyte series and the plasma cell series are distinct. Thoracic duct lymph cells appear to be able to form all of these immunoglobulins *in vitro* [88]. Biochemical data suggest that several forms of immunoglobulins can be found in the various lymphoid organs but that the synthetic rate for each globulin is different [89].

It has not yet been possible to determine with certainty the derivation of the pyroninophilic cells seen in the primary immune response in the splenic red pulp and medullary portion of the lymph nodes, some of which at least are identical with the antibody-containing cells identified with the immunohistochemical technique. Their origin has been traced to reticular cells by some investigators [5, 23, 51] and to lymphocytes by others [45] (Fig. 5-8). Considerable evidence based on both tissue culture and conventional morphological techniques indicates the multipotentiality of mesenchymal reticular cells [90]. There is less agreement concerning the developmental potential of the lymphocyte [91]. Although the large lymphocyte in the embryo may be capable of developing into granulocyte and erythrocyte precursors [92], this potential does not seem to exist in the normal adult animal [93]. Many have considered the small lympho-

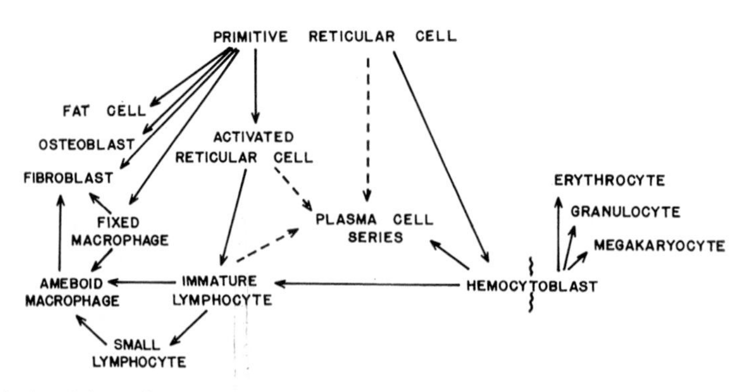

Fig. 5-8. Interrelationships of mesenchymal cells. *Solid arrows* indicate transformation about which there is general agreement; *broken arrows* indicate suggested transformations. In the adult animal, there are probably separate myeloid and lymphoid hemocytoblastic stem cells, both of which may be derived from primitive mesenchymal cells. The primary immune response is associated principally with proliferation of large pyroninophilic cells which are difficult to characterize by conventional histological methods. Most of them transform into cells morphologically indistinguishable from lymphocytes. Plasma cell proliferation is characteristic of the secondary immune response and is probably associated with production of 7S antibody.

cyte to be an "end stage" cell which has no mitotic potential. Separation of the lymphocyte cell series into three categories, large, medium, and small, is entirely arbitrary. Sainte-Marie and Leblond [94] described a developmental pattern for lymphocytes in the thymus in which a large lymphocyte as a result of eight divisions gives rise to 128 small lymphocytes. The first of these divisions is asymmetrical and all are accompanied by a decrease in cell size. Only the last generation of small lymphocytes seems to lack mitotic capabilities. Gowans *et al.* [76, 95] have clearly shown the immunological competence of cells from thoracic duct lymph. These cells, which apparently transform directly into larger pyroninophilic cells, have morphological characteristics of the smaller lymphocytes. It has not been determined, however, that these cells are in fact true lymphocytes. They may be identical with the immature plasma cells described by Braunsteiner in the thoracic duct lymph [47]. These two kinds of cells (if they really are different) cannot be separated by conventional histological methods [96]. In the future, refined techniques may permit positive identification of, and an improved terminology for, these immunological competent cells (Fig. 5-9).

Attempts to determine the origin of antibody-forming cells have included investigations of plasma cell development. Plasma cells have rather distinctive morphological characteristics best seen with electron microscopy [97]. These include abundant endoplasmic reticulum, highly developed centrospheres, and large mitochondria. Development of the plasma cell series has been traced to a fixed stem reticular cell which gives rise to free stem cells that have been known by various names [97, 98]. It must be noted, however, that these first stages in differentiation appear to be the same for all blood cells. A free stem cell destined to become a lymphocyte cannot be distinguished from one evolving toward a plasma cell. However, as the immature cells acquire denser cytoplasm containing rough-surfaced endoplasmic reticulum and a prominent Golgi zone, plasma cell differentiation is evident. The ultrastructure of the more mature elements of the plasma cell series resembles that of cells of protein-secreting glands such as the exocrine pancreas and is the morphological basis for assuming that its function is primarily that of producing and releasing protein. Indeed, specific antibodies have been shown recently within the lumina of the endoplasmic reticulum of plasma cells [99] (Fig. 5-10).

There is additional evidence concerning the cytogenesis of antibody-forming plasma cells found during the secondary response. In an elegant series of experiments, Nossal and Mäkelä [100] used tritium-labeled thymidine to mark cells capable of DNA synthesis. Rats previously immunized with *Salmonella* flagella were given a single injection of tritium-labeled thymidine. Two hours after the tracer injection, smears prepared from the regional lymph node demonstrated that 82 percent of the large lymphocytes and "plasmablasts" were labeled, as were 13 percent of medium lymphocytes. A second injection of antigen was then

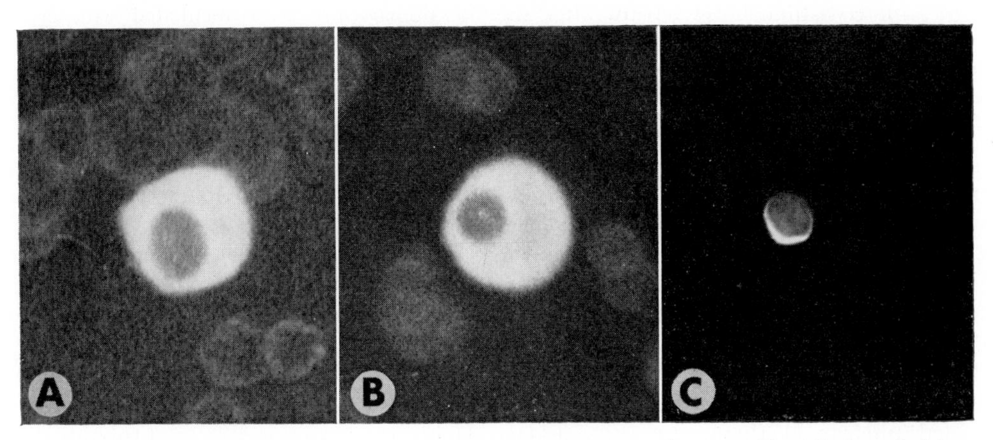

Fig. 5-9. Antibody-containing cells. (*A*) Pre-plasma cells; (*B*) plasma cell; (*C*) lymphokinetocyte. Immunohistochemical demonstration of antibody-containing cells in a brush-smear preparation of lymph node from rabbit hyperimmunized with bovine serum albumin. (*A, B* from J. J. Vasquez, courtesy *Lab. Invest.;* *C* from Vasquez, personal communication.)

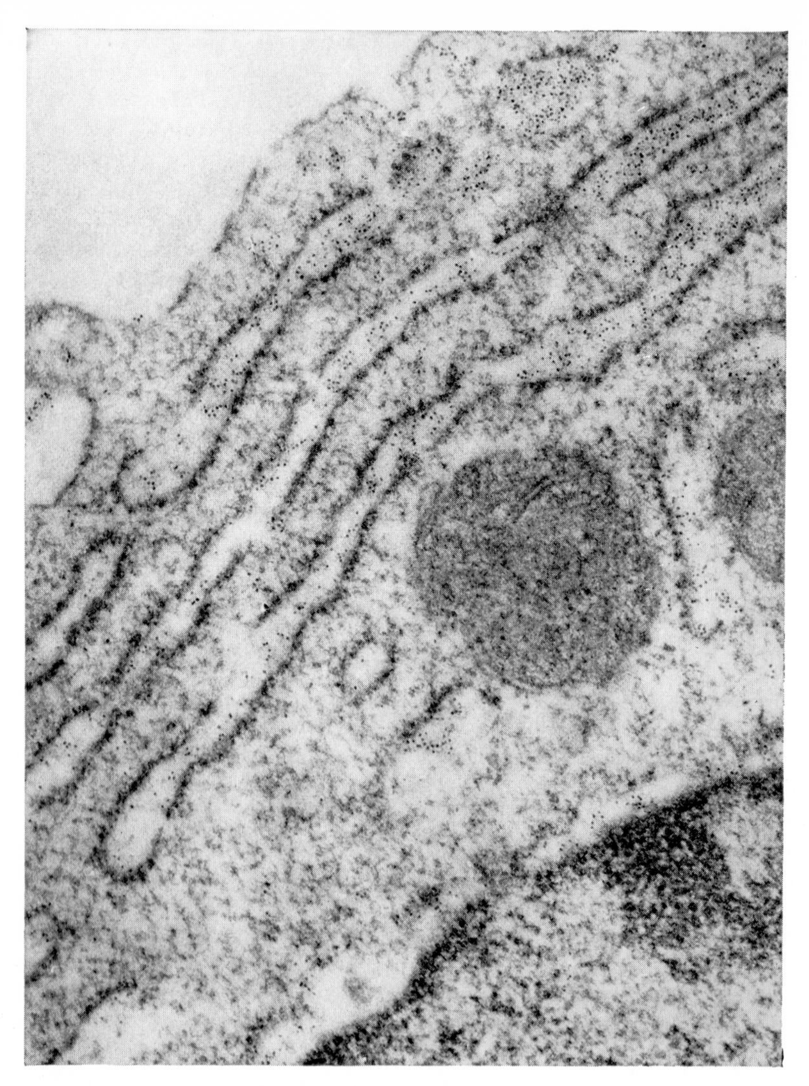

Fig. 5-10. Antibody with plasma cell. Isolated lymph node cells from an adult rabbit hyperimmunized with crystalline horse ferritin after suitable preparations were incubated with crystalline horse ferritin and sectioned for electron microscopy. Dense granules of ferritin are evident in the cisternae of the endoplasmic reticulum and in the perinuclear space. The nucleus is in the lower right corner. A detailed report of these studies was made by de Petris *et al.* [99]. (×90,000 before 30% reduction.) (Courtesy Dr. Benvenuto Pernis.)

given and animals were killed at intervals. Nearly 100 percent of the immature and mature "plasma cells" formed within the five or six days after infection were labeled. In contrast, during this same interval a maximum of 35 percent of the mature plasma cells were labeled in resting, previously stimulated rats, although nearly all immature plasma cells contained nuclear H^3-thymidine (Fig. 5-11). More striking, however, was the approximate doubling of the absolute number of labeled plasma cells in the secondarily stimulated animals. The number of labeled lymphocytes increased about 50 percent.

Thus there is a great increase in numbers of both plasma cells and lymphocytes in response to the second antigenic stimulation. Most of these newly formed cells were derived from cells which had been labeled with tritium-thymidine *before* the second antigen injection. Hence the plasma cells were probably descendants of either large or medium lymphocytes. Possible origin from fixed primitive reticular cells has not been excluded, since such cells

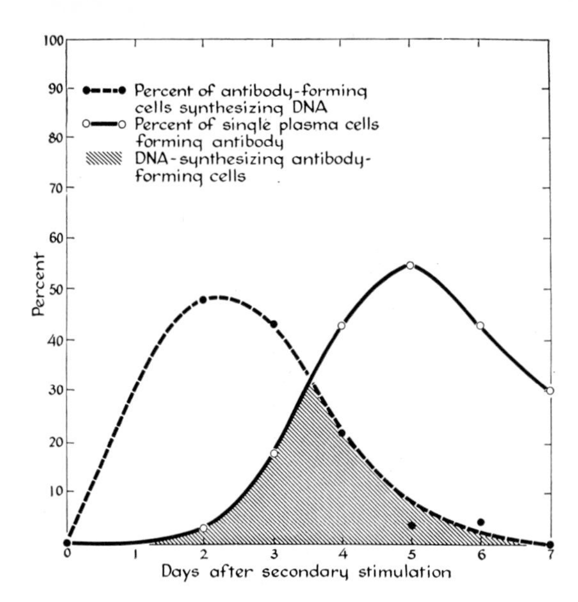

Fig. 5-11. DNA synthesis among antibody-forming cells. Most of the proliferation of potential antibody-producing cells precedes active antibody formation. (From Nossal, courtesy *Stanford Med. Bull.* 20:32, 1962.)

are not found intact in smears. This evidence suggests that immunological memory which results in the more rapid and extensive antibody formation seen in the secondary response depends on the persistence, following primary stimulation, of a continuously dividing stem line of lymphocytes reactive to further antigenic stimulation.

Mitosis and differentiation are integral parts of the primary immune response. On the other hand, the importance of mitosis in the secondary response has been questioned in the past. Earlier experiments suggested that lymph node or peritoneal exudate cells from secondarily stimulated animals might transform directly into antibody-forming plasma cells when transferred to x-ray-irradiated recipients [101, 102]. Recent studies, however, indicate that antibody-containing cells in transfer sites were possibly derived from those transferred cells capable of division, mainly large and medium lymphoid cells, although such cells constituted only a small proportion of the ones transferred [103, 103a].

Nearly all antibody-containing or -releasing cells formed after secondary stimulation are newly formed cells arising from division of a precursor sometime after antigen stimulation [104, 105]. The less mature antibody-containing cells are also able to divide (Fig. 5-12). However, the mature antibody-containing plasma cell does not appear to be capable of division, and studies with H^3-cytidine and H^3-leucine indicate that it has little if any RNA-synthesizing or protein-synthesizing ability [106]. The antibody which it does contain is presumably the remnant of that formed during its less mature stage.

The rate of division, of both lymphocytes and plasma cell precursors, is strikingly increased by secondary antigenic stimulation. Doubling time during the peak of mitotic activity is decreased from 24 to 12 hours [69, 105]. Accompanying this almost explosive production of cells, there is continuing transformation of some of them from immature forms into plasma cells. Makinodan and Albright [107] consider this differentiation process "suicidal" since the end cells of the five to seven somatic divisions of the secondary response are apparently nondividing and rather short-lived. Available evidence indicates that plasma cell formation does not explain the persistence of immunological memory, and it appears that

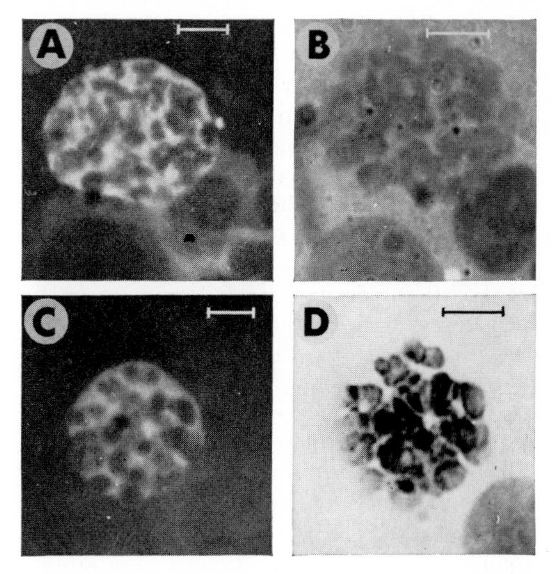

Fig. 5-12. Antibody-containing cells in mitosis. Lymph node cells from rabbit secondarily stimulated with bovine serum albumin. Cells have been cultured in diffusion chambers placed intraperitoneally in irradiated rabbits. Mitosis has been blocked with colchicine. Immunohistochemical technique demonstrates antibody (*A* and *C*). Chromosomes do not react in this method but do stain with methyl green (*B* and *D*). Scale marker, 5μ. (From Urso and Makinodan [105], courtesy *J. Immun.*)

the lymphocyte is more likely to carry immunological messages to future antibody-forming cells.

To account for the greater number of specifically responsive cells, it seems necessary to postulate either the asymmetrical somatic division of potentially competent cells or symmetrical somatic division and the existence of nonchromosomal autoregulating units. A provocative theoretical discussion of these aspects has been given by Talmage and Claman [108]. This problem of control of cell division and maturation is not unique to immunology. There are similar difficulties in interpreting erythropoiesis and granulopoiesis with transformation and differentiation of stem cells and eventual formation of erythrocytes [109–111] and granulocytes.

Various means have been used to suppress antibody formation. Some of these studies are helpful in interpreting the histological reactions of the immune response. Total body exposure to ionizing radiation before immunization results in severe impairment of antibody formation [112]. There appears to be little if any alteration of antigen fixation, but the cellular proliferation usually seen after antigen injection is suppressed [49]. The effect of total body irradiation after antigen injection appears to be different in various species of animals. Greater impairment of the immune response was noted in the rat [113, 114] and mouse [115] than in the rabbit [42, 116].

Suppression of the pyroninophilic cellular reaction in the splenic red pulp was correlated with impaired antibody formation in the rat given radiation up to four days after antigen injection [114]. In the rabbit, however, there is relatively slight impairment of the immune response if x-ray irradiation is done simultaneously with or shortly after antigen injection [116]. Proliferative changes such as those described by Langevoort were noted by Kuening *et al.* [116] in the spleen of rabbits immunized immediately before irradiation; antibody was formed even though the splenic lymphoid tissue showed the characteristic pattern of radiation damage. In none of these studies has the relative contribution of the different immunoglobulin molecular types to the total antibody level been determined.

It is possible that total body irradiation may adversely influence antibody formation by cells through several different mechanisms. The marked suppression of antibody response noted when antigen administration follows irradiation almost certainly is the result of damage to a vital portion of the inductive process. The less severe depression of antibody formation by irradiation after immunization is in all likelihood due to inhibition of mitosis of the antibody-forming cells.

Antimetabolites of various kinds have been used to interfere with antibody formation. Actinomycin administered to animals for several days after antigen injection greatly reduced the number of antibody-producing cells [117]. Addition of actinomycin to antibody-forming cells *in vitro* did not reduce the number of antibody-forming cells in short-term experiments [117]. Similar results have been obtained with chloramphenicol [118, 118a]. The presence of chloramphenicol during the first few days of incubation markedly suppressed antibody formation; or, if added after production was under way, little effect was noted. Actinomycin and chloramphenicol are thought to interfere with formation of messenger RNA. The results described above suggest that messenger RNA, once formed by antibody-forming cells, is effective during the periods in which antibody production has been studied even though its further formation is inhibited.

Protein depletion and administration of amino acid antagonists also suppress antibody production [119] and the related histological reaction [120, 121]. The mechanism of these types of inhibition is undoubtedly complex. Hibernation inhibits antibody formation, but some of the events of the induction period apparently occur during hibernation since the induction period after arousal is shorter than that found in nonhibernating animals [122]. Cold-blooded vertebrates apparently form antibody only when maintained at about room temperature: cooling of the animal terminates antibody production. It is of interest, however, that induction of the potential to form antibody can be acquired in the cold [123]. Only the production of antibody and concomitant release into the circulation appear to be temperature-dependent.

As mentioned before, formation of 19S antibody does not appear to prepare the animal for the secondary response, and repeated injections of a small quantity of bacteriophage ΦX174 or *Salmonella* O antigen result in production of similar amounts of 19S antibody after each injection. In this instance, there appears to be stimulation of the antibody-forming cells but with no formation of "immunological memory cells." On the other hand, as animals emerge spontaneously from the tolerant state, one may find enhanced immunological reactivity and in some instances spontaneous immunity with production of "highly avid," probably 7S, antibody [124, 125]. In this situation, apparently, immunological memory cells are produced, but antibody-producing (or -releasing) cells are not present.

If there are two functionally distinct cells, as postulated above, they may be also morphologically distinct and comprise separate cell lines. It is also possible that such functionally distinct cells may represent different developmental stages of the same cell line. Sercarz and Coons [126] have postulated the two-stage development of antibody-forming cells: The primary antigen contact would result in the priming of cells resulting in a state of readiness to produce antibody; a second antigen contact would then result in antibody formation by the cells for a finite time, followed by their exhaustion. The second antigen contact could also prime additional cells which by this time have reached the necessary stage of development. These suggestions would explain many aspects of the 7S immunoglobulin response. A somewhat similar sequence of cellular change has been suggested previously [7] (Fig. 5-13).

Obviously, there are great gaps in knowledge concerning the histological changes seen in the immune response. Both lymphocytes and plasma cells participate in the antigen-induced proliferation and maturation of cells. The histological reaction associated with 19S immunoglobulin response is associated with the formation of large basophilic, pyroninophilic lymphoid cells (transitional cells, anti-

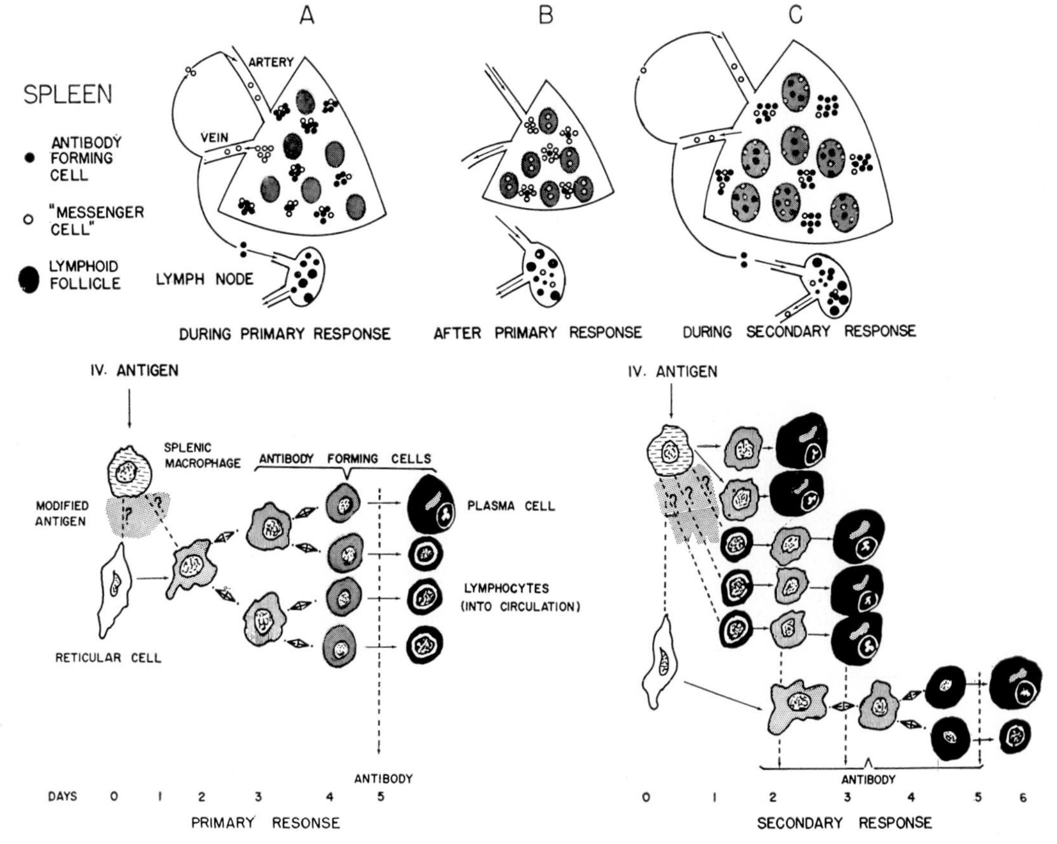

Fig. 5-13. Proposed cellular patterns during "primary" (*A*) and "secondary" (*C*) immune response following intravenous injection of particulate antigen. The "secondary" response pattern may follow the "primary" response pattern after a single injection of some antigens and be responsible for 7S antibody formation. The "primary" response pattern appears to be associated with production of 19S antibody. (From Wissler *et al.* [7], courtesy *Ann. N.Y. Acad. Sci.*)

body forming cells) which do not seem to transform into mature plasma cells. The 7S antibody response appears to be associated with proliferation of lymphocytes and the appearance of many mature plasma cells. Factors controlling proliferation and differentiation of antibody-forming lymphoid cells are largely unknown, as is true for most other constantly developing cell systems. Deciphering the regulatory mechanism of the cellular changes in the immune response may furnish the key for understanding other significant biological processes. Further study of antibody formation may also add considerable knowledge regarding stimulation and regulation of protein synthesis by mammalian cell systems.

REFERENCES

1. Taliaferro, W. H. The cellular basis of immunity. *Ann. Rev. Microbiol.* 3:159, 1949.
2. McMaster, P. D. Sites of Antibody Formation. In *The Nature and Significance of the Antibody Response.* Pappenheimer, A. M., Jr. (Ed.). New York: Columbia University Press, 1953.
3. Good, R. A. Morphological Basis of the Immune Response and Hypersensitivity. In *Host-Parasite Relationships in Living Cells.* Felton, H. M. (Ed.). Springfield, Ill.: Charles C Thomas, Publisher, 1957.
4. Harris, T. N., and Harris, S. The genesis of antibodies. *Amer. J. Med.* 20:114, 1956.
5. Wissler, R. W., Fitch, F. W., LaVia, M. F., and Gunderson, C. H. The cellular basis for antibody formation. *J. Cell. Comp. Physiol.* 50 (supp. 1):265, 1957.
6. Coons, A. H. The cytology of antibody formation. *J. Cell. Comp. Physiol.* 52(supp. 1):55, 1958.
7. Wissler, R. W., Fitch, F. W., and LaVia, M. F. The reticuloendothelial system in antibody formation. *Ann. N.Y. Acad. Sci.* 88:134, 1960.
8. McMaster, P. D. Antibody Formation. In *The Cell.* Brachet, J., and Mirsky, A. E. (Eds.). New York: Academic Press, Inc., 1961. Vol. 5.
9. Nossal, G. J. V. Genetic control of lymphopoiesis, plasma cell formation, and antibody production. *Int. Rev. Exp. Path.* 1:1, 1962.
10. Nossal, G. J. V. Cellular genetics of immune responses. *Advances Immun.* 2:163, 1962.
11. Sabesin, S. M. A function of the eosinophil: Phagocytosis of antigen-antibody complexes. *Proc. Soc. Exp. Biol. Med.* 112:667, 1963.
12. Cohen, S. G., Sapp, T. M., and Gallia, A. R. Experimental eosinophilia: V. Specificity of regional lymph node responses to antigen-antibody systems. *Proc. Soc. Exp. Biol. Med.* 113:29, 1963.
13. Speirs, R. S. Advances in the knowledge of the eosinophil in relation to antibody formation. *Ann. N.Y. Acad. Sci.* 73:283, 1958.
14. Pfeiffer, R., and Marx, Z. Die Bildungsstätte der Choleraschutzstoffe. Z. *Hyg. Infektionskra.* 27:272, 1898.
15. Metchnikoff, E. *Immunity in Infective Diseases* (tr. by F. G. Binnie), London: Cambridge University Press, 1905.
16. Sabin, F. R. Cellular reactions to a dye-protein with a concept of the mechanism of antibody formation. *J. Exp. Med.* 70:67, 1939.
17. Hartley, G. The local formation of antivaccinial antibodies by the skin. *J. Infect. Dis.* 66:44, 1940.
18. McMaster, P. D., and Hudack, S. S. The formation of agglutinins within lymph nodes. *J. Exp. Med.* 61:783, 1935.
19. Ehrich, W. E., and Harris, T. N. The formation of antibodies in the popliteal lymph node in rabbits. *J. Exp. Med.* 76:335, 1942.
20. Dougherty, T. F., Chase, J. H., and White, A. The demonstration of antibodies in lymphocytes. *Proc. Soc. Exp. Biol. Med.* 57:295, 1944.
21. Dougherty, T. F., Chase, J. H., and White, A. Pituitary-adrenal cortical control of antibody release from lymphocytes: An explanation of the anamnestic response. *Proc. Soc. Exp. Biol. Med.* 58:135, 1945.
22. Bjørneboe, M., and Gormsen, H. Experimental studies on the role of plasma cells as antibody producers. *Acta Path. Microbiol. Scand.* 20:649, 1944.
23. Fagraeus, A. Antibody production in relation to the development of plasma cells. *Acta Med. Scand.* 130(supp. 204):3, 1948.
24. Reiss, E., Mertens, E., and Ehrich, W. E. Agglutination of bacteria by lymphoid cells in vitro. *Proc. Soc. Exp. Biol. Med.* 74:732, 1950.
25. Moeschlin, S., and Demiral, B. Antikörperbildung der Plasmazellen *in vitro. Klin. Wschr.* 30:827, 1952.
26. Hayes, S. P., and Dougherty, T. F. Studies on local antibody production: Demonstration of agglutination by lymphocytes. *J. Immun.* 73: 95, 1954.
27. Mäkelä, O., and Nossal, G. J. V. Bacterial adherence: A method for detecting antibody production by single cells. *J. Immun.* 87:447, 1961.

27a. Nossal, G. J. V. Antibody production by single cells: III The histology of antibody production. *Brit. J. Exp. Path.* 40:25, 1959.

27b. Attardi, G., Cohn, M., Horibata, K., and

Lennox, E. S. Antibody formation by rabbit lymph node cells: IV. The detailed methods for measuring antibody synthesis by individual cells, the kinetics of antibody formation by rabbits, and the properties of cell suspensions. *J. Immun.* 92:372, 1964.

28. Coons, A. H. Histochemistry with labeled antibody. *Int. Rev. Cytol.* 5:1, 1956.
29. Hughes, W. L., Bond, V. P., Brecher, G., Cronkite, E. P., Painter, R. B., Quastler, H., and Sherman, F. G. Cellular proliferation in the mouse as revealed by autoradiography with tritiated thymidine. *Proc. Nat. Acad. Sci. U.S.A.* 44:476, 1958.

29a. Jerne, N. K., and Nordin, A. A. Plaque formation in agar by single antibody producing cells. *Science* 140:405, 1963.

29b. Attardi, G., Cohn, M., Horibata, K., and Lennox, E. S. Antibody formation by rabbit lymph node cells: II. Further observations on the behavior of single antibody-producing cells with respect to their synthetic capacity and morphology. *J. Immun.* 92:346, 1964.

30. Holtzer, H., and Holtzer, S. The *in vitro* uptake of fluorescein labelled plasma proteins: I. Mature cells. *C. R. Lab. Carlsberg* 31:373, 1960.
31. Thiery, J. P. Microcinematographic Contributions to the Study of Plasma Cells. In Wolstenholme, G. E., and O'Connor, M. (Eds.), *Cellular Aspects of Immunity.* Boston: Little, Brown, 1960.
32. Coons, A. H., Leduc, E. H., and Kaplan, M. H. Localization of antigen in tissue cells: VI. The fate of injected foreign proteins in the mouse. *J. Exp. Med.* 93:173, 1951.

32a. Wellensiek, H., and Coons, A. H. Studies on antibody production: IX. The cellular localization of antigen molecules (ferritin) in the secondary response. *J. Exp. Med.* 119:685, 1964.

33. Tranzer, J. P., Porte, A., Kempf, J., and Fruhling, L. Différenciation plasmocytaire d'éléments réticulaires après stimulation antigénique par de la ferritine hétérologue. *C. R. Acad. Sci.* (Paris) 256:823, 1963.
34. Cardinali, G., and Carrescia, P. M. Phagocytose plasmocytaire dans un cas de β-plasmocytome. *Sang* 27:682, 1956.
35. Richter, G. W. Electron microscopy: Proteins in experimental pathology. *Science* 141:834, 1963.
36. Fishman, M. Antibody formation *in vitro. J. Exp. Med.* 114:837, 1961.
37. Fishman, M., and Adler, F. L. Antibody formation initiated *in vitro:* II. Antibody synthesis in x-irradiated recipients of diffusion chambers containing nucleic acid derived from macrophages incubated with antigen. *J. Exp. Med.* 117:595, 1963.
38. Friedman, H. Persistence of antigen in nucleoprotein fractions of mouse spleen cells during antibody formation. *Nature* (London) 199:502, 1963.

38a. Nossal, G. J. V., Ada, G. L., and Austin, C. M. Antigens in immunity IV. Cellular localization of ^{125}J- and ^{131}J-labelled flagella in lymph nodes. *Aust. J. Exp. Biol. Med. Sci.* 42:311, 1964.

38b. Ada, G. L., Nossal, G. J. V., and Austin, C. M. Antigens in immunity V. The ability of cells in lymphoid follicles to recognize foreignness. *Ibid.,* p. 331.

39. Weigle, W. O. The Elimination of Heterologous Proteins from the Blood of Animals. In Holub, M., and Jarošková, L. (Eds.): *Mechanisms of Antibody Formation.* Prague: Publishing House of Czechoslovak Academy of Sciences; and New York: Academic Press, 1960.
40. Uhr, J. W., Finkelstein, M. S., and Baumann, J. B. Antibody formation: III. The primary and secondary antibody response to bacteriophage ΦX174 in guinea pigs. *J. Exp. Med.* 115:655, 1962.
41. Dixon, F. J., Talmage, D. W., and Mauer, P. H. Radiosensitive and radioresistant phases in the antibody response. *J. Immun.* 68:693, 1952.
42. Taliaferro, W. H., Taliaferro, L. G., and Janssen, E. F. The localization of x-ray injury to the initial phases of antibody response. *J. Infect. Dis.* 91:105, 1952.
43. Berglund, K. Studies on factors which condition the effect of cortisone on antibody production. *Acta Path. Microbiol. Scand.* 38:311, 1956.
44. Michaelides, M. C., and Coons, A. H. Studies on antibody production: V. The secondary response *in vitro. J. Exp. Med.* 117:1035, 1963.
45. Langevoort, H. L. The histophysiology of the antibody response: I. Histogenesis of the plasma cell reaction in rabbit spleen. *Lab. Invest.* 12:106, 1963.
46. Snook, T. A comparative study of the vascular arrangements in mammalian spleens. *Amer. J. Anat.* 87:31, 1950.
47. Braunsteiner, H., and Pakesch, F. Elektronenmikroskopische Untersuchungen zur Frage der Blutplasmazellen. *Wien. Z. Inn Med.* 41:58, 1960.
48. Gunderson, C. H., Juras, D., LaVia, M. F., and Wissler, R. W. Tissue and cellular changes associated with antibody formation in the rat spleen. *J. A. M. A.* 180:1038, 1962.
49. Fitch, F. W., Barker, P., Soules, K. H., and Wissler, R. W. A study of the antigen localization and degradation and the histologic reaction in the spleen of normal, x-irradiated, and spleen-shielded rats. *J. Lab. Clin. Med.* 42:598 1953.
50. LaVia, M. F., Fitch, F. W., Gunderson, C. H., and Wissler, R. W. The relation of antibody

formation to reticuloendothelial structure and function. In Heller, J. H. (Ed.), *Reticuloendothelial Structure and Function.* New York: Ronald Press Company, 1960.

50a. Cannon, D. A Study of the Cellular Migrations in the Antigenically Stimulated Rat Spleen and Other Immunological Implications. University of Chicago Ph.D. Thesis, 1964.

51. Marshall, A. H. E., and White, R. G. Reactions of the reticular tissues to antigens. *Brit. J. Exp. Path.* 31:157, 1950.
52. Ward, P. A., Johnson, A. G., and Abell, M. R. Studies on the adjuvant action of bacterial endotoxins on antibody formation: III. Histologic response of the rabbit spleen to a single injection of a purified protein antigen. *J. Exp. Med.* 109:463, 1959.
53. Ward, P. A., Johnson, A. G., and Abell, M. R. Histologic response of rabbits to two injections of purified protein antigen. *Lab. Invest.* 12:180, 1963.
54. Coons, A. H., Leduc, E. H., and Connolly, J. M. Studies on antibody production: I. A method for the histochemical demonstration of specific antibody and its application to the hyperimmune rabbit. *J. Exp. Med.* 102:49, 1955.
55. Leduc, E. H., Coons, A. H., and Connolly, J. M. Studies on antibody production: II. The primary and secondary responses in the popliteal lymph node of the rabbit. *Ibid.,* p. 61.
56. White, R. G. The Relation of the Cellular Responses in Germinal or Lymphocytopoietic Centers of Lymph Nodes to the Production of Antibody. Ref. 39.
57. Sussdorf, D. H. Quantitative changes in the white and red pulp of the spleen during hemolysin formation in x-irradiated and non-irradiated rabbits. *J. Infect. Dis.* 105:238, 1959.
58. Congdon, C. C., and Makinodan, T. Splenic white pulp alteration after antigen injection: Relation to time of serum antibody production. *Amer. J. Path.* 39:697, 1961.
59. Bauer, D. C., and Stavitsky, A. B. On the different molecular forms of antibody synthesized by rabbits during the early response to a single injection of protein and cellular antigens. *Proc. Nat. Acad. Sci. U.S.A.* 47:1667, 1961.
60. Bauer, D. C., Mathies, M. J., and Stavitsky, A. B. Sequences of synthesis of gamma$_1$-macroglobulin and gamma$_2$-globulin antibodies during primary and secondary response to proteins, *Salmonella* antigens, and phage. *J. Exp. Med.* 117:889, 1963.
61. Uhr, J. W., and Finkelstein, M. S. Antibody formation: IV. Formation of rapidly and slowly sedimenting antibodies and immunological memory to bacteriophage ΦX174. *Ibid.,* p. 457.
62. Talmage, D. W., Freter, G. G., and Taliaferro, W. H. Two antibodies of related specificity but different hemolytic efficiency separated by centrifugation. *J. Infect. Dis.* 98:300, 1956.
63. Bloch, K. J., Kourilsky, F. M., Ovary, Z., and Benacerraf, B. Properties of guinea pig 7S antibodies: III. Identification of antibodies involved in complement fixation and hemolysis. *J. Exp. Med.* 117:965, 1963.
64. Kenton, H. B. The Arthus phenomenon in the rat. *J. Infect. Dis.* 69:238, 1941.
65. Rowley, D. A. The effect of splenectomy on the formation of circulating antibody in the adult male albino rat. *J. Immun.* 64:289, 1950.
66. Taliaferro, W. H., and Taliaferro, L. G. The dynamics of hemolysin formation in intact and splenectomized rabbits. *J. Infect. Dis.* 87:37, 1950.
67. O'Brien, T. F., Michaelides, M. C., and Coons, A. H. Studies on antibody production: VI. The course, sensitivity, and histology of the secondary response *in vitro*. *J. Exp. Med.* 117:1053, 1963.
68. Fitch, F. W. Effect of splenectomy on the agglutinin response of the rat. *Fed. Proc.* 22:374, 1963.
69. Vasquez, J. J. Kinetics of Proliferation of Antibody Forming Cells. In Good, R. A., and Gabrielsen, A. E. (Eds.), *The Thymus in Immunobiology.* New York: Paul B. Hoeber, Inc., 1964.
70. Bridges, R. A., Condie, R. M., Zak, S. J., and Good, R. A. The morphologic basis of antibody formation development during the neonatal period. *J. Lab. Clin. Med.* 53:331, 1959.
71. Miyakawa, M., Iijima, S., Kobayashi, R. and Tajima, M. Observation on the lymphoid tissue of the germ-free guinea pig. *Acta Path. Jap.* 7:183, 1957.
72. Taliaferro, W. H., and Talmage, D. W. Antibodies in the rabbit with different rates of metabolic decay. *J. Infect. Dis.* 99:21, 1956.
73. Dixon, F. J., Talmage, D. W., Maurer, P. H., and Deichmiller, M. The half-life of homologous gamma-globulin (antibody) in several species. *J. Exp. Med.* 96:313, 1952.
74. Trowell, O. A. Re-utilization of lymphocytes in lymphopoiesis. *J. Biophys. Biochem. Cytol.* 3:317, 1957.
75. Hill, M. Re-utilization of lymphocyte remnants by reticular cells. *Nature* (London) 183:1059, 1959.
76. Gowans, J. L. The fate of parental strain small lymphocytes in F_1 hybrid rats. *Ann. N.Y. Acad. Sci.* 99:432, 1962.
77. Porter, K. A., and Cooper, E. H. Transformation of adult allogeneic small lymphocytes after transfusion into newborn rats. *J. Exp. Med.* 115:997, 1962.
78. Burtin, P. A Study of Serum Proteins Related to Immunity and Their Cellular Origins. Ref. 31.

79. Dutcher, T. F., and Fahey, J. L. Immunocytochemical demonstration of intranuclear localization of 18S gammamacroglobulin in macroglobulin in macroglobulinemia of Waldenström. *Proc. Soc. Exp. Biol. Med.* 103:452, 1960.
80. Kritzman, J., Kunkel, H. G., McCarthy, J., and Mellors, R. C. Studies of a Waldenström-type macroglobulin with rheumatoid factor properties. *J. Lab. Clin. Med.* 57:905, 1961.
81. Zucker-Franklin, D., Franklin, E. C., and Cooper, N. S. Production of macroglobulins *in vitro* and a study of their cellular origin. *Blood* 20:56, 1962.
82. Curtain, C. C., and O'Dea, J. F. Possible sites of macroglobulin synthesis: A study made with fluorescent antibody. *Aust. Ann. Med.* 8:143, 1959.
83. Cruchaud, A., Rosen, F. S., Craig, J. M., Janeway, C. A., and Gitlin, D. The site of synthesis of the 19S gamma-globulins in dysgammaglobulinemia. *J. Exp. Med.* 115:1141, 1962.
84. Mellors, R. C., Heimer, R., Corcos, J., and Korngold, L. Cellular origin of rheumatoid factor. *J. Exp. Med.* 110:875, 1959.
85. Smith, R. T. Response to Active Immunization of Human Infants during the Neonatal Period. Ref. 31.
86. Craig, J. M. The histology of antigenically stimulated lymph nodes in rabbits given ACTH or cortisone. *Amer. J. Path.* 28:629, 1952.
86a. Mellors, R. C., and Korngold, L. The cellular origin of human immunoglobulins (γ_2, γ_{1M}, γ_{1A}). *J. Exp. Med.* 118:387, 1963.
86b. Nossal, G. J. V., Szenberg, A., Ada, G. L., and Austin, C. M. Single cell studies on 19S antibody production. *J. Exp. Med.* 119:485, 1964.
87. Ortega, L. G., and Mellors, R. C. Cellular sites of formation of gamma globulin. *J. Exp. Med.* 106:627, 1957.
88. Asofsky, R., and Thorbecke, G. J. Sites of formation of immune globulins and of a component of C'_3: II. Production of immunoelectrophoretically identified serum proteins by human and monkey tissues *in vitro*. *J. Exp. Med.* 114:471, 1961.
89. Askonas, B. A., Humphrey, J. H., and Porter, R. R. On the origin of the multiple forms of rabbit gamma-globulin. *Biochem. J.* 63:412, 1956.
90. Maximow, A. A. The Lymphocytes and Plasma Cells. In Cowdry, E. V. (Ed.), *Special Cytology* (2nd ed.). New York: Paul B. Hoeber, Inc., 1928, Vol. I.
91. Trowell, O. A. The lymphocyte. *Int. Rev. Cytol.* 7:235, 1958.
92. Bloom, W. The Embryogenesis of Mammalian Blood. In Downey, H. (Ed.), *Handbook of Hematology*. New York: Paul B. Hoeber, Inc., 1938, Vol. 1.
93. Jacobson, L. O., Marks, E. K., Simmons, E. L., and Gaston, E. O. Immune response in irradiated mice with Peyer's patch shielding. *Proc. Soc. Exp. Biol. Med.* 108:487, 1961.
94. Sainte-Marie, G., and Leblond, C. P. Tentative pattern for renewal of lymphocytes in cortex of the rat thymus. *Proc. Soc. Exp. Biol. Med.* 97:263, 1958.
95. Gowans, J. L., Gesner, B. L., and McGregor, D. D. The immunological activity of lymphocytes. In Wolstenholme, G. E. W., and O'Connor, M. (Eds.), *Biological Activity of the Leucocyte,* Ciba Foundation Study Group No. 10, 1961. Boston: Little, Brown.
96. Braunsteiner, H., Höfer, R., and Sailer, S. The lymphocytes. *German Med. Month.* 6:273, 1961.
97. Bernhard, W., and Granboulas, N. Ultrastructure of Immunologically Competent Cells. Ref. 31.
98. Policard, A., Collet, A., Martin, J-C., and Prégermain, S. Cytologie infrastructurale: Étude au microscope életronique des premièrs stades de la formation des plasmocytes ganglionnaires. *C. R. Acad. Sci.* (Paris) 253:2027, 1961.
99. de Petris, S., Karlsbad, G., and Pernis, B. Localization of antibodies in plasma cells by electron microscopy. *J. Exp. Med.* 117:849, 1963.
100. Nossal, G. J. V., and Mäkelä, O. Autoradiographic studies on the immune response: I. The kinetics of plasma cell proliferation. *J. Exp. Med.* 115:209, 1962.
101. Roberts, J. C., Jr., Dixon, F. J., and Weigle, W. O. Antibody-producing lymph node cells and peritoneal exudate cells. *Arch. Path.* 64:324, 1957.
102. Neil, A. L., and Dixon, F. J. Immunohistochemical detection of antibody in cell-transfer studies. *Arch. Path.* 67:643, 1959.
103. Zlotnick, A., Vazquez, J. J., and Dixon, F. J. Mitotic activity of immunologically competent lymphoid cells transferred into x-irradiated recipients. *Lab. Invest.* 11:493, 1962.
103a. Sainte-Marie, G., and Coons, A. H. Studies on antibody production: X. Mode of formation of plasmocytes in cell transfer experiments. *J. Exp. Med.* 119:743, 1964.
104. Baney, R. N., Vazquez, J. J., and Dixon, F. J. Cellular proliferation in relation to antibody synthesis. *Proc. Soc. Exp. Biol. Med.* 109:1, 1962.
105. Urso, P., and Makinodan, T. The roles of cellular division and maturation in the formation of precipitating antibody. *J. Immun.* 90:897, 1963.
106. Schooley, J. C. Autoradiographic observations of plasma cell formation. *J. Immun.* 86:331, 1961.
107. Makinodan, T., and Albright, J. F. Cellular variation during the immune response: One possible model of cellular differentiation. *J. Cell. Comp. Physiol.* 60(supp. 1):129, 1962.
108. Talmage, D. W., and Claman, H. N. Cell

Potential—Its Mutation and Selection. Ref. 69.

109. Gurney, C. W., Wackman, N., and Filmanowicz, E. Studies on erythropoiesis: XVII. Some quantitative aspects of the erythropoietic response to erythropoietin. *Blood* 17:531, 1961.
110. Lajtha, L. G. Stem Cell Kinetics and Erythropoietin. In Jacobson, L. O., and Doyle, M. (Eds.), *Erythropoiesis*. New York: Grune & Stratton, Inc., 1962.
111. Erslev, A. J. Erythropoietin *in vitro*. *Ibid.*
112. Taliaferro, W. H., and Taliaferro, L. G. Effect of x-rays on immunity: A review. *J. Immun.* 66:181, 1951.
113. Kohn, H. I. Effect of x-rays upon hemolysin production in the rat. *Ibid.*, p. 525.
114. Fitch, F. W., Wissler, R. W., LaVia, M., and Barker, P. The timing of antigen injection relative to whole body x-irradiation and the development of circulating antibody and the splenic histologic reaction in the rat. *J. Immun.* 76:151, 1956.
115. Gengozian, N., and Makinodan, T. Relation of primary antigen injection to time of irradiation on antibody production in mice. *J. Immun.* 80:189, 1958.
116. Keuning, F. J., van der Meer, J., Nieuwenhuis, P., and Oudendijk, P. The histophysiology of the antibody response: II. Antibody responses and splenic plasma cell reactions in sublethally x-irradiated rabbits. *Lab. Invest.* 12:156, 1963.
117. Jerne, N. K., Nordin, A. A., and Henry, C. The Agar Plaque Technique for Recognizing Antibody-producing Cells. In Amos, B., and Koprowski, H. (Eds.), *Cell-Bound Antibodies*. Philadelphia: Wistar Institute Press, 1963.
118. Ambrose, C. T., and Coons, A. H. Studies on antibody production: VIII. The inhibitory effect of chloramphenicol on the synthesis of antibody in tissue culture. *J. Exp. Med.* 117:1075, 1963.

118a. Weisberger, A. S., Daniel, T. M., and Hoffman, A. Suppression of antibody synthesis and prolongation of homograft survival by chloramphenicol. *J. Exp. Med.* 120:183, 1964.

119. Cannon, P. R., Chase, W. E., and Wissler, R. W. The relationship of the protein-reserves to antibody-production: I. The effects of a low protein diet and of plasmapheresis upon the formation of agglutinins. *J. Immun.* 47:133, 1943.
120. LaVia, M. F., Barker, P. A., and Wissler, R. W. A study of the correlation of antigen phagocytosis and the splenic histological reaction with antibody formation in protein-depleted rats. *J. Lab. Clin. Med.* 48:237, 1956.
121. Wissler, R. W., Frazier, L. F., Soules, K. H., Barker, P., and Bristow, E. C., III. The acute effects of beta-3-thienylalanine in the adult male albino rat. *Arch. Path.* 62:62, 1956.
122. Jaroslow, B. N., and Smith, D. E. Antigen disappearance in hibernating ground squirrels. *Science* 134:734, 1961.
123. Bissett, K. A. The effect of temperature upon antibody production in cold-blooded vertebrates. *J. Path. Bact.* 60:87, 1948.
124. Thorbecke, G. J., Siskind, G. W., and Goldberger, N. The induction in mice of sensitization and immunological unresponsiveness by neonatal injection of bovine γ-globulin. *J. Immun.* 87:147, 1961.
125. Sorem, G. L., and Terres, G. The temporal relationship of acquired tolerance and the immune response following injection of bovine serum albumin into neonatal mice. *J. Immun.* 90:217, 1963.
126. Sercarz, E., and Coons, A. H. The Exhaustion of Specific Antibody Producing Capacity during a Secondary Response. In Hašek, M., Lengerová, A., and Vojtišková, M. (Eds.). *Mechanism of Immunological Tolerance.* Prague: Publishing House of Czechoslovak Academy of Sciences; and New York: Academic Press, 1962.

6. *Antibody Production and Specificity*

DAVID W. TALMAGE AND EDWARD P. COHEN

THE SYNTHESIS OF SPECIFICALLY REactive proteins following the injection of foreign antigens is a subject of major concern to the present volume. Antibody response is also of interest to other fields of clinical medicine, especially infectious disease, and to many basic biological disciplines, such as genetics, biochemistry, and cytology. Moreover, the induction of antibody formation provides a valuable, controllable model of induced protein synthesis. Thus a study of antibody synthesis lends insight into the cell differentiation and maturation from which this synthesis derives.

Because of the importance of the antibody response to both clinical medicine and molecular biology, a large number of theoretical attempts have been made to explain its underlying mechanisms. In this chapter we will indicate the major differences among these attempts and will stress the contributions of each to the development of biological and immunological concepts. The references will enable the interested reader to pursue this study at greater depth.

The various theories of antibody formation fall into three groups which differ in the role ascribed to antigen (Fig. 6-1): (1) direct template theories which postulate that antigen acts as a template or pattern for the synthesis or folding of the antibody protein molecule; (2) indirect template theories which postulate that antigen acts to alter the replicable nucleic acids of the cell, endowing them with the required information for specific antibody synthesis, and (3) natural selection theories which postulate that the antigen selects from among many pre-existing patterns of protein synthesis and stimulates the production of those proteins which combine with the antigen.

Direct and indirect template theories are sometimes linked under the term instructive theories. In contrast, natural selection theories are considered inductive. The term induction implies the activation of a naturally occurring, pre-existing synthetic process, and natural selection the selective multiplication of self-replicating units, for example, cells which have the inherited capacity for specific antibody synthesis. Both processes are implicit in the natural selection theories. This should be distinguished from the nonreplicative selection postulated in the direct template theory. Here the antigen selects from among many ways of folding a peptide chain, but the peptide chain cannot replicate.

A difference in the concept of antibody specificity associated with instruction and induction may be illustrated by analogy to the specific and complementary relationship between a lock and its key. There are two methods of obtaining a specific key to fit a lock (Fig. 6-2). One method is to tailor a key to the exact specifications of the lock (instruction). The other is to select from a large number of master keys one that fits the lock (selection). In general, the custom-made key should be the more specific, but the difference may be hard to detect from an examination of the keys. Either key may fit some other lock which is structurally related. According to the instructive theories, antibodies are custom made; according to inductive theories, the antibody is a master key.

EARLY MODELS

Perhaps the earliest concept which attempted to explain the immune response was proposed by Pasteur [1]. Based on the *in vitro* observation that a medium which previously supported the growth of a specific microorganism would no longer allow the further cultivation of that organism, Pasteur postulated that an essential, nonreplaceable nutrient had been exhausted. He further postulated that the same mechanism of immunity occurred *in vivo* and suggested that "the growth of the microorganism, by a previous culture, had eliminated from the muscle some prin-

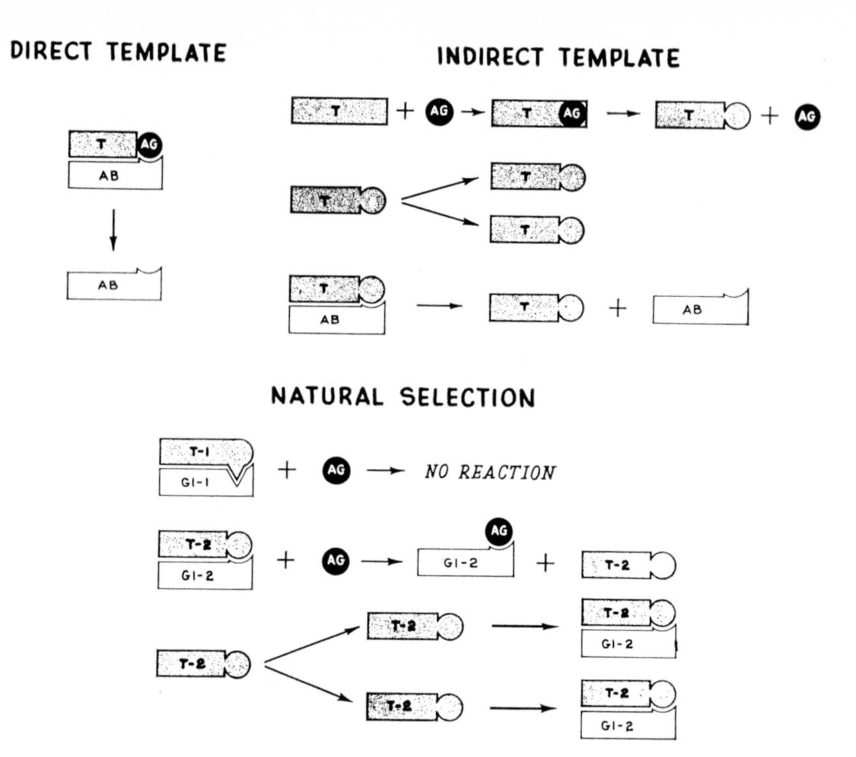

Fig. 6-1. The three groups of theories of antibody formation. In the direct template theories, the antigen (*Ag*) becomes a part of the template (*T*) synthesizing γ-globulin. In indirect template theories, the antigen changes a replicating globulin-synthesizing unit. In the natural selection theories, the antigen induces replication of preexisting patterns of globulin synthesis.

ciple that life does not bring back and whose absence prevents the development of the small organisms." This theory was quickly abandoned following the observation of Chauveau [2] that sheep, resistant to large numbers of anthrax bacilli, were fully susceptible to the injections of enormous numbers of the organisms.

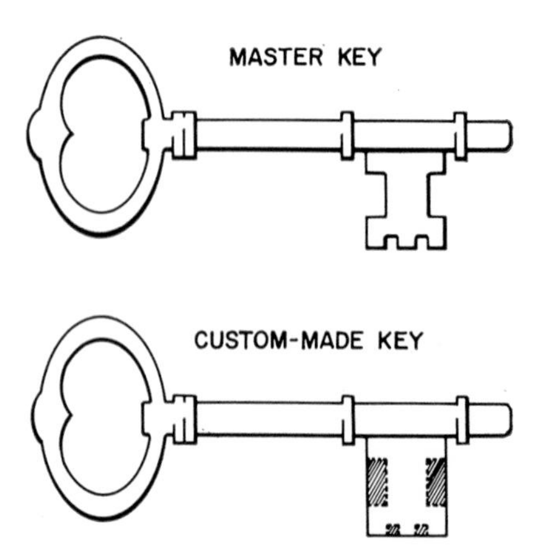

Fig. 6-2. The two concepts of antibody specificity implicit in selection (master key) and instruction (custom-made key).

Another early attempt to explain the immune response in some detail was published by Ehrlich [3] in 1900. In this classic paper, Ehrlich postulated that antibodies were preformed side chains attached to cells (Fig. 6-3). These side chains functioned as aids in the nutritive physiology of the cell. Some of them, perhaps fortuitously, had structures complementary to antigens. When an antigen reacted with these side chains, it interfered with their function. As a response, the cell then synthesized additional side chains identical to those which had combined with the antigen. Some of these would be released into the circulation and become the circulating antibody. The major significance of this early concept is twofold: (1) it emphasized the chemical nature of the antigen-antibody interaction, and (2) it suggested the existence of preformed, inherited antibody capable of being synthesized in large amounts in response to a foreign stimulus.

With the subsequent demonstrations by Landsteiner [4] that antibodies could be induced to form against a number of "artificial" antigens synthesized in the laboratory, the side

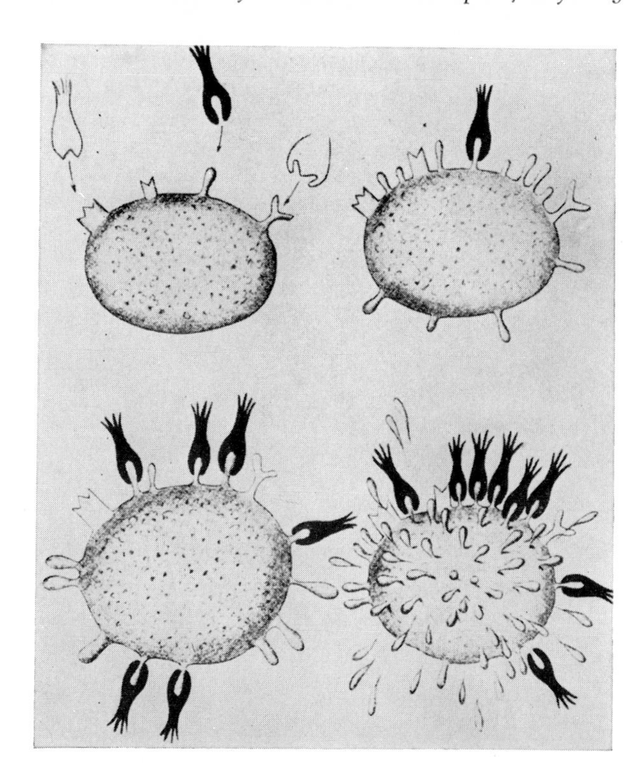

Fig. 6-3. Ehrlich's concept of the multiplication and shedding of natural cellular receptors after their combination with antigen. (From original paper by Ehrlich [3].)

chain theory fell into disrepute. Conceptually, it became difficult to understand the preexistence of molecules with combining specificities toward such a large number of antigens, some of which must be new to the organism. This difficulty arose in part from the teleological aspect of Ehrlich's theory, namely, his postulation that antibodies had a specific function as cellular side chains.

DIRECT TEMPLATE THEORIES

Perhaps as a reaction to these concepts, there followed the direct template theories. The first to ascribe a direct role of antigen in the formation of antibody were Breinl and Haurowitz [5] in 1930. Similar theories were advanced by Alexander [6] and Mudd [7] in 1932. In these theories, the antibody molecule was thought to form in direct contact with antigen which served as a pattern or template producing an antibody which was complementary in structure. Thus the problem of the specific formation of antibodies to thousands of different antigens (natural and synthetic) could be explained.

Pauling [8] in 1940 expressed essentially the same idea in a more detailed manner. He assumed that all antibodies have the same amino acid sequence and that an antibody molecule forms directly on the antigen. After the antibody is formed, it is released spontaneously. This concept is illustrated in Figure 6-4. Pauling's theory stresses the reversibility of the antigen-antibody reaction and has stimulated a large amount of research into the thermodynamics of this reaction.

Karush [9] has since provided a biochemical explanation of the mechanism by which a globulin molecule can be folded into a structure complementary to antigen. Karush showed experimentally that the critical bond in the folding of the antibody molecule responsible for maintenance of specificity was the disulfide bond between two cysteine residues in the polypeptide chain. He postulated that antibodies are first formed as a reduced polypeptide chain, capable of being folded in many ways. In the presence of the antigen, this precursor polypeptide assumes a configuration complementary to the antigen. This configuration becomes stabilized by formation of disulfide bonds, and the completed molecule dissociates from the antigen. Karush's model was the first to utilize information gained from an analysis of the structure of the antibody molecule in an attempt to draw

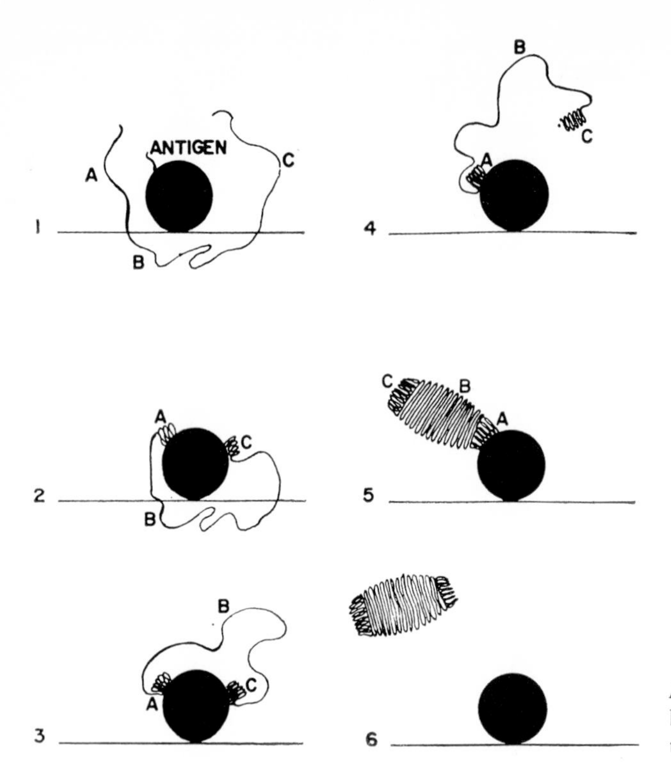

Fig. 6-4. Sequence of events postulated by Pauling [8] to occur during the formation of antibody.

conclusions concerning the mechanism of its synthesis.

Because it provides the simplest explanation of immunological specificity, the direct template theory is still held as a working hypothesis by many immunochemists (Chap. 2). Its greatest difficulties have been in explaining the specificity of cell memory (immunological tolerance and anamnesis), the efficiency of antibody synthesis by individual cells [10], and the cellular responses which are an integral part of the antibody response (Chap. 5).

Immunological tolerance and anamnesis have been explained as the effects of different ways of handling the antigen, either because of the presence of specific enzymes to destroy it (tolerance) or because of specific antibody to transport it (anamnesis).

INDIRECT TEMPLATE THEORIES

In 1941, Burnet and Fenner [11] published their classic monograph on antibody production. They felt that immunology had veered from the mainstream of biology. Since antibody is a protein synthesized by a biological organism, it was pertinent to consider how other adaptive proteins are synthesized. Burnet and Fenner based their theory on concepts current at that time concerning adaptive enzymes in bacteria. They postulated that when antigens enter an antibody-forming cell, changes are produced in the replicable enzymes responsible for synthesis of the antibody molecule. This theory introduced the concept of a replicable antibody-synthesizing unit which is inheritable on a cellular level. Thus the theory explained the anamnestic response, the efficiency of antibody synthesis, and the logarithmic rise of antibody levels in the serum following antigenic stimulation. It focused the interest of immunology on the antibody-forming cell and the characteristics of the immune response. Later, these authors [12] proposed that recognition of one's own antigens develops during embryonic life by means of a "self-marker." With progress in the knowledge of induced protein synthesis in bacteria, Burnet [13] modified the theory to implicate the desoxyribonucleic acids (DNA) in the inheritable units responsible for specific antibody synthesis. A similar theory, postulating specific mutations of DNA induced by antigen was advanced simultaneously by Schweet and Owen [14]. More recently, Goldstein [15] has described a theory involving modification of the ribonucleic acids (RNA) by antigen. However, it is difficult to explain the molecular mechanism by which an antigen produces a specific mutation in either DNA or RNA. This difficulty probably opened the way once again to the natural selection theories.

THEORIES OF NATURAL SELECTION

In 1955, Jerne [16] first used the term natural selection in connection with a systematic theory of antibody production. Jerne postulated that about 1 million different γ-globulin molecules are formed in embryonic life, perhaps by the thymus. Once formed, these molecules can be used by antibody-forming cells as models for the synthesis of identical molecules. Thus, in a sense, the γ-globulin molecule is considered a replicable unit. These molecules with reactivities to self-antigens are removed during fetal life before the appearance of antibody-forming cells. Antigen injected after birth combines selectively with certain γ-globulins possessing complementary configurations (antibodies) and increases the entry of these γ-globulins into antibody-forming cells. As a consequence, the antibody globulin is used preferentially as a model for the synthesis of new protein.

Jerne's theory introduced new concepts of immunological specificity and tolerance. It explained the presence of preformed "antibodies" to synthetic haptens by eliminating Ehrlich's concept of a specific function for each pre-existing antibody and substituting a concept of the randomized production of a wide variety of γ-globulins with overlapping reactivities. Jerne's theory was the first to provide a molecular explanation of immunological tolerance, i.e., the distinction between self and not-self. Previous explanations had at some point all required homocentric expression such as "self-recognition." In place of self-recognition Jerne substituted recognition of not-self and attributed the lack of antibodies to self to the absence of γ-globulin molecules with which to react.

The main objection to Jerne's theory is experimental evidence that immunological memory resides in the cells, not in the serum. This objection can be resolved by substituting cell potential for γ-globulin in the randomizing process. In 1957, cell selection theories were advanced almost simultaneously by Talmage [17] and by Burnet [18]. Subsequently, these concepts were described in more detail by Burnet [19] in *The Clonal Selection Theory of Acquired Immunity* which introduced the concept of the "forbidden clone" to explain autoimmunity. Cells with the capacity for the formation of antibody against a normal body protein were "forbidden" and eliminated during embryonic life. The assumptions of cell selection were stated explicitly by Lederberg [20]. The master key concept of specificity referred to earlier was discussed in detail by Talmage [21].

CONCEPTS OF CELL POTENTIAL

Recent developments in immunological theory have related primarily to the problems of cell potential, its mechanism, and its specificity.

Monod [22] suggested that immunological memory is similar to that produced by the permease system in *Escherichia coli.* In this case, an enzyme located in the cell membrane selectively increases the entry into the cell of its substrate. Monod postulated that antigen is selectively brought into cells previously exposed to the same antigen. Boyden [23] suggested that this specific concentrating mechanism is effected by cell-fixed antibody. Boyden further emphasized the importance of self-recognition in phagocytic phenomena which antedate antibody formation in the phylogenetic scale.

Both Monod and Boyden postulated that an altered handling of antigen by the immunized animal is responsible for the increased antibody synthesis of the secondary response. In support of this concept, Segre and Kaeberle [24] described experiments with colostrum-deprived pigs which indicated a stimulatory effect of specific antibody. It would appear that in antibody excess, antibody suppresses the antigenic stimulus, but in antigen excess, augmentation of the response occurs.

Although factors (including antibody) which affect the distribution and metabolism of antigen are undoubtedly important in determining the quantity of antibody produced, there is also evidence of the importance of the intrinsic and immediate potential of the cell to respond. Perhaps the most important evidence relates to the remarkable specificity of immunological memory. Among the first to recognize this specificity were Davenport *et al.* [25]

in connection with antibody responses to influenza viruses. They noted that individuals exposed to influenza virus frequently responded by synthesizing antibody directed most specifically against related strains to which they had been exposed many years before.

An experimental test of the specificity of immunological memory was performed by Dubert [26]. He prepared two cross-reacting antigens from the closely related haptens, metanilic and sulfanilic acids. Animals immunized with one antigen gave anamnestic responses on injection of the other. However, the antibody produced during the anamnestic response possessed a greater affinity for the antigen first injected than for the antigen which induced the recall response. These observations indicate that immunological memory involves more than an altered distribution of antigen, since the antibody produced during the secondary response reflects qualitative characteristics of the antigen first injected that are not present in the second antigen.

Evidence that the locus of immunological memory is associated with lymphoid cells is demonstrated by the ability to transfer this memory to immunologically inert recipients with lymphoid cells [27, 28] but not with serum [29]. Quantitatively, the antibody response of the recipient has been shown to be directly proportional to the number of cells transferred [30].

Another aspect of cell potential which has received considerable attention is the number of different antibodies a single cell can make. Lederberg [20] predicted that a cell with two sets of chromosomes may have two such potentials. Attardi *et al.* [31], using microdroplets containing single cells, demonstrated antibodies to both of two noncross-reacting bacteriophages in 2 to 3 percent of the examined cells. The remainder made either no antibody or only one of the two antibodies. The number of double producers detected by Nossal [32] in similar experiments with *Salmonella* antigens was a much smaller fraction of the total antibody-forming cells.

The failure of a cell to synthesize antibody to all the antigens to which it is exposed cannot be equated with the absence of these potentials in the originally responding cell. The expression of one potential may conceivably inhibit the others. For this reason it is necessary to consider experiments which attempt to determine the fraction of immunologically competent cells capable of making a response to an individual antigen.

The introduction of chicken peripheral buffy coat cells or a spleen suspension onto the chorioallantoic membrane (CAM) of the embryonated chick egg results in the formation of discrete focal collections of donor cells proliferating in the membrane [33]. If the adult chicken donor and the egg are inbred, fewer foci result [34]. This suggests that in the outbred cell transfer, immunologically competent donor cells with the predetermined capacity for recognition of foreign antigen are reacting against foreign antigenic determinants in the CAM of the immunologically inert egg host. This is an example of the graft-versus-host reaction and is probably analogous to the transfer of adult mouse spleen cells to newborn mice with the production of runting in the recipients (Chap. 13). Indeed, if the embryonated egg recipient is allowed to hatch, the newborn chick does not thrive but develops a runting type of syndrome which includes splenomegaly and hemolytic anemia [35]. On the basis that each focus derives from one immunologically competent cell, the Burnets [34] attempted to determine the minimal number of cells which must be transferred in order to cause the appearance of one cellular focus. Experimentally, one focus was produced for each 10,000 lymphoid cells transferred [36].

The interpretation of these findings depends on how many different immunological potentials the adult chicken is thought to possess and whether the small lymphocyte is considered to possess immunological potential. Since a great majority of lymphoid cells are small lymphocytes, an elimination of this cell type from the group of cells with antibody-forming potential would reduce greatly the number of such cells and necessarily increase the number of potentials per cell. However, if one accords immunological potential to the small lymphocyte (see later), the number of different potentials per cell is probably quite small, although not necessarily as low as 1.

The mechanism by which cells acquire the immediate potential to synthesize some but not all antibodies is unknown. On biological grounds, it would seem likely that differentiation of the antibody-forming precursor cell occurs by the same mechanisms that operate in the differentiation of cells destined to synthesize other specialized proteins, e.g., hemoglobin, serum albumin, insulin. In the case of antibodies, the large number of different potentials required would favor some sort of internal randomizing process. In the past, embryologists tended to think in terms of environmental inducers, but Flickinger [37] recently proposed a model in which the initial steps in differentiation are intrinsic.

IMMUNOLOGICAL MEMORY RELATED TO CELL DIFFERENTIATION, MATURATION, AND REPLICATION

If one accepts the concept of specific cell potential described in the foregoing discussion, immunological memory becomes a problem of cell differentiation and replication. Differentiation is used here to describe the process by which the immediate potential of one cell becomes different from another. According to instructive theories, this differentiation is produced by the antigen. According to natural selection theories, cell potential is randomized in the absence of antigen, and cells with potential for autoantibody production are purged as they are formed. Mackay and Burnet [38] proposed that the process of differentiation and purging takes place in the thymus and in support of this concept described thymic lesions in mice in which autoimmune disease had developed spontaneously. Miller [39] reported a prolongation of immunological suppression by x-ray irradiation of thymectomized animals, and Claman and Talmage [40] reported that thymectomy prolonged the state of immunological tolerance induced by antigen. Since the thymus has an environment relatively protected from antigen, its contribution to the development of competent cells in adult as well as newborn animals is a strong argument against antigen's playing a role in the differentiation of antibody-forming potential. Further evidence of the role of the thymus in the development of immunological potential is given in Chapter 4.

Contradictory evidence exists concerning the specific cell type which is the locus of immunological memory. On the basis of labeled thymidine studies, Nossal and Mäkelä [41] concluded that immunological memory resides in a large blast cell which is dividing almost continuously. Other workers have implicated the small lymphocyte as the locus of immunological memory. Gowans *et al.* [42] showed that the ability to produce graft-versus-host reactions with thoracic duct lymphocytes of rats correlated better with their content of small than with their content of medium or large lymphocytes. After transferring thoracic duct lymphocytes from which most of the medium and large lymphocytes had been removed, Gowans demonstrated both cell division of the donor lymphocytes and their antibody-forming capacity. From this he and his co-workers [43] concluded that the small lymphocyte on exposure to antigen enlarges, becomes pyroninophilic, and divides several times.

Another important related question is the mechanism by which immunological memory increases and decreases. Anamnestic responsiveness and immunological tolerance represent these opposite effects of antigen on immunological memory. In a recent theoretical discussion of this problem [44] it was suggested that during the steady state (memory neither increasing nor decreasing), replication of the blast cell is exactly matched by its maturation through a process of asymmetrical division. Under this concept, one daughter cell of each blast cell division is committed to maturation and eventual death, the other to immaturity and further division. Anamnestic responsiveness, according to this hypothesis, would be produced by a shift to symmetrical division (both cells remaining immature and dividing) and an expansion of the blast cell pool. Immunological tolerance, on the other hand, would be produced by maturation of all the memory cells in the blast cell pool capable of responding to that particular antigen. In support of this concept, Dresser [45] and Claman [46] both have produced immunological tolerance in adult mice by an injection of bovine γ-globulin. The additional injection of bacterial endotoxin which is known to stimulate division of lymphoid cells produced the opposite effect, namely, anamnestic responsiveness. Crowle [47] and Katsh *et al.* [48], using different systems, have produced an immunological tolerance in mice which was preceded by a period of increased responsiveness. This supports the concept that tolerance is the result of a suicidal commitment of all the memory cells to a limited period of antibody formation followed by cell death.

INFORMATION TRANSFER

According to present concepts [49], the information required for protein synthesis is inherited in the form of a one-dimensional

DNA code. Each triplet of nucleotides in the DNA chain specifies one amino acid in a peptide chain. The information in the DNA is translated into protein by means of a three-component system consisting of: (1) messenger RNA (containing information in the same triplet code as DNA), (2) a ribosome (or ribosomes), and (3) a set of adaptors called transfer RNA's and their activating enzymes. This scheme has been compared to an automated system in which information (from the DNA) is punched onto a tape (the messenger RNA) which directs a factory (the ribosomes) in the production of the finished products (protein). There is at least one transfer RNA and one activating enzyme for each of the 20 natural amino acids specified in the DNA and RNA code. The activating enzyme combines specifically with the appropriate amino acid and attaches it to the corresponding transfer RNA. In conjunction with the ribosomes and messenger RNA, the transfer RNA then adds this amino acid to the peptide chain but only at the appropriate place as specified in the messenger RNA triplet code. As the messenger RNA coded tape passes by or through the ribosomes, one amino acid is added for each nucleotide triplet until the entire tape has passed through and the peptide is complete.

A single antibody molecule, like many other proteins, is composed of a number of peptides derived from at least two different genes (Chap. 3). The synthesis of the different peptides is somehow coordinated, so that the completed protein is put together without significant excess of one of the peptides. To accomplish this, the messenger RNA, ribosomes, and transfer RNA must be synthesized in the nucleus and transported to the cytoplasm where the synthesis of protein takes place.

The antigen appears to act as an inducer of this synthetic process, since DNA and RNA synthesis increases following an injection of antigen (Chap. 5). The cytoplasm enlarges and becomes filled with ribosomes.

A major problem in the formulation of any molecular model of antibody formation is the explanation of the observed induction of DNA and RNA synthesis and thus the origin of the specific adaptors between DNA and an antigen with which the species has had no prior experience. In 1960, Szilard [50] described a model of selective induction of antibody synthesis which attempted to solve this problem and was the first to provide a molecular bridge between antigen and DNA. He postulated that cells of the lymphocytic series first exist in a multipotential state with respect to antibody production. At this time cells properly stimulated would be capable of making any of approximately 10,000 different globulins. The 10,000 globulins were thought to be derived from 10,000 enzymes, each controlled by a different specific repressor and coupling enzyme. The coupling enzymes, on the one hand, have specific affinity for antigen (similar to the antibody whose production it controls). On the other hand, the enzyme acts specifically with an RNA repressor, completing it to a form capable of suppressing a specific portion of DNA or gene. Thus the coupling enzyme and repressor act as a bridge between antigen and DNA in the same fashion as the transfer RNA and activating enzymes act as a bridge between messenger RNA and amino acids. According to Szilard, the antigen, as it enters the multipotential cell, would selectively precipitate or absorb the coupling enzyme and lock the cell into a permanent state of antibody production. The multiplication of these locked or committed cells was further postulated to be repressed by a complement-like enzyme. A second injection of antigen after forming complexes with the antibody in these cells absorbs or coprecipitates the complement-like repressor and stimulates cell division, thus producing an anamnestic response.

Szilard's model explains how a specifically adapted bridge is developed for each antibody to transmit the specific stimulus from antigen to DNA but does not explain how a perfect correspondence between repressor and antibody is maintained in the face of expected mutations. The enzymic origin of antibodies seems unlikely because, unlike different enzymes, all γ-globulins of the same species are remarkably similar in molecular weight, in amino acid composition, and probably in general structure.

Another attempt to describe a molecular bridge between antigen and DNA was made by Talmage and Pearlman [51]. They assumed that the initial reaction of antigen is with preformed antibody and that the next step in the chain of reactions leading to derepression of DNA might be either of two general types: (1) the displacement of specific inducers by antigen-antibody interaction, or (2) the displacement of preformed antibody from its site of synthesis. In the first case it was necessary to postulate that the gene for each peptide has its own specific inducer which also has a specific affinity for the completed peptide it controls. Antigen, by displacing the inducers from the antibody molecule, would derepress the right combination of genes and thus cause the formation of more of the same antibody. The number of different kinds of antibody one cell could make would be determined by the inducers it could synthesize. This would represent the cell's potential. It is conceivable, according to this model, that inducers released from one cell can stimulate antibody formation by an adjoining cell.

According to the second possible pathway of DNA derepression, the energy of the reaction between antigen and antibody was postulated to be sufficient to release both antibody and messenger RNA from a ribosome strategically located in the nuclear membrane. It was further postulated that as long as the antibody remains fixed to this ribosome, the messenger RNA molecules from which it was synthesized cannot pass into the cytoplasm. Thus the effect of the release of antibody by antigen is to increase the rate at which specific messenger RNA molecules are transported out of the nucleus. This would have the double effect of derepressing the right combination of genes and providing the cytoplasm with the information required for specific protein synthesis.

GENETICS OF ANTIBODY FORMATION

Experimental studies have shown that the amount of antibody produced in response to a specific antigen is at least partially controlled by inherited factors. Several reports [52–54] have noted a difference between strains of inbred mice in the quantity of antibody produced in response to the same antigenic stimulus. In a study of outbred rabbits a correlation was found between the antibody titers of parent and those of offspring [55]. The difficulty with these studies is the uncertainty concerning what is being inherited. The synthesis of even a small amount of antibody is evidence in favor of the inheritance of the structural genes containing the information to order the necessary peptides. The quantity of antibody produced may relate to cofactors involved in the induction of antibody synthesis. Even in congenital hypogammaglobulinemia, in which usually no antibody response can be detected, it is not known whether the defect is within the immunoglobulin peptides or in the inducing system.

A question of major interest is the number of gene loci which determine the peptides from which antibodies are synthesized. Chapter 3 describes two kinds of peptides which have been separated from the immunoglobulins by nonenzymatic methods, the A or heavy chains, and the B or light chains. Three classes of A chains have been identified which determine the classification of the immunoglobulins as IgG, IgM, and IgA. The antigenic determinants on the A chains appear to segregate in a way which suggests a single gene locus for each of the three classes.

The B chains appear to be very heterogeneous in every species studied except the horse. However, these heterogeneous B chains contain common antigenic determinants which are present in all three classes of immunoglobulin. In human beings there are at least two mutually exclusive antigenic determinants which derive from the B chains. Termed group I and group II, these have many differences in amino acid composition, which is strong evidence that they derive from distinct inherited genes (see Chap. 3). That is, they probably do not arise from somatic mutations of the same gene and certainly do not represent different ways of folding the same peptide. If the two groups of B chains derive from different genes, the evidence would indicate that the two groups arise from different genetic loci. This is because the inheritance of these two antigens does not segregate in the same fashion as other antigens of common locus, e.g., the ABO antigens of human red blood cells. Rather, the two antigens appear to be present in all individuals in a fairly constant ratio of about 2 : 1 [56]. One explanation of this surprising finding is that the two groups of peptides have arisen from gene duplication and subsequent gene mutation and that the structural requirements of the γ-globulin molecule have kept the process of diversification within the bounds of two major antigenic groups.

Whether all of the different B chains arise from hundreds of different loci or whether all of those of a single group arise from somatic mutation of the two genes at a single locus cannot be answered at this time. An answer will require information concerning the inheritance of individual B chain moieties.

ANTIBODY SPECIFICITY AND INFORMATION THEORY

In 1957, Jaroslow and Quastler [57] suggested that the antigen-antibody interaction has many of the aspects of information transfer and asked the question, "How many different antigens are there?" The reciprocal question, "How many different antibodies?" has been raised frequently in connection with the various theories of antibody formation.

Antibodies may be considered to give information concerning the antigens with which they react. A group or family of different antibody globulins all reacting with the same antigen gives more information about the antigen and is thus more specific for the antigen than any one member of the family acting alone. This concept of immunological specificity is illustrated on a two-dimensional level in Figure 6-5.

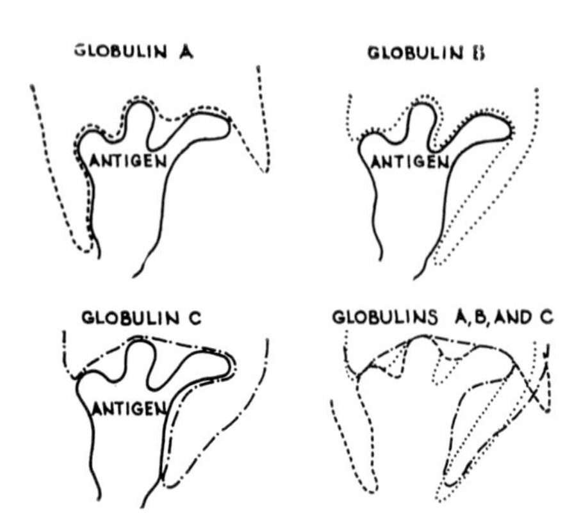

Fig. 6-5. Two-dimensional diagrams illustrating the concept that an antigen molecule may react with more than one antibody (globulin *A*, globulin *B*, and globulin *C*). The last diagram illustrates the concept that an antiserum with three different antibodies contains more information about the antigen and thus greater specificity than an antiserum with only one kind of antibody.

The number of families of different globulins that may be formed is much larger than the number of different globulins that make up the information system. The 26 letters of our alphabet make up several hundred thousand English words. As few as 500 different globulins may form 10^{11} different families containing 5 globulins and 10^{20} different families containing 10 globulins. In general the number of different families of a given size (F) which may be formed from N different globulins is given by the formula

$$\text{Number of families} = \frac{N!}{(N-F)!F!}$$

On the basis of the amount of information contained, 500 different globulins would seem quite adequate to recognize or distinguish between almost all of the different antigenic determinants that have been or could be synthesized. However, the immunological information system has two other properties which make 500 appear to be an inadequate number. These properties are specificity and universality.

Specificity may be represented mathematically by the statement that the probability of two randomly selected families having a common member is low. Universality implies that the probability of a randomly selected antigen having a family size of zero is low. Figure 6-6 and 6-7 illustrate how these two properties relate to the average family size in informational systems containing 500 and 8,000 different globulins. Specificity is represented by the probability of a cross-reaction between two randomly selected families which is given by the formula

$$\text{Probability of cross-reaction} = \frac{F^2}{N}$$

Universality is indicated by the probability of no reaction with a randomly selected antigenic determinant. This was calculated from the formula

$$\text{Probability of no reaction} = \left(1 - \frac{F}{N}\right)^N$$

The curves in Figures 6-6 and 6-7 reveal that increasing the family size has opposite effects on the two probabilities; it increases the probability of a cross-reaction and lowers the probability of no reaction. With 500 different globulins the curves cross at a probability of 3 percent, giving an optimal family size between 3 and 4. With higher or lower family size, the chance of either a cross-reaction or no reaction rises rapidly. With 8,000 globulins the curves cross at 0.3 percent and give an average family size of 6.

Perhaps the major biological value of im-

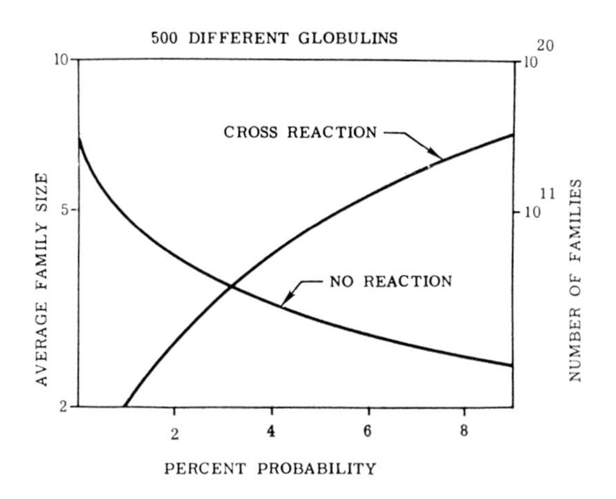

Fig. 6-6. Theoretical curves which relate the probabilities of cross-reaction and no reaction to the average family size in an information system containing 500 different globulins.

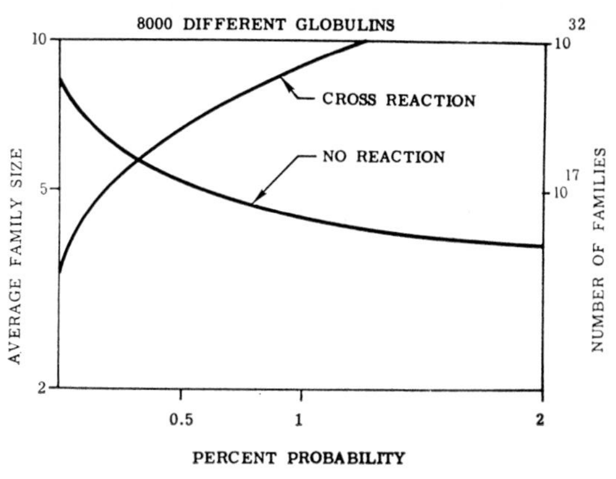

Fig. 6-7. Theoretical curves which relate the probabilities of cross-reaction and no reaction to the average family size in an information system containing 8,000 different globulins.

munological specificity is the ability to distinguish between self and not-self. As pointed out by Jerne [58] any set of immunoglobulins with randomized reactivity must first be purged of those globulins capable of reacting with self. Since there are undoubtedly many different self-antigens, a set of globulins which is too small in number and too nonspecific in its reactivity will become almost entirely purged by the preliminary reaction with self-antigens. This problem is illustrated in Figure 6-8. The percentage of globulins which would not be purged by 1,000 different self-antigens has been calculated from the formula

$$\text{Fraction of globulins not purged} = \left(1 - \frac{F}{N}\right)^{1,000}$$

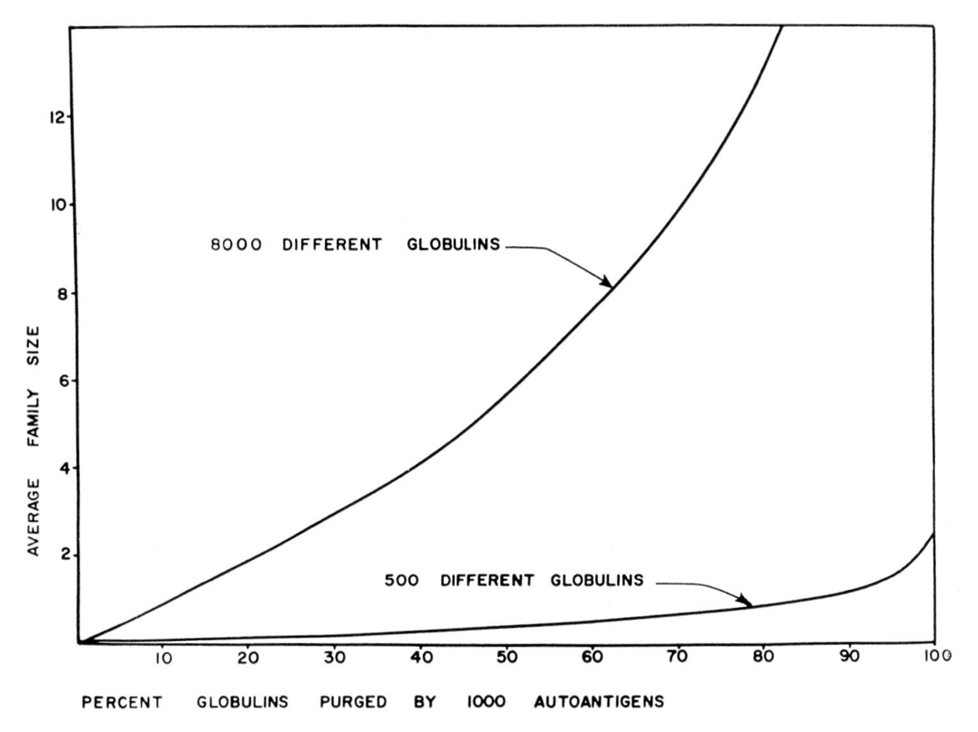

Fig. 6-8. The effect of purging by 1,000 autoantigens on information systems containing 500 and 8,000 different globulins.

It may be seen from Figure 6-8 that with 500 different globulins, less than 1 percent will be left if the average family size is near the optimal value of 3. However, approximately one-half of 8,000 globulins would be left at the optimal family size of 6.

At present it is impossible to set accurate values for any of the factors mentioned. The main value of approaching antibody specificity from the standpoint of information theory is that it illustrates the relationships of these various factors. It also states explicitly the biological advantage of a large as compared to a small number of different globulins.

The figure which is most likely to be determined from direct experimental observation is the average family size. When this is known, the order of magnitude of the other factors can then be estimated.

REFERENCES

1. Pasteur, L. *C. R. Acad. Sci.* (Paris) 90:247, 1880.
2. Chauveau, A. *C. R. Acad. Sci.* (Paris). *Ibid.,* p. 1526.
3. Ehrlich, P. On immunity with special reference to cell life. *Proc. Roy. Soc.* [*Biol.*] 66:424, 1900.
4. Landsteiner, K. *Die Spezifizität der serologischen Reaktionen.* Berlin: J. Springer, Verlag, 1933.
5. Breinl, F., and Haurowitz, F. Chemische Untersuching des Präzipitates aus Hämoglobin und Anti-Hämoglobin-Serum und Bemerkungen über die Natur der Antikörper. *Z. Physiol. Chem.* 192:45, 1930.
6. Alexander, J. Some intracellular aspects of life and disease. *Protoplasma* 14:296, 1932.
7. Mudd, S. A hypothetical mechanism of antibody formation. *J. Immun.* 23:423, 1932.
8. Pauling, L. A theory of the structure and process of formation of antibody. *J. Amer. Chem. Soc.* 62:2643, 1940.
9. Karush, F. Specificity of antibodies. *Trans. N.Y. Acad. Sci.* 20:581, 1958.
10. Nossal, G. J. V., and Mäkelä, O. Elaboration of antibodies by single cells. *Ann. Rev. Microbiol.* 16:53, 1962.
11. Burnet, F. M., and Fenner, F. *The Production of Antibodies.* London: Macmillan & Company, 1941.
12. Burnet, F. M., and Fenner, F. *Ibid.* (2nd ed.), 1949.
13. Burnet, F. M. *Enzyme, Antigen and Virus.* London: Cambridge University Press, 1956.
14. Schweet, R., and Owen, R. D. Concepts of protein synthesis in relation to antibody formation. *J. Cell. Comp. Physiol.* 50(supp. 1): 199, 1957.
15. Goldstein, D. J. Theoretical mechanisms of immunological tolerance. *Ann. Allerg.* 18:1081, 1960.
16. Jerne, N. K. The natural selection theory of antibody formation. *Proc. Nat. Acad. Sci. U.S.A.* 41:849, 1955.
17. Talmage, D. W. Allergy and immunology. *Ann. Rev. Med.* 8:239, 1957.
18. Burnet, F. M. A modification of Jerne's theory of antibody production using the concept of clonal selection. *Aust. J. Sci.* 20:67, 1957.
19. Burnet, F. M. *The Clonal Selection Theory of Acquired Immunity.* London: Cambridge University Press; and Nashville, Tenn.: Vanderbilt University Press, 1959.
20. Lederberg, J. Genes and antibodies. *Science* 129:1649, 1959.
21. Talmage, D. W. Immunological specificity. *Ibid.,* p. 1643.
22. Monod, J. Antibodies and Induced Enzymes. In Lawrence, H. S. (Ed.), *Cellular and Hormonal Aspects of the Hypersensitive State.* New York: Paul B. Hoeber, Inc., 1959.
23. Boyden, S. V. Antibody production. *Nature* (London) 185:724, 1960.
24. Segre, D., and Kaeberle, M. L. The immunologic behavior of baby pigs. *J. Immun.* 89:782 and 790, 1962.
25. Davenport, F. M., Hennessy, A.V., and Francis, T. Epidemiologic and immunologic significance of age distribution of antibody to antigenic variants of influenza virus. *J. Exp. Med.* 98:641, 1953.
26. Dubert, J. M. *Thèses à la Faculté des Sciènćes de l'Université de Paris.* Paris: Editions Cluron, 1959.
27. Harris, T. M., Harris, S., and Farber, M. B. Transfer to x-irradiated rabbits of lymph node cells incubated "in vitro" with *Shigella paradysenteriae. Proc. Soc. Exp. Biol. Med.* 86:549, 1954.
28. Roberts, J. C., and Dixon, F. J. The transfer of lymph node cells in the study of the immune response to foreign proteins. *J. Exp. Med.* 102:379, 1955.
29. Talmage, D. W., Freter, G. G., and Thomson, A. The effect of whole body x-radiation on the specific anamnestic response in the rabbit. *J. Infect. Dis.* 99:246, 1956.
30. Perkins, E. H., Robinson, M. A., and Makino-

dan, T. Agglutination response, a function of cell number. *J. Immun.* 86:533, 1961.

31. Attardi, G., Cohn, M., Horibata, K., and Lennox, E. S. The analysis of antibody synthesis at the cellular level. *Bact. Rev.* 23:213, 1959.
32. Nossal, G. J. V. Antibody production by single cells. *Brit. J. Exp. Path.* 41:89, 1960.
33. Boyer, G. Chorioallantoic membrane lesions produced by inoculation of adult fowl leucocytes. *Nature* (London) 185:327, 1960.
34. Burnet, M., and Burnet, D. Graft versus host reactions on the chorioallantoic membrane of the chick embryo. *Nature* (London) 188:376, 1960.
35. Simonsen, M. The impact on the developing embryo and newborn animal of adult homologous cells. *Acta Path. Microbiol. Scand.* 40:480, 1957.
36. Burnet, F. M. Cellular aspects of immunology as manifested in the Simonsen reaction. *Yale J. Biol. Med.* 34:207, 1961.
37. Flickinger, R. A. Cell differentiation: Some aspects of the problem. *Science* 141:608, 1963.
38. Mackay, J. R., and Burnet, F. M. *Autoimmune Diseases, Pathogenesis, Chemistry, and Therapy.* Springfield, Ill.: Charles C Thomas, Publisher, 1963.
39. Miller, J. F. A. P. Immunological significance of the thymus of the adult mouse. *Nature* (London) 195:1318, 1962.
40. Claman, H. N., and Talmage, D. W. Thymectomy: Prolongation of immunological tolerance in the adult mouse. *Science* 141:1193, 1963.
41. Nossal, G. J. V., and Mäkelä, O. Autoradiographic studies on the immune response. *J. Exp. Med.* 115:209, 1962.
42. Gowans, J. L., Gesner, B. M., and McGregor, D. D. In Wolstenholme, G. E. W., and O'Connor, M. (Eds.), *The Immunologic Activity of Lymphocytes,* Ciba Foundation Study Group No. 10. Boston: Little, Brown, 1961.
43. Gowans, J. L., McGregor, D. D., and Cowen, D. M. Initiation of immune responses by small lymphocytes. *Nature* (London) 196:651, 1962.
44. Talmage, D. W., and Claman, H. N. Cell Potential—Its Mutation and Selection. In Good, R. A., and Gabrielsen, A. E. (Eds.), *The Thymus in Immunobiology.* New York: Paul B. Hoeber, Inc., 1964.
45. Dresser, D. W. Specific inhibition of antibody production. *Immunology* 5:161 and 378, 1962.
46. Claman, H. N. Tolerance to a protein antigen in adult mice. *J. Immun.* 91:833, 1963.
47. Crowle, A. J. Immunologic unresponsiveness induced in hypersensitive mice. *J. Allerg.* 34:504, 1963.
48. Katsh, G. F., Talmage, D. W., and Katsh, S. Acceptance or rejection of male skin grafts by isologous female mice: Effect of injection of sperm. *Science* 143:41, 1964.
49. Watson, J. D. Involvement of RNA in the synthesis of proteins. *Science* 140:17, 1963.
50. Szilard, L. The molecular basis of antibody formation. *Proc. Nat. Acad. Sci. U.S.A.* 46:293, 1960.
51. Talmage, D. W., and Pearlman, D. S. The antibody response: A model based on antagonistic actions of antigen. *J. Theor. Biol.* 5:321, 1963.
52. Ipsen, J. Differences in primary and secondary immunizability of inbred mice strains. *J. Immun.* 83:448, 1959.
53. Rothberg, R., and Talmage, D. W. Circulating antibody and anaphylaxis in mice. *J. Immun.* 86:302, 1961.
54. Farr, R. S., Grey, H. M., Dickenson, W., and Rosenstein, D. H. Genetic influences of antibovine albumin (BSA) produced in mice. *Fed. Proc.* 22:265, 1963.
55. Sang, J. H., and Sobey, W. R. The genetic control of response to antigenic stimuli. *J. Immun.* 72:52, 1954.
56. Mannik, M., and Kunkel, H. G. Two major types of normal 7S gamma-globulin. *J. Exp. Med.,* 117:213, 1963.
57. Jaroslow, B. N., and Quastler, H. Antigenic specificity. In Yockey, H. (Ed.), *Symposium on Information Theory in Biology.* New York: Pergamon Press, 1958.
58. Jerne, N. K. Immunological speculations. *Ann. Rev. Microbiol.* 14:341, 1960.

7. The Suppression of Immune Responses by Nonspecific Agents

JOHN H. HUMPHREY

IN THIS CHAPTER WILL BE CONSIDERED some of the various ways in which it is possible to suppress the capacity of animals to respond to antigens, in terms either of antibody production or of delayed type hypersensitivity, by agents which are nonspecific in the sense that they may apply more or less equally to any antigen. They include x-rays, radiomimetic drugs, and antimetabolites and for convenience will be referred to collectively as immunosuppressive agents. In theory such procedures as thymectomy and bursectomy could also be included under this heading but will be omitted since they are discussed in Chapter 4. Specific immunological unresponsiveness (tolerance or paralysis) produced by administration of antigen to newborn or adult *normal* animals also will not be considered except where the induction of such unresponsiveness depends upon the temporary general suppression of immunological response by x-rays or drugs.

THE PURPOSE OF SUPPRESSING IMMUNE RESPONSES

The discovery that antibody production could be suppressed by a sufficient dose of x-rays appeared, at first, to be of purely theoretical interest. The idea that dangerous or annoying allergic conditions might be treated this way was considered, but on the whole dismissed because the immune response was regarded as being largely beneficial, and indeed essential to survival. However, with the recognition of crippling autoimmune diseases and of the immunological basis of homograft reactions, coupled with the realization that tolerance could be induced to certain specific antigens while the response to others remained largely unimpaired, there has been a sharp change of attitude. We are now witnessing an intensive search for means of suppressing immune responses by agents which can achieve this without excessively damaging other vital functions such as hemopoiesis and epithelial regeneration. Broadly, the main aims are twofold: (1) To suppress the immune response reversibly, for a limited but possibly prolonged period of time, e.g., during the course of an autoimmune disease or while a homograft is becoming established. Ideally, during this period a state of complete or partial tolerance should be produced to the relevant antigens (either autoantigens or graft antigens). (2) To destroy the capacity to produce an immune response permanently and completely. All the treatments known to accomplish this also destroy the hemopoietic capacity, and the latter must be restored by grafting hemopoietic cells from another animal (or preserved cells taken from the animal before treatment). There is no problem of a host-versus-graft reaction from the foreign hematopoietic cells, and such chimeric animals are readily obtained. However, since the chimera cannot exist indefinitely with its capacity to give an immune response permanently impaired, the graft must also include immunologically competent cells. Unless these are isogenic with the host they are likely to give rise to the graft-versus-host reaction (see Chaps. 13 and 21). In certain circumstances, however, the immune responses of the graft cells can also be temporarily suppressed so that tolerance of the host results, and this problem comes under category (1) above.

THE VULNERABLE STAGES OF IMMUNE RESPONSES

It is far from fully understood how immunosuppressive agents work, nor is such understanding likely until more is known about the fundamental mechanisms whereby antigens stimulate the cellular proliferation and differentiation which result in antibody production. However, a possible rational approach is to consider certain stages of the immune response at which nonspecific agents might be able to interfere. For this purpose schematic and simplified outlines of these stages as they occur in lymph nodes draining the site of antigen administration in primary and secondary antibody responses and in predominantly delayed-type responses will be given. The evidence on which these schemes are based comes partly from work done in our laboratory [1, 2] and partly from that of others (e.g., Ref. 3–7). If the schemes differ in detail from those put forward in other chapters this need occasion the reader no alarm, since they are intended primarily as an aid to the interpretation of the theme of this chapter.

It will be seen that in each response there is a stage which involves cell division, with concomitant synthesis of new desoxyribonucleic acid (DNA) and the ribonucleic acid (RNA) necessary to provide the mechanism for rapid protein synthesis. In the two primary responses there is also an inductive phase, during which the previously unstimulated immunologically competent cells are in some way altered by contact with antigen (or a derivative of it) so as to change to an active immature stem cell (hemocytoblast). This stage

STAGES IN PRIMARY ANTIBODY RESPONSE

LATENT OR INDUCTIVE PHASE

Unstimulated *immunologically competent cell* (? lymphocyte, ? blast cell, ? reticulum cell) at suitable stage in its life cycle—probably in prophase.

(contact with antigen or product of interaction of antigen with macrophage)

↓

hemocytoblast (stimulated immature cell)

PROLIFERATIVE AND PRODUCTIVE PHASE

(via one or more rapid cell divisions. Antibody-forming capacity becomes apparent in hemocytoblasts at the end of the period of DNA synthesis before final division)

Persisting 'blast' or reticulum cell (involved in immunological memory and perhaps making antibody at a very low level)

immature plasma cells—synthesize and secrete antibody

(probably without further cell division)

↓

mature plasma cells—synthesize and secrete antibody

STAGES IN SECONDARY ANTIBODY RESPONSE

Stages similar to those in the primary response occur, in which previously unstimulated immunologically competent cells are involved. In addition, the persisting 'blast' cells are stimulated by antigen to divide rapidly, without passing through a similar latent phase. The capacity to make large amounts of antibody again appears at the end of the period of DNA synthesis, and the daughter immature plasma cells are already secreting antibody.

STAGES IN PRIMARY RESPONSE LEADING TO DELAYED-TYPE HYPERSENSITIVITY

LATENT OR INDUCTIVE PHASE

Unstimulated *immunologically competent cell* (? lymphocyte)

(contact with antigen or hapten-protein conjugate)

↓

stimulated immature cell (*hemocytoblast*) in lymph node (via one or more rapid cell divisions)

persisting 'blast' or reticulum cell ← – – – *sensitized lymphocyte*

↘

circulation to blood and other lymph nodes

(N.B.: A concomitant stimulation of antibody synthesis usually also occurs. This is omitted from this scheme.)

presumably involves synthesis of new RNA but not necessarily of new DNA. Evidence of the existence of this stage has been discussed, among others, by Sterzl [7] and Makinodan and Albright [6]. The ultimate effector cells, plasma cells or sensitized lymphocytes, require no further cell division and may be sufficiently equipped with specific RNA to continue their function without much further RNA synthesis.

From these schemes it might be predicted, being wise by hindsight, that agents which interfere with synthesis of new DNA or RNA would be able to block immune responses, except perhaps at the very last stages.

ESTABLISHMENT OF IMMUNOLOGICAL UNRESPONSIVENESS

It is known that antigens introduced into animals during or before the neonatal period may readily produce a state of specific immunological unresponsiveness which can last indefinitely so long as contact with the antigen is repeated. The phenomenon has been recently reviewed [8, 9]. It is now recognized that in adult animals also the introduction of sufficient quantities of antigen may lead to a state of specific immunological unresponsiveness or "paralysis," but the amounts of antigen required to do this vary conspicuously with the nature of the antigen and the species of animal [8]. There appear to be no valid grounds for making any fundamental distinction between immunological tolerance induced in the newborn and paralysis induced in the adult, although the latter may require such large amounts of certain antigens as to be virtually impossible to achieve in normal animals. It is outside the scope of this chapter to attempt to explain how specific unresponsiveness comes about, but it can be stated as an empirical observation that when antigens are introduced into adult animals while they are subjected to procedures which reduce nonspecifically their capacity to give immune responses, amounts of antigens which would normally immunize cause instead a subsequent state of specific immunological unresponsiveness. In other words, the smaller the total number of immunologically competent cells, the smaller the amount of antigen required to produce immunological paralysis. This observation implies that such paralysis must depend on something more than the achievement and maintenance of a sufficient concentration of antigen in the environment of the immunologically competent cells [10]. It also implies that if the number of such cells is diminished by means of immunosuppressive agents, tolerance may be achieved in circumstances where it would otherwise not have been possible.

IMMUNOSUPPRESSIVE AGENTS

With the general background in mind we may consider some agents which have been found to suppress immune responses.

X-RAY IRRADIATION

Supralethal Doses. The fact that sufficient doses of whole body radiation could suppress the antibody response to antigens injected shortly afterward has been recognized for many years [11]. Because x-rays in high doses destroy the capacity of most cells to divide, including not only immunologically competent cells but hemopoietic cells and the lining cells of the intestinal mucous membrane—producing in fact radiation sickness and death—it was not possible until recent years to study the long-term effect of lethal doses of radiation on the antibody response. However, since the development of antibiotics and of techniques for transfusing hemopoietic tissues from animals of identical genetic constitution (isogenic) or of the same or a very closely related species (allogenic), it has become possible to maintain alive for a long time animals which have received an otherwise lethal dose of whole body radiation. (The fact that the whole body is irradiated must be stressed, since if parts of the animal such as the bone marrow, spleen, or appendix are shielded during irradiation they act as sources of cells from which the bone marrow and lymphoid tissues are rapidly repopulated [12].) Between 900 and 1,200 r is a suitable supralethal dose for such studies in most species. At higher doses, and sometimes at these, death is likely to occur from radiation sickness, pulmonary edema and electrolyte imbalance, despite transfusion of hemopoietic tissues.

Lethal doses of x-rays of the order mentioned must destroy the host's capacity to give an immune response, since long-term acceptance of grafted cells is the rule; in fact, unless these cells repopulated the host it could not survive. There is evidence that at the lower doses of radiation within the lethal range small numbers of host hemopoietic cells (and also leukemic cells) may survive and gradually repopulate the host, partially replacing the grafted cells [13]. When this occurs the surviving host cells are probably tolerant of the grafted cells, and vice versa. More usually the grafted cells colonize the hemopoietic and/or lymphoid tissues of the host completely, and, except in isogenic animals, there commonly arise complications due to graft-versus-host reactions by these cells. Attempts, sometimes successful for prolonged periods, have been made to control such graft-versus-host reactions by previous x-ray treatment of the graft [14] or by treatment with immunosuppressive drugs of the type discussed later [15, 16].

Sublethal Doses. When sublethal doses of x-rays are used (550-300 r) the immunological response to many antigens is depressed for long periods but not, in general, permanently. The situation in experimental animals has been reviewed by Taliaferro [17] and by Makinodan and Gengozian [18]. Most complete studies have been made on the antibody response in rabbits and mice to red cell antigens, but the results of these and of more limited studies with protein antigens are in general agreement. Generalization may therefore be permissible, although obviously the length of time during which any antigenic stimulus acts will be an important variable.

The main relevant cytological changes in lymphoid tissues following irradiation with less than 1 LD_{50} are inhibition of mitosis and disintegration of lymphocytes in the first few hours, followed by a period of phagocytosis of debris which is complete within twenty-four hours. There is next a period of inactivity, whose duration depends on the amount of radiation but may last for a week or more. Finally there is a period of active mitosis and proliferation of lymphoblasts, so that lymphoid tissue is restored fairly completely after three to four weeks. Macrophages, reticulum cells, and Hassal's corpuscles of the thymus are little damaged at these levels of irradiation.

The changes in immunological responsiveness can be summarized as follows:

Primary Responses to Irradiation. 1. The primary response is depressed, and may be abolished, when antigen is given 12 hours to 50 days after irradiation. Depression is manifested by a greatly delayed appearance of antibody and lower peak levels. The effect is greatest when antigen is given 24 to 48 hours after x-ray irradiation.

2. When antigen is given shortly before or a few hours after irradiation, the antibody response is delayed, but there is no constant change in peak levels compared with unirradiated controls.

3. When antigen is given more than 2 days before irradiation, there may be a delayed onset and slower rise in antibody production, but the peak level may be higher and the total amount of antibody formed is increased.

4. When large amounts of protein antigens are given during the phase of immunological depression following 400 or, better, 500 r, long-lasting specific unresponsiveness to these antigens may result [19, 20].

Secondary Responses to Irradiation. The secondary response is relatively resistant compared with the primary, and, regardless of the time relationship of antigen injection to x-ray irradiation, the peak levels of antibody are much the same. However, the interval between antigen administration and the appearance of antibody is lengthened. This is most pronounced when antigen is given during the twenty-four hours immediately preceding irradiation but is noticeable for up to two weeks afterward. Nevertheless the antibody response to a given standard secondary antigenic stimulus given during this period is prolonged and the total amount of antibody produced is actually increased.

Explanation of the Action of X-rays. In terms of the schemes outlined earlier, it is possible to produce a plausible, though undoubtedly superficial, explanation of the action of x-rays. Very large doses act by destroying both unstimulated immunologically competent cells and "memory" cells and preventing their regeneration. Smaller doses destroy most of the immunologically competent cells, although these are slowly regenerated. The induction of an immune response is thereby prevented or, after less drastic treatment, greatly delayed since even surviving cells do not multiply for some time. To explain the time relationships it must be assumed that once the process of antibody production has begun, and the initial stage of cell differentiation and perhaps the first mitosis is over, the cells now set upon the path of antibody formation are relatively radioresistant. This explanation has been advanced by Dixon and McConahey [21] to explain why primary antibody production may be greatly increased when 500 r is administered at a suitable time interval *after* the antigen. They suppose that the antigen-stimulated cells are able to multiply disproportionately and colonize the lymphoid tissue depleted of other cells by x-ray treatment. If memory cells are also relatively radioresistant (as already mentioned, reticulum cells appear to be so), a similar explanation probably applies to the increased secondary responses.

RADIOMIMETIC DRUGS

The term radiomimetic is applied to drugs whose general biological action resembles that of x-rays, although the detailed mechanisms whereby they act may be different and varied. In general they fall into the class of alkylating agents, which interfere with cell division by combining with DNA. It was shown long ago [22] that mustard gas administered to rabbits or dogs shortly before or simultaneously with (but not after) foreign red cells would delay and depress the antibody response. The depression, however, was only temporary and antibodies appeared after two to three weeks. Various nitrogen mustards studied since then appear to act similarly. At sublethal doses their effects resemble those of x-rays, insofar as they delay and depress rather than abolish the antibody response. The most interesting such agent at present appears to be cyclophosphamide, since it has been claimed in toxic but nonlethal doses to suppress immune responses in certain species more effectively than correspondingly toxic doses of x-rays and to do so even when first administered up to three days after the antigen [2, 23]. In general, immunosuppression lasts only during the period of administration of the drug, and responsiveness returns soon after this is stopped. However, there is evidence [24] that in guinea pigs a relatively lasting state of unresponsiveness can be produced by a moderately large dose of ovalbumin administered at the beginning of drug treatment. When Turk and Stone [2] examined the lymph nodes of guinea pigs draining the site of application of a chemical sensitizing agent, they found that cyclophosphamide completely prevented the cellular changes associated with the development of delayed type hypersensitivity. However, these changes occurred when drug treatment was stopped. Doses sufficient to effect immunosuppression also cause marked anemia and leukocytopenia.

CORTICOSTEROIDS

Cortisone, dehydrocortisone, and similar corticosteroids are used extensively in practice to depress immunological responses, but their mode of action is still a mystery. These drugs (referred to here for convenience collectively as cortisone) possess a powerful general anti-inflammatory activity; i.e., they markedly diminish the cellular invasion and accompanying tissue damage, irrespective of whether these are due to antigen-antibody reactions, delayed type hypersensitivity, or nonspecific irritants. It is possible that such activity is associated with the demonstrated capacity of these hormones to make cell lysosomes more resistant to agents which cause release of lysosomal enzymes [25]. In any event, by their anti-inflammatory action corticosteroids can undoubtedly minimize the pathogenic consequences of unwanted immunological responses. The extent to which they also cause actual suppression of the responses themselves is less certain.

Cortisone in large (toxic) doses causes lymphopenia and pronounced lymphocyte depletion in the lymphoid tissues of rabbits, rats, and mice. It is probable that in these species there is actual destruction of lymphocytes, and indeed a cytotoxic action of cortisone on lymphocytes has been demonstrated *in vitro* [26]. The mechanism whereby this occurs is not known. The effect of such large doses on the antibody response was reviewed some years ago [27, 28]. Both primary and secondary responses are diminished, and in respect to the timing of antigen administration relative to cortisone treatment the effect of this drug resembles that of moderate doses of x-rays [17].

Man, monkey, and the guinea pig are, however, relatively resistant to cortisone compared with the species mentioned [29], and in man ordinary therapeutic doses do not seem to diminish the antibody response [30], nor do they cause more than a transitory lymphopenia. Nevertheless large doses administered to patients with lymphatic leukemia have been found to lower the lymphocyte count, sometimes for long periods, and it must be assumed that sufficient cortisone can inhibit lymphopoiesis and perhaps in this way diminish immunological responses.

ANTIMETABOLITES

In the search for agents which will inhibit neoplasms, especially leukemias, a wide variety of substances have been tested which have in common the property of interfering with the synthesis of DNA or RNA, and thereby preventing cell division or new protein synthesis. The various agents found to have a sufficiently selective toxicity for rapidly dividing tumor cells to warrant clinical use exert their effects on several different biochemical pathways. Their modes of action were reviewed recently [31, 32]. Because immunological responses also involve a stage of rapid cell division, certain of these agents have been tested for their capacity to inhibit such responses and have shown considerable promise. It must be emphasized, however, that there are marked and unpredicted variations in their effects in different animal species and that generalizations from one to another are liable to be invalid. Some examples of different classes of antimetabolites will be discussed.

6-Mercaptopurine and Thioguanine (2-amino-6-mercaptopurine). Although the mode of action of these purine analogues has not been fully elucidated, a combination of studies on bacterial and mammalian cells, including resistant mutants, indicates that a necessary first step is conversion to the ribotide by an enzyme nucleotide pyrophosphorylase. The ribotides can block the interconversion of nucleotides within the cell, so that they could inhibit the synthesis of nucleic acids or of purine-containing enzymes, or of both. In sufficient doses the drugs depress bone marrow function severely, but in the rabbit they seem to have an even greater inhibitory action on the hemocytoblasts which are stimulated by antigen or on their precursor cells. There are striking differences among species in their tolerance of the drugs. Chickens and guinea pigs, for example, will stand relatively enormous doses (50 mg. per kg. daily or more), whereas rabbits may die at a dose level of 18 mg. per kg. if this is kept up for more than a few days. Such differences may be due to the presence in guinea pig bone marrow of an effective xanthine oxidase, which detoxifies 6-mercaptopurine (6-MP) by converting it to thiouric acid. Even between 6-MP and thioguanine there are pronounced but unexplained differences, for thioguanine is too toxic to use in rabbits [33], whereas in man there is little to choose between them. Such species differences may well account for apparently inconsistent findings by different workers.

Single large doses of 6-MP in mice can depress and delay primary antibody responses and significantly prolong the life of skin homografts if the drug is given simultaneously with or up to three or four days after the antigenic stimulus [34]. This timing contrasts with that of x-rays and radiomimetic drugs, which must be given before the antigen in order to be effective. Most studies have been made on animals given the drugs daily for a fortnight or even longer. In adult rabbits given 3 to 6 mg. 6-MP per kg. per day, antibody production to bovine or human serum albumin (BSA or HSA) is suppressed, provided that the drug is given from the day of antigen administration and is continued long enough. If it is stopped too soon, antibody production is delayed but eventually takes place, presumably because antigen is still present when the effect of the drug has worn off. At this dose level there is no evident effect on established antibody synthesis and little effect on a secondary response [35]. At higher levels (12 to 18 mg./kg. daily), however, even secondary responses to BSA can be prevented in rabbits [36]. More important, it now seems clear that complete, or almost complete, long-lasting specific immunological unresponsiveness can be produced in adult rabbits when antigens such as BSA are administered for the first time at the start of an intensive course of 6-MP [37, 20]. The proportion of rabbits which remain unresponsive after the drug is stopped increases sharply with the amount of antigen given, and quite large amounts (of the order of 70 mg. BSA/kg.) are required to obtain tolerance regularly [37]. Doses of 6-MP which prevent immune responses completely prevent the usual cytological changes in lymphoid tissue which follow antigenic stimulation. When a response occurs, despite drug treatment, it is characterized by an exaggerated outburst of blast cells, which are probably derived from drug-resistant clones [33].

In the guinea pig 6-MP can inhibit the development of delayed type hypersensitivity, even though antibody production may be little affected, and can delay the onset of or even suppress experimental allergic encephalomyelitis [38] or immune thyroiditis [39]. In man 6-MP and thioguanine, without combination with other drugs, have produced remissions, sometimes of long duration, in a proportion of patients with autoimmune hemolytic anemia [40].

Folic Acid Antagonists. The amino and aminoethyl pteroylglutamic acid derivatives aminopterin and amethopterin interfere with the conversion of folic acid to the active form tetrahydrofolic acid (folinic acid) by the enzyme dihydrofolic acid reductase. Synthesis of purines and of thymine requires folinic acid, and thus folic acid antagonists may prevent formation of new nucleic acid and inhibit mitosis (unless the cell already produces too much of the enzyme to be inhibited). These drugs, in doses which are reasonably well tolerated, have a marked suppressive effect on immune responses in guinea pigs, mice, and dogs but little or none in rabbits. Guinea pigs can withstand prolonged treatment with quite large amounts of amethopterin (10 to 15 mg./kg. on alternate days) without showing bone marrow depression or even lymphopenia. At this dose level antibody production, the development of delayed type hypersensitivity, and the production of experimental autoimmune diseases are prevented [41, 42, 39]. The effects are temporary, and, if the antigen is still present, delayed type hypersensitivity at least returns. (The effect on antibody production following large doses of antigens has not been reported, and it is not known whether tolerance can be produced by such means.) By transferring lymph node cells from amethopterin-treated (unresponsive) donors to untreated isogenic recipients, evidence has been obtained that the drug inhibits the proliferative rather than the inductive phase [43]. This agrees with observations on the cytological changes in lymph nodes draining skin painted with chemical sensitizers, in which it has been found that, unlike cyclophosphamide, amethopterin does not prevent the appearance of hemocytoblasts but appears to stop them from dividing further to give rise to sensitized lymphocytes [2].

In dogs amethopterin at lower doses (0.1 to 0.5 mg./kg. thrice weekly) can suppress antibody responses and greatly prolong homograft survival [44, 15]. In mice, at somewhat higher dose levels, not only was depression of the immune response produced to large amounts of allogeneic cells containing potent transplantation antigens but the mice would subsequently tolerate grafts containing these antigens [45].

OTHER IMMUNOSUPPRESSANT AGENTS

The agents discussed so far have been the subject of sufficient investigation for their activity to be considered established, at least in certain species. As a possible augury of things to come, we will mention briefly a few other agents for whose activities an apparently rational basis can be provided. Actinomycins C and D are extraordinarily potent inhibitors of RNA synthesis, by combining with and blocking DNA-primed RNA polymerase [46], and might be expected to interfere with immune responses. Actinomycin C has been used, apparently successfully, to reverse renal homograft rejection [47]. Azaserine (o-diazoacetyl-L-serine) and Duazomycin A (N-acetyl-6-diazo-5-oxo-L-norleucine) inhibit the biosynthesis of purines by interfering with the utilization of glutamine. Although in tolerated doses by themselves they are only moderately potent immunosuppressive agents, in combination with 6-MP they inhibit secondary antibody responses in rabbits almost completely [48]. It is not known whether or not immunological tolerance is also produced.

FUTURE OUTLOOK

The immunosuppressant agents discussed here undoubtedly hit at vital steps in the immunological response, but they do it indiscriminately and damage all dividing cells to a greater or lesser degree. For this reason they can, in general, be used only for limited periods of time. Even such limited use may be valuable to tide an animal over the most vulnerable stages in the establishment of a homograft, for example. So far as some agents, such as x-rays, cyclophosphamide, and 6-MP appear to be able to allow the establishment of specific immunological tolerance to antigens which are administered in sufficient quantities (and are not too foreign to the host), there is a hope that even temporary treatment with such agents will give a sufficiently permanent suppression of immune responses to be clinically useful both in homografting and in autoimmune diseases. Various combinations of treatments are being tested empirically, and it is possible that some will be found which still impair the immunological system while damaging less the body as a whole. The immune response, however, is not simply a matter of differentiation and division of immunologically competent cells. There must be something quite specific about the manner in which the antigen initiates these changes in the immune response or prevents them in immunological tolerance, although we are still woefully ignorant of the molecular mechanisms involved. It is probably not too much to hope that, with better understanding of these mechanisms, agents will be found which, though still immunologically nonspecific, can act selectively on some stage in them.

REFERENCES

1. Balfour, B. M., and Cooper, E. C. Morphological and kinetic studies of antibody-producing cells in rat lymph nodes. *Immunology* (in press).
2. Turk, J. L., and Stone, S. H. Implications of the Cellular Changes in Lymph Nodes during the Development and Inhibition of Delayed Type Hypersensitivity. In Amos, B., and Koprowski, H. (Eds.), *Cell-bound Antibodies.* Philadelphia: Wistar Institute Press, 1963.
3. White, R. G. The Relation of the Cellular Responses in Germinal Lymphocytopoietic Centres of Lymph Nodes to the Production of Antibody. In Holub, M., and Jarošková, L. (Eds.), *Mechanisms of Antibody Formation.* Prague: Publishing House of Czechoslovak Academy of Sciences; and New York: Academic Press, Inc., 1960.
4. Gowans, J. L., McGregor, D. D., Cowen, D. M., and Ford, C. E. Initiation of immune responses by small lymphocytes. *Nature* (London) 196:651, 1962.
5. Nossal, G. J. V. Genetic studies on immunologically competent cells. *Advances Immun.* 2:163, 1962.
6. Makinodan, T., and Albright, J. F. Cytokinetics of Antibody Response. In Grabar, P., and Miescher, P. A. (Eds.). *Immunopathology* (3rd International Symposium). Basel: Benno Schwabe & Co., 1963.
7. Sterzl, J. Quantitative and qualitative aspect of the inductive phase of antibody formation. *J. Hyg. Epidem.* (Praha) 7:301, 1963.
8. Smith, R. T. Immunological tolerance of nonliving antigens. *Advances Immun.* 1:67, 1961.
9. Hasek, M., Langerová, A., and Hrouba, T. Transplantation immunity and tolerance. *Ibid.*, p. 1.
10. Humphrey, J. H. Acquired Tolerance after Treatment by Physical or Chemical Agents. In Bussard, A. (Ed.), *La Tolérance Acquise et la Tolérance Naturelle à l'Égard de Substances Antigéniques Définies.* Paris: Centre National de la Réchèrches Scientifique, 1963.
11. Benjamin, E., and Sluka, E. Antikörperbildung nach experimentelle Schähdigung des hämatopoietischen Systems durch Röntgenstrahlen. *Wien. Klin. Woschr.* 21:311, 1908.
12. Süssdorf, D. H., and Draper, L. R. The primary hemolysin response in rabbits following shielding from x-rays or x-irradiation of the spleen, appendix, liver or hind legs. *J. Infect. Dis.* 99:129, 1956.
13. Thomas, E. D. Bone Marrow Transplantation in Man. In *Diagnosis and Treatment of Acute Radiation Injury.* Geneva: World Health Organization, 1961.
14. Argyris, B. F. Elimination of runt disease and induction of acquired tolerance by x-irradiated spleen cells. *Transplant. Bull.* 29:100, 1962.
15. Blumenstock, D. A., Collins, J. A., Hechtman, H. B., Thomas, E. D., and Ferrebee, J. W. Functioning homografts of the lung in dogs. *Ann. N.Y. Acad. Sci.* 99:882, 1962.
16. Mathé, G., Amiel, J. L., Schwarzenberg, L., Caltem, A., and Schneider, M. Haematopoietic chimera in man after allogeneic (homologous) bone-marrow transplantation. *Brit. Med. J.* 2:1633, 1963.
17. Taliaferro, W. H. Modification of the immune response by radiation and cortisone. *Ann. N.Y. Acad. Sci.* 69:745, 1957.
18. Makinodan, T., and Gengozian, N. X-ray Depression of the Recognition Mechanism of Antibody-Forming Cells. Ref. 3.
19. Weigle, W. O., and Dixon, F. J. Immunologic Unresponsiveness to Protein Antigens. In Shaffer, J. H., LoGroppo, G. A., and Chase, M. W. (Eds.), *Mechanisms of Hypersensitivity.* Boston: Little, Brown, 1959.
20. Nachtigal, D., and Feldman, M. Immunological unresponsiveness to protein antigens in rabbits exposed to x-irradiation and 6-mercaptopurine. *Immunology* 6:356, 1963.
21. Dixon, F. J., and McConahey, P. J. Enhancement of antibody formation by whole body radiation. *J. Exp. Med.* 117:833, 1963.
22. Hektoen, L., and Corper, H. J. Effect of mustard gas (dichloroethylsulphid) on antibody formation. *J. Infect. Dis.* 28:279, 1921.
23. Stender, H. S., Strauch, D., and Winter, H. Comparative studies on the inhibition of anti-

body production by x-rays and an N-mustard-phosphamide. *Strahlentherapie* 115:175, 1961.

24. Maguire, H. C., and Maibach, H. L. Specific immune tolerance to anaphylactic sensitization (egg albumin) in the guinea pig by cyclophoramide (cytoxan). *J. Allerg.* 32:406, 1961.
25. Weissman, G., and Thomas, L. Studies on lysosomes: I. The effects of endotoxin, endotoxin tolerance and cortisone on the release of acid hydrolases from a granular fraction of rabbit liver. *J. Exp. Med.* 116:433, 1962.
26. Feldman, J. D. *In vitro* reaction of cells to adrenal cortical steroids with special reference to lymphocytes. *Endocrinology* 46:552, 1950.
27. Fischel, E. E. Adrenal Hormones and the Development of Antibody and Hypersensitivity. In Schwartzman, G. S. (Ed.), *The Effect of ACTH and Cortisone upon Infection and Resistance.* New York: Columbia University Press, 1953.
28. Kass, E. H., and Finland, M. Adrenal cortical hormones in infection and immunity. *Ann. Rev. Microbiol.* 7:361, 1953.
29. Shewell, J., and Long, D. A. A species difference with regard to the effect of cortisone acetate on body weight, γ-globulin and circulating antitoxin levels. *J. Hyg.* (Cambridge) 54:452, 1956.
30. Mirick, G. S. The effects of ACTH and cortisone on antibodies in human beings. *Bull. Hopkins Hosp.* 88:332, 1951.
31. Henderson, J. F., and Mandel, H. G. Purine and pyrimidine antimetabolites in cancer chemotherapy. *Advances Pharmacol.* 2:297, 1963.
32. Schwartz, R. S. Alteration of Immunity by Antimetabolites. In *Conceptual Advances in Immunology and Onchology.* New York: Paul B. Hoeber, Inc., 1963.
33. André, J. A., Schwartz, R. S., Mitus, J. W., and Dameshek, W. The morphologic responses of the lymphoid system to homografts: II. The effect of antimetabolites. *Blood* 19:334, 1962.
34. Berenbaum, M. C. The effect of cytotoxic agents on the production of antibody to T.A.B. vaccine in the mouse. *Biochem. Pharmacol.* 11:29, 1962.
35. Schwartz, R., Eisner, A., and Dameshek, W. The effect of 6-MP on the primary and secondary immune response. *J. Clin. Invest.* 38: 1394, 1959.
36. La Plante, E. S., Condie, R. M., and Good, R. A. Prevention of secondary immune response with 6-mercaptopurine. *J. Lab. Clin. Med.* 59: 542, 1962.
37. Schwartz, R. S., and Dameshek, W. The role of antigen dosage in drug-induced immunologic tolerance. *J. Immun.* 90:703, 1963.
38. Hoyer, L. W., Good, R. A., and Condie, R. M. Experimental allergic encephalomyelitis: The effect of 6-mercaptopurine. *J. Exp. Med.* 116:311, 1962.
39. Spiegelberg, H. L., and Miescher, P. A. The effect of 6-mercaptopurine and aminopterin on experimental immune thyroiditis in guinea pigs. *J. Exp. Med.* 118:869, 1963.
40. Schwartz, R., and Dameshek, W. The treatment of auto-immune hemolytic anemia with 6-mercaptopurine and thioguanine. *Blood* 19: 483, 1962.
41. Friedman, R. M., Buckler, C. E., and Baron, S. The effect of aminomethylpteroylglutamic acid on the development of skin hypersensitivity and antibody formation in guinea pigs. *J. Exp. Med.* 114:173, 1961.
42. Brandriss, M. W. Methotrexate suppression of experimental allergic encephalomyelitis. *Science* 140:186, 1963.
43. Friedman, R. M., and Buckler, C. E. Methotrexate inhibition of tuberculin hypersensitivity in inbred guinea pigs. *J. Immun.* 91:846, 1963.
44. Thomas, E. D., Baker, J. A., and Ferrebee, J. W. The effect of methotrexate on the production of antibodies against distemper virus in the dog. *J. Immun.* 90:324, 1963.
45. Uphoff, D. E. Drug-induced immunological "tolerance" for homotransplantation. *Transplant. Bull.* 28:12, 1961.
46. Goldberg, I. H., and Rabinowitz, M. Actinomycin D inhibition of deoxyribonucleic acid-dependent synthesis of ribonucleic acid. *Science* 136:315, 1962.
47. Murray, J. E., Merrill, J. P., Harrison, J. H., Wilson, R. E., and Dammin, G. J. Prolonged survival of human-kidney homografts by immunosuppressive drug therapy. *New Eng. J. Med.* 268:1315, 1963.
48. Rosenberg, S., and Calabresi, P. Enhanced suppression of secondary immune response by combination of 6-mercaptopurine and "Duazomycin A." *Nature* (London) 199:1101, 1963.

8. Measurement of Antibody Production and Immune Responses*

DAVID W. TALMAGE AND HENRY N. CLAMAN

THE SUBJECT OF THIS CHAPTER IS the measurement of circulating antibody and the antibody responses to antigenic stimulation. There are many ways to measure antibody, and the characteristics of the response to antigen depend on the particular method used. We will describe first the principles and some general methods of antibody measurement, then attempt to evaluate critically the various types of response to antigen. Since this chapter is not intended to replace a laboratory manual, references are given which contain detailed descriptions of methods [1].

The *sine qua non* of antibody activity is the ability to combine specifically with antigen; measurements of antibody activity therefore involve measurements of combination with antigen and of the effects of this combination. Other measurements may be made, such as the size and structure of the antibody molecule, but these properties are not central to the definition of antibody activity and are discussed in Chapter 3. The reaction between antigen and antibody may occur *in vivo* or *in vitro* and may be quantitated by changes in concentrations of antigen, antibody, or antigen-antibody complexes or by some secondary phenomenon resulting from antigen-antibody interaction, such as agglutination of visible particles *in vitro* or anaphylaxis in the intact animal.

The various methods of measuring antibody may be divided arbitrarily into measurements of primary reactions and of secondary manifestations. The primary reactions involve determinations of free and bound antigen (or free and bound antibody). Because they disturb the processes of antigen-antibody interaction to a minimum and because of the precision permitted by well-defined conditions, some of these methods have been used to evaluate such immunochemical properties as the equilibrium and rate constants of the antigen-antibody interaction, and the valence of antigen and antibody. In the secondary reactions, a quantitation is made of some secondary manifestation of the antigen-antibody interaction. These methods have been extensively used to follow *in vivo* antibody production. A list of primary and secondary reactions appears in Table 8-1.

PRIMARY REACTIONS

Except in the study of the kinetics of antigen-antibody interaction, primary reactions are often carried out at equilibrium. The general nature of this equilibrium will be discussed to show what types of information it may give.

In its simplest form, the reaction between antigen and antibody may be written in the form of a reversible equation

$$\mathrm{Ag} + \mathrm{Ab} \rightleftharpoons \mathrm{AgAb}$$

The forward rate of reaction (V_1) equals the product of the concentrations of antigen (Ag) and antibody (Ab) multiplied by the rate constant of the forward reaction (k_1). In similar fashion, the velocity of the reaction to the left (V_2) equals the concentration of antigen-antibody complex (AgAb) times the rate constant of this reaction (k_2). By definition, the velocities of the forward and backward reactions are equal at equilibrium.

$$V_1 = k_1(\mathrm{Ag})(\mathrm{Ab}) = k_2(\mathrm{AgAb}) = V_2 \qquad (1)$$

By transposition

$$\frac{k_2}{k_1} = \frac{(\mathrm{Ag})(\mathrm{Ab})}{(\mathrm{AgAb})} = K \qquad (2)$$

* Supported by U.S. Public Health Service Grants No. AI 04152 and AI 03047.

TABLE 8-1. Methods of Antibody Measurement[a]

	Primary
Adsorption to paper	Virus neutralization
Equilibrium dialysis	Precipitation of globulin
Fluorescence quenching	Toxin neutralization
	Secondary
Precipitation	Immune disappearance [3]
Agglutination	Opsonization [4] and immune adherence [5]
Lysis	Anaphylaxis *in vitro* [6a] and *in vivo* [6b]
Complement fixation	Skin reactions [7]
Animal protection [2]	Histamine release [8]

[a] References suitable for the student and laboratory are given in brackets for methods not described in this chapter.

K is the equilibrium constant of the reaction. It may be expressed as the dissociation constant (K_D) as in its present form, or as the association constant (K_A), which is $\frac{1}{K_D}$.

The reaction takes place at antigen and antibody combining sites, and since there may be more than one such site on a molecule, it is most accurate to think in terms of the concentration of these sites. Free antigen sites may be designated (F) and bound antigen sites (B). The total concentration of antibody is (M), and the total concentration of antibody sites is (nM), where n is the valence of antibody. Since (B) is the concentration of bound antibody sites as well as bound antigen sites, then ($nM - B$) equals the concentration of free antibody sites. Equation (2) may be rewritten as

$$K_D = \frac{(F)(nM - B)}{(B)} \tag{3}$$

Solving for (B), which is the concentration of bound antigen, one obtains

$$(B) = nM - \frac{B}{F} K_D$$

This is a linear equation which shows that the concentration of bound antigen varies with the ratio of bound to free antigen. It is the equation of a straight line with a slope of $-K$. If measurements of B and F are made under conditions of constant antibody but varying antigen concentrations, B may be plotted against B/F. In extreme antigen excess, where $B/F \rightarrow 0$, the concentration of bound antigen equals nM, giving the concentration of antibody sites. If M is known, the plot yields the value of n, or the valence of antibody. The equilibrium constant obtained from the slope of the plot ($-K$) provides a measure of the average affinity of antigen for antibody. This method is valuable if either antigen or antibody is univalent. More detailed mathematical treatments are required if both antigen and antibody are multivalent [9].

ADSORPTION TO PAPER

Berson and Yalow [10] used the insulin-anti-insulin system and paper adsorption to study antigen-antibody interactions. In this method, varying amounts of I^{131}-insulin (univalent) were combined with varying amounts of antibodies to insulin. The mixtures were separated on chromatographic paper. Free insulin remained at the site of application because it was adsorbed to the paper, while antibody-bound insulin moved with the serum proteins. By use of I^{131}-tagged insulin, the amounts of bound and free insulin were determined. The graph of B/F versus B is shown in Figure 8-1. The slope of the line indicates that the equi-

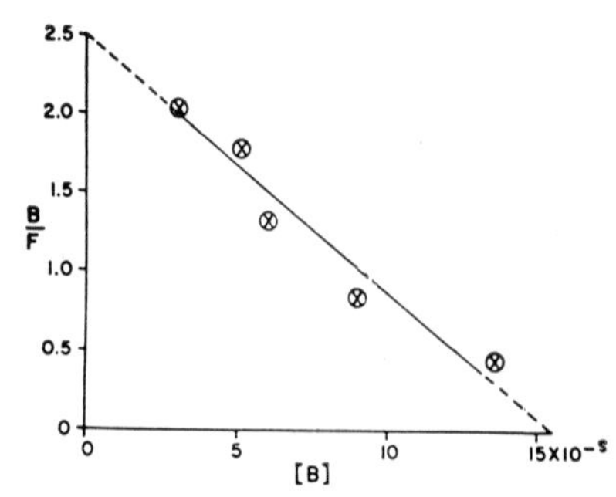

Fig. 8-1. A plot of the concentration of bound insulin (B) versus the ratio of bound to free insulin (B/F). (From Berson and Yalow [10].)

librium constant, K_D, is 6×10^{-9} moles per liter. This method is not often used, but it illustrates an application of the mathematical principles described earlier.

EQUILIBRIUM DIALYSIS

This method may be used if the antigen is small enough to diffuse freely through a membrane impervious to antibody globulin. Radioactive and dye-labeled haptens have been used [11]. In principle, a known concentration of antibody is placed on one side of a semipermeable membrane (usually inside a cellophane dialysis bag) and a known concentration of hapten on the other. Hapten then diffuses across the membrane. At equilibrium the concentration of free hapten is measured outside the membrane and is assumed to be equal on both sides of the membrane. Thus the amount bound to antibody may be calculated by subtracting the total free hapten on both sides from the total hapten added to the system at the beginning of the experiment. Because of nonspecific adsorption of haptens to other proteins and to the membrane, purified antibody must be used and correction made for adsorption to the membrane. If radioactively labeled haptens are used, this correction may be obviated since measurements of hapten may be made on both sides of the membrane.

FLUORESCENCE QUENCHING

This method is based on the facts that tryptophan residues of proteins will emit fluorescent energy when excited in the proper spectral range and that this energy yield is diminished when certain molecules attach to the protein. This change in fluorescence yield will occur if the adsorption spectrum of the attached molecule overlaps the emission spectrum of the protein; in these conditions a portion of the protein's energy of emission is transferred to the attached molecule, to be dissipated either as heat or at a different wavelength. The result is that the quantum fluorescence yield of the protein is diminished in proportion to the amount of molecular binding. The foregoing requirements are satisfied by antibody (emission maximum, 300 to 400 mμ). Thus the binding of hapten to antibody may be measured, giving values for B, B/F, n and K. Using this system, Velick *et al.* [12] concluded that the DNP-anti-DNP system involves antibody with 1.8 binding sites per molecule and a K_D of approximately 10^{-9} moles per liter.

The success of the system depends on purified antibody and is limited to haptens fulfilling the above spectral requirements.

VIRUS NEUTRALIZATION

Material to be assayed for virus-neutralizing antibody is incubated with virus, aliquots are removed at successive time intervals, and the fractions of surviving virus particles are determined. In the system using bacteriophage, each aliquot is mixed with host bacteria and plated on agar. A single phage particle produces a visible lytic plaque on the confluent growth of bacteria. The number of plaques and hence the number of free phage particles is easily counted [13]. Figure 8-2 shows a plot

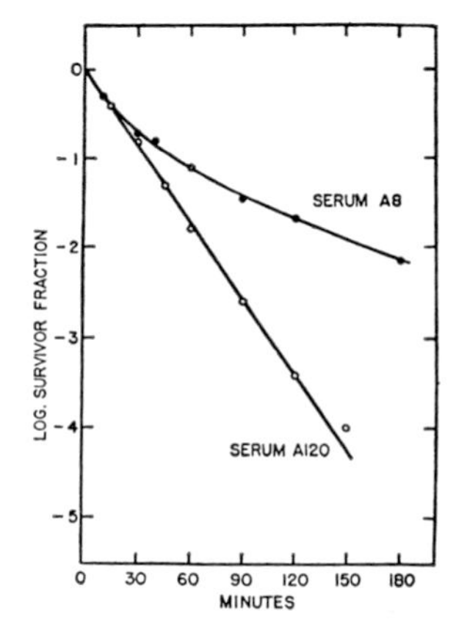

Fig. 8-2. Kinetics of neutralization of T-4 phage by two antisera obtained from early (serum A8) and late (serum A120) bleedings. Early antiserum is undiluted. Late antiserum is diluted 1/15,000. (From Jerne and Avegno [14].)

of the results of such an experiment in which the neutralization of virus follows an exponential path (serum A120) suggesting that a single antibody molecule is sufficient to neutralize one virus particle. The slope of the line is proportional to the antibody concentration, but an absolute measure of antibody concentration cannot be derived from these data. The method demonstrates clearly, however, that some samples of antibody (serum A8) show deviation from logarithmic neutralization. This suggests dissociation of virus from antibody and implies heterogeneity in the affinity between antigen and antibody. The affinity or avidity of antibody for antigen is frequently called the quality of the antibody, and Figure

8-2 shows that late or hyperimmune antibody (serum A120) has greater affinity for antigen than does early antibody [14].

This method has been used to determine antibody production in man and animals immunized with bacterial or animal viruses. In the case of animal viruses such as poliomyelitis and vaccinia, the method is similar in principle to that already described. Instead of bacteria, however, cultured cells or the chick chorioallantoic membrane is used as the host on which presence or absence of virus growth is visible [15]. Antiserum dilutions are either incubated with virus in a test tube or added at a fixed time interval after a standard amount of virus has been added to the host cells, and the number of free virus particles is estimated from virus growth. In this case the dilution of antiserum producing a given amount of virus neutralization (usually 50 percent) is used as a measure of antibody. Some virus antibody may only be detected by neutralization of virus in living animals, by using inhibition of death or illness as the end point. With certain viruses, particularly the influenza group, the presence of free virus can be quantitated by its capacity to agglutinate erythrocytes [16]. The amount of virus-neutralizing antibody is measured by the inhibition of this hemagglutination.

PRECIPITATION OF GLOBULIN

This method separates bound and free antigen by precipitating the globulins—and hence the antigen bound to antibody globulin—while leaving free antigen unprecipitated. The most specific method uses antiglobulin antiserum prepared in another species [17]. To measure human antibodies, for instance, one immunizes a rabbit with human γ-globulin (HGG). The rabbit anti-HGG is used to precipitate the HGG and the antigen bound to it from the antigen-antibody mixture. This method requires large quantities of expensive antiserum and freezes the antigen-antibody interaction too slowly to prevent some readjustment of the antigen-antibody equilibrium.

For practical purposes, 50 percent saturated $(NH_4)_2SO_4$ has been used to precipitate the globulin when the antigen is soluble in this reagent [18]. Antigen, usually an albumin, is labeled with radioactive iodine. Constant amounts of I*-antigen are added to varying dilutions of antiserum and incubated, $(NH_4)_2$-SO_4 is added to a concentration of 50 percent, and globulin together with bound I*-antigen is precipitated. The supernatant is separated, and the relative amount of I*-antigen in the precipitate compared with total I*-antigen added is calculated. The end point is generally taken to be that dilution of antiserum at which a constant fraction (usually 33 percent) of antigen is precipitated. This end point is reproducible to ± 10 percent. It must be noted that no direct measurement of antibody quantity is made: the test measures the ability of antiserum to bind antigen (antigen-binding capacity). This method may also be used to determine dissociation and rate constants of antigen-antibody interactions.

TOXIN NEUTRALIZATION

In this method, the amount of free antigen (toxin) is measured by its toxicity in living tissue, and the amount of antibody (antitoxin) by the neutralization of these toxic effects. A standard antitoxin is used as a reference, and a standard toxin is mixed both with aliquots of dilutions of this standard and with those of the unknown antiserum. After incubation, these toxin-antitoxin mixtures are tested *in vivo* either by lethality for guinea pigs or, more commonly, by intradermal injection into guinea pigs or rabbits. Carefully derived results permit estimates of free toxin concentration remaining in the mixture. Jerne [19] made important contributions concerning antibody avidity by this method.

SECONDARY MANIFESTATIONS

PRECIPITIN REACTIONS

When antigen is mixed with antiserum under certain conditions, a specific precipitate of insoluble antigen-antibody complexes may be formed. This reaction has been extensively investigated by Heidelberger, Kendall, Kabat, and others and is considered the cornerstone of quantitative immunology [20]. In this quantitative method, increasing amounts of antigen are added to replicate aliquots, each containing a constant amount of antiserum. The precipitates are allowed to form spontaneously and are spun down, washed, and their nitrogen content analyzed. If the antigen is a polysaccharide, the nitrogen content of the precipitate may be directly calculated. If the antigen itself contains nitrogen, the amount of antigen nitrogen in the precipitate is calculated from the difference between the antigen nitrogen added and that left in the supernatant.

If the antigen is not labeled in some way to permit the determination of its concentration in the supernatant, the assumption is frequently made that in the region of antibody excess all of the antigen is precipitated. This is approximately true in at least some antigen-antibody systems. The amount of antigen estimated to be in the precipitate is subtracted from the total nitrogen in the precipitate to give the antibody nitrogen precipitated. A typical result of such a series of measurements is shown in Figure 8-3.

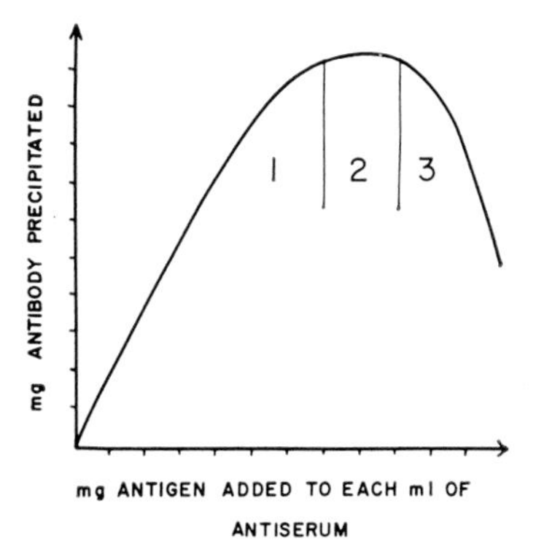

Fig. 8-3. The precipitin reaction. *Zone 1,* antibody excess; *zone 2,* equivalence (zone of maximum antibody precipitation); *zone 3,* antigen excess (soluble antigen-antibody complexes present). (Adapted from Raffel, S., *Immunity* [2nd ed.]. New York: Appleton-Century-Crofts, 1961.)

As increasing amounts of antigen are added, the amount of antibody nitrogen precipitated increases *(zone 1)* to a maximum *(zone 2)* and then decreases again *(zone 3)*. *Zone 1* is the region of antibody excess, while *zone 2* is the equivalence zone of maximal antigen-antibody precipitation.* *Zone 3* is the region of antigen excess where the formation of soluble antigen-antibody complexes (AgAb) prevents the lattice formation required for precipitation.

Other modifications of this method are numerous. An interfacial ring test is often used for rapid estimations of antiserum potency. The precipitation of radioactively tagged antigen obviates the need for frequent nitrogen determinations [21].

This method is sensitive enough to detect 10 to 20 μg. of antibody nitrogen. It provides a means of separating specific antibody and is therefore frequently used for the preparation of purified antibody. By definition, it detects precipitating antibody only, but nonprecipitating antibody may be estimated by the technique of coprecipitation. Because it was at first thought that the amount of antibody precipitated was independent of concentration, the antigen concentration is usually varied while the antiserum concentration is kept constant. It is now known, however, that antigen-antibody precipitation falls off with dilution. For this reason, it is preferable to use a low constant concentration of antigen and add varying dilutions of antiserum. This method insures that both antigen and antibody are constant at the chosen end point.

A powerful application of the principle of precipitation exists in the gel diffusion methods developed by Oudin, Ouchterlony, Elek, Oakley, and Fulthorpe (for review see Ref. 22). These techniques allow antigen and antibody to diffuse in gel media, and precipitation occurs in well-defined zones or bands. In single diffusion, either antigen or antibody may diffuse, but in double diffusion both reactants move. The test may be carried out in tubes or Petri dishes. It has been of greatest value in detecting components or multiple precipitin reactions coexisting in antigen-antibody systems. It is the most sensitive method of identifying antigenic mixtures. It has been modified to give semiquantitative information by using serial dilutions of one of the reactants, but this system must be calibrated by some other means of measurement.

A further application of the gel precipitation method is that of immunoelectrophoresis [22]. One component (usually antigen) is subjected to electrophoresis in agar in one direction. The fractions thus separated participate in a gel precipitation reaction with the other component (antiserum), which is placed in an elongated well parallel to the electrophoretically separated fractions.

AGGLUTININ REACTIONS

These methods are derived from the phenomenon of agglutination of bacteria by specific antiserums [23]. The principle is similar to that concerned with the building of an antigen-antibody lattice in the precipitin reaction, but in this case the antigen is attached to a visible inert indicator particle. Different

* In the equivalence zone, neither antigen nor antibody can be detected in the supernatant after the precipitate has been separated. The point of maximal antibody precipitation may be in slight antigen excess.

particles are linked by the combination of antibody with antigens, and in effect the particles behave as magnifiers of the process; i.e., an agglutination reaction may become visible because of the presence of relatively few antibody molecules. This reaction is shown in Figure 8-4.

The antigens may form an intrinsic part of the particle, as with the surface antigens of bacteria and the blood group antigens of erythrocytes. In this case, the mixture of antiserum with the untreated particle will cause agglutination. In the passive agglutination reaction, antiserum is prepared by immunization with any of a wide variety of antigens, and then inert particles are passively coated with the same antigen and used for agglutination indicators. The indicator particles used include erythrocytes, latex particles, and bentonite. Antigens used include polysaccharides, proteins, viruses, extracts of *Rickettsia,* bacteria, and protozoa. In some instances the antigen may be adsorbed directly (polysaccharides to erythrocytes), but in other cases treatment of the erythrocyte with formalin [24], tannic acid [25a], or both [25b] enhances the adsorption of proteins. A more stable bond between antigen and erythrocyte may be formed by coupling the two with a diazo link [26].

The agglutination reaction is ordinarily performed by adding a constant amount of coated particle suspension to serial dilutions of antiserum. Dilutions may be made in any fashion, but serial twofold dilutions are most frequently used. The end point occurs at the greatest dilution of antiserum in which definite agglutination takes place. The titer is usually expressed as the reciprocal of this dilution.

One of the greatest advantages of agglutination reactions is their extraordinary sensitivity. As little as 0.003 to 0.006 μg. of antibody nitrogen has been detected. Other advantages are the rapidity and simplicity of technique and the versatility of the method, which may be applied to a wide variety of antigen-antibody systems.

Difficulties arise, however, in quantitative aspects. As usually performed, the agglutination method indicates only a relative amount of antibody. Quantitative agglutination reactions have been devised, but these are often unsatisfactory, especially when dealing with weak antisera, the situation in which this sensitive test is most useful. In addition, the precision of the method is not as great as may be desired, since the end point in a doubling-dilution type of titration is precise by no more than a factor of 2. Nevertheless this is one of the most widely used methods of antibody detection.

A number of modifications have been made. In the reverse passive agglutination reaction, antibody rather than antigen is adsorbed to the particles [27]. Agglutination occurs when known amounts of antigen are then added. Another modification is the red cell-linked antigen test [28]. Here the antigen is coupled to nonagglutinating antibodies to sheep red cells. Then this unit is added to sheep erythrocytes so that the antigen is attached to the cells via the antisheep cell antibody intermediate. These coated cells will agglutinate in the presence of antibody to the antigen. This test was derived from the Coombs test, which

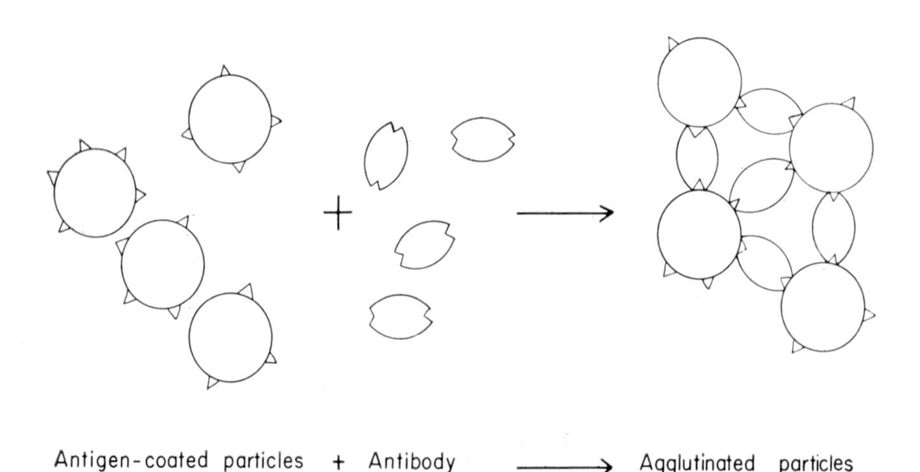

Fig. 8-4. The agglutinin reaction (active or passive).

measures nonagglutinating antibody to red cells [29]. This antibody is a γ-globulin, and it behaves as an antigen adsorbed to erythrocytes. The presence of the antibody is detected by an antiglobulin serum. This test has been applied to nonagglutinating antibodies to bacteria and tissue cells.

LYSIS

If complement is present, the addition of specific antibody to suspensions of some whole bacteria will cause lysis rather than agglutination. Although the bacteriolytic system is rarely used, the same principle has had wide application to the measurement of antibodies to red cells (hemolysin). Animals given injections of heterologous erythrocytes produce antibodies which, in the presence of complement, will lyse a sample of the same erythrocytes. The amount of antibody is determined by testing serial dilutions of antiserum against a standard amount of red cells. The end point usually taken is that dilution of antiserum which will produce lysis of 50 percent of the red cells. This method is sensitive, accurate, and reproducible [30].

Some forms of the passive erythrocyte agglutination test may be converted to lytic tests by the addition of complement.

This principle has been applied in an ingenious fashion by Jerne and Nordin [31] and Ingraham [32] to detect antibody production by single cells. Animals immunized with sheep red cells were killed, and suspensions of their spleen cells were mixed with sheep erythrocytes in dilute agar and plated on a Petri dish. Fresh complement was added which diffused into the red cell-spleen cell layer. Discrete plaques of hemolysis were found surrounding different spleen cells. Presumably these cells were producing hemolysin which diffused outward and adhered to the surrounding red cells, which were then lysed when complement attached to them. This method promises to be most useful in study of the cellular response to antigens.

COMPLEMENT FIXATION

Since complement is discussed at length in Chapter 14, it will suffice here to show in what ways complement fixation is used to measure antibody. The principle is that when antigen combines with antibody, complement may then combine with the antigen-antibody complex. Thus the removal of complement from a system is an indication that an Ag-Ab complex has been formed. The complement fixation method of measurement of antibody thus depends on an indicator system for the presence of free complement. The usual indicator system involves the sensitized erythrocyte, i.e., a sheep erythrocyte coated with rabbit antibody directed against sheep erythrocytes. These coated (sensitized) cells have insufficient antibody to permit spontaneous agglutination but will undergo lysis if complement is present. Therefore the absence of hemolysis of sensitized sheep erythrocytes indicates the absence of complement. The complete system comprises a reaction mixture containing antigen and the antibody in question, to which is added first a definite amount of complement and then some sensitized erythrocytes. The absence of hemolysis indicates the fixation of complement and hence an antigen-antibody interaction. It is imperative to control the system adequately, since either antigens or serum alone may have anticomplementary activity [33].

INHIBITION REACTIONS

Many of the foregoing methods may be converted to inhibition systems. In most instances, e.g., inhibition of precipitation or agglutination, these systems are used to measure incomplete antigen or hapten concentration by its capacity to inhibit the reaction of standard amounts of antibody and complete antigen [34]. In other instances, such as the reversed passive agglutination method, free antibody may be estimated by its ability to inhibit the agglutination system.

THE ANTIBODY RESPONSE

The pattern of antibody response to an antigenic stimulus is of great interest in at least three fields of study. In attempts to immunize man and animals against infectious agents, it is of course desirable to know what methods will be most effective. Similarly, patterns of antibody response give information concerning the pathogenesis of spontaneous and induced allergies, such as hay fever and serum sickness, and perhaps autoimmune diseases and tissue transplantation reactions. In addition, the antibody response is of critical interest in studies of protein synthesis, cellular metabolism, and genetics.

If an organism somewhat higher in the phylogenic scale than the hagfish receives a specific antigenic stimulus for the first time, it produces a primary antibody response. The characteristics are usually cited as a long induction period (delay before detection of circulating antibody), a slow to intermediate rate of rise to a moderate peak titer, and then a fall. After some time (days to years), reintroduction of the same antigen produces a secondary or anamnestic response. The characteristics of this are a short induction period, a rapid rise to a high peak titer, and then a fall [35]. Our purpose here is to analyze the forms of the antibody response and to show that they are profoundly influenced by a large variety of factors, alteration of only one of which may produce a very different picture. The number of variables is so large that it will be impossible to discuss each one systematically. Rather, a series of general topics will be discussed, with specific examples, to indicate the general nature of the problems involved.

THE HOST

Species Differences. These are important in the antibody response. Some species, e.g., rabbit, are good precipitin-formers; others, e.g., rat, are not. It is easy to produce anaphylaxis *in vivo* or *in vitro* in the guinea pig but more difficult to demonstrate anaphylaxis in the rabbit, rat, or mouse. The horse produces large quantities of high molecular weight antibodies (19S); the other species mentioned produce smaller quantities.

Strain Differences. Within the same species, strain differences may also be important. Farr and co-workers [36] found that A/Jax mice produce more antibody to a standard dose of bovine serum albumin (BSA) than do $C_{57}Bl_6$ mice and that F_1 hybrids (A/Jax × $C_{57}Bl_6$) produce an intermediate amount. Thus genetic differences in antibody-producing capacity probably exist.

Age. The age of the animal is also relevant. In general, young animals do not form antibody as easily as mature animals, but, on the other hand, antibody has been produced by baby opossums while still in the pouch.

Sex. Differences in sex are not important.

THE ANTIGEN

Chemical Type. The typical differences between the primary and secondary reactions are well illustrated by the response to BSA in the rabbit [37]. Here one sees the long induction period, moderate rise, and fall of antibody after the primary injection, with a short induction period, steep rise, and slower fall after the anamnestic dose (Fig. 8-5). Some polysaccharide antigens, e.g., the Forssman antigen of sheep erythrocytes given intravenously to rabbits [38] or pneumococcus polysaccharides given subcutaneously to human beings [39] may have a shorter induction period following a secondary stimulation but do not have a significantly higher peak titer after the booster injection. Also, the antibody level falls more slowly than it does with protein antigens. These features have been explained by suggesting that the "primary" responses are really secondary, since the ubiquity of polysaccharides in nature makes it likely that the animal had been "naturally" stimulated before the experiment. Since polysaccharides are more resistant to *in vivo* degradation, a single antigenic stimulus with polysaccharides has a more prolonged effect than a stimulus with protein antigens.

Physical Form. In general, particulate antigens are more effective than soluble antigens. In fact, soluble bovine γ-globulin (BGG) produces tolerance in the mouse (inhibition of antibody production), whereas the same amount of BGG adsorbed to bentonite and given by the same route produces a vigorous anti-BGG response [40]. Large molecules are more antigenic than small ones, perhaps because they contain more of the same antigenic determinants per molecule.

Route of Antigen Administration. The intravenous route is frequently used experimentally. It is probably the least effective route for soluble antigens, perhaps because of rapid dissipation and excretion of the antigen. It is effective with particulate antigens, but the status of the reticuloendothelial system is important. Splenectomy markedly inhibits the antibody response of rats given sheep red cells intravenously, but has no effect on antibody titers (as compared with unoperated controls) if the antigen is given intraportally, intraperitoneally, or intradermally [41]. In rabbits, on the other hand, the same antigen given intravenously induces substantial amounts of antibody even if the rabbit is first splenectomized, although the response is delayed compared to unoperated controls [38]. Intramuscular, intraperitoneal, and subcutaneous injections of antigen are likely to be more effective in producing antibody. If antigens are injected intradermally, only very small

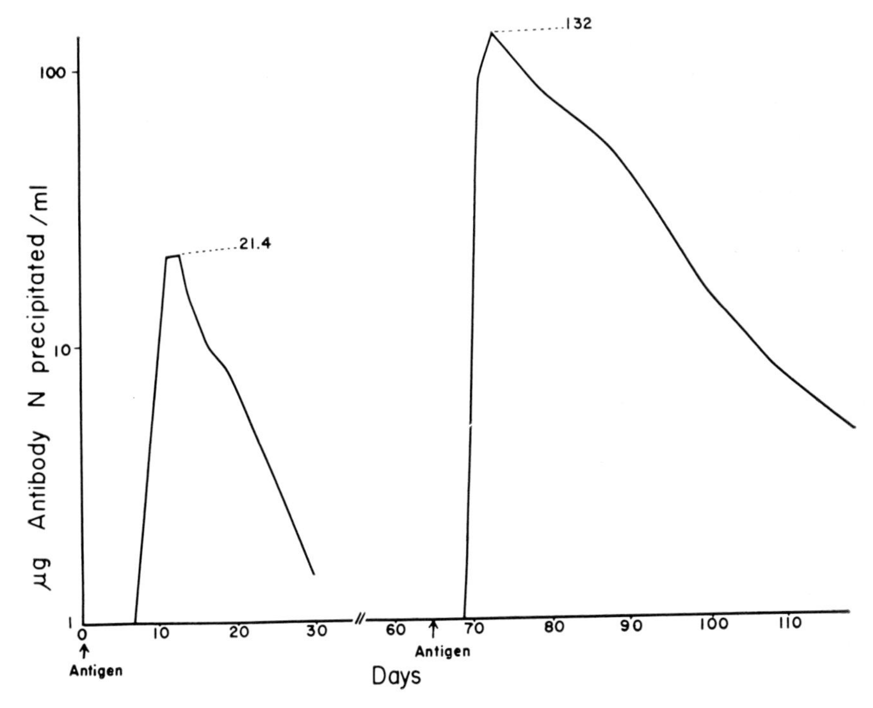

Fig. 8-5. Primary and secondary antibody responses. A rabbit was given 15 mg./kg. BSA intravenously on day 0 and day 65. Antibody activity present is represented on the ordinate, expressed as μg. I*BSA N precipitated by 1 ml. serum at 80 percent antigen precipitation. (Adapted from Dixon, *et al.* [37].)

quantities are necessary for the induction of antibody formation. This probably is the most efficient route of soluble antigen administration. Almost any route may be effective, however, including oral, nasal, pulmonary, mesenteric vein, epidermal (contact), conjunctival, and intraureteral.

Amount of Antigen. Very small amounts of antigen seldom lead to the production of detectable antibody. Above this threshold, larger single doses of antigen will produce larger amounts of antibody, especially in a primary reaction. In many instances, however, this applies only within a certain range. Doses of antigen in excess of that range may produce no increase or even a decrease in antibody production. This decrease is related to specific acquired tolerance in the newborn or adult [42]. Repeated administrations of antigen after the anamnestic dose may either further increase the antibody level or prolong the antibody response, or both.

ADJUVANT FACTORS

Recently it has become obvious that the magnitude and even the existence of an antibody response to a particular antigen may depend on factors other than the antigen itself. These factors are often described as nonspecific since they appear to be unrelated to the antigen used, and in general each adjuvant factor is effective with a wide variety of antigens. The importance of adjuvant factors was first demonstrated by Dienes [43], who found that the antigenicity of egg albumin is enhanced when it is injected into a guinea pig's tuberculous focus. Later, Freund [44] and his associates found that antibody production could be greatly increased by incorporating the antigen as a water-in-oil emulsion either with (Freund's complete) or without (Freund's incomplete) added killed *Mycobacteria.* Many other vehicles have been used as adjuvants, including peanut oil, beeswax, and paraffin. These emulsions were injected parenterally. It was demonstrated that slow absorption of antigen was not entirely responsible for the adjuvant effect because complete surgical excision of the injection site one and a half hours later did not prevent a considerable adjuvant response. Also, some effect is obtained if the adjuvant is injected separately from the antigen. In fact, two strong adjuvants, bacterial endotoxin and pertussis vaccine, are usually injected at different sites and produce a marked increase in antibody production [45]. It is important, however, that for maximal effect these bacterial adjuvants be given at the same time or within six hours after injection of antigen.

The mechanism of the adjuvant action of these diverse substances is obscure. Cell proliferation may be important. If antigen is given during recovery from whole body radiation, an event associated with rapid lymphoid cell regeneration, an adjuvant effect is seen [46].

It is important to note that in nearly all experimental systems which induce autoimmune disease, the antigen must be given in adjuvant form to cause the production of autoantibodies.

THE ANTIBODY

The form of the antibody response depends not only on the three broad groups of factors already outlined (host, antigen, adjuvant) but on the system of antibody detection itself. To take a simple example, a given antiserum might have no antibody detectable by the precipitin method, whereas a more sensitive agglutination system might show significant amounts. The problem is considerably more complicated, however. The unitarian hypothesis of Zinsser is no longer tenable since antibodies to a single antigen have been shown to be diverse in at least two respects, physicochemical characteristics and affinity for antigen. It has already been mentioned that late antibody binds more closely to antigen than early antibody. This has been partially correlated with the fact that in at least some systems, 19S antibody is produced at first, to be replaced by 7S antibody of higher avidity [47]. Therefore a method of antibody measurement which detects mainly low affinity antibody will show an immunization pattern different from that of a method detecting high affinity antibodies. As an example, one may notice the differences in antibody response in Figures

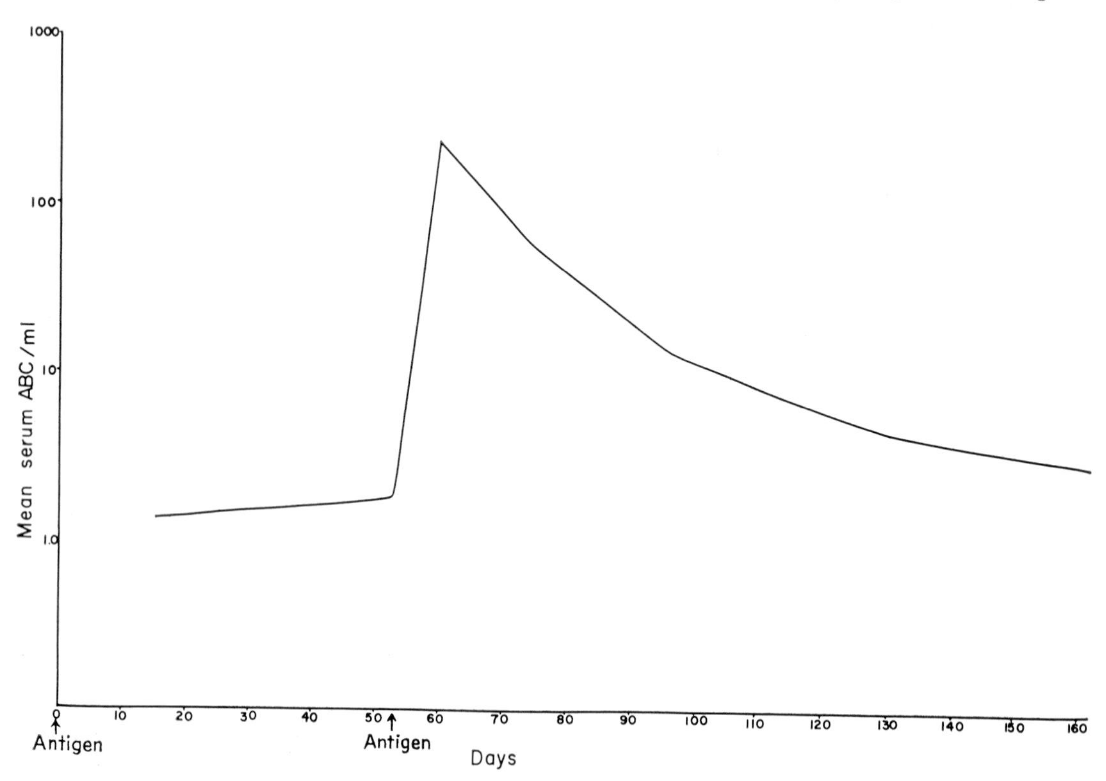

Fig. 8-6. Primary and secondary antibody responses. Three rabbits were given 15 mg./kg. BSA intravenously on day 0 and day 53. Antibody activity present is represented on the ordinate, expressed as mean serum antigen-binding capacity (ABC) per ml. (μg. I*BSA N/ml. serum bound at 33 percent binding, at antigen concentration of 0.1 μg. N/ml.). Antibody detection was by the ammonium sulfate precipitation method of Farr [18]. (Adapted from Claman [48].)

8-5 and 8-6. In these experiments, done in different laboratories to be sure, the host, the antigen, the form and amount of antigen, and the route of inoculation were identical; but the methods of antibody titration differed. Figure 8-5 shows that, using the precipitin test, there was a prompt rise to a peak primary response with a very rapid fall. The secondary response also showed a rapid rise and somewhat less rapid fall with little tendency to level off. Figure 8-6, however, shows that when the $(NH_4)_2SO_4$ precipitation method was used, a steady level of primary response was maintained until the anamnestic dose of antigen was given on day 53. Then there was a steep rise to the secondary peak followed by a fall, leveling off at the height of the primary response [48]. The differences in antibody curves are probably due to the fact that the two methods give different weights to antibodies of high and low affinity.

Recent investigations have suggested that the behavior of an antiserum in various serological reactions may depend not upon antigenic specificity but upon physicochemical structure. Stelos and Talmage [49] found that rabbit antiserum against sheep red cell Forssman antigen contained anti-Forssman activity in two components which differed both in electrophoretic mobility and in relative combining and hemolytic properties. Benacerraf and co-workers [50] found that guinea pig antibodies to dinitrophenol could be electrophoretically separated into slow (γ_2) and fast (γ_1) antibodies, both of the 7S variety. The slow component appeared first in animals immunized with antigen in adjuvant, and the fast component was mainly produced when adjuvants were not used. Gamma$_1$ antibodies mediated passive systemic or cutaneous anaphylaxis, but γ_2 components would inhibit the passive cutaneous anaphylactic reaction provoked by γ_1 antibodies. Gamma$_2$ components fixed complement in the presence of antigen and lysed antigen-coated red cells in the presence of complement.

REFERENCES

1. Books with good descriptions of methods include: (*a*) Kabat, E. A., and Mayer, M. M. *Experimental Immunochemistry* (2nd ed.). Springfield, Ill.: Charles C Thomas, Publisher, 1961. (*b*) Boyd, W. C. *Fundamentals of Immunology* (4th ed.). New York: Interscience Publishers, Inc., 1956. (*c*) Wilson, G. S., and Miles, A. A. In *Topley and Wilson's Principles of Bacteriology and Immunity*. Baltimore: Williams & Wilkins Company, 1955. (*d*) Ackroyd, J. F. (Ed.), *Immunological Methods*. Philadelphia: F. A. Davis Company, 1964.
2. Wilson and Miles. Ref. 1 (*c*), p. 1194.
3. (*a*) Talmage, D. W., Dixon, F. J., Bukantz, S. C., and Dammin, G. J. Antigen elimination from the blood as an early manifestation of the immune response. *J. Immun.* 67:243, 1951. (*b*) Paterson, R., Weigle, W. O., and Dixon, F. J. Elimination of circulating serum protein antigens as a sensitive measure of antibody. *Proc. Soc. Exp. Biol. Med.* 105:330, 1960.
4. (*a*) Elberg, S. S. Cellular immunity. *Bact. Rev.* 24:67, 1960. (*b*) Lancefield, R. C. Differentiation of group A streptococci with a common R antigen into three serological types. *J. Exp. Med.* 106:525, 1957.
5. (*a*) Lamanna, C. Adhesion of foreign particles to particulate antigens in the presence of antibody and complement. *Bact. Rev.* 21:30, 1957. (*b*) Turk, J. L. The Detection of Antibodies by Immune-adherence. Ref. 1(*d*).
6. (*a*) Coulson, E. J. The Schultz-Dale technique. *J. Immun.* 24:458, 1953. (*b*) Austen, K. F., and Brocklehurst, W. E. Anaphylaxis in chopped guinea pig lung. *J. Exp. Med.* 113: 521, 1961. (*c*) Boyd. Ref. 1(*b*), p. 385. (*d*) Kabat and Mayer. Ref. 1(*a*), p. 268. (*e*) Ovary, Z. Passive Cutaneous Anaphylaxis. In Brown, E. A. (Ed.), *Allergology* (Proc. 4th Internat. Congr.). New York: Pergamon Press, 1962.
7. (*a*) Cooke, R. A. *Allergy in Theory and Practice*. Philadelphia: W. B. Saunders Company, 1947. (*b*) Pepys, J. Skin Tests in Diagnosis. In Gell, P. G. H., and Coombs, R. R. A. (Eds.), *Clinical Aspects of Immunology*. Philadelphia: F. A. Davis Company, 1963.
8. (*a*) Noah, J. W., and Brand, A. Release of histamine in the blood of ragweed-sensitive individuals. *J. Allerg.* 25:210, 1954. (*b*) Van Arsdel, P. P., Jr., Middleton, E., Jr., Sherman, W. B., and Buchwald, H. A quantitative study on the *in vitro* release of histamine from leukocytes of atopic persons. *J. Allerg.* 29:429, 1958.
9. Talmage, D. W. The Measurement of Antibody. Ref. 6(*e*), p. 282.
10. Berson, S. A., and Yalow, R. S. Quantitative aspects of the reaction between insulin and insulin-binding antibody. *J. Clin. Invest.* 38: 1996, 1959.
11. (*a*) Marrack, J., and Smith, F. C. Aspects of immunity reactions: The combination of anti-

bodies with simple haptenes. *Brit. J. Exp. Path.* 13:394, 1932. (*b*) Nisonoff, A., and Pressman, D. Heterogeneity of antibody sites in their relative combining affinities for structurally related haptenes. *J. Immun.* 81:126, 1958. (*c*) Dubert, J. M. Études sur l'évolution de la spécificité des anticorps au cours du phénomène de rappel. Thesis presented to Faculty of Sciences. University of Paris Ph.D. Thesis, 1959.

12. Velick, S. F., Parker, C. W., and Eisen, H. N. Excitation energy transfer and the quantitative study of the antibody haptene reaction. *Proc. Nat. Acad. Sci. U.S.A.* 46:1470, 1960.
13. Adams, M. H. *Bacteriophages.* New York: Interscience Publishers, Inc., 1959.
14. Jerne, N. K., and Avegno, P. Development of phage-inactivating properties of serum. *J. Immun.* 76:200, 1956.
15. (*a*) Burnet, F. M., Keogh, E. V., and Lush, D. The immunological reactions of the filtrable viruses. *Aust. J. Exp. Biol. Med. Sci.* 15:227, 1937. (*b*) Dulbecco, R. Production of plaques in monolayer tissue cultures by single particles of an animal virus. *Proc. Nat. Acad. Sci., U.S.A.* 38:1747, 1952. (*c*) Dulbecco, R., Vogt, M., and Strickland, A. G. R. A study of the basic aspects of neutralization of two animal viruses. *Virology,* 2:162, 1956.
16. Kabat and Mayer. Ref. 1(*a*), p. 127.
17. (*a*) Smith, F. C., and Marrack, J. Diphtheria toxin-antitoxin floccules. *Brit. J. Exp. Path.* 11:494, 1930. (*b*) Skom, J. H., and Talmage, D. W. Nonprecipitating insulin antibodies. *J. Clin. Invest.* 37:783, 1958.
18. Farr, R. S. A quantitative immunochemical measure of the primary interaction between I-BSA and antibody. *J. Infect. Dis.* 103:239, 1958.
19. Jerne, N. K. A study of avidity. *Acta Path. Microbiol. Scand.* Supp. 28:87, 1951.
20. (*a*) Heidelberger, M., and Kendall, F. E. A quantitative theory of the preciptin reaction: III. The reaction between crystalline egg albumin and its homologus antibody. *J. Exp. Med.* 62:697, 1935. (*b*) Kabat and Mayer. Ref. 1(*a*).
21. (*a*) Eisen, H. N., and Keston, A. S. The immunologic reactivity of bovine serum albumin labeled with trace amounts of radioactive iodine. *J. Immun.* 63:71, 1949. (*b*) Talmage, D. W., and Maurer, P. H. I^{131}-labeled antigen precipitation as a measure of quantity and quality of antibody. *J. Infect. Dis.* 92:288, 1953.
22. Crowle, A. J. *Immunodiffusion.* New York: Academic Press, Inc., 1961.
23. Neter, E. Bacterial Hemagglutination and Hemolysis. *Bact. Rev.* 20:166, 1956.
24. Ingraham, J. S. Identification individuelle des cellules productrices d'anticorps par une réaction hémolytique locale. *C. R. Acad. Sci.* (Paris) 256:5005, 1963.
25. (*a*) Boyden, S. V. Adsorption of proteins on erythrocytes treated with tannic acid and subsequent hemagglutination by antiprotein sera. *J. Exp. Med.* 93:107, 1951. (*b*) Butler, W. T. Hemagglutination studies with formalinized erythrocytes: Effect of bis-diazo-benzidine and tannic acid treatment on sensitization by soluble antigen. *J. Immun.* 90:663, 1963.
26. (*a*) Pressman, D., Campbell, D. H., and Pauling, L. The agglutination of intact azo-erythrocytes by antisera homologous to the attached groups. *J. Immun.* 44:101, 1942. (*b*) Stavitsky, A. B., and Arquilla, E. R. Micromethods for the study of proteins and antibodies: III. *J. Immun.* 74:306, 1955.
27. Cua-Lim, F., Richter, M., and Rose, B. The reversed BDB technique. *J. Allerg.* 34:142, 1963.
28. Coombs, R. R. A., Howard, A. N., and Mynors, L. S. A serological procedure theoretically capable of detecting incomplete and non-precipitating antibodies to soluble protein antigen. *Brit. J. Exp. Path.* 34:525, 1953.
29. (*a*) Coombs, R. R. A., Mourant, A. E., and Race, R. R. A new test for the detection of weak and "incomplete" Rh agglutinins. *Brit. J. Exp. Path.* 26:255, 1945. (*b*) Stratton, F., and Renton, P. H. *Practical Blood Grouping.* Springfield, Ill.: Charles C Thomas, Publisher, 1958, p. 60.
30. Taliaferro, W. H., and Taliaferro, L. G. The dynamics of hemolysin formation in intact and splenectomized rabbits. *J. Infect. Dis.* 87:37, 1950.
31. Jerne, N. K., and Nordin, A. A. Plaque formation in agar by single antibody-producing cells. *Science* 140:405, 1963.
32. Ingraham, J. S., and Bussard, A. Application of a localized hemolysin reaction for specific detection of individual antibody-forming cells. *J. Exp. Med.* 119:667, 1964.
33. Kabat and Mayer. Ref. 1(*a*), p. 133.
34. *Ibid.,* p. 241.
35. Wilson and Miles. Ref. 1(*c*), p. 1261.
36. Farr, R. S., Grey, H. M., Dickinson, W., and Rosenstein, D. H. Genetic influences on antibovine albumin (BSA) produced in mice. *Fed. Proc.* 22:265, 1963.
37. Dixon, F. J., Maurer, P. H., and Deichmiller, M. P. Primary and specific anamnestic antibody responses of rabbits to heterologous serum protein antigens. *J. Immun.* 72:179, 1954.
38. Taliaferro, W. H., and Taliaferro, L. G. The role of the spleen and the dynamics of hemolysin production in homologous anamnesis. *J. Infect. Dis.* 90:205, 1952.
39. Heidelberger, M., MacLeod, C. M., Kaiser, S. J., and Robinson, B. Antibody formation in

volunteers following injection of pneumococci or their type-specific polysaccharides. *J. Exp. Med.* 83:303, 1946.

40. (*a*) Dresser, D. W. Specific inhibition of antibody production: II. Paralysis induced in adult mice by small quantities of protein antigen. *Immunology* 5:378, 1962. (*b*) Claman, H. N. Tolerance to a protein antigen in adult mice and the effect of nonspecific factors. *J. Immun.* 91:833, 1963.
41. Rowley, D. A. The effect of splenectomy on the formation of circulating antibody in the adult male albino rat. *J. Immun.* 64:289, 1950.
42. Smith, R. T. Immunological tolerance of nonliving antigens. *Advances Immun.* 1:67, 1961.
43. Dienes, L. Further observations concerning the sensitization of tuberculous guinea pigs. *J. Immun.* 15:153, 1928.
44. Freund, J. The mode of action of immunologic adjuvants. *Advances Tuberc. Res.* 7:130, 1956.
45. Kind, P., and Johnson, A. G. Studies on the adjuvant action of bacterial endotoxins on antibody formation. *J. Immun.* 82:415, 1959.
46. Dixon, F. J., and McConahey, P. J. Enhancement of antibody formation by whole body x-radiation. *J. Exp. Med.* 117:833, 1963.
47. Uhr, J. W., and Finkelstein, M. S. Antibody formation: IV. Formation of rapidly and slowly sedimenting antibodies and immunological memory to bacteriophage ØX-174. *Ibid.*, p. 457.
48. Claman, H. N. Decline of antibody and impaired anamnesis following x-ray. *J. Immun.* 91:29, 1963.
49. Stelos, P., and Talmage, D. W. The separation by starch electrophoresis of two antibodies to sheep red cells differing in hemolytic efficiency. *J. Infect. Dis.* 100:126, 1957.
50. (*a*) Benacerraf, B., Ovary, Z., Bloch, K. J., and Franklin, E. C. Properties of guinea pig 7S antibodies: I. Electrophoretic separation of two types of guinea pig 7S antibodies. *J. Exp. Med.* 117:937, 1963. (*b*) Ovary, Z., Benacerraf, B., and Bloch, K. J. Properties of guinea pig 7S antibodies: II. Identification of antibodies involved in passive cutaneous and systemic anaphylaxis. *Ibid.*, p. 951. (*c*) Bloch, K. J., Kourilsky, F. M., Ovary, Z., and Benacerraf, B. Properties of guinea pig 7S antibodies: III. Identification of antibodies involved in complement fixation and hemolysis. *Ibid.*, p. 965.

SECTION II. ANTIGEN-ANTIBODY INTERACTIONS

9. The Nature of Antigen-Antibody Interactions*

LISA A. STEINER AND HERMAN N. EISEN

. . . They were standing under a tree, each with an arm round the other's neck, and Alice knew which was which in a moment, because one of them had "DUM" embroidered on his collar, and the other "DEE."

Through the Looking Glass, and What Alice Found There, Lewis Carroll

IT IS IMPORTANT AT THE OUTSET to clarify the terms antigen, hapten, and ligand as used in this chapter. An *antigen* is defined in the usual manner as a substance which is immunogenic (stimulates the formation of antibodies) and which reacts with the antibodies whose formation it evokes. A *hapten* is not immunogenic but reacts specifically with certain antibodies. The term *ligand* will be used generically for both antigen and hapten. The distinction between antigen and hapten, based on immunogenicity, is largely irrelevant to the subject matter of this chapter. Furthermore, many conflicting reports in the literature testify to the fact that it is not always easy to decide whether a substance is a hapten or an antigen.

A review of the contents of this volume makes it clear that there are many ways of looking at the antigen-antibody reaction. For instance one may consider its biological consequences, its specificity, its application to the measurement of antibody and antigen levels. Here we wish only to consider the reaction in its elemental form, as the reversible reaction of an antibody molecule (Ab) with an antigen molecule (Ag) to form the antibody-antigen complex (AbAg)

$$\mathrm{Ab} + \mathrm{Ag} \rightleftharpoons \mathrm{AbAg} \tag{1}$$

Antibodies seem always to be bivalent, and antigens are nearly always multivalent. Hence the reaction rarely occurs in the simple form shown in (1). Instead, in most real situations the mixture of a solution of antigen with its corresponding antibodies leads to the formation of a variety of complexes. These are the products of many individual reactions such as

$$\begin{aligned} &\mathrm{Ab} + \mathrm{Ag} \underset{K_1'}{\overset{K_1}{\rightleftharpoons}} \mathrm{AbAg}, \\ &\mathrm{AbAg} + \mathrm{Ag} \underset{K_2'}{\overset{K_2}{\rightleftharpoons}} \mathrm{AbAg_2}, \\ &\mathrm{AbAg} + \mathrm{Ab} \underset{K_3'}{\overset{K_3}{\rightleftharpoons}} \mathrm{Ab_2Ag}, \text{ etc.} \end{aligned} \tag{2}$$

Given such a series of reactions, the distribution of complexes existing in solution at any time is determined by the initial concentration of reactants and the rate constants for the individual reactions. Conversely, the concentrations of all intermediates as a function of time establishes the rate constants for the separate reactions. In practice, however, for the reactions of antibodies with large antigens one does not know the number or types of possible complexes, let alone their concentrations. It is useful, therefore, to discuss first the reactions of antibodies with ligands of simple structure. Once such reactions are characterized, one can proceed to consider the inter-

* This work was supported, in part, by U.S. Public Health Service Grant No. AI-03231 from the National Institute for Allergy and Infectious Diseases and by a contract with the Research and Development Command, Department of Army.

TABLE 9-1. Classification of Antibody-Ligand Reactions According to Type of Ligand

Type of Interaction	Ligand Valency	Ligand Specificity	Examples
A	1	1	Anti-DNP : ε-DNP-L-lysine Anti-insulin : insulin[a]
B	1	>1	Anti-insulin : insulin[a]
C	>1	1	Anti-DNP-BγG : DNP-HSA
D	>1	>1	Anti-BSA : BSA

[a] The reaction of insulin with its antibodies is placed tentatively in both categories A and B because it is not clear whether there is one or more than one type of reactive group on the insulin molecule. See text for abbreviations.

actions with complex antigens of general biological interest.

For purposes of discussion we shall divide antibody-antigen interactions into four categories, according to the nature of the ligand. These are outlined in Table 9-1. The divisions in this table are based on the concepts of valency and specificity.

Valency refers to the number of functional groups per molecule of reactant (ligand or antibody). Thus the valence of the ligand is the maximum number of antibody molecules which 1 molecule of ligand can bind at one time. The valence of antibody is defined in similar fashion. Since the number of functional groups is determined operationally, the notion of valency has meaning only in reference to a particular ligand-antibody system. Although the possibility that univalent or multivalent (more than two) antibodies will be found cannot be excluded, in all systems so far examined antibodies have been bivalent. Ligand valences have, however, varied widely; some have a valence of 1, others a valence of 5 or 10, and some high molecular weight ligands have a valence of 100 or even higher. In fact, a given ligand may be univalent with respect to one population* of antibody molecules but bivalent or multivalent with respect to another.

It should be stressed that the concepts of valency and immunogenicity are not necessarily related. Thus haptens may be either univalent or multivalent, and antigens also may be either univalent or multivalent.

* A population of antibody molecules is defined by the capacity, common to all members of the population, to bind a given ligand.

Specificity refers to the nature of the functional groups. A ligand L_1 containing the group X is said to have specificity X with respect to a given antibody population if and only if the antibody reacts with L_1 and also with some other ligand L_2 which contains the same group X. Further, it must be established that the common reactivity of L_1 and L_2 is not due to some group, other than X, or in addition to X, which the two ligands also happen to have in common. The antibody is said to have specificity X and is often called "anti-X antibody." The following example illustrates the application of the definition.

The ligand ε-2,4-dinitrophenyl-L-lysine (DNP-lysine) is said to have DNP specificity since the antibody populations which react with it will in general react also with other ligands which contain the DNP group (e.g., 2,4-dinitroaniline). In this case, dinitroaniline also has DNP specificity. On the other hand, if DNP-lysine is the *only* DNP-containing compound with which a particular antibody population reacts, then DNP-lysine does *not* have DNP specificity with respect to this set of antibody molecules; it has DNP-lysine specificity. For the sake of completeness, we say that a ligand L_1 has specificity equal to itself if one can demonstrate antibodies which react with L_1 but not with some portion of it. In this case we waive the requirement that the antibody also react with L_1 as a portion of some *other* ligand. It is clear that the notion of ligand specificity depends both on the nature of the reference antibody population and on the method of detecting the antibody-ligand reaction.

Multiple specificity is defined in an analogous manner. A ligand L_1 has specificities X and Y if it satisfies the conditions for having both specificity X and specificity Y and if, in addition, it can be shown that X and Y are independent specificities; that is, X and Y are not part of a single specificity which we might designate X-Y. The latter requirement is met if the reference antibody population (e.g., in an antiserum) can be shown to react with some other ligand L_2 containing X but not Y (and vice versa). This definition places no limits on the nature of the groups X and Y. They may be as compact and chemically unambiguous as a benzene ring or as difficult to define as a cluster of amino acid residues whose spatial conformation is determined by the intact tertiary structure of a protein molecule.

It follows from the definition of specificity that for every ligand there must be at least one antibody population (e.g., an antiserum) with respect to which the ligand has a maximum number of specificities. Usually, but not necessarily, the immunizing antigen (that which is injected to stimulate antibody formation) is the ligand which has the greatest number of specificities with respect to the population of antibodies it evokes.

As has been mentioned already, the valency and specificity of ligands are defined in terms of the antibodies with which the ligands react. However, since the molecules in any given antibody population are not homogeneous with respect to reactivity with ligand, and since there is usually variation among populations as well, it may not be possible to define valency and specificity in an unambiguous manner. Nevertheless most ligands can be reasonably placed into one of the four categories of Table 9-1. We shall now discuss in more detail each of the antibody-ligand reactions in these categories. We consider first those reactions in which the ligand is restricted with respect to number and type of functional group. These reactions are then comparable to the interactions between other proteins, for example, enzymes, and their ligands (substrates, coenzymes, etc.) and can be studied by a variety of techniques such as equilibrium dialysis and fluorescence quenching. We shall find that many of the features of the reactions of relatively simple ligands with their antibodies will apply also to the reactions of more complex ligands.

REACTIONS OF ANTIBODIES WITH UNIVALENT LIGANDS OF A SINGLE SPECIFICITY

The binding by antibody (Ab) of a univalent ligand of specificity X can be represented by the following series of reactions:

$$\begin{gathered} \mathrm{Ab} + \mathrm{X} \underset{K_1'}{\overset{K_1}{\rightleftharpoons}} \mathrm{AbX} \\ \mathrm{AbX} + \mathrm{X} \underset{K_2'}{\overset{K_2}{\rightleftharpoons}} \mathrm{AbX_2} \\ \cdots \\ \mathrm{AbX}_{n-1} + \mathrm{X} \underset{K_n'}{\overset{K_n}{\rightleftharpoons}} \mathrm{AbX}_n \end{gathered} \tag{3}$$

Each K is an intrinsic rate constant describing the binding of the ligand molecules, and n is the number of binding sites (valence) per antibody molecule. If

$$K_1 = K_2 = \cdots = K_n, \text{ and}$$
$$K_1' = K_2' = \cdots = K_n'$$

the reaction can then be written in the simplified fashion

$$\mathrm{Ab} + \mathrm{X} \underset{K'}{\overset{K}{\rightleftharpoons}} \mathrm{AbX} \tag{4}$$

where (Ab) is now the concentration of antibody *sites* (equal to the product of n and molar antibody concentration). The concentrations of reactants and products as a function of time give the rate constants K and K', and the equilibrium constant K_A is defined as the quotient of these K/K'. The forward rates are, however, so very rapid that it is experimentally more feasible to obtain the equilibrium constant, K_A, from the concentrations of reactants when the reaction has gone to equilibrium. Thus

$$K_A = \frac{K}{K'} = \frac{(\mathrm{AbX})_e}{(\mathrm{Ab})_e(\mathrm{X})_e} \tag{5}$$

where the subscript e denotes concentrations at equilibrium. This last equation can also be written

$$r = \frac{Kc}{1 + Kc} \tag{6}$$

where at equilibrium r = fraction of antibody sites occupied, c = concentration of free (unbound) ligand, $K = K_A$, the association constant. If the equation is rewritten in the form

$$\frac{r}{c} = K - Kr \qquad (7)$$

it is apparent that a plot of r/c vs. r gives a straight line with slope $-K$.

In the case of a typical antibody-ligand reaction, however, one observes that r/c does *not* vary linearly with r. Figure 9-1, for example,

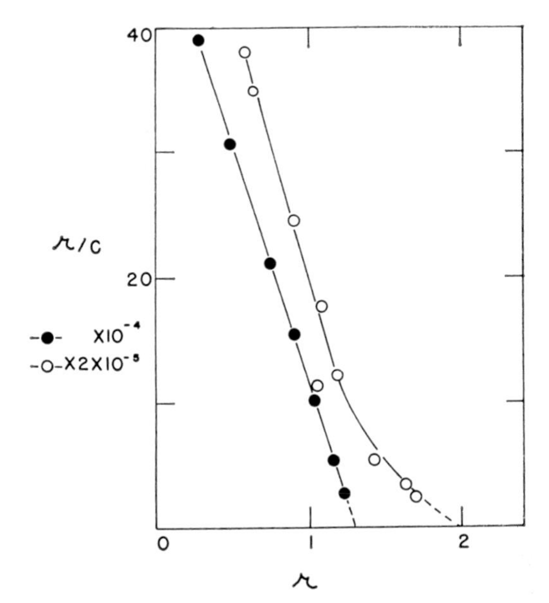

Fig. 9-1. o———o, binding of 1-C^{14}-2, 4-dinitroaniline by purified rabbit antibodies [1]. •———•, binding of TPNH by glutamic acid dehydrogenase. (Recalculated by J. R. Little, Jr., from data of C. Frieden, *J. Biol. Chem.* 238:3286, 1963.)

gives the plot of r/c against r for the reaction of anti-DNP antibodies with 1-C^{14}-2,4-dinitroaniline. The failure to conform to the linear relation predicted by equation (7) is consistent with other evidence that there is heterogeneity with respect to the equilibrium constant K_A, i.e., that some antibody sites have greater affinity for the ligand than do others. Other antibody-ligand systems almost invariably also show heterogeneity with respect to binding. Similar degrees of heterogeneity are observed if the binding studies are carried out with the crude globulin fraction of an antiserum or with antibodies specifically purified from such serum. Despite the heterogeneity, it is possible to define an average association constant as that K_A which satisfies equation (5) when at equilibrium half the antibody sites are occupied by ligand.

The heterogeneity with respect to affinities which is so typical of antibody-ligand interactions is not characteristic of the specific reactions of other proteins. For example, enzyme-substrate reactions are typically described by single association constants, indicating that the molecules of enzyme of a given specificity are uniform in their capacity to react with the substrate. Figure 9-1 illustrates the linearity of the relation of r/c and r for the binding of triphosphopyridine nucleotide (TPNH) by glutamic acid dehydrogenase.

Further examination of the interaction of DNP ligands with antibody has also revealed that different samples of antibody, each characterized by heterogeneity with respect to association constant, often have different *average* association constants. Indeed, two preparations of antibody each obtained from the same rabbit may have average association constants that differ more than a thousand fold. It was found, furthermore, that the average association constant of antibodies purified from the sera of individual rabbits increases systematically with time after immunization. Some typical values for these association constants for a number of rabbits are given in Table 9-2. (The change in average association constant in time seems not to be related in any simple fashion to the *amount* of circulating antibody.)

It is evident, therefore, that the interaction of antibody with even a univalent monospecific ligand is not as simple as one might have hoped. Indeed, one of the most striking features of these reactions is their variability, indicated both by heterogeneity of binding and by the change in average association constant. Our disappointment that antibody-antigen reactions do not conform to the model provided by other protein-ligand systems may reflect no more than disillusion with an expectation which may not have been reasonable in the first place. Much evidence indicates that any given antibody population may be composed of molecules of many different kinds, varying in size, charge, and perhaps even in amino acid composition. That such a collection of molecules differs from other proteins in the mode of ligand binding is perhaps, at least in retrospect, not surprising.

TABLE 9-2. Binding of ε-DNP-l-Lysine by Antibodies Isolated at Various Times after Injection of 2, 4-DNP-BγG

Rabbit No.	Amt. of DNP-BγG Injected[a]	Time after Injection of DNP-BγG 2 weeks K_A[b]	5 weeks K_A	8 weeks K_A
1	5 mg.	0.60	32	—
2	5 mg.	1.6	27	—
3	5 mg.	0.32	1.6	20
4	5 mg.	1.0	5.9	250
5	5 mg.	0.78	1.5	80

[a] DNP-BγG was injected in oil-in-water emulsion with *Mycobacteria* (complete Freund's adjuvant) into the four foot pads at zero time. Antibodies were purified by the method described by Farah *et al.* [2].

[b] K_A is defined in equation (5) in the text, and expressed in liters per mole $\times 10^{-6}$.

SOURCE: Eisen and Siskind [1].

REACTIONS OF ANTIBODIES WITH UNIVALENT LIGANDS OF MORE THAN ONE SPECIFICITY

If one applies the definition of valency and specificity to a given antibody-antigen reaction, one may find that the ligand has a valency of 1 but that its specificity is greater than 1. There are two major ways in which this may come about.

1. The ligand L is impure and consists of a mixture of distinct ligands $L_1, L_2, \ldots, L_n$, each of which is univalent and monospecific with respect to a given antibody population. The over-all valency of L with respect to a mixture of the antibody populations will be 1, but the specificity will be equal to the total number of distinguishable specificities present. A simple example of such a case is one in which the ligand is a mixture of 2,4-dinitrophenol and benzenearsonic acid and the antibody a mixture of anti-DNP and antibenzenearsonate. The requirement for chemical homogeneity of the ligand was not included in its definition, and since one often does not know whether or not a ligand is homogeneous, it is well to keep the definition as general as possible.

We stress again the determining role of the antibody in the definition of specificity. In the above example, if we consider the same mixed ligand but have available for testing only the population of anti-DNP molecules, the ligand will have a specificity of 1 rather than 2.

2. Even if the ligand is chemically homogeneous it is possible for it to be monovalent but to have more than one specificity. This could happen if there are a number of groups on the ligand each of which can react with a fraction of the testing antibody population, but that, at any time, no more than one antibody molecule can combine with a single ligand molecule. One can envision several reasons for such limitations on ligand reactivity, but perhaps the most likely is steric hindrance; that is, if the ligand is relatively small in size compared to the size of the antibody, then only one antibody molecule can be accommodated at any moment by the ligand, even though other ligand sites are unoccupied and potentially available for reaction with antibody. An example of a ligand which has a single valency but may have more than one specificity is provided by insulin. Berson and Yalow [3] have found that their data on the binding of insulin by its antibodies are compatible with the assumption that insulin is univalent and that there are two distinct types of antibody combining sites. As they point out, however, the binding studies do not exclude the possibility that there are two (or more) distinct antigenic sites and that steric restrictions prevent the binding by the relatively small insulin molecule of more than one antibody molecule at a time.

REACTIONS OF ANTIBODIES WITH MULTIVALENT LIGANDS OF A SINGLE SPECIFICITY

We shall use as model for this type of ligand a protein containing a number of DNP substituents, e.g., DNP-human serum albumin (DNP-HSA). This ligand can be prepared in such a manner that there are many DNP groups per molecule found almost exclusively on lysine side chains. We shall now consider the evidence that this ligand actually has multiple valency and single specificity.

1. The criterion of multiple valency is satisfied if we can demonstrate that on the average more than one antibody molecule can react at the same time with each ligand molecule. This is easily shown in this instance by the precipitin reaction. When DNP-HSA is mixed with a large molar excess of antibody, the resulting precipitate has a mole ratio of antibody : antigen greater than 1.

2. By single specificity we mean that with reference to a particular antibody population (i.e., an antiserum or a preparation of purified antibody) the ligand has one and *only* one specificity. Given an average anti-DNP serum, it is easy to demonstrate that the ligand has DNP specificity. (We need show only that DNP-HSA reacts with the serum and that the reaction can be inhibited by a simple DNP ligand, e.g., 2,4-dinitroaniline.) It is not a simple matter, however, to decide whether the ligand has *at most* one specificity with respect to the serum. One would have to rule out all other possible specificities of the ligand which are detectable by this serum. In practice, because of both the complexity of the ligand and the heterogeneity of antibody populations, this is not possible.

Despite the practical impossibility of obtaining a ligand with many functional groups all of which can be demonstrated to have exactly the same specificity, one can approximate this situation by judicious choice of ligand and antiserum. Thus, if the ligand is DNP-HSA, we can obtain the antiserum from an animal which has been immunized with another DNP-substituted protein, for instance, DNP-bovine-γ-globulin (DNP-BγG). The antibodies in such a serum are likely to react only with those portions of DNP-HSA that contain groups that are also found in DNP-BγG. Since HSA and BγG are themselves quite unrelated proteins, the use of such an antiserum amounts to restricting the specificity of DNP-HSA to the DNP group itself or to the DNP group plus the amino acid residue to which it is attached (usually lysine in both DNP-BγG and DNP-HSA). Although with respect to the anti-DNP-BγG serum, the ligand DNP-HSA approaches the desired characteristics of multiple valency and single specificity, it should be emphasized that the various individual DNP groups of this ligand doubtless have somewhat different reactivities with each antibody molecule. Furthermore, the various antibody molecules are not equivalent in their reactivity with any single functional group of the ligand.

Having pointed out the nonideality of the available multivalent monospecific ligands, we shall in the remainder of this discussion nevertheless assume that the many functional groups of the DNP-HSA ligand are of the same specificity when the antisera are anti-DNP-BγG. Let us now consider the reactions of such sera with DNP-HSA, as indicated by the precipitin curves in Figure 9-2 (upper set).

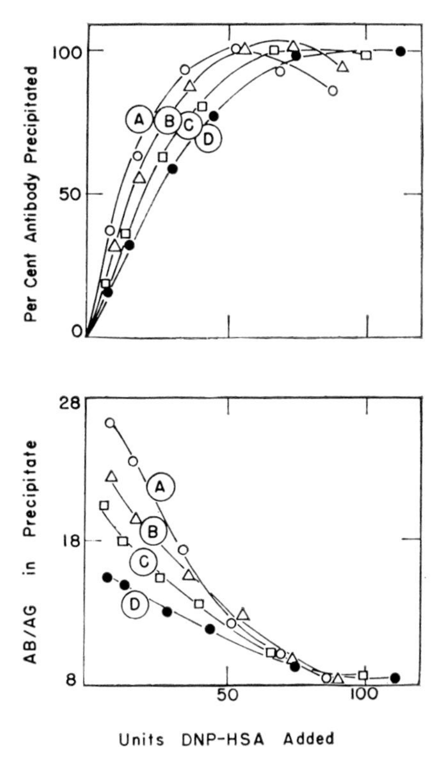

Fig. 9-2. Precipitin reactions of DNP-HSA with rabbit antisera obtained after a single injection of 2 mg. of DNP-BγG in complete Freund's adjuvant. Units DNP-HSA are expressed as milligrams of antigen added, normalized with respect to the maximum antibody precipitated. (*Upper*) Percentage of antibody precipitated vs. DNP-HSA added. (*Lower*) Weight ratio antibody : DNP-HSA in precipitate vs. DNP-HSA added. (*A*) Pooled sera 8 weeks, (*B*) 5 weeks, (*C*) 3 weeks, and (*D*) 10 days after immunization.

In each case, different amounts of antigen are required to reach equivalence, and the curves also vary in general shape. Another way to plot the precipitin data is shown in Figure 9-2 (lower set), where the weight ratio of antibody to antigen in the precipitates (the Ab : Ag ratio) is plotted against total antigen added. This method of plotting the data amplifies the differences in *A–D* already demonstrated in the upper set. In the region of antibody excess (to the left of the maximum or equivalence region), relatively more antibody is precipitated by a given amount of antigen in *A* than in *D*.

Suppose that we were given these data without any detailed information about the source of the sera or the specifications of the ligand preparations used. What are the possible explanations for the observed differences between these antibody-ligand pairs?

1. Ligand differences. The same antiserum but different ligands were used to obtain curves *A–D*.

The differences in the ligands can be classified into two types.

a. The concentration of reactive groups in the ligands varies; i.e., there are more DNP groups per mole ligand in *A* than in *D*. Therefore, for a given number of moles of ligand added, more antibody will be bound in *A* than in *D*.

b. The number of reactive groups per mole ligand is the same, but the intrinsic association constants of these groups in the reaction with antibody is greater for the ligand in *A* than in *D*. This might come about, for example, if the DNP-HSA used in precipitin reaction *A* were unfolded, thus exposing a larger portion of each reactive group. Therefore, for a given number of ligand groups, more antibody will be bound and precipitated in *A* than in *D*.

2. Antibody differences. The same ligand but different antisera were used to obtain *A–D*.

The differences in the antisera can be classified into two types.

a. Certain groups in the ligand can combine with some antibody molecules in *A* but with none of the antibody molecules in *D*. This means that the effective ligand concentration is greater in *A* than in *D*, although the molar ligand concentration is the same in both cases.

b. The average intrinsic association constant for the reaction of antibody molecules with DNP groups of the ligand is greater in *A* than in *D*.

Since the ligand and antibody are characterized operationally in terms of the other, one cannot distinguish between (1) and (2) by examining the precipitin curves alone. However, in any actual example we know of course if we are concerned with the reactions of a given antibody population with several distinct ligands or with the reactions of several antibody populations with a single ligand. In the case presented in Figure 9-2, for instance, it was variation in the antisera which was responsible for the differences in the shape of the precipitin curves. The sera in *A–D* were obtained from a group of rabbits at various intervals after immunization. The antigen solution was the same for each precipitin curve. In this instance, therefore, the differences in antigen-antibody reactions *A–D* are clearly due to variation in the antisera. Serum *A* is said to have the greatest "combining power" or "avidity" for antigen, and *D* the least.

In either category (1) or (2), (*a*) is concerned with the *number* of functional groups, while (*b*) is concerned with the *affinity* between groups. It is usually not possible to distinguish clearly between number and affinity. This is because the presence of a "reactive group" on either ligand or antibody will be revealed only if the energy of interaction is such that a given assay can determine that the reaction has actually occurred. From the point of view of most antigen-antibody reactions, functional groups are not either present or absent. They are more or less present according to their affinity and our methods of detection.

Again referring to the example in Figure 9-2, the greater ability of serum *A* to precipitate the antigen may be attributed either to a larger number of reactive groups on the antigen with which antibody molecules can combine or to a greater affinity of some or all of the antibodies in serum *A* for some or all of the ligand groups. The broadening of specificity which is generally observed with progressive immunization, e.g. [4], has usually been ascribed to the former mechanism, but it could just as well be due to the latter. On the other hand, the increasing avidity observed with progressive immunization, e.g. [5–8], seems to have been ascribed to the latter mechanism, but it could just as well be due to the former. With respect to the precipitin reaction alone, there is no way of distinguishing between these alternatives. In the case of the DNP system, however, it has been possible to obtain detailed information about the reactivity of antibody with specific functional groups.

As indicated earlier, heterogeneity of association constants was invoked to explain the interaction between anti-DNP antibodies and simple DNP ligands (Fig. 9-1). This heterogeneity was attributed to the antibody because with relatively simple ligands, such as DNP-lysine, it is much more reasonable to assume variability in the antibody population rather than in the ligand. By extrapolation, we assume that the antibody population is also heterogeneous in its reaction with more complicated ligands (e.g., DNP-HSA), although in these instances the ligand may contribute an additional source of heterogeneity.

The existence of more than one kind of anti-DNP molecule as expressed in the reaction of anti-DNP-BγG with DNP-HSA can, in fact, be demonstrated directly. If a relatively small amount of DNP-HSA is added to the antiserum, a portion of the antibody population is precipitated. This subpopulation of antibody molecules can be recovered in part from the precipitate and shown to have an average affinity for DNP-lysine which is higher than that of the average antibody molecule in the larger population from which it was precipitated. This experiment demonstrates that those antibody molecules in the antiserum which have the greatest tendency to combine and precipitate with the multivalent ligand DNP-HSA also have a relatively greater ability to combine with the univalent ligand DNP-lysine [1].

Another result discussed earlier is that the average association constant of serum antibodies for DNP-lysine increases systematically with time after immunization. The corresponding result for the multivalent ligand DNP-HSA is given in the two sets of curves in Figure 9-2. The source of the antiserum which yielded curve *D* was a serum pool obtained from rabbits 10 days after immunization with DNP-BγG. Serum *C* was obtained at three weeks, serum *B* at five weeks, and serum *A* at eight weeks after immunization. The later sera have a greater tendency to combine with antigen than do the earlier sera. The analogy between these results and those for the reaction with DNP-lysine was confirmed by purifying a portion of the antibodies in these sera and obtaining average association constants for the reaction with DNP-lysine of $> 10^8$, 1×10^7, 5×10^6, and 1×10^6 liters per mole for *A, B, C,* and *D,* respectively (unpublished data).

Thus the reactions of a simple univalent ligand, DNP-lysine, are an essential guide to an understanding of more complicated ligands such as DNP-HSA. The reactions of the latter, in turn, provide a model for the most complex type of antibody-ligand interaction, that of antibody with multivalent ligands of *multiple* specificity.

REACTIONS OF ANTIBODIES WITH MULTIVALENT LIGANDS OF MULTIPLE SPECIFICITY

Almost all naturally occurring antigens (e.g., globular proteins) fall into this class, and it was the explanation of the behavior of such substances that provided at least the original stimulus for most immunological investigations. Ligands such as bovine serum albumin (BSA), egg albumin, and the like, have many functional groups of various types, each of which can react with a heterogeneous set of antibody molecules. Despite, or perhaps more accurately because of, this increased complexity it is the reactions of this group of ligands which are of primary interest to the biologist. From a chemical point of view, however, the complex nature of the ligands in this class makes the detailed analysis of their reactions with antibodies extremely difficult.

Although we may find that the complexity of the whole is greater than the sum of the complexities of the parts, the general principles that govern the reactions of the functional groups of small ligands seem also to apply when the groups are located on larger and more complicated antigens. Thus the reversibility of the antigen-antibody reaction is generally easy to demonstrate. These reactions are also evidently heterogeneous, some antibody molecules having greater over-all tendency to combine with antigen than others. In addition, the average combining power of antisera resulting from the administration of complex antigens such as diphtheria toxin and BSA changes with time after immunization [5–8]. In the case of the reactions of the protein ligand DNP-HSA with antibodies formed in response to DNP-BγG (discussed earlier), one can approximate the reactions of the functional groups by studying the reactions of the antibodies with simple DNP ligands. With protein antigens generally, however, this is not possible since we do not know the nature of the reactive groups. Nevertheless, since some of the general features evident in the reactions of simple ligands with their antibodies can also be discerned in the reactions of protein antigens, it seems reasonable to suppose that the reactive groups on these antigens, were we able to study them, would react with their antibodies in an analogous fashion.

We have considered the reactions of ligands and antibodies with little regard for the specific chemical properties of the reactants. This approach is feasible in that the reactants themselves and many of their properties (e.g., valency, specificity) can be defined formally without reference to their specific structures or to the nature of the functional groups. Indeed, because of the symmetry of the definitions, with reference to the reacting system we cannot formally distinguish between antibody and ligand. Nevertheless it need hardly be pointed out that we are not primarily concerned with an abstract system. Antibodies are *not* the same as ligands, and by going beyond the interaction itself to the chemical properties of the reactants and to the notion of immunogenicity we have, in fact, no real difficulty in distinguishing between them. Thus antibodies are always proteins, and despite some variability, they have distinctive structural characteristics (see Chapter 3). Ligands, on the other hand, can be any of a vast variety of substances: proteins, nucleic acids, polysaccharides, lipids, synthetic polypeptides, small organic molecules, and so on. A knowledge of the properties of ligands and of antibodies will doubtless make clear certain limitations on their interactions which are not implied by the definitions themselves. In these terms then, one of the goals for immunology is to establish a correspondence between the formal system and the structural entities it describes.

REFERENCES

1. Eisen, H. N., and Siskind, G. W. Variations in affinities of antibodies during the immune response, *Biochemistry* 3:996, 1964.
2. Farah, F. S., Kern, M., and Eisen, H. N. The preparation and some properties of purified antibody specific for the 2,4-dinitrophenyl group, *J. Exp. Med.* 112:1195, 1960.
3. Berson, S. A., and Yalow, R. S. Quantitative aspects of the reaction between insulin and insulin-binding antibody, *J. Clin. Invest.* 38: 1996, 1959.
4. Heidelberger, M., and Kendall, F. E. A quantitative theory of the precipitin reaction: III. The reaction between crystalline egg albumin and its homologous antibody, *J. Exp. Med.* 62:697, 1935.
5. Jerne, N. K. A study of avidity based on rabbit skin responses to diphtheria toxin-antitoxin mixtures, *Acta Path. Microbiol. Scand.*, vol. 28, supp. 87, 1951.
6. Talmage, D. W., and Maurer, P. H. I^{131}-labeled antigen precipitation as a measure of quantity and quality of antibody, *J. Infect. Dis.* 92:288, 1953.
7. Farr, R. S. A quantitative immunochemical measure of the primary interaction between I*BSA and antibody, *J. Infect. Dis.* 103:239, 1958.
8. Grey, H. M. Studies on changes in the quality of rabbit-bovine serum albumin antibody following immunization, *Immunology* 7:82, 1964.

10. Experimental Anaphylaxis*

KIMISHIGE ISHIZAKA

GENERAL CONCEPTS

ACTIVE AND PASSIVE ANAPHYLAXIS

The phenomenon called anaphylaxis was first described by Richet and Portier in 1902 when they were studying the antitoxic immunity of dogs to the poison of sea anemone. They found that some dogs previously immunized with the poison exhibited severe shock symptoms and died on reinjection of an amount less than the minimal lethal dose. Since this phenomenon was contrary to immunity, in which animals are in a "prophylactic" state, they called the phenomenon *anaphylaxie.* Much work has been done on the mechanisms involved in anaphylaxis since then. It was found that the substance which induces anaphylactic shock is not necessarily a toxic or pathogenic agent and that anaphylactic shock can be induced in many animal species. For example, guinea pigs receiving an injection of crystalline ovalbumin, with no harmful effect, exhibit anaphylactic shock when the same substance is reinjected intravenously 10 days to 3 weeks later. The interval between the first and second injection of antigen necessary for the induction of anaphylaxis is in accord with the time of antibody formation. Anaphylaxis can also be induced passively by the administration of antiserum instead of by active immunization. If guinea pigs receive antibody followed by an intravenous injection of the corresponding antigen 24 hours later, anaphylactic shock results. These facts indicate that anaphylactic shock is one of the manifestations of the combination of antigen with antibody *in vivo.*

The anaphylactic state induced by active immunization (sensitization) of animals by antigen is called active anaphylaxis and that obtained by the administration of antibody is called passive anaphylaxis. In active anaphylaxis, the first injection of antigen is known as the sensitizing injection and the second injection, the shocking dose. Sensitizing antigen may be administered intravenously, subcutaneously, or intraperitoneally. Sensitization is accomplished even by inhalation of antigen dispersed as fine droplets [1]. The shocking dose should be administered intravenously for uniform results. If the dose is suitable, the shocking injection will produce anaphylactic death within ten minutes. Anaphylactic shock may be induced by subcutaneous or intracutaneous injection of antigen [2]. In these cases, however, a larger amount of antigen is required. The shock symptoms may be delayed, mild, or prolonged. Induction of anaphylaxis by inhalation is not as uniform as by intravenous injection, but the results are better than those obtained by either subcutaneous or intraperitoneal injections [3]. After receiving a sublethal shocking dose of antigen, sensitized guinea pigs may become completely and specifically refractory to the antigen used. This is called desensitization.

In passive anaphylaxis, antibody is generally administered to animals by intravenous or intraperitoneal injection, followed by an intravenous injection (shocking dose) of antigen 24 to 48 hours later. In some antigen-antibody systems, anaphylactic shock can be induced by the injection of antigen followed by an intravenous injection of antibody 1 to 2 days later. This type of reaction is called reversed passive anaphylaxis. In connection with reversed anaphylaxis, Forssman [4] found that the injection into normal guinea pigs of rabbit antiserum to sheep erythrocytes would produce symptoms and death similar to that of anaphylaxis. This phenomenon is due to the combination of the antibody with the Forssman antigen present in guinea pig tissues. However, symptoms in Forssman shock are slightly different from those of anaphylactic shock. Forssman antibody does not cause isolated uterine strips from normal guinea pigs to contract [5]. The heterophil antibody in-

* This work was supported in part by Research Grants E-3308 and AI-4985 from the U.S. Public Health Service.

jected intracutaneously into guinea pigs induces local hemorrhage but not cutaneous anaphylaxis [6]. It is therefore questionable that Forssman shock should be considered a form of anaphylaxis.

SYSTEMIC AND LOCAL ANAPHYLAXIS

Anaphylactic shock may be provoked in numerous animal species, including man. Guinea pigs exhibit the most rapid and severe anaphylactic responses, characterized by restlessness, chewing, rubbing of the nose and ears, dyspnea, convulsions, and frequently death. Decreases in blood pressure and body temperature are also characteristic. Best responses are obtained in guinea pigs in the weight range of 250 to 300 gm.

Regardless of the species, the shock symptoms are based on two underlying physiological responses: an increase in the permeability of capillaries and small vessels, and contraction of smooth muscle. Thus anaphylactic reactions can be observed locally by measuring these responses. Representative examples of local anaphylaxis commonly utilized in animal experiments are cutaneous anaphylaxis and Schultz-Dale reactions. If a shocking injection is administered intracutaneously to actively or passively sensitized guinea pigs, and if a dye such as Evans blue (5 mg.) is injected intravenously immediately after the injection of antigen, the dye accumulates at the skin site [6]. The leakage of dye is due to the increased capillary permeability resulting from the antigen-antibody interaction. Maximal localization of blue dye occurs within fifteen minutes after the injection of antigen. Intensities of the reactions are determined by measuring the diameter of the blue spot on the inner surface of the skin. Care must be taken to avoid solutions of antigen which are irritating to the skin of unsensitized animals.

Cutaneous anaphylaxis is also observed when the local skin site is sensitized by an intracutaneous injection of antibody and a mixture of antigen and dye is injected intravenously 3 to 6 hours later [6]. Or both antigen and antibody may be injected into the same skin site for the induction of cutaneous anaphylaxis. Regardless of which method is used, the reaction is called passive cutaneous anaphylaxis (PCA) if the antibody is injected before the antigen. If the antigen is injected first, the reaction is called reversed PCA. A nonspecific irritation may occur from the antiserum but this generally does not last more than 1 hour. Thus if antigen is injected intravenously 3 to 6 hours after an intracutaneous injection of antiserum, the skin-irritating activities of both antiserum and antigen may be avoided. For this reason, as well as because of its high sensitivity for detecting antibody, this sequence of injections is the most frequently used in studies involving PCA. The PCA reaction is also observed in mice and rats [6], in which the maximal reaction is not reached until 30 minutes after the injection of antigen. The sensitivity of the reaction in these animals is much lower than in guinea pigs.

Another representative anaphylactic reaction is contraction of isolated uterine or intestinal strips from sensitized animals on contact with antigen (Schultz-Dale reaction). Originally, Dale used uterine horns from female guinea pigs, but intestinal strips gave more reproducible results [7]. Jejunum is much less sensitive than ileum. The strips are thoroughly washed with Tyrode's solution and suspended in a Dale bath containing Tyrode's solution at 37° C. Oxygen is continuously bubbled in the bath. When antigen solution is added, the ileum contracts. The intensity of the contraction can be recorded with a kymograph. Passive sensitization of isolated guinea pig ileum can be accomplished *in vitro* by incubation of the isolated ileum from normal guinea pigs with antibody diluted in Tyrode's solution [8]. As will be described, *in vitro* sensitization of the isolated guinea pig ileum is an important technique for quantitative studies of the anaphylactic reaction.

Local anaphylactic reactions have been observed in guinea pig lung tissues [9a]. Chopped lung from a sensitized guinea pig is suspended in Tyrode's solution. The intensity of the anaphylactic reactions is determined by measuring the quantity of histamine liberated on contact of the tissues with antigen. Recently, *in vitro* sensitization of normal lung tissues with antibody was reported [10]. Release of histamine and slow-reacting substance from lung tissues is discussed in Chapter 15.

Vasoactive amines such as histamine and serotonin play an important role in the induction of anaphylaxis. Mast cells of the isolated mesenteries of sensitized guinea pigs are damaged by the addition of antigen. Granules of the cells which contain histamine are lost as the result of the antigen-antibody interaction [11]. A close correlation between damage of mast cells and the occurrence of anaphylactic shock has been demonstrated by Humphrey and Mota [12]. Since rabbit platelets contain a large amount of histamine and serotonin, the effect of an antigen-antibody interaction on the platelets was studied by Humphrey and Jacques [13]. Platelets from sensitized rabbits liberated these amines when antigen was added. It was also found that serum components other than antibody were necessary for the reaction.

SITE OF ANTIGEN-ANTIBODY INTERACTION IN ANAPHYLAXIS

Since anaphylaxis can be produced in normal animals by passive transfer of antiserum from a sensitized animal, it is evident that the antibody involved in anaphylaxis is present in the antiserum. But the site of the antigen-antibody interaction which induces anaphylaxis is probably not in the circulation. In actively sensitized animals, the amount of circulating antibody has no correlation with the degree of anaphylactic sensitivity [14]. For passive anaphylaxis, an interval between sensitization and shock is required. Although the level of circulating antibody is highest immediately after the injection of antiserum, severe anaphylactic shock does not occur if the antigen is injected then. However, if the antigen is injected 24 hours after the passive sensitization, when the antibody level in the circulation is much less, severe shock appears. The reverse is true in the Arthus reaction, which can also be transferred by antiserum. In the Arthus type of reaction, the effect of an injection of antigen is more severe immediately after passive transfer of the antiserum than 24 hours later. The presence of a latent period in both systemic and local anaphylaxis indicates that antigen-antibody interactions in tissues rather than in the circulation induce both forms of anaphylaxis. This is especially clear in the case of the latent period observed with PCA, in which the antibody concentration in the skin site is highest immediately after the injection. It is generally accepted that antibody in passive anaphylaxis is fixed to some tissue constituent or cell and that anaphylactic reactions are induced by the combination of antigen to this fixed antibody.

CONDITIONS FOR ESTABLISHING A SENSITIZED STATE

ACTIVE SENSITIZATION

Antigens which induce the formation of serum antibodies usually induce active sensitization. Guinea pigs are actively sensitized with various kinds of foreign protein antigens but not with haptens. Sensitization of guinea pigs can be induced with as little as 10^{-6} ml. of horse serum [15] or with 0.05 μg. of crystalline ovalbumin. In most experiments, however, larger amounts of an antigen are used for sensitization. A single injection of 0.1 to 1 mg. of protein antigen is usually sufficient. More uniform results are obtained by repeated subcutaneous injections (four times) of antigen at three to four day intervals. Sensitization, as stated, has also been effected by inhalation of antigen dispersed as fine droplets [1]. Sensitivity, once established, persists for several months or longer.

Mice and rats may also be actively sensitized for anaphylactic shock. However, fatal anaphylaxis rarely occurs unless the sensitizing antigen is incorporated in Freund's adjuvant [16–18]. For mice, 1 mg. of bovine serum albumin (BSA), 0.05 to 0.25 mg. of alum-precipitated BSA [17], and 0.1 mg. of the antigen in Freund's adjuvant are optimal sensitizing doses [18]. Anaphylactic shock can be obtained by injecting 1 to 2 mg. of the antigen 24 to 35 days later. The effect of *Hemophilus pertussis* on anaphylaxis in mice and rats is interesting. If the antigen is mixed with *H. pertussis* cells, active anaphylactic sensitivity in mice can be induced with a single injection of a minute amount of antigen [19, 20]. The maximal effect in mice is obtained by intraperitoneal injection of 250 million (phase 1) *H. pertussis* [21]. *Hemophilus pertussis* also increases the susceptibility of mice to passive anaphylaxis, indicating that an adjuvant effect is not the only factor [22]. Injection of the bacilli into mice increases susceptibility to histamine [23], serotonin [24], and endotoxin [25] (Chap. 16). However, active anaphylaxis can be produced at a time when serotonin and histamine hypersensitivity have disappeared [25]. The increased susceptibility to passive anaphylaxis disappears at a time when histamine and serotonin sensitivity is still present [21]. Although CF-1 mice do not develop hypersensitivity to histamine, they become more sensitive to anaphylaxis after treatment with *H. pertussis* [26]. It may be concluded that the increase in susceptibility to vasoactive amines by *H. pertussis* does not correlate with its enhancing effect on anaphylaxis. *Brucella abortus* also increases the susceptibility of the mouse to histamine and to anaphylaxis but is less effective than *H. pertussis* [27]. It was also found that adrenalectomized mice become susceptible to histamine [28], serotonin, and anaphylaxis [16].

PASSIVE SENSITIZATION

Latent Period and Persistence of Sensitivity. An interval between the sensitizing and shocking injections is required for passive anaphylaxis. This latent period is a function of the sensitizing dose of antibody, as described by Benacerraf and Kabat [29]. If the shocking dose of antigen was constant (1 mg. of ovalbumin), an interval of 5 hours was necessary for anaphylactic death when guinea pigs received 30 μg. of rabbit antibody N. With a very large dose of antibody (2 mg. N), fatal shock occurred without a latent period. Similar results were obtained in PCA reactions by Ovary and Bier [30]. When guinea pig skin was sensitized by an intracutaneous injection of 1 μg. of antibody N, definite skin reactions were obtained, even when antigen was injected 30 minutes later, whereas 1 to 3 hours were necessary following the injection of 0.01 μg. of antibody N (Table 10-1). In mice, the latent period was not so marked, but the greatest skin reactions were observed when the antigen was injected intravenously 3 hours after an intracutaneous injection of antibody [31]. A latent period was also observed in the sensitization of guinea pig ileum *in vitro*. Halpern *et al.* [8] found that only 0.25 μg. of antibody N per ml. of Tyrode's solution was sufficient to sensitize guinea pig ileum if the antibody was incubated with the ileum for 120 minutes. To obtain a contraction of comparable intensity with 15 minutes' incubation, as much as 16 μg. of antibody N per ml. was required. A linear relationship was obtained between the reciprocal of time of incubation and the concentration of antibody used.

In passive anaphylaxis, persistence of the sensitized state is limited. In guinea pigs, sensitivity following intravenous injections of 30 to 100 μg. of rabbit antibody N persisted for 8 days but disappeared by 12 days [6]. After intracutaneous injection of 0.025 μg. of antibody N, sensitivity disappeared after 24 hours. If 0.25 μg. was injected, a strong reaction was observed after 24 hours, but not at 48 hours. With guinea pig antibody, both systemic and passive cutaneous sensitivity persisted for a longer period. Fatal anaphylaxis occurred 28 days after intravenous injection of 30 μg. of guinea pig antibody N [32]. Passive cutaneous sensitization persisted 72 hours after local injection of 0.03 μg. of guinea pig antiovalbumin N. In PCA reactions in mice, sensitivity obtained with rabbit antibody disappeared 24 hours after the sensitization even when ten times as much or more antibody than the threshold amount was used [31]. Even with mouse antibody, sensitivity diminished 24 hours after passive sensitization [33].

Nature and Quantities of Antibody for Passive Sensitization. Passive sensitization depends on the species from which the antibody is derived. Guinea pig, rabbit, dog, human, and monkey antibodies can sensitize guinea pigs for anaphylactic reactions, whereas horse, cow, goat, rat, and chicken antibodies do not

TABLE 10-1. Relationship between Latent Period of PCA and Amount of Intradermally Injected Rabbit Antiovalbumin

Antibody N Injected i.d., μg.	13 mg. Ovalbumin in 1 Ml. Saline Injected i.v. with Dye after[a]							
	0 min.	30 min.	1 hr.	2 hr.	3 hr.	6 hr.	24 hr.	48 hr.
1.00	0 0	3 3	3 2	4 4	4 4	4 4	4 4	4 4
0.10	0 0	2 2	2 1	3 3	4 3	4 4	3 4	0 0
0.05	0 0	1 1	2 1	3 3	4 3	4 4	1 2	0 0
0.02	0 0	½ ½	2 2 1	1 2 2	4 4 4	2 2 1	0 0 0	0 0 0
0.01	0 0	0 ½	1 1 ½	½ 1 1	2 2 2	2 2 ½	0 0 0	0 0 0
0.005	0 0	0 0	½ ½ ½	0 0 ½	0 0 0	0 0 0	0 0 0	0 0 0

[a] Results graded from 0 (no reaction) to 4 (blue spot larger than 20 mm. in diameter).
SOURCE: Ovary and Bier [30].

[6, 34–36]. Kabat and Boldt [37] showed that guinea pig and rabbit antibodies have a comparable capacity to sensitize guinea pigs. Thirty μg. of antiovalbumin N from both animal species sensitized guinea pigs to fatal anaphylaxis. Intravenous injections of 1 mg. (0.16 mg. N) of ovalbumin 48 hours later resulted in shock and death. When guinea pigs were sensitized with smaller amounts of antibody (6 to 25 μg. of antibody N), anaphylactic shock occurred but was not always fatal, even when large amounts of antigen were used for the shocking dose (Table 10-2). In PCA reactions in guinea pigs, an intracutaneous injection of 0.003 to 0.01 μg. of antibody N from these species, followed by an intravenous injection of 1 mg. of ovalbumin 3 to 6 hours later, induced a definite skin response [6], whereas 0.1 to 0.2 μg. of human antibody N was required for this. Evidently human antibody has less sensitizing activity than rabbit or guinea pig antibody in guinea pigs. Munoz and Anacker [33, 38] made similar observations in anaphylactic reactions in mice. Both rabbit and mouse antibodies sensitized mice. In pertussis-treated mice, 160 μg. of rabbit antibody N and 6.2 μg. of mouse antibody N were required for the induction of fatal anaphylaxis. The minimal amounts of these antibodies for PCA sensitization were 4.8 μg. N and 0.009 μg. N, respectively.

The Schultz-Dale reaction and degranulation of mast cells of guinea pigs are more readily induced with the antiserum of some species than of others [34]. Goat, chicken, rat, and horse antibodies failed to sensitize guinea pig cells. To induce a definite contraction of guinea pig intestine in the Schultz-Dale reaction, 30 μg. or more of rabbit antibody N must be injected 24 hours before the intestine is taken out [39]. Halpern *et al.* [8] have shown that *in vitro* sensitization of guinea pig intestine with as little as 0.1 μg. of antibody N per ml. of rabbit antiovalbumin in Tyrode's solution was enough to sensitize the isolated intestine after a 4-hour incubation. Uniform results may be obtained by incubation of the intestine for 30 minutes in 1 μg. of antibody N per ml. of rabbit antibody.

The ability of antibody to sensitize guinea pigs passively also depends on its physicochemical properties. Ovary *et al.* [40] have demonstrated that guinea pig γ_2-globulin antibody does not sensitize guinea pig skin for PCA reactions, whereas γ_1 antibody does. It was also found [41a] that human 19S γ-globulin (IgM) antibody failed to sensitize guinea pig skin, whereas 7S γ_2-globulin (IgG) antibody did. Rabbit 19S γ-globulin antibody also lacks sensitizing activity in guinea pigs. Many efforts have been made to detect human reaginic antibody by PCA reactions in guinea pigs, but a definite result has never been obtained [6]. Recently, evidence has been accumulated that reaginic antibody may be associated with γ_{1A}-globulin (IgA) but not with γ_2-globulin [42–44]. As described later, the lack of sensitizing activity of human reaginic

TABLE 10-2. Passive Sensitization of Guinea Pigs with Varying Amounts of Rabbit Antiovalbumin

Antibody N Injected, Mg.	No. of Guinea Pigs Used	Results[a]			
		Deaths	Severe Reactions	Slight Reactions	No Reactions
0.0019	4	0	0	2	2
0.0038	4	0	1	3	
0.0057	5	0	3	2	
0.0064	1	1			
0.0075	4	0	3	1	
0.0113	6	4	2		
0.023; 0.024	5	3	2		
0.034; 0.036	6	6			
0.048	2	2			
0.060	8	8			
0.072	1	1			

[a] Guinea pigs shocked with 1 mg. ovalbumin intravenously 48 hours after sensitizing injection.

SOURCE: Kabat and Landow [76b].

antibody in guinea pigs may be due to the fact that it is not γ_2 globulin (IgG).

The sensitizing activity of antibody does not correlate with its behavior in precipitin reactions. Precipitating antibody and nonprecipitating antibody are equally capable of provoking passive anaphylaxis [45] and PCA reactions [6, 46].

The ability of rabbit antibody to sensitize guinea pigs can be diminished by chemical treatment. Papain- or pepsin-digested antibody does not sensitize guinea pig skin. Porter's piece I or a mixture of pieces I and II, which contain the combining sites for antigen (Chap. 3), do not induce PCA reactions [47]. These fragments specifically inhibit the reaction if mixed with the original undigested antibody. The inhibition is transitory because the fragments do not stay in the tissues for a long time. Reduction of rabbit antibody in 0.1 M mercaptoethanol followed by alkylation, which results in irreversible cleavage of some disulfide bonds in the antibody molecule, reduces its sensitizing power without impairing its behavior as a precipitin [48].

Type of Antigen Required in Reversed Passive Anaphylaxis. Anaphylactic reactions are generally observed when antibody is present *in vivo* before the shocking dose of antigen is introduced. If antigens, such as serum albumin, ovalbumin, hemocyanin, and polysaccharides, are injected into guinea pigs, followed by an intravenous injection of antibody one to two days later, no anaphylactic reaction is obtained. Reversed passive anaphylaxis, in which antigen is first introduced, can be observed only with antigens capable of fixing to skin. Bier and Siqueira [49] produced cutaneous anaphylaxis by intracutaneous injections of rabbit γ-globulin followed by an intravenous injection of guinea pig antirabbit γ-globulin. Humphrey and Mota [34] demonstrated that human γ-globulin, as well, can passively sensitize guinea pigs. They injected 10 mg. of rabbit γ-globulin or human γ-globulin into normal guinea pigs. When these animals received guinea pig or rabbit antibody two days later, they developed systemic anaphylaxis. Intestines from guinea pigs which had received γ-globulin contracted on contact with homologous antibody. In reversed PCA in which the antigen is first injected intracutaneously, both human and rabbit 7S γ_2-globulin (IgG) can induce skin responses in the guinea pig, even with horse, chicken, or sheep antisera [50, 51]. As described previously, these antibodies were unable to sensitize the guinea pig skin directly, but when the γ-globulin antigens are injected before the antibody, characteristic anaphylactic reactions are obtained. The minimal amounts of human and of rabbit γ-globulins required to produce reversed PCA reactions in guinea pigs are 0.1 μg. N and 0.01 μg. N, respectively, which are comparable to the minimal doses of human and rabbit antibody for sensitizing guinea pig skin [50]. Reversed PCA reactions in guinea pigs could not be demonstrated if goat, cattle, or chicken γ-globulin were used as antigens. In general, the γ-globulin of a species whose antibodies can passively sensitize the guinea pig can induce reversed passive anaphylaxis even with antibodies of those species which cannot themselves sensitize the guinea pig passively. It was also found that both human 19S γ-globulin (IgM) and γ_{1A} (IgA) failed to cause reversed PCA reactions [41].

The ability of human and rabbit γ-globulins to give reversed passive sensitization is affected by some chemical treatments. Porter's pieces I and II obtained from papain-digested rabbit γ-globulin do not induce reversed PCA reactions with either sheep or chicken antiserum to rabbit γ-globulin. It is of interest that piece III can induce reversed passive sensitization [47]. Lack of the reversed PCA reactions with pieces I and II is not due to the absence of major antigenic determinants of rabbit γ-globulin in these fragments. Rabbit γ-globulin induced reversed PCA reactions with anti-piece III and anti-(I+II) chicken antibody, whereas piece I or II did not cause the skin reaction with anti-(I+II) [51]. The ability of human and rabbit γ-globulins to induce reversed passive sensitization is diminished by partial reduction of the γ-globulins with mercaptoethanol followed by alkylation, without changing their specificity as antigens [48]. These findings indicate that the type of antigen required for sensitizing guinea pigs in reversed passive anaphylaxis is quite similar to the type of antibody required for sensitization in direct passive anaphylaxis and suggests that the same mechanisms are involved in both processes.

Blocking of Passive Sensitization with γ-Globulin. In PCA reactions, the sensitizing ability of antiserum does not parallel its antibody concentration. With weak antisera, large amounts of antibody are required to sensitize guinea pig skin [6]. Ovary and Bier [52], for instance, found that 0.5 μg. of rabbit antiovalbumin N was required for minimal PCA sensitization when the antiserum was diluted with normal rabbit serum. This is fifty times as much as the minimal sensitizing dose of the same antiserum diluted with saline. Human serum also has this inhibitory effect on the sensitization of guinea pig skin with rabbit antibody. The inhibitory activity in these sera is associated with the γ-globulin [53, 54]. Other proteins such as albumin and α- and β-globulins of normal rabbit serum do not have this inhibitory effect [55, 56]. Biozzi *et al.* [54] studied the quantitative relationship between the amount of antibody used for passive sensitization and the amount of normal γ-globulin required to block the sensitization and found that 16 to 20 μg. of normal rabbit γ-globulin N per ml. were required to block PCA sensitization of guinea pig skin with 0.1 μg. of rabbit antibody N per ml. Forty μg. of human γ-globulin N per ml. were required to give the same effect. They also found that horse, cattle, and chicken γ-globulins cannot block the sensitization with rabbit antibody. Guinea pig 7S γ_1-globulin, but not γ_2-globulin, showed the blocking effect [40]. Similar observations were made in passive sensitization for systemic anaphylaxis and *in vitro* sensitization of the isolated guinea pig intestine. Human and rabbit γ-globulins completely protected guinea pigs against fatal anaphylaxis when injected before or simultaneously with sensitization [57]. These γ-globulins, when added to the incubating medium containing rabbit antibody, inhibited *in vitro* sensitization of isolated guinea pig ileum [58a]. The blocking effect in guinea pigs of the γ-globulins from many species decreases in the following order: rabbit> man> dog> guinea pig> rat> horse> cattle> pig> chicken> goat [58a]. Halpern *et al.* [58b] reported that incubation of the sensitized isolated guinea pig ileum with normal rabbit γ-globulin resulted in desensitization. With labeled antibody used for *in vitro* sensitization, part of the antibody in the sensitized tissues is liberated by incubation with normal unlabeled γ-globulin.

The blocking effect of γ-globulin depends not only on the species of γ-globulin but also on its physicochemical properties. Neither human 19S γ- nor γ_{1A}-globulin blocked passive sensitization of guinea pig skin with rabbit antibody [44]. It appears that the same physicochemical properties are required for the blocking of passive sensitization by normal γ-globulin as are required for sensitization by antibody. This suggests that the normal γ-globulins have affinity for the same guinea pig tissue constituent with which antibody combines upon sensitization.

It was also found that Porter's piece III of rabbit γ-globulin, but not piece I or II, blocked passive sensitization with rabbit antibody [59]. This finding, as well as the fact that piece III can sensitize guinea pig skin for reversed PCA reactions [47], indicates that this fragment contains the structures essential for passive sensitization. Olins and Edelman [60] and Porter [61] have shown that piece III is the major part of the heavy chain (A chain) in the γ-globulin molecule and that pieces I and II are composed of the light chain (B chain) and a part of the heavy (A) chain. It is therefore evident that the structures essential for passive sensitization are present in the heavy chain. Evidence has been presented [62–64] that the heavy chains in human γ_2-, 19S γ-, and γ_{1A}-globulin molecules are different from each other, whereas a difference in the light chains of these three classes of γ-globulins has never been detected. The lack of sensitizing ability of human 19S γ-globulin and γ_{1A}-globulins in guinea pigs might be explained by the difference in structure of the heavy chains in these molecules from that of γ_2-globulin.

Antibody in Sensitized Tissues. As the anaphylactic reactions are caused by antigen-antibody interactions in the tissues, the actual concentration of antibody in sensitized tissues has to be considered. By using I^{131}-labeled antibody for passive sensitization *in vivo,* it was found that the minimal rabbit anti-BSA concentration per gm. of intestinal strip required for a Schultz-Dale response was 0.08 to 0.1 μg. N [39]. For *in vitro* sensitization, Nielsen *et al.* [65] found that 0.12 μg. of AbN per gm. of tissues was the approximate minimal ratio required to induce a Schultz-Dale reaction. It is possible, however, that all of the antibody in sensitized tissue is not involved in the anaphylactic reaction. This possibility was suggested by Humphrey and Mota's finding that horse antibody (which does not sensitize the guinea pig ileum) is adsorbed by guinea pig mesentery to as great an extent as rabbit antibody [34, 66]. By *in vitro* sensitization of guinea pig intestine, Feigen *et al.* [67] separated the process of sensitization from that of adsorption. They found that neither the velocity of adsorption nor the amount of antibody bound was affected by the temperature of incubation, whereas the amount of histamine released was regularly increased with increased temperature during incubation. It was suggested that certain cells on the surface of the tissues have the capacity to release active agents when antigen combines with the fixed antibody and that other cells may combine with the antibody but not be involved in the anaphylactic reaction.

Mechanisms involved in the fixation of antibody to certain animal tissues are unknown. It is of interest, however, that *in vitro* sensitization of guinea pig ileum occurs much more rapidly with a given quantity of antibody when carried out in a salt-free medium [68]. Addition of a variety of electrolytes slowed the rate of fixation. In a salt-free medium containing glucose and $NaHCO_3$, as little as 0.002 μg. of antibody N per ml. caused sensitization of isolated guinea pig ileum in eight hours. Urea at a concentration of 0.8 M also increased the rate of antibody fixation to the tissues [69].

INDUCTION OF ANAPHYLACTIC REACTIONS

NATURE AND DOSE OF THE SHOCKING INJECTION

The substance used for shocking injections does not necessarily induce the formation of serum antibodies. Kabat and Landow [76b] showed that pneumococcus polysaccharide, which does not induce antibodies in guinea pigs, can cause anaphylactic reactions in guinea pigs passively sensitized with rabbit antiserum to pneumococcus. Synthetic polyvalent hapten, such as resorcinol R'_3, can induce anaphylactic reactions in animals sensitized against arsanyl-azoprotein [70]. The only antigen which cannot induce anaphylactic reactions is a simple hapten having one determinant group. If administered shortly before the shocking dose of antigen, simple haptens inhibit systemic anaphylaxis [71], Schultz-Dale reactions, and cutaneous anaphylaxis. In PCA reactions in guinea pigs, Ovary and Karush [72] found that 85 mg. of lactose administered twenty minutes before 5 μg. N of lactoside-human fibrinogen inhibited PCA reactions in the sites sensitized with 0.8 μg. of anti-lac antibody N. It was also found by Ovary [73] that ε-dinitrophenyl (DNP)-lysine did not induce PCA reactions in a site that received anti-DNP rabbit antibody, whereas ε-, α-DNP-lysine did. Since the latter hapten contains two determinant groups in a molecule, the results indicate that the presence of two or more antigenic determinants in an antigen molecule is an essential property for the induction of anaphylactic reactions. The ε, α-DNP-lysine does not induce precipitin reactions with antibody. Thus an antigen need not be able to produce a precipitin reaction in order to induce an anaphylactic reaction.

The dose of antigen required to induce an anaphylactic reaction depends on the amount of antibody used for passive sensitization. A reciprocal relationship has been established between the amount of antigen and the amount of antibody necessary to elicit systemic anaphylaxis [76], the Schultz-Dale reaction [74], and passive cutaneous anaphylaxis. Data on PCA reactions are shown in Table 10-3 [75]. By using I^{131}-labeled guinea pig and

TABLE 10-3. Passive Cutaneous Anaphylactic Reactions in Guinea Pig Elicited by Varying Amounts of Ovalbumin and Two Levels of Rabbit Ovalbumin[a]

Antigen N μg., i.v.	1.0 μg. Antibody N, i.d.								0.02 μg. Ovalbumin N, i.d.							
0.5	50	0	0	0	0	0	0	0	not done							
0.1	20	28	50	78	0	0	0	0	not done							
0.2	78	254	153	490	490	315	315	0	not done							
0.4	78	176	254	153	176	315	706	706	not done							
0.625	not done								63	28	38	0	0	0	0	0
0.8	706	380	490	615	706	615	615	706	not done							
1.25	not done								79	50	7	154	0	0	0	0
2.5	not done								113	79	28	663	79	20	0	0
5.0	not done								79	132	94	50	132	132	25	0
10.0	not done								201	154	417	79	19	28	201	113
50.0	490	380	452	380	490	706	706	314	132	226	176	38	176	113	154	154

[a] Area in mm^2.
SOURCE: Ovary [75].

rabbit antibody, Ishizaka *et al.* [39, 74] found that a hyperbolic relationship exists between the amount of antibody present on guinea pig intestine and the concentration of antigen necessary to produce a given intensity of Schultz-Dale response (Fig. 10-1).

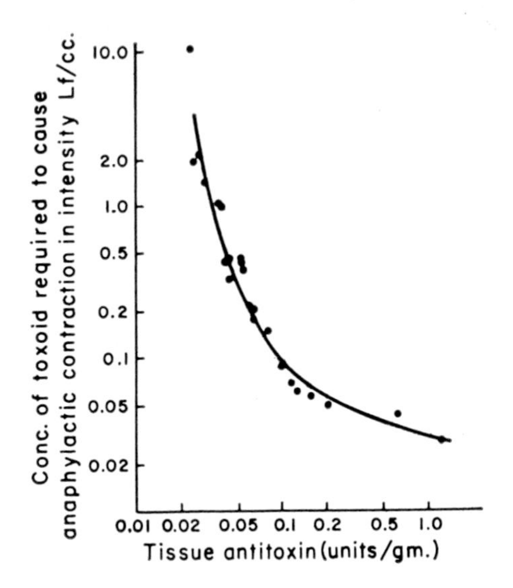

Fig. 10-1. Relation between concentration of antibody in intestine and concentration of antigen required to induce a given intensity of Schultz-Dale response. When anaphylactic contraction was comparable in intensity to that caused by acetylcholine in concentration of 10^{-8} gm./ml., the relation between antibody (X) and antigen (Y) concentrations fit the following curve: $(\log X + 2.32)(\log Y + 2.48) = 2.06$. (From Ishizaka *et al.* [74].)

The amount of antigen needed to induce systemic anaphylaxis also depends on the antigen-antibody system. In the tobacco mosaic virus-antibody system, much more antigen was required than was needed with the ovalbumin- or pneumococcus-polysaccharide system [76a]. This might be expected from its high molecular weight and high antigen : antibody weight ratio at the equivalence point. In PCA reactions in guinea pigs, Leskowitz and Ovary [77] studied this problem systematically by using seven different antigen-antibody systems. They confirmed that the weight of antigen needed to elicit a reaction, at a given antibody level, increases with its molecular weight. When the number of moles of antigen required at each level of antibody was calculated, these values fell approximately within the same general range. They also computed the product of the antigen and antibody molar concentrations needed to cause a positive reaction and suggested that the results in the various antigen-antibody systems were fairly constant. This finding is in accord with the hyperbolic relationship between the concentration of antibody in tissues and the concentration of antigen required to produce a given intensity of anaphylactic reaction. It seems that the product of the antigen concentration and the antibody concentration may relate to the minimal number of collisions of antigen and antibody required for the induction of an anaphylactic reaction.

ANAPHYLAXIS AND COMPLEMENT

It has been demonstrated repeatedly that antigen-antibody interactions *in vivo* are associated with a fall of serum complement (C′) levels [78]. Thus the possibility has been considered that C′ may participate in anaphylactic reactions through a possible role in the activation of serum protease [79]. Osler *et al.* [80, 81] reported that an induced C′ deficiency in albino rats was associated with a diminished reactivity to PCA. They also indicated that the injection of hemolytically active serum into C′-deficient rats was accompanied by a partial restoration of PCA. Enhancement of PCA in normal rats was observed with C′ component reagents containing C'_3 activity [80]. They also indicated that C′ is involved in the formation of "anaphylatoxin" *in vitro* [82]. These findings support the idea that C′ is involved in anaphylactic reactions in rats. Similar experiments have been made by Christian and Thurer [83] in guinea pigs. However, a decrease in serum C′ titer did not correlate with a diminished reactivity to anaphylaxis. Moreover, it has been shown that reversed PCA reactions are induced by antigen-antibody systems which lack C′-fixing properties. For example, rabbit γ-globulin-chicken antibody or sheep antibody systems do not show C′ fixation but may induce a reversed PCA reaction [50, 51]. Reversed PCA reactions were also observed with the human γ-globulin-pepsin-digested rabbit antibody system which fails to fix C′ [84]. Recently it was shown that guinea pig γ_1-globulin antibody which participates in anaphylaxis does not fix C′ with antigen, whereas γ_2-globulin antibody which fixes C′ does not induce anaphylactic reactions [40, 85]. It is unlikely that C′ components are essential for the induction of PCA reactions in guinea pigs, although it is possible that C′

may enhance anaphylactic reactions in some antigen-antibody systems and in other animal species.

BIOLOGICAL ACTIVITIES OF SOLUBLE ANTIGEN-ANTIBODY COMPLEXES AND IMMUNE MECHANISMS OF ANAPHYLACTIC REACTIONS

Anaphylactic reactions involve an antigen-antibody combination which results in a disturbance of the cells on which antibody or antigen is fixed. Regarding the mechanisms involved in the initiation of the cellular reactions, two possibilities may be suggested: the antigen-antibody combination may stimulate the tissues mechanically, or more generally the antigen-antibody complexes formed on the tissues may have a biological activity which is lacking for either antigen or antibody alone and thus the formation of such complexes *in vivo* may induce allergic reactions. In regard to the latter idea, Germuth and McKinnon [86], Trapani *et al.* [87], and Ishizaka and Campbell [88] established the fact that the soluble antigen-antibody complexes formed in excess antigen can induce anaphylactic shock, cause contraction of isolated smooth muscle from normal guinea pigs, and increase the permeability of skin capillaries in a manner similar to that obtained in PCA. The amount of antigen and antibody contained in the minimal skin reactive dose of preformed soluble antigen-antibody complexes is of the same order of magnitude as the threshold amount of antibody required to elicit a skin reaction when challenged as quickly as possible by the antigen [89]. This indicates that the intensity of the skin reaction is independent of whether the preformed complexes were injected or antigen and antibody were injected separately, and suggests that antigen-antibody complexes themselves are toxic as far as the increased permeability of guinea pig skin capillaries is concerned. It was also found that soluble complexes formed at the equivalence point and in excess antibody with nonprecipitating antibody have skin-reactive properties [46].

Subsequent experiments on skin reactions produced by soluble antigen-antibody complexes indicate that the activity of the complexes depends on the nature of the antibody [90]. Rabbit antibodies generally form skin-reactive complexes with antigen, irrespective of whether the antigen is protein, polysaccharide, or synthetic precipitating dye hapten, whereas neither horse nor chicken antibodies were able to form skin-reactive complexes. Rabbit γ-globulin-chicken antibody complexes are the exception; they induce skin reactions in normal guinea pigs [48]. As described previously, the rabbit γ-globulin-chicken antibody system can induce reversed PCA. An essential property of antigen for the formation of skin-reactive complexes is that the antigen molecules have two or more determinant groups. As in the case of PCA reactions, ϵ-, α-DNP-lysine, which is divalent, can form skin-reactive complexes with rabbit antibody, whereas simple haptens, such as ϵ-DNP-lysine and sodium arsanilate cannot [90, 91]. The skin reactivity of soluble antigen-antibody complexes parallels the behavior of the same antigen-antibody systems in PCA reactions, suggesting that the PCA reactions are caused by the formation of skin-reactive complexes *in vivo*. In connection with this idea, it was found that a skin reaction with soluble antigen-antibody complexes is inhibited by the presence of normal human or rabbit γ-globulin with the complex preparation, suggesting that there is competition between soluble complexes and the γ-globulin for fixation to animal tissues [92]. This competition between soluble complexes and γ-globulin was confirmed by the inhibition of PCA sensitization with heterologous antigen-antibody complexes. When rabbit diphtheria antitoxin was diluted with BSA-anti-BSA complexes, instead of saline, and used for sensitization, the PCA reaction by the diphtheria toxin-antitoxin system was inhibited. These findings suggest that the soluble complexes have an affinity for the same tissue constituents with which antibody combines in sensitization. Soluble complexes lacking the blocking effect on PCA sensitization with heterologous antibody did not have skin reactivity. It seems that the fixation of soluble complexes with tissues is one of the necessary processes in the skin reaction.

It was also found that a complex composed of two antigens and one antibody molecule, i.e., Ag_2Ab, did not have skin reactivity, but the complexes containing two or more antibody molecules did [84]. This is in agreement with the fact that simple hapten-antibody complexes do not induce skin reactions and indicates that two antibody molecules are necessary for the formation of skin-reactive complexes. Perhaps the molecular configuration of the antibody molecule is changed to a toxic configuration when two or more antibody molecules combine with one antigen and the skin reaction is caused by the combination with the tissues of such altered antibody molecules. Or two or more antibody molecules combined with the same antigen might interact with each other, and the antibody-antibody interaction and/or consequent changes in the antibody molecules might result in the production of skin-reactive properties. If this is correct, one might expect that the interaction of human and rabbit antibody (γ-globulin) molecules induced by a reagent other than specific antigen might also be accompanied by the development of skin reactivity. In fact, nonspecifically aggregated γ-globulins from the rabbit and man induce skin reactions in guinea pigs [93, 94]. Quantitatively, the minimal skin-reactive doses of the aggregated γ-globulins are comparable to those of soluble antigen-antibody complexes. It was also found that nonspecifically aggregated γ-globulins induced Arthus-like reactions in normal guinea pigs [92], inactivated complement *in vitro* [93, 95], and were capable of releasing histamine and serotonin from rabbit blood [93]. One might speculate that the induction of anaphylactic reactions, as well as the fixation of complement, are characteristic not of antigen-antibody systems per se but of the interaction between γ-globulin molecules.

As is the case with soluble antigen-antibody complexes, the skin-reactivity and complement-fixing properties of aggregated γ-globulin depend on the species from which the γ-globulin is obtained. Aggregated horse, cattle, and chicken γ-globulins do not induce these activities in guinea pig skin or with guinea pig complement [92]. Neither aggregated α- nor aggregated β-globulins from rabbit serum induce skin reactivity. The γ-globulins from certain animal species may possess an essential structure for the induction of skin reactivity. In order to learn about the essential structures, each of three fragments obtained by papain digestion of rabbit γ-globulin was aggregated by coupling with bis-diazotized benzidine. As shown in Table 10-4, only aggregated piece III gave skin reactions and complement fixation [59]. It is apparent that piece III contains some structure essential to the induction of these biological activities.

TABLE 10-4. Complement-fixing and Skin-reactive Properties of γ-Globulin Fragments and of Their Aggregated Products

Preparation	Ultracentrifuge[a]	$C'F_{50}$[b] (μg. N)	Min. Skin-reactive Dose[c] (μg. N)
Whole γ-globulin		624	32
Benzidine azo-γ-globulin	Pellet	5.6	1.0
	Supernate	341	4.0
Piece I		> 800	> 35
Benzidine azo-	Pellet	> 800	> 49
Piece I	Supernate	>> 800	> 39
Piece II		>> 800	> 35
Benzidine azo-	Pellet	>> 800	> 41
Piece II	Supernate	>> 800	> 42
Supernate (piece I + II)		>> 800	> 70
Benzidine azo-	Pellet	>> 800	> 100
(Piece I + II)	Supernate	>> 800	> 82
Piece III		>> 800	> 16
Benzidine azo-	Pellet	7.8	2.0
Piece III	Supernate	137	15.0

[a] At 100,000 g for five hours.
[b] Quantity of protein N required to inactivate 50 $C'H_{50}$ out of 100.
[c] These values indicate the minimal quantity required to induce a definite skin bluing average diameter more than 8 mm.
SOURCE: Ishizaka *et al.* [59].

In summarizing the data obtained on antigen-antibody complexes, aggregated γ-globulin, and passive sensitization, one might speculate about the molecular bases of anaphylactic reactions as follows: During sensitization, antibody molecules are fixed on certain tissue cells by a region of the antibody surface corresponding to piece III. As a result of the antigen-antibody combination, antigen-antibody complexes are formed on the cells, and antibody molecules combining with the same antigen may interact with each other. A structural alteration in the piece III segment may occur as a result of the antibody-antibody interaction and produce the cellular disturbance which is manifest as the allergic reaction.

REFERENCES

1. Chase, M. W. The Allergic State. In Dubos, R. (Ed.), *Bacterial and Mycotic Disease of Man*. Philadelphia: J. B. Lippincott Company, 1958. P. 149.
2. Stone, S. F. Anaphylaxis in passively sensitized guinea pigs after subcutaneous eliciting injection. *Science* 128:1090, 1958.
3. Kallos, P., and Kallos-Deffner, L. Die experimentellen Grundlagen der Erkennung und Behandlung der allergischen Krankheiten. *Ergebn. Hyg. Bakt. Immunitätsforsch.* 19:178, 1937.
4. Forssman, J. Der Ursprung des anaphylaktischen Schockes. *Biochem. Z.* 110:133, 1920.
5. Redfern, W. W. A study of the primary toxicity of heterophile immune rabbit serum for guinea pigs and its apparent relation to the phenomenon of anaphylaxis. *Amer. J. Hyg.* 6:278, 1926.
6. Ovary, Z. Immediate reactions in the skin of experimental animals provoked by antigen-antibody interaction. *Progr. Allerg.* 5:459, 1958.
7. Kendall, A. T., and Schumate, F. O. A quantitative response of intestine from sensitized guinea pigs to homologous protein and to histamine. *J. Infect. Dis.* 47:267, 1930.
8. Halpern, B. N., Liacopoulos, P., Liacopoulos-Briot, M., Binaghi, R., and Van Neer, F. Patterns of the *in vitro* sensitization of isolated smooth muscle tissue with precipitating antibody. *Immunology* 2:351, 1958.
9. Monger, J. L., and Schild, H. O. Inhibition of the anaphylactic reaction. *J. Physiol.* 135:301, 1957.

9a. Monger, J. L., and Schild, H. O. Effect of temperature on the anaphylactic reaction. *J. Physiol.* 132:320, 1957.

10. Monger, J. L., and Schild, H. O. A study of the mechanism of passive sensitization. *J. Physiol.* 150:546, 1960.
11. Mota, I. Mast cell and anaphylaxis. *J. Physiol.* 140:6P, 1958.
12. Humphrey, J. H., and Mota, I. The mechanism of anaphylaxis: Specificity of antigen-induced mast cell damage in anaphylaxis in the guinea pig. *Immunology* 2:31, 1959.
13. Humphrey, J. H., and Jacques, R. The release of histamine and 5-hydroxy-tryptamine (serotonin) from platelets by antigen-antibody reactions (*in vitro*). *J. Physiol.* 128:9, 1955.
14. Baserga, R., and Bergamini, F. Quantitative studies on anaphylaxis: Deallergization and desensitization, *J. Immun.* 71:397, 1953.
15. Rosenau, M. J., and Anderson, J. F. The specific nature of anaphylaxis. *J. Infect. Dis.* 4: 552, 1907.
16. Weiser, R., Gloub, O. J., and Hamre, J. J. Studies on anaphylaxis in the mouse. *J. Infect. Dis.* 68:97, 1941.
17. Solotorovsky, M., and Winsten, S. Anaphylaxis in the mouse produced with crystalline bovine albumin. *J. Immun.* 71:296, 1953.
18. Morgan, P., Sherwood, N. P., and Werder, A. A. Studies on anaphylactic shock in the mouse. *J. Immun.* 79:46, 1957.
19. Malkiel, S., and Hargis, B. J. Anaphylactic shock in the pertussis-vaccinated mouse. *J. Allerg.* 23:352, 1952.
20. Malkiel, S., and Hargis, B. J. Histamine sensitivity and anaphylaxis in the pertussis-vaccinated rat. *Proc. Soc. Exp. Biol. Med.* 81:689, 1952.
21. Munoz, J., Schuchardt, L. F., and Verwey, W. F. Anaphylaxis in *Hemophilus pertussis*-treated mice: I. Passive anaphylaxis with heterologous rabbit antibody. *J. Immun.* 80:77, 1958.
22. Kind, L. S. Relationship of the anaphylaxis sensitizing and adjuvant properties of *Hemophilus pertussis* vaccine. *J. Immun.* 79:238, 1957.
23. Parfentjev, I. A., and Goodline, M. Histamine shock in mice sensitized with *Hemophilus pertussis* vaccine. *J. Pharm. Exp. Ther.* 92:411, 1948.
24. Munoz, J. Effect of *H. pertussis* on sensitizing of mice to serotonin. *Proc. Soc. Exp. Biol. Med.* 95:328, 1957.
25. Kind, L. S. Sensitivity of pertussis inoculated mice to endotoxin. *J. Immun.* 82:32, 1959.
26. Munoz, J., and Schuchardt, L. F. Studies on the sensitivity of mice to histamine following injection of *Hemophilus pertussis*: I. Effect of strain and age of mice. *J. Allerg.* 24:330, 1953.
27. Malkiel, S., and Hargis, B. Enhancement of histamine and anaphylactic shock in mice by *Brucella abortus*. *J. Allerg.* 29:524, 1958.

28. Munoz, J., and Schuchardt, L. F. Sensitivity to histamine of adrenalectomized mice from different strains. *J. Allerg.* 25:125, 1954.
29. Benacerraf, B., and Kabat, E. A. A quantitative study of passive anaphylaxis in the guinea pig: V. The latent period in passive anaphylaxis in its relation to the dose of rabbit ovalbumin. *J. Immun.* 62:517, 1949.
30. Ovary, Z., and Bier, O. G. Quantitative studies on passive cutaneous anaphylaxis in the guinea pig and its relationship to the Arthus phenomenon. *J. Immun.* 71:6, 1953.
31. Ovary, Z. Passive cutaneous anaphylaxis in the mouse. *J. Immun.* 81:355, 1958.
32. Chandler, M. H., Rosenberg, L. T., and Fishel, E. E. Persistence of passively administered homologous and heterologous antibody in the guinea pig. *J. Immun.* 82:103, 1959.
33. Munoz, J., and Anacker, R. L. Anaphylaxis in *Bordetella pertussis*-treated mice: III. Passive cutaneous anaphylaxis. *J. Immun.* 83:640, 1959.
34. Humphrey, J. H., and Mota, I. The mechanism of anaphylaxis: Observations on the failure of antibodies from certain species to sensitize guinea pigs in direct and reversed passive anaphylaxis. *Immunology* 2:19, 1959.
35. Benacerraf, B., and Kabat, E. A. A quantitative study of the Arthus phenomenon induced passively in the guinea pig. *J. Immun.* 64:1, 1950.
36. Kuhns, W. J., and Pappenheimer, A. M., Jr. Immunochemical studies of antitoxin produced in normal and allergic individuals hyperimmunized with diphtheria toxoid. *J. Exp. Med.* 95:363, 375, 1952.
37. Kabat, E. A., and Boldt, M. H. A quantitative study of passive anaphylaxis. *J. Immun.* 48:181, 1944.
38. Munoz, J., and Anacker, R. L. Anaphylaxis in *Bordetella pertussis*-treated mice: II. Passive anaphylaxis with homologous antibody. *J. Immun.* 83:502, 1959.
39. Ishizaka, K., Ishizaka, T., Sugahara, T., and Matsunaga, S. Quantitative studies on anaphylaxis *in vitro:* III. Comparison between Schultz-Dale reaction and serological reactions *in vitro*. *Jap. J. Med. Sci. Biol.* 10:329, 1957.
40. Ovary, Z., Benacerraf, B., and Bloch, K. J. Properties of guinea pig 7S antibodies: II. Identification of antibodies involved in passive cutaneous and systemic anaphylaxis. *J. Exp. Med.* 117:951, 1963.
41. (*a*) Ovary, Z., Fudenberg, H. H., and Kunkel, H. G. Anaphylactic reactions in the skin of the guinea pig with high and low molecular weight antibodies and gamma globulins. *J. Exp. Med.* 112:953, 1960. (*b*) Franklin, E. C., and Ovary, Z. On the sensitizing properties of some normal and pathologic human immune globulins and fragments obtained by papain or pepsin digestion. *Immunology* 6: 434, 1963.
42. Heremans, J. F., and Vaerman, J. P. β_{2A}-globulin as a possible carrier of allergic reaginic activity. *Nature* (London) 193, 1091, 1962.
43. Fireman, P., Vannier, W. E., and Goodman, H. C. The association of skin sensitizing antibody with the β_{2A}-globulins in sera from ragweed sensitive patients. *J. Exp. Med.* 117:603, 1963.
44. Ishizaka, K., Ishizaka, T., and Hornbrook, M. M. Blocking of Prausnitz-Küstner sensitization with reagin by normal human β_{2A}-globulin. *J. Allerg.* 34:395, 1963.
45. Kabat, E. A., and Benacerraf, B. A quantitative study of passive anaphylaxis in the guinea pig: IV. Passive sensitization with non-precipitating or univalent rabbit antiovalbumin. *J. Immun.* 86:590, 1961.
46. Ishizaka, K., Ishizaka, T., and Sugahara, T. Biological activity of soluble antigen-antibody complexes: VI. Complexes in equivalence and in excess antibody. *J. Immun.* 86: 590, 1961.
47. Ovary, Z., and Karush, F. Studies on the immunologic mechanism of anaphylaxis: II. Sensitizing and combining capacity *in vivo* of fractions separated from papain digests of antihapten antibody. *Ibid.,* p. 146.
48. Ishizaka, K., Ishizaka, T., and Sugahara, T. Molecular bases of passive sensitization: I. Role of disulfide linkages in γ globulin molecule. *J. Immun.* 87:548, 1961.
49. Bier, O. G., and Siqueira, M. Passive reverse cutaneous anaphylaxis to protein antigens: Preliminary report. *Int. Arch. Allerg.* 6:391, 1955.
50. Ovary, Z. Reverse passive cutaneous anaphylaxis in the guinea pig with horse, sheep or hen antibodies. *Immunology* 3:19, 1960.
51. Ishizaka, K., Ishizaka, T., and Sugahara, T. Biologic activity of soluble antigen-antibody complexes: VIII. Complexes of chicken antibodies. *J. Immun.* 91:257, 1963.
52. Ovary, Z., and Bier, O. G. Action empéchante du sérum normal de lapin sur l'anaphylaxie cutanée passive de cobaye. *Ann. Inst. Pasteur* (Paris) 84:443, 1953.
53. Fisher, J. P., and Cooke, R. A. Passive cutaneous anaphylaxis (PCA) in the guinea pig. *J. Allerg.* 28:150, 1957.
54. Biozzi, G., Halpern, B. N., and Binaghi, R. The competitive effect of normal serum proteins from various animal species on antibody fixation in passive cutaneous anaphylaxis in the guinea pig. *J. Immun.* 82:215, 1959.
55. Halpern, B. N. Le Processus de Sensibilisation. In Brown, E. A. (Ed.), *Allergology* (Proc. 4th Internat. Congr.). New York: Pergamon Press, 1962. P. 50.

56. Sugahara, T., Ishizaka, K., and Ishizaka, T. Biologic activities of aggregated γ globulin: VI. Aggregated products of rabbit serum proteins. *J. Immun.* 90:960, 1963.
57. Halpern, B. N., and Frick, O. L. Protection against fatal anaphylactic shock with γ globulins in guinea pigs and mice. *J. Immun.* 88:683, 1962.
58. (*a*) Binaghi, R., Liacopoulos, P., Halpern, B. N., and Liacopoulos-Briot, M. C. Interference of non-specific gamma globulins with passive *in vitro* anaphylactic sensitization of isolated guinea pig intestine. *Immunology* 5:204, 1962. (*b*) Halpern, B. N., Liacopoulos, P., Liacopoulos-Briot, M. C., and Binaghi, R. Modalités de la sensibilisation passive des organes isolés en survie à l'aide d'anticorps du type précipitant in vitro. *C. R. Acad. Sci.* (Paris) 247:1798, 1958.
59. Ishizaka, K., Ishizaka, T., and Sugahara, T. Biological activity of soluble antigen-antibody complexes: VII. Role of an antibody fragment in the induction of biological activities. *J. Immun.* 88:690, 1962.
60. Olins, D. E., and Edelman, G. M. The antigenic structure of the polypeptide chains of human γ globulin. *J. Exp. Med.* 116:635, 1962.
61. Porter, R. R. The Structure of Gamma Globulin and Antibodies. In Gellhorn, A., and Herschberg, E. (Eds.), *Basic Problems in Neoplastic Disease.* New York: Columbia University Press, 1962. P. 177.
62. Cohen, D. S. Properties of the separated chains of human γ globulin. *Nature* (London) 197:253, 1963.
63. Heremans, J. F., Carbonara, A. O., Mancini, G., and Lontie, R. Studies on normal and pathological γ_{1A}-globulins and their subunits. *Protides of the Biological Fluids* 11:45, 1964.
64. Edelman, G. M., and Benacerraf, B. On structural and functional relation between antibodies and proteins of the γ system. *Proc. Nat. Acad. Sci. U.S.A.* 48:1035, 1962.
65. Nielsen, C. B., Treffers, G., and Feigen, G. A. Adsorption of antibody *in vitro* and magnitude of the Schultz-Dale reaction of guinea pig ileum. *Science* 130:41, 1959.
66. Ishizaka, K., Ishizaka, T., and Sugahara, T. Quantitative studies on anaphylaxis *in vitro*: II. Studies on the species difference of diphtheria antitoxin in sensitizing activity. *Jap. J. Med. Sci.* 10:93, 1957.
67. Feigen, G. A., Nielsen, C. B., and Treffers, G. Effect of antibody concentration and temperature upon physical adsorption and histamine release. *J. Immun.* 89:717, 1962.
68. Binaghi, R., Liacopoulos, P., Halpern, B. N., Liacopoulos-Briot, M. C., and Bloch, C. Influence of the ionic strength of the medium on the velocity of passive anaphylactic sensitization *in vitro. J. Immun.* 87:269, 1961.
69. Binaghi, R., Halpern, B. N., Liacopoulos, P., and Neveu, T. Promoting effect of urea on the *in vitro* passive sensitization of isolated plain muscles with precipitating antibody. *Nature* (London) 184:1805, 1959.
70. Campbell, D. H., and McCasland, G. E. *In vitro* anaphylactic response to polyhaptenic and monohaptenic simple antigens. *J. Immun.* 49:315, 1944.
71. Landsteiner, K., and Van der Scheer, J. Anaphylactic shock by azodyes: II. *J. Exp. Med.* 67:79, 1938.
72. Ovary, Z., and Karush, F. Studies on the immunologic mechanism of anaphylaxis: I. Antigen-hapten interactions studied by passive cutaneous anaphylaxis in the guinea pig. *J. Immun.* 84:409, 1960.
73. Ovary, Z. Activité des substances à faible poids moléculaire dans les réactions antigène-anticorps *in vivo* et *in vitro. C. R. Acad. Sci.* (Paris) 253:582, 1961.
74. Ishizaka, K., Ishizaka, T., and Sugahara, T. Quantitative study on anaphylaxis *in vitro:* I. Proportion of antigen concentration to tissue antibody concentration in toxin anaphylaxis of diphtheria. *Jap. J. Med. Sci.* 9:191, 1956.
75. Ovary, Z. Passive cutaneous anaphylaxis in the guinea pig: Degree of reaction as a function of the quantity of antigen and antibody. *Int. Arch. Allerg.* 14:18, 1959.
76. (*a*) Kabat, E. A., Coffin, G., and Smith, D. J. A quantitative study of passive anaphylaxis in the guinea pig: III. *J. Immun.* 56:377, 1947. (*b*) Kabat, E. A., and Landow, M. J. A quantitative study of passive anaphylaxis in the guinea pig. *Ibid.* 44:69, 1942.
77. Leskowitz, S., and Ovary, Z. The relation between molecular weight of antigen and antibody to elicit passive cutaneous anaphylaxis. *Immunology* 5:1, 1962.
78. (*a*) Stavisky, A. B., Hackel, D. B., and Heymann, W. Reduction of serum complement following *in vivo* tissue antigen-antibody reactions. *Proc. Soc. Exp. Biol. Med.* 85:593, 1954. (*b*) Seltzer, G., Baron, S., and Fusco, J. A method for removing complement *in vivo* and its rate of return. *J. Immun.* 69:367, 1952.
79. Ungar, G., Damgaard, E., and Hummel, F. P. Activation of profibrinolysin by antigen-antibody reaction and by anaphylactoid agent: Its relation to complement. *J. Exp. Med.* 98: 291, 1953.
80. Osler, A. G., Hawrisiak, M. M., Ovary, Z., Siqueira, M., and Bier, O. G. Studies on the mechanism of hypersensitivity phenomena: II. The participation of complement in passive cutaneous anaphylaxis of the albino rat. *J. Exp. Med.* 106:811, 1957.
81. Osler, A. G. Functions of complement system. *Advances Immun.* 1:131, 1961.
82. Osler, A. G., Randall, M. G., Hill, B. H., and Ovary, Z. Studies on the mechanism of hy-

persensitivity phenomena: III. The participation of complement in the formation of anaphylatoxin. *J. Exp. Med.* 110:311, 1959.

83. Christian, C. L., and Thurer, R. J. Studies of anaphylaxis: Effect of decomplementation with aggregated γ globulin. *J. Immun.* 88:93, 1962.
84. Ovary, Z., and Taranta, A. Passive cutaneous anaphylaxis with antibody fragments. *Science* 140:193, 1963.
85. Bloch, K. J., Kourilsky, F. M., Ovary, Z., and Benacerraf, B. Properties of guinea pig 7S antibodies: III. Identification of antibodies involved in complement fixation and hemolysis. *J. Exp. Med.* 117:965, 1963.
86. Germuth, F. G., Jr., and McKinnon, G. E. Studies on the biological properties of antigen-antibody complexes: I. Anaphylactic shock induced by soluble complexes in unsensitized normal guinea pigs. *Bull. Hopkins Hosp.* 101:13, 1957.
87. Trapani, I. L., Garvey, J. S., and Campbell, D. H. Stimulating action of soluble antigen-antibody complexes on normal guinea pig smooth muscle. *Science* 127:700, 1957.
88. Ishizaka, K., and Campbell, D. H. Biological activity of soluble antigen-antibody complex: I. Skin reactive properties. *Proc. Soc. Exp. Biol. Med.* 97:635, 1958.
89. Ishizaka, K., Ishizaka, T., and Campbell, D. H. Biological activity of soluble antigen-antibody complex: II. Physical properties of soluble complexes having skin-irritating activity. *J. Exp. Med.* 109:127, 1959.
90. Ishizaka, K., Ishizaka, T., and Campbell, D. H. Biological activity of soluble antigen-antibody complex: III. Various antigen-antibody systems and the probable role of complement. *J. Immun.* 83:105, 1959.
91. Ishizaka, K., Ishizaka, T., and Banovitz, J. Biological activity of soluble antigen-antibody complexes: IX. Soluble complexes of rabbit antibody with univalent and divalent haptens. *J. Immun.* 93:1001, 1964.
92. Ishizaka, K., and Campbell, D. H. Biological activity of soluble antigen-antibody complex: IV. The inhibition of the skin reactivity of soluble complexes and the PCA reaction by heterologous complexes. *J. Immun.* 83:116, 1959.
93. Ishizaka, K. Gamma globulin and molecular mechanisms in hypersensitivity reactions. *Progr. Allerg.* 7:32, 1963.
94. Christian, C. L. Studies on aggregated gamma globulin: II. Effect *in vivo*. *J. Immun.* 84:117, 1960.
95. Christian, C. L. Studies on aggregated gamma globulin. I. Sedimentation and electrophoretic properties. *Ibid.*, p. 112.

11. Delayed (Cellular) Hypersensitivity

SIDNEY RAFFEL

UNTIL A FEW YEARS AGO, INTEREST in the nature or even the existence of delayed hypersensitivity was limited to some members of the fraternity of immunologists and perforce to allergists and dermatologists who must deal with clinical aspects of this reactive state. This situation changed sharply with the recent surge of interest in the grafting of tissues and in a variety of afflictions which are strikingly accompanied by—perhaps in some cases caused by—immune responses. The concepts and terminology associated with delayed hypersensitivity are now the province of investigators in a variety of medical and biological fields, from surgery to genetics. The floodgates of literature are open, viewpoints and methods of study cascade through, and the fabrication of a fair story of the current status of this subject is not an easy task.

GENERAL FEATURES OF DELAYED HYPERSENSITIVITY

Delayed hypersensitivity may still be exemplified by two classic prototypes: one, the reactivity induced by infection, and the second, termed contact sensitivity, resulting from exposure of skin to a variety of substances ranging from oily resins of plants to simple chemicals employed for domestic, industrial, and medical purposes, e.g., penicillin [1]. The designation "delayed" is applied to these states on the basis of characteristics of elicited reactions, not because of any special chronological facet of induction, which shows the same general sequence as is seen in any immunological process. Whereas in "immediate" reactions a response in the sensitive subject may come on in seconds or minutes, in the delayed type it gets under way after several hours and is apt to reach a maximum after two or three days. This temporal distinction reflects underlying differences in mechanism which will be discussed.

Delayed reactions may be local or systemic. The former can be occasioned by exposure of the skin or other tissue to an antigen through natural contact or by the application of a test dose. In the skin, a relatively slowly developing area of erythema and induration is seen, often vesiculated in man exposed to contact agents (dermatitis venenata). The systemic reaction may also come about spontaneously, as through the spillage of infectious material from a local lesion into the blood stream or into hitherto uninvolved areas of an organ. This may happen, for example, in the case of the softened necrotic content of a tuberculous abscess in the lung. Such an event can be duplicated experimentally by the systemic injection of antigen in large quantities. The reaction is marked by lassitude and collapse, accompanied by fluctuation in body temperature, leukopenia particularly of the monocytic elements, hemorrhages in the lungs, lymph nodes, intestines, and other abdominal viscera, and sometimes death in several hours or a day or longer [2–4].

As with other biological phenomena, there are wide variations in susceptibility to induction of this hypersensitive state, depending on individual as well as strain and species factors. The individual aspect is most difficult to assess critically, but it is readily seen in work with groups of experimental animals. In human beings, wide fluctuations in reactivity to tuberculin in tuberculous subjects has been frequently described, and even more apparent differences have been noted with respect to the contact reactants; for example, poison ivy apparently sensitizes about three fourths of the individuals who are exposed to it, and many of the simpler chemical agents also affect only some members of the population [5].

Some strains of animals are more readily sensitized than others [6]. Among the species used in the laboratory, the mouse and rat have been regarded as relatively impervious to sensitization of this kind, although under certain conditions they appear to be susceptible [4].

Various factors and circumstances influence the delayed hypersensitive state or the expression of its reactivity. Thus it is well known that tuberculin reactivity may be suppressed during measles and scarlet fever, presumably because of vascular changes which may favor the rapid elimination of injected test antigens from skin sites [7, 8]. However, the administration of measles vaccine is said similarly to influence this reactivity even when no obvious cutaneous lesions are induced by it [9]. Extraneous influences may also have significant effects; total body irradiation [10], nitrogen mustard [11], and corticosteroids [12] are among the agents which modify the induction or expression of these states. It is difficult to know in some instances whether the observed effects owe to interference with an immunological process or to a side issue such as modification of the capacity to develop an inflammatory response.

ESTABLISHMENT OF DELAYED REACTIVITY

Infection hypersensitivity, also referred to as of tuberculin type, probably accompanies all infections, but it is more strikingly evident in some, including tuberculosis, brucellosis, lymphogranuloma venereum, mumps, and vaccinia. All of these are instances in which empirical observation long ago led to the adoption of skin tests as aids to diagnosis or assessment of the immunological status of the individual. In most cases in which the chemical nature of the sensitizing constituent of the agent is known, this is found to be protein, but polysaccharides appear to be the effective elicitors of reactions in subjects sensitive to several of the fungi which cause systemic infections, including *Blastomyces, Histoplasma,* and *Coccidioides* [13, 14].

In contact hypersensitivity, effective inducing substances are those which are able to combine with proteins of the epidermis either a priori or after being modified by the metabolic processes of the subject [1, 15]. For example, studies with various dinitrophenyl compounds have shown clearly that combination occurs with the terminal amino groups of lysine or the sulfur of cystine or cysteine [16–20].

Certain factors are related to induction of these hypersensitive states in ways which are not entirely clear. One of these is the route by which antigens gain access to the tissues [21]. As suggested by the common occurrence of contact reactivity, the dermal portal is the one most likely to result in reactivity of this kind to simple chemical compounds. The sensitizing agents sensitize very poorly if they are administered by avenues that circumvent the skin.

Another factor which seems to enter into the establishment of these reactivities is the nature of the "envelope" in which an antigen presents itself to the tissues. Thus, in the case of infectious agents, route of access is of subsidiary importance, perhaps because substances helpful to the sensitizing process are present in the microbes. This has been studied most extensively in the case of the *Mycobacteria,* which, in addition to sensitizing against their own protein constituents, favor the development of delayed reactivity to other antigens administered in a mixture with them [22, 23], preferably in an oily emulsion [24]. The influence of the bacterium resides in a lipopolysaccharide constituent [25, 26]. The *Mycobacteria* or their lipoidal component are active as adjuvants in the induction of antibodies also; they cause proliferation of lymphoid cells which are associated with various immunological responses. This influence on cell proliferation may be the important one in bringing the delayed hypersensitizing activity of antigens to the fore, or some other potentiality of the mycobacterial entity may be concerned, e.g., an alteration of the permeability of potentially responding cells to antigens. Not all granuloma-inducers acting as adjuvant for antibody production are proficient in assisting the development of delayed sensitivity [27].

It is interesting that in the case of the contact sensitizers, the special circumstance of route of entry into the tissues can be "substituted" for by the use of the mycobacterial emulsion as a vehicle; noncutaneous administration then results in contact hypersensitivity. Perhaps this can be explained on the basis that sensitivity to a contact agent is directed against a considerable portion of the protein molecule with which the substance conjugates in the skin, and the injection of such substances into other areas of the body may result in the formation of protein complexes which are not structurally identical to those that are subsequently formed in the skin test site [28]. The concomitance of an adjuvant which increases the response may then favor the detection of cross-reactivity. It is conceivable also that the skin may itself provide an analogous adjuvant activity to account for its importance as a route for sensitization. Other tissue cells have been found to possess a related effect [29, 30].

In the face of these considerations which stress the importance of routes of access to the tissues and of adjuvants influencing the development of delayed hypersensitivity, it is well established that soluble proteins administered by any route and without adjuvant can engender a type of delayed hypersensitive reactivity in man and animals. The earliest observations of this were made by Dienes and Mallory [31] and others [32, 33], and the subject has been explored in detail in recent years [34]. The failure of some investigators to equate reactivity induced by the simple application of proteins with those of infection and contact type possibly owes to the circumstances of induction of reactivity and elicitation of reactions, which differ in some respects from those pertinent to infection and contact reactivity. For the demonstration of delayed sensitivity induced by proteins, it is most appropriate to administer antigen in small doses [35, 36], or complexed with an excess of antibody [34], or conjugated with a simple chemical hapten [37]. Frequently, the reactive states tend to be short-lived in contrast to those established by infectious or contact agents, although this is not always the case. The transitory nature of this state has been especially well seen in the cornea, where a primary injection of antigen leads after several days to a reaction expressed by clouding, which soon disappears. About nine or more days later, a typical precipitative reaction occurs in the cornea caused by the interaction of newly appearing antibody with persisting *residual* antigen [37].

There may be other distinctions as well between this protein-induced state, for which the eponym Jones-Mote reactivity has been proposed [35], and the other reactive states described. Thus: (1) Elicited reactions tend to disappear more quickly, showing a peak of induration at 24 hours with subsidence at 48. (2) There may be a greater susceptibility of newborn animals (guinea pigs) to induction of protein sensitivity than to that of the tuberculin type [39–42]. (3) Desensitization is effected with greater ease in the case of protein reactivity [43, 44]. (4) There appear to be differences in retention of antigen at the sites of reaction in the two cases [45]. (5) Jones-Mote reactivity has not thus far been established by polysaccharides [37], while, as mentioned earlier, reactivity to these occurs in certain of the systemic fungal infections. (6) Although protein-induced reactions have been described as being cytologically identical to those of infection type (see later), we believe that they differ significantly in two respects. First, small lymphocytes constitute a larger part of the infiltrate in reactions of the infection type, and, second, the late cellular picture at about a week after application of antigen is one of preponderance of plasmacytes in the protein reaction and of macrophages in the infection type test site, suggesting the developmental transition of different initial cell types [46]. (7) There are differences in susceptibility of the inductive process to total body irradiation; tuberculin reactivity is modified by this, as mentioned earlier, whereas protein-induced reactivity appears not to be [47], and similar observations have been made with cortisone [37]. (8) Necrosis, sometimes at a microscopical level, appears frequently even in moderately severe tuberculin reactions and is not seen as a component of relatively severe protein-induced reactions.

These differences are perhaps stressed beyond their actual significance, but until they have been clarified, it seems reasonable to retain reservations about the mechanistic identity of these reactive states. There exists a considerable heterogeneity of the circulating antibody response which may well be associated with a parallel disparity of cellular source, and an analogous situation could obtain here.

ANTIGENIC DETERMINANTS IN DELAYED HYPERSENSITIVITY

An interesting aspect of delayed reactivity concerns the relative molecular dimensions of the antigenic determinants to which the response is made and the reaction occurs. This information comes from studies of contact and Jones-Mote reactivity; comparable work has not been carried out with fragments of the proteins or polysaccharides involved in infection hypersensitivity.

In these reactive states the response is directed against larger structures of an antigen than are recognized by humoral antibodies. Thus, in antibody induction, a small hapten (e.g., dinitrobenzene) conjugated to a carrier protein incites the synthesis of globulins which react against the hapten and a small area of contiguous amino acid, so that cross-reactions occur widely with the same hapten attached to a variety of unrelated proteins. In contrast, the delayed reaction to hapten-protein complexes is directed largely against the modified carrier protein, as revealed by weak cross-reactivity to hapten-heterologous protein [28, 48, 49]. But it is an interesting fact that for the *induction* of antibody formation the *recognition* of antigen by synthesizing cells appears also to require areas of the conjugated molecule considerably larger than the hapten portion. For example, if dinitrobenzene-bovine serum albumin is used as a primary immunizing antigen, antibodies with specificity directed toward the hapten are obtained. On subsequent injection of the dinitrobenzene attached to ovalbumin, however, no secondary response to the hapten occurs [50, 51]. Yet the antibodies elaborated in response to either of these antigens cross-react well with each other by virtue of their antihapten specificity. Thus, while macromolecular recognition seems to be concerned both in induction and in elicitation of delayed reactivities, it is most important to the inductive phase in the case of antibody synthesis.

Perhaps the narrower specificity of antibodies reflects the capacity of molecules to combine with smaller molecular structures than can cells, which appear to be directly involved in delayed hypersensitive reactions [28]; or entirely different cells and processes may be responsible for the two states. There is some evidence that protein-induced delayed reactivity may more readily develop against some determinants on protein molecules while antibodies are preferentially produced against others, as suggested by work with native and denatured substances [52, 53].

CYTOLOGIC FEATURES OF DELAYED REACTIONS

A number of chronological studies of the histological aspects of delayed reactions agree that during the early hours after exposure to antigen the area of reaction is marked by the appearance of numbers of monocytic cells, in vessels of the dermis and infiltrating the surrounding tissues, and this becomes progressively more intense during the succeeding 24 to 48 hours, accompanied to some extent by proliferation of local reticulum cells. Some investigators stress infiltration during the earlier phases of the reaction by appreciable numbers of polymorphonuclear cells also; the quantitative aspects of this response are in some dispute. But all agree on the characteristic early appearance of monocytes [31, 54–56].

It is common opinion that one or more among these cell types is probably implicated directly in the delayed reactive state, i.e., that certain cells themselves react with antigen. Questions which follow from this assumption are: Which of the cell types is concerned? What is the nature of the attraction which brings them to an area containing antigen? In what way does tissue damage result from the immunological events which occur there?

CELLS AS MEDIATORS OF DELAYED HYPERSENSITIVE REACTIONS

As a preface to the consideration of these questions, the pros and cons of the central issue whether delayed reactivity is indeed of cellular kind should be assessed. Several considerations strongly suggest that cells rather than blood proteins are the reactive elements:

1. Delayed reactivity cannot be transferred from a sensitive to a normal subject by means of serum, but it can be passed by cells obtained from lymphoid tissue, peritoneal exudate, or peripheral blood [26, 57]. In animals, particularly guinea pigs, which have been much used for such studies, viable cells seem to be required; neither dead cells nor extracts from them appear to be satisfactory for the purpose [58], although some successes with these have been reported [59, 60]. In the case of human beings, however, the supernatant fluids of disrupted perhipheral blood leukocytes can transfer reactivity to other human subjects [61, 62]. The nature of the transfer factor is unknown; it resists destruction by ribonuclease and trypsin, and whether it in some way instigates activity on the part of cells of the recipient is not clear.

2. Lymphoid cells derived from sensitive subjects are adversely affected by exposure to appropriate soluble antigen *in vitro* [3, 26, 63,

64]. (They are also more vulnerable to other influences [118–120].) When animals have been induced to reject homologous tissue cells, a reactive state which is probably an analogue of delayed hypersensitivity, their cells *in vitro* have been seen to make contact with those bearing the responsible antigens, with fatal issue to both [65–68].

3. In certain clinical states dichotomies exist between the ability to synthesize circulating antibodies and the ability to develop delayed hypersensitive reactivity. Thus in hypogammaglobulinemia, antibody production may be virtually undetectable while delayed sensitivity can be induced [69–71]. On the contrary, in Hodgkin's disease [72] and in sarcoidosis [73, 74], the reverse of this situation often obtains.

ANTIBODIES AS MEDIATORS OF DELAYED HYPERSENSITIVE REACTIONS

This evidence favoring cell reactivity does not close the issue entirely, for it is possible that antibody of humoral origin may be adsorbed to cells which themselves have no specific quality. Thus Boyden *et al.* [75] have observed "cytophilic" antibodies with special adsorptive capacities, while disrupted peripheral blood leukocytes of tuberculin-sensitive human subjects have been found to liberate antibodies which enter into the hemagglutination reaction with tuberculin-treated erythrocytes [76], and a factor has been described as being shed into plasma by lymphoid cells of tuberculin-sensitive animals which may make normal cells vulnerable to the injurious action of tuberculin [77]. Further, an α-globulin of serum has been reported to transfer delayed reactivity between animals [78, 79], although in this instance no serologically active antibody was concomitantly detected [80]. The latter experiments with serum transfer have not yet been affirmed [81].

It has been suggested that the reactive elements in delayed hypersensitivity may be antibodies of high combining affinity for antigen but present in the blood in very small amount [82]. Such antibodies might accumulate slowly in an area of antigen deposition to provide the sluggish picture of the developing reaction. The general failure of serum transfer in this view is attributable to the small quantities of antibodies present in any reasonable sample with which this could be attempted, and successful transfer by cells is laid to the capacity of some of these to continue synthesis of antibodies in the recipient.

Most students of these hypersensitive states favor the concept that they are cell-mediated, while keeping alive the alternative viewpoint until more definitive information becomes available.

SPECIFIC CELLS CONCERNED IN DELAYED HYPERSENSITIVITY

The first question now becomes one of determining which cells may be specifically concerned in this reactivity. It is quite apparent that humoral antibodies are largely or entirely the products of plasmacytes, but no one has seriously imputed to these cells a role in the delayed reaction, for transfers of reactivity may be made with cell suspensions which contain few if any such elements. Unquestionably, however, the cells which are concerned in delayed reactivity are characterizable as of "lymphoid origin"; those successful in transfer are derivable from lymphoid tissues per se, from induced exudates of serosal cavities [57], and from cells of the thoracic duct lymph [83], as mentioned before, whereas other cell types from a sensitive donor, e.g., such specialized entities as kidney tubular epithelium, fail in this respect [84]. A variety of evidence suggests that the active cells are probably small lymphocytes. It is difficult to establish this as a fact because of the virtual impossibility of preparing suspensions of a single cell type from any of the sources mentioned. However, some cytological studies suggest a role for these cells: appreciable numbers of them are seen to accumulate in the developing tuberculin reaction [46], and in a type of graft rejection phenomenon (runt disease), isotopically labeled cells from thoracic duct lymph which were active upon recipient tissues were identified as small lymphocytes. These apparently developed in the recipient into large pyroninophilic cells [85, 86].

Recent efforts to ascertain by more direct means which cells have the capacity to react specifically with antigen have been rewarding. It was mentioned that lymphocytes derived from sensitized animals have affinity *in vitro* for homologous cells against which they are directed [65, 66], and analogous studies have been made with soluble antigens. Iodine^{131}-labeled tuberculin has been observed to have a predilection for the lymphocytes of sensitive animals *in vitro* [88], although large mononuclear cells were also implicated in this reactivity. Similar evidence of participation of small lymphocytes in delayed reactivity has been gained from studies with the fluorescence technique in tuberculin sensitivity [89] and in allergic encephalomyelitis, in this case by use of a protein antigen derived from spinal cord [90].

As is true of most of the evidence in this field, there are alternative views to be reckoned with here. It was mentioned earlier that in one of the studies with labeled tuberculin, large monocytes were seen to have an apparent specific affinity for antigen. Waksman [54] also believes that histiocytes are concerned in such reactions, while Weiser [91] has clearly implicated such cells in an acquired response against isolated tumor cells. There may indeed be some as yet undefined relationship between these large monocytic cells and small lymphocytes, as suggested by the description [85, 86] of the emergence of large pyroninophilic cells from small lymphocytes, as well as by older histological thought concerning the potentialities of lymphocytes, and by a somewhat tenuous association which has been found to occur between delayed reactivity in certain infectious processes and macrophagic immunity to infectious agents, as will be discussed.

The Thymus in Relation to the Cells Concerned in Delayed Hypersensitivity. The thymus is an enigmatic organ containing many lymphocytes which for many years has eluded efforts to discover its reason-for-being. Straightforward efforts to implicate it in immune responses have been made repeatedly for the obvious reason provided by its content of lymphocytes and because of the uncommonly frequent association of thymomas with human diseases associated with striking immunological characteristics, such as the dysproteinemias and systemic lupus erythematosus. Attempts to transfer the antibody-synthesizing process, or delayed reactivity, from sensitized animals to normal recipients by means of thymocytes have been generally disappointing [92, 93], although some successes have been recorded in both respects [4, 94, 95].

Insight into the immunological potentialities of this organ has come from recent experiments entailing ablation of the organ in newborn animals. In such animals the subsequent development of lymphoid tissue throughout the body is impaired [96, 97], and they become markedly deficient in their capacities to respond to various antigenic stimuli, including soluble and particulate injected antigens as well as tissue grafts [96, 98, 99]. Removal of the organ from the adult has little or no influence on either the cytological or the immunological potentialities of the animal. The thymus is thought to exert a directive influence on immunologically responding tissues, perhaps by populating them with cells bearing the potentiality to develop into clones of reactive entities against various antigens [96, 100–102]. Whether or not this influence pertains equally to all immunological reactivities is not yet clear; in newborn mammals, thymectomy affects subsequent antibody synthesis as well as homograft rejection and delayed hypersensitivity [103, 104], but in fowl these responses seem to be dissociable. Chickens possess, in addition to a thymus, an analogue to it in the region of the cloaca, called the bursa of Fabricius. This may be suppressed in its development by administration of androgenic steroids to the newly hatched animal. Suppression of the bursa alone has been found to interfere with subsequent antibody formation [105], whereas thymectomy impedes the development of homograft rejectivity [106] but affects antibody synthesis only to a small degree [107]. Removal of both organs results in the loss of all of these capacities [105, 108].

A further implication of the thymus in immunological events is suggested by recent findings of Mowbray [109] that the injection into animals of an α-2 glycoprotein of plasma along with antigen can suppress antibody synthesis strikingly and the capacity for homograft rejection to some degree. Of a variety of tissues examined as possible sources of origin of this factor, only the thymus yielded it [110].

Although the precise interrelationships of the properties of the thymus are not clear, these suggestions that it may suppress as well as guide immunological function are fertile ones for future study.

ATTRACTION OF CELLS TO SITES OF ANTIGEN DEPOSITION

A second question concerning cells as instruments in the delayed hypersensitive reaction has to do with the way in which such reactions are initiated, i.e., how the appropriate cells manage to appear in areas of tissue where antigen is deposited. There are several obvious possibilities to account for this. The reactive cells may be attracted to such areas through some kind of specific chemotaxis exerted by the antigen. This hypothesis has been tested by the transfer of isotopically labeled cells from hypersensitive donors to normal recipients, with results which at first suggested that this explanation might be borne out [111]. However, subsequent observations contradict this point of view: labeled cells appear in numbers consonant with the proportion which they constitute of the total circulating cells of the recipient. Further, the same relative numbers of these infiltrate sites of nonspecific antigen deposition. In brief, no specific attraction seems to obtain [112, 113], or if it does, considerable clarification will be required to establish this [47].

A second thesis is that blood- and lymph-borne reactive cells in passing through an area of antigen deposition combine with it, that this causes a mild inflammatory reaction (toxic products of such combinations have been described [114, 115]), and as a result extravasation of more cells occurs, among which randomly represented hypersensitive elements could slowly amplify the reaction to a local climax.

Finally, one might assume that the triggering of the response depends on a reaction with antigen of ordinary antibodies present in the body fluids, perhaps in small quantities. This is not to be confused with the hypothesis discussed before in which small quantities of antibodies with high qualities of association are considered to be responsible for the entire sequence of the delayed reaction. In the present instance, antibodies of indifferent avidity interacting with antigen could release small quantities of the pharmacological mediators associated with immediate hypersensitive reactions, which cause dilatation and increased permeability of capillaries. Among the cells exuded from these vessels would be sensitive ones, and again, once begun, the reaction could progress on the basis of cell-antigen interaction. Experiments in which an intravenously administered dye has been used to detect such changes in capillaries at the onset of the tuberculin reaction suggest that in the sensitive guinea pig an initial effect of this kind may occur, the antibodies concerned being probably directed against polysaccharide constituents of tuberculin [116]. We have carried out tests in animals sensitized with BCG vaccine and studied early after sensitization when antibodies readily demonstrable by serological tests are not present. With an electrophoretically isolated protein fraction of tuberculin to which antibodies could not be revealed in the sensitized subjects, we were unable to find any initial increase in capillary dilatation, but despite this the delayed reaction proceeded in the usual fashion [117].

It is not possible now to do more than outline the nature of thought and evidence on this question; conclusions are not yet at hand.

TISSUE DAMAGE IN DELAYED REACTIONS

The third question raised earlier deals with the rationale for the occurrence of general tissue damage which is frequently seen in sites of delayed hypersensitive reactions. To illustrate, a pulmonary lesion in tuberculosis soon undergoes allergic necrosis which encompasses a variety of cytological elements of the lung parenchyma. Since available evidence implicates only specifically reactive lymphoid cells as vulnerable to exposure to antigen, the widespread damage must be accounted for on some other basis. One can speculate that antigen may be adsorbed to various cells and structures, and these might then be attacked by sensitized cells, as has been seen to occur with homologous cells employed in the *in vitro* studies described earlier. This hypothesis is attractive for its reasonableness, but it was not justified when tested by immersing renal tubular epithelial cells in tuberculin *in vitro* and subjecting them to lymphoid cells of tuberculin-sensitive animals. The tubular epithelium proceeded to proliferate unimpeded over several days of observation [121].

Alternatively, a release of toxic substances from injured lymphocytes is a possibility, but it has not been clearly substantiated [114, 115]. The renal epithelial studies might have revealed the presence of cytotoxins also, for in some experiments tuberculin was not washed out of the culture medium containing both the target cells and the sensitized lymphoid elements, but here too the epithelial cells were not manifestly damaged. It may be that toxins deriving from such a reaction are effective on blood vessels and are consequently not revealed by maneuvers performed away from the body. In that case, generalized tissue damage may follow from what has been described as a vasculonecrotic reaction [122, 123].

TOLERANCE IN DELAYED REACTIVITY

Immunological tolerance denotes a specific state of "anti-immunity," i.e., the circumstance in which a subject is incapable of responding to one or more antigens while retaining the general capacity to react against others in normal fashion. The conditions under which this state may occur are discussed in other chapters; briefly, these include exposure to antigen of the fetus in its later stages of development, or of the newborn, or even of the adult if the dosage of antigen is large, and especially if antimetabolic drugs or total body irradiation are employed during the time when the exposure occurs [26].

If the state of homograft rejectivity is accepted as an example of delayed hypersensitivity, the occurrence of tolerance in the latter is not far to seek, for its classic example comes from studies of homologous tissue interactions [124]. If we turn to those states with which this chapter has dealt, the best documented example comes from studies of some of the chemical contact agents [125]. The feeding of picrylchloride to guinea pigs, for example, renders them incapable of responding to subsequent exposure of the skin to this substance with either delayed hypersensitivity or antibody formation [126]. The latter incapacity may be overcome by injection of the hapten conjugated to a protein foreign to the subject, but the failure to develop contact reactivity is not made good by this procedure. These occurrences are in part related to the earlier discussion concerning the dimensions of molecular entities required for recognition by responding cells and for elicitation of reactions. Presumably the prefed animal develops an incapacity to respond in any manner to hapten autoprotein. The introduction of the hapten attached to a foreign substance changes the total molecular pattern sufficiently to permit its recognition as a "new" antigen by the antibody-synthesizing mechanism, and antibodies with antihapten specificity are produced. The delayed response fails to occur because elicitation requires that the protein component be homologous to that participating in induction of the state, and tolerance to this has not been by-passed by the new conjugate employed.

In the case of tuberculin reactivity, tolerance of variable degree has been described as occurring in some animals given pre- and postnatal injections of *Mycobacteria* [41, 127]. In similar trials in which we injected avirulent bacilli of "human type" into chick embryos, we were unable to accomplish this.

In protein-induced reactive states (Jones-Mote hypersensitivity), injections of antigens into fetal guinea pigs have resulted in postnatal unresponsiveness [128–130], although newborn animals are amenable to sensitization [39–42].

DESENSITIZATION

The art of converting sensitive subjects to a nonreactive state by means of repeated injections of antigens to which they are responsive has been exploited especially in the case of the spontaneously occurring immediate hypersensitive states in human beings. In such antibody-mediated reactivities it is rational to suppose that the effect of repeated injections of antigen might be to reduce the level of circulating antibodies to a relatively harmless range of concentration. But the explanation seems not to be as simple as this [26]; desensitization may in fact depend on the development by the treated subject of antibodies with lesser capacity for anchoring to tissues than those responsible for hypersensitivity, but with equal or greater avidity for antigen [131, 132].

In delayed reactivity, desensitization can also be accomplished, although in both infection and contact reactivity, general experience suggests that this is a process which requires multiple treatments with increasing doses of antigen over a considerable period of time [3, 133]. As an example of the application of this process to human subjects, Madigan [134] has desensitized tuberculous patients with Old Tuberculin and a killed tubercle bacillary emulsion by adhering to a schedule of daily injections of increasing quantities for a period of forty-nine days. In almost all instances these subjects became unreactive to large quantities of concentrated tuberculin, up to several million times the amount which would ordinarily induce a local skin reaction. In attempted treatment of analogous kind in human subjects sensitive to contact reactants, results have been variably successful [135–137].

In Jones-Mote sensitivity, desensitization is much more readily attained: a single administration of the responsible antigen is said to abolish reactivity for variable periods of time [138a]. This has been mentioned before as a possible point of distinction between this reactive state and those of infection and contact types.

DELAYED HYPERSENSITIVITY IN RESISTANCE TO DISEASE AGENTS

The foregoing discussion has been almost wholly concerned with the injurious aspects of delayed hypersensitive reactivity. One would expect that this kind of reactivity has evolved and persisted in many orders of the vertebrates because it serves some useful function. Observations dealing with tissue graft rejection support this view. However, the transfer of cells or tissues between individuals is not a natural occurrence, and it has been proposed [138b] that this mechanism may perhaps be concerned under spontaneous conditions in discouraging cells arising as neoplasia which, experiments have shown, may be antigenically different from the normal tissues of the host.

With regard to infectious agents, the case for a protective function of delayed reactivity is not clear. It has been pointed out frequently that patients with hypogammaglobulinemia are able to fend off many of the infectious agents despite the paucity of their antibodies and that they possess the capacity to develop delayed hypersensitivity. This information is suggestive, but it is beset by pitfalls, such as the facts that the very small quantities of antibodies which many, perhaps all, of these patients can synthesize may suffice for protection and that in the case of viral infections interferon may have a decisive role in terminating the disease process.

To turn to a few specific examples about which there is sufficient information for discussion, in tuberculosis it is quite well established that antibodies elicited by infection or vaccination are not concerned in acquired resistance [26]. By default, cells have been considered to account for immunity, and a number of workers have implicated macrophages as the responsible ones [139–142], although this has not been a universal observation [26]. Such cells or lysates of them have been found, furthermore, to transmit immunity to several normal recipients seriatim, as if a specific factor in the donor's cells could transfer itself widely to similar cells of the recipient [143]. In recent interesting work, Mackaness [144] has found that macrophages of animals vaccinated with intracellularly localizing bacteria (*Listeria*), and rendered immune as well as hypersensitive, possess macrophages with unusual morphological and functional characteristics, the latter expressed in a greater capacity to inhibit and destroy bacteria which they may engulf. The test microbes need not be of the species employed for vaccination; thus cells obtained from animals treated with tubercle bacillus vaccine may act on *Listeria* or *Brucella,* and vice versa [87]. This demonstration correlates with a considerable body of information indicating that cross-immunities exist in animals which have been vaccinated with tubercle bacilli and that other vaccines may induce degrees of resistance to tuberculosis, presumably through an activating effect on cells of the reticuloendothelial system [145–147]. There may be a relationship also with the description by Myrvik and colleagues [148, 149] of the appearance in the lungs of tuberculin-sensitive animals re-exposed to bacilli intravenously of enormous numbers of macrophages which yield extracts with striking tuberculostatic activity; with observations of the ability of large mononuclear cells of sensitized animals to take up tuberculin [88]; and with a phenomenon of "macrophage disappearance" which has been observed in the peritoneal cavities of tuberculin-sensitive animals after administration of very small doses of tuberculin [150]. These observations have in common the fact that activities or responses on the part of macrophages of the sensitized subject with immunity have been noted.

The difficulty in judging whether these interesting pieces of information signify that delayed hypersensitive reactivity provides a basis for immunity lies in such points as these: that animals vaccinated with tubercle bacilli can be desensitized to tuberculin without losing their acquired resistance [151], and that most studies of the cells implicated in delayed hypersensitivity have designated these as lymphocytes rather than as macrophages. A path through this bog may eventually be found to rest on such grounds as the possibility that small lymphocytes can give rise to macrophages [152] or to "large pyroninophilic cells" [85], or in the further possibility that ribonucleic acid may be transferred between cell types, as has been suggested by experiments dealing with the synthesis of antibody [153].

In vaccinia infection, there is evidence to support the view that immunity resides in the possession of humoral antibodies, in animals as well as in man [26]. However, Kempe [154] has found that an infant with generalized vaccinal infection was not helped by large doses of human immune serum, while peripheral blood leukocytes from the same donor successfully overcame the infection. The apparent participation of cells in this process does not necessarily imply that the same cells are also concerned in delayed hypersensitivity.

Lymphocytic choriomeningitis virus produces fatal infections in young mice. If these animals are rendered tolerant to the virus through prenatal exposure, subsequent challenge results in multiplication of the virus without signs of disease. In this instance, it appears that failure of the animal to respond to the agent with delayed reactivity is in itself a protective device [155].

In the protein-induced delayed type of reactivity instigated by neutralized mixtures of diphtheria toxin and antitoxin, delayed reactivity to toxin in the absence of antibodies has been found not to be accompanied by an ability to neutralize the toxic effects of this substance.

REFERENCES

1. Davies, G. E. Chemical Structure and Pharmacodynamic Action in Relation to Drug Sensitivity. In Rosenheim, M. L., and Moulton, R. (Eds.), *Sensitivity Reactions to Drugs.* Oxford: Blackwell Scientific Publications, 1958. P. 149.
2. Salvin, S. B. Specificity of allergic reactions: V. Observations on the systemic delayed reaction in guinea pigs sensitized to purified protein-conjugates. *J. Immun.* 89:910, 1962.
3. Rich, A. R. *The Pathogenesis of Tuberculosis* (2nd ed.). Springfield, Ill.: Charles C Thomas, Publisher, 1951.
4. Crowle, A. J. *Delayed Hypersensitivity in Health and Disease.* Springfield, Ill.: Charles C Thomas, Publisher, 1962.
5. Grolnick, M. Contact allergy of the skin. *Ann. N.Y. Acad. Sci.* 50:718, 1949.
6. Chase, M. W. Inheritance in guinea pigs of the susceptibility to skin sensitization with simple chemical compounds. *J. Exp. Med.* 73: 711, 1941.
7. Berzton, J. W. The effect of certain infectious diseases on tuberculin allergy. *Tubercle* 34:34, 1953.
8. Pepys, J. The relationship of nonspecific and specific factors in the tuberculin reaction. *Am. Rev. Tuberc.* 71:49, 1955.
9. Mellman, W. J., and Wetton, R. Depression of the tuberculin reaction by attenuated measles virus vaccine. *J. Lab. Clin. Med.* 61: 453, 1963.
10. Cummings, M. M., Hudgins, P. C., Patnode, R. A., and Besack, S. R. The influence of x-irradiation on the passive transfer of tuberculin hypersensitivity in the guinea pig. *J. Immun.* 74:142, 1955.
11. Pepys, J. The effect of nitrogen mustard on the tuberculin reaction. *Int. Arch. Allerg.* 5: 233, 1954.
12. Ebert, R. H. *In vivo* observations on the effect of cortisone on experimental tuberculosis, using the rabbit ear chamber technique. *Amer. Rev. Tuberc.* 65:64, 1952.
13. Edwards, P. Q., Knight, R. A., and Marcus, S. Skin sensitivity of human beings to *Histoplasma capsulatum* and *Blastomyces dermatitidis* polysaccharide antigens. *Amer. Rev. Resp. Dis.* 83:528, 1961.
14. Hassid, W. Z., Baker, E. E., and McCready, R. M. An immunologically active polysaccharide produced by *Coccidioides immitis* Rixford and Gilchrist. *J. Biol. Chem.* 149:303, 1943.
15. Chase, M. W. Chemical considerations of drug hypersensitivity. In Brown, E. A. (Ed.), *Allergology* (Proc. 4th Internat. Congr.). London: Pergamon Press, 1962. P. 92.
16. Landsteiner, K., and Jacobs, J. L. Studies on the sensitization of animals with simple chemical compounds. *J. Exp. Med.* 61:643, 1935.
17. Landsteiner, K., and Jacobs, J. L. Studies on the sensitization of animals with simple chemical compounds: II. *J. Exp. Med.* 64:625, 1936.
18. Brownlie, I. A., and Cumming, W. M. Tetryl

dermatitis: 2. The interaction of aromatic nitro-compounds with amino acids and proteins. *Biochem. J.* 40:640, 1946.
19. Eisen, H. N., Orris, L., and Belman, S. Elicitation of delayed allergic skin reactions with haptens: The dependence of elicitation on hapten combination with protein. *J. Exp. Med.* 95:473, 1952.
20. Eisen, H. N., and Belman, S. Studies of hypersensitivity to low molecular weight substances: II. Reactions of some allergenic substituted dinitrobenzenes with cysteine or cystine of skin proteins. *J. Exp. Med.* 98:533, 1953.
21. Leskowitz, S., and Waksman, B. H. A guinea pig potency test for adenovirus vaccine. *J. Immun.* 84:58, 1960.
22. Dienes, L., and Schoenheit, E. W. Certain characteristics of the infectious processes in connection with the influence exerted on the immunity response. *J. Immun.* 19:41, 1930.
23. Landsteiner, K., and Chase, M. W. Studies on the sensitization of animals with simple chemical compounds: VII. Skin sensitization by intraperitoneal injections. *J. Exp. Med.* 71:237, 1940.
24. Ben-Efraim, S., Fuchs, S., and Sela, M. Hypersensitivity to a synthetic polypeptide: Induction of a delayed reaction. *Science* 139:1222, 1963.
25. Choucroun, N. Sur un antigène sensibilisant extrait du bacilli tuberculeux. *C. R. Acad. Sci.* 83:505, 1929.
26. Raffel, S. *Immunity* (2nd ed.). New York: Appleton-Century-Crofts, Inc., 1961.
27. Salvaggie, J. E., Flax, M., and Leskowitz, S. The adjuvant effect of beryllium on production of antibody and delayed hypersensitivity. *Fed. Proc.* 22:267, 1963.
28. Gell, P. G. H., and Benacerraf, B. Studies of hypersensitivity: IV. The relationship between contact and delayed sensitivity; A study on the specificity of cellular immune reactions. *J. Exp. Med.* 113:571, 1961.
29. Block, H., and Nordin, A. A. Production of tuberculin sensitivity. *Nature* (London) 187:434, 1960.
30. Messina, V. P., and Rosenberg, L. T. Enhancement by normal cells of an immunological response. *Proc. Soc. Exp. Biol. Med.* 110:893, 1962.
31. Dienes, L., and Mallory, T. B. Histological studies of hypersensitive reactions. *Am. J. Path.* 8:689, 1932.
32. Jones, T. D., and Mote, J. R. The phases of foreign protein sensitization in human beings. *New Eng. J. Med.* 210:120, 1934.
33. Simon, F. A., and Rackemann, F. M. The development of hypersensitiveness in man: I. Following intradermal injection of the antigen. *J. Allerg.* 5:439, 1934.
34. Uhr, J. W., Salvin, S. B., and Pappenheimer, A. M., Jr. Delayed Hypersensitivity: II. Induction of hypersensitivity in guinea pigs by means of antigen-antibody complexes. *J. Exp. Med.* 105:11, 1957.
35. Raffel, S., and Newel, J. M. The "delayed hypersensitivity" induced by antigen-antibody complexes. *J. Exp. Med.* 108:823, 1958.
36. Becker, R. J., Sparks, D. B., Feinberg, S. M., Patterson, R., Pruzansky, J. J., and Feinberg, A. R. Delayed and immediate skin reactivity in man after the injection of antigen emulsion. Cell transfer of the delayed sensitivity. *J. Allerg.* 32:229, 1961.
37. Salvin, S. B. Delayed Hypersensitivity to Protein Antigens. Ref. 15, p. 209.
38. Parks, J. J., Liebowitz, H. M. I., and Maumenee, A. E. A transient stage of suspected delayed sensitivity during the early induction phase of immediate corneal sensitivity. *J. Exp. Med.* 115:867, 1962.
39. Salvin, S. B., Gregg, M. B., and Smith, R. F. Hypersensitivity in newborn guinea pigs. *J. Exp. Med.* 115:707, 1962.
40. Hunziker, N., and Schinos, G. Expériences sur cobayes nouveau-nés: Eczema au dinitrochlorobenzène. *Dermatologica* 124:235, 1962.
41. Lithander, A. Studies of pathogenic staphylococci among the staff in a department of medicine and infectious diseases. *Acta Path. Microbiol. Scand.* 49:165, 1960.
42. Uhr, J. W. Development of delayed-type hypersensitivity in guinea pig embryos. *Nature* (London) 187:957, 1960.
43. Sell, S., and Weigle, W. O. The relationship between delayed hypersensitivity and circulating antibody induced by protein antigens in guinea pigs. *J. Immun.* 83:257, 1959.
44. Pappenheimer, A. M., Jr., Scharff, M., and Uhr, J. W. Delayed Hypersensitivity and Its Possible Relation to Antibody Formation. In Shaffer, J. H., LoGrippo, G. A., and Chase, M. W. (Eds.), *Mechanisms of Hypersensitivity*. Boston: Little, Brown, 1959. P. 417.
45. Oort, J., and Turk, J. L. The fate of [^{131}I] labelled antigens in the skin of normal guinea pigs and those with delayed-type hypersensitivity. *Immunology* 6:148, 1963.
46. Martins, A. B., and Raffel, S. Cellular activities in hypersensitive reactions: I. Comparative cytology of delayed, "Jones-Mote" and Arthus reactions. *J. Immun.* in press, 1964. II. Plasmapoiesis in delayed and "Jones-Mote" reaction sites. *Ibid.*
47. Salvin, S. B., and Smith, R. F. Delayed hypersensitivity in the development of circulating antibody: The effect of x-irradiation. *J. Exp. Med.* 109:325, 1959.
48. Landsteiner, K. *The Specificity of Serological Reactions* (2nd ed.). Cambridge: Harvard University Press, 1945.

49. Haurowitz, F. Separation and determination of multiple antibodies. *J. Immun.* 43:331, 1942.
50. Ovary, Z., and Benacerraf, B. Contribution of the hapten and the carrier protein to the anamnestic response of rabbits primarily immunized with 2,4-dinitrophenyl bovine gamma globulin (DNP-BGG). *Fed. Proc.* 22:266, 1963.
51. Amkraut, A. Induction and Properties of Anti-hapten Antibody. Stanford University Ph.D. Thesis, 1963.
52. Benacerraf, B., and Gell, P. G. H. Studies on hypersensitivity: II. Delayed hypersensitivity to denatured proteins in guinea pigs. *Immunology* 2:64, 1959.
53. Leskowitz, S. Immunochemical study of antigenic specificity in delayed hypersensitivity. *J. Immun.* 89:435, 1962.
54. Waksman, B. H. A Comparative Histopathological Study of Delayed Hypersensitive Reactions. In Wolstenholme, G. E. W., and O'Connor, M. (Eds.), *Cellular Aspects of Immunity*. Boston: Little, Brown, 1960. P. 280.
55. Kaplan, M. H., and Dienes, L. The Cellular Response in Forms of Delayed- and Immediate-Type Skin Reactions in the Guinea Pig. Ref. 44, p. 435.
56. Gell, P. G. H., and Hinde, I. T. Observations on the histology of Arthus reaction and its relation to other known types of skin hypersensitivity. *Int. Arch. Allerg.* 5:23, 1954.
57. Chase, M. W. The cellular transfer of cutaneous hypersensitivity to tuberculin. *Proc. Soc. Exp. Biol. Med.* 59:134, 1945.
58. Bloom, B. R., Chase, M. W., and Goldstein, G. Failure to transfer delayed-type hypersensitivity to chemical allergens in the guinea pig by cell extracts. *Bact. Proc.*, M24, 1961.
59. Jeter, W. S., Tremaine, M. M., and Seebohm, P. M. Passive transfer of delayed hypersensitivity to 2,4-dinitrochlorobenzene in guinea pigs with leucocytic extracts. *Proc. Soc. Exp. Biol. Med.* 86:251, 1954.
60. Turk, J. L. Passive transfer of contact sensitivity to picryl chloride in guinea pigs, with subcellular material. *Nature* (London) 191: 915, 1961.
61. Lawrence, H. S. The Transfer of Hypersensitivity of the Delayed Type in Man. In *Cellular and Humoral Aspects of the Hypersensitive States*. New York: Paul B. Hoeber, Inc., 1959. P. 279.
62. Lawrence, H. S., Rapoport, F. T., Converse, J. M., and Tillett, W. S. Transfer of delayed hypersensitivity to skin homografts with leukocyte extracts in man. *J. Clin. Invest.* 39:185, 1960.
63. Holst, P. M. Studies on the effects of tuberculin. *Tubercle* 3:337, 1922.
64. Hall, H. E., and Scherago, M. The development of leukocytic sensitivity to tuberculin in guinea pigs experimentally infected with *Mycobacterium tuberculosis* $H_{37}R_v$. *Am. Rev. Tuberc.* 76:888, 1957.
65. Rosenau, W., and Moon, H. D. Effect of splenic homogenates on homologous cells *in vitro*. *Lab. Invest.* 11:1260, 1962.
66. Rosenau, W., and Moon, H. D. Lysis of homologous cells by sensitized lymphocytes in tissue culture. *J. Nat. Canc. Inst.* 27:471, 1961.
67. Koprowski, H., and Fernandes, M. V. Autosensitization reaction in vitro: Contactual agglutination of sensitized lymph node cells in brain tissue culture accompanied by destruction of glial elements. *J. Exp. Med.* 116:467, 1962.
68. Sinkovics, J. G., Howe, C. D., and Schullenberger, C. C. Mechanisms of immunological tissue damage. *Med. Rec. Ann.* 56:133, 1963.
69. Janeway, C. A. Hypogammaglobulinemia and Immunological Responses. Ref. 15, p. 241.
70. Porter, H. M. Immunologic studies in congenital agammaglobulinemia with emphasis on delayed hypersensitivity. *Pediatrics* 20:958, 1957.
71. Good, R. A., Varco, R. L., Aust, J. B., and Zak, S. Transplantation studies in patients with agammaglobulinemia. *Ann. N.Y. Acad. Sci.* 64:882, 1957.
72. Aisenberg, A. C., and Leskowitz, S. Antibody formation in Hodgkin's disease. *New Eng. J. Med.* 268:1269, 1963.
73. Rostenberg, A., Jr. Etiologic and immunologic concepts regarding sarcoidosis. *Arch. Dermat.* 64:385, 1951.
74. Israel, H. L., Sones, M., Stein, S. C., and Aronson, J. D. BCG vaccination in sarcoidosis. *Am. Rev. Tuberc.* 62:408, 1950.
75. Boyden, S. V., Sorkin, E., and Spärck, J. V. Observations on the Antibodies Associated with Spleen Cells at Different Stages of Immunization. In Holub, M., and Jarošková (Eds.), *Mechanisms of Antibody Formation*. Prague: Publishing House of Czechoslovak Academy of Sciences; and New York: Academic Press, Inc., 1960. P. 237.
76. Freedman, S. O., Turcotte, R., Fish, H. A., and Sehon, A. H. The *in vitro* detection of "cell-fixed" hemagglutinating antibodies to tuberculin purified protein derivative (PPD) in humans. *J. Immun.* 90:52, 1963.
77. Miller, J. M., and Favour, C. B. The lymphocytic origin of a plasma factor responsible for hypersensitivity *in vitro* of tuberculin type. *J. Exp. Med.* 93:1, 1951.
78. Rauch, H. C., and Favour, C. B. Passive transfer of allergic reactions to tuberculin with plasma protein fractions from hypersensitive guinea pigs. *Ann. N.Y. Acad. Sci.* 87:231, 1960.
79. Cole, L. R., Paldino, R. L., Henderson, R. W.,

and West, A. F. Passive transfer of a delayed type of skin reactivity to tuberculin PPD. *Amer. Rev. Resp. Dis.* 80:398, 1959.

80. Cole, L. R., Matloff, J. J., and Farrell, V. R. A method for coupling protein antigens to erythrocytes: II. Use of the method in the diagnosis of tuberculosis. *J. Exp. Med.* 102:647, 1955.
81. Ehrenkranz, N. J., and Waksman, B. H. Failure to transfer tuberculin sensitivity passively with plasma fractions containing alpha globulin. *J. Exp. Med.* 104:935, 1956.
82. Karush, F., and Eisen, H. N. A theory of delayed hypersensitivity: The main features of this phenomenon are explicable in terms of high-affinity humoral antibody. *Science* 136: 1032, 1962.
83. Wesslén, T. Passive transfer of tuberculin hypersensitivity by viable lymphocytes from the thoracic duct. *Acta Tuberc. Scand.* 26:38, 1952.
84. Messina, V. P., and Raffel, S. To be published.
85. Gowans, J. L. The fate of parental strain small lymphocytes in F_1 hybrid rats. *Ann. N.Y. Acad. Sci.* 99:432, 1962.
86. Porter, K. A., and Cooper, E. H. Transformation of adult allogenic small lymphocytes after transfusion into newborn rats. *J. Exp. Med.* 115:997, 1962.
87. Mackaness, G. B. The Behaviour of Microbial Parasites in Relation to Phagocytic Cells *in vitro* and *in vivo.* In Smith, H., and Taylor, J. (Eds.), *Microbial Behaviour* in vivo *and* in vitro (Soc. Gen. Microb., 14th symposium). London: Cambridge Univ. Press, 1964. P. 213.
88. Kay, K., and Rieke, W. O. Tuberculin hypersensitivity: Studies with radioactive antigen and mononuclear cells. *Science* 139:487, 1963.
89. Martins, A. B., Moore, W. D., Dickinson, J. B., and Raffel, S. Cellular activities in hypersensitive reactions: III. Specifically reactive cells in delayed hypersensitivity: Tuberculin hypersensitivity. *J. Immun.* in press, 1964.
90. Rauch, H., and Raffel, S. Immunofluorescent localization of encephalatogenic protein in myelin. *J. Immun.* 92:452, 1964.
91. Weiser, R. S. Hypersensitivity and the Homograft Reaction. In *Proceedings of the Conference on Immuno-Reproduction.* La Jolla, Calif., September, 1962. P. 193.
92. Thorbecke, A. J., and Keuning, F. J. Antibody and gamma globulin formation *in vitro* in hemopoietic organs. *J. Infect. Dis.* 98:157, 1956.
93. Fagraeus, A. *Antibody Production in Relation to the Development of Plasma Cells.* Stockholm: Esselte, A. B., 1948.
94. Stoner, R. D., and Hale, W. M. Antibody production by thymus and Peyer's patches intraocular transplants. *J. Immun.* 75:203, 1955.
95. Hapthausen, H. Studies on the role of the lymphocytes as "transmitter" of the hypersensitiveness in allergic eczema. *Acta Dermatovener.* 27:275, 1947.
96. Miller, J. F. A. P. Immunological function of the thymus. *Lancet* 2:748, 1961.
97. Parrott, D. M. V., and East, J. Role of the thymus in neonatal life. *Nature* (London) 195:347, 1962.
98. Archer, O. K., and Pierce, J. C. Role of thymus in development of the immune response. *Fed. Proc.* 20:26, 1961.
99. Martinez, C., Kersey, J., Papermaster, B. W., and Good, R. A. Skin homograft survival in thymectomized mice. *Proc. Soc. Exp. Biol. Med.* 109:193, 1962.
100. Congdon, C. C., and Duda, D. B. Prevention of bone marrow heterografting: Use of isologous thymus in lethally irradiated mice. *Arch. Path.* 71:311, 1961.
101. Auerbach, R. Genetic control of thymus lymphoid differentiation. *Proc. Nat. Acad. Sci. U.S.A.* 47:1175, 1961.
102. Ruth, R. F. Derivation of antibody-producing cells from ectodermal-endodermal epithelia. *Anat. Rec.* 139:270, 1961.
103. Arnason, B. G., Janković, B. D., and Waksman, B. H. Effect of thymectomy on "Delayed" hypersensitive reactions. *Nature,* 194: 99, 1962.
104. Arnason, B. G., Janković, B. D., Waksman, B. H., and Wenersten, C. Role of the thymus in immune reactions in rats: II. Suppressive effect of thymectomy at birth on reactions of delayed (cellular) hypersensitivity and the circulating small lymphocyte. *J. Exp. Med.* 116: 177, 1962.
105. Chang, T. S., Glick, B., and Winter, A. P. The significance of the bursa of Fabricius of chickens in antibody production. *Poult. Sci.* 34:1187, 1955.
106. Aspinall, R. L., Meyer, R. K., Graetzer, M. A., and Wolfe, H. R. Effect of thymectomy and bursectomy on the survival of skin homografts in chickens. *J. Immun.* 90:873, 1963.
107. Graetzer, M. A., Wolfe, H. R., Aspinall, R. L., and Meyer, R. K. Effect of thymectomy and bursectomy on precipitin and natural hemagglutinin production in the chicken. *Ibid.,* p. 878.
108. Szenberg, A., and Warner, N. L. Immunological function of thymus and bursa of Fabricius. *Nature* (London) 194:146, 1962.
109. Mowbray, J. F. Ability of large doses of an $alpha_2$ plasma protein fraction to inhibit antibody production. *Immunology* 6:217, 1963.
110. Mowbray, J. F. Personal communication, 1963.
111. Najarian, J. S., and Feldman, J. D. Passive transfer of tuberculin sensitivity by tritiated

thymidine-labeled lymphoid cells. *J. Exp. Med.* 114:779, 1961.

112. Hamilton, L. D., and Chase, M. W. Labelled cells in the cellular transfer of delayed hypersensitivity. *Fed. Proc.* 21:40, 1962.
113. Turk, J. L., and Oort, J. A histological study of the early stages of the development of the Tuberculin reaction after passive transfer of cells labelled with [^{3}H] thymidine. *Immunology* 6:140, 1963.
114. Johanovsky, J. Production of pyrogenic substances in the reaction of cells of hypersensitive guinea pigs with antigen *"in vitro." Immunology* 3:179, 1960.
115. Hall, C. H., Jr., and Atkins, E. Studies on tuberculin fever: I. The mechanism of fever in tuberculin hypersensitivity. *J. Exp. Med.* 109:339, 1959.
116. Voisin, G. A., and Toullet, F. Modifications of Capillary Permeability in Immunological Reactions Mediated Through Cells. Ref. 54, p. 373.
117. Dedrick, C. T., and Raffel, S. Unpublished observations, 1963.
118. Patnode, R. A., and Hudgins, P. C. Sonic fragility of leukocytes from guinea pigs vaccinated with BCG. *Amer. Rev. Tuberc.* 79: 323, 1959.
119. O'Neill, E. F., and Favour, C. B. Tissue culture analysis of tuberculin hypersensitivity in man. *Amer. Rev. Tuberc.* 72:577, 1955.
120. Lasfargues, E., Boquet, P., and Delaunay, A. Cultures de tissus appliquées à la solution de problèmes immunologiques: IV. Réactions Tuberculiniques. *Ann. Inst. Pasteur* (Paris) 73:169, 1947.
121. Messina, V. P., Martins, A. B., and Raffel, S. To be published.
122. Gell, P. G. H. Cytologic Events in Hypersensitivity Reactions. Ref. 61, p. 43.
123. Waksman, B. H. Tissue Damage in the "Delayed" (Cellular) Type of Hypersensitivity. In Grabar, P., and Miescher, P. (Eds.), *Second International Symposium on Immunopathology*. Basel: Benno Schwabe, 1962. P. 146.
124. Billingham, R. E., Brent, L., and Medawar, P. B. Quantitative studies on tissue transplantation immunity: III. Actively acquired tolerance. *Phil. Trans. Roy. Soc.* [Biol.] 239: 357, 1956.
125. Sulzberger, M. B. Hypersensitiveness to arsphenamine in guinea pigs: I. Experiments in prevention and in desensitization. *Arch. Derm.* 20:669, 1929; II. Experiments demonstrating the role of the skin, both as originator and as site of the hypersensitivenss. *Ibid.* 22:839, 1930.
126. Chase, M. W., and Battisto, J. R. Immunologic Unresponsiveness to Allergenic Chemicals. Ref. 44, p. 507.
127. Weiss, D. W. Inhibition of tuberculin skin hypersensitivity in guinea pigs by injection of tuberculin and intact tubercle bacilli during fetal life. *J. Exp. Med.* 108:83, 1958.
128. Humphrey, J.H., and Turk, J. L. Immunological unresponsiveness in guinea pigs: I. Immunological unresponsiveness to heterologous serum proteins. *Immunology* 4:301, 1961.
129. Turk, J. L., and Humphrey, J. H. Immunological unresponsiveness in guinea pigs: II. The effect of unresponsiveness on the development of delayed type hypersensitivity to protein antigens. *Ibid.*, p. 310.
130. Gregg, M. B., and Salvin, S. B. Immunologic unresponsiveness to purified proteins in guinea pigs. *J. Immun.* 90:368, 1963.
131. Cooke, R. A., Barnard, J. H., Hebold, S., and Stull, A. Serological evidence of immunity with coexisting sensitization in a type of human allergy (hay fever). *J. Exp. Med.* 62:733, 1935.
132. Loveless, M. H. Immunological studies of pollinosis: I. The presence of two antibodies related to the same pollen-antigen in the serum of treated hay-fever patients. *J. Immun.* 38:25, 1940; IV. The relationship between thermostable antibody in the circulation and clinical immunity. *Ibid.* 47:165, 1943.
133. Chase, M. W. Models for Hypersensitivity Studies. Ref. 61, p. 251.
134. Madigan, D. G. Desensitization in Man: The Hypersensitive State in Human Tuberculosis: The use of tuberculin and bacillary emulsion as desensitizing agents. *Report to Mississippi Valley Conference on Tuberculosis,* Minneapolis, October, 1953.
135. Epstein, W. L. Rhus dermatitis: Fact and fiction. *Kaiser Fdn. Med. Bull.* 6:197, 1958.
136. Shaffer, B., and Strauss, M. B. Oral prophylaxis against poison ivy dermatitis with Aqua Ivy tablets: I. A controlled experiment and preliminary clinical report. *J. Allerg.* 30:130, 1959.
137. Kligman, A. M. Hyposensitization against rhus dermatitis. *Arch. Derm.* 78:47, 1958.

138a. Uhr, J. W. Specific desensitization of guinea pigs with delayed hypersensitivity to protein antigens. *Ann. N.Y. Acad. Sci.* 73:753, 1958.

138b. Burnet, F. M. *Integrity of the Body.* Cambridge, Mass.: Harvard Univ. Press, 1962. P. 179.

139. Suter, E. Letter to the editor. *Amer. Rev. Tuberc.* 69:1060, 1954.
140. Lurie, M. B. Studies on the mechanism of immunity in tuberculosis: The fate of tubercle bacilli ingested by mononuclear phagocytes derived from normal and immunized animals. *J. Exp. Med.* 75:247, 1942.

141. Berthrong, M., and Hamilton, M. A. Tissue culture studies on resistance in tuberculosis: II. Monocytes from normal and immunized guinea pigs infected with virulent human tubercle bacilli. *Amer. Rev. Resp. Dis.* 79:221, 1959.
142. Fong, J., Schneider, P., and Elberg, S. S. Studies on tubercle bacillus-monocyte relationship: II. Induction of monocyte degeneration by bacteria and culture filtrate; Specificity of serum and monocyte effects on resistance to degeneration. *J. Exp. Med.* 105: 25, 1957.
143. Fong, J., Chin, D., and Elberg, S. S. Studies on tubercle bacillus-histiocyte relationship: V. Passive transfer of cellular resistance. *J. Exp. Med.* 115:475, 1962.
144. Mackaness, G. B. Cellular resistance to infection. *J. Exp. Med.* 116:381, 1962.
145. Nyka, W. Enhancement of resistance to tuberculosis in mice experimentally infected with *Brucella abortus. Amer. Rev. Tuberc.* 73:251, 1956.
146. Elberg, S. S., Schneider, P., and Fong, J. Cross-immunity between *Brucella melitensis* and *Mycobacterium tuberculosis:* Intracellular behavior of *Brucella melitensis* in monocytes from vaccinated animals. *J. Exp. Med.* 106:545, 1957.
147. Rees, R. J. W. The chemotherapeutic activity of Triton WR 1339 and Macrocyclon in murine leprosy. *Amer. Rev. Tuberc.* 76:915, 1957.
148. Oshima, S., Myrvik, Q. N., and Leake, E. The demonstration of lysozyme as a dominant tuberculostatic factor in extracts of granulomatous lungs. *Brit. J. Exp. Path.* 42: 138, 1961.
149. Myrvik, Q. N., Leake, E. S., and Oshima, S. A study of macrophages and epithelioid-like cells from granulomatous (BCG-induced) lungs of rabbits. *J. Immun.* 89:745, 1962.
150. Nelson, D. S., and Boyden, S. V. The loss of macrophages from peritoneal exudates following the injection of antigens into guinea-pigs with delayed-type hypersensitivity. *Immunology* 6:264, 1963.
151. Rothschild, H., Friedenwald, J. S., and Bernstein, C. The relation of allergy to immunity in tuberculosis. *Bull. Hopkins Hosp.* 54: 232, 1934.
152. Trowell, O. A. The lymphocyte. *Int. Rev. Cytol.* 7:235, 1958.
153. Fishman, M., Hammerstrom, R. A., and Bond, V. P. *In vitro* transfer of macrophage RNA to lymph node cells. *Nature* (London) 198: 549, 1963.
154. Kempe, H. C. Studies on smallpox and complications of smallpox vaccination. *Pediatrics* 26:176, 1960.
155. Hotchin, J., and Weigand, H. Studies of lymphocytic choriomeningitis in mice: I. The relationship between age at inoculation and outcome of infection. *J. Immun.* 86:392, 1961.

*12. Experimental Serum Sickness**

FRANK J. DIXON

EXPERIMENTAL SERUM SICKNESS IS of considerable interest for several reasons. First, it corresponds closely to clinical serum sickness, a not uncommon iatrogenic complication of serum therapy, and has provided a useful model for the study of this disease. Second, the signs, symptoms, and morphological lesions of serum sickness bear close resemblance to some of the changes seen in various poorly understood human diseases of the connective tissues and certain drug reactions. Third, the pathogenic mechanisms which have been defined in studies of experimental serum sickness also may be operative in those clinical diseases which it resembles. The resemblance between serum sickness and seasonal allergy, urticaria, postscarlet fever nephritis, tuberculosis, syphilis, and several other infectious diseases originally led von Pirquet to suggest that, like serum sickness, these diseases were entirely, or in part, manifestations of antigen-antibody interactions [1]. Later, pathologists such as Klinge [2] and Rich [3] pointed out morphological similarities between lesions of serum sickness and those of rheumatoid arthritis, rheumatic fever, disseminated lupus erythematosus, glomerulonephritis, polyarteritis, and certain purpuras. Although an immunological basis for these clinical disorders is now considered likely, the precise pathogenic mechanisms are still unknown. However, recent work on experimental serum sickness has helped in defining these mechanisms [4].

Usually, experimental serum sickness is produced by one or several closely spaced, relatively large injections of heterologous serum protein into an animal with little or no pre-existing homologous antibody. In the case of the initial exposure to a given foreign protein, there is no pre-existing antibody and the disease develops one to two weeks after injection; if it is a repeated exposure, some pre-existing antibody may be present and the disease develops sooner, as would be expected in an anamnestic response. In either case, disease appears as antibody formation begins. The early work of von Pirquet [1], Longcope and Rackemann [5], Mackenzie and Leake [6], and the later studies of Rich [3], Hawn and Janeway [7], and Germuth [8, 9] established beyond much doubt that serum disease results from an antigen-antibody interaction. Further work on its pathogenesis has suggested that the essence of serum sickness is the protracted interaction between antigen and antibody in the circulation with the formation of antigen-antibody complexes in an environment of antigen excess and associated inflammatory and proliferative lesions in the connective tissues [4, 10]. (Immediate reactions between pre-existing antibodies and injected foreign serum protein antigens do not differ from other immediate anaphylactic reactions in animals and should be properly considered to be anaphylaxis, not serum sickness.) The particular immunological sequences of serum sickness are achieved only with antigens capable of remaining in the circulation for long periods, i.e., until antibody formation to them occurs. The antigens best suited to prolonged persistance in the circulation are native or near-native serum proteins. Serum protein molecules, homologous or heterologous, are removed from the circulation at exponential rates by nonimmune means that are incompletely understood. The rates are characteristic for a given protein-host combination but vary considerably from one combination to another [11]. Most nonserum protein antigens are rapidly cleared from the circulation of nonimmune subjects by renal excretion and/or action of phagocytic cells and therefore are not available to react in the circula-

* This work was supported in part by U.S. Public Health Service Grant AI-03897 and an Atomic Energy Commission contract.

tion with antibody made by the host some days after their injection.

The temporal relationships of the better recognized immunological and pathological events transpiring in serum sickness are illustrated in Figure 12-1. Data for this figure were

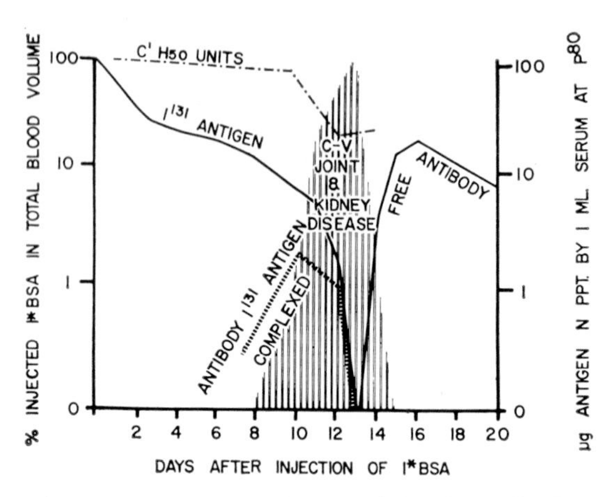

Fig. 12-1. Sequence of events following injection of 250 mg. I*BSA/kg. body weight in rabbits. Elimination of I^{131} antigen indicated by solid line relating to log scale at left. Amount of free antibody in the circulation relates to log scale at right. Antigen-antibody complexes plotted as percent of total I*BSA injected. Level of complement indicated as percent of normal. Incidence of cardiovascular, joint and kidney disease indicated by shaded area, reaching 100 percent on day 13.

obtained from previously unimmunized rabbits given intravenous injections of 0.25 gm. of I^{131}-labeled bovine serum albumin (I*BSA) per kilogram of body weight [10]. Except for differences in the speed of the response, these observations apply to human or experimental serum sickness induced with a large dose of virtually any serum protein antigen. The solid line indicating the level of I^{131}-antigen in the blood shows a rapid fall during the first two days as the intravenously injected antigen equilibrates between intra- and extravascular components of the serum protein pool. There follows a relatively slow, nonimmune decline lasting a little more than a week, and then the remaining antigen is rapidly eliminated from the circulation within two days. Following the elimination of circulating antigen, free antibody promptly appears in the serum. As far as is known, there is nothing peculiar about the antibody produced by animals with serum sickness. These antibodies usually will form antigen-antibody precipitates and will fix complement, although occasional exceptions have been noted. The rapid, final elimination of circulating antigen is caused by the production of antibody which combines with circulating antigen, forming antigen-antibody complexes which are removed from the circulation. The amounts of detectable circulating complexes are indicated by the dash line beginning about seven days after administration of antigen and increasing to a maximum at ten days, just prior to the beginning of rapid, immune elimination of antigen. The initial accumulation of complexes in the circulation probably consists of very small complexes formed in extreme antigen excess by the first small amounts of antibody formed. Such complexes will remain in the circulation for prolonged periods [12]. As more antibody becomes available, the complexes enlarge and their proportion of antibody increases. They then react with serum complement and finally become so large that they are rapidly removed from the circulation. Simultaneously with the formation of sizable complexes in the circulation, two other events transpire. The level of serum complement (C′) falls abruptly to levels less than half those existing prior to the antibody response, and there develop acute exudative and proliferative focal inflammatory lesions in the connective tissues.

The tissues primarily involved are the heart, arteries, joints, and kidneys [7, 8, 10]. The cardiac lesions include endocardial proliferation and infiltration by inflammatory cells, the formation of verrucous valvular vegetations, and mononuclear focal or diffuse myocarditis and pericarditis. The arterial lesions which occur most often in the coronaries are focal, necrotizing, and inflammatory processes involving often all layers of the arterial wall (Fig. 12-2). The lesions may show an acute inflammatory exudate, necrosis of the arterial wall, and fibrinoid material or may be primarily a mononuclear reaction. The presence of fibrinoid material (i.e., an amorphous eosinophilic material having some of the tinctorial qualities of fibrin) has been considered by many to indicate a type of necrosis characteristic of hypersensitivity reactions. However, it seems more likely that fibrinoid is largely a protein-rich exudate which may form in a variety of inflammatory and/or degenerative lesions. The kind of proteins in fibrinoid

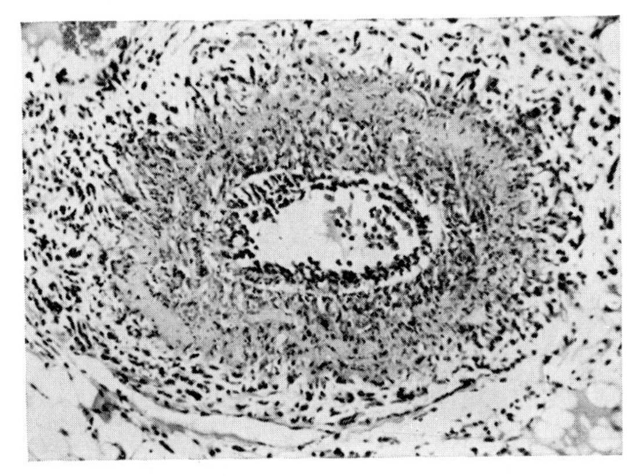

Fig. 12-2. Hematoxylin-eosin stained paraffin section of medium-sized coronary artery of rabbit with serum sickness on day of antigen elimination. There is considerable proliferation and infiltration of endothelium. Muscular media is almost entirely replaced by fibrinoid. There is a moderate infiltration by polymorphonuclear leukocytes and mononuclear cells in the media and adventitia.

varies greatly from one condition to another [13]. The joints are less regularly involved. They have focal mononuclear infiltrates with edema and fibrinoid formation in the synovial tissues. The kidneys show extensive uniform endothelial proliferation of glomerular capillaries with slight basement membrane thickening (Figs. 12-3 to 12-6). These are the lesions Klinge and Rich likened to those of rheumatic fever, polyarteritis nodosa, rheumatoid arthritis, lupus erythematosus, glomerulonephritis, and so on. The incidence of these lesions increases rapidly so that about the time of elimination of complexes and antigen from the circulation, virtually every rabbit will have one or more of these lesions, the most common being glomerulonephritis and endocarditis. After the elimination of complexes from the circulation, the lesions rapidly disappear, and in most instances healing is complete.

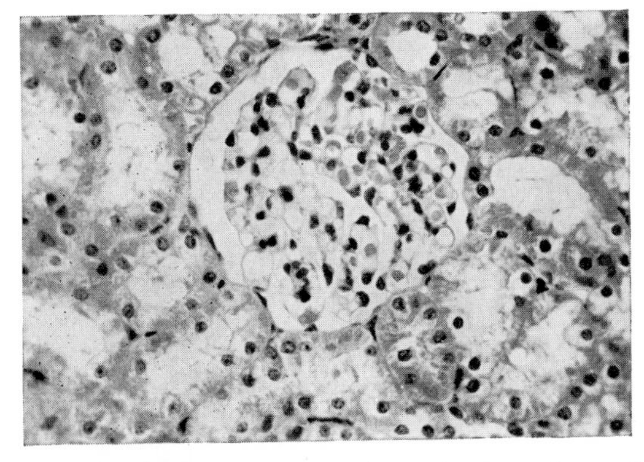

Fig. 12-3. Hematoxylin-eosin stained section of normal glomerulus from control rabbit. Note widely patent capillaries containing some erythrocytes and normal number of nucleated glomerular cells.

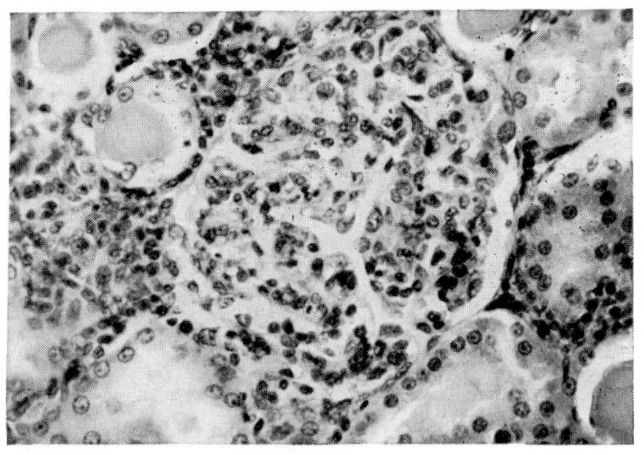

Fig. 12-4. Hematoxylin-eosin stained section of glomerulus from rabbit with serum sickness on day of antigen elimination. Glomerulus is swollen and avascular. It is filled with an increased number of endothelial and, to a lesser extent, epithelial cells.

Rarely, animals are found in which antibodies to the foreign serum protein are produced and complexes appear in the serum, but there is no rapid elimination of complexes and no detectable utilization of complement [14]. In such animals, moderate serum sickness lesions may develop, but florid disease has not been observed. It seems likely that in these instances the quality of the antibody is different and the consequent antigen-antibody interaction is a less efficient inflammatory agent than is usually the case. This type of persisting complex may be related to the occasional extremely protracted serum disease which is seen clinically.

By what means might serum protein antigen-antibody interaction in the circulation lead to damage of the host's tissues? Numerous experiments suppressing the host's antibody response have demonstrated the lack of any primary toxicity of foreign serum antigens themselves; thus the interaction of antigen and antibody appears essential to the production of disease. There is little to suggest that the initial antigen-antibody interaction itself takes place in the sites of the lesions. Certainly there is no reason to believe that there is any specific immunological relationship between host antibody formed in serum sickness

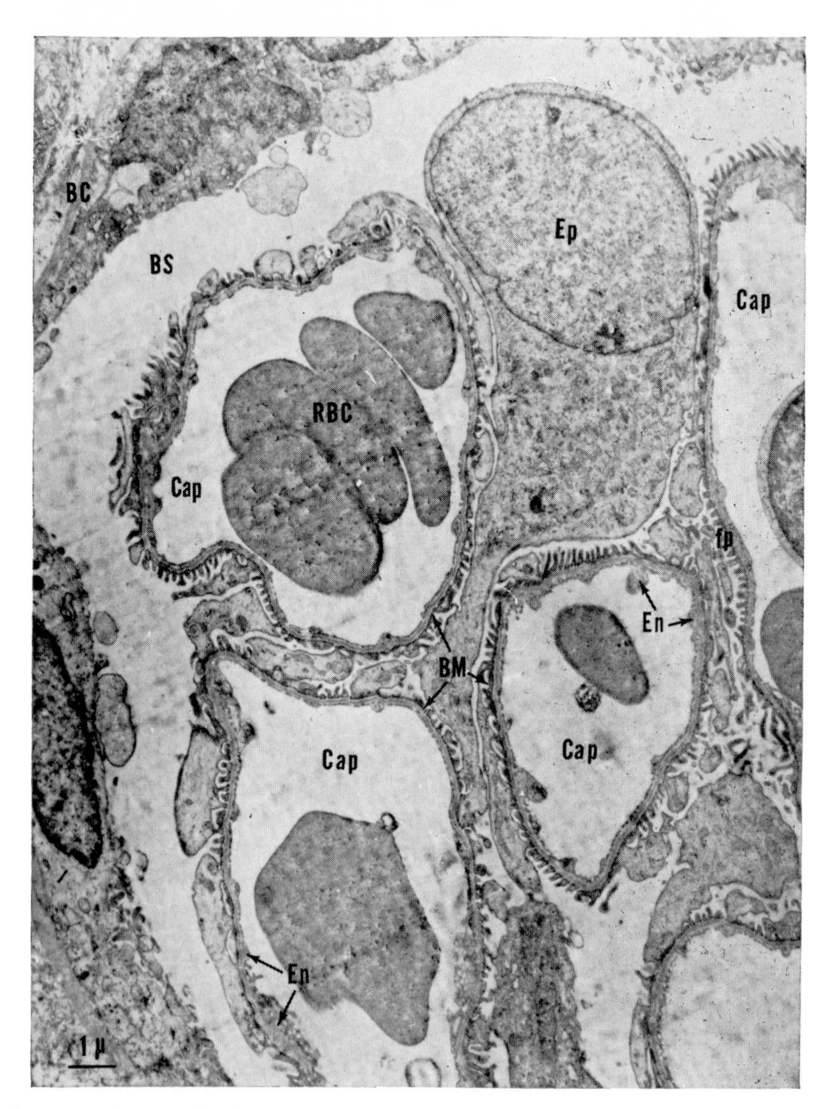

Fig. 12-5. Electron micrograph of normal rabbit glomerulus. Note open capillaries (*Cap*) containing red cells (*RBC*), thin, frequently perforated endothelial cytoplasm (*En*), regular basement membrane (*BM*), and epithelial cells (*Ep*) attached by fine foot processes (*fp*) to the outer aspects of the basement membrane. Bowman's space (*BS*) and Bowman's capsule (*BC*) seen at left.

and the injured tissues, i.e., an antitissue autoantibody, since a wide variety of serum protein antigens induces similar lesions. It has been postulated that soon after injection, some of the foreign serum proteins might fix in the connective tissues destined to develop lesions and persist there until antibody is formed which would then react with the tissue-bound foreign protein [7, 15]. However, no evidence has been obtained of such a tissue fixation of antigen. Early workers employing whole serum as antigen found coexistence of antigen and antibody in the circulation in significant amounts during serum sickness and postulated that this mixture of antigen and antibody in the circulation resulted in the formation of a toxic compound which caused the disease [1]. Actually, they were observing not the antigen-antibody complexes or homologous antigen-antibody systems but antibody to some of the serum globulin antigens which call forth an early antibody response coexisting with serum albumin antigens which are slower to initiate antibody formation and therefore persist longer in the circulation. In spite of their misleading observations, their

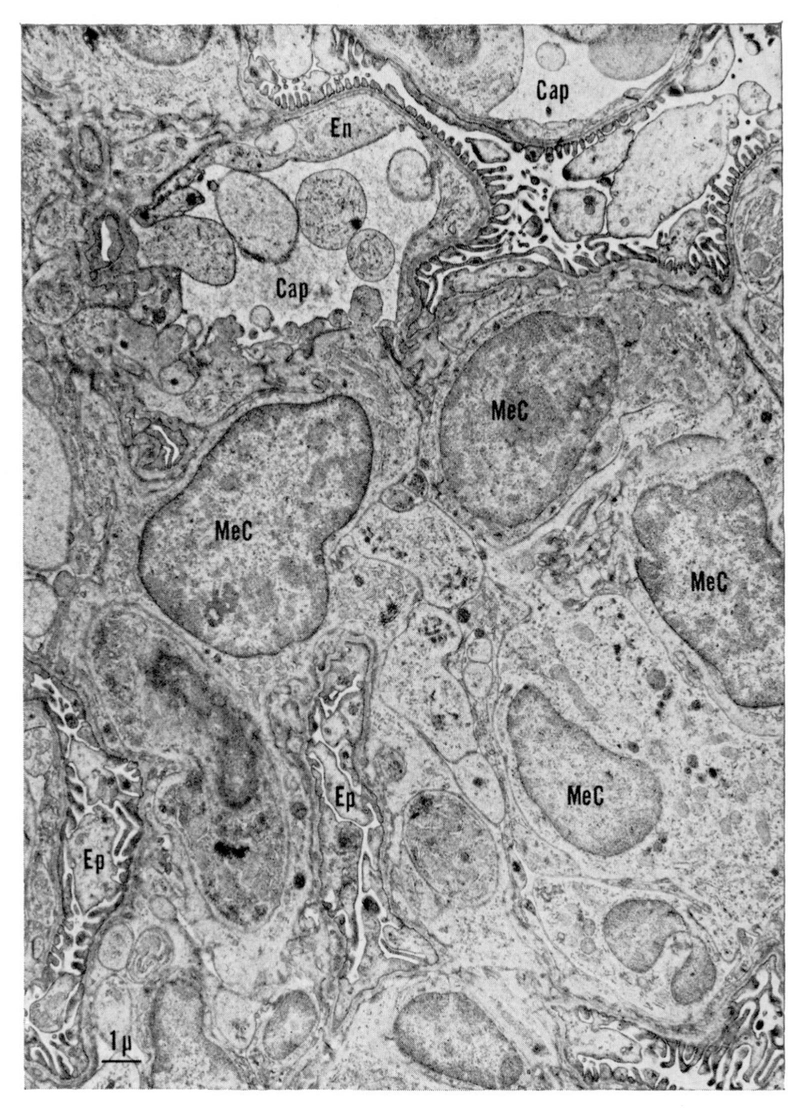

Fig. 12-6. Electron micrograph of glomerulus from rabbit with serum sickness taken on day of antigen elimination. (Abbreviations as for Fig. 12-5.) Capillary lumens are narrowed by proliferating endothelial cells and mesangial cells (*MeC*) in axial region of glomerular tuft. Many of the epithelial cell foot processes are broadened and irregular.

postulation of a toxic compound, i.e., antigen-antibody complex, in the circulation now has been adequately demonstrated by specific techniques [10]. A number of recent experiments have shown that antigen-antibody complexes similar to those present in the circulation in serum sickness are themselves phlogogenic agents capable of inducing a wide variety of inflammatory and degenerative responses without regard to the antigenic constitution of the tissues involved.

The phlogogenic properties of antigen-antibody complexes would appear to be adequate to account for the various lesions of serum sickness. It has been shown that under certain conditions antigen-antibody complexes can induce systemic anaphylaxis [16] and local inflammation [17, 18]. To get these effects, complexes formed in moderate antigen excess are most effective. Most active complexes contain antibody capable of fixing in tissues and of reacting with complement (C′), although the latter property may not be essential [19]. Such antigen-antibody complexes can react with normal serum constituents to release active esterase from C′1, which is, in part, a proesterase [20], fibrinolysin [21], anaphylatoxin [22], and peptides such as bradykinin [23]. The role of these and no doubt other substances liberated by antigen-antibody interactions in serum sickness remains to be determined. At a cellular level, complexes either directly or indirectly have the ability to: (1) cause mast cell degranulation and presumably liberate pharmocologically active substances [24], (2) react with and agglutinate leukocytes and platelets [25, 26], and liberate histamine from the latter [27], (3) cause contraction of smooth muscle [28], (4) increase vascular permeability [29], (5) induce endothelial proliferation [30], and (6) attract polymorphonuclear leukocytes by chemotaxis [31]. Thus the action of soluble complexes in tissues is extensive, and it seems logical that they could initiate the various lesions observed in serum sickness.

In serum sickness, not only are antigen-antibody complexes similar to those described earlier found in the circulation but also, by immunohistochemical techniques, antigen, host C′ and host γ-globulin, presumably in complex form, are found to localize specifically in tissue lesions simultaneously with their development [10] and thus appear to be etiological agents of tissue injury. Whether the earliest phlogogenic stimulus initiating the focal inflammatory lesions in serum sickness results from antigen-antibody interaction in the circulation, causing systemic liberation of active pharmacological agents which act locally, or from the initial, fortuitous focal deposition of small amounts of complexes in the tissue to be injured cannot be said with certainty. However, it is likely that the continuing accumulation of complexes from the circulation into the developing lesions, e.g., as a result of increasing vascular permeability, causes the snowballing inflammatory reaction observed.

Although, traditionally, serum sickness is produced by one or a few closely spaced large injections of foreign serum proteins, other schemes of foreign serum administration can also induce the essential pathogenic mechanism of serum sickness, i.e., formation of circulating antigen-antibody complexes. One such modification was devised to produce the chronic persistence of antigen-antibody complexes in the circulation [32]. In these experiments, rabbits were given injections daily for many months of a given heterologous serum protein. When possible, the amount of antigen given was calculated to exceed slightly the antibody-forming capacity of the recipient, thereby causing the repeated daily formation of antigen-antibody complexes in the circulation in an environment of moderate antigen excess. In those animals in which complexes were maintained in the circulation for weeks or months, chronic progressive glomerulonephritis developed but other tissues did not appear to suffer ill consequences. The glomerulonephritis appeared early as a membranous lesion, i.e., thickening of the glomerular capillary basement membrane (Fig. 12-7). Later, destruction of glomeruli and scarring ensued (Fig. 12-8). The diseased glomeruli revealed

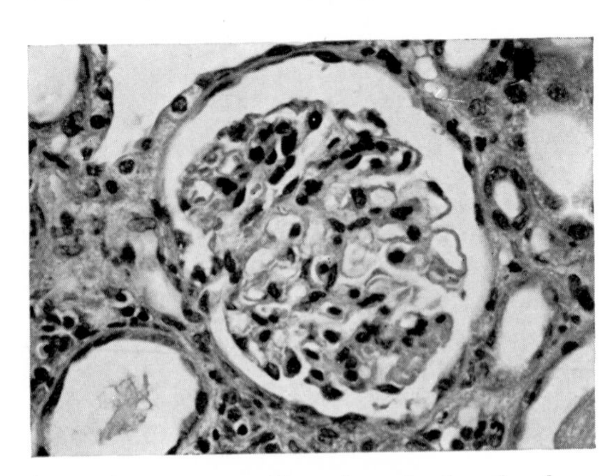

Fig. 12-7. Hematoxylin-eosin stained section from chronic membranous glomerulonephritis in rabbit given daily injections of BSA. Capillary lumens are widely patent, but the capillary walls show hyaline thickening. Number of fixed glomerular cells is normal or only slightly increased.

a deposition of antigen, C′, and host γ-globulin (Fig. 12-9) presumably in complex form along the outer aspect of the capillary basement membranes (Figs. 12-10 and 12-11). This deposition was regularly associated with the morphological thickening of the basement membrane, proteinuria, and other evidence of renal malfunction.

The chronic membranous glomerulonephritis produced by long-standing low levels of circulating complexes was quite different from the acute, proliferative glomerulonephritis associated with one-shot serum sickness, yet the antigen used and the antibody formed by the hosts in each instance were, as far as could be determined, identical. The chronic presence

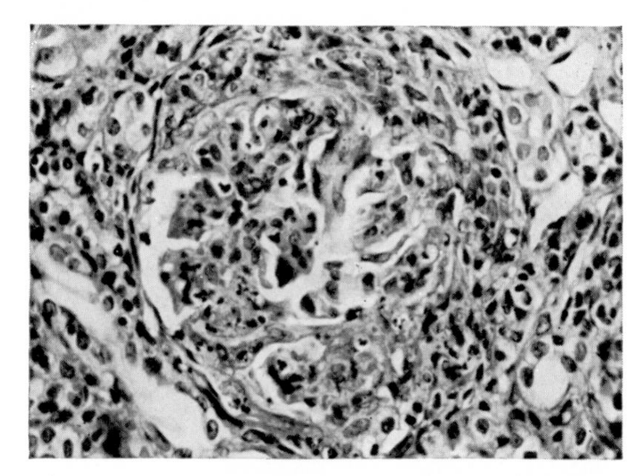

Fig. 12-8. Hematoxylin-eosin stained section from glomerulus of rabbit given daily injections of BSA. This glomerulus has undergone prolonged inflammation and is now virtually obliterated by scarring. Capillary lumens are occluded and the normal glomerular capillary tufts are no longer visible. Some nuclear fragments and other cell debris are visible.

of complexes in small amounts did not visibly injure nonrenal tissues. In the kidneys the change was hyaline basement membrane thickening, which is usually associated with a degenerative rather than an inflammatory process. It may be that the kidneys are particularly susceptible to injury by low levels of complexes because of their extensive blood supply and their normal filtering function which might serve to trap and concentrate the complexes. It is apparent that disease produced by administration of heterologous serum proteins

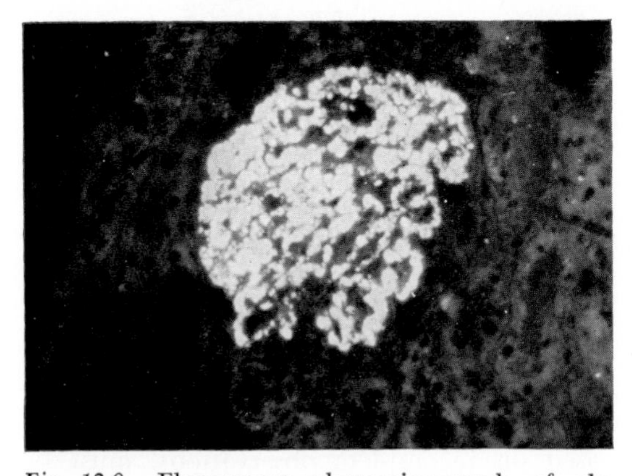

Fig. 12-9. Fluorescent photomicrograph of glomerulus similar to that in Figure 12-7. Stained with fluorescent anti-BSA. A lumpy fluorescent deposit is scattered along the glomerular capillary walls. Fluorescent staining for host γ-globulin gave comparable results. The gray tubular autofluorescence is barely visible around the glomerulus.

may vary considerably from an acute, necrotizing inflammatory process to a noninflammatory degenerative process as the amount and duration of antigen-antibody interaction is varied, although the mechanism of producing tissue injury, i.e., the formation of circulating antigen-antibody complexes, appears to be similar in all situations.

It is tempting to try to apply these pathogenic mechanisms involving circulating antigen-antibody complexes to those clinical diseases which bear a resemblance to serum sickness, and indeed there are observations consistent with such an application. Clinically, reactions to drugs such as penicillin may be identical to serum sickness, and a similar pathogenic mechanism seems likely. *In vivo,* penicillin is changed to several potent haptens, penicilloyls, and penicillinates, which react with most proteins to form complete antigens [33, 34]. Antibodies and/or specific sensitivity to these materials have been demonstrated in patients with serum disease-like reactions to penicillin. If, in these cases, the penicillin haptens combined with serum proteins, all of the conditions would exist to cause serum sickness to a circulating antigen composed of drug hapten and autologous serum protein. In the clinical connective tissue diseases, comparison with serum sickness must be on a different basis. In these diseases, the offending antigen is rarely known, so that immunological demonstration of antigen-antibody complexes or reactions is difficult. Rather, the relatively insensitive procedure of ultracentrifugation must be relied on to show molecular aggregates of abnormal size in the serum. However, this tool has revealed a variety of γ-globulin-containing complexes behaving like antigen-antibody complexes in the sera of patients with rheumatoid arthritis [35], systemic lupus erythematosus [36], macroglobulinemia [35], Sjögren's disease [37], purpura [35], untreated subacute bacterial endocarditis [38], and several less well-defined entities. These complexes had sedimentation rates either in the 9S to 17S range, presumably made up of 7S γ-globulin, or in the 22 + S range perhaps containing 7S or 19S γ-globulins, or both. In some cases of lupus erythematosus in which circulating complexes of host nuclear material and autoantibody to nuclear material were suspected, suggestive immunological observations have supported this suspicion. The morpho-

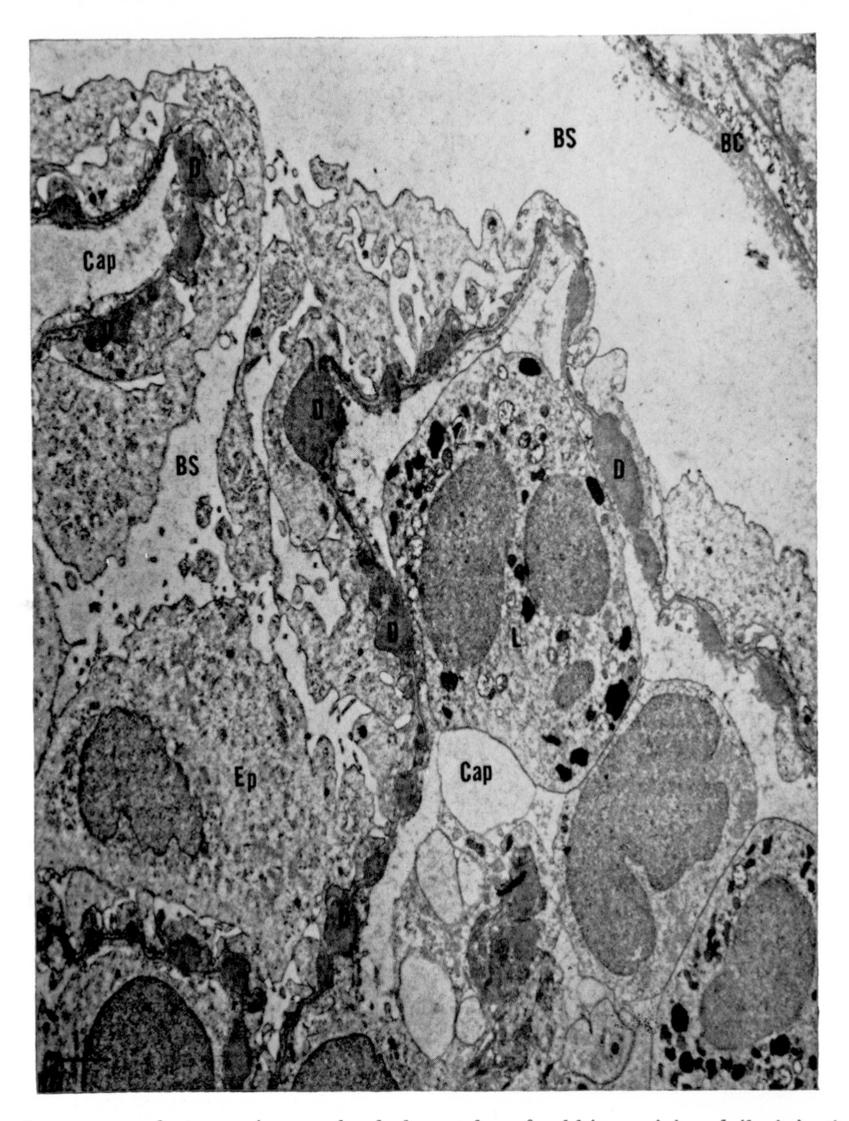

Fig. 12-10. Low power electron micrograph of glomerulus of rabbit receiving daily injections of BSA. In comparison with normal structure shown at a comparable power in Figure 12-5 (q.v. for abbreviations), this glomerulus shows numerous electron dense deposits (*D*) scattered along the capillary basement membranes. These deposits correspond to the location of antigen, host complement, and host γ-globulin revealed by the fluorescent antibody technique. Associated with the deposits, the epithelial cells have lost their normal foot processes attached to the basement membrane. Several granular leukocytes (*L*) are trapped in one of the capillary lumens. Endothelial cells show relatively little change.

logical and immunohistochemical characteristics of the various types of serum sickness glomerulonephritis are reproduced faithfully in the various stages of clinical glomerulonephritis and the nephritis of lupus erythematosus [4]. The electron dense deposits of antigen-antibody complexes along the outer aspect of the glomerular capillary basement membrane in chronic experimental serum sickness correspond exactly to morphologic structures containing immunoglobulins and complement in the clinical entities. Analogies such as these, bridging species barriers and based on incomplete observations, must be considered tentative at best. However, they provide one of our most promising leads to the understanding of a group of baffling diseases and as such may yet be the most valuable fruit borne by the study of experimental serum sickness.

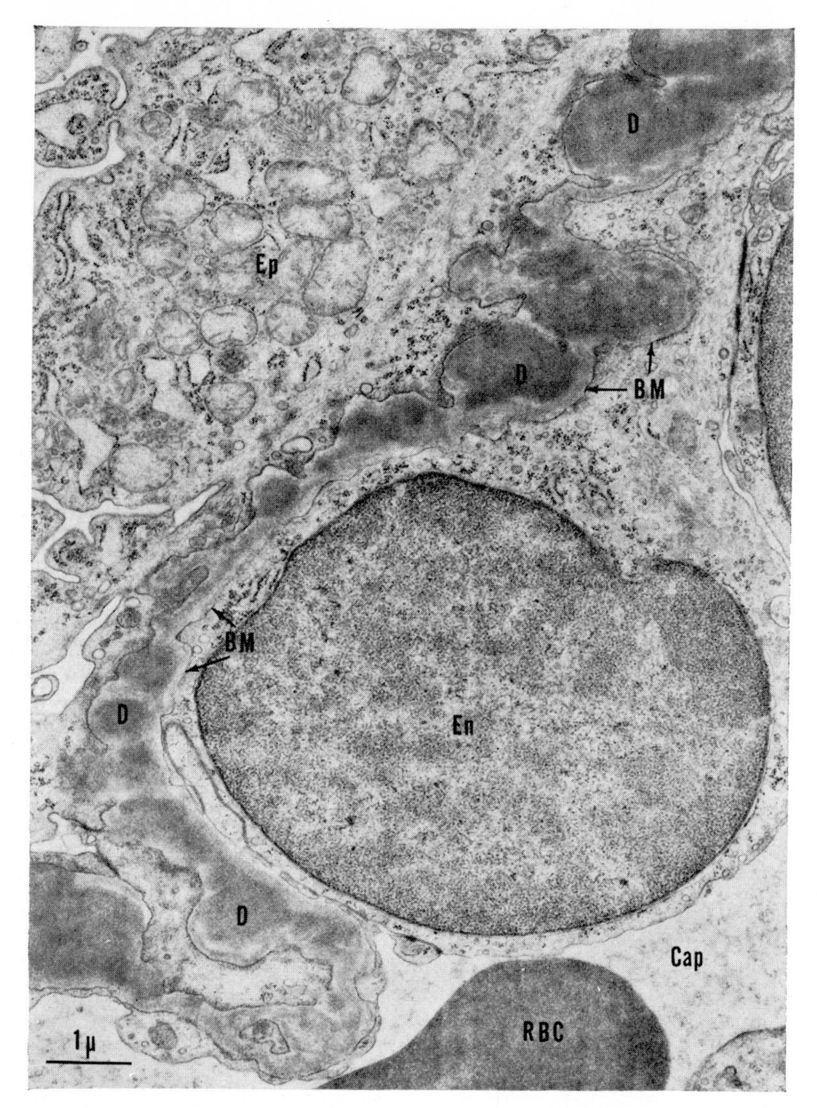

Fig. 12-11. Electron micrograph of higher power than Figure 12-10, showing relation of dense immunological deposits to basement membrane in a rabbit similar to that in Figure 12-10. The basement membrane can be visualized as a lightly staining band covered for the most part on its inner aspect by endothelial cell cytoplasm. Studded along the outer part of the basement membrane are the dense deposits which, in some places, appear to be discrete and, in other places, appear to fuse with the basement membrane. The epithelial cell visible here has lost all of its foot processes but contains a complex multistructured cytoplasm. Both endothelial and epithelial cells show a moderate number of darkly staining small ribosomes scattered in their cytoplasm.

REFERENCES

1. Von Pirquet, C. E. Allergy. *Arch. Int. Med.* 7:259, 1911.
2. Klinge, F. Die Eiweissüberempfindlichkeit (Gewebsanaphylaxie) der Gelenke: Experimentelle pathologischanatomische Studien zur Pathogenese des Gelenkrheumatismus. *Beitr. Path. Anat.* 83:185, 1929.
3. Rich, A. Hypersensitivity in disease, with especial reference to periarteritis nodosa, rheumatic fever, disseminated lupus erythematosus and rheumatoid arthritis. *Harvey Lect.* 42:106, 1947.
4. Dixon, F. J. The role of antigen-antibody complexes in disease. *Harvey Lect.* 58:21, 1963.

5. Longcope, W. T., and Rackemann, F. M. The relation of circulating antibodies to serum disease. *J. Exp. Med.* 27:341, 1918.
6. Mackenzie, G. M., and Leake, W. H. Relation of antibody and antigen to serum disease susceptibility. *J. Exp. Med.* 33:601, 1921.
7. Hawn, C. V., and Janeway, C. A. Histological and serological sequences in experimental hypersensitivity. *J. Exp. Med.* 85:571, 1947.
8. Germuth, F. G., Jr. A comparative histologic and immunologic study in rabbits of induced hypersensitivity of the serum sickness type. *J. Exp. Med.* 97:257, 1953.
9. Germuth, F. G., Jr., Pace, M. G., and Tippett, J. C. Comparative histologic and immunologic studies in rabbits of induced hypersensitivity of the serum sickness type: II. The effect of sensitization to homologous and cross-reactive antigens on the rate of antigen elimination and the development of allergic lesions. *J. Exp. Med.* 101:135, 1955.
10. Dixon, F. J., Vazquez, J. J., Weigle, W. O., and Cochrane, C. G. Pathogenesis of serum sickness. *Arch. Path.* 65:18, 1958.
11. Weigle, W. O. The elimination of heterologous serum proteins and associated antibody responses in guinea pigs and rats. *J. Immun.* 79:24, 1957.
12. Weigle, W. O. Elimination of antigen-antibody complexes from sera of rabbits. *J. Immun.* 81:204, 1958.
13. Vazquez, J. J., and Dixon, F. J. Immunohistochemical analysis of lesions associated with fibrinoid change. *Arch. Path.* 66:504, 1958.
14. Weigle, W. O., and Dixon, F. J. The relationship of circulating antigen-antibody complexes, antigen elimination and complement fixation in serum sickness. *Proc. Soc. Exp. Biol. Med.* 99:226, 1958.
15. Mellors, R. C., Arias-Stella, J., Seigel, M., and Pressman, D. Analytical pathology: II. Histopathologic demonstration of glomerular-localizing antibodies in experimental glomerulonephritis. *Amer. J. Path.* 31:687, 1955.
16. Germuth, F. G., and McKinnon, G. E. Studies on the biological properties of antigen-antibody complexes: I. Anaphylactic shock induced by soluble antigen-antibody complexes in unsensitized normal guinea pigs. *Bull. Hopkins Hosp.* 101:13, 1957.
17. Benacerraf, B., Potter, J. L., McCluskey, R. T., and Miller, F. J. The pathologic effects of intravenously administered soluble antigen-antibody complexes: II. Acute glomerulonephritis in rats. *J. Exp. Med.* 111:195, 1960.
18. Cochrane, C. G., and Weigle, W. O. The cutaneous reaction to soluble antigen-antibody complexes: A comparison with the Arthus phenomenon. *J. Exp. Med.* 108:591, 1958.
19. Ishizaka, K., Ishizaka, T., and Sugahara, T. Biological activity of soluble antigen-antibody complexes: VII. Role of an antibody fragment in the induction of biological activities. *J. Immun.* 88:690, 1962.
20. Lepow, I. H., Ratnoff, O. D., and Pillemer, L. Elution of an esterase from antigen-antibody aggregates treated with human complement. *Proc. Soc. Exp. Biol. Med.* 92:111, 1956.
21. Ungar, G., and Mist, S. H. Observations on the release of serum fibrinolysin by specific antigen, peptone, and certain polysaccharides. *J. Exp. Med.* 90:39, 1949.
22. Osler, A. G., Randall, H. G., Hill, B. M., and Ovary, Z. Studies on the mechanism of hypersensitivity phenomena: III. The participation of complement in the formation of anaphylatoxin. *J. Exp. Med.* 110:311, 1959.
23. Brocklehurst, W. E., and Lahiri, S. C. The production of bradykinin in anaphylaxis. *J. Physiol.* 160:15, 1962.
24. Mota, I. Mechanism of action of antigen-antibody complexes: Their effect on mast cells. *Nature* (London) 191:572, 1961.
25. Miescher, P., and Straessle, R. Experimentelle Studien über den Mechanismus der Thrombocytenschädigung durch Antigen-Antikorper Reaktionen. *Vox Sang.* 1:83, 1956.
26. Miescher, P. The Pathogenesis of Visceral Lupus Erythematosus as Reflected in the Sero-Reactions. In Grabar, P., and Miescher, P. (Eds.), *Immunopathology* (2nd Internat. Symp.) Basel: Benno Schwabe & Co., 1958.
27. Barbaro, J. F. The release of histamine from rabbit platelets by means of antigen-antibody precipitates: II. The role of plasma in the release of histamine. *J. Immun.* 86:377, 1961.
28. Trapani, I. L., Garvey, J. S., and Campbell, D. Stimulating action of soluble antigen-antibody complexes on normal guinea pig smooth muscle. *Science* 127:700, 1958.
29. Ishizaka, K., and Campbell, D. Biological activity of soluble antigen-antibody complexes: I. Skin reactive properties. *Proc. Soc. Exp. Biol. Med.* 97:635,1958.
30. Feldman, J. D. Electron microscopy of serum sickness nephritis. *J. Exp. Med.* 108:957, 1958.
31. Boyden, S. The chemotactic effect of mixtures of antibody and antigen on polymorphonuclear leucocytes. *J. Exp. Med.* 115:453, 1962.
32. Dixon, F. J., Feldman, J. D., and Vazquez, J. J. Experimental glomerulonephritis: The pathogenesis of a laboratory model resembling the spectrum of human glomerulonephritis. *J. Exp. Med.* 113:899, 1961.
33. Parker, C. W., Shapiro, J., Kern, M., and Eisen, H. N. The hypersensitivity to penicillinic acid derivatives in human beings with penicillin allergen. *J. Exp. Med.* 115:821, 1962.
34. Levine, B. B., and Ovary, Z. Studies on the

mechanism of the formation of the penicillin antigen: III. The N-(D-α-benzylpenicilloyl) group as an antigenic determinant responsible for hypersensitivity to penicillin. *J. Exp. Med.* 114:875, 1961.

35. Kunkel, H. G., Müller-Eberhard, H. J., Fudenberg, H. G., and Tomasi, T. B. Gamma-globulin complexes in rheumatoid arthritis and certain other conditions. *J. Clin. Invest.* 40: 117, 1961.
36. Christian, C. L., Hatfield, W. B., and Chase, P. H. Systemic lupus erythematosus: Cryoprecipitation of sera. *J. Clin. Invest.* 42:823, 1963.
37. Tomasi, T. B., Fudenberg, H., and Finby, N. Possible relationship of rheumatoid factors and pulmonary disease. *Amer. J. Med.* 33:243, 1962.
38. Williams, R. C., Jr., and Kunkel, H. G. Rheumatoid factors and their disappearance following therapy in patients with subacute bacterial endocarditis. *Arthritis Rheum.* 5:126, 1962.

*13. Immunological Aspects of Tissue Transplantation**

R. E. BILLINGHAM AND WILLYS K. SILVERS

. . . Nor can it be supposed that the diversity of chemical structure and process stops at the boundary of the species, and within that boundary, which has no real finality, rigid uniformity reigns. Such a conception is at variance with any evolutionary conception of the nature and origin of species. The existence of chemical individuality follows of necessity from chemical specificity, but we should expect the differences between individuals to be still more subtle and difficult of detection.

—Garrod [1].

THE TRANSPLANTATION OF LIVING cells, tissues, or organs for experimental or therapeutic purposes entails problems of two distinct kinds. The first are concerned directly with the act of transplantation itself and are largely of a technological nature. They are associated with the procurement, preparation, temporary storage, and relocation of the grafted tissues or organs in such a manner that the normal healing processes suffice to insure their continued viability and conservation of normal structure and function. In experimental animals and in man the feasibility of replacement, by grafting, of bone marrow, extensive areas of skin, kidneys, hearts, lungs, liver, and perhaps even limbs, is no longer in doubt, indicating that adequate, if not completely satisfactory, solutions to these problems have been achieved [2–4].

The second category of problems, by far the more formidable, stems from the phenomenon of incompatibility of *homografts* (i.e., grafts transplanted from one individual to another of the same species). This has an immunological basis and constitutes the subject matter of this chapter.

Homografts normally fail where *autografts* (grafts of which the donor is also the recipient) of the same tissue or organ, transplanted in exactly the same manner, are permanently successful. For example, if free skin autografts and homografts are placed on a common bed on the side of a rabbit's trunk, the autografts undergo a phase of minor reparative changes, including epidermal hyperplasia, and then reassume their original condition with a high degree of perfection. The homografts heal in, acquire a rich blood supply, and behave just like autografts at first, but soon they become inflamed and edematous and their dermis becomes heavily infiltrated by mononuclear leukocytes, principally small lymphocytes and histiocytes. There are cessation of blood flow and lymphatic drainage, disruption of vessel walls accompanied by distintegration, and separation of the entire epidermis [5–7]. Finally, the entire graft is transformed into a necrotic scab. This process of destruction, called the *homograft reaction,* is usually complete within two weeks.

An essentially similar fate overtakes homografts of all other solid tissues (normal or malignant) or organs that establish vascular connections with their hosts of their own accord or have them established surgically by vascular anastomoses.

This phenomenon of homograft incompatibility seems to occur in all species of vertebrates, and the reaction displays a remarkable degree of uniformity in histological detail and tempo [8]. Rather surprisingly, goldfish can destroy homografts even more rapidly than mammals [9].

Destruction of homografts is an immunological phenomenon, a conclusion reached independently from studies conducted on normal tissues, especially of skin, on the one hand, and of malignant tissues on the other [10–12]. Among the more "classic" lines of evidence are the following: (1) Sensitivity or

* Some of the work described here was supported by U.S. Public Health Service Grant No. CA-05927.

resistance to homografts is not innate; homografts enjoy a brief latent period of apparent well-being, during which their cells may proliferate freely. (2) There is a definite though weak dosage effect, tiny skin homografts having a longer expectation of survival than large ones. (3) Once called into being, the sensitivity evoked by homografts is systemic, i.e., generalized throughout all parts of the body supplied by blood vessels. The existence of a state of homograft immunity is revealed in terms of the accelerated or peremptory manner in which "second-set" homografts are destroyed by a host previously exposed to tissues or cells from the same donor. (4) Homograft destruction in many species, including man, mice, rabbits, chickens, and fish, is usually accompanied by the appearance of humoral antibodies in the host's serum, capable of reacting with donor cells, particularly erythrocytes, in various ways.

GENETIC BASIS OF HOMOGRAFT INCOMPATIBILITY

Soon after the beginning of this century, pioneer studies conducted with tumor homografts in mice established the principle that homograft incompatibility is genetic in origin [13]. The demonstration that skin grafts exchanged between identical human twins are permanently accepted, just like autografts, provided confirmatory evidence. Indeed, subject to one qualification (see p. 179), skin grafting provides a valid test for distinguishing between monozygotic and dizygotic twins. A small number of identical twins suffering from loss of skin through burning, or from acute renal disease, have been able to enjoy the benefits of having a compatible graft donor available [14]. It may be mentioned that grafts exchanged between individuals of identical genetic constitution, such as monozygotic twins, are known as *isografts.* These behave in all respects like autografts.

A prerequisite for the detailed analysis of the genetic basis of tissue incompatibility in any species is the availability of inbred or *isogenic* strains, i.e., populations of individuals of identical genetic constitution. These are produced and maintained by a strict regimen of inbreeding [15].

Because of its convenient size, short gestation period, fertility, and so on, the mouse has always been the animal of choice for this work, and many different isogenic strains have long been available [16]. Only in the last few years have some preliminary studies been conducted on the few strains of inbred fish, chickens, guinea pigs, rats, and Syrian hamsters which have so far been developed [17].

In the mouse, the application of standard breeding procedures with various isogenic strains, in conjunction with test grafting with homografts of both malignant and normal tissue, especially of skin, has revealed in considerable detail the extremely complex nature of the genetic determination of *transplantation antigens,* i.e., the cellular isoantigens responsible for provoking homograft reactions [12, 13, 18]. The discriminatory power of these analyses has been greatly heightened by the application of serological agents (i.e., humoral antibodies produced in response to homografts of various types, especially of certain tumors). These antibodies are directed against certain antigens present on red cells and leukocytes as well as on fixed tissues [12, 19, 20].

The determinants of transplantation antigens, designated *histocompatibility genes,* have chromosomal locations known as *histocompatibility loci.* At each of these loci a series or family of alternative genes, or alleles, may occur. The genetic basis for permanent acceptance of a graft is simply that each of the donor's complement of histocompatibility genes must also be represented in the host, so that it is not confronted with any alien *transplantation isoantigens.* This requirement is met if donor and recipient are identical twins or if they are members of the same isogenic strain. Another situation in which it is satisfied is when grafts from either of two unrelated isogenic parental strains are transplanted to their F_1 hybrids. This follows since histocompatibility genes are codominant, i.e., they express themselves when in the heterozygous condition, so that each hybrid has all the transplantation antigens of *both* of its parents.

In both rats and mice the total number of histocompatibility loci is certainly not less than 15, and probably more [21]. In mice, only 7 of these loci have been identified [12]. In this species the development of very closely related isogenic strains, differing only with respect to an allele at a single histocompatibility locus, have played an important role in elucidating the relative "strengths" of the products of these different loci [22]. Not all of the antigens determined by different histocompatibility loci are of equal potency, so that we refer to *major* and *minor* loci, with corresponding strong and weak transplantation antigens. A difference between donor and host with respect to a single strong antigen (or allele at a major locus) is usually sufficient to elicit a homograft reaction of near-maximal intensity, so that a skin homograft is destroyed within about 11 days. On the other hand, a difference at a minor locus may enable a skin homograft to live in a state of apparent normality for upward of 100 days before it is eventually overcome by its host. Where non-inbred populations are concerned, the survival times of homografts vary enormously, being inversely related to the genetic disparity between donor and host.

In mice, one major histocompatibility locus, the H-2, seems to predominate above all others in terms of the potency of its products. No less than 20 different H-2 alleles have been identified, and more will probably be found [23]. Since, in addition to determining tissue incompatibility, this locus determines cellular antigens that elicit the formation of humoral antibodies, its products have been subjected to extensive serological analyses. These have revealed the existence of upward of 33 distinct specificities which collectively characterize this locus. A given serologically detectable specificity may be associated with the product of a single allele or it may be shared in common by the products of 2 or more alleles. The complexity of this locus may stem from its having a composite structure, being made up of a series of closely linked genes, or pseudoalleles, having similar effects or determining similar specificities, rather like the Rh system in man.

Suggestive evidence has been obtained that when differences at several minor loci are involved, there is a synergistic effect.

The simplest conceivable *histoincompatibility* situation expresses itself in certain inbred strains of mice and rats. In both species there seems to be a weak histocompatibility locus on the Y chromosome which is lacking in the female [21, 24]. This explains the finding that in some isogenic strains, grafts from male donors are rejected by females after periods ranging from 15 to 100 days (median survival time about 30 days). Males, on the other hand, do not reject female skin isografts.

Thus, like most other inborn differences between individuals, the histocompatibility differences are due not to unique endowments of antigenic material but to unique combinations of endowments. In any species in which the number of histocompatibility loci is high and in which multiple alleles exist at many of them, the homograft reaction is unsurpassed as a means of discriminating between individuals of different genotypes.

At present there is practically no worthwhile information concerning the number of histocompatibility loci in man. If the situation in this species is as complex as in mice, even if means are eventually devised for typing individuals with respect to their transplantation antigens, the combinatorial possibilities are so great that the likelihood of discovering a compatible donor for a given recipient is very small. However, this certainly does not invalidate histocompatibility grouping of individuals. If donors can be selected which are compatible with their hosts so far as *major* histocompatibility loci are concerned, procedures are already known (see below) that will effectively suppress the homograft reactions evoked by weak histoincompatibilities.

DISTRIBUTION AND NATURE OF TRANSPLANTATION ANTIGENS

There is no evidence of any tissue specificity in transplantation immunity. The full spectrum of antigens corresponding to an animal's histocompatibility genes seems to be present in *all* living, nucleate cells of its body. Each of a wide variety of tissues, or "cellular" homografts prepared therefrom, will sensitize a host in respect of the others. Furthermore, animals made tolerant (see below) as a consequence of inoculation in early life with living homologous cells derived from one type of tissue are completely and specifically incapable of reacting against *any* other type of tissue or organ graft from the donor of the tolerance-conferring stimulus or from another donor of similar genetic constitution [25].

However, it would be very surprising if cells of different tissues did not differ quantitatively in their contents of transplantation antigens and in their capacity to release these substances [26]. Effective transplantation antigens are certainly present in the cells of very early avian and mammalian embryos [18].

Although the serologically detectable specificities of the erythrocytes of mice, and probably of rats, include some that are determined by important histocompatibility genes, there is no evidence that these cells can elicit sensitivity to normal tissue homografts. Possibly they are ineffective vehicles for the transportation of antigens to immunologically reactive sites, or their specificities may be inadequately represented or inappropriately located [27, 28]. The basis of this apparent shortcoming needs clarification, especially in the light of recent evidence that transplantation antigens are present in the nucleate red cells of chickens [27]. There is suggestive evidence that transplantation antigens are present in the blood platelets of rabbits and guinea pigs but not in those of the rat [29, 30].

Elucidation of the chemical nature of the gene-determined substances, or specificities, responsible for inciting homograft sensitization remains one of the most important objectives in transplantation immunology. At present, practically all the information available derives from studies on extracts of lymphoid tissues of mice and relates to products of the H-2 locus [12, 18]. The most exacting test for the presence of H-2 antigenic specificity in an extract is, of course, its ability to sensitize animals against subsequent test skin homografts. However, ability of extracts to elicit the formation of hemagglutinins with H-2 specificity, to inhibit specifically the hemagglutinating activity of H-2 antisera, and to enhance (see Ref. 64 and p. 177) the growth of appropriate test tumors in mice constitutes important ancillary assay procedures.

There is strong evidence that the antigenic specificity determined by the H-2 locus is associated with lipoproteins present in the microsomal fraction of homogenized lymphoid cells [18, 31, 32]. Although preparations capable of provoking homograft sensitization are serologically active, the two activities are separable, sensitizing activity being the more labile. It may be noted here that whereas intact viable cells elicit both modalities of response, repeated freezing and thawing or lyophilization of cells seems to abolish their sensitizing but not their serological reactivity or ability to provoke humoral responses. Most authorities are agreed that a single antigenic determinant is probably responsible for these two responses. Whether the antigenic specificities determined by each of the different families of histocompatibility alleles are associated with macromolecules of similar biochemical constitution has yet to be discovered. Possibly these specificities are borne by different "carrier" molecules in different cell types.

The physical form in which these antigens are released from homografts of living tissue, and very probably from the tissues of intact animals as a normal physiological process, is completely unknown, as is their functional significance. They may even be associated with the debris of wear and tear [33], a likely possibility if histocompatibility genes are concerned with the production of cell membranes [34].

MECHANISM OF HOMOGRAFT REJECTION

ROLE OF LYMPHOID CELLS

The principal seats of response to solid tissue homografts are the regional or draining lymph nodes. Although re-establishment of lymphatic connections between a homograft and its bed is apparently not a prerequisite for sensitization, the presence of draining lymphatics in the bed is required [35, 36].

All forms of homograft reactivity leading to destruction of solid tissues or organs are almost invariably associated with an infiltration of the foreign tissue by mononuclear cells of the lymphocytic series which precedes and accompanies the appearance of lesions. The plausible hypothesis that these cells are in some way responsible for the pathogenic changes was seriously considered by several investigators at the beginning of the century [10]. Subsequently, this hypothesis was greatly strengthened when it became firmly established that sensitivity to solid tissue homografts is not transferable by means of putatively immune sera, even in large amounts, but can be transferred "adoptively" by means of *living* cells from the regional nodes of specifically immunized animals [37–39]. Recently it has been shown that whole blood, leukocyte concentrates, peritoneal exudate cells, and thoracic duct cells (almost exclusively lymphocytes, predominantly of the small variety) are highly effective in transferring sensitivity [40]. (It need hardly be mentioned that for successful adoptive transfer of sensitivity both the donor and the recipient of the cellular "vehicles" of the sensitivity *must* be histocompatible.)

These facts constitute the cardinal pieces of an impressive body of evidence sustaining the prevalent view that homograft sensitivity is closely related to drug and bacterial delayed sensitivity and experimental autoimmune diseases. All of these are mediated by blood-borne, immunologically activated cells of the lymphocyte series, in contradistinction to humoral antibodies [41–43].

The final step in establishing that homograft reactivity is a delayed hypersensitivity phenomenon was the demonstration that guinea pigs sensitized by skin homografts respond to subsequent intradermal challenge with living donor cells, or antigenic extracts, with a delayed inflammatory response just like a classic tuberculin reaction [43]. Syrian hamsters behave similarly [44]. In both guinea pigs and rabbits, if a suspension of immunologically activated lymphoid cells from a specifically sensitized recipient is injected intradermally into the donor, a similar reaction ensues [43, 45]. This is referred to as the *transfer reaction* and is interpreted as the result of a local interaction between the immunologically activated cells and the transplantation antigens of the donor. This reaction furnishes the basis of a sensitive test for sensitized lymphoid cells.

Cell transfer studies indicate that activated lymphoid cells, identified as small lymphocytes, enter the circulation very rapidly after their formation in the regional nodes and that they persist in the blood stream for hundreds of days [40]. In the light of Gowans' [46] evidence that small lymphocytes have a long life span and constantly recirculate from blood to lymph via the nodes, this provides a satisfactory explanation of the long persistence of homograft sensitivity evoked by skin homografts. It also strengthens the view that the second-set reaction is an expression of a *pre-existing* state of sensitivity rather than a reawakened one. Nevertheless an anamnestic response is demonstrable in transplantation immunology [47].

Until fairly recently it was believed that immunologically competent cells were located only in the various lymphoid tissues of the body. However, studies on graft-versus-host reactions (see below) in mammals and birds revealed that normal peripheral blood also contains immunologically competent cells. These have been unequivocally identified as small lymphocytes [48–50]. On the basis of their evidence that gross depletion of a rat's small lymphocytes greatly impairs its ability to react against skin homografts and other antigens and that this impairment can be made good by injection of thoracic duct cells from which large lymphocytes had been eliminated, McGregor and Gowans [51] have postulated that the primary immunological response is initiated by contact of small lymphocytes with antigen. The "primed" cells subsequently become fixed in the lymphoid tissues. It is conceivable, therefore, that the antigenic stimulus may be transported from a homograft to the regional nodes by small lymphocytes which, after gaining admission to the graft via its blood vessels, leave by the afferent lymphatics. From studies on the fate of isotopically and cytologically tagged small lymphocytes of rats injected into F_1 hosts or x-ray irradiated mice (where they were stimulated by host antigens), Gowans and his associates [52] have suggested that, when a node is stimulated antigenically by a homograft, some of the small lymphocytes respond by differentiating into large pyroninophilic cells. These, in turn, produce more small lymphocytes which circulate in the blood and invade the graft, procuring its destruction. The fact that nearly all of the infiltrating cells in a skin homograft are of *new* formation is consistent with this interpretation [52, 53].

The proximate cause of death of a homograft remains unknown. Waksman [54] has recently concluded that two processes contribute: (1) local accumulation of mononuclear cells both inside and outside vessel walls, and (2) a direct cytopathic action of these cells on the foreign cell population of the graft, whether in vessel walls, connective tissue, or epidermis.

Studies with several different simple experimental systems *in vivo* have established that sensitization may occur *locally,* and sometimes be accompanied by tissue destruction, if normal, immunologically competent cells are introduced into the parenchyma of a target tissue under appropriate conditions [55, 56]. Sequestration of lymph node cells together with homologous skin in cell-impermeable Millipore membrane chambers, inserted intraperitoneally into homologous hosts, may also lead to sensitization of the cells [57].

It is difficult to escape the conclusion that the homograft reaction is the outcome of some form of local engagement between tissue antigens and sensitized lymphoid cells.

Several findings strongly suggest that specifically sensitized lymphoid cells can damage or destroy homologous target cells *in vivo* [58, 59]. More convincing still are the results of recent *in vitro* studies on the influence of exposing monolayers of homologous "target" cells to the action of splenic, lymph node, or thoracic duct cells from specifically sensitized animals [60, 61]. Here, aggregation and contact of the immune lymphocytes with the target cells seem to lead to degeneration and destruction of the latter in the absence of added humoral antibody or complement.

How immunologically activated lymphocytes mediate their postulated effect remains unknown. Whether cell-bound antibodies are involved or whether these cells release some potent, nonspecific, pharmacologically active agent(s) [62] on being triggered immunologically, through exposure to antigen, are only two of several possibilities.

At present one serious weakness of the hypothesis that infiltrating mononuclear cells are the principal agents of homograft destruction is the inability to demonstrate their specific localization in test skin homografts when sensitivity is transferred adoptively by means of labeled cells [18]. This applies not only to transfer of homograft sensitivity but, with one exception, to other forms of delayed hypersensitivity as well. McCluskey *et al.* [63] have recently suggested that only a small number of specifically sensitized cells are required at an antigen test site to give a delayed reaction, so that it is unnecessary to postulate any specific mechanism for localization. However, this certainly does not exclude the possibility that the abundant unsensitized host cells play some role.

ROLE OF HUMORAL ANTIBODIES

The possible role of the humoral isoantibodies which are usually formed as part of the host's response against homografts is still uncertain [12, 41, 59, 64] and will only be treated briefly here. In general, cell suspensions of lymphoid tissues, bone marrow, and leukemic tumors are susceptible to the action of antibodies, in the presence of complement, *in vitro,* and resistance to cellular homografts of these tissues can be transferred passively by means of serum [59, 65]. Complement seems to be responsible for the destruction of these cells [66]. With few exceptions, nonlymphohemopoietic tissues are practically insusceptible to the action of these humoral antibodies, although *dissociated suspensions* of their cells may sometimes display weak susceptibility. According to Winn [67] the differences in susceptibility of cells to humoral antibodies are probably quantitative and dependent on the concentration of antigenic sites on the cell surface. The existence of a few carefully studied immunogenic situations in which skin homograft rejection appears to have been accelerated by antiserum must not be neglected [68]. So far, however, no one has succeeded in bringing about the destruction of an established skin homograft on a *tolerant* host by means of antiserum—the *experimentum crucis,* in our opinion.

It is not possible at present to appraise the significance of experiments purporting to show that sensitivity to skin homografts can be transferred adoptively to normal hosts, either by means of densely packed sensitized lymphoid cells sequestered in cell-impermeable Millipore chambers, which are inserted intraperitoneally or subcutaneously into the hosts [69–72], or by means of *extracts* of these cells [73]. Again, the important question is whether tolerance can be abolished by these artifices.

In the light of all the evidence available, it is extremely difficult to sustain the view that humoral isoantibodies normally play a significant role in the destruction of solid grafts of nonlymphoid tissues.

One of the most interesting properties of these humoral antibodies is their ability to impair the development of an effective cellular immunity against tissue homografts or antigenic extracts, the basis of the phenomenon known as *immunological enhancement* [12, 64, 74, 75].

SPECIAL SITES AND TISSUES

There are certain "privileged" or favored sites in the body in which homografts may acquire a blood supply yet may long be accepted by a host [3, 76, 77]. Familiar examples are the brain [78], the submucosal tissue of the hamster's cheek pouch [76], probably certain subcutaneous fat pads [79], and the testis [80]. Other privileged sites, in which implanted tissue grafts do not usually acquire a blood supply, include the anterior chamber of the eye and the substantia propria of the cornea [81]. The uniqueness of each of these sites depends on the incompleteness of the physiological pathways necessary for either the induction or the expression of a state of sensitivity. In other words, there is a break in either the afferent or the efferent pathway of the immunological reflex. For example, the privileged status of the brain seems to result from the absence of lymphatic vessels, so that there is no pathway for transmission of an antigenic stimulus to a seat of response. However, an existing sensitivity is fully effective in the brain.

The only known examples of immunologically privileged tissues are the "skin" that constitutes the hamster's cheek pouch [76], and cartilage [82]. The privilege of the former seems to turn upon peculiar properties of its connective tissue which impairs the escape of transplantation antigens, despite the vascularity of the grafts. The long-term survival of cartilage homografts is well documented [82, 83]. These grafts are unique in that they will normally survive even in specifically sensitized hosts [82]. Their lack of blood vessels and distinctive physicochemical properties of the ground substance are held responsible for the invulnerability of the chondrocytes.

The mammalian fetus is, of course, an example of a relatively large homograft that *is* consistently successful and apparently completely invulnerable to attempts to procure its rejection by sensitization of the mother [18]. As emphasized earlier, fetal cells most certainly do contain transplantation antigens. The success of the fetus as a homograft seems to depend primarily on the complete separation of its blood circulation from that of the mother, and secondarily on peculiar properties of the fetal trophoblast cells that separate maternal from fetal tissues [84]. These cells behave as if they lack transplantation antigens.

It must be pointed out that most of our knowledge of homograft reactivity is based on the study of grafts of skin transplanted orthotopically or of tumor tissues implanted subcutaneously, and that a comparative study of other graft sites might reveal the existence of differences in the facility with which they allow grafts of different types of tissue to elicit sensitization [85].

INFLUENCE OF ROUTE OF IMMUNIZATION AND PHYSICAL FORM OF THE ANTIGENIC STIMULUS

Both the route and the form in which the antigenic stimulus is administered are important in determining the time of onset, duration [86–88], and the nature of the response, for in special circumstances it may be exactly the opposite of sensitization (see below).

Dissociated suspensions of lymphoid cells and particulate antigenic extracts injected intraperitoneally or intravenously evoke homograft sensitivity much more rapidly than orthotopic skin homografts. In guinea pigs, sensitivity can come into force within two to three days of inoculation of homologous cells by the intravenous route [87], and graft-versus-host reactions (see below) are extremely rapid in onset.

The latent period of apparent well-being enjoyed by solid tissue homografts probably reflects the need to establish vascular connections before their antigenic stimulus can take effect. However, the duration of sensitivity provoked by an orthotopic skin graft is much greater than that elicited by equivalent or much greater quantities of splenic cells or antigenic extracts injected intraperitoneally [87, 88].

For unknown reasons the intravenous and intraperitoneal routes are not always similar in effect. In rabbits, intravenous injection of living epidermal cells or leukocytes (but not spleen cells [86]) does not sensitize but may considerably *weaken* the animals' ability to react against subsequent homografts [89]. In mice, studies with antigenic extracts have shown that the intravenous route is less effective for sensitization than the intraperitoneal and that the intravenous administration of semisoluble preparations may prolong homograft survival [90].

These empirical discoveries that antigens can be administered in such a form or by such a route that, instead of eliciting transplantation immunity, they may excite transplantation tolerance are important for their therapeutic possibilities. Even solid tissue homografts transplanted to sites where they become vascularized, yet fail to evoke sensitivity, sometimes "condition" the host so that it behaves as if transplantation tolerance has been induced [91].

IMMUNOLOGICAL TOLERANCE

Many treatments are known which will prolong the life of homografts. Some are nonspecific in the sense that they depress a host's response to homografts in general, and usually affect responses to other classes of antigens as well. They include whole body irradiation [92], the injection of certain colloidal substances such as trypan blue [64], treatment with certain corticosteroid hormones such as cortisone [93], the injection of certain serum proteins [94] or metabolic analogues [90], neonatal thymectomy which results in a gross functional impairment of the lymphoid tissue [95, 96], and depletion of circulatory lymphocytes [51].

Other treatments, such as "enhancement" [74], are specific in that they depress only certain pathways of immunological response—against certain antigens only—leaving the animal with a perfectly useful immunological defense mechanism. Most important of these is that based on the principle of "immunological tolerance" [25, 97–99]. Not only does injection into embryonic or newborn animals of living lymphohemopoietic cellular homografts render the recipient incapable of rejecting the foreign cells and the descendants of these cells (so that they remain cellular chimeras), but the recipient after it has grown will also accept, or *tolerate,* subsequent tissue homografts of the same genotype as the tolerance-conferring inoculum. "Acquired tolerance" is brought about naturally in dizygotic twins which establish vascular anastomoses *in utero* or *in ovo* (in nearly every case in twin cattle, and probably in twin chickens and marmosets [100], but only exceptionally in human twins). Such twins are normally chimeric with respect to their red cells and probably their leukocytes and are tolerant of grafts of each other's tissues [25].

Extensive studies, conducted principally on mice and rats, have shown that inoculation (the intravenous route is the most effective) of newborn hosts with homologous cell suspensions derived from tissues of a variety of histological types, including spleen, bone marrow, blood leukocytes, and thymocytes, will induce tolerance of skin, adrenal, ovarian, thyroid, and other homografts. This constitutes evidence that there is no tissue specificity in tolerance [26, 97, 98].

However, the various cellular inocula cited above are not all equivalent in their ability to induce tolerance. For example, when major histoincompatibilities are involved, lymph node and splenic cells are more effective than marrow cells in mice, whereas in rats the situation is exactly the opposite. In both species, thymocytes constitute a very poor tolerance-conferring stimulus [26].

It seems that transplantation tolerance can only be consistently conferred by inoculation of cells of the erythropoietic, myeloid, or lymphoid series (i.e., those most readily prepared in suspension form). With cells of other types, successes have been very fitful even when high dosage inocula have been employed. It may be added that cells from early chick or mammalian embryos will confer tolerance [18]. No one has been able to induce tolerance with cells which have been propagated *in vitro,* although Terasaki [101] induced tolerance in chickens with monocytes which had been temporarily maintained *in vitro.* Exposure of cells to radiation greatly impairs or abolishes their tolerance-conferring capacity [26], and few successes have attended attempts to make neonatal animals tolerant by inoculation with antigenic extracts [102, 103]. On the basis of this sort of evidence it is generally believed that the prerequisites for a persisting tolerance-conferring inoculum are that the cells be capable of migrating and proliferating and of becoming permanently established *of their own accord* in the host's seats of immunological response. The fact that transplanted lymphoid cells "home" to anatomically appropriate sites [50] probably accounts for their remarkable tolerance-conferring efficacy.

Apart from the type of cell in an inoculum, the dosage of cells is a crucially important factor in determining whether tolerance will be conferred and whether it will be complete or partial, for tolerance is not an all-or-none phenomenon [26, 104]. All degrees of tolerance are found, ranging from an apparently total and persistent inability to reject homografts to a trivial impairment of the ability to destroy grafts with the usual tempo. Tolerance may also be induced and maintained to nonliving antigens if the antigen persists or is repeatedly injected [105].

Acquired tolerance is highly specific, extending only to foreign cells or grafts having the same genetic constitution as the tolerance-conferring inoculum. For example, if a neonatal A strain mouse is inoculated with CBA cells at birth, it will subsequently accept grafts of CBA skin but will promptly reject grafts of skin from a completely unrelated AU strain. However, if the second donor happened to be a strain, such as C3H, which shares some important transplantation antigens with the CBA strain, the A strain mouse that is tolerant of CBA tissue will also display an enfeebled ability to reject grafts of C3H skin.

ABOLITION OF TOLERANCE

A state of tolerance can be abolished quite rapidly, as evident from destruction of a hitherto healthy-appearing skin homograft and abolition of cell chimerism if the tolerant animal is inoculated with a suspension of lymph node cells, splenic cells, leukocytes, or thoracic duct cells from a normal, i.e., unsensitized, donor of its own strain [40, 97]. The speed with which this is effected depends on the dosage of lymphoid cells injected. This shows (1) that homografts on tolerant animals retain their antigenic specificity, i.e., tolerance does not depend on adaptation of the graft, and (2) that there is no impediment in the efferent pathway of the immunological reflex. Tolerance is the outcome of a specific *central* failure of the *host's* machinery of immunological response. Transfer of normal isologous lymph node cells simply re-equips the tolerant host with a functional machinery of response which is confronted not only by the antigens of tolerated grafts but also by those of the disseminated cells responsible for its chimerism. As one would anticipate, tolerance is abolished with greater promptitude if the transferred lymphoid cells are derived from donors presensitized to the antigens to which the host is tolerant.

INDUCTION OF TOLERANCE IN ADULT ANIMALS

Early analyses of the principle of acquired tolerance suggested that it turned upon exposure of the host's lymphopoietic system to antigens at a very early stage in its maturation; exposure of older animals resulted in sensitization. However, in the light of more recent findings this concept has become untenable [18]. A wealth of evidence has accumulated that a state of unresponsiveness to homografts, closely resembling, if not indistinguishable from, tolerance as originally procured by treatment of very young animals, can be induced in adult animals as well [18]. When only minor histocompatibility differences are involved, consistent results are obtainable, but when the differences involve more powerful antigens, induction of tolerance in an adult host presents a much more formidable problem. Induction of tolerance in adult animals requires their exposure to massive doses of antigen in living cellular form. This may be achieved (1) by a single very large dosage inoculum [106, 107], or (2) more effectively, by *repeated* administration of high dosages of cells [108, 109], or (3) by maintaining the intended subject in parabiotic union with a foreign partner, usually an F_1 hybrid, as a chronic and abundant source of the cellular antigens to which it is to become tolerant [110–112].

The conferment of tolerance in adult animals can to some extent be facilitated by treatment with certain metabolic antagonists, or by sublethal x-ray irradiation, in conjunction with administration of the homologous cellular inoculum. Of potential clinical significance is the recent report that some degree of tolerance can be induced in adult mice by intravenous inoculation with semisoluble antigenic extracts [90]. Although at present most of the experimental evidence indicates the necessity of massive exposure of adult hosts to antigen in order to confer tolerance, there are some indications that chronic exposure to exceedingly small dosages of antigen may also be able to achieve the same end result [91].

Similarities between the unresponsiveness induced by inoculation of young animals, on the one hand, and of adult animals, on the other, include: (1) both may be complete, or only partial; (2) both types of unresponsive animals are cellular chimeras, and maintenance of the unresponsiveness seems to require persistence of the homologous isoantigens; (3) both categories of tolerant animals do not possess hemagglutinating antibodies directed against donor cells; (4) both depend on a central failure of the host's immunological response machinery as evident from their abolition following transfer of normal isologous lymphoid cells, and (5) both are most easily produced by intravenous inoculation.

In conclusion, it seems that the only meaningful distinction that can be drawn between transplantation tolerance arrived at by these two different procedures is a quantitative one. This is best exemplified by the finding that even the highly tolerance-responsive neonatal mouse or rat can become *sensitized,* instead of tolerant, if confronted with very low dosages of homologous cells [26, 113, 114].

Theories of immunological tolerance are discussed in Chapter 6 in connection with the various theories of antibody formation.

GRAFT-VERSUS-HOST REACTIONS

A serious complication of attempts to induce tolerance of homografts by procedures entailing the inoculation of suspensions of cells derived from lymphohemopoietic tissues of adult donors into fetal or infant hosts is the intervention of a peculiar wasting disease or syndrome, usually referred to as *runt disease* on purely descriptive grounds [115, 116]. In rodents this disease may vary greatly in its time of onset and severity. Its onset is usually marked by an abrupt cessation of growth, often accompanied by diarrhea and the appearance of abnormalities of the integument. In rats, for example, there may be progressive dermatitis and erythema of the extremities [48, 117]. In the acute form these symptoms usually appear within a week or so after inoculation, and the victims usually die shortly thereafter. Occasionally, however, grossly emaciated individuals may struggle on for a few months. Milder, chronic forms of the disease can occur, with complete recovery after weeks or months. An essentially similar disease follows the injection into embryonic or very young chickens of homologous adult blood, or splenic cells [118–121].

The pathology of runt disease has been studied in detail in mice [115], rats [48, 117], rabbits [122], and chickens [118], and the salient features are closely similar. The earliest lesions appear in the host's lymphohemopoietic tissues, the spleen and nodes usually undergoing striking hyperplasia followed by atrophy, accompanied by loss of follicular organization. The thymus undergoes complete atrophy, and dyscrasia of the bone marrow and blood occurs. There is frequently evidence of hemolytic anemia with a positive reaction to the antiglobulin test [118, 123, 124].

There is overwhelming evidence that runt disease is an immunological disease caused by the reaction of inoculated mature, immunologically competent cells against the foreign transplantation antigens confronting them in their new host; i.e., it is a *graft-versus-host* reaction. Findings that sustain this interpretation include the following: (1) Both the incidence and the severity of the disease are proportional to the genetic disparity between donor and host strains; if these are closely related, the disease may never express itself. (2) The ability of a given type of cellular inoculum to cause the disease depends on its content of lymphoid cells. Thoracic duct cells, leukocytes, lymph node cells, and spleen cells are highly effective, whereas bone marrow, which contains relatively few lymphoid cells, is usually innocuous. (3) The *dosage* of the inoculum required to cause this syndrome is a crucial factor [104]. (4) The onset of the disease is more rapid if lymphoid cells from *sensitized* donors are inoculated [48, 115]. (5) The disease is not caused by embryonic cells or by adult cells of such a genetic constitution (e.g., F_1 hybrids) that makes them incapable of reacting against host antigens [119].

The last two findings constitute formal proof that runt disease is not causally related to tolerance, although the induction of some degree of tolerance probably predisposes to it by giving the attacking cells some degree of exemption from destruction by their host.

Other syndromes, closely resembling runt disease, have been discovered independently in adult animals and have also been shown to be the outcome of graft-versus-host reactions. They may occur in the following situations: (1) When genetically tolerant F_1 hybrid individuals are inoculated with lymphoid cells from adult donors of one of their parental strains [50, 125, 126]. (2) If massive dosages of normal or sensitized lymphoid cells are inoculated into adult hosts of a different strain (here, the induction of some degree of tolerance is almost certainly necessary to give the cellular homograft exemption from prompt attack by the host [127, 128]). (3) When an F_1

hybrid individual is united parabiotically to a parental strain partner in such a manner that vascular interconnections are established (the F_1 animal is always the victim, and the disease is referred to as parabiosis intoxication). Parabiotic union of genetically unrelated individuals may also result in this syndrome [119, 129, 130]. (4) When heavily x-ray irradiated mice have been rehabilitated by replacement of their depleted marrow by large numbers of bone marrow cells from donors of another strain [92] (these cellular homografts are not rejected because of the weakening of the animals' immunological defenses by the irradiation).

The occurrence and severity of all of these runt disease-like syndromes, or *homologous diseases* as they are sometimes designated, are determined by the genetic disparity between donor and host, and in all of them the tissues principally affected are the host's lymphoid tissues.

In addition to the foregoing, in which the *entire* host is involved in the graft-versus-host reaction, *localized* manifestations of graft-versus-host reactivity occur (1) if lymphoid cell suspensions are scattered over the chorioallantoic membranes of chick embryos [131], and (2) if lymphoid cells are deposited beneath the renal capsules of genetically or immunologically tolerant hosts [55, 56] or are injected intradermally into chickens [120, 121] or guinea pigs [132]. Indeed, the latter type of reactivity has recently been made the basis of an effective test for selecting the most compatible donor from a panel of guinea pigs for a particular recipient [132].

MECHANISM OF GRAFT-VERSUS-HOST REACTIONS

Inoculated immunologically competent cells behave as if they settle out very promptly and electively in anatomically appropriate tissues of the host where they proliferate at least initially, contributing to the observed hyperplasia of the nodes and spleen in runt disease [115, 133]. However, it has been clearly established that the *host* cells make the major contribution to this hyperplasia [134–136]. Gowans [50] has presented compelling evidence from studies of homologous disease in adult F_1 hybrid rats that some (but certainly not the majority) of the inoculated *small* lymphocytes which lodge in the host's lymphoid tissue are responsible for initiating the disease. These cells transform into large pyroninophilic cells which divide. These changes take place very rapidly after inoculation of the host.

The hosts' lymphohemopoietic tissues appear to bear the brunt of the graft-versus-host attack, and it is widely believed that many of the pathological and clinical features of these homologous diseases are secondary. Massive destruction of cells or tissues in runts has never been observed. A satisfactory interpretation of the syndrome is still awaited, and the proximate cause of death of afflicted individuals is unknown.

Since the wasting disease that follows neonatal thymectomy in mice closely resembles runt disease in many of its clinical and pathological features, the possibility cannot be excluded that these two conditions are the common end result of two different processes which procure depletion of a host's lymphoid tissue [137, 138].

PREVENTION OF RUNT DISEASE

There are several ways of preventing runt disease, some of which are also applicable to the other homologous disease syndromes. They include: (1) utilization of inocula prepared from very young donors or from donors whose cells are genetically tolerant of the antigens of the intended hosts; (2) treatment of the hosts with certain antimetabolites such as amethopterin, which may either destroy the immunologically competent cells present in the inoculum or allow them to become tolerant of their host [139]; and (3) treatment of the hosts with specific isoantisera, which probably destroy most of the dissociated homologous cells [140–142]. Obviously if a satisfactory method of inducing tolerance by means of antigenic extracts can be devised, this will be the tolerance-conferring stimulus of choice since it eliminates all risk of graft-versus-host reactivity.

Clinicians must certainly take cognizance of the possible occurrence of graft-versus-host reactions in certain surgical contexts, e.g., in the grafting of tissues containing relatively large numbers of immunologically competent cells. The possibility has also been raised that an accidental leakage of maternal lymphocytes across the placental barrier might result in an immunological attack on the fetus from *within* [116].

Not only does runt disease, or indeed do the other manifestations of graft-versus-host reactivity, furnish a plausible model of an autoimmune disease in the sense that the cells responsible for it are anatomically part of the host [124, 143], but it hints at the possible consequences if indigenous lymphoid tissues, or their malignant derivatives, underwent a change such as the loss of a transplantation isoantigen so that they became liable to antigenic stimulation by the host [144].

From the immunologist's point of view, the importance of graft-versus-host reactions, especially runt disease, turns upon their application as research tools. Already these have facilitated the recognition and identification of the immunologically competent cells in the blood, and the elucidation of a variety of basic problems in immunology [119].

Acknowledgments: The authors are indebted to Dr. Darcy B. Wilson for helpful criticism and to Miss Barbara A. Hodge for assistance in preparing this manuscript.

REFERENCES

1. Garrod, L. P. Inborn errors of metabolism. *Lancet* 2:1, 1908.
2. Peer, L. A. (Ed.) *Transplantation of Tissues.* Baltimore: Williams & Wilkins Company, 1955 and 1959. Vols. 1 and 2.
3. Woodruff, M. F. A. *The Transplantation of Tissues and Organs.* Springfield, Ill.: Charles C Thomas, Publisher, 1960.
4. Billingham, R. E., and Silvers, W. K. (Eds.) *Transplantation of Tissues and Cells.* Philadelphia: Wistar Institute Press, 1961.
5. Gibson, T., and Medawar, P. B. The fate of skin homografts in man. *J. Anat.* 77:299, 1943.
6. Medawar, P. B. The behaviour and fate of skin autografts and skin homografts in rabbits. *J. Anat.* 78:176, 1944.
7. Medawar, P. B. A second study of the behaviour and fate of skin homografts in rabbits. *J. Anat.* 79:157, 1945.
8. Medawar, P. B. The homograft reaction. *Proc. Roy. Soc.* [Biol.] 149:145, 1958.
9. Hildemann, W. H. Scale homotransplantation in goldfish (*Carrassius auratus*). *Ann. N.Y. Acad. Sci.* 64:775, 1957.
10. Medawar, P. B. The immunology of transplantation. *Harvey Lect.* 52:144, 1956–57.
11. Snell, G. D. The homograft reaction. *Ann. Rev. Microbiol.* 11:439, 1957.
12. Snell, G. D. The Immunology of Tissue Transplantation. In *Conceptual Advances in Immunology and Oncology.* New York: Paul B. Hoeber, Inc., 1962. P. 323.
13. Stimpfling, J. H. Genetics of tissue transplantation in mice and men. *J.A.M.A.* 177:484, 1961.
14. Murray, J. E., Merrill, J. P., and Harrison, J. H. Kidney transplantation between seven pairs of identical twins. *Ann. Surg.* 148:343, 1958.
15. Silvers, W. K. Definition and Maintenance of Inbred Strains. Ref. 4, p. 133.
16. Snell, G. D., Staats, J., Lyon, M. F., Dunn, L. C., Gruneberg, H., Hertwig, P., and Heston, W. E. Standardized nomenclature for inbred strains of mice: Second listing. *Cancer Res.* 20: 145, 1960.
17. Billingham, R. E., and Silvers, W. K. Inbred animals and tissue transplantation immunity. *Transplant. Bull.* 6:399, 1959.
18. Billingham, R. E., and Silvers, W. K. Sensitivity to homografts of normal tissues and cells. *Ann. Rev. Microbiol.* 17:531, 1963.
19. Gorer, P. A. Some recent work on tumor immunity. *Advances Cancer Res.* 4:149, 1956.
20. Amos, D. B. Some Iso-antigenic Systems of the Mouse. In Begg, R. W. (Ed.), *Proceedings of the Third Canadian Cancer Conference.* New York: Academic Press, Inc., 1959. P. 241.
21. Billingham, R. E., Hodge, B. A., and Silvers, W. K. An estimate of the number of histocompatibility loci in the rat. *Proc. Nat. Acad. Sci. U.S.A.* 48:138, 1962.
22. Snell, G. D. Histocompatibility genes of the mouse: II. Production and analysis of isogenic resistant lines. *J. Nat. Cancer Inst.* 21:843, 1958.
23. Stimpfling, J. H., and Snell, G. D. Histocompatibility Genes and Some Immunogenetic Problems. In Cristoffanini, A. P., and Hoecker, G. (Eds.), *International Symposium on Tissue Transplantation Problems.* Santiago: Universidad de Chile, 1962. P. 37.
24. Eichwald, E. G., Silmser, C. R., and Wheeler, H. The genetics of skin grafting. *Ann. N.Y. Acad. Sci.* 64:737, 1957.
25. Billingham, R. E. Actively Acquired Tolerance and Its Role in Development. In McElroy, W. D., and Glass, B. (Eds.), *A Symposium on the Chemical Basis of Development.* Baltimore: Johns Hopkins Press, 1958. P. 575.
26. Billingham, R. E., and Silvers, W. K. Some factors that determine the ability of cellular inocula to induce tolerance of tissue homografts. *J. Cell. Comp. Physiol.* 60 supp. 1: 183, 1962.
27. Kinsky, R., and Mitchison, N. A. Tolerance

of skin induced by erythrocytes in poultry. *Transplantation* 1:224, 1963.
28. Möller, G. Survival of mouse erythrocytes in histoincompatible recipients. *Nature* (London) 199:573, 1963.
29. Borel, Y., Baldini, M., and Ebbe, S. Iso-immunity to blood platelets in the rabbit. *Blood* 21:674, 1963.
30. Wilson, D. B. Blood platelets and transplantation antigens. *Transplantation* 1:318, 1963.
31. Brent, L., Medawar, P. B., and Rusziewicz, M. Studies on transplantation antigens. In Wolstenholme, G. E. W., and Cameron, M. P. (Eds.), *Transplantation*. Boston: Little, Brown, 1962. P. 6.
32. Manson, L. A., Foschi, G. V., and Palm, J. An association of transplantation antigens with microsomal lipoproteins of normal and malignant mouse tissues. *J. Cell. Comp. Physiol.* 61: 109, 1963.
33. Gowans, J. L. The Immunology of Tissue Transplantation. In Florey, H. W. (Ed.), *General Pathology*. Philadelphia: W. B. Saunders Company, 1962. P. 965.
34. Snell, G. D. Histocompatibility and Cellular Immunity. In Tyler, A. (Ed.), *Proceedings of the Conference on Immuno-Reproduction*. New York: Population Council, 1962. P. 161.
35. Scothorne, R. J. Lymphatic repair and the genesis of homograft immunity. *Ann. N.Y. Acad. Sci.* 73:673, 1958.
36. McKhann, C. F., and Berrian, J. H. Transplantation immunity: Some properties of induction and expression. *Ann. Surg.* 150:1025, 1959.
37. Mitchison, N. A. Passive transfer of transplantation immunity. *Proc. Roy. Soc.* [Biol.] 142:72, 1954.
38. Mitchison, N. A. Studies on the immunological response to foreign tumor transplanted in the mouse: I. The role of lymph node cells in conferring immunity by adoptive transfer. *J. Exp. Med.* 102:157, 1955.
39. Billingham, R. E., Brent, L., and Medawar, P. B. Quantitative studies on tissue transplantation immunity: II. The origin, strength and duration of actively and adoptively acquired immunity. *Proc. Roy. Soc.* [Biol.] 143: 58, 1954.
40. Billingham, R. E., Silvers, W. K., and Wilson, D. B. Further studies on adoptive transfer of sensitivity to skin homografts. *J. Exp. Med.* 118:397, 1963.
41. Lawrence, H. S. Homograft sensitivity. *Physiol. Rev.* 39:811, 1959.
42. Waksman, B. H. A Comparative Histopathological Study of Delayed Hypersensitive Reactions. In Wolstenholme, G. E. W., and O'Connor, M. (Eds.) *Cellular Aspects of Immunity*. Boston: Little, Brown, 1960. P. 280.
43. Brent, L., Brown, J. B., and Medawar, P. B. Quantitative studies on tissue transplantation immunity: VI. Hypersensitivity reactions associated with the rejections of homografts. *Proc. Roy. Soc.* [Biol.] 156:187, 1962.
44. Ramseier, H., and Billingham, R. E. Delayed cutaneous hypersensitivity reactions and transplantation immunity in Syrian hamsters. *Ann. N.Y. Acad. Sci.* 120:379, 1964.
45. Dvorak, H. F., Kosunen, T. U., and Waksman, B. H. The "transfer reaction" in the rabbit: I. A histologic study. *Lab. Invest.* 12:58, 1963.
46. Gowans, J. L. The recirculation of lymphocytes from blood to lymph in the rat. *J. Physiol.* 146:54, 1959.
47. Steinmuller, D. Evidence of a secondary response in transplantation immunity. *J. Immun.* 85:398, 1960.
48. Billingham, R. E., Defendi, V., Silvers, W. K., and Steinmuller, D. Quantitative studies on the induction of tolerance of skin homografts and on runt disease in neonatal rats. *J. Nat. Cancer Inst.* 28:365, 1962.
49. Porter, K. A., and Cooper, E. H. Transformation of adult allogeneic small lymphocytes after transfusion into newborn rats. *J. Exp. Med.* 115:997, 1962.
50. Gowans, J. L. The fate of parental strain small lymphocytes in F_1 hybrid rats. *Ann. N.Y. Acad. Sci.* 99:432, 1962.
51. McGregor, D. D., and Gowans, J. L. The antibody response of rats depleted of lymphocytes by chronic drainage from the thoracic duct. *J. Exp. Med.* 117:303, 1963.
52. Gowans, J. L., McGregor, D. D., Cowen, D. D., and Ford, C. E. Initiation of immune responses by small lymphocytes. *Nature* (London) 196:651, 1962.
53. Porter, K. A., and Calne, R. Y. Origin of the infiltrating cells in skin and kidney homografts. *Transplant. Bull.* 26:458, 1960.
54. Waksman, B. H. The pattern of rejection in rat skin homografts, and its relation to the vascular network. *Lab. Invest.* 12:46, 1963.
55. Wheeler, H. B., Corson, J. M., Coyne, J., and Dammin, G. J. Use of spleen-splice homografts in the study of graft-versus-host reactions. *Nature* (London) 197:712, 1963.
56. Elkins, W. L. Invasion and destruction of homologous kidney by locally inoculated lymphoid cells. *J. Exp. Med.* 120:329, 1964.
57. Dvorak, H., and Waksman, B. H. Primary immunization of lymph node cells in millipore chambers by exposure to homograft antigen. *J. Exp. Med.* 116:1, 1962.
58. Winn, H. J. Immune mechanisms in homotransplantation: II. Quantitative assay of the immunologic activity of lymphoid cells stimulated by tumor homografts. *J. Immun.* 86:228, 1961.
59. Billingham, R. E. Immunological Mechanisms

in Homograft Rejections. In Brown, E. A. (Ed.), *Allergology* (Proc. 4th Internat. Congr.). New York: Pergamon Press, 1962. P. 227.
60. Rosenau, W. Interaction of Lymphoid Cells with Target Cells in Tissue Culture. In Amos, D. B., and Koprowski, H. (Eds.), *Cell Bound Antibodies.* Philadelphia: Wistar Institute Press, 1963. P. 75.
61. Wilson, D. B. The reaction of immunologically activated lymphoid cells against homologous target tissue cells *in vitro. J. Cell. Comp. Physiol.,* 62:273, 1963.
62. Willoughby, D. A., Boughton, B., Spector, W. G., and Schild, H. O. A vascular permeability factor extracted from normal and sensitized guinea pig lymph node cells. *Life Sci.* 7:347, 1962.
63. McCluskey, R. T., Benacerraf, B., and McCluskey, J. W. Studies on the specificity of the cellular infiltrate in delayed hypersensitive reactions. *J. Immun.* 90:466, 1963.
64. Brent, L., and Medawar, P. B. Quantitative studies on tissue transplantation immunity: V. The role of antiserum in enhancement and desensitization. *Proc. Roy. Soc.* [Biol.] 155: 392, 1961.
65. Winn, H. J. The Immune Response and the Homograft Reaction. National Cancer Institute Monograph No. 2, 1960. P. 113.
66. Winn, H. J. Immune mechanisms in homotransplantation: I. The role of serum antibody and complement in the neutralization of lymphoma cells. *J. Immun.* 84:530, 1960.
67. Winn, H. J. The participation of complement in isoimmune reactions. *Ann. N.Y. Acad. Sci.* 101:23, 1962.
68. Steinmuller, D. Passive transfer of immunity to skin homografts in rats. *Ann. N.Y. Acad. Sci.* 99:629, 1962.
69. Najarian, J., and Feldman, J. D. Passive transfer of transplantation immunity: I. Tritiated lymphoid cells; II. Lymphoid cells in millipore chambers. *J. Exp. Med.* 115:1083, 1962.
70. Najarian, J. S. Mechanism of homograft rejection. *Plast. Reconstr. Surg.* 30:359, 1962.
71. Najarian, J. S., and Feldman, J. D. Passive transfer of transplantation immunity: III. Inbred guinea pigs. *J. Exp. Med.* 117:449, 1963.
72. Kretschmer, R. R., and Pérez-Tamayo, R. The role of humoral antibodies in rejection of skin homografts in rabbits: II. Passive transfer of transplantation immunity by sensitized lymph node cells within diffusion chambers. *J. Exp. Med.* 116:879, 1962.
73. Najarian, J. S., and Feldman, J. D. The Effect of an Extract of Sensitized Lymphoid Cells on the Homograft Reaction. Ref. 60, p. 61.
74. Kaliss, N. Immunological enhancement of tumor homografts in mice. *Cancer Res.* 18:992, 1958.
75. Snell, G. D., Winn, H. J., Stimpfling, J. H., and Parker, S. J. Depression by antibody of the immune response to homografts and its role in immunological enhancement. *J. Exp. Med.* 112:293, 1960.
76. Billingham, R. E., and Silvers, W. K. Studies on Cheek Pouch Skin Homografts in the Syrian Hamster. Ref. 31, p. 80.
77. Amos, D. B. The use of simplified systems as an aid to the interpretation of mechanisms of graft rejection. *Progr. Allerg.* 6:468, 1962.
78. Medawar, P. B. Immunity to homologous grafted skin: III. The fate of skin homografts transplanted to the brain, to subcutaneous tissue, and to the anterior chamber of the eye. *Brit. J. Exp. Path.* 29:58, 1948.
79. Krohn, P. L. Personal communication, 1964.
80. Russell, P. S. Endocrine Grafting Techniques. Ref. 4, p. 35.
81. Billingham, R. E., and Boswell, T. Studies on the problem of corneal homografts. *Proc. Roy. Soc.* [Biol.] 141:392, 1953.
82. Craigmyle, M. B. L. A study of cartilage homografts in rabbits sensitized by a skin homograft from the cartilage donor. *Transplant. Bull.* 26:150, 1960.
83. Gibson, T., Davis, W. B., and Curran, R. C. Long-term survival of cartilage homografts in man. *Brit. J. Plast. Surg.* 11:177, 1958.
84. Simmons, R. L., and Russell, P. S. The immunologic problem of pregnancy. *Am. J. Obst. Gynec.* 83:583, 1963.
85. Parrott, D. M. V. The effect of site of implantation on host reaction to ovarian homografts. *Immunology* 3:244, 1960.
86. Billingham, R. E., Brent, L., and Mitchison, N. A. The route of immunization in transplantation immunity. *Brit. J. Exp. Path.* 38: 467, 1957.
87. Billingham, R. E., Brent, L., Brown, J. B., and Medawar, P. B. Time of onset and duration of transplantation immunity. *Transplant. Bull.* 6:410, 1959.
88. Steinmuller, D., and Weiner, L. J. Evocation and persistence of transplantation immunity in rats. *Transplantation* 1:97, 1963.
89. Billingham, R. E., and Sparrow, E. M. The effect of prior intravenous injections of dissociated epidermal cells and blood on the survival of skin homografts in rabbits. *J. Embryol. Exp. Morph.* 3:265, 1955.
90. Medawar, P. B. The use of antigenic tissue extracts to weaken the immunological reaction against skin homografts in mice. *Transplantation* 1:21, 1963.
91. Billingham, R. E., and Silvers, W. K. Studies on homografts of foetal and infant skin and further observations on the anomalous prop-

erties of pouch skin grafts. *Proc. Roy. Soc. Lond., B,* 161:168, 1964.
92. Koller, P. C., Davies, A. J. S., and Doak, S. M. A. Radiation chimeras. *Advances Cancer Res.* 6:181, 1961.
93. Medawar, P. B. Reactions to Homologous Tissue Antigens in Relation to Hypersensitivity. In Lawrence, H. S. (Ed.), *Cellular and Humoral Aspects of the Hypersensitive States.* New York: Paul B. Hoeber, Inc., 1959. P. 504.
94. Mowbray, J. F. Effect of large doses of α_2-glycoprotein fraction on the survival of rat skin homografts. *Transplantation* 1:15, 1963.
95. Miller, J. F. A. P., Marshall, A. H. E., and White, R. J. The immunological influence of the thymus. *Advances Immun.* 2:111, 1962.
96. Levey, R. H., Trainin, N., and Law, L. W. Evidence for function of thymic tissue in diffusion chambers implanted in neonatally thymectomized mice: Preliminary report. *J. Nat. Cancer Inst.* 31:199, 1963.
97. Billingham, R. E., Brent, L., and Medawar, P. B. Quantitative studies on tissue transplantation immunity: III. Actively acquired tolerance. *Phil. Trans. Roy. Soc.* 239:357, 1956.
98. Hašek, M., Lengerová, A., and Hraba, T. Transplantation immunity and tolerance. *Advances Immun.* 1:1, 1961.
99. Medawar, P. B. Immunological tolerance. *Science* 133:303, 1961.
100. Benirschke, K., Anderson, J .M., and Brownhill, L. E. Marrow chimerism in marmosets. *Science* 138:513, 1962.
101. Terasaki, P. I. Tolerance of skin grafts produced by various adult cells, soluble extracts, and embryonic cells. *J. Embryol. Exp. Morph.* 7:409, 1959.
102. Billingham, R. E., and Silvers, W. K. Studies on tolerance of the Y chromosome antigen in mice. *J. Immun.* 85:14, 1960.
103. Billingham, R. E., Manson, L. A., and Silvers, W. K. Unpublished data, 1963.
104. Billingham, R. E., and Silvers, W. K. Quantitative studies on the ability of cells of different origins to induce tolerance of skin homografts and cause runt disease in neonatal mice. *J. Exp. Zool.* 146:113, 1961.
105. Smith, R. T. Immunological Tolerance of Non-living Antigens. *Advances Immun.* 1:67, 1961.
106. Guttmann, R. D., and Aust, J. B. Acquired tolerance to homografts produced by homologous spleen cell injection in adult mice. *Nature* (London) 192:564, 1961.
107. Wigzell, H. Studies of Prolonged Survival of Skin Homografts in Adult Mice. In Hašek, M., Lengerová, A., and Vojtišková, M. (Eds.), *Mechanisms of Immunological Tolerance.* Prague: Publishing House of Czechoslovak Academy of Sciences, 1962. P. 267.
108. Shapiro, F., Martinez, C., Smith, J. M. and Good, R. A. Tolerance of skin homografts induced in adult mice by multiple injection of homologous spleen cells. *Proc. Soc. Exp. Biol. Med.* 106:472, 1961.
109. Brent, L., and Gowland, G. Induction of tolerance of skin homografts in immunologically competent mice. *Nature* (London) 196: 1298, 1962.
110. Rubin, B. A. Tolerance of skin homografts of adult mice after parabiosis. *Nature* (London) 184:205, 1959.
111. Martinez, C., Shapiro, F., Kelman, H., Onstad, T., and Good, R. A. Tolerance of F_1 hybrid skin homografts in the parent strain induced by parabiosis. *Proc. Soc. Exp. Biol. Med.* 103:266, 1960.
112. Nakić, B., Kaštelan, A., and Avdalović, N. Induction of Specific Tolerance in Adult Rats by the Method of Parabiosis. Ref. 31, p. 328.
113. Howard, J. G., Michie, D., and Woodruff, M. F. A. Transplantation Tolerance and Immunity in Relation to Age. Ref. 31, p. 138.
114. Brent, L., and Gowland, G. Immunological competence of newborn mice. *Transplantation* 1:372, 1963.
115. Billingham, R. E., and Brent, L. Quantitative studies on tissue transplantation immunity: IV. Induction of tolerance in newborn mice and studies on the phenomenon of runt disease. *Phil. Trans. Roy. Soc.* 242:439, 1959.
116. Billingham, R. E. Reaction of grafts against their hosts. *Science* 130:947, 1959.
117. Nisbet, N. W., and Heslop, B. F. Runt disease. *Brit. Med. J.* 1:129 and 206, 962.
118. Simonsen, M. The impact on the developing embryo and newborn animal of adult homologous cells. *Acta Path. Microbiol. Scand.* 11: 480, 1957.
119. Simonsen, M. Graft versus host reactions: Their natural history, and applicability as tools of research. *Progr. Allerg.* 6:349, 1962.
120. Cock, A. G., and Simonsen, M. Immunological attack on newborn chickens by injected adult cells. *Immunology* 1:103, 1958.
121. Terasaki, P. I. Identification of the type of blood-cell responsible for the graft-versus-host reactions in chicks. *J. Embryol. Exp. Morph.* 7:394, 1959.
122. Porter, K. A. Graft-versus-host reactions in the rabbit. *Brit. J. Cancer* 14:66, 1960.
123. Porter, K. A. Immune hemolysis: A feature of secondary disease and runt disease in the rabbit. *Ann. N.Y. Acad. Sci.* 87:391, 1960.
124. Oliner, H., Schwartz, R., and Dameshek, W. Studies in experimental autoimmune disorders: I. Clinical and laboratory features of autoimmunization (runt disease) in the mouse. *Blood* 17:20, 1961.

125. Gorer, P. A., and Boyse, E. A. Pathological changes in F_1 hybrid mice following transplantation of spleen cells from donor of the parental strains. *Immunology* 2:182, 1959.
126. Fiscus, W. G., Morris, B. T., Session, J., and Trentin, J. J. Specificity, host-age effect, and pathology of homologous disease induced in unirradiated F_1 hybrid mice by transplantation of parental lymphoid tissue. *Ann. N.Y. Acad. Sci.* 99:355, 1962.
127. Castermans, A. Re-evaluation of a pre-treatment given to adult animals to modify their responsiveness to skin homografts. *Transplant. Bull.* 5:381, 1958.
128. Najarian, J. S., and Feldman, J. D. Induction of runt disease in adult mice by presensitized homologous lymphoid cells. *Proc. Soc. Exp. Biol. Med.* 110:16, 1962.
129. Nakić, B., Silobrčić, V., Nakić, Z., and Bunarević, A. Competitive tolerance of skin homografts in adult separated rat parabionts. *Brit. J. Exp. Path.* 42:63, 1961.
130. Eichwald, E. J., Lustgraaf, E. C., Fuson, R. B., and Weissman, I. Parabiotic anemia-polycythemia. *Proc. Soc. Exp. Biol. Med.* 106:441, 1961.
131. Burnet, F. M., and Boyer, G. S. The chorioallantoic lesion in the Simonsen phenomenon. *J. Path. Bact.* 81:141, 1961.
132. Brent, L., and Medawar, P. B. Tissue transplantation: A new approach to the "typing" problem. *Brit. Med. J.* 2:269, 1963.
133. Nowell, P. C., and Defendi, V. Distribution of proliferating donor cells in runt disease in rats. *Transplantation,* 2:375, 1964.
134. Biggs, P. M., and Payne, L. N. Cytological identification of proliferating donor cells in chick embryos injected with adult chicken blood. *Nature* (London) 184:1594, 1959.
135. Davies, A. J. S., and Doak, S. M. A. Fate of homologous adult spleen cells injected into newborn mice. *Nature* (London) 187:610, 1960.
136. Fox, M. Cytological estimation of proliferating donor cells during graft-versus-host disease in F_1 hybrid mice injected with parental spleen cells. *Immunology* 5:489, 1962.
137. Parrott, D. M. V., and East, J. Role of the thymus in neonatal life. *Nature* (London) 195:347, 1962.
138. Miller, J. F. A. P. Role of the thymus in transplantation immunity. *Ann. N.Y. Acad. Sci.* 99:340, 1962.
139. Russell, P. S. Modification of Runt Disease in Mice by Various Means. Ref. 31, p. 350.
140. Siskind, G. W., and Thomas, L. Studies on the runting syndrome in newborn mice. *J. Exp. Med.* 110:511, 1959.
141. Voisin, G. A., and Kinsky, R. Protection against runting by specific treatment of newborn mice, followed by increased tolerance. Ref. 31, p. 286.
142. Garver, R. M., and Cole, L. J. Passive transfer of bone marrow homotransplantation immunity with specific antisera. *J. Immun.* 86: 307, 1961.
143. Stastny, P., and Ziff, M. Homologous disease in the adult rat: A model for autoimmune disease. *Ann. N.Y. Acad. Sci.* 99:663, 1962.
144. Kaplan, H. S., and Smithers, D. W. Autoimmunity in man and homologous disease in mice in relation to the malignant lymphomas. *Lancet* 27:1, 1959.

SECTION III. BIOCHEMICAL CONSEQUENCES OF THE ANTIGEN-ANTIBODY INTERACTION

*14. Serum Complement and Properdin**

IRWIN H. LEPOW

THE SYNTHESIS OF ANTIBODY AND its specific combination with antigen are the cornerstones of immunological phenomena. It is clear, however, that these crucial processes may be only initial steps in a chain of humoral and cellular reactions leading to ultimate immunopathological expression. The union of antigen and antibody is, of itself, frequently an innocuous event. Its injurious potential may be realized only through the subsequent participation of accessory or effector mechanisms which, although initiated by an immunochemically specific reaction, function in a broadly specific or nonspecific manner. It is the purpose here to describe serum complement as one such effector system.

In general terms, complement (C′) may be defined as a group of factors present in fresh normal serum and capable of entering into many antigen-antibody interactions. The number of components which comprises the complement system is not certain. Four components, designated C′1, C′2, C′3, and C′4, have been recognized for many years, but recent data have demonstrated the further complexity of C′1 and C′3. Considerable progress has been made in the separation, purification, and characterization of complement components, and all have thus far proved to be protein in nature, representing trace or minor constituents of normal serum. In addition, two divalent cations, Ca^{++} and Mg^{++}, should be considered part of the complement system.

The concept of complement as a mediator of immune cellular injury is an important one and worthy of emphasis at the outset. For convenience, we may define the formation of the antigen-antibody complex as a primary event and its interaction with complement as a secondary event leading to various sequelae. In these terms, immune hemolysis, immune bacteriolysis, and immune cytotoxicity are examples of secondary events resulting in *direct* injury of cells by antibody and complement. However, in other situations, the secondary event is not accompanied by direct lysis or killing but leads to *indirect* injury as, for example, following phagocytosis or immune adherence. It is also conceivable that the products of direct injury of cells could mediate indirect injury by provoking an inflammatory response. These concepts, introduced only for purposes of orientation and as a basis for later amplification, are depicted in Figure 14-1 (p. 201).

The mechanism of hemolysis of sheep erythrocytes sensitized with rabbit antibody is the most intensively studied and best understood model of direct cellular injury mediated by complement. It is a convenient system which can be manipulated with precision to yield information which may be transposable to injury of other cells of the host or to microorganisms. Guinea pig and human sera have been the most widely investigated sources of complement and will be used exclusively in the discussion that follows on the measurement of hemolytic complement, the nature of the components, and their mechanism of action.

* The author is recipient of a Research Career Award of the U.S. Public Health Service. The personal investigations reviewed here were conducted, in part, under the auspices of the Commission on Immunization, Armed Forces Epidemiological Board, and supported by the Office of the Surgeon General, Department of the Army, Washington, D.C., and by a grant (AI-01255) from the National Institute of Allergy and Infectious Diseases, National Institutes of Health, Bethesda, Md.

MEASUREMENT OF TOTAL HEMOLYTIC COMPLEMENT

Immune hemolysis was first described by Bordet [1] following Pfeiffer's observations on immune bacteriolysis of *Vibrio cholerae* [2]. Subsequent advances in technology and in appreciation of the role of divalent cations have led to the development of accurate methods for measurement of the total hemolytic complement activity of normal serum. The procedures have been presented in detail by Mayer [3], and only the principles will be outlined here.

The over-all reaction which is being followed may be written in the terminology of Mayer [3]

$$EA + C' \xrightarrow[Mg^{++}]{Ca^{++}} \text{ghost} + \text{hemoglobin}$$

EA refers to sheep erythrocytes sensitized with an optimal concentration of rabbit antibody, and C′ designates a suitable dilution of fresh normal guinea pig or human serum. Incubation of a standardized concentration of EA with dilutions of C′ in the presence of optimal Ca^{++} and Mg^{++} results in various extents of hemolysis which can be quantified by measuring the absorption of the released hemoglobin at an appropriate wavelength. In practice, 5×10^8 EA in a final reaction volume of 7.5 ml. is frequently employed, but adjustments to meet special requirements are possible. The pH is maintained at 7.4 by use of suitable isotonic buffers, such as barbital-saline or triethanolamine-saline, to which have been added optimal concentrations of Ca^{++} (1.5×10^{-4} M) and Mg^{++} (5×10^{-4} M). Incubation is performed at 37° C. for 60 to 90 minutes for guinea pig complement and at 32° C. for 60 minutes for human complement. The mixtures are then centrifuged and the absorption of the clear supernatant fluids is measured at 541 mμ or, for greater sensitivity, at 412 mμ. A plot of the percentage of cells hemolyzed as obtained from absorption data versus the concentration of complement in an appropriate range reveals the sigmoidal dose-response curve of immune hemolysis. This function is described by the von Krogh equation

$$x = K\left(\frac{y}{1-y}\right)^{1/n}$$

in which x is the volume of diluted serum which produces hemolysis of y fraction of the total cells, and n is a constant which should remain unchanged for a given set of experimental conditions. The constant K defines the 50 percent hemolytic unit of complement ($C'H_{50}$); when one half of the cells are hemolyzed, $\frac{y}{1-y} = 1$ and $x = K$. The logarithmic form of the von Krogh equation

$$\log x = \log K + \frac{1}{n}\log\left(\frac{y}{1-y}\right)$$

is useful in expressing experimental data. A plot of $\log x$ versus $\log\left(\frac{y}{1-y}\right)$ should yield a straight line of slope $1/n$ and intercept log K, providing a graphic solution for the $C'H_{50}$ titer. In the procedure given above, guinea pig serum usually contains about 200 $C'H_{50}$ units per ml. and human serum about 40 $C'H_{50}$ units per ml.

THE MULTIPLE COMPONENT NATURE OF COMPLEMENT

Although total hemolytic complement in serum can be measured operationally in a single step, the release of hemoglobin represents only a final event in sequential action of components of a complex biological system. The multiple component nature of complement was recognized in 1907 by Ferrata [4], who showed that the euglobulin (midpiece) and pseudoglobulin (endpiece) fractions of guinea pig serum were each hemolytically inactive but could be combined to restore hemolytic activity. In current terminology, Ferrata succeeded in precipitating C′1 with the serum euglobulins and separating it from C′2, a pseudoglobulin. In contrast, C′3 was demonstrated in 1912 and C′4 in 1926 by selective inactivation procedures rather than by fractionation. Cobra venom [5], yeast [6], and zymosan [7], an insoluble cell wall carbohydrate of yeast, destroy hemolytic complement by inactivating C′3, while ammonia [8] and certain primary amines [9] inactivate C′4. Thus the numbering of the components is in the order of their discovery and does not signify the sequence of their action.

Serum reagents selectively deficient in C′1, C′2, C′3, and C′4 are termed R1, R2, R3, and

TABLE 14-1. Classic Components and Complement Reagents[a]

Treatment of Fresh Human Serum	Serum Reagent	Complement Components Present
Dialysis or dilution to pH 5.5, $\mu = 0.02$ at 1° C.		
Supernatant	R1	C′2, C′3, C′4
Precipitate	R2	C′1, C′3, C′4
2–3 mg. of zymosan/ml., 37° C., 1 hr.	R3	C′1, C′2, C′4
0.02–0.03 M hydrazine, 37° C., 1 hr.	R4	C′1, C′2, C′3
56° C., 30 min.	Heated serum	C′3 (±), C′4

[a] Modified from Lepow *et al.* [10].

R4, respectively, and may be prepared by the methods of separation and inactivation indicated earlier. Since all of the components are required for immune hemolysis, it is apparent that each of the R reagents should be inert but that any two of the six possible combinations should be hemolytically active.

The increasing order of thermal stability of the four classic components is C′2, C′1, C′3, and C′4. The commonly employed procedure of inactivating complement by heating at 56° C. for thirty minutes yields a serum reagent lacking C′1 and C′2 but containing small amounts of C′3 and larger amounts of C′4. Heated serum will therefore at least partially restore hemolytic activity to R3 or R4 but not to R1 or R2 and may, in fact, be employed to increase the C′3 and C′4 concentration of R1 or R2. Salient information on the classic components and reagents is summarized in Table 14-1.

The serum reagents provided evidence of the multiple component nature of complement and at the same time supplied the first approaches to measurement of individual components. The C′1 titer of a serum or serum fraction, for example, can be estimated by determining the greatest dilution of sample which will result in 50 percent hemolysis of EA in the presence of a standardized concentration of R1. Such assay procedures, described in greater detail elsewhere [3, 11], are based on the assumption of Hegedus and Greiner [12] that the reagent supplies three of the components in excess and that hemolysis is limited only by the concentration of the component being measured. Experimental data and theoretical considerations have demonstrated the lack of validity of this assumption and the impossibility of obtaining precise estimates of complement components by this approach [3]. Nevertheless the classic reagents have contributed enormously to accumulation of knowledge of the nature and mechanism of action of complement and retain utility in investigations in which qualitative, as opposed to absolute, changes may suffice to describe the existence of a phenomenon or to provide clues to mechanism. For example, the sequence of action of the components and the enzymatic nature of C′1 were first deduced from studies employing R reagents.

Some progress was made in the purification of C′1, C′2, C′3, and C′4 by methods of protein separation based on differential solubility in dilute salt solutions, ammonium sulfate, or alcohol [13–15], but column chromatography provided the necessary tool with which to attack these problems satisfactorily. This coupled with concurrent advances in methods of measurement has made it possible to obtain preparations of the components which are separated one from the other. C′4 and two of the several C′3 components now known to exist have been obtained as homogeneous proteins. The complex, macromolecular nature of C′1 has been demonstrated, and two of the three subunits now recognized have been highly purified. The enzymatic nature of C′1 has been documented, and insights into biochemical mechanisms of immune hemolysis have been obtained. These encouraging advances, the results of work in many laboratories, will be discussed further.

MECHANISM OF ACTION OF COMPLEMENT

Hemolysis of sheep erythrocytes (E) in the presence of rabbit antibody (A) and guinea pig or human complement proceeds according to the following descriptive reactions

$$E + A \longrightarrow EA \quad (1)$$
$$EA + C'1 \xrightarrow{Ca^{++}} EAC'1 \quad (2)$$
$$EAC'1 + C'4 \longrightarrow EAC'1, 4 \quad (3)$$
$$EAC'1, 4 + C'2 \xrightarrow{Mg^{++}} EAC'1, 4, 2 \quad (4)$$
$$EAC'1, 4, 2 + C'3 \text{ components} \longrightarrow E^* \quad (5)$$
$$E^* \longrightarrow \text{ghost} + \text{hemoglobin} \quad (6)$$

This scheme, based primarily on the extensive studies of Mayer and his associates [3], forms a convenient basis for examining the sequential events of immune hemolysis.

REACTION (1) : $E + A \longrightarrow EA$

Rabbit antisera to sheep erythrocytes contain both 7S and 19S antibodies which differ in their hemolytic characteristics. In the presence of excess complement, the rate of hemolysis with high molecular weight, γ_{1M}-globulin antibody is a function of the square of the antibody concentration [16], whereas with lower molecular weight γ_2-globulin the rate is a function of the fourth power of the antibody concentration [17, 18]. This suggests that sensitization of a site, S, on the erythrocyte involves the formation of a complex, SA_2 for γ_{1M} antibody and SA_4 for γ_2 antibody, in accordance with the lower hemolytic efficiency of γ_2 antibody.

Dissociation of antibody from the EA complex and its reassociation at other erythrocyte sites has been reported to occur with some antisera but not with others [19]. Transfer from site to site would increase the hemolytic potential of a given dose of antibody, permitting sensitization of new sites during the course of complement action.

The practical problem arises of determining, for a given antiserum, the concentration of antibody which will optimally sensitize erythrocytes to the action of complement. With antisera to intact sheep erythrocytes, containing a mixture of anti-isophil and antiheterophil antibodies, it is essentially impossible to define this optimum, since increasing concentrations of antiserum in the presence of a fixed, limited concentration of complement result in progressively increasing hemolysis [20]. On the other hand, antisera to boiled sheep erythrocyte stromata, prepared according to the procedures of Rapp [3], contain largely or exclusively 19S antiheterophil antibodies which usually produce a plateau in the antibody titration curve above a critical concentration. Thus, in the latter instance, an optimal hemolysin concentration can be defined, but this optimum by no means implies that the erythrocytes are maximally sensitized, since higher levels of hemolysis may be reached by use of large doses of a mixed anti-isophil, antiheterophil serum. A pragmatic solution of this dilemma is to employ antiheterophil sera yielding "optimally sensitized" cells and to exclude, by absorptions, for example, any additional contribution of hemolysin in the complement source [3].

Commercial hemolysins are of the mixed antibody type and are glycerinated for stabilization. They may contribute small amounts of C'1 and possibly other components of complement which are still present. Glycerin stabilizes C'1 to inactivation by heating at 56° C. for thirty minutes, but attachment of C'1 can be prevented by preparing EA in the presence of ethylenediaminetetraacetic acid (EDTA) [21].

It is apparent that there are unsolved problems in the first step of immune hemolysis, even before the participation of a component of complement. Of great theoretical interest are the questions of why the interaction of erythrocyte and antibody provides a structure which permits further interaction with complement and why a wide variety of immunochemically unrelated antigens form complexes with antibody which provide the same or similar structure. An important lead has come from the work of the Ishizakas [22] and Christian [23] who have shown that complement is fixed by γ_2-globulin which has been aggregated into high molecular weight complexes by heat. This suggests that the common structure resides in aggregates of γ-globulin and that the function of antigen is to permit such aggregation to occur. Such hypotheses are in conceptual agreement with earlier suggestions of Heidelberger *et al.* [24] and the experiments of Talmage and co-workers [16–18] which indicate more than 1 antibody molecule per erythrocyte site. Current structural studies on γ-globulins are also providing data on the portions of the molecule which are required for aggregation and interaction with complement, as discussed elsewhere in this volume.

$$\text{REACTION (2)}: \text{EA} + \text{C}'1 \xrightarrow{Ca^{++}} \text{EAC}'1$$

The initial interaction between sensitized erythrocytes and complement involves the first component, C′1. The intermediate complex EAC′1 may be prepared by reaction of EA with a source of C′1 lacking or deficient in C′4. This has been achieved with an EDTA eluate from complexes containing C′1 [25, 26] (see below), ether-treated serum [27], R4 [25, 28, 29], and chromatographically separated fractions of guinea pig and human C′1 [29–32]. Formation of the complex EAC′1 may be detected by subsequent hemolysis in a source of C′2, C′3, C′4 and Mg^{++}, such as R1. Serum diluted in the presence of Na_2Mg-EDTA is also a useful source of these components since the action of C′1 in the serum is blocked by chelation of Ca^{++}. EAC′1 can also be detected and measured by sequential reactions with chromatographically separated C′4, C′2, and C′3 components [3].

It is clear from these experiments that C′1 is the first known component of complement to react with EA. However, in 1961 it was independently reported by Müller-Eberhard and Kunkel [33] and Taranta *et al.* [34] that a previously unrecognized constituent of human serum, designated the 11S factor on the basis of its sedimentation constant, reacted with aggregated γ-globulin in the presence of EDTA and was required for immune hemolysis. The 11S factor, obtained as a homogeneous protein, appeared to be distinct from C′1 and to react with EA very early in immune hemolysis, presumably before C′1 [35]. These findings appeared to necessitate introduction of a new reaction between reactions (1) and (2) above (viz., EA + 11S factor ⟶ EA – 11S).

Further insight into these observations was provided by chromatographic studies on human C′1 by Lepow *et al.* [29]. When a euglobulin fraction of human serum was eluted with diethylaminoethyl (DEAE) cellulose in the presence of EDTA, C′1 was resolved into three distinct activities, designated C′1q, C′1r, and C′1s in order of their elution. All three activities were required for formation of the complex EAC′1 from EA as well as for other activities of C′1 to be discussed subsequently. It was further shown that C′1q was indistinguishable from the 11S factor. Thus the activity classically designated C′1 appeared to consist of at least three separate substances.

Recent investigations of Naff *et al.* [36] have led to a return to the original concept of C′1 as a single substance reacting with EA in a single reaction, as depicted in reaction (2). Kinetic and ultracentrifugal experiments have revealed that C′1 activity is associated with the serum macroglobulins, with an apparent sedimentation constant on sucrose density gradients of about 19S. Macromolecular C′1 can be dissociated into C′1q, C′1r, and C′1s by EDTA, and upon recalcification, macromolecular C′1 is reformed. Thus, C′1q, C′1r, and C′1s, with apparent sedimentation constants of 11S, 7S, and 4S, respectively, may be considered subunits of a macromolecule functioning as a single biologically active substance rather than as separate components of complement. This is a situation conceptually analogous to the subunits or substructures of antibody which have been obtained by reductive cleavage or enzymatic treatment. In the case of C′1, dissociation has been effected by EDTA, explaining the basis for the original isolation of the 11S factor and C′1q, C′1r, and C′1s. In these terms, the subcomponents of C′1 are artefacts of preparation which provide valuable tools for probing further into the biochemical mechanism of action of C′1.

Partially purified preparations of human and guinea pig C′1 have been described recently by Borsos and Rapp [31, 37]. Under the conditions of separation employed, C′1 was recovered in a single area of the chromatogram. In the case of guinea pig C′1, the fraction was obtained in a hemolytically active state (C′1a), while human C′1 was in a precursor form (see below). A precise assay for C′1 activity on a molecular basis was also developed. It would appear that the partial purification of C′1 by Borsos and Rapp, performed in the absence of Na_3H-EDTA, did not result in the dissociation phenomenon described by Naff *et al.* [36] and that the former procedure is an approach to isolation of more highly purified, native C′1. The apparent discrepancy in results may be related to differences in procedural details in the two laboratories, and resolution of this problem should contribute to further understanding of the structure and function of C′1.

The biochemical event associated with the interaction of sensitized cells and C′1 is the activation of a precursor form of C′1 to an active enzyme variously designated as activated C′1, converted C′1, C′1a, or C′1 esterase [10, 14, 26, 38–45]. The term C′1 esterase will be used here. C′1 esterase appears to be distinct from previously described serum enzymes and may be functionally characterized with respect to two recognized types of activity: (1) esterolysis of a limited spectrum of amino acid esters, including N-acetyl-L-tyrosine ethyl ester (ATE) and p-toluenesulfonyl-L-arginine methyl ester (TAMe), and (2) interaction with the fourth and second components of complement. Extensive purification of human C′1 esterase has failed to dissociate these properties, and it appears probable that they are functions not only of the same molecular species but of the same catalytic site [32]. The effect of C′1 esterase on C′4 and C′2 is discussed later.

Purified human C′1 esterase participates in the formation of EAC′1, but it is emphasized that this can be demonstrated only in the presence of C′1q and C′1r [32]. Thus C′1 esterase can be substituted for C′1s in the reaction of EA with C′1 subcomponents. It is apparent, therefore, that the preparation of purified C′1 esterase which has been obtained represents an enzymatically active portion of the C′1 macromolecule described earlier. Indeed, mixture of C′1q, C′1r, and C′1s under appropriate conditions results in generation of C′1 esterase activity [29] and dissociation of the macromolecular complex with EDTA then yields an enzymatically active subcomponent (C′1 esterase) rather than its precursor, C′1s (C′1 proesterase). The mechanism of this activation process is poorly understood, but it is crucial to a biochemical understanding of the initiation and control of complement function. Advances on this fundamental problem should be forthcoming in the next several years.

C′1 is not irreversibly bound by EA. In the case of EAC′1 made with human C′1, spontaneous dissociation occurs merely by cooling the intermediate complex, and reassociation can be effected by rewarming the reaction mixture [28]. Dissociation of C′1 from intermediate complexes is also inhibited at decreased ionic strengths, substituting sucrose or mannitol to maintain isotonicity [46]. This is in part an explanation of the increased hemolytic activity of complement at reduced ionic strengths, since C′1 which dissociates is in the enzymatically active form and is capable of inactivating C′4 and C′2 in solution [14, 40].

Normal serum of several species, including man and the guinea pig, contains an inhibitor of C′1 esterase [41, 47–49]. The inhibitor is an α_2-globulin having a sedimentation constant of 3S and a molecular weight of about 90,000. It is largely destroyed by heating at 56° C. for thirty minutes and is labile at slightly acid pH and in the presence of ether [50]. The inhibitor has been highly purified and stoichiometrically blocks the esterolytic activity of C′1 esterase and also inhibits interaction of the enzyme with C′4 and C′2. This inhibitor is probably responsible for the rapid decay of EAC′1 which occurs when this intermediate complex is made with R4 as a source of C′1 [25] since the serum inhibitor of C′1 esterase is present in this reagent. On the other hand, EAC′1 made in the presence of R2 or ether-treated serum [27], reagents which lack C′1 esterase inhibitor, does not demonstrate this marked decay reaction. More direct evidence of inhibition of C′1 esterase associated with intermediate complexes has been provided by studies with purified inhibitor in immune hemolysis of sheep erythrocytes [51, 52], immune human hemolysis in the Donath-Landsteiner reaction of paroxysmal cold hemoglobinuria [53], immune cytotoxicity [54], and complement fixation [55]. These experiments have contributed to the conclusion that C′1 esterase is a functional requirement for complement action. It is emphasized, however, that inhibition can be clearly demonstrated only when intermediate complexes are permitted to react with the inhibitor prior to addition of all of the components required for the complement function under investigation. This reflects the rapidity of reaction of C′1 esterase with C′4 and C′2, as compared with the rate of reaction of low concentrations of C′1 esterase with serum inhibitor, and serves to resolve the apparent paradox of the presence of both complement activity and a potent complement inhibitor in normal serum.

Despite extensive investigation in several laboratories, the precise role of Ca^{++} in the reaction of EA with C′1 is incompletely defined. It seems unlikely that Ca^{++} functions as an enzyme cofactor since the esterolytic activity of C′1 esterase is unimpaired by EDTA [32, 41]. At least part of the role of Ca^{++} appears to be related to the increased stability of C′1 at 37° C. in the presence of this cation [56, 57]. Indeed, a reagent satisfying requirements for R1 may be prepared by incubation of serum for a period of hours in the presence of Na_3H-EDTA or Na_2Mg-EDTA [58]. An additional function of Ca^{++}, as a ligand in the binding of C′1 by EA, has been postulated by Laporte and co-workers [25] and Becker [26]. This concept has arisen primarily from the observation that the C′1 activity of intermediate complexes may be eluted by EDTA and restored to sensitized cells by recalcification. An alternative explanation is now to be considered in view of the observation that EDTA can dissociate macromolecular C′1 into subcomponents which are incapable of forming EAC′1 until they are recalcified and reform the macromolecule [36]. It would seem that Ca^{++} may be an integral part of macromolecular C′1 and that the *absolute* requirement for Ca^{++}, demonstrated with EDTA [59, 60] but not with a cation exchange resin [38], may be referable to maintenance of macromolecular structure rather than chelation of *free* Ca^{++} [36].

REACTION (3) : EAC′1 + C′4 ⟶ EAC′1, 4

After formation of EAC′1, the next step of immune hemolysis involves a reaction with C′4 to form the intermediate complex EAC′1,4 [25, 27, 44]. There is no divalent cation requirement. In the case of guinea pig complement, the reaction is stoichiometric at 0° C., but the rate is enhanced at 37° C. [30]. C′1 in enzymatically active form must be present on the sensitized cell before C′4 activity can be expressed. Inhibition of EAC′1 with diisopropylfluorophosphate (DFP) [44, 61] or antibody to C′1 esterase [32] prevents the reaction. However, after C′4 has reacted, C′1 may be eluted with EDTA without affecting C′4 activity on the cell. Thus, although enzymatically active C′1 is required, C′1 is probably not the receptor for C′4. It has been postulated, therefore, that the action of C′1 esterase on C′4 may result in a covalent bond between C′4 and a receptor on the cell membrane or the sensitizing antibody [61].

Human C′4 has been obtained as a highly purified protein by Müller-Eberhard and Biro [61]. It has a sedimentation constant of 10S and, on the basis of immunoelectrophoretic behavior, has been designated β_{1E}-globulin. A specific antiserum has been prepared which inhibits C′4 on sensitized cells and which can be used to detect the presence of C′4 on antigen-antibody complexes. Purified β_{1E}-globulin is inactivated by hydrazine and, in all respects, fulfills criteria for C′4.

This important contribution by Müller-Eberhard and Biro now makes possible a biochemical attack on the nature of the reaction between C′1 esterase and C′4, using purified proteins. A key question to be answered is the basis for the inactivation of C′4 by C′1 esterase in solution [14, 32] versus the functionally fruitful reaction between C′1 esterase and C′4 which occurs on the sensitized cell. Investigation of this problem should lead to a better definition of the biochemical events associated with this step of complement function.

REACTION (4) :

$$\text{EAC}'1,4 + \text{C}'2 \xrightarrow{Mg^{++}} \text{EAC}'1,4,2$$

(with a return arrow from EAC′1,4,2 back to EAC′1,4)

The participation of C′2 in immune hemolysis at a step after the reactions of C′1 and C′4 and before C′3 was shown in 1942 by Pillemer and co-workers [13, 62] by means of R reagents. A large body of kinetic data and significant biochemical observations has since emerged, largely through the work of Mayer and associates [3] on guinea pig complement. Comparable kinetic studies on human complement by Leon [63–65] have revealed close similarities in the behavior of the two systems.

Borsos *et al.* [66] have shown with partially purified guinea pig C′2 [67] that C′2 reacts with the intermediate complex EAC′1,4 in the presence of Mg^{++} without time lag, implying that conversion of a single site on the complex EAC′1,4 to the state EAC′1,4,2 will lead to hemolysis in the presence of C′3. Similar kinetic arguments at other steps of complement action have led Mayer [3] to a theory of immune hemolysis as a one-hit or noncumulative process conceptually analogous to infection of one cell by a single virus particle. The theory, in turn, has led to methods for measuring complement components on an absolute molecular basis.

C′2 activity on the complex EAC′1,4,2 decays as a function of time and temperature, as first shown by Mayer and co-workers [68]. Unequivocal demonstration that a product of this decay reaction is a complex in the state EAC′1,4 has been provided by experiments of Borsos *et al.* [66] in which EAC′1,4,2 was cyclically decayed and regenerated with partially purified C′2. It is apparent, therefore, that the relative rates of formation and decay of EAC′1,4,2 determine, in part, the extent of hemolysis which can be achieved.

Both C′1 and C′4 must be present on the sensitized cell before C′2 can react, and C′1 must be in its enzymatically active form. Removal of C′1 from EAC′1,4 with EDTA or blocking of its enzymatic activity with DFP, serum inhibitor of C′1 esterase, or antibody to C′1 esterase, as described earlier, prevents interaction with C′2. This is in keeping with the ability of C′1 esterase to interact with C′2 in solution [14, 32]. However, as with C′1 esterase and C′4 in solution, this reaction leads to inactivation of hemolytic activity. On the other hand, the reaction of C′1 esterase on the complex EAC′1,4 with C′2 is expressed by the presence of C′2 activity on the sensitized cell. Although the nature of the reaction in free solution remains to be explored, evidence is now available that cleavage of C′2 is effected by the EAC′1,4 complex, resulting in release into the fluid phase of an inactive fragment or fragments and retention on the cell surface of an active portion of C′2, designated C′2a [69]. The dependence of this cleavage reaction on enzymatic activity of C′1 esterase present on EAC′1,4 [70], coupled with earlier evidence already cited, strongly suggests that C′2 is a natural substrate of C′1 esterase. It also implies that the enzyme can function both as an esterase and as a peptidase. The nature and function of C′2a and the roles of C′4 and Mg^{++} in this step of immune hemolysis are not known.

REACTION (5) :
EAC′1,4,2 + C′3 COMPONENTS ⟶ E*

The final steps of complement action in immune hemolysis involve sequential reaction of the complex EAC′1,4,2 (or EAC′1a,4,2a, to indicate known activated states) with C′3 components, in the absence of divalent cations, to yield an injured erythrocyte designated E*. It is noteworthy that once the complex EAC′1,4,2 has been formed, the function of C′1 esterase has been fulfilled, as shown first by Becker [44]. Inhibition or physical removal of C′1 activity from this intermediate, by the various means described previously, does not prevent hemolysis by C′3 components. Thus enzymatically active C′1 is required for formation of EAC′1,4,2 but does not directly influence the subsequent reactions of immune hemolysis.

Evidence of the multiple component nature of C′3, previously thought to be a single activity, has emerged from several laboratories in recent years [15, 71–79a]. The number of C′3 components is still unsettled, and their nomenclature is particularly confusing, some workers designating them in the order of elution from columns, others in the order of function, and others on the basis of immunoelectrophoretic behavior.

The four components of guinea pig C′3 separated by Linscott and Nishioka [78] react in the sequence C′3c, C′3b, C′3a, C′3d, yielding the complex EAC′1,4,2,3cbad(E*). C′3c is the component of C′3 which is inactivated by hydrazine or ammonia but is most heat-stable. Decay of EAC′1,4,2 is prevented after C′3c and C′3b have reacted.

The three components of human C′3 thus far recognized by Taylor and Leon [75] have been named C′3a, C′3b, and C′3c in the order of their reaction. Since EAC′1,4,2,3a, as defined by Leon, is a stable intermediate and his C′3a is hydrazine-sensitive, it might be inferred that Leon's C′3a, C′3b, and C′3c are functionally equivalent to Linscott and Nishioka's C′3c plus C′3b, C′3a, and C′3d, respectively. However, direct comparisons of preparations from these two laboratories have not been made.

A highly purified human serum protein, β_{1C}-globulin, isolated by Müller-Eberhard and Nilsson [76], is functionally active as a C′3 component. Since it is hydrazine-sensitive and, as originally prepared, was capable of converting EAC′1,4,2 to a stable intermediate, it appeared to be analogous to the C′3a of Leon and the C′3c plus C′3b of Linscott and Nishioka. In subsequent work Müller-Eberhard prepared β_{1C}-globulin by a modified procedure and obtained a product which combines with EAC′1,4,2 but does not produce a stable intermediate until *two* additional proteins are added, designated β_{1F}-globulin and C′6 [79a]. The former has been obtained in a highly purified state as a thermolabile euglobulin with a sedimentation constant of 9.4S. Employing numerical nomenclature in the order of function, β_{1C}-globulin has been referred to as C′3 and β_{1F}-globulin as C′5. In addition to C′6 at least two further factors, C′7 and C′8, are necessary for hemolysis. This area of research is in rapid flux, and more definitive equating of the components obtained in various laboratories must await further investigations.

The β_{1C}-globulin of Müller-Eberhard and

Nilsson [76] is highly antigenic, and the antiserum has proved to be very useful for detecting this C′3 component on antigen-antibody complexes and in tissue lesions. On aging human serum, β_{1C}-globulin undergoes slow conversion to a new immunoelectrophoretic species, β_{1A}-globulin, which is antigenically closely related to β_{1C}-globulin. Formation of β_{1A}-globulin is associated with a chemical alteration of a glycoprotein of sedimentation constant 9.5S (β_{1C}-globulin) to a protein of similar carbohydrate content but lower sedimentation constant (6.9S). On the other hand, incubation of β_{1C}-globulin with cells in the state EAC′1, 4, 2 results in appearance of an inactive product, β_{1G}-globulin, which resembles β_{1A}-globulin immunoelectrophoretically but is indistinguishable from β_{1C}-globulin ultracentrifugally [79b]. Since conversion of β_{1C}- to β_{1G}-globulin depends on the presence of cell bound, active C′2 and appears to proceed catalytically, it has been proposed that C′2 functions as an enzyme in this reaction [79b].

Further investigation is required in order to elucidate the biochemical mechanism of action of the C′3 components. Many years ago Pillemer [13] suggested that C′3 might function as a terminal enzyme in immune hemolysis, and more recently Rommel [79] has proposed that the C′3a and C′3d components of Linscott and Nishioka might be enzymatic in their action. Indirect evidence that the final step of immune hemolysis may be mediated by enzymatic production of lysolecithin has been brought forward by Fischer and Haupt [80]. However, direct demonstration of enzymatic activity of any of the C′3 components and their biochemical characterization has not been accomplished.

REACTION (6) :

$$E^* \longrightarrow \text{GHOST} + \text{HEMOGLOBIN}$$

As shown by Mayer and Levine [81], sequential reaction of all of the components of complement with sensitized erythrocytes results in an injured cell, E*, which undergoes an intrinsic cellular reaction expressed by release of hemoglobin and formation of erythrocyte ghosts. This final lytic step proceeds at a measurable rate which is more rapid at 37° C. than in the cold but is independent of the presence of complement components in the fluid phase.

The pathophysiology and pathological anatomy of cells corresponding to the state E* have been described by Green *et al.* [82–84], employing rabbit antibody and rabbit complement with Krebs ascites tumor cells or mouse erythrocytes. In the presence of antibody alone, electron microscopy reveals invagination and interdigitations of the cell membrane without other effect on the morphology of the cell or discernible disturbance of electrolyte physiology. On addition of complement, however, the mitochondria and membranous system of the Krebs cell undergo marked swelling and there is an increase in the size of perinuclear pores. Holes or pores in the cell membrane were not visualized, but their existence could be inferred. With both Krebs cells and erythrocytes, adding complement gives an early loss of K^+, amino acids, and ribonucleotides from the cell and a failure to exclude Na^+. This derangement of normal control of permeability then results in osmotic swelling and osmotic lysis, with release of macromolecules, such as hemoglobin, other cytoplasmic proteins, and ribonucleic acid. Osmotic lysis can be prevented by increasing the osmotic pressure of the medium, but the electrolyte disturbance is still present. These studies demonstrate that lysis is a secondary event which may or may not follow the primary cytotoxic injury.

Direct visualization of lesions in erythrocyte membranes caused by immune hemolysis has recently been achieved, employing negative staining techniques and electron microscopy [84a]. Nearly circular holes, 80 to 100 A in diameter, were observed in numbers corresponding closely to those predicted from mathematical calculations of damaged sites. This elegant investigation has provided direct evidence for the one-hit theory of immune hemolysis [3] and morphological description of the primary lesion produced by sequential action of all of the components of complement.

A brief framework is presented in Table 14-2 of the reactions of immune hemolysis and their associated known biochemical events. This represents a partial summary of the preceding complex discussion and serves to emphasize both the encouraging nature of recent advances and the incompleteness of current knowledge on the mechanism of action of complement.

TABLE 14-2. Correlation of Intermediate Reactions and Biochemical Events in Immune Hemolysis[a]

Reactants and Intermediate Complexes	Biochemical Events
1. E + A ⟶ EA	—
2. EA + C′1 —(Ca++)⟶ EAC′1	Generation of C′1 esterase from a macromolecular precursor (C′1)
3. EAC′1 + C′4 ⟶ EAC′1, 4	Interaction of C′1 esterase with C′4; firm attachment of C′4 activity at a site other than C′1; nature of reaction unknown
4. EAC′1, 4 + C′2 —(Mg++)⟶ EAC′1, 4, 2 (arrow returning to EAC′1)	Interaction of C′1 esterase with C′2; enzymatic cleavage of C′2 with retention of an active fragment at a site other than C′1, fulfillment of function of C′1 esterase
5. EAC′1, 4, 2 + C′3 components ⟶ E* 6. E* ⟶ ghost + hemoglobin	Unknown biochemical role of C′3 components (one or more enzymes?), resulting in holes in cell membrane, loss of permeability control, and osmotic lysis

[a] Modified from Lepow *et al.* [29].

COMPLEMENT FIXATION

The ability of complement to react with and be fixed by a wide variety of antigen-antibody complexes makes possible the use of complement for the detection and measurement of antigen or antibody. The underlying principle of complement fixation procedures is relatively simple, although proper performance requires close attention to technical details and controls.

Soluble or particulate antigens, in the presence of specific, complement-fixing antibodies, will react with the components of complement by a mechanism which appears to be very similar to that just described for immune hemolysis. As a result of these reactions, complement components are consumed. Addition of sensitized erythrocytes and further incubation will indicate that fixation of complement occurred in the initial reaction. Thus complement fixation tests involve two distinct steps:

(1) Antigen + antibody + complement —(Ca++, Mg++)⟶ complement fixation

(2) Reaction mixture (1) + sensitized erythrocytes —(Ca++, Mg++)⟶ no hemolysis

If antigen or antibody is not present in reaction (1), complement fixation will not occur and hemolysis will be observed in reaction (2). A positive result of the complement fixation test is indicated by the absence of hemolysis in reaction (2). Alternatively, the fixation of complement can be detected by a second reaction employing antibodies to one or more components of complement, but the indicator system of sensitized erythrocytes is of more general utility for detection and quantification of antigen or antibody *in vitro*.

The amount of complement (usually guinea pig serum) used in reaction (1) may be varied to meet special needs but is frequently 5 $C'H_{50}$. If present, complement in the antibody source is inactivated by heating at 56° C. for thirty minutes. Five $C'H_{50}$ represents a practical balance between good sensitivity of detection of an antigen-antibody complex and nonspecific fixation or inactivation of complement by antigen or antibody alone. The latter refers to the anticomplementary activity of many antigens and of antisera or their γ-globulin fractions, necessitating controls of antigen+complement and antibody+complement as well as the control of complement alone.

In general terms, it is emphasized that complement fixation is a function of both antigen and antibody concentrations and that it is necessary to define the optimal concentration of one to be used for detection of the other. The anticomplementary activity of antigen or antiserum may place practical limitations on achieving the desired optima, and further purification may sometimes be required. As an alternative to the use of a small concentration of complement (e.g., 5 $C'H_{50}$) and definition of complement fixation titers in terms of the greatest dilution of antigen or antibody which effects incomplete or absent hemolysis in reaction (2), quantitative complement fixation analyses may be performed for more precise purposes. In this procedure, a large excess of complement is employed (e.g., 100 $C'H_{50}$), and the actual titer of residual complement after completion of reaction (1) is determined by methods outlined earlier.

The long-standing and continued widespread use of complement fixation tests for clinical and research purposes attests to their general utility and important position in the armamentarium of serological methods. However, further discussion would devolve largely on procedural details which are beyond the scope of this chapter and which have been presented in a single source by Mayer [3].

COMPLEMENT AS MEDIATOR OF DIRECT IMMUNOLOGICAL INJURY

The role of complement as a mediator of immunological injury was emphasized at the beginning of this chapter and the concept of direct and indirect injury was introduced for convenience of discussion. Direct cellular injury refers to the cytotoxic action of antibody and complement on a cell which contains the antigen to which the antibody is directed. The sequential reactions of complement function may then lead directly to death of the cell, with or without lysis. Additional discussions of the role of complement in cytotoxic phenomena will be found in a review by Osler [85]. Only a brief synopsis will be presented here.

Immune Hemolysis. The participation and mechanism of action of human and guinea pig complement in hemolysis of sheep erythrocytes sensitized with rabbit antibody have been presented as a model of direct cytotoxic injury. Studies on paroxysmal cold hemoglobulinuria (PCH) by Hinz and co-workers [53] reveal a mechanism of immune human hemolysis which differs from that of the sheep erythrocyte model only in specific detail and not in over-all pathway. Hemolysis is best demonstrated in the two-stage Donath-Landsteiner (D-L) reaction. (See equation at bottom of page.)

The cold phase of the D-L reaction, step (1), can be completed by human C′1 in the absence of other components at cold temperatures. Indeed, more recent data indicate that only the 11S factor (C′1q) will suffice [86]. If the cold phase is performed as shown in step (1), a product is obtained which is analogous to EAC′1 and which can be inhibited by serum inhibitor of C′1 esterase or hemolyzed by the remaining components of human complement in a second reaction at 37° C. The sequence of action of the components and the reactions in which Ca^{++} and Mg^{++} participate are the same as for the sheep erythrocyte system, demonstrating both the biological validity of the latter model and a mechanism of hemolysis in an acquired hemolytic anemia associated with intravascular hemolysis.

Immune Cytotoxicity of Nucleated Mammalian Cells. The ability of specific antibody and fresh normal serum to kill a wide variety of normal and neoplastic nucleated cells *in vitro* has been amply demonstrated [85]. In most instances, the participation of complement has been inferred from the heat lability of the factors supplied by normal serum. Employing human amnion cells, rabbit antibody, and normal human serum, Ross and Lepow [54, 87] have shown that, at least with this system, cytotoxicity is mediated by the components of complement. So far as studied, the mechanism of action of comple-

$$\text{(1) Human erythrocyte} + \text{PCH} - \text{antibody} + C'1 \xrightarrow[0^\circ\ C.]{Ca^{++}} EAC'1$$

$$\text{(2) } EAC'1 + C'4 + C'2 + C'3 \text{ components} \xrightarrow[37^\circ\ C.]{Mg^{++}} \text{hemolysis}$$

ment was entirely analogous to that in immune hemolysis. These data do not imply, however, that other mediators of cytotoxicity, unrelated to complement, may not also exist in normal serum.

A role for complement as a mediator of direct immunological injury of fixed tissue cells *in vivo* is attractive but still largely inferential. Suggestive evidence includes: (1) *in vitro* data, cited above, and the further demonstration that destruction of thyroid cells in tissue culture by autoimmune antibodies [88] or lymphoma cells by isoimmune antibodies [89] is complement-dependent; (2) observation of tissue-bound complement in lesions of human acute glomerulonephritis, systemic lupus erythematosus, and several other suspected immunological diseases [90], and (3) correlation of appearance of lesions in experimental nephrotoxic nephritis with bound complement in the kidney [91]. This incomplete listing suffices to emphasize that the mediation of direct cytotoxic injury by complement *in vivo* is probable but unproved. The evidence rests either on extrapolation of *in vitro* information or on correlations which cannot satisfactorily distinguish between primary and secondary events in pathogenesis. The difficulties of manipulating complement levels *in vivo* and maintaining markedly depressed titers for sufficient periods of time have hindered more incisive approaches to this crucial question. An encouraging advance has been the preliminary development by Rother [79] of a strain of rabbits genetically deficient in a component of C′3. If sufficient numbers of such animals can be bred, they will provide invaluable material for direct investigation of the role of complement in experimental immunological diseases.

Immune Destruction of Microorganisms. The requirement of both specific and nonspecific factors for the lysis or killing of many microorganisms was the key observation which led to the discovery of serum complement. The lethal action of antibody and complement on microorganisms may be viewed as a further example of direct cellular injury, modified in concept from the preceding discussions only in that the target cell or particle is of extrinsic rather than host origin. As with host-directed manifestations of cellular injury, it is difficult to assess rigorously the significance of complement as a mediator, in this case, of resistance to infection *in vivo*. Again, argument is mainly by transposition of data obtained *in vitro*.

The participation of complement in immune lysis, killing, or neutralization of susceptible bacteria, viruses, protozoa, and spirochetes *in vitro* has been further documented in recent years [85, 92]. The possibility of qualitative differences between hemolytic and bactericidal complement has been considered [93, 94] but seems unlikely at the present time. We will have more to say about immune destruction of microorganisms in the discussion of the properdin system.

COMPLEMENT AS MEDIATOR OF INDIRECT IMMUNOLOGICAL INJURY

The interaction of antigen-antibody complexes with complement may result in indirect injury of cells or tissues, rather than in the direct cytotoxic manifestations already outlined. In the former situations, the antigen may be rendered more susceptible to destruction by phagocytic cells of the blood and reticuloendothelial system (RES). Additional serum constituents, such as conglutinin and immunoconglutinin, may also combine with antigen-antibody-complement complexes to produce aggregates which are readily cleared by the RES. Finally, the interaction of antigen, whether cellular, particulate, or soluble, with antibody and complement may initiate a chain of humoral and cellular events culminating in an acute inflammatory response. These manifestations of indirect immunological injury mediated by complement (or serum constituents resembling components of complement) will be considered briefly. More complete discussions and bibliography will be found in reviews by Osler [85], Austen and Humphrey [95], and Coombs *et al.* [96].

Phagocytosis and Erythrophagocytosis. The participation of normal serum factors in phagocytosis and their possible relation to components of hemolytic complement have been under investigation for more than 50 years [93]. Among the more definitive experiments in the older literature are those of Ward and Enders [97], who showed that the *rate* of phagocytosis of encapsulated pneumococci in the presence of immune serum was markedly increased by fresh but not heated normal serum. However, the same final result was achieved, much more slowly, without addition of fresh normal serum. Such an effect on rate alone could be of critical importance in natural infection, but this again is an inference rather than a direct conclusion from experimental data. More recent studies have not led to a completely satisfactory definition of the role of complement in phagocytosis of bacteria or particles such as starch granules. Lack of participation has been suggested in some experimental systems, while in others an effect varying from enhancement to requirement has been reported [85]. The probable identity of normal serum factors with components of complement is most suggestive in the case of phagocytosis of starch granules [98, 99]. Further assessment of the function of complement in phagocytosis awaits direct experiments which are now possible with purified components.

More definitive progress has been made in studies on erythrophagocytosis. In extension of previous studies [100], Gerlings-Petersen and Pondman [101] demonstrated a marked enhancing effect of complement on phagocytosis of sheep erythrocytes and further concluded that the intermediate EAC′1,4,2 or EAC′1,4,2,3a (terminology of Taylor and Leon [75]) is the susceptible complex. Linden *et al.* [102], working with an entirely human system and a different experimental approach, were unable to find a requirement for C′2 and suggested that the susceptible complex is EAC′1,4. Despite these uncertainties, it seems clear that completion of at least the first two steps of complement action produces an erythrocyte-antibody-complement complex which can be engulfed by phagocytic cells far more readily than the erythrocyte-antibody complex alone, a conclusion of relevance to immunological mechanisms of erythrocyte destruction.

Conglutination. The term conglutination was given by Bordet and Streng to a property of normal serum of cows and other ruminants capable of strongly agglutinating antigen-antibody-complement complexes. Recent experiments by Lachmann [103] indicate that complexes similar to EAC′1,4,2,3a are clumped by conglutinin in the presence of Ca^{++}, a cation requirement shown earlier by Leon [104].

Immunization of rabbits or man with antigen-antibody-complement complexes or with materials which can form such complexes *in vivo* results in appearance of a serum property designated immunoconglutinin [96]. Immunoconglutinin also agglutinates complexes analogous to EAC′1,4,2,3a (terminology of Taylor and Leon [75]), but unlike the naturally occurring conglutinin of ruminants does not require Ca^{++} for its activity. The two activities are also antigenically and electrophoretically distinguishable [103].

Neither conglutinin nor immunoconglutinin will react with complement in solution, but both require for their action the presence of complement components on the antigen-antibody complex. It has therefore been proposed that these properties are directed to one or more components of complement which have been altered in the process of fixation. In these terms, immunoconglutinin has been viewed as autoantibody to such modified components [96].

As shown by Coombs and co-workers, conglutination is a useful and sensitive serological technique for the detection and estimation of complement-fixing antibodies. However, the physiological and pathological significance of conglutinin and immunoconglutinin are not clear. It is reasonable to assume that expression of these activities would lead to rapid clearance of an antigen-antibody complex and that, in the case of microorganisms, this could be reflected by increased resistance to infection. Indeed, Coombs *et al.* [96] have presented initial data in support of the latter hypothesis.

Immune Adherence. This phenomenon refers to the ability of antigen-antibody-complement complexes to adhere to a variety of unsensitized particles, such as erythrocytes, platelets, bacteria, and starch granules. The antigen may itself be particulate, such as a bacterium or a spirochete, or it may be soluble. Unsensitized primate erythrocytes are frequently used as the indicator particle.

The studies of Lamanna and Hollander [105], Nelson [98, 106, 107], and Turk [108, 109] have firmly established that the cation requirements and sequence of action of complement components are the same in immune adherence and immune hemolysis. However, whereas hemolysis requires the participation of all of the components of complement, adherence occurs with complexes which have reacted with only one of the four recognized components of C′3, e.g., with complexes in a state analogous to EAC′1,4,2,3c (terminology of Nishioka and Linscott [77, 78]).

Immune adherence can be a very sensitive

method for the detection of antibody. The lower limit of 0.01 μg. of antibody nitrogen compares favorably with such highly sensitive techniques as hemagglutination and passive cutaneous anaphylaxis [98, 107]. The occurrence of immune adherence *in vivo* appears to be well established [98], and its possible significance in resistance to infection, the generalized Schwartzman reaction, and hypersensitivity reactions has been reviewed recently by Nelson [110].

Adherence of antigen-antibody-complement complexes to primate erythrocytes *in vivo* could well enhance their phagocytosis. Indeed, adherence of such complexes to phagocytic cells could account for the enhancing effect of complement on phagocytosis. It will be of interest to see if further investigations in these areas will reveal an intermediate such as EAC'1,4,2,3c as the common complex susceptible to the various indirect phenomena discussed thus far and indicate a final common pathway of injury referable to phagocytosis.

The Inflammatory Response. The role of complement in the initiation of increased vascular permeability, peripheral vasodilatation, smooth muscle contraction, and subsequent events of the inflammatory response is a central question in our incomplete understanding of mechanisms of immunological injury and immunological diseases. Limitations of space permit only a brief outline of concepts. More detailed information will be found in recent reviews [85, 95, 111].

In general terms, there are several possible pathways by which complement might be a mediator of inflammation. Direct cytotoxic injury of cells by antibody and complement could result in liberation of constituents of the damaged cells capable of initiating an inflammatory response. Similar considerations could apply to indirect cytotoxic injury, as in phagocytosis. The interaction of antigen-antibody complexes with complement could, of itself, produce a humoral factor (e.g., anaphylatoxin) acting on a cell (e.g., the mast cell) to liberate a pharmacological mediator of increased vascular permeability (e.g., histamine). This could represent a general pathway to initiation of inflammation, independent of the nature of the antigen. The ability of complement to increase the state of aggregation of antigen-antibody complexes and to precipitate soluble complexes [85, 111] could localize or enhance the injurious potential of such complexes. These suggested pathways are neither exhaustive nor mutually exclusive, and the possibility of two or more mechanisms acting in concert, in appropriate situations, could be entertained. For simplicity, only some of these hypotheses are depicted in Figure 14-1.

Experimental evaluation of complement as a mediator of inflammation has been hindered by technical problems of depressing complement levels *in vivo* for protracted periods without inducing ancillary effects, such as leukopenia and thrombocytopenia. Also potentially

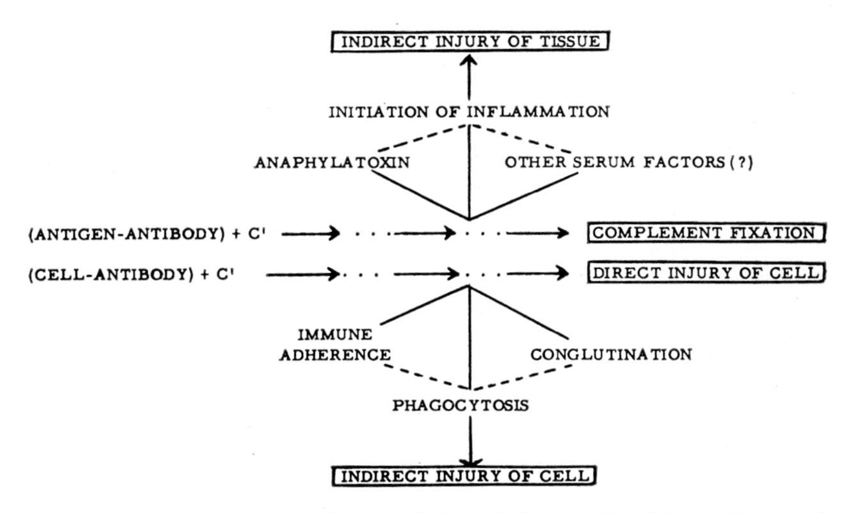

Fig. 14-1. Several possible pathways of cellular and tissue injury mediated by antibody and complement. *Horizontal arrows* symbolize the multiple steps of complement action leading to direct injury. *Vertical arrows,* arising from a reaction stage prior to utilization of all of the components of complement, indicate possible mechanisms of indirect injury. The figure is presented for conceptual purposes only.

present are the problems of low levels of complement sufficing for some reactions and of sequestered or tissue-bound complement not revealed by circulating titers. Experimental approaches have, of necessity, been limited to models which can yield an *in vivo* result rapidly or can be manipulated *in vitro* prior to testing *in vivo*.

Passive cutaneous anaphylaxis in the rat and the generation of anaphylatoxin from normal rat serum by antigen-antibody complexes fulfill these criteria. The extensive studies of Osler and his associates indicate that, at least in this species, complement can mediate increased vascular permeability and smooth muscle contraction [85], although recent data of Block and co-workers [112] appear to be inconsistent with this view.* The relative rapidity of the passive Arthus reaction has also led to investigation of the effect of decomplementation with unrelated antigen-antibody complexes on the pathogenesis of this inflammatory lesion. Although Bier and Siqueira [113] succeeded in preventing passive Arthus reactions in decomplemented guinea pigs, their results were interpreted as correlating with the concomitant thrombocytopenia rather than with the levels of circulating complement. On the other hand, preliminary experiments by Rother [79] with his strain of rabbits genetically deficient in a C′3 component have revealed failure of development of passive Arthus lesions. The relation of this observation to the complement deficiency, rather than to other factors, is suggested by the positive Arthus reactions obtained when a source of C′3 is injected at the same time as the test reagents. It is to be hoped that it will soon be possible to extend this approach to other inflammatory lesions in which a role for complement is suspected but unproved, such as serum sickness, experimental autoimmunity, and the homograft reaction.

Ratnoff and Lepow [114] made another approach to the evaluation of complement as a mediator of increased vascular permeability, employing normal guinea pigs and by-passing the use of antigen-antibody complexes and their possible effects on constituents other than complement. Since the activation of C′1 to C′1 esterase is an early event in the mechanism of action of complement, it was reasoned that if complement is a mediator of inflammation induced by antigen-antibody reactions, purified human C′1 esterase might be capable of inducing such a response. It was, in fact, found that the purified enzyme increased vascular permeability in guinea pig skin and that this property was referable to enzymatic activity and blocked by prior treatment of the test animals with an antihistaminic drug.

In addition to providing a useful experimental system for studying the mechanism of enhancement of vascular permeability by complement, these studies also bear on the pathogenesis of hereditary angioneurotic edema. Patients with this rare familial disease have repeated attacks of severe localized edema involving particularly the skin, gastrointestinal tract, and larynx. The serum of such individuals is deficient in an inhibitor of permeability globulins shown to be identical with serum inhibitor of C′1 esterase [115–117]. A link between the complement system and initiation of enhanced vascular permeability appears, therefore, to have been established in both an animal model and a human disease. The biological generality and significance of these findings remain to be determined.

COMPLEMENT TITERS IN HUMAN DISEASE

A large body of work has been directed toward determination of hemolytic complement titers in pathological sera, with the object of obtaining data which might prove useful in diagnosis or prognosis or provide insights into pathogenesis of human disease. In the main, these efforts have been unrewarding. Circulating hemolytic complement levels may be elevated, normal, or depressed in a given disease, and it is usually not possible to make useful interpretations. The subject has been amply reviewed [85, 118, 119], and a cataloguing of the available, sometimes conflicting, data will not be presented here.

There are a few noteworthy exceptions to the foregoing generalization. The finding of elevated complement titers in sera from patients with *acute* rheumatic fever led Fischel *et al.* [120–122] to examine sera from patients with a variety of acute inflammatory processes, including myocardial infarctions. The results of these studies suggested that complement behaved as an acute phase reactant. The elevation and return to normal levels of the

* For additional discussion of complement in anaphylaxis see Chapter 10.

complement titer essentially paralleled the corresponding patterns of other acute phase factors, such as C-reactive protein and erythrocyte sedimentation rate. This appeared to obtain either during the natural history of the inflammatory state or during intervention with anti-inflammatory agents, such as cortisone and salicylates. The pathological significance of these interesting observations has not yet emerged.

There is general agreement that serum complement titers are significantly depressed in serum sickness, acute glomerulonephritis, and disseminated lupus erythematosus. Use of these observations to support the concept that complement mediates the tissue injury in these diseases is tempered by the findings that in diseases frequently presumed to be on a similar etiological basis, complement levels tend to be elevated. These include dermatomyositis, polyarteritis nodosa, and rheumatoid arthritis. Complement titers can, therefore, be of some differential diagnostic aid in this group of diseases, although the underlying basis of these empirical findings is unknown.

COMPLEMENT SYNTHESIS

The restoration of serum complement levels within several hours following decomplementation procedures in experimental animals has been mentioned. The rapidity of regeneration suggests the possible existence of depots of preformed complement components, but the relative importance of release and *de novo* synthesis is not clear.

The cellular sites of synthesis of complement components are only beginning to be explored. A technique has been developed which depends on incorporation of C^{14}-labeled amino acids by tissues *in vitro,* followed by autoradiography of immunoelectrophoretic patterns of the culture fluid and carrier protein [123]. By this method, the synthesis of a C′3 component (β_{1C}-globulin) has been demonstrated with mouse spleen [123], monkey spleen, lymph nodes, and bone marrow, and human lymph node, bone marrow, and ileum [124]. Synthesis was not observed in monkey liver, thymus, kidney, and several other organs. Although no conclusions can be drawn from these studies concerning the cell type in lymphoid tissue which is responsible for the observed synthesis, it is noteworthy that some tissues which make at least one complement component also synthesize the three immunoglobulins. This is of particular interest in view of the proposed regulatory role of complement in antibody synthesis [125]. It would be of further interest to attempt to correlate the ontogenesis of immunological competence and complement synthesis in various species, particularly man, but data on fetal complement are not available.

THE PROPERDIN SYSTEM

The nature of properdin and of the properdin system has been the subject of a large literature and considerable controversy since the first publication on this subject by Pillemer and co-workers [126] in 1954. An attempt will be made here to summarize briefly the current status of the problem. More detailed presentations and historical development will be found in several reviews [3, 85, 127, 128] and the original references cited therein.

Properdin was originally described by Pillemer and associates as a serum factor which participated in the inactivation of C′3 by zymosan. In addition to zymosan, C′3, and properdin, this reaction required Mg^{++} and other normal serum constituents which resemble components of complement. The sum of these serum requirements was termed the properdin system. It was found that properdin participated in many other immunological activities of normal serum. Human serum depleted of properdin by absorption with zymosan at 17° C. (RP) lost most of its ability to kill susceptible bacteria, neutralize susceptible viruses, and hemolyze the abnormal erythrocytes from patients with paroxysmal nocturnal hemoglobinuria (PNH). These properties could be restored by addition to RP of partially purified properdin. Thus the concept rapidly emerged of properdin as a nonspecific factor functioning as part of a nonspecific system. The possible importance of properdin and the properdin system in phenomena of natural resistance led to a resurgence of interest in this previously neglected field.

Alternate views on the nature of properdin and the properdin system were soon expressed. Nelson [129] presented data which were consistent with the hypothesis that properdin was antibody to zymosan and that inactivation of C′3 by zymosan proceeded by way of a conventional complement fixation reaction. In these terms, neither properdin nor the properdin system was unique or nonspecific in function. The ability of properdin to react with a variety of apparently unrelated antigens was explained on the basis of cross-reactivity among closely related polysaccharides assumed to be widely distributed in nature.

The original concept of nonspecificity of the properdin system was further challenged by several investigations which clearly indicated serological specificity in the bactericidal and virus-neutralizing activities of normal human serum [130–133]. Accordingly, the properdin system could no longer be considered a nonspecific mechanism, but the question of the nature of properdin itself remained unresolved. At least two possibilities existed: (1) RP could be a source of complement, and properdin an antibody; (2) RP could be a source of antibody and complement-like factors, and properdin a nonspecific accessory factor required to complete a bactericidal or virus-neutralizing system. Studies by Wedgwood [134] indicated a requirement for both properdin and specific antibody for bactericidal activity of normal human serum and provided evidence for the second of the above hypotheses. Suggestive evidence of a similar dual requirement for inactivation of C′3 by zymosan has been reported by Blum [135].

It has been clear for some time that a completely satisfactory resolution of the properdin controversy depends on the isolation of properdin in a highly purified state and a direct evaluation of its properties. This goal has recently been attained by Pensky and coworkers [136]. Partially purified properdin, obtained by elution from zymosan [137], was resolved into a homogeneous protein peak by column chromatography on DEAE cellulose and CM-Sephadex. The final fraction, obtained in a yield of 2 mg. per liter of human serum, sedimented as a single boundary in the analytical ultracentrifuge ($S_{20} = 5.2$). The molecular weight of properdin was 230,000 calculated from sedimentation and diffusion constants and 216,000 by approach to equilibrium ultracentrifugation. The zymosan eluate had previously been found to contain four sedimenting species in the ultracentrifuge, with sedimentation constants of about 6S, 9S, 12S, and 18S. By direct sampling of the centrifuge cell, properdin activity was associated with heavy components [138]. It is apparent from the recent data on highly purified preparations that properdin is *not* a macroglobulin and that the earlier results could have represented either association of properdin with impurities under the conditions of ultracentrifugation or a sampling error. The latter possibility, although recognized, seems unlikely in view of the consistency of the results obtained.

Highly purified human properdin formed a single characteristic line in the slow β-globulin region on immunoelectrophoresis with unabsorbed rabbit antiserum to partially purified properdin [139]. In contrast, the zymosan eluate used as antigen for immunization and starting material for chromatography formed four lines. Absorption of the antiserum with RP, which contains the known immunoglobulins and components of complement, yields a serum which gives a single line with partially purified properdin [138]. The single line obtained with highly purified properdin and unabsorbed antiserum was not affected by absorption of the antiserum with RP [136].

These experiments were in agreement with previous work indicating that properdin was antigenically distinct from 7S and 19S γ-globulins [140]. The conclusion has been confirmed by immunoelectrophoretic analyses with rabbit antisera to γ_2-, γ_{1A}-, and γ_{1M}-globulins [136]. These antisera reacted with partially purified properdin but failed to give a detectable reaction with highly purified properdin. A discard fraction from the CM-Sephadex column had no properdin activity and behaved immunologically as γ_2-globulin.

Highly purified properdin restored activity to RP in the zymosan, bactericidal, and PNH assays for properdin, the only systems tested thus far [136]. In the bactericidal assay with *Shigella dysenteriae,* specific or heterologous antibody failed to restore the activity of RP. On the other hand, the bactericidal activity of human serum absorbed at 0° C. with the test organism could be restored by specific antibody but not by purified properdin or heterologous antibody. Finally, absorption of purified properdin with the test organism did not significantly affect its ability to restore bactericidal activity to RP. The lack of identity of properdin with specific antibody was apparent from these studies.

The current status of the properdin problem may be summarized as follows. *Properdin is a distinct serum protein which is physicochemically and immunologically distinct from the known immunoglobulins and which par-*

ticipates in a nonspecific manner in a variety of immunological reactions of normal serum. The *properdin system* is a group of substances in normal serum, comprising properdin itself, Mg^{++}, factors resembling components of complement, and naturally occurring specific antibody. The properdin system is serologically specific, but the expression of its activity requires a group of nonspecific factors, including properdin. In *concept,* this is analogous to the action of specific antibody and nonspecific complement components in immune hemolysis. Thus the nonspecific factors of the properdin system may be viewed as an effector mechanism for producing immunological injury.

These general statements represent a useful preliminary resolution of the properdin controversy. It should be emphasized, however, that serological specificity in the properdin system has been demonstrated directly only in the bactericidal assay [134, 136] and possibly in the zymosan assay [135]. Specificity in the virus-neutralizing system rests on only indirect evidence at present, and all attempts to demonstrate a specific antibody in PNH hemolysis have been unsuccessful. Furthermore, the identity of the nonspecific factors of the properdin system, aside from properdin, and their relation to complement components are still uncertain. Satisfactory solution of this problem will undoubtedly require direct isolation and characterization. Thus a completely satisfactory definition of the nature of the properdin system and its mechanism of action await further investigation. The existence of properdin and its participation in immunological injury are sufficient reasons to continue such investigation.

REFERENCES

1. Bordet, J. *Résumé of Immunity: Studies in Immunity* (collected and translated by F. Gay). New York: John Wiley & Son, 1909.
2. Pfeiffer, R. Weitere Untersuchungen über das Wesen der Choleraimmunität und über specifisch bactericide Processe, *Z. Hyg.* 18:1, 1894; Die Differentialdiagnose der Vibrionen der Cholera asiatica mit Hülfe der Immunisirung. *Ibid.* 19:75, 1895; Weitere Mittheilungen über die specifischen Antikörper der Cholera. *Ibid.* 20:198, 1895.
3. Mayer, M. M. Complement and Complement Fixation. In Kabat, E. A., and Mayer, M. M. (Eds.), *Experimental Immunochemistry* (2nd ed.). Springfield, Ill.: Charles C Thomas, Publisher, 1961, Chap. 4.
4. Ferrata, A. Die Unwirksamkeit des kompletten Hämolyse in salzfreien Lösungen und ihre Ursache. *Berlin. Klin. Wschr.* 44:366, 1907.
5. Ritz, H. Ueber die Wirkung des Cobragiftes auf die Komplemente: III. Mitteilung. Zugleich ein Beitrag zur Kenntnis der hämolytischen Komplemente. *Z. Immunitaetsforsch.* 13: 62, 1912.
6. Coca, A. F. A study of the anticomplementary action of yeast, of certain bacteria and of cobravenom. *Z. Immunitaetsforsch.* 21:604, 1914.
7. Pillemer, L., and Ecker, E. E. Anticomplementary factor in fresh yeast. *J. Biol. Chem.* 137:139, 1941.
8. Gordon, J., Whitehead, H. R., and Wormall, A. The action of ammonia on complement: The fourth component. *Biochem. J.* 20:1028, 1926.
9. Pillemer, L., Seifter, J., and Ecker, E. E. The effect of amino compounds on the fourth component of complement. *J. Immun.* 40:89, 1940.
10. Lepow, I. H. Complement: A Review (Including Esterase Activity). In Shaffer, J. H., LoGrippo, G. A., and Chase, M. W. (Eds.), *Mechanisms of Hypersensitivity.* Boston: Little, Brown, 1959. Chap. 18.
11. Wedgwood, R. J. Measurement of the components of complement by the reagent titration technique. *Z. Immunitaetsforsch.* 118:358, 1959.
12. Hegedus, A., and Greiner, H. Quantitative Bestimmung der Komplementbestandteile. *Z. Immunitaetsforsch.* 92:1, 1938.
13. Pillemer, L. Recent advances in the chemistry of complement. *Chem. Rev.* 33:1, 1943.
14. Lepow, I. H., Ratnoff, O. D., Rosen, F. S., and Pillemer, L. Observations on a pro-esterase associated with partially purified first component of human complement (C'1). *Proc. Soc. Exp. Biol. Med.* 92:32, 1956.
15. Arday, F. R., Pillemer, L., and Lepow, I. H. The properdin system and immunity: VIII. Studies on the purification and properties of the third component of human complement. *J. Immun.* 82:458, 1959.
16. Weinrach, R. S., Lai, M., and Talmage, D. W. The relation between hemolysin concentration and hemolytic rate as measured with chromium^{51}-labeled cells. *J. Infect. Dis.* 102: 60, 1958.
17. Talmage, D. W., Freter, G. G., and Taliaferro, W. H. Two antibodies of related specificity but different hemolytic efficiency separated by centrifugation. *J. Infect. Dis.* 98:300, 1956.
18. Stelos, P., and Talmage, D. W. The separa-

tion by starch electrophoresis of two antibodies to sheep red cells differing in hemolytic efficiency. *J. Infect. Dis.* 100:126, 1957.
19. Bowman, W. M., Mayer, M. M., and Rapp, H. J. Kinetic studies on immune hemolysis: II. The reversibility of red cell-antibody combination and the resultant transfer of antibody from cell to cell during hemolysis. *J. Exp. Med.* 94:87, 1951.
20. Osler, A. G., Strauss, J. H., and Mayer, M. M. Diagnostic complement fixation: I. A method. *Amer. J. Syph.* 36:140, 1952.
21. DeLooze, L. L., Ransby, A., and Leon, M. Activity of C′1 in rabbit anti-sheep hemolysin. *Proc. Soc. Exp. Biol. Med.* 109:393, 1962.
22. Ishizaka, T., and Ishizaka, K. Biological activities of aggregated gamma globulin: I. Skin reactive and complement-fixing properties of heat denatured gamma globulin. *Proc. Soc. Exp. Biol. Med.* 101:845, 1959.
23. Christian, C. L. Studies of aggregated γ-globulin: I. Sedimentation, electrophoretic and anticomplementary properties; II. Effect *in vivo*. *J. Immun.* 84:112 and 117, 1960.
24. Heidelberger, M., Weil, A. J., and Treffers, H. P. Quantitative chemical studies on complement or alexin: II. The interrelation of complement with antigen-antibody compounds and with sensitized red cells. *J. Exp. Med.* 73: 695, 1941.
25. Laporte, R., Hardré de Looze, L., and Sillard, R. Contribution à l'étude du complément: II. Premier stades de l'action hémolytique du complément; Rôle particulièr du premier composant. *Ann. Inst. Pasteur* (Paris) 92:15, 28, and 33, 1957.
26. Becker, E. L. Concerning the mechanism of complement action: IV. The properties of activated first component of guinea pig complement. *J. Immun.* 82:43, 1959.
27. Klein, P. G. Studies on immune hemolysis: Preparation of a stable and highly reactive complex of sensitized erythrocytes and the first component of complement (EAC′1); Inactivation of cell-fixed C′1 by some complement reagents. *J. Exp. Med.* 111:77, 1960.
28. DeLooze, L. L., and Leon, M. A. Reversibility of reaction between human C′1 and sensitized sheep erythrocytes. *Proc. Soc. Exp. Biol. Med.* 112:817, 1963.
29. Lepow, I. H., Naff, G. B., Todd, E. W., Pensky, J., and Hinz, C. F., Jr. Chromatographic resolution of the first component of human complement into three activities. *J. Exp. Med.* 117: 983, 1963.
30. Hoffmann, L. G. Unpublished data quoted in Ref. 3.
31. Borsos, T., and Rapp, H. J. Chromatographic separation of the first component of complement and its assay on a molecular basis. *J. Immun.* 91:851, 1963.
32. Haines, A. L., and Lepow, I. H. Studies on human C′1-esterase: I. Purification and enzymatic properties; II. Function of purified C′1-esterase in the human complement system; III. Effect of rabbit anti-C′1-esterase on enzymatic and complement activities. *J. Immun.* 92:456, 468, and 479, 1964.
33. Müller-Eberhard, H. J., and Kunkel, H. G. Isolation of a thermolabile serum protein which precipitates γ-globulin aggregates and participates in immune hemolysis. *Proc. Soc. Exp. Biol. Med.* 106:291, 1961.
34. Taranta, A., Weiss, H. S., and Franklin, E. C. Precipitating factor for aggregated γ-globulin in normal human sera. *Nature* (London) 189: 239, 1961.
35. Müller-Eberhard, H. J. Isolation and description of proteins related to the human complement system. *Acta Soc. Med. Upsal.* 66:1, 1961.
36. Naff, G. B., Pensky, J., and Lepow, I. H. The macromolecular nature of the first component of human complement. *J. Exp. Med.* 119:593, 1964.
37. Borsos, T., Rapp, H. J., and Walz, U. L. Action of the first component of complement: Activation of C′1a in the hemolytic system. *J. Immun.* 92:108, 1964.
38. Lepow, I. H., Wurz, L., Ratnoff, O. D., and Pillemer, L. Studies on the mechanism of inactivation of human complement by plasmin and by antigen-antibody aggregates: I. The requirement for a factor resembling C′1 and the role of Ca^{++}. *J. Immun.* 73:146, 1954.
39. Lepow, I. H., and Pillemer, L. Studies on the mechanism of inactivation of human complement by plasmin and by antigen-antibody aggregates: II. Demonstration of two distinct reaction stages in complement fixation. *J. Immun.* 75:63, 1955.
40. Lepow, I. H., Ratnoff, O. D., and Pillemer, L. Elution of an esterase from antigen-antibody aggregates treated with human complement. *Proc. Soc. Exp. Biol. Med.* 92:111, 1956.
41. Ratnoff, O. D., and Lepow, I. H. Some properties of an esterase derived from preparations of the first component of complement. *J. Exp. Med.* 106:327, 1957.
42. Lepow, I. H., Ratnoff, O. D., and Levy, L. R. Studies on the activation of a proesterase associated with partially purified first component of human complement. *J. Exp. Med.* 107: 451, 1958.
43. Becker, E. L. Inhibition of complement activity by di-isopropyl fluorophosphate. *Nature* (London) 176:1073, 1955.
44. Becker, E. L. Concerning the mechanism of complement action: I. Inhibition of complement activity by diisopropylfluorophosphate; II. The nature of the first component of guinea pig complement; V. Early steps in im-

mune hemolysis. *J. Immun.* 77:462 and 469, 1956; *ibid.* 84:299, 1960.
45. Levine, L. Inhibition of immune hemolysis by diisopropylfluorophosphate. *Biochem. Biophys. Acta* 18:283, 1955.
46. Rapp, H. J., and Borsos, T. Effects of low ionic strength on immune hemolysis. *J. Immun.* 91:826, 1963.
47. Levy, L. R., and Lepow, I. H. Assay and properties of serum inhibitor of C′l-esterase. *Proc. Soc. Exp. Biol. Med.* 101:608, 1959.
48. Pensky, J., Levy, L. R., and Lepow, I. H. Partial purification of a serum inhibitor of C′l-esterase. *J. Biol. Chem.* 236:1674, 1961.
49. Pensky, J., Hughes, G., and Lepow, I. H. Unpublished data.
50. Donaldson, V. H. Studies on the activation of a serum esterase with ether and its relationship to C′l-esterase. *J. Clin. Invest.* 40:673, 1961.
51. Lepow, I. H., and Leon, M. A. Interaction of a serum inhibitor of C′l-esterase with intermediate complexes of the immune haemolytic system: I. Specificity of inhibition of C′l activity associated with intermediate complexes. *Immunology* 5:222, 1962.
52. Leon, M. A., and Lepow, I. H. Interaction of a serum inhibitor of C′l-esterase with intermediate complexes of the immune haemolytic system: II. Kinetics and mechanism of the interaction. *Ibid.,* p. 235.
53. Hinz, C. F., Jr., Picken, M. E., and Lepow, I. H. Studies on immune human hemolysis: I. The kinetics of the Donath-Landsteiner reaction and the requirement for complement in the reaction; II. The Donath-Landsteiner reaction as a model system for studying the mechanism of action of complement and the role of C′l and C′l esterase. *J. Exp. Med.* 113: 177 and 193, 1961.
54. Lepow, I. H., and Ross, A. Studies on immune cellular injury: II. Functional role of C′l esterase in immune cytotoxicity. *J. Exp. Med.* 112:1107, 1960.
55. Lepow, I. H. Inhibition of human C′l esterase by its partially purified serum inhibitor. *Fed. Proc.* 19:76, 1960 (abst.).
56. Lepow, I. H., Pillemer, L., and Ratnoff, O. D. The influence of calcium ions on the inactivation of human complement and its components by plasmin. *J. Exp. Med.* 98:277, 1953.
57. Laporte, R., Hardré de Looze, L., and Sillard, R. Contribution à l'étude de complément: I. Inactivation spontanée dans les conditions de l'hémolyse; Action protectrice des ions calcium. *Ann. Inst. Pasteur* (Paris) 89:16, 1955.
58. Young, F. E., and Lepow, I. H. Further studies on the effect of Ca^{++} on the first component of human complement. *J. Immun.* 83:364, 1959.
59. Levine, L., Cowan, K. M., Osler, A. G., and Mayer, M. M. Studies on the role of Ca^{++} and Mg^{++} in complement fixation and immune hemolysis: I. Uptake of complement nitrogen by specific precipitates and its inhibition by ethylene diamine tetra acetate. *J. Immun.* 71:359, 1953.
60. Levine, L., Cowan, K. M., Osler, A. G., and Mayer, M. M. Studies on the role of Ca^{++} and Mg^{++} in complement fixation and immune hemolysis: II. The essential role of calcium in complement fixation. *Ibid.,* p. 367.
61. Müller-Eberhard, H. J., and Biro, C. E. Isolation and description of the fourth component of human complement. *J. Exp. Med.* 118: 447, 1963.
62. Pillemer, L., Seifter, S., Chu, F., and Ecker, E. E. Function of components of complement in immune hemolysis. *J. Exp. Med.* 76:93, 1942.
63. Leon, M. A. Quantitative studies on the properdin-complement system. *J. Exp. Med.* 103:285, 1956.
64. Leon, M. A. Kinetics of human complement: III. Intermediates in the reaction between human complement and sensitized cells; V. Decay of the intermediate complex $EAhuC'_A$. *J. Immun.* 79:480, 1957; *ibid.* 83:291, 1959.
65. Taylor, A. B., and Leon, M. A. Kinetics of human complement: IV. Kinetics of the inactivation of the C′3 complex by hydrazine. *J. Immun.* 83:284, 1959.
66. Borsos, T., Rapp, H. J., and Mayer, M. M. Studies on the second component of complement: I. The reaction between EAC′1,4 and C′2: Evidence on the single site mechanism of immune hemolysis and determination of C′2 on a molecular basis; II. The nature of the decay of EAC′1,4,2. *J. Immun.* 87:310 and 326, 1961.
67. Borsos, T., Rapp, H. J., and Cook, C. T. Studies on the second component of complement: III. Separation of the second component from guinea pig serum by chromatography on cellulose derivatives. *Ibid.,* p. 330.
68. Mayer, M. M., Levine, L., Rapp, H. J. and Marucci, A. A. Decay of EAC′1,4,2, fixation of C′3, and other factors influencing the hemolytic action of complement. *J. Immun.* 73:443, 1954.
69. Mayer, M. M., Asher, E. T., and Borsos, T. Inhibition of guinea pig C′2 by rabbit-anti-C′2. *Fed. Proc.* 21:17, 1962 (abst.).
70. Stroud, R. M., Austen, K. F., and Mayer, M. M. Immune hemolysis: Kinetics of enzymatic activation and fixation of C′2 by activated C′l (C′la). *Fed. Proc.* 22:613, 1963 (abst.).
71. Amiraian, K., Plescia, O. J., Cavallo, G., and Heidelberger, M. Complex nature of the step in immune hemolysis involving third component of complement. *Science* 127:239, 1958.

72. Rapp, H. J. Mechanism of immune hemolysis: Recognition of two steps in the conversion of EAC'1, 4, 2 to E*. *Ibid.* p. 234.
73. Rapp, H. J., Sims, M. R., and Borsos, T. Separation of components of guinea pig complement by chromatography. *Proc. Soc. Exp. Biol. Med.* 100:730, 1959.
74. Taylor, A. B., and Leon, M. A. Third component of human complement: Resolution into two factors and demonstration of a new reaction intermediate. *Proc. Soc. Exp. Biol. Med.* 101:587, 1959.
75. Taylor, A. B., and Leon, M. A. Isolation of three components of the C'3 complex. *Fed. Proc.* 20:19, 1961 (abst.).
76. Müller-Eberhard, H. J., and Nilsson, U. Relation of a β_1-glycoprotein of human serum to the complement system. *J. Exp. Med.* 111:217, 1960.
77. Nishioka, K., and Linscott, W. D. Components of guinea pig complement: I. Separation of a serum fraction essential for immune hemolysis and immune adherence. *J. Exp. Med.* 118:767, 1963.
78. Linscott, W. D., and Nishioka, K. Components of guinea pig complement: II. Separation of serum fractions essential for immune hemolysis. *Ibid.*, p. 795.
79. Rapp, H. J., and Borsos, T. Complement and hemolysis: Summary of the Complement Workshop. *Science* 141:738, 1963.
79a. Nilsson, U., and Müller-Eberhard, H. J. Isolation of β_{1F}-globulin and its characterization as a complement component. *Fed. Proc.* 23:506, 1964 (abst.).
79b. Müller-Eberhard, H. J., Calcott, M. A., and Mardiney, M. R. Conversion of β_{1c}-globulin by C'2a. *Fed. Proc.* 23:506, 1964 (abst.).
80. Fischer, H., and Haupt, I. Das cytolysierende Prinzip von Serum Komplement. *Z. Naturforsch.* [B] 16b:321, 1961.
81. Mayer, M. M., and Levine, L. Kinetic studies on immune hemolysis: III. Description of a terminal process which follows the Ca^{++} and Mg^{++} reaction steps in the action of complement on sensitized erythrocytes. *J. Immun.* 72: 511, 1954.
82. Goldberg, B., and Green, H. The cytotoxic action of immune gamma globulin and complement on Krebs ascites tumor cells: I. Ultrastructural studies. *J. Exp. Med.* 109:505, 1959.
83. Green, H., Fleischer, R. A., Barrow, P., and Goldberg, B. The cytotoxic action of immune gamma globulin and complement on Krebs ascites tumor cells: II. Chemical studies. *Ibid.*, p. 511.
84. Green, H., Barrow, P., and Goldberg, B. Effect of antibody and complement on permeability control in ascites tumor cells and erythrocytes. *J. Exp. Med.* 110:699, 1959.
84a. Borsos, T., Dourmashkin, R. R., and Humphrey, J. H. Lesions in erythrocyte membranes caused by immune hemolysis. *Nature* (London) 202:251, 1964.
85. Osler, A. G. Functions of the complement system. *Advances Immun.* 1:131, 1961.
86. Hinz, C. F., Jr., and Mollner, A. M. Studies on immune human hemolysis: III. Role of 11S component in initiating the Donath-Landsteiner reaction. *J. Immun.* 91:512, 1963.
87. Ross, A., and Lepow, I. H. Studies on immune cellular injury: I. Cytotoxic effects of antibody and complement. *J. Exp. Med.* 112: 1085, 1960.
88. Irvine, W. J. An investigation of the pathogenesis of Hashimoto's disease by thyroid tissue culture. *Endocrinology* 20:83, 1960.
89. Winn, H. J. Immune mechanisms in homotransplantation: I. The role of serum antibody and complement in the neutralization of lymphoma cells. *J. Immun.* 84:530, 1960.
90. Lachmann, P. J., Müller-Eberhard, H. J., Kunkel, H. G., and Paronetto, F. The localization of *in vivo* bound complement in tissue sections. *J. Exp. Med.* 115:63, 1962.
91. Vogt, A., and Kochem, H. G. Immediate and delayed nephrotoxic nephritis in rats: The role of complement fixation. *Amer. J. Path.* 39:379, 1961.
92. Wardlaw, A. C. The complement-dependent bacteriolytic activity of normal human serum: I. The effect of pH and ionic strength and the role of lysozyme. *J. Exp. Med.* 115:1231, 1962.
93. Zinsser, H., Enders, J. F., and Fothergill, L. D. *Immunity: Principles and Applications in Medicine and Public Health* (5th ed.). New York: Macmillan Company, 1939. Chap. 7 and 11.
94. Jordan, F. L. J. Complement bij hemolytische anemie. *Nederl. T. Geneesk.* 101:2316, 1957.
95. Austen, K. F., and Humphrey, J. H. *In vitro* studies of the mechanism of anaphylaxis. *Advances Immun.* 3:1, 1963.
96. Coombs, R. R. A., Coombs, A. M., and Ingram, D. G. *The Serology of Conglutination and Its Relation to Disease.* Oxford: Blackwell Scientific Publications, 1961.
97. Ward, H. K., and Enders, J. F. An analysis of the opsonic and tropic action of normal and immune sera based on experiments with the pneumococcus. *J. Exp. Med.* 57:527, 1933.
98. Nelson, R. A., Jr. The immune-adherence phenomenon: A hypothetical role of erythrocytes in defence against bacteria and viruses. *Proc. Roy. Soc. Med.* 49:55, 1956.
99. Ludány, G., Döklen, A., and Toth, E. Die Beeinflussung der Leukozytenphagozytose mit Phlorrhizin. *Experientia* 13:409, 1957.
100. Mabry, D. W., Wallace, J. H., Dodd, M. C., and Wright, C. S. Opsonic factors in normal and immune sera in the differential phagocytosis of normal, trypsinized and virus-

treated human and rabbit erythrocytes by macrophages in tissue culture. *J. Immun.* 76:62, 1956.

101. Gerlings-Petersen, B. T., and Pondman, K. W. Erythrophagocytosis: A study of the antigen-antibody-complement reaction. *Vox. Sang.* 7: 655, 1962.
102. Linden, D. A., Junglas, D. W., and Hinz, C. F., Jr. Personal communication.
103. Lachmann, P. J. A comparison of some properties of bovine conglutinin with those of rabbit immuno-conglutinin. *Immunology* 5:687, 1962.
104. Leon, M. A. Role of cations in conglutination and in formation of properdin zymosan complex from bovine serum. *Proc. Soc. Exp. Biol. Med.* 96:202, 1957.
105. Lamanna, C., and Hollander, D. H. Demonstration of particulate adhesion of the Rieckenberg type with the spirochete of syphilis. *Science* 123:989, 1956.
106. Nelson, R. A., Jr. The immune-adherence phenomenon: An immunologically specific reaction between microorganisms and erythrocytes leading to enhanced phagocytosis. *Science* 118:733, 1953.
107. Nelson, R. A., Jr., and Nelson, D. S. On the mechanism of immune adherence: II. Analogy to mixed aggregation of sensitized antigens in the presence of complement; immune adherence with animal platelets. *Yale J. Biol. Med.* 31:201, 1959.
108. Turk, J. L. The relationship between complement and antibodies of different animals in the immune-adherence phenomenon. *Immunology* 2:127, 1959.
109. Turk, J. L. The immune-adherence activity of normal serum. *Brit. J. Exp. Path.* 40:97, 1959.
110. Nelson, D. S. Immune Adherence. *Advances Immun.* 3:131, 1963.
111. Weigle, W. O. Fate and biological action of antigen-antibody complexes. *Advances Immun.* 1:283, 1961.
112. Block, K. J., Kourilsky, F. M., Ovary, Z., and Benacerraf, B. Properties of guinea pig 7S antibodies: III. Identification of antibodies involved in complement fixation and hemolysis. *J. Exp. Med.* 117:965, 1963.
113. Bier, O. G., and Siqueira, M. Prevention by intravenous injection of antigen and antibody of passive Arthus reaction to unrelated immune system. *Proc. Soc. Exp. Biol. Med.* 101:502, 1959.
114. Ratnoff, O. D., and Lepow, I. H. Complement as a mediator of inflammation: Enhancement of vascular permeability by purified human C′1 esterase. *J. Exp. Med.* 118: 681, 1963.
115. Landerman, N. S., Webster, M. E., Becker, E. L., and Ratcliffe, H. Hereditary angioneurotic edema: II. Deficiency of inhibitor for serum globulin permeability factor and/or plasma kallikrein. *J. Allerg.* 33:330, 1962.
116. Donaldson, V. H., and Evans, R. R. A biochemical abnormality in hereditary angioneurotic edema: Absence of serum inhibitor of C′1-esterase. *Amer. J. Med.* 35:37, 1963.
117. Kagan, L. J., and Becker, E. L. Inhibition of permeability globulins by C′1 esterase inhibitor. *Fed. Proc.* 22:613, 1963 (abst.).
118. Ecker, E. E., Seifter, S., Dozois, T. F., and Barr, L. Complement in infectious disease in man. *J. Clin. Invest.* 25:800, 1946.
119. Brückel, K. W., Schultze, H. E., and Schwick, G. Das Properdin-Komplement-System bei verschiedenen Krankheiten. *Deutsch. Med. Wschr.* 82:1898, 1957.
120. Boltax, A. J., and Fischel, E. E. Serologic tests for inflammation: Serum complement, C-reactive protein and erythrocyte sedimentation role in myocardial infarction. *Amer. J. Med.* 20:418, 1956.
121. Fischel, E. E. Manifestations of acute inflammation in the plasma. *Med. Clin. N. Amer.* 41:685, 1957.
122. Fischel, E. E., Frank, C. W., Boltax, A. J., and Arcasoy, M. Observations on the treatment of rheumatic fever with salicylate, ACTH and cortisone: II. Combined salicylate and corticoid therapy and attempts at rebound suppression. *Arthritis Rheum.* 1:351, 1958.
123. Hochwald, G. M., Thorbecke, G. J., and Asofsky, R. Sites of formation of immune globulins and of a component of C′3: I. A new technique for the demonstration of the synthesis of individual serum proteins by tissues *in vitro*. *J. Exp. Med.* 114:459, 1961.
124. Asofsky, R., and Thorbecke, G. J. Sites of formation of immune globulins and of a component of C′3: II. Production of immunoelectrophoretically identified serum proteins by human and monkey tissues *in vitro*. *Ibid.*, p. 471.
125. Talmage, D. W., and Pearlman, D. S. The antibody response: A model based on antagonistic actions of antigen. *J. Theor. Biol.* 5: 321, 1963.
126. Pillemer, L., Blum, L., Lepow, I. H., Ross, O. A., Todd, E. W., and Wardlaw, A. C. The properdin system and immunity: I. Demonstration and isolation of a new serum protein, properdin, and its role in immune phenomena. *Science* 120:279, 1954.
127. Lepow, I. H. The Properdin System: A Review of Current Concepts. In Heidelberger, M., Plescia, O. J., and Day, R. A. (Eds.), *Immunochemical Approaches to Problems in Microbiology*. New Brunswick, N.J.: Rutgers University Press, 1961. Chap. 19.
128. Nelson, R. A., Jr. The Properdin System: Methods of Measurement and Inactivation of

Human Complement Components. Ref. 127, Chap. 20.

129. Nelson, R. A., Jr. An alternative mechanism for the properdin system. *J. Exp. Med.* 108: 515, 1958.
130. Muschel, L. H., Chamberlin, R. H., and Osawa, E. Bactericidal activity of normal serum against bacterial cultures: I. Activity against *Salmonella typhi* strains. *Proc. Soc. Exp. Biol. Med.* 97:376, 1958.
131. Osawa E., and Muschel, L. H. The bactericidal action of normal serum and the properdin system. *J. Immun.* 84:203, 1960.
132. Cowan, K. M. Interpretation of properdin levels determined by phage neutralization technique. *Science* 128:778, 1958.
133. Toussaint, A. J., and Muschel, L. H. Neutralization of bacteriophage by normal serum. *Nature* (London) 183:1825, 1959.
134. Wedgwood, R. J. Antibody requirement for interaction of properdin and bacteria. *Fed. Proc.* 19:79, 1960 (abst.).
135. Blum, L. Evidence for immunological specificity of the properdin system: Demonstration, isolation and properties of a serum factor which interacts with zymosan and other polysaccharides at 0° C. *J. Immun.* 92:61, 1964.
136. Pensky, J., Hinz, C. F., Jr., Todd, E. W., Wedgwood, R. J., and Lepow, I. H. Properties of highly purified human properdin. *Fed. Proc.* 23:505, 1964 (abst.).
137. Todd, E. W., Pillemer, L., and Lepow, I. H. The properdin system and immunity: IX. Studies on the purification of human properdin. *J. Immun.* 83:418, 1959.
138. Lepow, I. H., Pillemer, L., Schoenberg, M. D., Todd, E. W., and Wedgwood, R. J. The properdin system and immunity: X. Characterization of partially purified human properdin. *Ibid.,* p. 428.
139. Pillemer, L., Hinz, C. F., Jr., and Wurz, L. Preparation and properties of antihuman properdin rabbit serum. *Science* 125:1244, 1957.
140. Hinz, C. F., Jr., Wedgwood, R. J., Todd, E. W., and Pillemer, L. The properdin system and immunity: XIV. The injection of human properdin into rabbits and the production of antibodies to properdin. *J. Immun.* 85:547, 1960.

15. Histamine and Other Mediators of Allergic Reactions

K. FRANK AUSTEN *

THE SYMPTOM COMPLEX WHICH APpears immediately after the parenteral administration of antigen into a suitably sensitized animal or man results largely from the discharge of pharmacologically active materials. These are apparently released from a rather small number of cell types, and their action on other cells or tissues, mainly smooth muscle and vascular, produce the symptom complex termed systemic anaphylaxis. The pronounced species variation in this symptom complex resides in a number of factors: the *relative proportion* of the four recognized mediators of the anaphylactic reaction, namely, histamine, slow-reacting substance, serotonin, and plasma kinins; the particular host organ, termed *shock organ,* most susceptible to damage because of a unique distribution or concentration of mediator or smooth muscle; the *sensitivity* or reactivity of host smooth muscle and vascular tissue to each of these mediators; the rate at which each species *degrades* them, and the extent of direct participation by antigen-antibody *complexes.*

Because of the complexity of the systemic anaphylactic reaction, it is difficult to establish securely a definite role for a given mediator in a particular species; it is even more difficult to deny the possible contribution of a potential mediator. Positive evidence would include: an *effective concentration* of the mediator in the shock organ before or as a result of the antigen-antibody interaction; evidence that the mediator is pharmacologically *active* against the shock organ and not merely stored; abolition or significant *suppression* of the consequences of the antigen-antibody interaction by a rather specific inhibitor of the mediator in question or by removal of this mediator from the tissue prior to the antigen-antibody interaction; and finally, but not by itself, the demonstration that the mediator alone or in combination with other alleged mediators *mimics* the anaphylactic reaction in the species under consideration. Results of *in vivo* or *in vitro* studies in which a mediator is *released* from sensitized tissue by antigen-antibody interaction are admissible evidence, especially if the tissue is the shock organ of the species in question.

Although *in vivo* experiments are necessary to establish the role of a given mediator, quantitative experiments which study the mechanism by which the antigen-antibody interaction releases these materials cannot be adequately performed in the whole animal. However, their release *in vitro* from replicate samples of sensitized tissue can be quantitated and has been used to investigate the steps in their release. *In vitro* experiments in which the tissue is thoroughly washed permit a study of the reaction between antigen and antibody fixed to tissue in the absence of gross serum factors. The use of a homogeneous suspension of cells capable of discharging some mediator in the presence of an antigen-antibody interaction further refines the system by eliminating nonparticipating cell types, but it must be kept in mind that such a refinement of the *in vitro* test system may eliminate a cell type which gives rise to an important mediator of the *in vivo* reaction.

This chapter is divided into three parts dealing with (1) the nature of the chemical mediators, (2) the evidence that their release by antigen-antibody interaction is responsible

* Recipient of a research career-development award from the National Institute of Allergy and Infectious Diseases, Bethesda, Md.

for the anaphylactic symptom complex, and (3) the mechanism of their release by antigen-antibody interaction *in vitro*.

PROPERTIES OF THE PHARMACOLOGICAL MEDIATORS

This section is concerned with the nomenclature, structure, tissue location, synthesis, degradation, pharmacology, and physiology of the four recognized mediators of the anaphylactic symptom complex.

HISTAMINE

Histamine (β-imidazolylethylamine) is widely distributed in mammalian tissue [1], but the concentration in a given organ has great species variation. Much of the tissue histamine is associated with the granules of the mast cell [2], and the histamine content per mast cell is reasonably constant in normal tissue, ranging from 7 to 40 μμg. in the dog [3], 21 to 34 in the guinea pig [4], and 10 to 59 in the rat [5, 6]. The mast cells, located mainly in connective tissue in relation to blood vessels [7], are not the only cells containing histamine. Histamine has been found in platelets [8] and in basophilic leukocytes [9, 10]; it is present in high concentration in fetal liver [11] and in the parietal region of the stomach [1] even though mast cells are virtually nonexistent in these sites. Regardless of whether or not the tissue histamine is contained in mast cells, it is formed from L-histidine and degraded either by oxidation or by methylation such that the principal excretion products are imidazoleacetic acid-riboside or 1-methyl imidazoleacetic acid, respectively [12, 13]. Schayer [13] has observed an increase in histidine decarboxylase activity in tissues not necessarily rich in mast cells in response to a variety of nonspecific stimuli and refers to the alleged product of this adaptive enzyme activity as induced histamine to distinguish it from that stored in mast cells.

Some of the established pharmacological actions of histamine include increase of capillary permeability, bronchiolar and other smooth muscle constriction, and stimulation of the glands of exocrine secretion. Despite this diverse activity and its widespread distribution, the physiological role of histamine is not established. It has recently been proposed that *stored histamine* plays an important role in anabolic events such as growth and repair by increasing capillary permeability and stimulating phagocytosis of the mucopolysaccharide contained in the same mast cell population [11, 14], and that *induced histamine,* allegedly synthesized in the cells of the vascular system, is an important regulator of the microcirculation [13]. Much of the data presented for and against a role for histamine depend on the action of antihistamines, which unfortunately are not entirely specific; antihistamines antagonize both acetylcholine and 5-hydroxytryptamine and have a local anesthetic effect [15].

SLOW-REACTING SUBSTANCE

The term slow-reacting substance (SRS) refers to material or materials which contract smooth muscle, usually guinea pig ileum, more slowly than histamine or acetylcholine. Feldberg and Kellaway [16] introduced this term to describe a substance obtained from guinea pig lung during perfusion with cobra venom, and a similar material was subsequently detected in the effluent collected during anaphylactic shock of the same tissue [17]. In both experiments the effluent produced a more prolonged contraction of the guinea pig ileum than was produced by histamine alone. Brocklehurst [18] used antihistamines to abolish the response of the ileum to histamine and obtained direct evidence of the anaphylactic release of a slow-reacting substance, termed SRS-A to indicate that it appeared as a result of antigen-antibody interaction. The chemical properties of the SRS produced by the lecithinase A in cobra venom are consistent with those of an unsaturated fatty acid [19]. The material released from sensitized guinea pig lung by antigen (SRS-A) is also acidic but may not be a true lipid [15, 20]; partially purified SRS-A is highly water-soluble but associates readily with lipids, thereby assuming the solubility characteristics of a lipid.

Evidence has been offered that SRS arises from the mast cells of the rat or guinea pig [21, 22], but there are also compelling data to the contrary. Austen and Humphrey [23] detected no slow-reacting material during reversed anaphylaxis of a suspension of rat peritoneal mast cells even though up to 80 percent of the histamine was released from the cells. The ratio of histamine (μμg.) to SRS (standard units) released by 48/80 or antigen from the perfused cat's paw, isolated guinea pig lung, and isolated rat peritoneal mast cells is, respectively, 5 : 1, 4 : 1, and 240 : 1 [24]. The poor release of SRS relative to histamine from the isolated mast cell preparation favors the view that the source of SRS in the tissues is not the mast cell. Finally, Rapp [25] has found that the intraperitoneal injection of antigen into rats previously passively sensitized by the intraperitoneal administration of rabbit antibody consistently releases large quantities of SRS in the absence of mast cell damage or histamine release.

SRS-A is present in shocked, perfused guinea pig lung and in the effluent therefrom, but only trace amounts are detected in the unshocked tissue and none in the effluent [18]. This would indicate that, in general, SRS-A is formed as well as released by antigen-antibody interaction. In the sensitized guinea pig the major source of SRS-A release has been the lung, but appreciable amounts have also been detected in the aorta and great veins. Antigen-induced release of a slow-reacting material has also been obtained *in vitro* with sensitized rabbit, monkey, and human lung but not with horse or goat lung [18]. The *in vivo* release of a slow-reacting material following antigen-antibody interaction has been demonstrated only in the rat [25]. In contrast to the findings in most species, a slow-reacting substance indistinguishable from SRS-A has been obtained from normal swine lung [26].

SRS-A contracts only a limited number of isolated smooth muscle preparations. These include the guinea pig ileum, rabbit jejunum, fowl rectal cecum, and human bronchiole, but not the rat colon, rat uterus, or bronchiole of the rabbit, dog, or cat [18, 20]. The bronchoconstrictor action of SRS-A in the guinea pig has been demonstrated with isolated tissue and in the whole animal following intravenous injection [27]. This bronchoconstrictor activity can be suppressed by acetylsalicylic acid. SRS-A (guinea pig) administered by aerosol has very limited bronchoconstrictor activity in asthmatic patients and none in normal subjects [28].

SEROTONIN

In mammalian tissue, serotonin (5-hydroxytryptamine) is localized primarily in the mucosal layer of the gastrointestinal tract and to a lesser extent in brain tissue [29]. Species variation in the serotonin content of the remaining organs is marked. Rat, mouse, and rabbit lung contain appreciable amounts of serotonin, whereas it is virtually absent from dog, cat, guinea pig, or human lung [30, 31]. Only the rat and mouse have a significant skin concentration. In the gastrointestinal tract, serotonin is presumably in the enterochromaffin cells [32], while in the skin of the rat and mouse it is contained in the mast cells [33], the concentration in the rat peritoneal mast cell ranging from 0.2 to 6 $\mu\mu$g. per cell [6]. Serotonin is not present in the mast cells of dog, cat, cow, and man [34, 35], but has been identified in the platelets of most species, including horse, ox, goat, dog, guinea pig, and rabbit [36]. Serotonin is derived from the amino acid, tryptophan, by the introduction of a hydroxyl group into the 5 position and decarboxylation [37]; 5-hydroxytryptophan decarboxylase activity has been noted in the mast cells of the rat and mouse [38]. Detoxification by deamination to 5-hydroxyindoleacetic acid is accomplished by amine oxidase, an enzyme present in many tissues [39].

Serotonin increases capillary permeability [40] and constricts smooth muscle [41], but the species variation is great [30, 31, 42]. The smooth muscle of the rat is very sensitive to serotonin and relatively insensitive to histamine, and so the isolated rat colon or estrus rat uterus have been widely used in the bioassay of this material. Pharmacological identification is also facilitated by demonstrating inhibition with small amounts of lysergic acid [43]. The physiological role of serotonin is not clear. There is no convincing evidence that it plays a role in hemostasis [36], and its possible role in central nervous system function and gastrointestinal physiology is still to be elucidated [41].

PLASMA KININS

In 1930, Kraut, Frey, and Werle [44] demonstrated that the intravenous injection of pancreatic extract into dogs produced hypotension and termed the active principle kallikrein. *In vitro* experiments revealed that kallikrein reacted with plasma to form a smooth muscle-stimulating principle, kallidin, from an α-globulin termed kallidinogen [45]. During the same period, Rocha e Silva *et al.* [46] reported that trypsin and some snake venoms also released a hypotensive, smooth muscle-stimulating principle referred to as bradykinin from an α-globulin in plasma. Bradykinin was subsequently shown to be a nonapeptide by degradation studies [47], while kallidin was identified as a decapeptide differing only in the presence of an N-terminal lysine [48]. Synthesis of the nonapeptide [49], bradykinin or kallidin I, and the decapeptide [50], kallidin II, has now been accomplished. Glandular kallikrein, salivary or pancreatic, and urinary kallikrein produce kallidin II, which is converted to kallidin I by an aminopeptidase in plasma whereas plasma kallikrein yields kallidin I directly [48, 51]. The kallidins are rapidly inactivated in plasma by a basic carboxypeptidase which cleaves the peptide bond of the C-terminal arginine [52]. The kallidins and related polypeptides have been grouped under the generic term, plasma kinins [53].

Three enzymes capable of elaborating a permeability-producing factor have been identified in plasma, i.e., plasma kallikrein, plasmin [54], and a permeability-producing globulin activated by dilution, PF/dil [55]. Each is associated with esterase activity against p-toluenesulfonyl-L-arginine methyl ester (TAMe) and is inhibited by diisopropylfluophosphate (DFP) or the trypsin inhibitor from soy beans [51, 56]. Plasmin is distinguished by its marked fibrinolytic and relatively poor kinin-forming activity. The other two would seem to have been separated by chromatographic and electrophoretic differences, kallikrein being a γ-globulin and PF/dil a β-globulin [57]. Margolis [58] demonstrated that the surface-activated factor involved in blood clotting, Hageman factor, is required for the activation of plasma kallikrein, and it seems likely that PF/dil is also a distinct part of the plasma system leading to the elaboration of a kinin [59, 60].

Using the pure nonapeptide, kallidin I or bradykinin, Elliott *et al.* [61] demonstrated five pharmacological activities: smooth muscle stimulation, vasodilatation, increase in capillary permeability, migration of leukocytes, and stimulation of pain fibers. The decapeptide, kallidin II, has similar pharmacological activity which differs in degree depending on the assay [51]. On intravenous administration, both kallidin I and II increase the resistance of the lungs of the anesthetized guinea pig to inflation [62]; this bronchoconstrictor activity is antagonized by analgesic antipyretics, such as acetylsalicylic acid, which exhibit no antagonism against the other pharmacological activities of the kallidins [62]. Kallidin I by aerosol has no bronchoconstrictor effect in the guinea pig or in normal man but does initiate bronchoconstriction in the asthmatic [63]. There is evidence that a physiological role of kallikrein is the mediation of functional vasodilatation in glands [64, 65].

Table 15-1 summarizes some of the properties of the mediators just considered. An important point to keep in mind is that two of them, histamine and serotonin, exist in tissue in their pharmacologically active *final form,* whereas the other two must be *elaborated* as well as released by antigen-antibody interaction.

EVIDENCE OF ROLE OF PHARMACOLOGICAL MEDIATORS IN ANAPHYLAXIS

To be discussed here are the findings *in vivo* and *in vitro* which implicate pharmacological mediators in anaphylactic reactions, each evaluated according to the five criteria noted in the introduction. The species to be considered are guinea pig, rat, mouse, rabbit, dog, and man. The anaphylactic symptom complex peculiar to each species is reviewed briefly under histamine.

HISTAMINE

Guinea Pig. Dyspnea due to acute bronchiolar constriction is the predominant sign of anaphylactic shock in the guinea pig after intravenous challenge with antigen; on post-mortem examination the lungs are found to be markedly distended and bloodless due to acute hyperinflation [66]. The same acute bronchiolar constriction and emphysema can be produced *in vitro* by perfusing the sensitized guinea pig lung with antigen [67] and is associated with the release of histamine [68]. In 1910, Dale and Laidlow [69] pointed out the many resemblances and some differences between histamine shock and anaphylactic shock in the guinea pig, and in 1939 histamine was detected *in vivo* during anaphylaxis in the guinea pig [70]. More recently, Mota and Vugman [71] showed that fatal anaphylaxis in

TABLE 15-1. Pharmacological Mediators

Material	Cell Source	Form	Chemistry	Identification
Histamine	Mast cell Platelet Unknown	Final	Amine	Inhibition by antihistamine
SRS-A	Unknown	Precursor	Acid	Constriction of human bronchiole Resistant to antihistamine Resistant to chymotrypsin Inactive on rat uterus
Serotonin	Enterochromaffin cell Mast cell Platelet	Final	Amine	Contraction of rat uterus Inhibition by lysergic acid Tachyphylaxis of guinea pig ileum
Kallidin I and II	Unknown	Precursor (α-globulin)	Nona- or decapeptide	Contraction of rat uterus Destruction by chymotrypsin

the guinea pig was associated with a pronounced reduction of the stainable mast cell population of the emphysematous lung; emphysema from histamine shock did not diminish the mast cell count, whereas guinea pigs protected against fatal anaphylaxis by antihistamines had degranulation without much emphysema when subsequently killed. Boreus [72, 73] performed quantitative mast cell counts on biopsy specimens of guinea pig nasal mucosa before and after systemic anaphylaxis and observed a gross correlation between the disappearance of stainable mast cells and the intensity of shock. Mast cell degranulation can also be produced *in vitro* by incubating sensitized lung or mesentery with antigen [74]. The data on the release of histamine from the shock organ, *in vivo* or *in vitro* [68, 71], the sensitivity of the guinea pig bronchiole to histamine [42], and protection *in vivo* by antihistamines [71, 75] secure the role of histamine as the principal mediator of the anaphylactic reaction in this species. In general, the actively sensitized guinea pig produces two populations of antibodies of identical molecular weight but different electrophoretic mobility: the γ_1 antibody rather than the γ_2 is responsible for the systemic anaphylactic reaction mediated by histamine [76].

Rat. Circulatory collapse and increased peristaltic activity are prominent during anaphylactic shock in the rat, and the small intestine has been proposed as the shock organ [77, 78]. Systemic anaphylaxis in rats, sensitized by the intraperitoneal injection of various protein antigens, together with killed *Bordetella pertussis* in the smooth phase, is regularly accompanied by generalized mast cell disruption and histamine release [78]. On the other hand, passively sensitized rats pretreated with *B. pertussis* undergo passive systemic anaphylaxis without showing mast cell disruption, even when the antiserum is obtained from a rat actively sensitized with antigen plus *B. pertussis* [79]. Mesentery from rats actively sensitized with antigen plus *B. pertussis* show mast cell disruption when exposed to antigen *in vitro,* whereas mesentery from passively sensitized rats [80] or from rats actively sensitized without *B. pertussis* but with antigen emulsified in Freund's adjuvant [23] do not. Apparently the rat produces at least two types of antibody which can be distinguished in terms of their capacity to produce mast cell sensitization and hemagglutination [81]. By the sixth day after injection of *B. pertussis* vaccine and antigen, the antiserum has the capacity to sensitize rat mast cells *in vitro* or *in vivo* to subsequent antigen-induced histamine release. This capacity disappears from the antiserum as the hemagglutination titer rises with repeated booster doses of antigen.

Antigen-induced histamine release from the small intestine of rats sensitized with *B. pertussis* and antigen has been demonstrated *in vitro* [82]; and animals sensitized in this manner experience mast cell disruption and histamine release *in vivo* following antigen challenge [78]. Such histamine release may contribute to the anaphylactic reaction in the rat but is certainly not critical. Active [5] and passive systemic anaphylaxis [79] occur without mast cell disruption, rat smooth muscle is rather insensitive to histamine, and antihistamines afford little protection even in the animal sensitized with *B. pertussis and antigen* [78, 82].

Mouse. Anaphylaxis in the mouse sensitized with *B. pertussis* and antigen is characterized by respiratory distress [83] and prostration [84], but whether the shock organ is lung or intestine is not established. Local anaphylaxis is associated with mast cell degranulation [85], and an increase in blood and lung histamine has been observed during the systemic reaction [83]. The relative insensitivity of mouse smooth muscle to histamine is somewhat reversed by *B. pertussis* [83], but there is no evidence that the increased reactivity to histamine is sufficient to mark this amine as the principal mediator and the lung the shock organ. Furthermore, antihistamines fail to protect against systemic anaphylaxis [86], and antigen does not release histamine *in vitro* from mouse lung even when histamine is released *in vitro* from skin or intestine [83].

Rabbit. As early as 1911 [87, 88], postmortem data suggested that the anaphylactic circulatory collapse of the rabbit was related to acute dilatation of the right heart. The mechanism of the responsible acute pulmonary hypertension has been repeatedly investigated since then and appears to be a combination of mechanical and pharmacological factors. Histamine has been released into the plasma from sensitized rabbit blood *in vitro* on the addition of antigen [89], and rabbit smooth muscle is responsive to histamine [42]. In the whole animal, anaphylaxis is associated with an increase in plasma histamine, but there is a decrease in total blood histamine due to the deposition of platelet-leukocyte clumps in the lung [90, 91]. Antigen-antibody aggregates have also been identified in the pulmonary capillaries of rabbits experiencing systemic anaphylaxis [92, 93]. Whether trapped antigen-antibody aggregates initiate the formation of the platelet-leukocyte clumps which presumably release their pharmacological contents directly into the pulmonary circulation is unknown; anaphylaxis has been produced in rabbits by soluble antigen-antibody complexes without obvious pulmonary embolization [94]. In view of the combined nature of the insult to the pulmonary circulation which undoubtedly represents the shock organ, it is virtually impossible to evaluate the contribution of a single pharmacological agent such as histamine, and it is not surprising that antihistamines have not proved beneficial [75].

Dog. Circulatory collapse is the predominant clinical manifestation of anaphylaxis in the dog, and a grossly congested liver without stasis in the kidney or spleen is the most striking postmortem finding [95]. If the liver is excluded from the general circulation, the anaphylactic reaction is aborted [96, 97]. That the hepatic veins and liver are the shock organ and histamine is the principal mediator is indicated by a variety of evidence: histamine has been identified in the thoracic duct lymph and peripheral blood during anaphylactic shock in the dog [70, 98]; in comparison with that of other species, dog liver contains a relatively large amount of histamine (8–100 μg./gm.) [1] and the hepatic veins a unique abundance of smooth muscle [99]; histamine can be released from the isolated liver of the sensitized dog by perfusion with antigen [100], and pretreatment with 48/80 so as to reduce liver histamine by more than 40 percent abolishes the anaphylactic reaction to antigen for at least seventeen days [101]. The fact that antihistamines fail to prevent the antigen-induced increase in portal pressure [75] may mean that histamine is not the sole mediator or may merely reflect their limitations.

Man. Severe respiratory distress and profound shock without respiratory difficulty are the two commonest patterns of anaphylactic shock in man. Acute pulmonary emphysema was a striking postmortem finding in the early reviews of this subject [102, 103] and was present in all seven cases of fatal anaphylaxis reported by Vance and Strassman [104]. More recently, Lewis and Austen [105] studied six cases of fatal anaphylaxis in which the interval between injection of antigen and onset of the symptoms leading to death was known. In five, the principal symptom was respiratory, and death was attributed to obstructing laryngeal edema or acute pulmonary emphysema, or both, with the first being more significant in three cases. Circulatory collapse without respiratory symptoms predominated in the sixth case, and on postmortem examination no anatomical cause of death was evident. The assertion in the older literature [106, 107] that anaphylaxis in man resembles not only that of the guinea pig but also that of the rabbit or the dog is not substantiated by review of the available postmortem data; according to Popper [108], man even lacks the muscle bundles in the hepatic veins which make the liver the shock organ in the dog. The respiratory tract, upper or lower, or both, is the commonest shock organ in man, and the extensive involvement of the upper respiratory tract may be an important species characteristic.

Histamine has been released *in vitro* from the white cells or lung tissue of allergic individuals [109, 110], and the human bronchiole is highly sensitive to the histamine released [111]. Insight into the possible role of histamine in *in vivo* anaphylaxis comes from the studies of Lecomte [112, 113] on endogenous histamine release by chemical histamine releasors. The reaction is characterized by pruritus, skin erythema, urticaria, a reduction of blood pressure, a feeling of retrosternal oppression, and angioneurotic edema. Despite a two- to threefold rise in plasma histamine, circulatory collapse was not observed or bronchospasm apparent on physical examination. It is not clear whether the subjective respiratory difficulty was upper or lower respiratory tract in origin. In any event, histamine would seem to account for only some of the manifestations of anaphylaxis in man.

THE OTHER MEDIATORS

Histamine appears to be the principal mediator of the systemic anaphylactic reaction in the guinea pig and dog and an important contributor to the reaction in man. Its role in the rabbit, mouse, and rat is not yet secure, but most probably is not great. Accordingly, it is pertinent to evaluate the possible contribution of the other potential mediators.

Slow-Reacting Substance. Slow-reacting substance (SRS-A) is released *in vitro* by perfusing sensitized guinea pig lung with antigen [17, 18], but there is no evidence that it contributes significantly to the systemic anaphylactic reaction. It has little [27] or no [20] action on the isolated guinea pig bronchiole and fails to increase the resistance of the lungs of the normal anesthetized guinea pig to inflation when given by aerosol, although intravenous administration of SRS-A does produce some increase in resistance [27, 28]. Slow-reacting substance is also released *in vitro* from the sensitized lung of the rabbit [18] or rat [114] and *in vivo* by antigen-antibody interaction in the rat peritoneal cavity [25]. Although rabbit jejunum reacts to guinea pig SRS-A, neither rabbit bronchiole nor the smooth muscles of the rat (bronchiolar, colonic, and uterine) respond to the guinea pig product, and the available data simply do not permit judgment as to the possible role of SRS in the anaphylactic reaction of these two species. There are no data on antigen-induced SRS in the mouse or dog.

Brocklehurst [18, 115] has demonstrated the release of SRS from perfused segments of lung of two pollen-sensitive individuals and from a bronchial ring preparation which contracted in response to the specific antigen. In addition, human bronchiolar tissue is the only bronchiolar tissue known to be very sensitive to guinea pig SRS-A [20]. However, crude guinea pig SRS-A administered by aerosol has no effect in normal man and only limited bronchoconstrictor action in the asthmatic [28]. A judgment as to the role of SRS in antigen-induced bronchoconstriction in man is premature in the absence of a specific inhibitor and while the only test material available is the crude guinea pig product. The activity of the guinea pig material in the asthmatic is also not informative inasmuch as the asthmatic bronchiole is hyperactive to a variety of pharmacological agents [116].

Serotonin. There are no compelling data to implicate serotonin in the anaphylactic reaction of guinea pig, dog, or man, and the extent of its contribution to the reaction in the rabbit cannot be specified. Serotonin constricts the guinea pig bronchiole *in vitro* [42] or *in vivo* [117], but the concentration of serotonin in the guinea pig lung is negligible [31]; serotonin has not been identified in the effluent from perfused, shocked lung *in vitro*

[20], and lysergic acid diethylamide has no protective effect in systemic anaphylaxis [117]. Although the dog liver contains an appreciable concentration of serotonin, neither systemic anaphylaxis nor the addition of antigen to sensitized dog liver *in vitro* releases serotonin [101]. Human lung contains virtually no serotonin, and the mast cells of man, like those of most other species, are devoid of this amine. The isolated human bronchiole is resistant to serotonin [42], and inhalation by aerosol has no effect in normal man [117]; the bronchoconstrictor action of the aerosol in some asthmatics [117] merely reflects the general hyperactivity of the asthmatic bronchiole. Rabbit lung has an appreciable serotonin concentration [31] which increases during systemic anaphylaxis due to the deposition of platelet-leukocyte clumps [90, 91]; simultaneously, there is a fall in total blood serotonin and an increment in plasma serotonin. Serotonin has also been released *in vitro* from rabbit platelets by antigen-antibody interaction [8]. The sensitivity of the rabbit pulmonary vasculature to serotonin is unknown, but the bronchial smooth muscle is rather resistant [42]. Serotonin depletion by reserpine administration does not ameliorate the anaphylactic reaction in the rabbit [118], and the contribution of serotonin, if any, is not proved.

In the rat and mouse there are data to implicate serotonin as a significant mediator of the anaphylactic reaction. Rat smooth muscle (bronchiole, uterus, colon) and connective tissue are very susceptible to the contractile and permeability-increasing effects of serotonin [40, 42, 119]. Benditt *et al.* [120] have observed a marked increase in intestinal capillary permeability during rat anaphylaxis, particularly in relation to the distribution of the enterochromaffin cells, presumed to contain serotonin, and serotonin has been released from the sensitized ileum *in vitro* on exposure to antigen [82]. The combination of 2-bromolysergic acid and an antihistamine has been reported to be ineffective against systemic anaphylaxis in the rat [121], minimally effective [78], and substantially protective [82]. Since the protected rats [82] exhibited much less hemorrhage in the small intestine, the apparent shock organ, than controls dying of anaphylaxis, it may well be that serotonin plays a significant role.

Serotonin has also been implicated in anaphylaxis in the mouse. This is based on protection studies with lysergic acid [122], with reserpine, which releases the serotonin from tissue prior to antigenic challenge [84, 122], and with 3, 4-dihydroxyphenyl-1-α-methylalanine (methyl DOPA), which prevents serotonin synthesis [84]. The reserpine protection was associated with depletion of chromaffin material in the enterochromaffin cells of the bowel, and a similar depletion was characteristic of the systemic anaphylactic reaction, suggesting that material from this site, presumably serotonin, mediated the reaction [84]. This view is supported by the release of serotonin *in vitro* from the intestine of the sensitized mouse on the addition of antigen [83]. On the negative side has been the failure to find a change in the intestinal content of serotonin or an increase in blood or lung serotonin as a result of systemic anaphylaxis [83].

Plasma kinin. Kinin activity has been identified in the plasma of the dog [123], guinea pig, rat, and rabbit [124] in association with anaphylactic shock; and in the guinea pig and rabbit, the plasma substrate from which kinin is formed has been shown to be depleted [125, 126]. Nonetheless, the contribution of kinin activity to the anaphylactic symptom complex even in these four species remains to be established. In the dog, the magnitude of the kinin activity does not correlate well with the severity of the shock [123]. A kinin-forming enzyme has been released *in vitro* from perfused, shocked guinea pig lung [124], and intravenous administration of kallidin I or II does increase the resistance of the lung of the anesthetized guinea pig to inflation [62]; however, kallidin has no bronchoconstrictor activity in the guinea pig when given by aerosol. Kallidin I by aerosol has no action in normal man, and the response of the asthmatic [63] may well be nonspecific. The protective action of ϵ-amino caproic acid against anaphylaxis in the mouse has been attributed to the prevention of kinin elaboration [127], but the specificity of this inhibitor for this system is not established.

The kinins not only merit consideration in regard to the well-recognized patterns of anaphylaxis already examined in detail but must be considered in reference to the occasional reaction in man characterized by vascular collapse without respiratory distress and the so-called protracted shock syndrome in the guinea pig [128]. If a large amount of antigen is deposited subcutaneously, the sensitized guinea pig does not experience respiratory distress; instead, shock is protracted over many hours and leads to death. On postmortem examination the lungs are not distended, but the abdominal viscera reveal marked hyperemia and hemorrhages. Antihistamines are of no benefit, and this reaction pattern has been shown to be associated with appreciable kinin formation [124].

Table 15-2 summarizes the data on the *in vitro* and *in vivo* release of pharmacological mediators just presented. *In vitro* release does not necessarily refer to the shock organ. There is still much to be learned about the relative contribution of these mediators in a particular species, and there are no secure data which would move SRS-A or kinin into the column with primary or contributory mediators. Still other mediators may yet be recognized. Nor are there firm data to indicate that acetylcholine and heparin merit consideration as mediators. Acetylcholine has not been detected in the effluent from perfused shocked guinea pig lung [15] or heart [129], and the small amount released from the shocked ileum has not been considered significant [130]. The incoagulability of dog blood during anaphylactic shock has been recognized since 1909, and the responsible material, heparin, was isolated from the blood in crystalline form in 1941 [131], but it does not seem to contribute to the severity of the reaction in this species.

MECHANISM OF RELEASE OF PHARMACOLOGICAL MEDIATORS

The available information on the mechanism whereby antigen-antibody interaction releases the mediators of the anaphylactic reaction from tissue or cells *in vitro* has been reviewed in detail by Austen and Humphrey [132]. Only four tissue or cell systems have received appreciable attention, namely, chopped guinea pig lung, rat mesentery or peritoneal mast cells, rabbit platelets, and human leukocytes. In each instance, histamine release has been of primary concern; there are only meager data on the mechanism of release of serotonin from rabbit platelets [8] or SRS-A from guinea pig lung [133–135] and none on the elaboration of plasma kinin. In general, the findings with these four systems have been remarkably similar and support the assumption that despite species variation in the anaphylactic symptom complex, the mecha-

TABLE 15-2. Evidence of Role of Pharmacological Mediators in Anaphylaxis

Species	Shock Organ	Release of Mediator		Role of Mediator	
		In vitro	In vivo	Primary	Contributory
Guinea pig	Lung (bronchioles)	Histamine SRS-A Serotonin Kinin	Histamine Kinin	Histamine	
Rat	Intestine	Histamine SRS Serotonin	Histamine SRS Kinin		Serotonin
Mouse	Intestine/lung	Histamine Serotonin	Histamine		Serotonin
Rabbit	Heart (pulmonary vasculature)	Histamine SRS Serotonin	Histamine Serotonin Kinin		Histamine Serotonin AgAb aggregate
Dog	Hepatic (hepatic vein)	Histamine	Histamine Kinin	Histamine	
Man	Lung (bronchiole) and/or larynx Unknown	Histamine SRS			Histamine

nism whereby the mediators are released is basically the same. Since antigen-induced histamine release has been most extensively investigated in chopped guinea pig lung and the lung does represent the shock organ in this species, it seems appropriate to summarize the known characteristics of the reaction in this tissue.

The mechanism required for the *in vitro* anaphylactic release of histamine from perfused, chopped, guinea pig lung has the following characteristics: The reaction specifically requires calcium ion [136], has a pH optimum of 7.5 to 7.9 [136], and is very sensitive to the ionic strength of the containing medium [137]. The reaction proceeds optimally at 38 to 40° C. and requires a heat-labile tissue factor which is irreversibly inactivated at 45° C. [138]. The reaction does not require cytochrome-mediated aerobic metabolism [137], but is prevented by the combination of anoxia and glucose lack [139] or by thiol alkylating or oxidizing agents [134, 140], implying a need for the glycolytic pathway. The reaction involves activation of an esterase which can be inhibited by DFP [141]. The reaction is inhibited by synthetic substrates of chymotrypsin [134]. It is markedly influenced by compounds normally present in mammalian tissue—certain dibasic acids, succinic or maleic, produce enhancement while the monobasic fatty acids from valeric to dodecanoic are inhibitory [135]. The reaction is not augmented in any manner by the presence of fresh guinea pig serum. By no permissible stretch of the imagination can these findings be integrated into a unified reaction scheme at present, but they do imply that antigen-induced histamine release involves the activation and participation of one or more enzymatic activities.

Calcium ion is required for antigen-induced histamine release from guinea pig lung [136], rat mesentery [80] or mast cells [5], rabbit platelets [8], and human leukocytes [142], and there is some evidence that the calcium-dependent step follows immediately upon the antigen-antibody interaction. The ileum of the sensitized guinea pig fails to respond to antigen *in vitro* when suspended in a calcium-free buffer [143] but will contract without further addition of antigen if the tissue is washed and placed in a calcium-containing buffer within the next thirty minutes. Lack of calcium ion apparently does not prevent antigen-antibody interaction but does block the activation of some, presumably intermediate, subsequent step.

The anaphylactic release of histamine from guinea pig lung [138], rat mesentery [80], and human leukocytes [144] is abolished by preheating the tissue or cells at 45° C. Of equal interest is the finding that exposure of guinea pig lung [138] or rat mast cells [5] to the antigen-antibody interaction at 17° C. produces no histamine release until the reaction mixture is warmed; the longer the tissue or cells are held at 17° C., the less the histamine release on warming back to 37° C. Apparently at 17° C. the antigen-antibody interaction activates a factor, possibly enzymatic, which, though unable to act at that temperature, can be dissipated.

The conclusion that cytochrome-mediated aerobic metabolism is not a prerequisite of antigen-induced histamine release is based on the failure of carbon monoxide to inhibit it [137] and on the observation that anoxia due to a nitrogen atmosphere is not inhibitory unless glucose is lacking from the buffer [139]. Whether the ability of glucose to reverse anoxic inhibition depends on some energy requirement met by the glycolytic pathway is not known; however, a requirement for an intact glycolytic pathway would also explain the irreversible inhibition produced by the thiol alkylating and oxidizing agents.

DFP prevents antigen-induced histamine release by blocking an antigen-antibody activated esterase which exists in tissue in a DFP-resistant precursor state until its activation by the antigen-antibody interaction [134, 141]. DFP prevents the anaphylactic release of histamine from guinea pig lung [134], rat mast cells [23], human leukocytes [145], and rabbit platelets [146], but there is insufficient evidence to conclude that the same esterase is involved in each reaction. In the guinea pig lung, antigen-induced histamine release is prevented by synthetic ester substrates of chymotrypsin but not by substrates of the other peptidases [134]. However, recent evidence indicates that DFP and the chymotrypsin substrates block at different sites in the reaction sequence [147, 148].

In vitro anaphylactic histamine release occurs readily with well-washed guinea pig lung [18] and with human white cells [142], and there is no evidence of an absolute requirement of free serum factors. Reversed anaphylaxis of the rat peritoneal mast cell suspension occurs in the absence of fresh serum but is strikingly enhanced by its presence [5]; this enhancement is abolished if the serum is heated at 56° C. for thirty minutes or "decomplemented" by serial absorption with a preformed immune aggregate [148]. The release of histamine from rabbit platelets has an absolute serum or plasma requirement [8], but its identity with serum complement has not been established [149]. The fact that some *in vitro* systems do not require gross serum factors or are not enhanced by them does not exclude the possibility that complement factors in part or in the whole are already present in or on the tissue. An alternative to the concept of "tissue complement," adsorbed or manufactured therein, arises from recent studies demonstrating that the guinea pig produces two populations of antibodies capable of mediating recognizable cell damage on interaction with the same antigen. The interaction of the γ_2 antibody with antigen activates the complement sequence, producing immune hemolysis, but the same aggregation will not release histamine from guinea pig mast cells; γ_1 antibody will sensitize guinea pig mast cells so that subsequent interaction with antigen releases histamine but will not activate the complement sequence [76, 150, 151]. Since both immune hemolysis and histamine release are blocked by DFP and involve an antigen-antibody activated enzyme sequence(s), it may well be that variation in the gross serum requirements for *in vitro* histamine release merely reflects different biological capabilities of the antibody involved. Using the phosphonate series of inhibitors, Becker and Austen [147, 148] have recently concluded that the organophosphorus inhibitable, antigen-antibody activated esterases, respectively involved in the guinea pig complement and histamine-releasing sequence, are similar but not identical. Thus physiochemically different antibodies, guinea pig γ_1 and γ_2, reacting with the same antigen, initiate different enzyme sequences leading respectively to cytotoxic (complement-dependent) and anaphylactic immune injury.

REFERENCES

1. Feldberg, W. Distribution of Histamine in the Body. In Wolstenholme, G. E. W., and O'Connor, C. M. (Eds.), *Histamine.* Boston: Little, Brown, 1956.
2. Riley, J. F., and West, G. B. The presence of histamine in tissue mast cells. *J. Physiol.* 120: 528, 1953.
3. Graham, H. T., Lowry, O. H., Wahl, N., and Priebat, M. K. Mast cells as sources of tissue histamine. *J. Exp. Med.* 102:307, 1955.
4. Boreus, L. O., and Chakravarty, N. The histamine content of guinea pig mast cells. *Experimentia* 16:1, 1960.
5. Humphrey, J. H., Austen, K. F., and Rapp, H. J. *In vitro* studies of reversed anaphylaxis with rat cells. *Immunology* 6:226, 1963.
6. Moran, N. C., Uvnas, B., and Westerholm, B. Release of 5-hydroxytryptamine and histamine from rat mast cells. *Acta Physiol. Scand.* 56:26, 1962.
7. Riley, J. F. The effects of histamine-liberators on the mast cells of the rat. *J. Path. Bact.* 65:471, 1953.
8. Humphrey, J. H., and Jaques, R. The release of histamine and 5-hydroxytryptamine (serotonin) from platelets by antigen-antibody reactions (*in vitro*). *J. Physiol.* 128:9, 1955.
9. Graham, H. T., Wheelwright, F., Parish, H. H., Marks, A. R., and Lowry, O. H. Distribution of histamine among the blood elements. *Fed. Proc.* 11:350, 1952 (abst.).
10. VanArsdel, P. P., Middleton, E., Sherman, W. B., and Buchwald, H. Quantitative study on the *in vitro* release of histamine from leukocytes of atopic persons. *J. Allerg.* 29:429, 1958.
11. Kahlson, G. A place for histamine in normal physiology. *Lancet* 1:67, 1960.
12. Schayer, R. W. Catabolism of physiological quantities of histamine *in vivo. Physiol. Rev.* 39:116, 1959.
13. Schayer, R. W. Histidine decarboxylase in mast cells. *Ann. N.Y. Acad. Sci.* 103:164, 1963.
14. Riley, J. F. Functional significance of histamine and heparin in tissue mast cells. *Ibid.,* p. 164.
15. Brocklehurst, W. E. Pharmacological Mediators of Hypersensitivity Reactions. In Gell, P. G. H., and Coombs, R. R. A. *Clinical Aspects of Immunology.* Philadelphia: F. A. Davis Company, 1963.
16. Feldberg, W., and Kellaway, C. H. Liberation of histamine and formation of a lysocithin-like substance by cobra venom. *J. Physiol.* (London) 94:187, 1938.

17. Kellaway, C. H., and Trethewie, E. R. The liberation of a slow-reacting smooth muscle stimulating substance in anaphylaxis. *Quart. J. Exp. Physiol.* 30:121, 1940.
18. Brocklehurst, W. E. The release of histamine and formation of a slow-reacting substance (SRS-A) during anaphylactic shock. *J. Physiol.* (London) 151:416, 1960.
19. Vogt, W. Naturally occurring lipid-soluble acids of pharmacological interest. *Pharmacol. Rev.* 10:407, 1958.
20. Brocklehurst, W. E. Slow reacting substance and related compounds. *Progr. Allerg.* 6:539, 1962.
21. Uvnas, B., and Thon, I. Isolation of biologically intact mast cells. *Exp. Cell Res.* 18:512, 1959.
22. Boreus, L. O., and Chakravarty, N. Tissue mast cells, histamine, and slow reacting substance in anaphylactic reaction in guinea pig. *Acta Physiol. Scand.* 48:315, 1960.
23. Austen, K. F., and Humphrey, J. H. Mechanism of the Anaphylactic Release of Histamine and Slow Reacting Substance. In Grabar, P., and Miescher, P. (Eds.), *Mechanism of Cell and Tissue Damage Produced by Immune Reactions.* Basel: Benno Schwabe & Co., 1962.
24. Uvnas, B. Lipid spasmogens appearing in connection with histamine liberation. *Biochem. Pharmacol.* 12:439, 1963.
25. Rapp, H. J. The release of a slow reacting substance (SRS) in the peritoneal cavity of rats by antigen-antibody interaction. *J. Physiol.* (London) 158:35P, 1961.
26. Linn, B. O., Shunk, C. H., Folkers, K., Ganley, O., and Robinson, H. J. SRS-S concentrates from normal swine lung without anaphylaxis. *Biochem. Pharmacol.* 8:339, 1961.
27. Berry, P. A., Collier, H. O. J., and Holgate, J. A. Bronchoconstrictor action *in vivo* of slow reacting substance (SRS-A) in anaphylaxis and its antagonism. *J. Physiol.* (London) 165: 71P, 1963.
28. Herxheimer, H., and Stresemann, E. The effect of slow reacting substance (SRS-A) in guinea pigs and in asthmatic patients. *Ibid.,* p. 78P.
29. Erspamer, V. Pharmacology of indolealkylamines. *Pharmacol. Rev.* 6:425, 1954.
30. Parratt, J. R., and West, G. B. 5-Hydroxytryptamine and tissue mast cells. *J. Physiol.* (London) 137:169, 1957.
31. Udenfriend, S., and Waalkes, T. P. On the Role of Serotonin in Anaphylaxis. In Shaffer, J. H., Lo Grippo, G. A., and Chase, M. W. (Eds.), *Mechanisms of Hypersensitivity.* Boston: Little, Brown, 1959.
32. Benditt, E. P., and Wong, R. L. On the concentration of 5-hydroxytryptamine in mammalian enterochromaffin cells and its release by reserpine. *J. Exp. Med.* 105:509, 1957.
33. Benditt, E. P., Wong, R. L., Arase, M., and Roeper, E. 5-Hydroxytryptamine in mast cells. *Proc. Soc. Exp. Biol. Med.* 90:303, 1955.
34. Sjoerdsma, A., Waalkes, T. P., and Weissbach, H. Serotonin and histamine in mast cells. *Science* 125:1202, 1957.
35. West, G. B. Tissue mast cells and tissue amines. *J. Pharm. Pharmacol.* 11:513, 1959.
36. Zucker, M. B. Serotonin (5-hydroxytryptamine): Hematologic aspects. *Progr. Hemat.* 2:206, 1959.
37. Clark, C. T., Weissbach, H., and Udenfriend, S. 5-HT decarboxylase: preparation and properties. *J. Biol. Chem.* 210:139, 1955.
38. Lagunoff, D., and Benditt, E. P. 5-Hydroxytryptophan decarboxylase activity in rat mast cells. *Amer. J. Physiol.* 196:993, 1959.
39. Udenfriend, S., Titus, E., Weissbach, H., and Peterson, R. E. Biogenesis and metabolism of 5-hydroxyindole compounds. *J. Biol. Chem.* 219:335, 1956.
40. Rowley, D. A., and Benditt, E. P. 5-Hydroxytryptamine and histamine as mediators of the vascular injury produced by agents which damage mast cells in rats. *J. Exp. Med.* 103: 399, 1956.
41. Page, I. H. Serotonin (5-Hydroxytryptamine): The last four years. *Physiol. Rev.* 38: 277, 1958.
42. Brocklehurst, W. E. The Action of 5-Hydroxytryptamine on Smooth Muscle. In Lewis, G. P. (Ed.), *5-Hydroxytryptamine.* New York: Pergamon Press, 1958.
43. Gaddum, J. H., and Hameed, K.A. Drugs which antagonize 5-HT. *Brit. J. Pharmacol.* 9: 240, 1954.
44. Kraut, H., Frey, E. K., and Werle, E. Der Nachweis eines Kreislaufhormons in der Pankreasdrüse: IV. Mitteilung uber dieses Kreislaufhormon. *Z. Physiol. Chem.* 189:97, 1930.
45. Werle, E. The Chemistry and Pharmacology of Kallikrein and Kallidin. In Gaddum, J. H. (Ed.), *Polypeptides Which Stimulate Plain Muscle.* Edinburgh: E. & S. Livingstone, Ltd., 1955.
46. Rocha e Silva, M., Beraldo, W. T., and Rosenfield, G. Bradykinin, a hypotensive and smooth muscle stimulating factor released from plasma globulin by snake venoms and by trypsin. *Amer. J. Physiol.* 156:261, 1949.
47. Elliot, D. F., Lewis, G. P., and Horton, E. W. The structure of bradykinin—a plasma kinin from ox blood. *Biochem. Biophys. Res. Commun.* 3:87, 1960.
48. Pierce, J. V., and Webster, M. E. Human plasma kallidins: Isolation and chemical studies. *Biochem. Biophys. Res. Commun.* 5:353, 1961.
49. Boissonnas, R. A., Guttmann, St., and Jaquenoud, P. A. Synthèse de la L-arginyl-L-prolyl-L-prolyl-glycyl-L-phénylalanyl-L-seryl-L-prolyl-

phénylalanyl-L-arginine, un nonapeptide présentant les propriétés de la bradykinine. *Helv. Chim. Acta* 43:1349, 1960.
50. Nicolaides, E. D., Dewald, H. A., and McCarthy, D. A. The synthesis of a biologically active decapeptide having the structure proposed for kallidin II. *Biochem. Biophys. Res. Commun.* 6:210, 1961.
51. Webster, M. E., and Pierce, J. V. The nature of the kallidins released from human plasma by kallikreins and other enzymes. *Ann. N.Y. Acad. Sci.* 104:91, 1963.
52. Erdos, E. G., Renfrew, A. G., Sloane, E. M., and Wohler, J. R. Enzymatic studies on bradykinin and similar peptides. *Ibid.*, p. 222.
53. Elliot, D. F. Introductory remarks. *Ibid.*, p. 4.
54. Lewis, G. P. Formation of plasma kinin by plasmin. *J. Physiol.* (London) 140:285, 1958.
55. Mackay, M. E., Miles, A. A., Shachter, C. B. E., and Wilhelm, D. L. Susceptibility of the guinea pig to pharmacological factors in its own serum. *Nature* (London) 172:714, 1953.
56. Webster, M. E., and Pierce, J. V. Action of the kallikreins on synthetic ester substrates. *Proc. Soc. Exp. Biol. Med.* 107:186, 1961.
57. Kagen, L. J., Leddy, J. P., and Becker, E. L. The presence of two permeability globulins in human serum. *J. Clin. Invest.* 42:1353, 1963.
58. Margolis, J. The interrelationship of coagulation of plasma and the release of peptides. *Ann. N.Y. Acad. Sci.* 104:133, 1963.
59. Mason, B., and Miles, A. A. Globulin permeability factors without kininogenase activity. *Nature* (London) 196:587, 1962.
60. Webster, M. E., and Ratnoff, O. D. Role of Hageman factor in the activation of vasodilator activity in human plasma. *Nature* (London) 192:180, 1961.
61. Elliot, D. F., Horton, E. W., and Lewis, G. P. Actions of pure bradykinin. *J. Physiol.* (London) 153:473, 1960.
62. Collier, H. O. J. The action and antagonism of kinins on bronchioles. *Ann. N.Y. Acad. Sci.* 104:290, 1963.
63. Herxheimer, H., and Stresemann, E. The effect of bradykinin aerosol in guinea pigs and in man. *J. Physiol.* (London) 158:38P, 1961.
64. Lewis, G. P. Pharmacological actions of bradykinin and its role in physiological and pathological reactions. *Ann. N.Y. Acad. Sci.* 104: 236, 1963.
65. Hilton, S. M. A discussion of the evidence for kinins as the agents of vasodilator reactions. *Ibid.*, p. 275.
66. Auer, J., and Lewis, P. A. The physiology of the immediate reaction of anaphylaxis in the guinea pig. *J. Exp. Med.* 12:151, 1912.
67. Dale, H. H. The anaphylactic reaction of plain muscle in the guinea pig. *J. Pharmacol. Exp. Ther.* 4:167, 1912.
68. Bartosch, R., Feldberg, W., and Nagel, E. Das Freiwerden eines histaminähnlichen Stoffes bei der Anaphylaxie des Meerschweinchens. *Pflueger. Arch. Ges. Physiol.* 230:129, 1932.
69. Dale, H. H., and Laidlaw, P. P. The physiological action of B iminazolyl ethylamine. *J. Physiol.* (London) 41:318, 1910.
70. Code, C. F. The histamine content of the blood of guinea pigs and dogs during anaphylactic shock. *Amer. J. Physiol.* 127:78, 1939.
71. Mota, I., and Vugman, I. Effects of anaphylactic shock and compound 48/80 on the mast cells of the guinea pig lung. *Nature* (London) 177:427, 1956.
72. Boreus, L. O. Quantitative studies on the anaphylactic mast cell reaction *in vivo* in the guinea pig. *Acta Physiol. Scand.* 48:431, 1960.
73. Boreus, L. O. A study of the anaphylactic mast-cell reaction *in vivo* following desensitization of sensitized guinea pigs. *Acta Physiol. Scand.* 50:375, 1960.
74. Mota, I. Effect of antigen and octylamine on mast cells and histamine content of sensitized guinea-pig tissues. *J. Physiol.* (London) 147:425, 1959.
75. Reuse, J. J. Antihistamine Drugs and Histamine Release, Especially in Anaphylaxis. Ref. 1.
76. Ovary, Z., Benacerraf, B., and Bloch, K. Properties of guinea pig 7S antibodies: II. Identification of antibodies involved in passive cutaneous and systemic anaphylaxis. *J. Exp. Med.* 117:951,1963.
77. West, G. B. Some factors involved in anaphylactic shock. *Int. Arch. Allerg.* 15:231, 1959.
78. Mota, I. Mast cells and anaphylaxis. *Ann. N.Y. Acad. Sci.* 103:264, 1963.
79. Mota, I. Failure of rat and rabbit antiserum to passively sensitize normal and pertussis-treated rats and mice so as to induce mast cell damage and histamine release on later contact with antigen. *Immunology* 5:11, 1962.
80. Mota, I., and Ishii, T. Inhibition of mast cell disruption and histamine release in rat anaphylaxis *in vitro:* Comparison with compound 48/80 *Brit. J. Pharmacol.* 15:82, 1960.
81. Mota, I. Biol. characterization of "mast cell sensitizing" antibodies. *Life Sci.* 7:465, 1963.
82. Garcia-Arocha, H. Liberation of 5-hydroxytryptamine and histamine in the anaphylactic reaction of the rat. *Canad. J. Biochem. Physiol.* 39:403, 1961.
83. Waalkes, T. P., and Coburn, H. The role of histamine and serotonin during anaphylaxis in the mouse. *J. Allerg.* 31:151, 1960.
84. Gershon, M. D., and Ross, L. L. Studies on the relationship of 5-hydroxytryptamine and the enterochromaffin cell to anaphylactic shock in mice. *J. Exp. Med.* 115:367, 1962.
85. Carter, P. B., Higginbotham, R. D., and

Dougherty, T. J. The local response of tissue mast cells to antigen in sensitized mice. *J. Immun.* 79:259, 1957.
86. Malkiel, S., and Hargis, B. J. Anaphylactic shock in the pertussis-vaccinated mouse. *J. Allerg.* 23:352, 1952.
87. Auer, J. Lethal cardiac anaphylaxis in the rabbit. *J. Exp. Med.* 14:476, 1911.
88. Scott, W. H. Anaphylaxis in the rabbit: The mechanism of the symptoms. *J. Path. Bact.* 15: 31, 1911.
89. Katz, G. Histamine release from blood cells in anaphylaxis *in vitro. Science* 91:221, 1940.
90. Waalkes, T. P., Weissbach, H., Bozicevich, J., and Udenfriend, S. Serotonin and histamine release during anaphylaxis in the rabbit. *J. Clin. Invest.* 36:1115, 1957.
91. Waalkes, T. P., and Coburn, H. The role of platelets and the release of serotonin and histamine during anaphylaxis in the rabbit. *J. Allerg.* 30:394, 1959.
92. Dixon, F. J. The use of I^{131} in immunologic investigations. *J. Allerg.* 24:547, 1953.
93. McKinnon, G. E., Andrews, E. C., Heptinstall, R. H., and Germuth, F. G. An immunohistologic study on the occurrence of intravascular antigen-antibody precipitation and its role in anaphylaxis in the rabbit. *Bull. Hopkins Hosp.* 101:258, 1957.
94. Weigle, W. O., Cochrane, C. G., and Dixon, F. J. Anaphylactogenic properties of soluble antigen-antibody complexes in the guinea pig and rabbit. *J. Immun.* 85:469, 1960.
95. Pearce, R. M., and Eisenbrey, A. B. The physiology of anaphylactic shock in the dog. *J. Infect. Dis.* 7:565, 1910.
96. Manwaring, W. H. Serophysiologische Untersuchungen: I. Der physiologische Mechanismus des anaphylaktischen Shocks. *Z. Immunitaetsforsch* 8:1, 1910.
97. Voegtlin, C., and Bernheim, B. M. The liver in its relation to anaphylactic shock. *J. Pharmacol. Exp. Therap.* 2:507, 1911.
98. Dragstedt, C. A., and Gebauer-Fuelnegg, E. Studies in anaphylaxis: The appearance of a physiologically active substance during anaphylactic shock. *Amer. J. Physiol.* 102:512, 1932.
99. Arey, L. B., and Simonds, J. P. The relation of the smooth muscle in the hepatic veins to shock phenomena. *Anat. Rec.* 18:219, 1920.
100. Scroggie, A. E., and Jaques, L. B. The release of histamine and heparin by antigen from the isolated perfused liver of the sensitized dog. *J. Immun.* 62:103, 1949.
101. Akcasu, A., and West, G. B. Anaphylaxis in the dog. *Int. Arch. Allerg.* 16:326, 1960.
102. Lamson, R. W. Sudden death associated with the injection of foreign substances. *J.A.M.A.* 82:1091, 1924.
103 Scheppe, W. M. Fatal anaphylaxis in man. *J. Lab. Clin. Med.* 16:372, 1930.
104. Vance, B. M., and Strassman, G. Sudden death following injection of foreign protein. *Arch. Path.* 34:849, 1942.
105. Lewis, J. P., and Austen, K. F. Fatal systemic anaphylaxis in man. *New Eng. J. Med.* 270: 597, 1964.
106. Dean, H. R. The histology of a case of anaphylactic shock occurring in man. *J. Path. Bact.* 25:305, 1922.
107. Rocha e Silva, M. *Histamine—Its Role in Anaphylaxis and Allergy.* Springfield, Ill.: Charles C Thomas, Publisher, 1955.
108. Popper, H. Über Drosselvorrichtungen an Lebervenen. *Klin. Wschr.* 10:2129, 1931.
109. Katz, G., and Cohen, S. Experimental evidence of histamine release in allergy. *J.A.M.A.* 117:1782,1941.
110. Schild, H. O., Hawkins, D. F., Mongar, J. L., and Herxheimer, H. Reactions of isolated human asthmatic lung and bronchial tissue to a specific antigen. *Lancet* 2:376, 1951.
111. Schild, H. O. Histamine Release and Anaphylaxis. Ref. 1.
112. Lecomte, J. Endogenous Histamine Liberation in Man. Ref. 1.
113. Lecomte, J. Liberation of endogenous histamine in man. *J. Allerg.* 28:102, 1957.
114. Chakravarty, N. Observations on Histamine Release and Formation of a Lipid-soluble Smooth-muscle Stimulating Principle (SRS) by Antigen-Antibody Reaction and Compound 48/80. Karolinska Institute, Stockholm, Academic Thesis, 1959.
115. Brocklehurst, W. E. A Slow Reacting Substance in Anaphylaxis-SRS-A. Ref. 1.
116. Curry, J. J., and Lowell, F. C. Measurement of vital capacity in asthmatic subjects receiving histamine and acetyl-beta-methyl-choline: A clinical study. *J. Allerg.* 19:9, 1948.
117. Herxheimer, H. The 5-hydroxytryptamine shock in the guinea pig. *J. Physiol.* (London) 128:435, 1955.
118. Fisher, P., and Lecomte, J. Choc anaphylactique chez le lapin traité par réserpine. *C. R. Soc. Biol.* (Paris) 150:1026, 1956.
119. Sparrow, E. M., and Wilhelm, D. L. Species differences in susceptibility to capillary permeability factors, histamine, 5-hydroxytryptamine, and 48/80. *J. Physiol.* (London) 137:51, 1957.
120. Benditt, E. P., Holcenberg, J., and Lagunoff, D. The role of serotonin (5-hydroxytryptamine) in mast cells. *Ann. N.Y. Acad. Sci.* 103:179, 1963.
121. Sanyal, R. K., and West, G. B. The relationship of histamine and 5-hydroxytryptamine to anaphylactic shock in different species. *J. Physiol.* (London) 144:525, 1958.
122. Fox, C. L., Einbinder, J. M., and Nelson,

C. T. Comparative inhibition of anaphylaxis in mice by steroids, tranquilizers, and other drugs. *Amer. J. Physiol.* 193:241, 1958.

123. Beraldo, W. T. Formation of bradykinin in anaphylactic and peptone shock. *Amer. J. Physiol.* 163:283, 1950.
124. Brocklehurst, W. E., and Lahiri, S. C. The production of bradykinin in anaphylaxis. *J. Physiol.* (London) 160:15P, 1962.
125. Brocklehurst, W. E., and Lahiri, S. C. Formation and destruction of bradykinin during anaphylaxis. *J. Physiol.* (London) 165:39P, 1963.
126. Diniz, C. R., and Carvalho, I. F. A micromethod for determination of bradykinogen under several conditions. *Ann. N.Y. Acad. Sci.* 104:77, 1963.
127. Zweifach, B. W., Nagler, A. L., and Troll, W. Some effects of proteolytic inhibitors on tissue injury and systemic anaphylaxis. *J. Exp. Med.* 113:437, 1961.
128. Stone, S. H. Anaphylaxis in passively sensitized guinea pigs after subcutaneous eliciting injection. *Science* 128:1090, 1958.
129. Feigen, G. A., Williams, E. M., Peterson, J. K., and Nielsen, C. B. Histamine release and intracellular potentials during anaphylaxis in the isolated heart. *Circ. Res.* 8:713, 1960.
130. Geiger, W. B., and Alpers, H. S. The mechanism of the Schultz-Dale reaction. *J. Allerg.* 30:316, 1959.
131. Jaques, L. B., and Waters, E. T. The identity and origin of the anticoagulant of anaphylactic shock in the dog. *J. Physiol.* (London) 99:454, 1941.
132. Austen, K. F., and Humphrey, J. H. *In vitro* studies of the mechanism of anaphylaxis. *Advances Immun.* 3:1, 1963.
133. Chakravarty, N., and Uvnas, B. Histamine and a lipid-soluble smooth-muscle stimulating principle (SRS) in anaphylactic reaction. *Acta Physiol. Scand.* 48:302, 1959.
134. Austen, K. F., and Brocklehurst, W. E. Anaphylaxis in chopped guinea pig lung: I. Effect of peptidase substrates and inhibitors. *J. Exp. Med.* 113:521, 1961.
135. Austen, K. F., and Brocklehurst, W. E. Anaphylaxis in chopped guinea pig lung: II. Enhancement of the anaphylactic release of histamine and slow reacting substance by certain dibasic aliphatic acids and inhibition by monobasic fatty acids. *Ibid.*, p. 541.
136. Mongar, J. L., and Schild, H. O. The effect of calcium and pH on the anaphylactic reaction. *J. Physiol.* (London) 140:272, 1958.
137. Austen, K. F., and Brocklehurst, W. E. Anaphylaxis in chopped guinea pig lung: III. Effect of carbon monoxide, cyanide, salicylaldoxime, and ionic strength. *J. Exp. Med.* 114:29, 1961.
138. Mongar, J. L., and Schild, H. O. Effect of temperature on the anaphylactic reaction. *J. Physiol.* (London) 135:320, 1957.
139. Diamant, B. Observations on anaphylactic and compound 48/80-induced histamine release from guinea pig and rat lung tissue *in vitro*. *Acta Physiol. Scand.* 55:11, 1962.
140. Mongar, J. L., and Schild, H. O. Inhibition of the anaphylactic reaction. *J. Physiol.* (London) 135:301, 1957.
141. Austen, K. F., and Brocklehurst, W. E. Inhibition of the anaphylactic release of histamine from chopped guinea pig lung by chymotrypsin substrates and inhibitors. *Nature* (London) 186:866, 1960.
142. Middleton, E., and Sherman, W. B. Relationship of complement to allergic histamine release in blood of ragweed-sensitive subjects. *J. Allerg.* 31:441, 1960.
143. Huidobro, H., and Valette, G. Du rôle de l'ion calcium dans le déclenchement de la reaction anaphylactique *in vitro*. *C. R. Acad. Sci.* (Paris) 250:1375, 1960.
144. Middleton, E., Sherman, W. B., Fleming, W., and VanArsdel, P. Some biochemical characteristics of allergic histamine release from leukocytes of ragweed-sensitive subjects. *J. Allerg.* 31:448, 1960.
145. Lichtenstein, L. M., and Osler, A. G. Unpublished observations, 1962.
146. Barbaro, J. F. Reported by Becker, E. L., The Possible Significance of a Particular Group of Serine Esterases in Pathological Permeability Changes. In Grabar, P., and Miescher, P. (Eds.), *Mechanism of Cell and Tissue Damage Produced by Immune Reactions.* Basel: Benno Schwabe & Co., 1962.
147. Becker, E. L., and Austen, K. F. A comparison of the specificity of inhibition by phosphonate esters of the first component of complement and the antigen-induced release of histamine from guinea pig lung. *J. Exp. Med.* 120:491, 1964.
148. Austen, K. F., and Bloch, K. J. Differentiation *In Vitro* of Antigen-Induced Histamine Release from Complement-dependent Immune Injury. In Humphrey, J. H. (Ed.), *Complement.* Boston: Little, Brown, 1965.
149. Barbaro, J. F. The release of histamine from rabbit platelets by means of antigen-antibody precipitates: II. The role of plasma in the release of histamine. *J. Immun.* 86:377, 1961.
150. Bloch, K. J., Kourilsky, F. M., Ovary, Z., and Benacerraf, B. Properties of guinea pig 7S antibodies: III. Identification of antibodies involved in complement fixation and hemolysis. *J. Exp. Med.* 117:965, 1963.
151. Baker, A. R., Bloch, K. J., and Austen, K. F. *In vitro* passive sensitization of chopped guinea pig lung by guinea pig 7S antibodies. *J. Immun.* (in press).

*16. Effect of Bacterial Products on Responses to the Allergic Mediators**

ANDOR SZENTIVANYI AND CHARLES W. FISHEL

IT IS THE OBJECTIVE IN THIS CHAPter to discuss the effects of bacterial products on the response to the chemical mediators of the immediate forms of allergic reactions. These mediators have been described in detail in Chapter 15.

Among the immediate forms of allergy, the atopic group occupies a unique position in that the mechanism of atopy appears to involve an abnormal reactivity to the allergic mediators as well as the immunological basis for their release. For instance, anaphylactic reactivity of sensitized guinea pig depends on the immunological release of an amount of chemical mediator sufficient to be toxic for every member of the same species. In contrast, there is much evidence to indicate that atopic individuals possess an abnormal reactivity to otherwise nontoxic concentrations of chemical mediators [1–14]. This hyperreactivity appears to be qualitatively as well as quantitatively abnormal. It is limited to the target cells of one or more shock organs instead of affecting all the target cells uniformly, and the mediator is capable of eliciting responses which are different from its usual pharmacological effects. In asthmatics, for example, the injection of an otherwise nontoxic amount of histamine induces wheezing but not hives [1–4, 14]. In individuals with chronic urticaria, it induces hives but not wheezing [4, 14]. In atopic dermatitis, the histamine flush appears at the cutaneous sites of characteristic predilection, whether or not the disease is active at the time of testing [12]. Given an individual with any of the atopic disorders, a trace amount of intradermally injected acetylcholine may produce local blanching ("delayed blanch"), i.e., a vasoconstrictor instead of the usual vasodilator effect [13].

Another difference between atopic and other immediate hypersensitivities is the major contributory role played by infection in atopy. This is best exemplified by "intrinsic, intractable, or infectious" asthma, in which bacteria are held responsible for many of the clinical manifestations of the disease [15]. Infection has not been shown to be causally related to anaphylaxis, the Arthus reaction, or serum sickness.

While the importance of infection in atopic allergy is readily acknowledged, its precise role is not clear, nor is it known whether this role is the same in different atopic diseases or in different individuals suffering from the same disease. It is thought that in some cases the various microorganisms, their components, or products may act as antigens or as adjuvants enhancing antibody production to unrelated antigens.

Another possible reason for the close relation between infection and atopic allergy is that some bacterial products may modify the threshold and the quality of the responses of target cells to the immunologically released chemical mediators. The evidence of this effect of bacteria will be reviewed without implying that this is their only important effect on atopic allergy. Nor is the abnormality of response to chemical mediators seen in atopic allergy thought to arise solely from exposure to bacterial products.

CHEMICAL MEDIATORS OF THE ALLERGIC RESPONSE

The chemical mediators known to be involved in immediate hypersensitivities can be separated into two groups: (1) three small chemically defined compounds: histamine, serotonin, and acetylcholine, and (2) a group

* Supported by U.S. Public Health Service Grant AI-04193 and National Science Foundation Research Grant GE-1490.

of larger compounds, the so-called slow-reacting substances and plasma kinins [16].

In addition, the catecholamines (epinephrine, norepinephrine) might be considered a third group of mediators of the allergic response. Their inclusion is justified since each of the first group and most of the plasma kinins release or are capable of releasing the catechols [17–20]. Thus the latter are at least among the potential participants of the allergic reaction. In this capacity, the catecholamines occasionally have a harmful effect. In many tissues of most species the catecholamines are the principal natural antagonists of most of the first two groups of mediators and thus play a major role in determining the nature of reactivity of the target cells to these substances [16]. In this discussion, the catecholamines and the first group of allergic mediators will be called amine mediators.

IDENTITY BETWEEN PRINCIPAL TARGET CELLS OF THE ALLERGIC MEDIATORS AND EFFECTOR CELLS OF THE AUTONOMIC NERVOUS SYSTEM

Following release, the mediators elicit their individually characteristic effect through the activation of cells which are their specific targets and could be called, therefore, "target cells." It is generally believed that the target cells possess a receptive substance, or "receptor," with a steric configuration complementary to the mediator in question [21–28].

All of the allergic mediators act on the same target cells, which include smooth muscle, exocrine gland, and some nerve cells [16]. This is important because these are the same cells which are commonly referred to as the effector cells of the autonomic nervous system [22, 29].

The nervous system is composed of highly specialized elements, the nerve cells or neurons. A neuron is a cell, the protoplasm of which is extended into several processes. In normal conditions, one process (the axon) of each neuron conveys impulses away from the perikaryon. The remaining process or processes (dendrites) receive impulses and convey them to the perikaryon. Thus the nerve impulse generated within the nerve cell travels away from the perikaryon along the axon and its branches until it reaches an anatomical end formation, the so-called terminal button. At this point, the impulse must cross a gap between the terminal button and a succeeding non-nervous cell or the perikaryon of a second neuron. This method of joining cellular elements is commonly referred to as a junction. There are two types of junctions: (1) a "synapse" involving two nervous elements and (2) a "neuroeffector junction" between a nerve ending and a non-nervous effector cell (muscle or gland cell) [29]. Because of the lack of anatomical continuity at all central and peripheral levels of the nervous system [30], nerve impulses are transmitted from one cell to another by chemical substances called neurotransmitters [31].

"Transmission" of the nerve impulse refers to the chemical transfer of a stimulus from the nerve terminal to the succeeding unit, whether the latter is a neuron or an effector cell. At both categories of junctions, the second unit should be regarded as an effector cell regardless of its nervous or non-nervous nature. Thus in the autonomic nervous system there are three types of effector cells: at the synaptic junctions the nerve cells, and at the neuroeffector junctions, the smooth muscle and exocrine gland cells. These are the principal target cells of the allergic mediators.

MEDIATORS OF THE ALLERGIC RESPONSE AS NATURAL CHEMICAL ORGANIZERS OF AUTONOMIC ACTION

The identity of the neuroeffector cells and the principal target cells of allergic mediators immediately suggests that these substances may participate in impulse transmission. Indeed, acetylcholine and the catecholamines have long been associated with chemical transmission at the periphery [21, 22, 29, 35], and there is evidence that they may participate in central transmission as well [21, 31, 35]. Acetylcholine is believed to play a crucial role also in conduction of the nerve impulse [32, 33]. Transmission at various levels of the nervous system may also involve substances other than acetylcholine and the catecholamines. For reasons discussed in detail elsewhere [16], histamine and serotonin are believed to possess such a neurotransmitter role. However, in mammals, histaminergic and serotonin-mediated synapses have not been identified.

The activities of the amine mediators need not be conceived only in terms of impulse conduction or its transmission from one neuron to the other; they may be released from nerve terminals in small quantities without nerve stimulus. It is thought that this "resting" secretion maintains the sensitivity of the effector cell at a level optimal for the succeeding stimulus [34]. The amine mediators may also act on the effector cells after being released from specialized cells which do not stand in a junctional relationship with neurons, thus subserving some local, autonomous function [35]. The classical neurotransmitter, acetylcholine, is believed to initiate and maintain the rhythmic contractions of the atrium and the tone and motility of the gut independently of nerve impulses from the central nervous system [36]. Present knowledge of the action of serotonin in the intestinal tract would seem to make it more reasonable to consider this amine an autonomous neurohumor of the gut than a conventional neurotransmitter [21, 35]. Also, histamine and epinephrine released without neural stimulus have been postulated to be the natural regulators of microcirculation in mammals [37]. It would seem, therefore, that the amine mediators should be regarded not in the restrictive sense of neurotransmitters but more broadly as the natural chemical organizers of autonomic action [16].

The physiological role of the slow-reacting substances and plasma kinins cannot be assessed at present.

THE RECEPTOR AS THE PHARMACOLOGICALLY SPECIFIC COMPONENT OF THE TARGET CELL

From the standpoint of specificity of action, the important component of the effector or target cell is the receptor. Because of a natural affinity, the immunologically released mediator is thought to combine with a complementary receptor site, thereby initiating a chain of biochemical reactions of undetermined nature culminating in the observable biological response [21–28].

The best available evidence indicates that the cellular receptors for the amine mediators are enzymes, and it is possible that some or all of them are phosphorylated proteins [16, 21]. Since the exact nature of the various amine receptors is not known, they are designated either by the effector response resulting from their activation or by their specific blocking agents. By the use of such specific blocking agents and by comparison of the activities of amines with those of their synthetic or natural analogues, the distribution of many of the amine receptors and the natural functions associated with each of them have been plotted throughout the body [16, 21].

On this basis, there appear to be two principal types of adrenergic receptors, termed alpha and beta [24]. Receptors blocked by ergotoxin, dibenamine, and phenoxybenzamine (and others) are called alpha receptors; those blocked by dichloroisoproterenol (DCI) and Nethalide are beta receptors. Norepinephrine acts mainly on alpha receptors, isoproterenol mainly on beta receptors, with epinephrine possessing dualistic action [21, 23–26]. At least three types of acetylcholine receptors can be distinguished: atropine-sensitive, tetraethylammonium-sensitive, and curare-sensitive, which are equivalent to the postganglionic, cholinergic, and neuromuscular (striated muscle) junctions, respectively [22]. Different receptors may exist also for serotonin, as evident from the presence of two types of serotonin receptors in the guinea pig ileum. One, the "nervous receptor" (M-receptor), can be blocked by morphine, atropine, cocaine, and methadone; the other type, the "smooth muscle receptor" (D-receptor), is blocked by dibenzyline, D-lysergic acid diethylamide, and others [21, 27, 28]. Concerning histamine, the failure of antihistamines to prevent its action on atria and on gastric secretion indicates that these receptors may be different from those involved in the action of the amine on smooth muscle and sympathetic ganglia [28].

No information is available on the cellular receptors of slow-reacting substances and plasma kinins.

METHODS OF PRODUCING ALTERED RESPONSES TO ALLERGIC MEDIATORS

Before the mechanisms by which bacteria induce abnormal responses to allergic mediators are discussed, a number of methods will be described by which similar abnormal responses have been produced surgically or chemically. The advantage of such an approach lies in the fact that in these conditions the biological effect of the surgical or chemical intervention is fairly well understood. It is hoped that this analysis will be valuable in the subsequent interpretation of altered reactivity induced by bacteria.

We shall discuss these procedures separately and in succession as though the resultant conditions were mechanistically distinct entities. In reality, there is no clear borderline between them, and each contains elements shared by the others. Because of the interrelated effects of the various amine mediators in the maintenance of normal autonomic regulation, the altered responsiveness in each of these conditions can be explained on the basis of an imbalance of autonomic regulation at the amine receptor level [16, 38].

INHIBITION OF THE SPECIFIC ENZYME NORMALLY INACTIVATING THE MEDIATOR

Although enhancement or prolongation of effector response to any of the amine mediators may be obtained by inhibition of its specific catabolizing enzyme, some distinction must be made between acetylcholine and the other amines. Thus suppression of cholinesterase activity results in a rather consistent enhancement of acetylcholine action, regardless of the species and effector response tested or which of the anticholinesterases is employed [22]. In contrast, results of similar procedures concerning catechols, histamine, and serotonin vary with all of these factors [21, 39–42]. This disparity might in part be attributed to the several different and competing degradative pathways available for each of the latter amines. Selective blockade of one of them may be compensated by an increase in the catabolic contribution of the alternative pathways [21, 43]. Furthermore, the relative importance of noncatabolic processes in inactivating some of the latter mediators seems to be greater than is the case with acetylcholine [44, 45].

SURGICALLY OR PHARMACOLOGICALLY INDUCED "DENERVATION SUPERSENSITIVITY"

Small amounts of neurotransmitters are released continually by the nerve terminals during the resting state of the neuron, and in much greater amounts following the arrival of an impulse. Apparently the function of the resting secretion, which is too small to activate the effector cell, is to keep the sensitivity of the effector at a low level [34]. When the effector cell is deprived of this resting secretion, it acquires within a few days a hypersensitivity to its specific neurotransmitter. For example, surgical interruption of the final neuron results in degeneration of the distal portion of the axon and cessation of its resting secretion. In the case of an adrenergic nerve ending, this results in a hypersensitivity to epinephrine in the succeeding effector cell. In many instances, a hypersensitivity of the effector ensues also to other natural neurohumors (serotonin, histamine) and to a number of similar as well as unrelated chemicals. When acetylcholine is used as a test substance and the striated muscle as an indicator tissue, the order of magnitude of the level of sensitivity so produced is within the range of 20 to 200 times* that of the normal level [46]. A less pronounced hypersensitivity develops after the penultimate neuron, i.e., the presynaptic neuron, is cut. In this case, the effector is deprived only of the transmitter released by the incoming impulses. Regeneration of the neuron or local application of the transmitter restores the normal level of sensitivity. Although the precise molecular mechanism of the hypersensitivity is not understood, it is probably due to the local and prolonged unavailability of the neurotransmitter [34, 45, 47, 48].

Denervation hypersensitivity can also be produced by pharmacological means. Drugs having as their main effect the interruption of impulse transmission at any point and which are allowed to act for an extended period, can produce a hypersensitivity essentially identical with that caused by surgical denervation [34, 45]. In general, it would appear that any natural constituent or foreign substance capable of blocking the synthesis, storage, release, or action of the transmitter, and thereby depriving the effector cell of its specific controlling agent, can produce a denervation supersensitivity.

DEPLETION OF NONJUNCTIONAL MEDIATOR STORES

It is implicit in the foregoing concept of denervation supersensitivity that the lacking transmitter is normally derived from a store (i.e., synaptic vesicles) which stands in a junctional relationship with the effector cell. However, an alteration in sensitivity of the effector

* Under appropriate conditions of testing, the increase in the level of sensitivity may reach 100,000 [126].

to a mediator can also be produced when the action of the mediator is preceded by depletion of its specific, though nonjunctional, stores. For instance, neuronal histamine stores are quite insulated from the action of otherwise highly potent chemical histamine liberators, and repeated administration of such agents for over thirty days fails to remove the neuronal histamine. Mobilization of the latter can be accomplished only at the high concentrations of the liberator obtainable by direct perfusion of the neuron through its own vascular supply [49]. Therefore parenteral administration of the liberator will presumably result in release of histamine from nonjunctional stores only. When 48/80 or n-octylamine was administered parenterally, a hypersensitivity to histamine coincided with the periods during which tissue levels of histamine are known to remain low after treatment with 48/80 or n-octylamine, or both [50, 51]. This suggested an inverse relationship between sensitivity to histamine and tissue concentration of the same amine. Although available information does not permit a detailed comparison between this altered reactivity and that produced by denervation, it seems that, in contrast to denervation, this hypersensitivity may develop more rapidly and is limited to the mediator whose tissue stores were previously depleted.

SELECTIVE BLOCKADE OF ONE OF TWO ANTAGONISTIC SETS OF RECEPTORS SPECIFICALLY ACTIVATED BY THE SAME MEDIATOR

If at the time of action of a mediator there is a shift in the relative availability of its two functionally antagonistic sets of specific receptors, the normal response to that mediator will be quantitatively or qualitatively altered [16, 19, 23–26, 38, 52–55].

For instance, in the tracheobronchial tract, the normal balance between the alpha adrenergic and beta adrenergic receptor systems appears to favor a beta adrenergic response of the smooth musculature to epinephrine. If, however, the beta adrenergic receptors are blocked by DCI, bronchoconstriction occurs instead of the usual relaxation, exemplifying a qualitatively abnormal response to the mediator [52]. In certain segments of the vascular system, where the normal receptor distribution seems to favor adrenergic contracting effects, the same pharmacological beta blockade results in a qualitatively normal but quantitatively enhanced response to epinephrine, i.e., exaggerated vasoconstriction of the small cutaneous vessels [55].

In the foregoing examples, the two antagonistic receptors may be components of the same target cell [25]. Similar considerations apply to those situations in which the two receptors are associated with two different cell systems which have a common function with respect to the organism as a whole. For instance, hyperglycemia to epinephrine is the net result of a combination of adrenergic effects: (1) hepatic glycogenolysis leading to the release of free glucose into the extracellular space, and (2) a simultaneous reduction of glucose uptake by the muscle and other extrahepatic cells [56]. In the mouse, hepatic glycogenolysis appears to be an alpha adrenergic function. When the beta receptors of the mouse are blocked by DCI, the blood sugar level fails to rise following epinephrine administrations and this occurs despite increased hepatic glycogenolysis [19, 54]. This illustrates a quantitatively and qualitatively abnormal response to a mediator produced by the selective blockade of one of its receptors.

Selective blockade of one receptor system, however, can modify the target cell response not only to the specific activator of the receptor affected but also to unrelated amines. An example is the DCI-induced hypersensitivity of mice to both histamine and serotonin. Within a certain dose range, this beta adrenergic blockade can increase the normal sensitivity of mice to histamine and serotonin about 50- and 10-fold, respectively [53]. This nonspecificity is similar to pharmacological or surgical denervation of the salivary glands. Normally, the secretion of these glands is stimulated by both adrenergic and cholinergic impulses. When the cholinergic receptors of the cat's submaxillary gland cells are blocked for a long time by chronic atropinization, they become hypersensitive to epinephrine and to a number of other sympathomimetics as well as to adrenergic nerve stimulation. The same hypersensitivity to adrenergic agents arises following section of the chorda [34].

HORMONAL DEPRIVATION AND OVERDOSAGE

The reactivity of the target cell to the allergic mediators may depend on the hormonal balance within the body. The most striking illustration of this is the effect of bilateral adrenalectomy in various laboratory species. Adrenalectomy increases the sensitivity to a variety of stressful stimuli and pharmacologically active agents, including histamine and serotonin.

For instance, cats without adrenals are 13 to 60 times as sensitive to histamine as intact animals [57], and in adrenalectomized mice the corresponding figure for serotonin is about 30 [58]. Since in most reported studies, response after medullectomy or total sympathectomy has not been tested, it is not possible to assess the relative role of catechol versus corticosteroid deficit in these conditions. Nevertheless, in general, the sympathectomized animal occupies an intermediate position between the normal and the adrenalectomized.

The adrenal corticosteroids and the catecholamines appear to operate largely as a functional unit. The sites of action and character of target cell responses to these two natural substances are strikingly similar. The corticosteroids seem to be required for target cell responses to catechols, but there is no evidence of interchangeability between these groups. Although the molecular mechanism underlying the catecholamine-corticosteroid relationship remains obscure, it is well established that in the absence of steroids the receptor threshold for catechols may be raised, occasionally to the point of complete unresponsiveness [59]. Therefore corticosteroid deprivation can clinically simulate either an indiscriminate or a selective adrenergic blockade, depending on the types of effector responses tested [19, 59]. Conversely, even a pharmacologically established blockade in an intact animal can be overcome with an excess amount of corticosteroid [19]. This seems to imply that the corticosteroids not only support the target cell responses to catechols but, under certain conditions, are also capable of sensitizing these cells to the action of these amines.

The sensitizing effects of thyroxin and triiodothyronine to histamine and serotonin do not require separate discussion, since their effects appear to be indirect and mediated through the adrenal steroids. Hyperthyroidism causes a temporary state of cortical deficiency, whereas hypothyroidism results in a temporary accumulation of corticosteroids in tissues [60].

Excess amounts of insulin are also known to increase the responses of the target cells to the allergic mediators. The mechanism of this sensitizing effect is not known but might be related to the physiological action of this hormone, since an increased peripheral uptake of glucose occurs in some conditions in which hypersensitivity to the mediators has been demonstrated [54, 61–64].

REFLEXLY AND CENTRALLY INDUCED HYPOTHALAMIC IMBALANCE

There are two reciprocally antagonistic divisions in the hypothalamus: the anterior hypothalamus, which mediates mainly cholinergic responses, and the posterior hypothalamus, the stimulation of which results largely in adrenergic responses [65]. A balance between these antagonistic divisions is thought to be important in maintaining the normal autonomic functions, e.g., blood pressure. The activity of the posterior hypothalamus is normally suppressed by inhibitory impulses transmitted from the sino-aortic baroreceptors. Pressure is the physiological stimulus of the baroreceptors, and because of the constant stimulus of the blood pressure on these pressure-sensitive devices, nerve impulses at low frequency are continually traveling up through their connecting afferent pathways to the medullary and hypothalamic centers. These inhibitory impulses, among others, keep the posterior hypothalamus in check.

When histamine or acetylcholine is given under appropriate conditions, the systemic blood pressure falls, and consequently the sino-aortic tension decreases, causing a reduction in the frequency of inhibitory impulses traveling to the higher centers. This relieves the suppression of the posterior hypothalamus and results in a shift to sympathetic activity. Accordingly, a general increase in rate of firing of peripheral adrenergic structures, including the adrenal medullary cells, follows, leading to the release of catechols. In these circumstances, the normal balance of the hypothalamus is shifted to the adrenergic side, which tends to correct and limit the blood pressure drop [66]. Conversely, when catecholamines are given systemically, the blood pressure rises and the increased rate of upward discharges shifts the hypothalamic balance to the cholinergic side [66].

Although in these examples we are dealing

with a reflexly induced hypothalamic imbalance, it is possible to produce imbalance of the hypothalamus by applying histamine, acetylcholine, or catecholamines directly on hypothalamic structures, by the electrolytic removal or electrical stimulation of one of the divisions of the hypothalamus, and by many other stimuli [66–70].

The reflexly or locally induced hypothalamic imbalance leads not only to an increased excitability of one hypothalamic division but to simultaneous inhibition of the antagonistic division. Consequently the action of either a parasympathomimetic stimulus (acetylcholine, histamine) or a sympathomimetic stimulus (catechols) may be reduced by a counteracting imbalance induced in the hypothalamus. If, therefore, at the time of action of an exogenously administered or endogenously released allergic mediator the hypothalamus is already in a state of imbalance for any reason, the capacity of the hypothalamus to counteract and control the stimuli will be markedly reduced. In this way the action of the mediator may be profoundly modified both quantitatively and qualitatively even to the complete reversal of its usual pharmacological activity [66–70].

MECHANISM OF ALTERED RESPONSES TO ALLERGIC MEDIATORS INDUCED BY BACTERIAL PRODUCTS

We have described surgical and pharmacological methods for altering responses to the allergic mediators. Numerous examples of similar alterations following the injection of bacterial products are known, and some of these will now be described. The difficulty in determining the mechanism of action of the bacterial products arises from the complexity of the substances injected and lack of knowledge concerning their structure or pharmacological action. Thus at this time it is necessary to speculate concerning the mechanism of action of the bacterial products and consider in each case a number of hypotheses. It is hoped that by looking for similarities between the altered responses produced by definitive surgical and pharmacological methods and those produced by bacterial products the investigator will be led to a hypothesis which is experimentally testable.

EFFECT OF BACTERIAL EXOTOXINS ON ALLERGIC MEDIATORS

It appears that most of the well-known bacterial exotoxins produce some alteration in the response to the chemical mediators. However, this alteration is not a significant part of the symptomatic effect of these toxins but rather appears to be a harmless by-product. In addition, since many of the exotoxins are a cause of relatively rare and self-limited diseases, they play an insignificant role in clinical allergy. A discussion of the exotoxins is included here for completeness and because they form an intermediate step between the definitive experimental procedures of the preceding discussion and the extremely complex actions of the bacterial endotoxins.

Two of these toxins, the botulinus and tetanus toxins, are rather similar, being produced by related species of the *Clostridium* genus. Both are proteins and have essentially the same qualitative composition of amino acids, the relative proportions of which are in marked contrast with those of other proteins. Both toxins show an extraordinarily high and selective affinity for cholinergic terminals. It is thus possible that the active groups of the two toxins are closely related. Both can produce muscle paralysis, but in the case of tetanus, tonic contractions are predominant [71].

Impulse conduction in a nerve trunk bathed in high concentrations of the botulinus toxin was found to be unimpaired [72], as was the activity of choline acetylase and other essential components of the choline acetylating system such as coenzyme A, adenosine triphosphate, and adenosinetriphosphatase [71, 73]. Direct measurements of the activity of "true" and "pseudo" cholinesterases were in the normal range [73, 74], and anticholinesterases failed to decrease or reverse the paralysis [73, 75, 76]. Blockade or some other malfunctioning of the cholinergic receptor can be excluded, since completely paralyzed muscles respond to exogenous acetylcholine and potent anticurare drugs have no effect on the nerve-muscle preparation poisoned by the toxin. In addition, the botulinus toxin preparation exhibited normal tetanic responses and summation curves in contrast to the curarized preparation [71]. No destructive damage of the effector cell was demonstrable, since the end plate region did not show specific histological changes [76], and the muscle response to direct stimulation was unaffected by the toxin [71]. No change in the ultrastructure of the nerve terminals was detected following botulinus intoxication [77].

Botulinus toxin appears to block the junctional transmission of the impulse. The selective localization of ferritin-labeled botulinus toxin in the subsynaptic apparatus suggests that the toxin prevents the release of acetylcholine [78]. In agreement with this, the spontaneous miniature potentials were absent in toxin-poisoned nerve-muscle preparations. Nerve stimulation does not produce an end plate potential [34], and following nerve stimulation, the output of acetylcholine was markedly reduced [73].

If botulinus toxin blocks impulse transmission, it should produce a denervation hypersensitivity. Thus in poisoned muscle fibers the area responsive to acetylcholine is increased beyond the boundaries of the end plate as seen in denervated fibers, and the time development of this phenomenon was the same in the two conditions [79, 91]. Recordings of mechanical and electrical responses of intoxicated muscle to acetylcholine showed that the quick mechanical response immediately following the action potential is gradually replaced by a secondary tonic contraction associated with complete electrical silence [79]. These are the characteristic responses of chronically denervated muscle fibers [22]. Furthermore, the sensitizing effects of the toxin and surgical denervation appear to be additive on the same structure, implying that similar or identical mechanisms are at work [34, 92]. The nonspecific character of denervation hypersensitivity can be duplicated with botulinus toxin in the salivary glands, which acquire a hypersensitivity to both sympathomimetic and parasympathomimetic agents [80]. Although the toxin does not interfere with the smooth muscle-contracting effect of serotonin, the possibility has been raised that it is capable of preventing the anaphylactic release of the amine from the same smooth muscle preparation [81]. The toxin is reported to block the activity of serotonin in transporting calcium across the neuronal cell membrane [82].

The action of the neurotoxin of *Clostridium tetani* in many respects also resembles the early changes seen in denervation hypersensitivity. The release of acetylcholine is considerably depressed by the toxin, although no specific morphological changes can be detected in nerve tissue and the toxin has no effect on choline-acetylase or on other components of the acetylcholine synthesizing system. Injection of the toxin into the anterior chamber of the eye is followed by persistent mydriasis which is refractory to reflex stimuli, indicating that cholinergic transmission to the sphincter pupillae is paralyzed. The normal response, however, can be at least partially restored by instillation of a cholinesterase blocker into the conjunctival sac [71]. An increase in cholinesterase activity, however, does not appear to be responsible for the paralysis, since cholinesterase activity does not seem to be affected by the toxin. The iris of the intoxicated eye was found to be hypersensitive to application of carbaminocholine, a stable acetylcholine analogue, and the period required for recovery in local tetanus is within the range of time needed for repair of a crushed nerve [71].

A number of other exotoxins, including one each from staphylococcus [85, 86], *Cl. welchii* [87] and cholera [88] are known to cause the liberation of histamine. Although these toxins have never been shown to produce a hypersensitivity to histamine, this would not be unexpected since the pharmacological histamine liberators have this effect, among them the frequently used polymyxins, which are bacterial products as well [89, 90].

Recently it has been shown that diphtheria toxin has a specific effect on peripheral blood vessels, reducing their sensitivity to norepinephrine. This abnormality seems to be due to a loss of the supportive action of corticosteroids on alpha adrenergic receptors resulting from the diphtheritic lesions in the zona fasciculata of the adrenal cortex [83].

The exotoxin of *Shigella dysenteriae* produces paralytic symptoms, a fact which is responsible for its classification as a neurotoxin. Despite the fact that the lesions most commonly observed following the administration of this toxin are in the intestinal mucosa, the toxin appears to act through the central nervous system. Thus direct contact of the toxin and intestinal mucosa produces no lesion, whereas its intravenous injection causes the appearance of a number of focal lesions in the intestinal tract. These lesions reveal changes in permeability of the intestinal vascular bed which are believed to be primarily due to an exaggerated vasospasm in the involved areas. This enhanced alpha adrenergic response together with other symptoms of a general activation of the adrenergic system can be prevented by drugs which block the transmission in sympathetic ganglia [84].

BORDETELLA PERTUSSIS-INDUCED HISTAMINE AND SEROTONIN HYPERSENSITIVITY

The injection of *B. pertussis* organisms increases the normal sensitivity of certain strains of mice and rats to histamine in the order of magnitude of 30- to 300-fold. Rabbits and guinea pigs do not seem to be affected, but an increased cutaneous sensitivity to histamine following pertussis infection has been reported in man [93, 96]. This histamine-sensitizing property is not shared by most other bacteria. The hypersensitivity to histamine reaches a maximum about five days after pertussis administration and then declines [93, 94].

By the same procedure, mice and rats are rendered hypersensitive to serotonin, though the time course of the development and disappearance of the sensitivity may differ slightly from that to histamine. The increase in sensitivity to serotonin is about 20- to 50-fold [93, 94].

The various hypotheses which have been offered to explain the mechanism of the pertussis-induced histamine and serotonin hypersensitivity can be classified into one of the following general categories: (1) impairment of the normal rapid detoxification of these amines; (2) adrenal insufficiency; (3) abnormal production of excessive amounts of the amines and thus continued exposure and sensitization of the target cells to these agents, and (4) localized hyperreactivity of some of the target cells to otherwise nontoxic concentrations of these substances, resulting from an imbalance between the two adrenergic effector systems.

The first hypothesis was based on the *in vitro* demonstration of decreased histaminase (diamine oxidase) activity in various tissues of pertussis-inoculated rats and mice [97, 98]. However, the resistance of the pertussis-sensitized mouse was found to be unaltered to agmatine, which is also inactivated by diamine oxidase [53]. The histamine sensitivity of mice and rats could not be increased by histaminase inhibitors [42], and pertussis sensitizes these animals to serotonin, which is not a substrate for the enzyme [21, 99]. Finally, no gross abnormality in the degradation pattern of radioactive histamine or serotonin, or both, could be detected in the highly sensitive animal [53]. Inadequate detoxifying processes, therefore, do not seem to be involved in the mechanism of the hypersensitivity.

Bordetella pertussis does not appear to alter the function of the adrenal gland. In fact, this organ appears to be intact morphologically [100], secretion of corticosteroids seems normal [93, 100], and the adrenal medullary tissue is capable of storing normal amounts of catecholamines and of releasing them in response to various stimuli [19]. Moreover, a strain of mice was found which became hypersensitive to histamine following pertussis inoculation but not after adrenalectomy [101]. Nor can the beneficial effects of cortisone in pertussis-induced sensitivity be used as a valid argument in support of the second hypothesis. These effects might well be pharmacological in nature (i.e., sensitization of the adrenergic receptors) and do not necessarily imply hormonal replacement. On the other hand, however, it is recognized that pertussis action may occur at a level beyond the adrenal gland by an interference with the utilization of steroids, by increasing their inactivation or by altering the tissue requirements for these hormones. The altered resistance to histamine following pertussis can be only partially restored by cortisone [102], whereas it can be completely restored by administration of progressively increasing amounts of histamine and serotonin, but not of agmatine [53]. These findings suggest that the sensitive state is induced through some mechanism other than impairment of adrenal function or steroid deficiency.

The third hypothesis is based on the observation that the tissue histidine decarboxylase activity in the hypersensitive animals increases parallel to the development of the hypersensitivity [37, 99]. Histidine decarboxylase is an important enzyme which converts histidine to histamine, and its increase might lead to an increased production of histamine. To explain this observation it was assumed that continued exposure of the target cells to histamine causes the hypersensitivity. As a rule, however, the repeated acute or prolonged exposure of target cells to an amine mediator results in tachyphylaxis or tolerance, i.e., increased resistance [103–108, 112]. In fact, hypersensitivity to an amine seems generally to be associated with a reduced, not an increased, availability of the amine [34, 45, 50, 51]. Furthermore, this hypothesis fails to account for the pertussis-induced hypersensitivity to serotonin. Finally, the restoration of normal resistance to both histamine and serotonin by the administration of progressively increasing amounts of either amine, together with the success of cross-desensitization [53], makes such a hypothesis even more difficult to entertain.

Originally, the fourth hypothesis was based mainly on the fact that pertussis-inoculated mice could be protected from the lethal effects of histamine and serotonin by the administration of an alpha adrenergic blocking agent (dibenzyline), and, conversely, normal animals could be rendered hypersensitive to both amines by the injection of a beta blocker [DCI]. Furthermore, DCI administration to normal animals resulted in a bimodal dose-response curve to histamine similar to the type elicited by pertussis vaccination. For this reason, it has been said that the pertussis-sensitized mouse behaves as though it were beta adrenergically blocked [53].

In the pertussis-sensitized mouse, no hyperglycemia follows the administration of histamine and serotonin, presumably because of the blockade of the beta receptors. The lack of epinephrine responsiveness is confined to selective areas of epinephrine action, since the hepatic glycogenolytic activity is not only retained but exaggerated in the pertussis-sensitized animal. The combination of exaggerated responses in one area of epinephrine activity and failure of response in another area is itself a strong indication of a selective adrenergic blockade. That in the pertussis-sensitized animal a selective blockade or some other malfunctioning of the beta adrenergic receptors may be responsible for the failure of hyperglycemia is suggested by the fact that DCI produces the same split pattern of epinephrine activity in the normal mouse [19].

The beta adrenergic receptors normally associated with the inhibition of peripheral uptake of glucose are blocked in the pertussis-sensitized animal. Such blockade, then, leads to a reduction in the degree of antagonism to insulin which exists in normal circumstances. Relative hyperinsulinism occurs largely because of this effect, and consequently hypoglycemia may follow. This glycemic maladjustment does not appear to be a trivial by-product of the beta adrenergic blockade but might influence the induction of the hypersensitive state. Two lines of evidence support this assumption. Both alloxan diabetes and long-term as well as acute administration of glucose restore the normal resistance of the pertussis-sensitized mouse to serotonin, whereas insulin sensitizes normal mice to both histamine and serotonin [54].

Based on these observations, the pathogenesis of the pertussis-induced hypersensitive state could be conceived as follows. The pertussis organism possesses either a component or causes the host to elaborate a substance which inhibits the function of the beta adrenergic receptors. When such an animal is challenged with histamine or serotonin, the antagonistic action of the released catecholamines is blocked at the beta receptor level, leaving the alpha adrenergic activities unopposed. According to this hypothesis, the altered or increased sensitivity of the pertussis-inoculated mouse to histamine and serotonin stems from an acquired functional imbalance of the two adrenergic effector systems [19, 53–55].

BACTERIAL ENDOTOXINS AND REACTIVITY TO THE CHEMICAL MEDIATORS

Endotoxin is the term conventionally used to designate a class of high molecular weight phospholipid-polysaccharide-protein complexes which comprise the somatic portion of gram-negative bacteria. These endotoxins (or at least the complexes with which they are associated) show sharp serological specificity for the species of origin. Nevertheless they all bring about strikingly identical pathological effects, in contrast to the individually characteristic effects produced by the exotoxins [84, 109, 110].

The pattern of responses produced by endotoxins includes: fever, sometimes followed by hypothermia, diarrhea and intestinal congestion; hyperglycemia, sometimes followed by hypoglycemia; depletion of hepatic glycogen; elevated blood levels of inorganic phosphates and lactic and pyruvic acids; short-lived leukopenia with subsequent leukocytosis; endothelial damage resulting in hemorrhages and leading to focal necrosis in various tissues; fibrinoid necrosis in arterial walls, and, finally, profound circulatory disturbances leading eventually to irreversible shock without specific morphological findings at autopsy [84, 110]. This pattern of responses can also be produced by components of certain gram-positive bacteria and by constituents of a wide variety of plant and animal tissues, although in the latter instance there is some question of bacterial contamination [109, 119].

The fundamental similarity in the action of all of these substances is seen again when attempts are made to immunize against them. The resistance so produced is never of a high order, and it is short-lived despite the relative ease with which high titers of precipitating sera can be obtained [84]. It may be added that, while some of the biological effects of the endotoxins may depend on their antigenicity [109], it is probable that the nonantigenic lipid component is responsible for most of their toxic effects [111].

Many of the biological effects of endotoxin can be accentuated by injecting it in two doses separated by a period of several hours to a day [116]. If the first injection is made intradermally, a second intravenous injection will produce a hemorrhagic necrotic lesion at the site of the first injection. This is the local Shwartzman reaction [121]. If both injections are given intravenously, bilateral cortical necrosis of the kidneys predominates (generalized Shwartzman or Sanarelli phenomenon) [110, 121].

Although there have been many hypotheses concerning the mechanism of action of bacterial endotoxin, convincing evidence cannot be marshaled in favor of any single primary mechanism. We believe that the unusual biological activity of these substances can best be explained by postulating at least two different but synergistic actions. In the neurophysiological frame of reference of this chapter, it is suggested that these two actions lie in the general areas of a modification in the responsiveness to the chemical mediators, and in the liberation of these mediators from their cellular stores. Such a hypothesis best explains the enhancement produced by dividing the endotoxin into two separate doses. It also explains the immediate and local effects of endotoxin and the ability to substitute epinephrine and adrenergic blocking agents for one or both of the injections of endotoxin.

It is generally agreed that one of the earliest effects of endotoxin on the whole animal (manifest in certain tissues within 15 to 35 seconds following application [117]) is a violent and prolonged arteriolar and metarteriolar constriction alternating with brief periods of vasodilation [110, 113–117]. These early vascular responses are not associated with evidence of damage to the endothelial wall or basement membrane of capillaries and venules or of any alteration in their permeability [116]. If shock-producing doses are given, the constrictor phase gives way later to an extreme vasodilatation leading eventually to irreversible vasoparalysis [113]. The initial constrictor phase can be prevented by prior depletion of the catechol stores with reserpine [120] or by pretreatment with adrenergic blocking agents of the alpha variety [110].

The so-called "epinephrine lesion" can be briefly described as follows. When an animal is given an intravenous injection of 1 μg. of purified endotoxin, followed at any time during the next four hours by the intradermal injection of 10 μg. of epinephrine, hemorrhagic necrosis of considerable proportions develops at the injected site. In contrast, no evidence of tissue destruction can be detected when even as large a dose as 100 to 200 μg. of epinephrine is repeatedly injected into the same skin site of a normal member of the same species [114]. A similar lesion can also be produced by norepinephrine following the administration of endotoxin, but not by ephedrine [110]. That this lesion is due not to the systemic activity of the endotoxin but to its local effect is demonstrated by the intradermal injection of an endotoxin-epinephrine mixture which is capable of producing the same hemorrhagic necrosis [114]. In these circumstances the endotoxin is not absorbed and consequently has no opportunity to act systemically.

A better insight into the mechanism of this necrotizing activity can be obtained by employing the isolated rabbit ear for measuring resistance to perfused fluid and by studying the reactions of terminal vessels in the exteriorized mesoappendix of the rat. For instance, perfusion of a small amount of endotoxin (0.5 μg.) into the isolated rabbit ear is followed within a few minutes by a 200- to 800-fold increase in the vasoconstrictor response to epinephrine. Similarly, even a 1,000-fold potentiation of epinephrine activity by endotoxin can be seen to occur in the mesoappendix [115]. It is of further interest that blockade of the reticuloendothelial system by Thorotrast or denatured protein, i.e., an intervention which is known to render the animal highly sensitive to the subsequent administration of endotoxin, produces itself a moderate degree of the same type of hyperreactivity to epinephrine and serotonin, a response which is magnified when the endotoxin is injected [116].

These observations indicate that the systemic effects of endotoxin are due primarily to an enhanced response of the adrenergic effector cells to the catechols and not to an increased activity of the sympathoadrenal system. The inefficacy of ephedrine [110] and the fact that none of the naturally occurring vasoconstrictor agents, by themselves, can reproduce the vascular sequelae of bacterial endotoxins [118] point in the same direction. Furthermore, a comparison of the *in vitro* responsiveness of arterial strips from endotoxin-treated versus normal rabbits to chemical and electrical stimuli shows profound qualitative differences. While the normal strip, following a maximal contraction, must undergo relaxation before it can respond again, the endotoxin-treated strip is incapable of complete relaxation so that the next stimulus is superimposed on the residual tone, leading to a complete contracture [118]. It is permissible to conclude, therefore, that following endotoxin there is a quantitatively and qualitatively abnormal response of the effector cell to catechols. However, an over-all hyperactivity of the adrenergic nervous system brought about by an induced hypothalamic imbalance [65, 66] as well as by a peripheral depletion of catechols [117] may also contribute to the general symptoms of toxemia.

At the receptor level, such a quantitatively and qualitatively abnormal response of the vascular smooth muscle cells could be due either to a hypersensitivity of the alpha adrenergic receptors or to a functional deficiency of the beta receptor system. The aforementioned *in vitro* observations with arterial strips suggest that the lesion must be associated with the relaxation mechanism of the cell [118]. It is of more than passing interest, therefore, that a lesion grossly resembling the "epinephrine lesion" may be produced in the skin of both guinea pigs and rabbits following the injection of a mixture of a selective beta blocker (DCI) and epinephrine [55].

Serotonin cannot substitute for epinephrine in the cutaneous necrotizing action of endotoxin [114], but in the mesoappendix after systemic exposure to endotoxin it does produce an unusually exaggerated response [116]. Furthermore, a mixture of epinephrine and serotonin causes dermal necrosis in rabbits and also brings about disproportionately strong venous constriction in rat mesentery [122]. Since serotonin is capable both of sensitizing the alpha adrenergic receptors [123] and of releasing catechols [18, 19], the synergistic action can be explained through either of these mechanisms.

The reactivity of the target cells to histamine following endotoxin administration does not seem to be altered [93, 116]. This is surprising in view of the manifold similarities between pertussis and endotoxin phenomena. It is possible, however, that this histamine disparity is due to a different pattern of selective involvement of the adrenergic receptors in the two phenomena.

Intensified adrenergic vasoconstriction appears to be involved also in the local and generalized Shwartzman reactions. Adrenergic blocking agents such as SY-28 and dibenamine are capable of inhibiting the local reaction; conversely, the lesion can be produced by vasoconstrictor drugs when used either in place of endotoxin in the provocative challenge or injected into the prepared skin site [124]. In the generalized form, dibenamine and sympathectomy protect the kidney against necrosis [125], and necrosis is also inhibited in epinephrine-tolerant animals [112].

Although this review outlines complex experiments and observations, the implied results of these studies are comparatively simple and straightforward. The autonomic nervous system provides the body with regulatory mechanisms, the primary function of which is to help to maintain a constant internal environment. The most important elements so regulated include the blood pressure, body temperature, tissue blood flow, and blood glucose concentration. The antagonistic actions of the amine mediators (histamine, serotonin, acetylcholine, and the catecholamines) are an essential part of this system of checks and balances.

Antigen-antibody reactions, probably through cell injury, cause the release of unphysiological amounts of the amine mediators. Thus most of the symptoms of the immediate types of allergy are characteristic of the actions of these mediators. In addition, bacterial products have the capacity to interfere with the complex workings of the nervous system. This interference varies from the specific and restricted action of potent exotoxins to a broad pattern of effects common to the endotoxins. Endotoxins appear to have the synergistic properties of releasing the amine mediators and simultaneously increasing the responsiveness of the effector cells (cells on which the mediators act). Thus not only do they produce directly the symptoms of autonomic derangement such as fever, shock, and hypoglycemia but they enhance the nonspecific sequels of subsequent antigen-antibody interactions. In other words, the endotoxins are potentially important augmenters of the allergic reaction.

REFERENCES

1. Weiss, S., Robb, G. P., and Ellis, L. B. The systemic effects of histamine in man: With special reference to the responses of the cardiovascular system. *Arch. Int. Med.* 49:360, 1932.
2. Samter, M. Bronchial asthma and sensitivity to histamine. *Z. Ges. Exp. Med.* 89:24, 1933.
3. Rose, B., Rusted, I., and Fownes, A. Intravascular catheterization studies of bronchial asthma: I. Histamine levels in arterial and mixed venous blood of asthmatic patients before and during induced attacks. *J. Clin. Invest.* 29:1113, 1950.
4. Rose, B. Role of histamine in anaphylaxis and allergy. *Amer. J. Med.* 3:545, 1947.
5. Curry, J. J. Comparative action of acetyl-beta-methyl choline and histamine on the respiratory tract in normals, patients with hay fever, and subjects with bronchial asthma. *J. Clin. Invest.* 26:430, 1947.
6. Curry, J. J. The action of histamine on the respiratory tract in normal and asthmatic subjects. *J. Clin. Invest., Ibid.,* p. 785.
7. Curry, J. J. The effect of antihistamine substances and other drugs on histamine bronchoconstriction in asthmatic subjects. *J. Clin. Invest.* 25:792, 1946.
8. Tiffeneau, R. *Examen Pulmonaire de l'Asthmatique: Déductions Diagnostiques, Prognostiques et Thérapeutiques.* Paris: Masson et Cie, 1957.
9. Melon, J., and Lecomte, J. Étude comparée des éffets de la bradykinine et des réactions anaphylactiques locales chez l'homme. *Int. Arch. Allerg.* 21:89, 1962.
10. Scherbel, A., and Harrison, J. Serotonin hypersensitivity in collagen diseases. *Bull. Rheum. Dis.* 9:179, 1959.
11. Hajos, M. K. Clinical studies on the role of serotonin in bronchial asthma. *Acta Allerg.* 17:358, 1962.
12. Baer, R. L. *Atopic Dermatitis.* New York: New York University Press, 1955.
13. West, J. R., Johnson, L. A., and Winkelmann, R. K. Delayed-blanch phenomenon in atopic individuals without dermatitis. *Arch. Derm.* (Chicago) 85:107, 1962.
14. Halpern, B. N. Histamine and Processes of Histamine Liberation. In Prigal, S. J. (Ed.), *Fundamentals of Modern Allergy.* New York: McGraw-Hill Book Company, Inc., 1960.
15. Hampton, S. F. Infection in Bronchial Asthma. Chapter 50, this volume.
16. Szentivanyi, A., and Fishel, C. W. The Amine Mediators of the Allergic Response and the Reactivity of their Target Cells. In Filipp, G. (Ed.), *Kausale Therapie der allergischen Krankheiten. Grundprinzipien und Experimentelle Grundlagen.* Stuttgart: Ferdinand Enke (in press).
17. Satake, Y. Secretion of adrenaline and sympathins. *Tokohu J. Exp. Med.,* Vol. 60, supp. II, 1954.
18. Hagen, P. The storage and release of catecholamines. *Pharmacol. Rev.* 11:361, 1959.
19. Szentivanyi, A., Fishel, C. W., and Talmage, D. W. Adrenaline mediation of histamine and serotonin hyperglycemia in normal mice, and the absence of adrenaline-induced hyperglycemia in pertussis-sensitized mice. *J. Infect. Dis.* 113:86, 1963.
20. Rocha e Silva, M. The physiological significance of bradykinin. *Ann. N.Y. Acad. Sci.* 104:190, 1963.
21. Robson, J. J., and Stacey, R. S. *Recent Advances in Pharmacology* (3rd ed.). Boston: Little, Brown, 1962.
22. Riker, W. F. Cholinergic Drugs. In Drill, V. A. (Ed.), *Pharmacology in Medicine* (2nd ed.). New York: McGraw-Hill Book Company, Inc., 1958.
23. Nickerson, M. Blockade of the actions of adrenaline and noradrenaline. *Pharmacol. Rev.* 11:443, 1959.
24. Ahlquist, R. P. A study of the adrenotropic receptors. *Amer. J. Physiol.* 153:586, 1948.
25. Furchgott, R. F. The pharmacology of vascular smooth muscle. *Pharmacol. Rev.* 7:183, 1955.
26. Furchgott, R. F. Receptors for Sympathomimetic Amines. In Vane, J. R., Wolstenholme, G. E. W., and O'Connor, M. (Eds.), *Ciba Foundation Symposium on Adrenergic Mechanisms.* Boston: Little, Brown, 1960.
27. Gyermek, L. 5-Hydroxytryptamine antagonists. *Pharmacol. Rev.* 13:399, 1961.
28. Green, J. P. Binding of some biogenic amines in tissues. *Advances Pharmacol.* 1:349, 1962.
29. Röthlin, E., and Berde, B. The structure and function of the autonomic nervous system. *Aerztl. Monatsh.* 5:865, 1953.
30. Eccles, J. C. Problems of plasticity and organization at simplest levels of mammalian central nervous system. *Perspect. Biol. Med.* 1:379, 1958.

31. Crossland, J. Chemical transmission in the central nervous system. *J. Pharm. Pharmacol.* 12:1, 1960.
32. Nachmansohn, D. *Chemical and Molecular Basis of Nerve Activity*. New York: Academic Press, Inc., 1959.
33. Nachmansohn, D. Chemical factors controlling nerve activity. *Science* 134:1962, 1961.
34. Emmelin, N. Supersensitivity following "pharmacological denervation." *Pharmacol. Rev.* 13:17, 1961.
35. Koelle, G. B. Neurohumoral Agents as a Mechanism of Nervous Integration. In Bass, A. D. (Ed.), *Evolution of Nervous Control from Primitive Organisms to Man*. Washington, D.C.: American Association for the Advancement of Science, 1959.
36. Burn, J. H. Relation of motor and inhibitor effects of local hormones. *Physiol. Rev.* 30:177, 1950.
37. Schayer, R. W. Induced synthesis of histamine, microcirculatory regulation and the mechanism of action of the adrenal glucocorticoid hormones. *Progr. Allerg.* 7:187, 1963.
38. Pearlman, D. S., and Szentivanyi, A. Excessive Reactivity of Defense Mechanisms—Allergy. In Cook, R. E. (Ed.), *Biologic Basis of Pediatric Practice*. New York: McGraw-Hill Book Company, Inc. (in press).
39. Johnson, G. E., and Sellers, E. A. The influence of iproniazid and pyrogallol on the thermogenic effects of noradrenaline. *Canad. J. Biochem. Physiol.* 40:631, 1962.
40. Vanov, S. Effect of monoamine oxidase inhibitors and pyrogallol on the pressor response to adrenaline, noradrenaline, normetanephrine, and tyramine in the rat. *Arch. Int. Pharmacodynam.* 138:51, 1962.
41. Wylie, D. W., Archer, S., and Arnold, A. Augmentation of pharmacological properties of catecholamines by o-methyl transferase inhibitors. *J. Pharm. Exp. Ther.* 130:239, 1960.
42. Angelakos, E. T., and Loew, E. R. Histamine toxicity in mice and rats following treatment with histaminase inhibitors. *J. Pharm. Exp. Ther.* 119:444, 1957.
43. Schayer, R. W. Catabolism of physiological quantities of histamine in vivo. *Physiol. Rev.* 39:116, 1959.
44. Koelle, G. B. Possible mechanisms for the termination of the physiological actions of catecholamines. *Pharmacol. Rev.* 11:381, 1959.
45. Trendelenburg, U. Supersensitivity and subsensitivity to sympathomimetic amines. *Pharmacol. Rev.* 15:225, 1963.
46. Buchthal, F., and Kahlson, G. Effect of acetylcholine and adenosine triphosphate on denervated muscle. *Acta Physiol. Scand.* 11:284, 1946.
47. Cannon, W. B. A law of denervation. *Amer. J. Med. Sci.* 198:737, 1939.
48. Cannon, W. B., and Rosenblueth, A. *The Supersensitivity of Denervated Structures*. New York: Macmillan Company, 1949.
49. West, G. B. Histamine in Nervous Tissue. In Richter, D. (Ed.), *Metabolism of the Nervous System*. New York: Pergamon Press, 1957.
50. Harvey, J. A. Modification of histamine sensitivity after 48/80 treatment. *J. Pharm. Pharmacol.* 13:61, 1961.
51. Guth, P. S., Byron, J. W., and Ambrus, J. L. Histamine releasers and histamine sensitivity. *Ibid.*, p. 254.
52. Castro de la Mata, R., Penna, M., and Aviado, D. M. Reversal of sympathomimetic bronchodilation by dichloroisoproterenol. *J. Pharm. Exp. Ther.* 135:197, 1962.
53. Fishel, C. W., Szentivanyi, A., and Talmage, D. W. Sensitization and desensitization of mice to histamine and serotonin by neurohumors. *J. Immun.* 89:8, 1962.
54. Fishel, C. W., and Szentivanyi, A. The absence of adrenaline-induced hyperglycemia in pertussis-sensitized mice and its relation to histamine and serotonin hypersensitivity. *J. Allerg.* 34:439, 1963.
55. Fishel, C. W., Szentivanyi, A., and Talmage, D. W. Adrenergic Factors in Pertussis-Induced Histamine and Serotonin Hypersensitivity of Mice. In Landy, M., and Braun, W. (Eds.), *Bacterial Endotoxins*. New Brunswick, N.J.: Rutgers University Press, 1964.
56. Ellis, S. The metabolic effects of epinephrine and related amines. *Pharmacol. Rev.* 8:485, 1956.
57. Dale, J. H. Conditions which are conducive to the production of shock by histamine. *Brit. J. Exp. Path.* 1:103, 1920.
58. Higginbotham, R. D. Influence of adrenalectomy and cortisol on resistance of mice to histamine, serotonin, anaphylactic and endotoxin shocks. *J. Allerg.* 33:35, 1962.
59. Ramey, E. R., and Goldstein, M. S. The adrenal cortex and the sympathetic nervous system. *Physiol. Rev.* 37:155, 1957.
60. Spencer, P. S. J., and West, G. B. Further observations on the relationship between the thyroid gland and the anaphylactoid reaction in rats. *Int. Arch. Allerg.* 20:321, 1962.
61. Adamkiewicz, V. W., and Langlois, Y. Sensitization by insulin to the dextran "anaphylactoid" reaction. *Canad. J. Biochem. Physiol.* 35:251, 1957.
62. Adamkiewicz, V. W., Langlois, Y. L., and Poirier, L. J. Sensitization by insulin to dextran anaphylactoid inflammation in spinal rats. *Amer. J. Physiol.* 195:635, 1958.
63. Sanyal, R. K., Spencer, P. S. J., and West, G. B. Insulin and hypersensitivity. *Nature* (London) 185:2020, 1959.
64. Sanyal, R. K. The effect of insulin on hyper-

sensitivity reactions in the rat. *Allerg. Asthma* 6:317, 1960.

65. Hess, W. R. *Diencephalon, Autonomic and Extrapyramidal Functions.* New York: Grune & Stratton, Inc., 1954.
66. Gellhorn, E. *Autonomic Imbalance and the Hypothalamus.* Minneapolis: University of Minnesota Press, 1957.
67. Szentivanyi, A., and Szekely, J. Wirkung der konstanten Reizung hypothalamischer Strukturer durch Tiefenelekroden auf den histaminbedingten und anaphylaktischen Schock des Meerschweinchens. *Acta Physiol. Hung.* 11 (supp.):41, 1957.
68. Szentivanyi, A., and Filipp, G. Anaphylaxis and the nervous system: Part II. *Ann. Allerg.* 16:143, 1958.
69. Filipp, G., and Szentivanyi, A. Anaphylaxis and the nervous system: Part III. *Ibid.,* p. 306.
70. Szentivanyi, A., and Szekely, J. Anaphylaxis and the nervous system: Part IV. *Ibid.,* p. 389.
71. Stevenson, J. W. Bacterial neurotoxins. *Amer. J. Med. Sci.* 235:317, 1958.
72. Bishop, G. H., and Bronfenbrenner, J. J. The site of action of botulinum toxin. *Amer. J. Physiol.* 117:393, 1936.
73. Surgen, A. S. V., Dickens, F., and Zatman, L. J. The action of botulinum toxin on the neuro-muscular junction. *J. Physiol.* (London) 109:10, 1949.
74. Strömblad, B. C. R. Cholinesterase activity in skeletal muscle after botulinum toxin. *Experientia* 16:458, 1960.
75. Edmunds, C. W., and Keiper, G. F. Further studies on the action of botulinus toxin. *J.A.M.A.* 81:542, 1923.
76. Guyton, A. C., and MacDonald, M. A. Physiology of botulinus toxin. *Arch. Neurol. Psychiat.* 57:578, 1947.
77. Thesleff, S. Nervous control of chemosensitivity in muscle. *Ann. N.Y. Acad. Sci.* 94:337, 1961.
78. Zacks, S. I, Metzger, J. F., Smith, C. W., and Blumberg, J. M. Localization of ferritin-labeled botulinus toxin in the neuromuscular junction of the mouse. *J. Neuropath. Exp. Neurol.* 21:610, 1962.
79. Thesleff, S. Supersensitivity of skeletal muscle produced by botulinum toxin. *J. Physiol.* (London) 151:598, 1960.
80. Emmelin, N. Supersensitivity of salivary gland caused by botulinum toxin. *J. Physiol.* (London) 156:121, 1961.
81. Geiger, W. B., and Alpers, H. S. Mode of action of antigen and other smooth muscle stimulants. *Science* 125:1141, 1957.
82. Boroff, D. A. Chemistry and biological activity of the toxin of *Clostridium botulinum:* Research report. *J. Albert Einstein Med. Center* 11:5, 1963.
83. Arseculeratne, S. N. The effects of diphtheritic toxaemia on blood vessels. *J. Path. Bact.* 85:21, 1963.
84. Dubos, R. J. *Biochemical Determinants of Microbial Diseases.* Cambridge, Mass.: Harvard University Press, 1954.
85. Feldberg, W., and Kellaway, C. H. The liberation of histamine by staphylococcal toxin and mercuric chloride. *Aust. J. Exp. Biol. Med. Sci.* 16:249, 1938.
86. Feldberg, W., and Keogh, E. V. Liberation of histamine from the perfused lung by staphylococcal toxin. *J. Physiol.* (London) 90:280, 1937.
87. Kellaway, C. H., Trethewie, E. R., and Turner, A. W. The liberation of histamine and of adenyl compounds by the toxin of *Cl. welchii* type *P. Aust. J. Exp. Biol. Med. Sci.* 17:253, 1940.
88. Panse, M. V., and Dutta, N. K. Release of histamine by cholera toxin. *Arch. Int. Pharmacodyn.* 145:479, 1963.
89. Norton, S., and de Beer, E. J. Effect of some antibiotics on rat cells *in vitro. Arch. Int. Pharmacodyn.* 102:352, 1955.
90. Bushby, S. R. M., and Green, A. F. The release of histamine by polymyxin B and polymyxin E. *Brit. J. Pharmacol.* 10:215, 1955.
91. Axelsson, J., and Thesleff, S. A study of supersensitivity in denervated mammalian skeletal muscle. *J. Physiol.* (London) 147:178, 1959.
92. Hilton, S. M., and Lewis, G. P. The cause of vasodilatation in the submandibular gland on stimulation of the chorda tympani. *J. Physiol.* (London) 128:235, 1955.
93. Kind, L. S. The altered reactivity of mice after inoculation with *Bordetella pertussis* vaccine. *Bact. Rev.* 22:173, 1958.
94. Sanyal, R. K., and West, G. B. Sensitizing properties of *Haemophilus pertussis* vaccine in laboratory animals. *Int. Arch. Allerg.* 14:241, 1959.
95. Parfentjev, I. A., and Goodline, M. A. Histamine shock in mice sensitized with *Hemophilus pertussis* vaccine. *J. Pharm. Exp. Ther.* 92:411, 1948.
96. Sanyal, R. K. Histamine sensitivity in man. *Int. Arch. Allerg.* 18:197, 1961.
97. Kind, L. S., and Woods, E. F. Inactivation of histamine by lung tissue from histamine sensitive and histamine resistant mice. *Proc. Soc. Exp. Biol. Med.* 84:601, 1954.
98. Niwa, M., Yamadeya, Y., Matsui, T., and Kuwajima, Y. Reduced activity of histaminase in rats sensitized by *Bordetella pertussis. Nature* (London) 183:755, 1959.
99. Schayer, R. W., and Ganley, O. H. Relationship of increased histidine decarboxylase activity to *Bordetella pertussis* vaccine sensitization of mice. *J. Allerg.* 32:204, 1961.

100. Malkiel, S. Anaphylactic shock in the mouse vaccinated with *Hemophilus pertussis. J. Allerg.* 27:445, 1956.
101. Gauthier, G. F., Loew, E. R., and Jenkins, H. J. Histamine sensitivity of adrenalectomized and pertussis treated mice. *Proc. Soc. Exp. Biol. Med.* 90:726, 1955.
102. Kind, L. S. Inhibition of histamine death in pertussis-inoculated mice by cortisone and Neoantergan. *J. Allerg.* 24:52, 1953.
103. Katzenstein, R. Histamine tolerance. *Yale J. Biol. Med.* 16:325, 1944.
104. Essex, H. E., and Horton, B. T. Observations on development of resistance to histamine in the guinea pig. *Proc. Mayo Clin.* 16:603, 1941.
105. Herxheimer, H. The 5-hydroxytryptamine shock in the guinea pig. *J. Physiol.* (London) 128:435, 1955.
106. Bulbring, E., and Burnstock, G. Membrane potential changes associated with tachyphylaxis and potentiation of the response to stimulating drugs in smooth muscle. *Brit. J. Pharmacol.* 15:611, 1960.
107. Axelsson, J., and Thesleff, S. The "desensitizing" effect of acetylcholine on the mammalian motor end-plate. *Acta Physiol. Scand.* 43:15, 1958.
108. Maslinski, C., Maslinski, S. M., and Weinrauder, H. The effect of inhalatory adaptation to histamine on histamine shock and the anaphylactic shock. *Experientia* 12:258, 1963.
109. Stetson, C. A., Jr. Endotoxins and Bacterial Allergy. In Lawrence, H. S. (Ed.), *Cellular and Humoral Aspects of the Hypersensitive States.* New York: Paul B. Hoeber, Inc., 1959.
110. Thomas, L. Mechanisms Involved in Tissue Damage by the Endotoxins of Gram Negative Bacteria. *Ibid.,* p. 451.
111. Westphal, O., and Luderitz, O. Chemische Erfärschung von lipopolysacchariden gramnegativer Bakterien. *Angew. Chem.* 66:407, 1954.
112. Brunson, J. G. Relationships between Endotoxin and Sympathomimetic Amines. Ref. 55.
113. Gilbert, R.P. Mechanisms of the hemodynamic effects of endotoxin. *Physiol. Rev.* 40: 245, 1960.
114. Thomas, L. The role of epinephrine in the reactions produced by the endotoxins of gram-negative bacteria: I. Hemorrhagic necrosis produced by epinephrine in the skin of endotoxin-treated rabbits. *J. Exp. Med.* 104: 865, 1956.
115. Zweifach, B. W., Nagler, A. L., and Thomas, L. The role of epinephrine in the reactions produced by the endotoxins of gram-negative bacteria: II. The changes produced by endotoxin in the vascular reactivity to epinephrine, in the rat mesoappendix and the isolated, perfused rabbit ear. *Ibid.,* p. 881.
116. Zweifach, B. W. Vascular Effects of Bacterial Endotoxin. Ref. 55.
117. Hinshaw, L. B. The Release of Vasoactive Agents by Endotoxin. Ref. 55.
118. Zweifach, B. W. Discussion to Chapter 12. Ref. 109, p. 446.
119. Merler, P., Perrault, A., Trapani, R. J., Landy, M., and Shear, M. J. Absence of endotoxic activity in materials derived without bacterial contamination from mammalian tissue. *Proc. Soc. Exp. Biol. Med.* 105:443, 1960.
120. Gourzis, J. T., Hollenberg, M. W., and Nickerson, M. Involvement of adrenergic factors in the effects of bacterial endotoxin. *J. Exp. Med.* 114:593, 1961.
121. Shwartzman, G. *Phenomenon of Local Tissue Reactivity.* New York: Paul B. Hoeber, Inc. 1937.
122. Thomas, L., Zweifach, B. W., and Benacerraf, B. Mechanisms of tissue damage and shock by endotoxins. *Trans. Ass. Amer. Physicians* 70:54, 1957.
123. Innes, I. R. An action of 5-hydroxytryptamine on adrenaline receptors. *Brit. J. Pharmacol.* 19:427, 1962.
124. Rall, D. P., and Kelly, M. G. The role of vasoconstriction in the local Shwartzman reaction. *J. Exp. Med.* 105:643, 1957.
125. Palmerio, C., Ming, S. C., Frank, E., and Fine, J. The role of the sympathetic nervous system in the generalized Shwartzman reaction. *J. Exp. Med.* 115:609, 1962.
126. Thesleff, S. Effects of motor innervation on the chemical sensitivity of skeletal muscle. *Physiol. Rev.,* 40:734, 1960.

17. Eosinophils*

MAX SAMTER

EOSINOPHILS HAVE A COLORFUL HISTORY. Since their discovery in 1846 [1] they have been controversial components of circulating blood and tissues. Their distinctive appearance has been a constant reminder to imaginative investigators, but in spite of continuing efforts, even the most basic questions about their origin, their disposal, and the possible reasons for their existence are only partially solved or not solved at all.

It is a peculiar distinction of the eosinophils that they participate conspicuously in allergic reactions. In fact, they are major instruments of diagnosis even though their actual function is obscure, whereas lymphocytes, which have a definite and established function, are rarely considered essential to the diagnosis of allergic diseases.

The history of eosinophils has a number of important landmarks. Jones's description of the unstained cell, prominent because of its double-refractory granules, did not cause much excitement: most of the work was initiated after Ehrlich discovered the glamorous stain by which they are so readily identified [2, 3].

It is strange to read the early literature, which contains heated arguments about their structure, e.g., the notion, encouraged by the appearance of their granules, that eosinophils are scavenger cells which dispose of erythrocytes. Charcot-Leyden crystals, the product of disintegrating eosinophils [4, 5], were thought to consist of spermin phosphate, and even though this did not prove to be true, their chemical structure is still unknown.† The entire literature up to 1914 has been admirably summarized by Schwarz [6], whose review, written in German, reports and digests a wealth of observations.

Origin. The origin of eosinophils is still uncertain. Most authors believe that they originate in the bone marrow, are released into the circulation, and migrate into the tissue in which the antigen-antibody interaction has taken place [7–11]. This opinion, however, is not unanimous: a number of investigators maintain that eosinophils develop in tissues [12, 13] and that those found in the circulation represent an overflow, e.g., for the disposal of waste products; it has been suggested, for instance, that they remove histamine from the site of the antigen-antibody interaction [14].

Distribution. This is controlled by specific and nonspecific factors. If specific factors, i.e., tissue "demand" for eosinophils, promote their release from the bone marrow and consequently their increase in the peripheral blood, there must be some communication between bone marrow and tissue which has not been recognized. Speirs [15] speculates about the manner in which such information might be transmitted (and considers it likely "that the antigen or some specific material formed by the antigen could be carried back to the bone marrow by cells"), but the actual mechanism is unknown. It is our suspicion that the nonspecific response, for instance, their adherence to the vascular wall induced by adrenocortical hormones, their fluctuation in laboratory animals as the result of simple handling, or their shift after administration of autonomic drugs [16–18], has been a major reason for the contradictory findings which complicate the interpretation of their behavior.

Function. This is still uncertain, but recent studies have brought forth a number of promising leads. It is probably fair to state that the hypotheses about their role in allergic reactions can be divided into two groups: (1) those which attribute to them a role in the immunological sequence, i.e., in the handling

* Supported in part by U.S. Public Health Service Research Grant No. AI-1855-07.

† Recently Hornung has contributed some evidence that they are polypeptides and that tyrosine is one of their major components (*Proc. Soc. Exp. Biol. Med.* 110:119, 1962).

of antigen or in the synthesis of antibodies, and (2) those which assume that they are involved in tissue changes that develop as the result of the antigen-antibody interaction, e.g., the removal and neutralization of histamine [19, 20]* or the handling of other components of the tissue in which the antigen-antibody interaction occurs [21].

In 1915, Weinberg and Séguin [22, 23] suggested that eosinophils absorb antigen and synthesize antibodies after absorption. In an extension of their studies, Godlowski [24] concluded that eosinophils (which may originate in the bone marrow or in nonhemopoetic tissues) are cells which are invaded by foreign protein. "Eosinophilization" occurs if the intracellular enzyme system is unable to dispose of the intruding molecule; if the invading protein is antigenic, eosinophils become antigen carriers.

The concept of the eosinophil as an antigen carrier implied more or less that it might play a role in antibody formation, a concept which was proposed by Speirs as the result of a series of startling observations. Speirs' [25] early concept was very similar to Godlowski's: Speirs formerly believed that eosinophils react with antigen which induces specific enzymatic changes within the cell. Subsequently, they are incorporated into reticuloendothelial cells which utilize the enzyme to form antibody. Speirs [26] has now modified this concept by the addition of an intermediate step:

> The presence of antigen in the tissues produces an inflammatory response which varies quantitatively depending upon previous exposure of the animal to that antigen. During the early stages, the antigen is engulfed primarily by neutrophils. Later, necrotic neutrophils, as well as antigen, are engulfed by activated lymphocytemacrophage cells. As the inflammation subsides, these cells are stimulated to undergo DNA synthesis and to divide and form medium and small lymphocytes. Some of the mononuclear cells taking part in the inflammatory reaction are specifically injured by the antigen. These cells become highly swollen and form numerous vesicles. Eosinophils are attracted to these injured cells, penetrating their plasma membranes and causing a disruption of their cytoplasm. Later, macrophages engulf the cellular fragments with adherent antigen as well as the eosinophils associated with these fragments. The macrophages then cease their phagocytic activity and undergo morphologic transformation into antibody-producing cells.

Speirs' [27] concepts are stimulating, indeed, and have encouraged a fundamental debate on the subject. Until a few years ago it had been our impression that "the majority of experimental and clinical findings seem to support the belief that eosinophils appear as a result rather than in anticipation of an antigen-antibody interaction" [28], but it seems likely that studies now in progress will modify these conclusions.

The evidence which has been added in recent years supports the belief that antigen-antibody complexes or their sequelae induce eosinophilia. Litt [29, 30] studied lymph nodes which drain the foot pads of guinea pigs after injection of hemocyanin or heterologous protein into the foot pads. Eosinophils invaded lymph nodes within twenty-four hours after a primary antigenic stimulus. His current experiments reconfirm the impression that the early eosinophilia occurs at lymph nodes, not at the site of antigen deposition: antigen and antibody are required to produce eosinophilia in nonlymphoid tissue. On the basis of ingenious experiments with multiple fluorescence, Litt [31] has concluded that eosinophils probably phagocytize antigen-antibody complexes.

Cohen's group [32, 33] is inclined to believe that nonimmunological and immunological mechanisms might be "eosinotactic," but if nonimmunological mechanisms are involved, they appear to require macromolecular complexes of critical qualities rather than micromolecular chemical mediators.

Cohen and Sapp examined the popliteal lymph nodes of the rabbit four hours after injection of polysaccharides into the foot pad. Glycogen, starch, laminarin, and high molecular weight dextran produced significant infiltration by eosinophils, but low molecular weight dextran, dextrose, levulose, polyvinylpyrrolidone, stilbamidine, peptone, and trypsin did not. They emphasize that it is uncertain whether the eosinophilia is caused by a

* The possibility that eosinophils detoxify histamine has been proposed by several investigators. It has been strongly supported by Archer, who studied the eosinophils of the horse. Feldberg, in a foreword to Archer's monograph [20], calls attention to what he considers the major findings of the comprehensive study: (1) that histamine attracts eosinophils, and (2) that suspensions of extracts of equine eosinophils block the action of histamine and, to some extent, of serotonin.

chemotactic or an immunological mechanism, but inhibitors of histamine, serotonin, and heparin had no effect on the development of localized eosinophilic infiltration.

The results of our own studies are similar to those of Litt and Cohen. Initially, we used *Ascaris* keratin, since the response to *Ascaris* and its components has been documented by numerous investigators [34–36]. We succeeded in producing massive pulmonary eosinophilia by injecting it into the anterior vena cava of guinea pigs and hogs. We have confirmed the early appearance of eosinophils in lungs (which might reasonably be called a lymphoid tissue), but the eosinophils, unlike Litt's, were not limited to areas of contact with lymphocytes. Like Litt and Cohen, we have used a reproducible technique: injection of antigenic and nonantigenic substances in a repository vehicle directly into the lung. If this is done, a number of antigens and some nonantigens produce massive tissue eosinophilia but no eosinophilia in the circulating blood.

Voorhorst [37] had previously observed that in mice infected with *Ascaris* there is a good correlation between blood eosinophils and eosinophils in the bone marrow. At the same time, his findings indicate that a sizable increase in circulating eosinophils does not occur until after antigen-antibody interactions have taken place.

It is true that we have never been able to find partially ingested eosinophils or eosinophilic granules incorporated into other cells, but we have very little doubt, on the basis of a comprehensive correspondence which we have carried on with Cohen, Litt, Speirs, and others in anticipation of this review, that it will be possible to reconcile differences in our experimental findings. It is obvious that we differ in interpretation. Litt, for instance, finds eosinophils in lymph nodes after an exceedingly short interval following antigen injection. Since he believes that antigen-antibody complexes induce eosinophilia, he concludes that antibody formation must begin at an astonishingly early moment.

The finding that comparatively simple nonantigens can induce eosinophilia in tissues is not surprising: the antigen-antibody complex might attract eosinophils not per se but by the activation of unknown chemical mediators. The chemicals which have been shown to induce eosinophilia do not seem to have a common denominator. Only one fact is certain and continues to emerge from a variety of old and new techniques [38]: the antigen-antibody complex is the most reliable eosinotactic factor and, as Litt says, probably one of the keys to the mystery. It seems certain that the recognition that eosinophils participate in very early stages of the immunological sequence, an observation for which we owe credit to Speirs, will be an important step toward the long-overdue clarification of their role in allergic events.

REFERENCES

1. Jones, W. T. The blood corpuscle considered in its different phases of development in the animal series, *Phil. Trans. Roy. Soc.* 1:82, 1846.
2. Ehrlich, P. Über die spezifischen Granulationen des Blutes, *Arch. Anat. Physiol.* P. 571, 1879.
3. Ehrlich, P., and Lazarus, A. Die Anaemie. In Nothnagel, H. (Ed.), *Spezielle Pathologie,* 2nd ed., vol. VIII, part I. Vienna: A. Hölder, 1909.
4. Samter, M. Charcot-Leyden crystals. *J. Allerg.* 18:221, 1947.
5. Ayres, W. W., and Starkey, N. M. Studies on Charcot-Leyden crystals. *Blood* 5:254, 1950.
6. Schwarz, E. Die Lehre von der allgemeinen und örtlichen "Eosinophilie." *Ergebn. Allg. Path.* 17:137, 1914.
7. Homma, E. Pathologische und biologische Untersuchungen über die eosinophil Zellen und die Eosinophilie. *Virchow. Arch. Path. Anat.* 233:11, 1921.
8. Hajos, K. Beiträge zur Eosinophilie-Frage: II. Mitteilung. Die Verteilung der eosinophilen Zellen nach Proteininjektionen und in anaphylaktisierten Meerschweinchen. *Z. Ges. Exp. Med.* 59:383 and 389, 1928.
9. Hajos, K., and Mazgon, R. Beiträge zur Eosinophiliefrage: IV. Mitteilung. Die Desensibilisierungseosinophilie. *Z. Ges. Exp. Med.* 68:767, 1929.
10. Samter, M. The role of the formed elements of the blood in allergy and hypersensitivity: A symposium. *J. Allerg.* 26:219, 261, 1955.
11. Samter, M. The response of eosinophils in the guinea pig to sensitization, anaphylaxis and various drugs. *Blood* 4:217, 1949.
12. Ringoen, A. R. The origin of the eosinophil leucocytes of mammals. *Fol. Haemat. Arch.* 27:10, 1921.
13. Godlowski, Z. Z. The fate of eosinophils in hormonally induced eosinopenia and its significance. *J. Endocrinol.* 8:102, 1952.

14. Vaughn, J. The function of the eosinophile leukocyte, *Blood* 8:1, 1953.
15. Speirs, R. S. Production of Antibody in the Reticulo-Endothelial System Initiated by Eosinophils. Presented at International Symposium of the Reticulo-Endothelial Society, Rapallo, Italy, Aug. 29, 1958.
16. von Neusser, E. Haematologische Mitteilungen:I. *Wien. Klin. Wschr.* 41:64, 1892.
17. Bertelli, G., Falta, W., and Schweeger, O. Über die Wechselbeziehung der Drüsen mit innerer Sekretion: III. Über Chemotaxis. *Z. Klin. Med.* 75:77, 1912.
18. Camp, W. J. R. The effect of drugs on the number of circulating white cells. *J. Lab. Clin. Med.* 13:206, 1927.
19. Code, C. F. The mechanism of anaphylactic and allergic reactions: An evaluation of the role of histamine in their production. *Ann. Allerg.* 2:457, 1944.
20. Archer, R. K. *The Eosinophil Leucocytes.* Oxford: Blackwell Scientific Publications, 1963.
21. Samter, M., Kofoed, M. A., and Pieper, W. A factor in lungs of anaphylactically shocked guinea pigs which can induce eosinophilia in normal animals. *Blood* 8:1078, 1953.
22. Weinberg, M., and Séguin, P. Récherches biologiques sur l'éosinophilie. *Ann. Inst. Pasteur* (Paris) 28:470, 1914.
23. Weinberg, W., and Séguin, P. Récherches biologiques sur l'éosinophilie: II. Propriétés phagocytaires et absorption de produits vermineux. *Ann. Inst. Pasteur* (Paris) 29:323, 1915.
24. Godlowski, Z. Z. Allergy and Anaphylaxis as Metabolic Error. *Dual Response to Antigenic Stimulation.* Chicago: Immuno-metabolic Press, 1962. Vol. I.
25. Speirs, R. S. A theory of antibody formation involving eosinophils and reticuloendothelial cells. *Nature* (London) 181:681, 1958.
26. Speirs, R. S. Cells involved in hypersensitivity and immunity, *Blood* 22:363, 1963.
27. Speirs, R. S. Chemotactic Responses of Eosinophils to Antigen-Containing Cells. In *Conceptual Advances in Immunology and Oncology.* New York: Paul B. Hoeber, Inc., 1963. P. 251.
28. Samter, M. On eosinophils, *Allerg. Asthma* 6:195, 1960.
29. Litt, M. Studies in experimental eosinophilia: IV. Determinants of eosinophil localization. *J. Allerg.* 33:532, 1962.
30. Litt, M. Studies in experimental eosinophilia: V. Eosinophils in lymph nodes of guinea pigs following primary antigenic stimulation. *Amer. J. Path.* 42:529, 1963.
31. Litt, M. Eosinophils and Antigen-Antibody Reactions. Presented at Conference on the Acute Inflammatory Response, New York Academy of Sciences, November, 1963.
32. Cohen, S. G., Sapp, T. M., and Gallia, A. R. Experimental eosinophilia: V. Specificity of regional lymph node responses to antigen-antibody systems. *Proc. Soc. Exp. Biol. Med.* 113: 29, 1963.
33. Cohen, S. C., and Sapp, T. M. Experimental eosinophilia: IV. Eosinotactic influences of polysaccharides. *Exp. Molec. Path.* 2:74,1963.
34. Campbell, D. H. Relationship of the eosinophil response to factors involved in anaphylaxis. *J. Infect. Dis.* 72:42, 1943.
35. Gross, R. Zu den Beziehungen zwischen Blut- und Organeosinophilen, besonders bei allergisch-entzündlichen Erkrankungen und unter Corticoiden. *Verhand. Deutsch. Ges. Inn. Med.*, Kongr. 60, p. 736, 1954.
36. Gross, R. Die eosinophilen Leukocyten. In Braunsteiner, H. (Ed.), *Physiologie und Physiopathologie der Weissen Blutzellen.* Stuttgart: Georg Thieme, 1959.
37. Voorhorst, R. *Basic Facts of Allergy.* Leiden: Stenfert Kroese N.V., 1962.
38. Eidinger, D., Raff, M., and Rose, B. Tissue eosinophilia in hypersensitivity reactions as revealed by the human skin window. *Nature* (London) 196:683, 1962.

PART TWO: THE IMMUNOLOGICAL SYSTEM IN MAN

Bram Rose, Editor

Introduction

BRAM ROSE

IN THIS PART AN ATTEMPT IS MADE to present in logical sequence, the origin of antibody and antibody-like substances in man, a discussion of those diseases which influence their production, and finally their role in the manifestations of hypersensitivity to infectious agents.

The two types of immunological reactions with which we are concerned are those mediated by conventional or circulating antibody and those mediated by cells as exemplified by the tuberculin reaction. The latter appear to be of importance not only in infectious processes but also in homograft rejection and in diseases of "autoimmunity." The term "antibody-like" is used by some since it is not precisely known what the mediating factor is in delayed sensitivity. However, if antibody is defined as a substance which arises as a consequence of antigenic stimulation and which is capable of combining specifically with the antigen responsible, then the term "antibody" should be acceptable.

Section I deals in part with a consideration of the lymphatic system as it pertains to the synthesis of antibody and the physicochemical nature of the eight immunoglobulins which have been described thus far. It is of particular interest that the small lymphocyte is thought to be the cell responsible for delayed or cell-bound immunity as well as the precursor of the "immunocyte" and plasma cell from which the immunoglobulins are derived.

These points are discussed again in Section II, where diseases which may affect the normal physiology of the immunological system are considered. It is this group of diseases which Dr. Good is so fond of calling "experiments of nature," particularly the hypogammaglobulinemias, myeloma, and macroglobulinemia, which have provided such a wealth of material for studies on the immunoglobulins. Here we see plasma cells related to γ-globulins of the 7S variety and lymphocytoid cells giving rise to macroglobulins, as suggested by Waldenström. In both myeloma and macroglobulinemia, it is of interest that no antibody activity has yet been demonstrated in the excessive protein characteristic of each condition. A marked lowering of resistance to the bacterial infections is characteristic of the hypogammaglobulinemias. However, positive skin reactions of both the immediate and the delayed variety have been described. With reference to the former, it has recently been suggested that reagin (skin-sensitizing antibody) is a γ_A-globulin. However, Kunkel and, more recently, Loveless have described the appearance of skin-sensitizing antibody in the sera of individuals devoid of this globulin. Clearly, the site of origin of this vexing antibody system is still obscure. Studies in patients with Hodgkin's disease and sarcoidosis may well provide the key to the basic mechanisms involved in delayed sensitivity. One curious and as yet unexplained phenomenon is the effect of cortisol locally on delayed sensitivity in patients with sarcoidosis. The reaction which may be suppressed by cortisol in normal subjects is apparently enhanced in patients with sarcoidosis.

Although in Section III we are concerned mainly with immune responses which produce diseases in man, it is apparent that these are only one aspect of the natural response to infection. That group of factors which in one manner or another provide man with the ability to overcome an invasion of some foreign agent such as the viruses, fungi, bacteria, and parasites may be collectively termed "host resistance." The majority of these do not appear to play any role in hypersensitivity or allergy. Apart from fever and leukocytosis, one might list such entities as lysozyme, properdin, phagocytin, and interferon, to mention a few. However, it is entirely possible that one or more may be found to influence or even participate in hypersensitivity mechanisms. It seems apparent that hypersensitivity in many instances is part of the normal response, again best illustrated by the reaction to the tubercle bacillus or its components. In the absence of any disease interfering with the immune response, virtually 100 percent of individuals will develop delayed sensitivity on exposure. Although this is called allergy, it is in sharp contrast to the incidence of the so-called poststreptococcal diseases and the common forms of allergy in which only a small percentage of exposed individuals develop disease. For example, what are the host factors which predispose individuals infected with the β-hemolytic streptococcus to one of the poststreptococcal diseases such as glomerulonephritis and rheumatic carditis? It has been suggested that these may be contingent on the identity of some tissue antigens (genetically acquired) with those of the invading organism, but even here there is no unanimity of opinion and many more theories have been suggested. As one considers delayed skin reactions and immune responses mediated by circulating antibody, their significance varies considerably from one disease to another. Take, for example, the interpretation of the delayed skin reaction in coccidioidomycosis, as compared to that in histoplasmosis. Disappearance of skin reactivity in the former may indicate a marked lowering of resistance to subsequent infection, whereas in histoplasmosis, the reverse appears to be the case.

One is tempted to speculate on the nature of the response of the host in terms of the invading agent. The variety of reactions, such as exanthematous rashes, urticaria, parenchymal lesions, and central nervous system manifestations, would seem to be somewhat dependent on the invading organism. Viruses, the smallest of which are made up only of an outer shell of protein and an inner core of nucleic acid, appear to be much less complex than, for example, the metazoan parasites, such as *Ascaris*. The number of antigenic determinants in the latter are surely legion. It is of interest in this connection that in the latter, immediate type reactions associated with circulating reagin, eosinophilia, and many of the common forms of allergy in the classic sense abound. Does this have to do with the size or with the physical make-up of the antigen?

Whether cell-mediated phenomena related to "transfer factor" will prove to be more important than circulating antibody remains an open question. It is hoped that the clarity and vigor of the chapters making up Part Two, as presented by the authors whom we were fortunate enough to enlist, will do much to stimulate the reader and provide many avenues for future exploration.

SECTION I. RESPONSES OF ANTIBODY-FORMING CELLS

18. Lymphoid Tissues: Their Morphology and Role in the Immune Response

WILLIAM E. EHRICH

THE LYMPHOID TISSUES WHICH OCcur in man range from diffuse infiltrates of lymphoid cells to highly developed lymphoid organs. All contain a matrix consisting largely of reticulum cells and lymphoid cells. But whereas in the thymus this matrix is homogeneous (diffuse lymphoid tissue) (Figs. 18-1, *A,* and 18-2), in the mucosa, spleen, and lymph nodes it usually contains "follicles" (nodular lymphoid tissue) (Fig. 18-1, *B* and *C*). In the spleen, the follicles (Fig. 18-1, *B, b*) develop in the white pulp, that is, the lymphoid sheaths which surround the central arteries (Fig. 18-1, *B, a*). In the lymph nodes, they arise in the cortex (Fig. 18-1, *C*). Nodular lymphoid tissue is distinguished by the presence of specialized veins whose inner lining is crowded with high endothelial cells (*postcapillary veins*) (Figs. 18-1, *C, e,* and 18-3). These do not occur in the thymus and have not been seen in the spleen.

The follicles of lymphoid tissue have been divided into primary, secondary, and tertiary nodules [1]. The primary nodules (solid secondary nodules) consist largely of small lymphocytes (Figs. 18-1, *C, b,* and 18-4). As they are the first to appear in ontogeny (see below), the term primary nodule seems to be appropriate. The secondary nodules are characterized by the presence of so-called germinal centers consisting of large lymphoid cells (Figs. 18-1, *B, b,* and *C, c,* and 18-5). Although some of these may originate primarily in the diffuse lymphoid matrix [1, 2], most of them seem to arise in primary nodules (hence the term secondary nodules). After they have been present for a few weeks, both primary and secondary nodules usually undergo dissolution, but some may develop into tertiary nodules (pseudosecondary nodules) (Figs. 18-1 *C, d,* and 18-6). These, like the primary nodules, contain abundant small lymphocytes. They differ in that they are larger and are the chief sites of postcapillary veins. Primary, secondary, and tertiary nodules do not normally occur in the thymus, nor have tertiary nodules been seen in the spleen.

The lymphoid organs which contain nodular lymphoid tissue also develop plasma cells, but in the spleen these appear chiefly in the red pulp (Figs. 18-1, *B, c,* and 18-7) and in the lymph nodes in the medullary cords (Figs. 18-1, *C, f,* and 18-8) [3–5]. They do not normally occur in the thymus.

Phylogeny. Organized lymphoid tissues are found only in vertebrates. Lymph nodes with "germinal centers" were first noted in birds [3].

Ontogeny. It is agreed that the thymus and, in birds, the bursa of Fabricius* develop before other lymphoid organs.

In the human thymus, lymphopoiesis is first seen in the ninth week of gestation [9]. Cortex and medulla are well differentiated at the end of the second month [10]. The first lymph nodes are found in the third month [3, 11] and are well developed at midgestation [3, 4, 12].

* The bursa of Fabricius is a lymphoepithelial organ peculiar to birds. The saclike structure arises as a posterior diverticulum from the cloaca. The lymphoid tissue, like that of the thymus, forms lobules rather than "follicles." It resembles the thymus also in that it is divided into a central medulla and peripheral cortex, and has therefore been called the "cloacal thymus" [6–8].

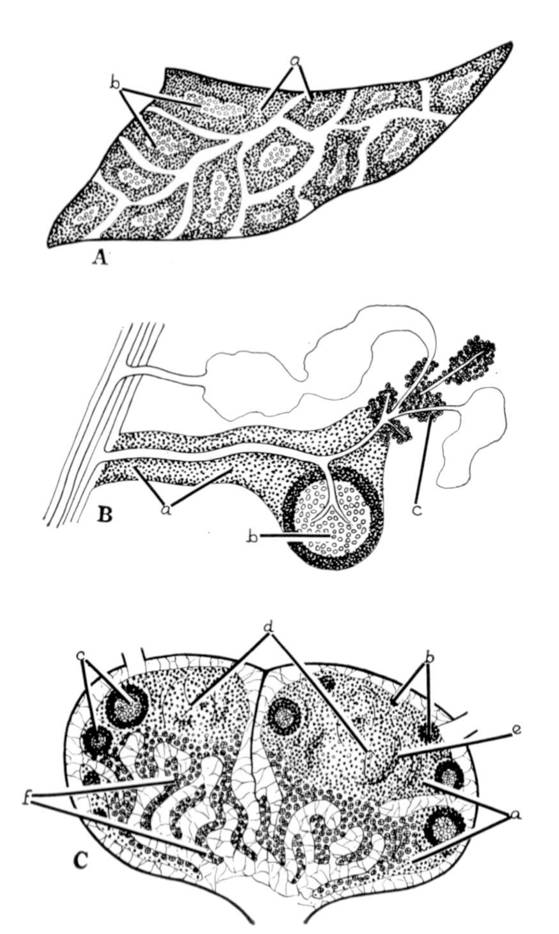

Fig. 18-1. (*A*) Diagram of thymus. Lobules consist of cortex (*a*) and medulla (*b*). The cortex is diffusely infiltrated by lymphocytes. (*B*) Diagram of lymphoid tissue of spleen. Lymph sheaths (*a*) are diffusely infiltrated by lymphocytes. In places, they contain follicles which may have germinal centers (secondary nodules) (*b*). Note that plasma cells, if present, develop in the red pulp (*c*). (*C*) Diagram of lymph node. Cortex (*a*) contains several follicles, e.g., primary nodules consisting of small lymphocytes (*b*), secondary nodules containing germinoblasts (*c*), and large tertiary nodules (*d*). The last contain specialized postcapillary veins (*e*). Medullary cords (*f*) are crowded with plasma cells.

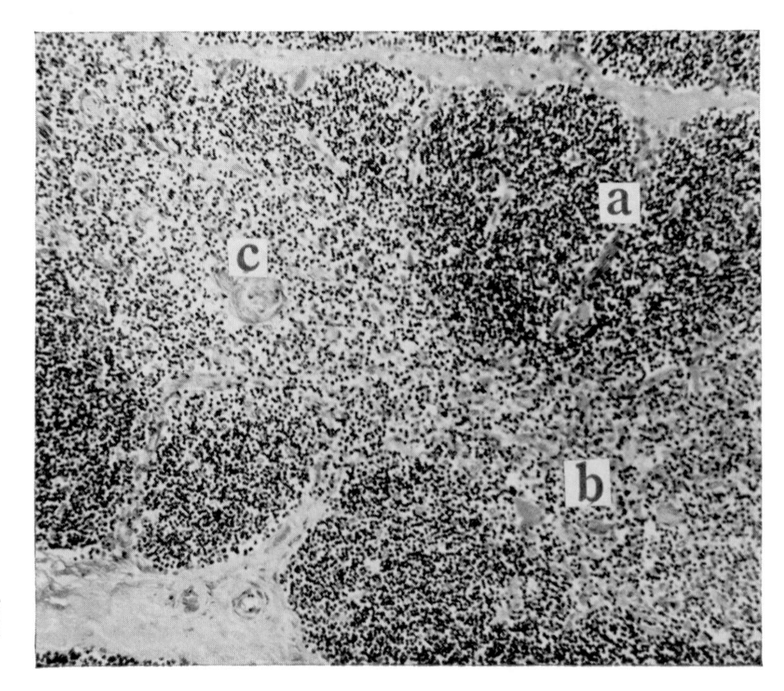

Fig. 18-2. Thymus showing cortex (*a*), medulla (*b*), and Hassall's bodies (*c*).

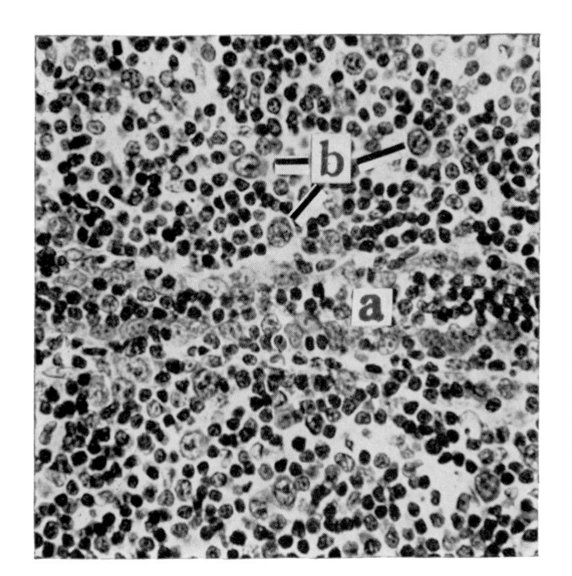

Fig. 18-3. Postcapillary vein in cortex of lymph node. Lumen is crowded with emigrating small lymphocytes (*a*). Note blast forms (*b*) in surrounding lymphoid tissue. (×600, before 25% reduction.) (From Ehrich [125]; courtesy of the publisher.)

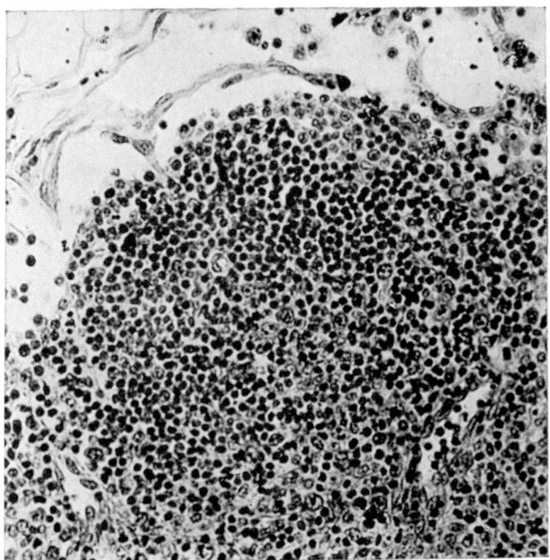

Fig. 18-4. Primary nodule in cortex of lymph node consisting largely of small lymphocytes. (×350, before 25% reduction.) (From Ehrich [2]; courtesy of the publisher.)

Primary and tertiary nodules, the first follicles to appear in ontogeny, are found in axillary lymph nodes as early as the twenty-first week of gestation (Fig. 18-9) [12]. Secondary nodules with germinal centers and plasma cells, on the other hand, appear normally only several months after birth [12, 13].

In the chicken, lymphopoiesis in the thymus is observed first on the twelfth day of incubation [14], in the bursa on the fifteenth to eighteenth day [6, 14, 15], whereas "lymphoid follicle development" in spleen and gut occurs only after hatching [14].

Involution. The relative weight of the thymus (gm./kg. of body weight) increases in fetal life and until the neonatal period, then decreases. The cortex undergoes involution more rapidly than the medulla [9, 16–18]. Its absolute weight is said to double its birth weight by age 2 years, triple it by 11 years, then decrease slowly to about birth size in senility. Hammar's classic data from human beings (Fig. 18-10) and similar data from rabbits [19] (Fig. 18-11) are the best available but

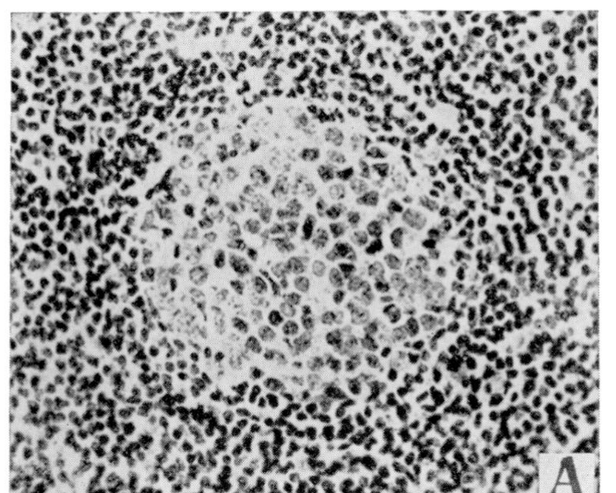

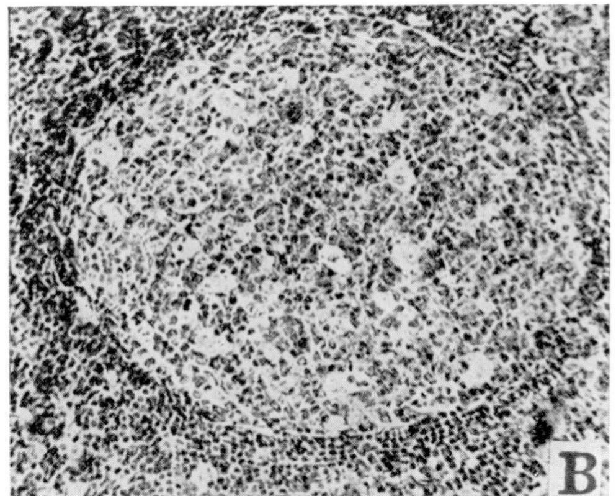

Fig. 18-5. (*A*) Initial stage of secondary nodule (germinal center). Macrophages with tingible bodies are still absent. (*B*) Fully developed secondary nodule. Note numerous macrophages with tingible bodies (nuclear debris). (From Mottura [111]; courtesy of the publisher.)

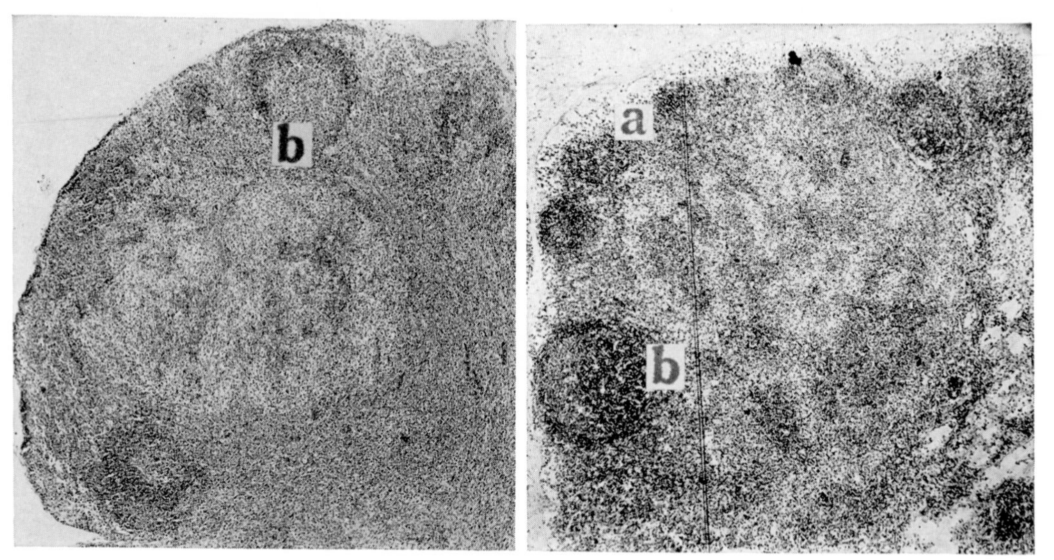

Fig. 18-6. Tertiary nodules in cortex of lymph nodes. In the periphery note primary (*a*) and secondary (*b*) nodules. (×60, before 25% reduction.) (From Ehrich [1, 124]; courtesy of the publishers.)

show remarkable variations, due apparently to failure to exclude glands of individuals or animals who were exposed to stress [20].

Involution of the bursa parallels that of the thymus [6]. Jolly is said to have stated in 1911 and 1913 that it begins "precisely" at puberty [9]. According to Ruth [15], the bursa of all but the most primitive birds involutes completely during sexual maturation. In the chicken, involution begins between 7 and 13 weeks [7].

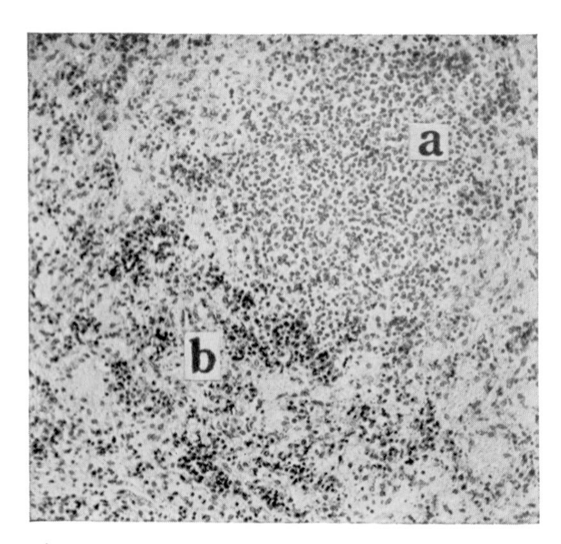

Fig. 18-7. Spleen, showing a follicle (*a*) and nests of plasma cells (*b*); note that the latter are in the red pulp. (From Ehrich [140]; courtesy of the publisher.)

Knowledge of the involution of the nodular lymphoid tissues in lymph nodes, spleen, and mucosa is very incomplete. It appears that they reach their greatest weight later than the thymus and undergo involution less rapidly [3, 4, 21–23].

CELLS OF THE LYMPHOID TISSUES

The cells which characterize the lymphoid tissues consist of fixed and free cells. The fixed cells are known as reticulum cells, the free cells as lymphoid cells.

RETICULUM CELLS

The reticulum cells form a spongelike meshwork whose spaces are filled with lymph and lymphoid cells (Fig. 18-12). Most reticulum cells are capable of ingesting colloidal substances (athrocytosis) and formed particles (phagocytosis). The reticulum cells having this capability were included by Aschoff [24, 25] in his "reticuloendothelial system." Hence they are spoken of also as reticuloendothelial (RE) cells. It should be emphasized, however, that Aschoff meant only those cells which were active phagocytes. The decisive criterion in his own words was "the intensity, the frequency of phagocytosis" [24]. Aschoff did not include the granulocytes in this system, but did include the monocytes of Pappenheim and Ferrata (the large mononuclear cells and

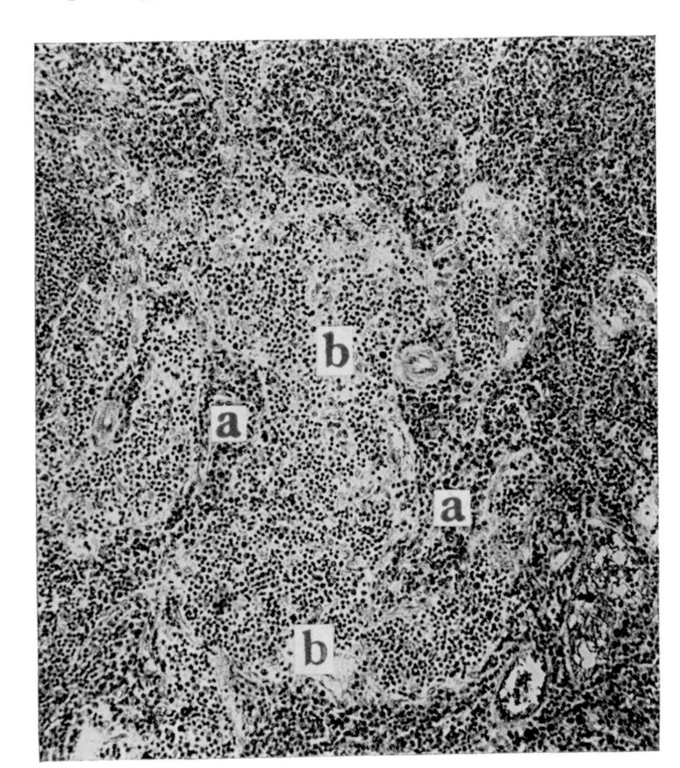

Fig. 18-8. Lymph node, showing plasma cells in the medullary cords (*a*) and emigration through the sinuses of small lymphocytes (*b*). (×170, before 25% reduction.) (From Ehrich [2]; courtesy of the publisher.)

transition forms of Ehrlich) and the histiocytes of Kiyono (the phagocytic mononuclear cells of the tissues). He thus meant the same cells called macrophages by Metchnikoff since 1883 [26]. The term reticuloendothelial cells, like the term macrophages, is therefore a functional one, referring to cells with a special function. The term reticulum cells, on the other hand, is a morphological one, referring to the fixed cells of the blood-forming organs.

The identity of the reticulum cells is not certain. Most writers [27–36] seem to believe that they are the same as the RE cells or macrophages. They postulate that athrocytosis and phagocytosis may be temporary functions during their development and that after completing these functions, they may change into lymphocytes, plasma cells, granulocytes,

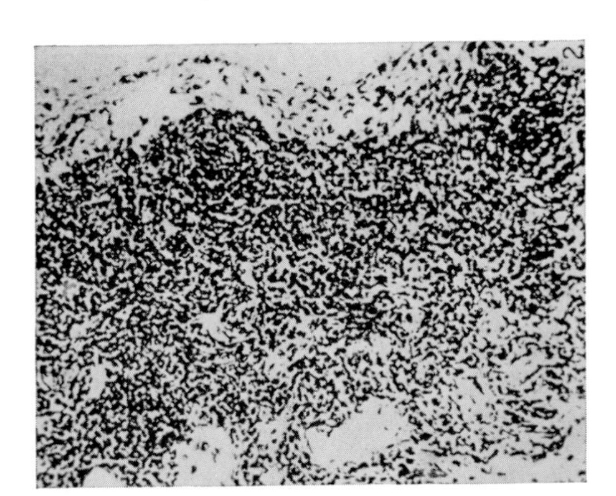

Fig. 18-9. Primary nodules in cortex of an axillary lymph node of a 26-week fetus. (From Ehrich [12]; courtesy of the publisher.)

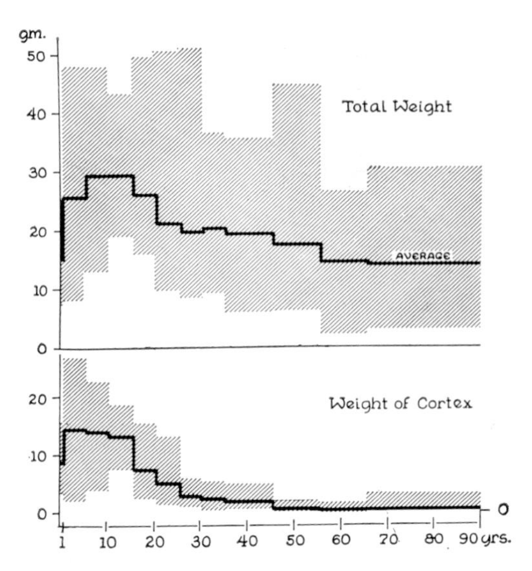

Fig. 18-10. Weights of 345 "normal" thymus glands of persons who died soon after injury. (Drawn after data of Hammar [9, 16].)

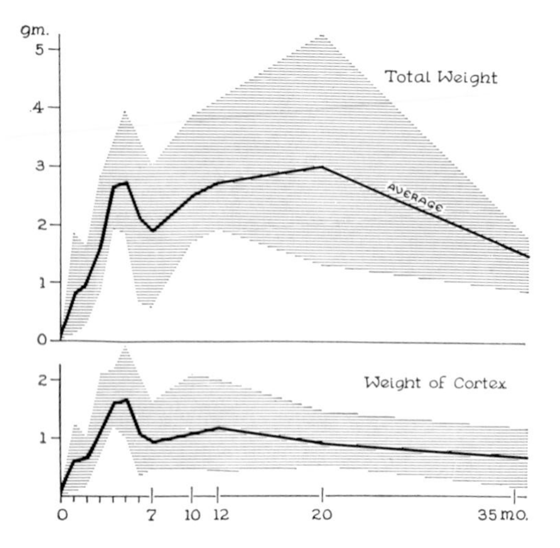

Fig. 18-11. Weights of 120 "normal" thymus glands of "normal" rabbits. (Drawn after data of Gedda [19].)

and other mesenchymal elements. According to this view, they are undifferentiated mesenchymal cells (stem cells) as well as phagocytes.

In fact, some investigators have suggested that these two functions are interdependent, i.e., that the second function, differentiation into other cells, depends on the first function, the athrocytosis and phagocytosis. Thus Fagraeus [31] believed that differentiation of RE cells into plasma cells was initiated by their phagocytosis of antigen. Similarly, Trowell [33, 37] postulated that transformation in the germinal centers of macrophages into lymphoblasts was due to their uptake of disintegrating lymphocytes.

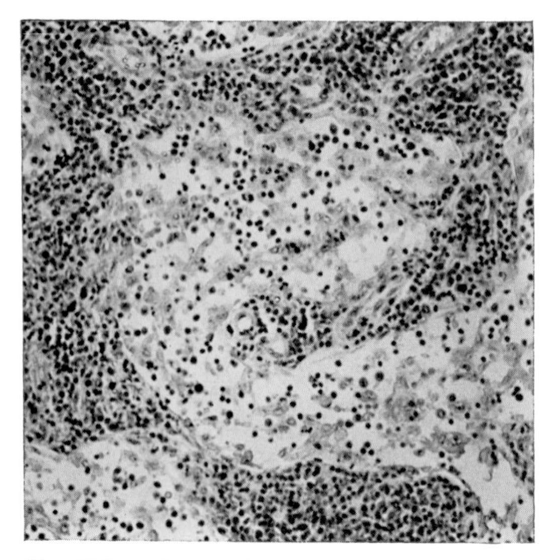

Fig. 18-12. Sinuses of lymph node with activated reticulum cells. (×230, before 25% reduction.) (From Ehrich [2]; courtesy of the publisher.)

Amano [38], Japan's outstanding histohematologist, and his pupil Tanaka [39] concluded from extensive phase contrast and electron microscopic studies that all reticulum cells, in either the proliferative or functional phase, perform athrocytosis and phagocytosis, the difference in this activity being quantitative rather than qualitative. But they insisted that the reticulum cells in proliferative phase are not pluripotential and can give rise only to "lymphogonia," the mother cells of the lymphocytes. Therefore they spoke of lymphoreticular cells.

It should be emphasized that Aschoff never claimed that his RE system was a pluripotential cell system. Maximow [40], who first thought that the macrophages were undifferentiated stem cells, later [41, 42] stated emphatically that the macrophages were end forms which could not differentiate into other cells. He then agreed with Marchand [43, 44] and his pupil Herzog [45–47] that the phagocytosing reticulum cells are associated with inconspicuous cells which lack the power of phagocytosis but are capable of differentiating into macrophages and other mesenchymal cells (Fig. 18-13). As these cells were most conspicuous in the adventitia of small blood vessels, Marchand called them adventitial cells. However, some of the cells that Marchand called adventitial cells could well have been migrating lymphocytes (Fig. 18-14, *A*) [5], and some of those that Herzog called adventitial cells could have been histiocytes (Fig. 18-14, *B*)

If all of the reticulum cells were undifferentiated stem cells as well as phagocytes, it would be difficult to understand why, after lethal irradiation, the RE cells are incapable of repopulating the blood-forming tissues with myeloid or lymphoid cells (see below), although they appear to be well preserved and retain their capability of phagocytosis [48].

The view of Marchand, Herzog, and Maximow that the reticulum cells are not all the same and that they include undifferentiated remnants of the primitive mesenchyme which prevailed early in life is shared by many authors [49–54]. It must be admitted that this view has not been proved. At least, some of the cells which were looked on as undiffer-

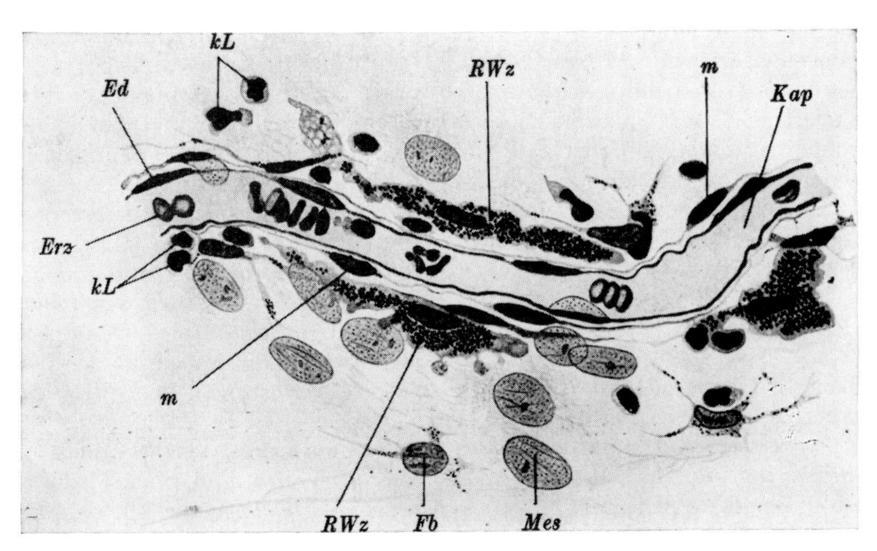

Fig. 18-13. Drawing by Maximow [42] showing undifferentiated mesenchymal cells (*m*) in adventitia of a capillary (*Kap*), macrophages filled with carmine (*RWz*), endothelial cells (*Ed*), fibrocytes (*Fb*), mesothelium (*Mes*), and small lymphocytes (*kL*). (Courtesy of the publisher.)

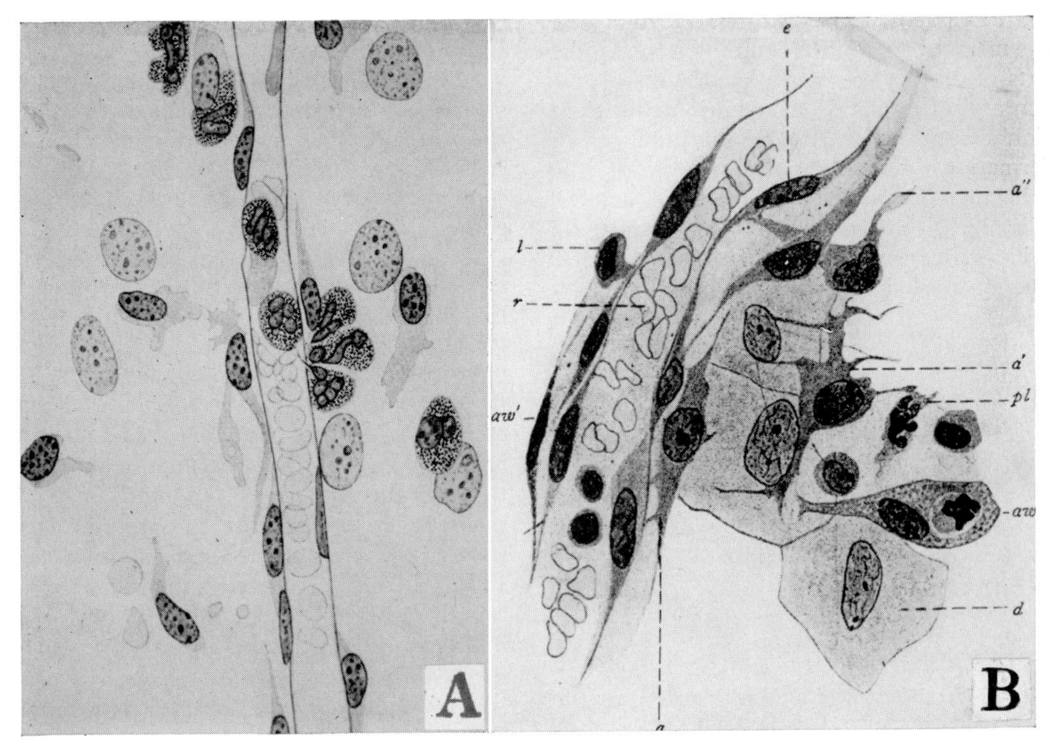

Fig. 18-14. (*A*) Drawing by Marchand [44] showing activation of "adventitial cells." Activated cells resemble small lymphocytes. (*B*) Drawing by Herzog [45] showing activation of "adventitial cells" (*aw'*). Activated cells (*a, a'*) resemble macrophages.

entiated mesenchymal cells might well have been migrating small lymphocytes or some other mesenchymal elements. It seems best, at present, to assume that the reticulum cells present a heterogeneous population of ontogenetically and functionally different cells and that they possibly include undifferentiated stem cells and all stages of development between these cells and fully differentiated macrophages.

ROLE OF MACROPHAGES IN THE IMMUNE RESPONSE

Metchnikoff [26] believed that the macrophages were cellular sources of serum antibodies. This view seemed to be supported by the observation that the formation of such antibodies could be depressed through "blockage" of the macrophages by colloids or formed particles [55]. Subsequent studies, however, have shown that blockage interferes with the ingestion and digestion of the antigen by the macrophages but not with the synthesis of serum antibodies by the antibody-forming cells [56] (see below).

The evidence now indicates that the role of the macrophages in the immune response consists of athrocytosis and phagocytosis of antigen and of preparation, retention, and excretion of substances capable of inducing the formation of immunologically competent cells, including antibody-forming plasma cells (Fig. 18-15) [5, 57–60]. It is possible that this preparatory function is the cause of the induction period of antibody formation.

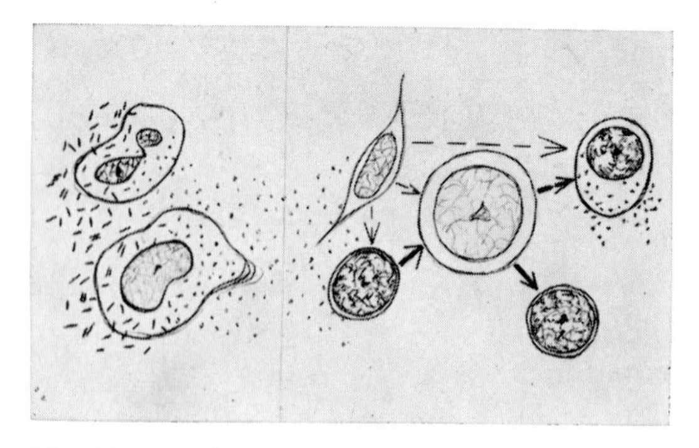

Fig. 18-15. Diagram showing, from left to right: phagocytes ingesting bacteria and excreting material which induces a small lymphocyte (and undifferentiated mesenchymal cell) to change into a large blast form which, in turn, changes into plasma cells and again into small lymphocytes. Transformation indicated by the broken line has not been proved.

The nature of the substances which induce antibody formation is not known. We first believed that the macrophages converted bacteria and other corpuscular antigens into soluble molecules [5, 57], but it now appears that they modify soluble antigen as well [59, 61]. Antigenic ferritin molecules, which can be seen in the electron microscope, disappear during this preparation [62]. It appears that they are broken down into fragments which may not be larger than a specific antigenic determinant measuring 1,000 sq. A, i.e., equivalent to four simple amino acids [61]. These observations suggest that the inducing substances are either fractions of antigen or mediators formed by the cell in response to the antigenic stimulation. Tissue culture experiments by Fishman [60] suggest that they are ribonuclease-sensitive.

The capacity of macrophages to retain antigenic material for long periods has been demonstrated by several workers [63–65]. According to Campbell and Garvey [61], such material is intimately associated with ribonucleic acid (RNA).

LYMPHOID CELLS

The lymphoid cells in mammals include several distinct entities. Outstanding among them are the lymphocytes, plasma cells, and cells of the germinal centers. Because of their controversial nature, the last have been called germinoblasts [66].

It is generally agreed that these three types of cells originate in blast forms. Confirmation has been obtained through studies with tritiated thymidine, a nucleotide incorporated only in the desoxyribonucleic acid (DNA) of the chromosomes. If lymphoid cells are exposed to a single injection of this material, radioactive granules appear first in the blasts, then in medium-sized cells, and finally in small cells, the number of granules being reduced to one-half at each division (Fig. 18-16) [67–74]. Whereas the blasts were rapidly labeled, it took three weeks of 12-hourly injections to label up to 40 percent of the small lymphocytes [75].

The identity of the blasts is not certain. Ehrlich and Lazarus, Naegeli, Marchand [44], Aschoff and Kiyono [76], Schilling [77], and others believed that each series of leukocytes had their own blast (myeloblast, lymphoblast, monoblast)—the *polyphyletic theory.* Pappenheim [78], Ferrata [79], and later Sabin and

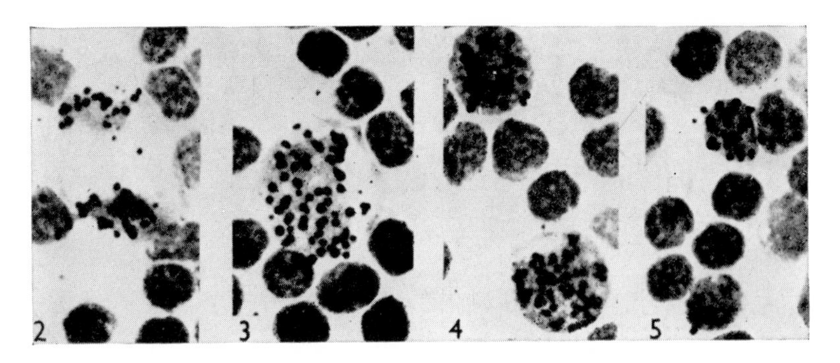

Fig. 18-16. Tritiated thymidine-labeled thoracic duct lymphocytes. From left to right: large lymphocyte dividing (*2*); large lymphocyte (*3*); two medium lymphocytes (*4*); and small lymphocyte (*5*). (From Gowans [70]; courtesy of the publisher.)

her pupils [49] shared this view but felt that the various blasts were preceded by a polyvalent blast, the "large lymphocyte" of Pappenheim, later called "hemocytoblast" by Ferrata—the *neopolyphyletic theory*. On the other hand, Maximow [40–42, 80], Weidenreich [27], Downey [28, 29, 81], and others postulated that all blasts were uniformly polyvalent and that the small lymphocyte was also a blast with similar if not identical potentialities—the *monophyletic theory*. Therefore Maximow recommended replacement of the terms myeloblast, lymphoblast, and monoblast by Ferrata's term, hemocytoblast, although this term was coined to designate another cell, as mentioned earlier. The view that the lymphocyte was not an end form but was capable of transforming into macrophages had previously been advocated by Metchnikoff [30].

The term "polyblast" was introduced by Maximow to designate "inflammatory macrophages." He chose this term not because he thought that they were polyvalent but because of their pleomorphic shape [42]. The identity of these cells is not clear. Maximow thought that they were derivates of small lymphocytes, monocytes, and histiocytes, but Downey [30] identified them with the histiocytes (resting wandering cells of Maximow).

PLASMA CELLS

The plasma cells have long been known to aggregate around small blood vessels (Fig. 18-17*) [5, 27, 42, 82–84]. In the spleen they are found in the red pulp, and in the lymph nodes, in the medulla. It is agreed that the plasma cells originate in plasmablasts (Fig. 18-18†) and that plasmacytogenesis is associated with considerable mitotic activity [5, 52, 88, 89]. The formation of plasma cells through mitotic division of blasts has been confirmed through studies with tritiated thymidine [70, 90]. The origin of the plasmablasts is still uncertain. The fact that plasma cells aggregate around small blood vessels has been interpreted to signify that they are derivates of adventitial cells (undifferentiated stem cells) [5, 38, 84, 91]. Recent studies, however, have led to a revival of Marschalko's theory [82] that they are derivates of small lymphocytes (see below).

Experiments with tritiated thymidine indicate that the maturation time of the plasma cells is less than twelve hours. Their life span was estimated to range from two to four days after the last mitosis [90].

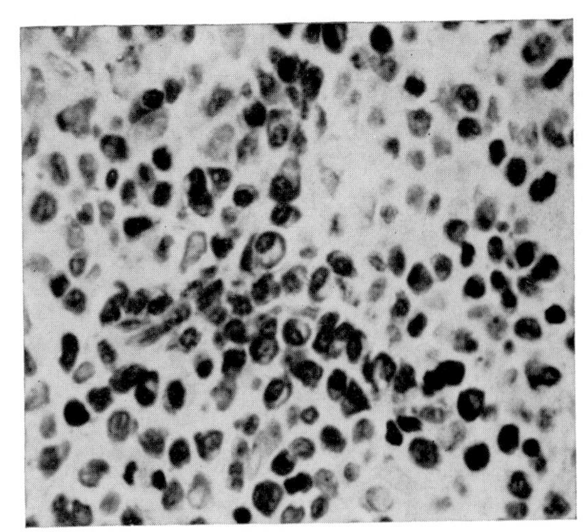

Fig. 18-17. Perivascular aggregation of plasma cells in human bone marrow. (From Ehrich [5]; courtesy of the publisher.)

* An excellent illustration of the perivascular aggregation of antibody-forming plasma cells shown by the fluorescent antibody technique was published by Vazquez [85].

† Excellent photographs showing abundant blasts among developing plasma cells were furnished by Fagraeus [31], Thorbecke [86], and Movat [87].

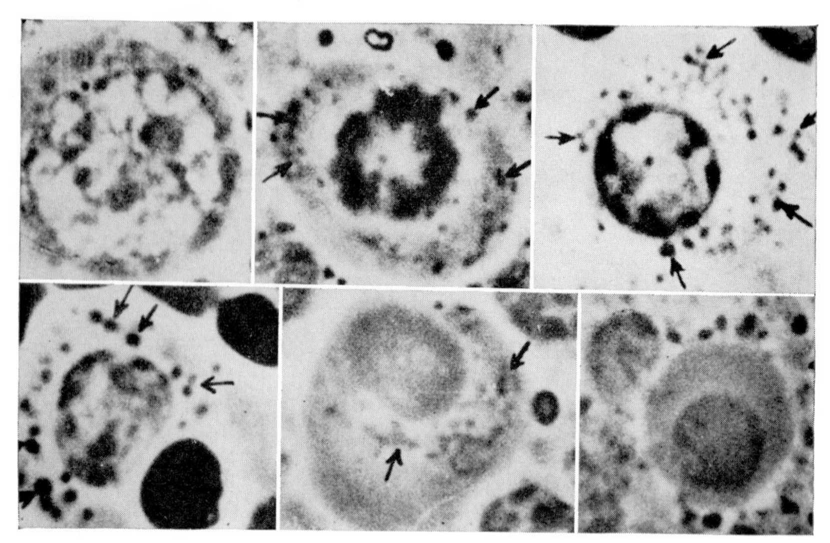

Fig. 18-18. Plasmablasts, proplasmacytes and plasma cells as seen through the phase microscope. (From Moeschlin, Pelaez and Hugentobler [243]; courtesy of the publisher.)

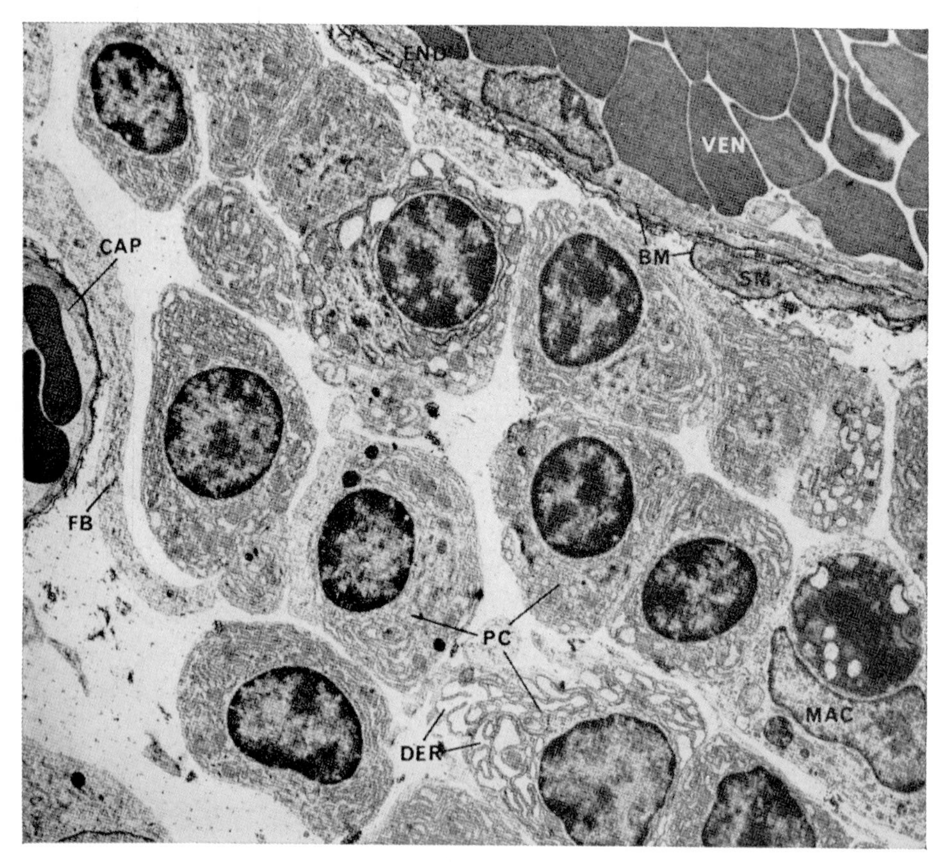

Fig. 18-19. Plasma cells with distinct endoplasmic reticulum (*PC*) and a macrophage without this reticulum (*Mac*). (From Movat and Fernando; courtesy of the publisher.)

ROLE IN THE IMMUNE RESPONSE

We know that plasma cells form serum antibodies and other γ-globulins. The evidence is (1) morphological, (2) clinical, and (3) experimental.

1. Plasma cells resemble other protein-secreting cells in that their cytoplasm is crowded with roughly surfaced endoplasmic reticulum (ergastoplasm) (Fig. 18-19) [92, 93]. Macrophages are similarly furnished with such reticulum, but of different quantity [38, 39]. The lymphocytes, like other nonprotein-secreting cells, contain no such reticulum [92].

2. Patients with a rise in γ-globulins have a corresponding increase in plasma cells, the highest levels being seen in patients with plasma cell tumors (multiple myelomas) [5, 94]. Conversely, newborn animals and human beings, and patients with agammaglobulinemia, who lack the ability to form serum antibodies and other γ-globulins, do not have plasma cells [95–98] while their macrophages and lymphocytes are usually normal [99, 100].

3. If lymphoid cells were removed from lymph nodes that were forming serum antibodies and were mixed on a slide with the bacteria with which antibody formation was induced, we [101] observed that the bacteria agglutinated on the surface of cells resembling plasma cells but not on macrophages or lymphocytes (Fig. 18-20). This observation has been confirmed by several investigators [74, 90]. If two different bacteria were used simultaneously, some plasma cells agglutinated only one species, others only the other species, while still others did not agglutinate at all. This was interpreted to indicate that plasma cells usually form only one serum antibody, the plasma cell being as specific as the antibody which it forms, and that antibody formation is initiated during mobilization of plasmablasts from their stem cells, the synthesis of antibody, like that of hemoglobin, being accomplished during differentiation or maturation of the protein-forming cell [58].

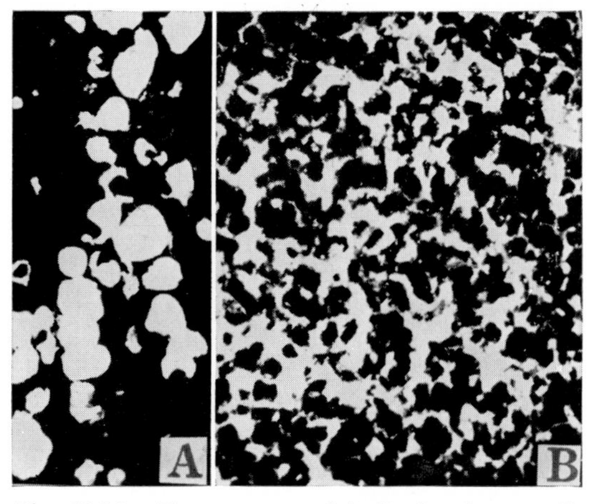

Fig. 18-21. Fluorescent γ-globulin in plasma cells (*A*) and germinoblasts (*B*). (From Ortega and Mellors [128]; courtesy of the publisher.)

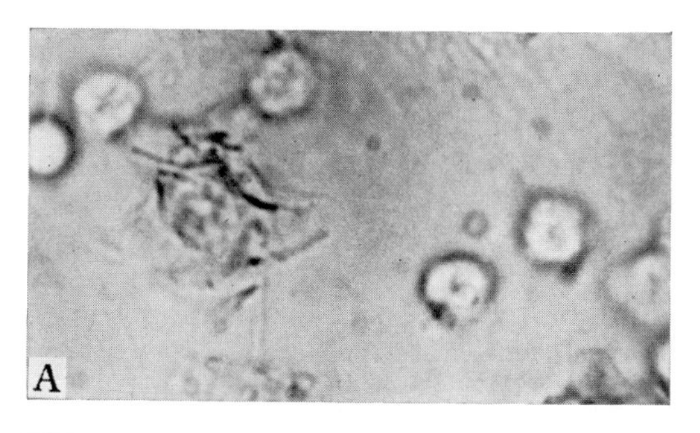

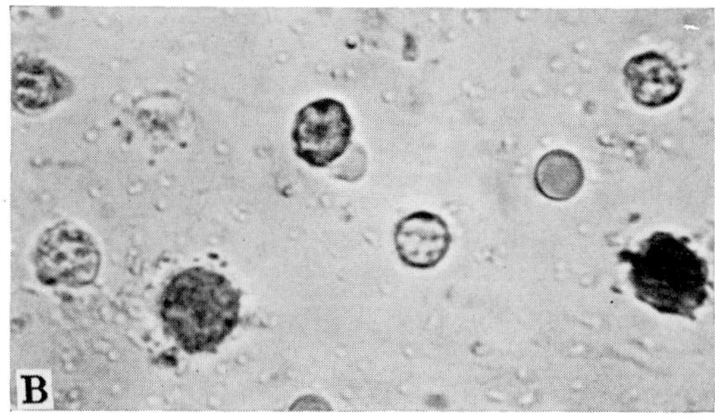

Fig. 18-20. Agglutination of typhoid bacilli (*A*) and *Brucella* bacilli (*B*) by antibody-forming plasma cells. Note that the lymphocytes are not involved. (From Reiss *et al.* [101]; courtesy of the publisher.)

Similar results were later obtained by Coons *et al.* [88, 102, 103] by means of Coons's fluorescent antibody technique (Fig. 18-21, *A*) and by Nossal [104, 105] through observation of immobilization of flagellae of *Salmonella* by antibodies formed *in vitro* by isolated lymphoid cells. But whereas in 1,399 experiments with two different flagellar antigens the plasma cells formed only one or the other antibody or no antibody at all [106], in experiments in which antibody production against flagellar and somatic antigens was tested simultaneously by immobilization of flagellae and by surface agglutination of bacteria, 7 of 658 plasma cells were found to be "double-producers" in that they produced two antibodies simultaneously [74]. But as no one had observed production of more than two antibodies by one cell, Nossal and Mäkelä [74] concluded that it is not necessary to assume that "more than one gene locus in diploid cells is involved in antibody specificity."

It has long been known that the antibody response to a second injection of soluble antigen (secondary response) is much faster and stronger than the response to the first (primary response) [108]. This has been explained by the presence during the secondary response of specific antibody-containing plasmablasts or proplasmacytes and their rapid division caused by the precipitation of antigen on their surface [107, 109].

It has recently been shown that drainage of the thoracic duct and the resulting loss of lymphocytes from the tissues cause severe depression of the primary antibody response but not of the second [110]. This seems to show that the first response requires new formation of plasma cells from stem cells, while the second response is a function of "sensitized" plasma cells which, in contrast to lymphocytes, do not enter the circulation and so are retained in the tissues [90, 110].

These and other observations have led to the suggestion that the formation of serum antibodies by plasma cells is primarily a function of the genetic apparatus of the immunologically competent cells, antibody production being induced by the interaction of specific inducing substances (see p. 90) with the DNA contained in the chromosomes of these cells (genetic theory of antibody formation) [58, 107]. If antibody formation were primarily due to an interaction with RNA such as the messenger RNA, there would be no reason why one plasma cell should not form any number of different antibodies.

GERMINOBLASTS

The germinoblasts of the germinal centers are quite homogeneous in appearance (Fig. 18-5). They are characterized by marked mitotic activity. One-half hour after a single injection of tritiated thymidine, as many as 50 to 60 percent of all germinoblasts were found to be labeled [112]. Their DNA synthesis time was estimated at approximately five hours, their generation time, i.e., the interval between successive mitoses, at 13.4 hours or less [75].

Fully developed germinal centers are distinguished by the presence in their macrophages of numerous disintegrating nuclei (tingible bodies) (Figs. 18-5, *B*, and 18-22). This led Heiberg [113] and others [1] to postulate that they were graveyards of small lymphocytes. However, recent studies with tritiated thymidine by Fliedner *et al.* [75] leave little doubt that Cottier [114] was right when he suggested that the tingible bodies originated not from small lymphocytes but from the germinoblasts themselves. The significance of this turn-over is not clear. It possibly plays a role in nucleoprotein metabolism [20, 115–118].

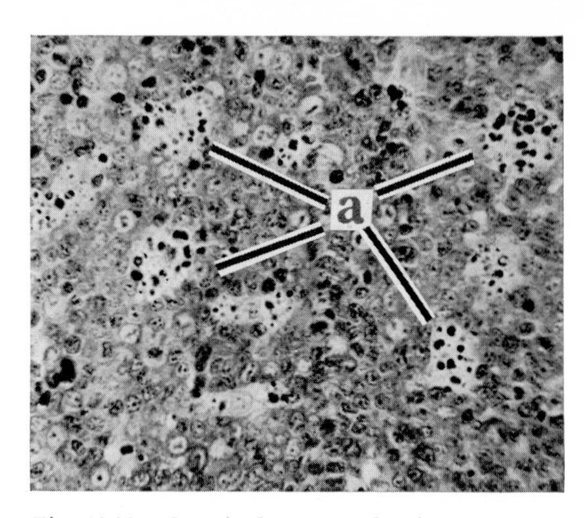

Fig. 18-22. Germinal center, showing numerous macrophages containing tingible bodies (disintegrating nuclei) (*a*).

Histochemically, the germinoblasts differ from other lymphoid cells and from macrophages in that they are adenosine triphosphatase-negative but rich in 5-nucleotidase. Also, they lack esterase and acid and alkaline phosphatase [119].

The usual fate of germinal centers is dissolution [1, 2, 28]. The morphological appearance of occasional germinal centers (plate 11 of Ref. 4) and of some tertiary nodules (Fig. 18-6) suggests, however, that occasionally they may give rise to tertiary nodules.

ROLE IN THE IMMUNE RESPONSE

While some authorities [33, 90, 120–122] still believe with Flemming [123] that the germinal centers are chief centers of lymphopoiesis, others [1, 5, 75, 113, 124–127] think that the multiplication of these cells does not necessarily lead to the formation of small lymphocytes, but that they constitute a special tissue with an immunological function, as first suggested by Hellman [3, 4, 13, 21, 22]. It can hardly be doubted that certain elements in the germinal centers can give rise to lymphocytes, just as they can give rise to plasma cells [23, 28, 42, 128] and to myelocytes [42, 50, 129, 130]. But this must not be taken to indicate that the germinoblasts are lymphoblasts or hemocytoblasts. In fact, the myelocytes in germinal centers have been traced to the "adventitial cells" of the blood vessels contained in these centers [50].

Nossal [90], who was one of the last to defend Flemming's theory, felt that its validity was confirmed by autoradiographic studies with tritiated thymidine [122, 131, 132]. However, positive labeling merely shows that the germinoblasts divide by mitosis. It does not illuminate their nature. Fliedner *et al.* [75, 112], studied active germinal centers with tritiated thymidine and found no evidence of migration of lymphocytes from the centers into the surrounding mantle zone. Also, they collected grain-count data in the germinal centers and in their mantle zone which were incompatible with Flemming's theory.

Hellman's view that the germinoblasts may be special cells with an immunological function received strong support by the recent observation of Ortega and Mellors [128] and of White [133], in that they may reveal the presence of serum antibodies and other γ-globulins if treated by Coons's fluorescent antibody technique (Fig. 18-21, *B*). The production of plasma cells and serum antibodies during the primary antibody response commences after 2 to 3 days, reaches its peak after 4 to 6 days, then subsides [1, 134–138]. The germinal centers, in contrast, make their appearance first after 4 to 6 days, reach their peak after 6 to 10 days, and subside after 2 to 3 weeks [1, 125–127, 133, 134, 138, 139]. For this and similar reasons it is difficult to believe that the function of the germinoblasts is primarily one of formation of serum antibodies. As the germinoblasts were found to contain antibodies only during the secondary response [133], the possibility cannot be ruled out that the presence of antibodies in these cells is accidentally due to uptake of antigenically induced messenger RNA from disintegrating antibody-forming plasma cells [140].

How ever this may be, it cannot be doubted that the reaction of the germinal centers during the primary and secondary responses is initiated by contact of the host with antigen [134]. Whether or not the reaction of the centers is specifically due to antigenic stimulation remains to be seen, for it has been observed also following the injection of benzene or turpentine oil [2].

LYMPHOCYTES

The concept of the lymphocyte was introduced in 1884 by Ehrlich through Einhorn. Weidenreich [27], describing the history of this concept, pointed out that Ehrlich was in error when he credited Virchow with the concept. Naegeli, who, like Ehrlich, distinguished lymphogenic and myelogenic cells, meant by lymphocytes only the small lymphocytes. Both Ehrlich and Naegeli considered the "large mononuclear cells and transitional forms" of Ehrlich to be myelogenous cells, while Pappenheim and Weidenreich counted them with the lymphocytes. These cells were later called monocytes by Pappenheim and Ferrata [141].

Mature lymphocytes are small cells with little cytoplasm containing one or several Gall bodies but lacking endoplasmic reticulum and a complex Golgi apparatus [50, 92, 142]. They rarely, if at all, divide by mitosis [37]. Recent experiments with labeled small lymphocytes, however, leave little doubt that Maximow [40–42] was right in believing that at least some small lymphocytes can change into large blasts resembling the hemocytoblasts of Ferrata or the lymphogonia of Amano and then begin to divide again (discussed below).

The life span of small lymphocytes is usually given as 4 to 7 days [37, 143, 144], but recent studies seem to show that they may live for weeks or months [54, 90, 145]. In fact, Little *et al.* [146] concluded from their studies with continuous infusion of tritiated thymidine that the life span was in excess of 100 days. Others, however, believe that there are two different populations of small lymphocytes, one short- and one long-lived [68, 69, 115, 117, 147, 148]. The latter, according to Cronkite *et al.* [69], differ from the former by their intensively basophilic cytoplasm and loose chromatin network. The view that the small lymphocytes might not be all the same had previously been considered by Aschoff and others [5].

LYMPHOPOIESIS

The origin of the lymphocytes is being vigorously studied. It is agreed that the small lymphocytes are derivates of blast forms (lymphoblasts) (Fig. 18-23) and that lymphopoiesis is a function of all lymphoid tissues.

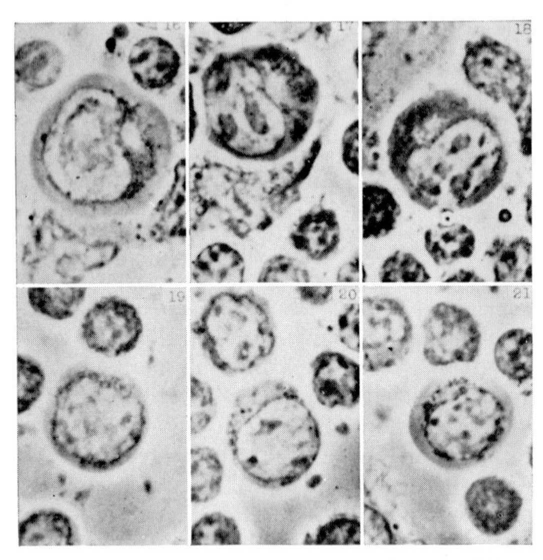

Fig. 18-23. Lymphogonia (lymphoblasts) and lymphocytes as seen through the phase contrast microscope. (From Unno *et al.* [32]; courtesy of the publisher.)

In 1894, Beard postulated that the lymphocytes originate primarily in the thymus and that after maturation they enter the blood to furnish the developing nodular lymphoid tissues with lymphoid cells [40]. This theory was later extended to include the bursa of Fabricius and is now widely accepted [6, 15, 149–152]. The evidence for Beard's view is impressive: (1) It has been shown that the thymus and, in birds, the bursa develop prior to the other lymphoid organs. (2) The thymus and bursa in young animals seem to be the most active sites of lymphopoiesis [149, 153–155]. (3) Removal of the thymus or bursa in young animals causes a reduction of the number of circulating lymphocytes and weight of the nodular lymphoid tissues [8, 152, 156–162]. Conversely, in thymectomized mice grafted with active thymus tissue, the nodular lymphoid tissues developed normally [152].

The evidence for Beard's theory, however, is not conclusive [152, 159, 163], for the facts on which it is based may be explained as well by the view that the thymus and bursa furnish humoral building stones, energy, or other stimulating factors rather than lymphocytes [20, 164]. The presence in the thymus of such substances was demonstrated by Metcalf [165]. Their effectiveness is apparent from the observation by Levey *et al.* [166, 167] and Osoba and Miller [168] that the lymphoid apparatus and immunological competence in thymectomized mice develop normally if the removed thymus tissue is returned to the animals in cell-impermeable Millipore diffusion chambers.* In accordance with this view, Nossal [169] found it possible in guinea pigs to label 50 percent of the thymus lymphocytes without the appearance of more than a rare labeled lymphocyte in the other lymphoid structures, even when stimulated with antigen. These various observations are difficult to reconcile with Beard's theory.

Whatever the answer, we can be sure that small lymphocytes are formed not only in the thymus and bursa but in other lymphoid organs. This is apparent from the facts that their formation continues and that there is no significant depression in the number of circulating lymphocytes after the thymus and bursa have involuted.

ORIGIN OF LYMPHOBLASTS

Some 50 years ago it seemed to be established that the first lymphoid cells in the thymus and bursa were large lymphocytes (blast forms), and that lymphopoiesis in these organs was preceded by the formation of large lymphocytes elsewhere in the mesenchyme [9, 15, 16, 40, 42, 170]. It was thought, therefore, that the "thymocytes" were not epithelial in origin, as formerly believed [6, 9, 40], but were derivates of the undifferentiated mesenchyme and arrived in the epithelial primordium of thymus and bursa from without [9, 16, 40, 42, 170].

The theory that the lymphoblasts of thymus and bursa are of epithelial origin has recently been revived [6, 15, 171–174]. Jankovic *et al.* [173] have stated categorically that "the Mammalian thymus contains, at first, reticular cells of epithelial origin and later cells resembling small lymphocytes which have been shown to

* These chambers are made of material permeable for colloids but not for cells. After being loaded, the chambers can be implanted into the peritoneal cavity of small animals. As the cells cannot escape and no cells can enter the chamber, this method combines the advantages of both the *in vitro* and the *in vivo* technique.

be derived from these epithelial precursors." The bursa "also produces small lymphocytes derived from epithelial precursors." If one looks at the sources on which these statements were based, however, one finds only one argument which can be called upon to support this view—the observation by Auerbach [172] that the lymphocytes which develop in combined cultures of thymus epithelium of mouse embryos and of chicken mesenchyme look like mouse lymphocytes rather than chicken lymphocytes. This observation would be weightier if it could be reinforced by chromosome studies.

CIRCULATION OF LYMPHOCYTES

A dog weighing 10 kg. contains about 1 liter of blood. The number of lymphocytes contained in the blood is approximately 2,500 per cu. mm. Therefore there circulate at a given time some 2.5 billion lymphocytes. The volume of lymph which flows through the thoracic duct of such a dog approximates 20 ml. per hour, or 0.5 liter per day. The number of lymphocytes contained in such lymph averages 10,000 per cu. mm. Therefore there enter into the blood through this duct some 5 billion lymphocytes per day, or twice the number that circulate in the blood. These figures show conclusively that in dogs the lymphocytes leave the circulating blood on the average in less than 12 hours [175].

If the lymph which flows through the thoracic duct is permitted to drain away, the number of lymphocytes of lymph and blood rapidly drops to several 100 per cu. mm. [53]. If the lymph is reinfused intravenously, on the other hand, the lymphocytes of lymph and blood rapidly return to a normal level [176]. These observations were interpreted by Gowans [176] as proof that Sjövall [177] was right when, some thirty years earlier, he concluded that many of the small lymphocytes which leave the blood return to the lymphoid organs and then recirculate.

When these experiments were repeated in animals treated with tritiated thymidine, Gowans [70] found that only a small percentage of the lymphocytes of the thoracic duct became labeled. From this he concluded that at least 90 percent of the thoracic duct lymphocytes are in the process of recirculation.

While in the nodular lymphoid tissues the lymphocytes enter the blood largely through the lymphatics (Fig. 18-8), in the thymus and probably the bursa, lymphatics are difficult to demonstrate [9]. As the veins in these organs are often crowded with lymphocytes, whose migration through the vessel walls is readily observed, Dantschakoff in 1909 concluded that in these organs the small lymphocytes enter the circulation via the blood vessels [166].

The routes by which the lymphocytes return to the nodular lymphoid tissues have been demonstrated by labeled lymphocytes [71]. In lymph nodes they entered the cortex through the postcapillary veins, as first suggested by Sjövall [177]. In the spleen, they appeared first in the lymph sheaths (? via the splenic sinuses). No labeled lymphocytes were found in the germinal centers, casting doubt on the graveyard theory of Heiberg mentioned earlier. Nor were they found in the medullary cords of lymph nodes or the red pulp of the spleen, where the plasma cells are located. Nor did labeled small lymphocytes return to the thymus or bursa. This and the fact that these organs lack the postcapillary veins of nodular lymphoid tissues support the view that traffic of the lymphocytes from thymus to the circulation is one-way [71, 178–180].

THE FATE OF LYMPHOCYTES

While the polyphyleticists believe that the small lymphocytes are end forms, the "extreme" monophyleticists consider them immature stem cells which can give rise to erythrocytes, to "polyblasts," monocytes, and histiocytes, to plasma cells, and to other elements.

The theory that the small lymphocytes give rise to erythrocytes [122, 150, 153, 181, 182] is at variance with certain clinical observations [5]. Also, it is difficult to reconcile with the scarcity in the marrow of tritiated thymidine-labeled lymphocytes in parabiotic and cross-transfused rats [183], with the lack in marrow of transitions between tritiated adenosine-labeled lymphocytes and large pyroninophilic cells in rabbits [180], and with the observation that shielding of a Peyer's patch during whole body radiation will assure rapid repopulation of lymphoid tissues but not of the marrow [184].

It is true that, in contrast to previous observations [185–188], Delorme [189] has demonstrated that the bone marrow and the circulating blood cells after destruction by irradiation can be repopulated with isogenic thoracic duct lymphocytes. It was cautiously pointed out, however, that the newly formed blood cells were not necessarily derived from the donor lymph cells, but that these might have acted as stimuli to inactive host stem cells which then recovered and repopulated the blood-forming tissues, or that the lymphocytes prevented death by combating bacterial invasion.

Fliedner *et al.* [190] studied the fate of transfused tritiated thymidine-labeled bone marrow cells in lethally irradiated recipients and reported that regeneration of the myeloid cells commenced from unlabeled elements, suggesting that the "stem cell population" was relatively quiescent, awaiting a stimulus (erythropoietin; hypoxia) to divide and differentiate. They considered the possibility that certain lymphocytes might be omnipotent but would give rise to hemopoiesis only under certain conditions such as inflammation or extramedullary hemopoiesis, as first suggested by Maximow.

The theory that small lymphocytes can differentiate into "polyblasts," monocytes, and histiocytes [28, 30, 40–42] is supported especially by Rebuck [191–193]. By the application of an elegant coverglass method to the study of acute inflammation of the skin, he believes he has shown that during the first 12 to 24 hours of the experiment small lymphocytes migrate into the field of inflammation, where they differentiate or modulate into macrophages. This interpretation is shared by several workers [194–197]. Others [5, 140, 198], however, have pointed out that Rebuck's illustrations of cells which he calls lymphocytes show monocytes rather than lymphocytes. Amano [199], who repeated Rebuck's experiment with Ikuta's coverglass method, also spoke of monocytes. Similarly, Marchesi [200], a co-worker of Gowans, reported that in the electron-microscope only granulocytes and monocytes but no lymphocytes are seen to migrate into the field of inflammation.

Recently, Rebuck [193] and others [201] reported that the mononuclear cells under the coverglass take up colloidal dyes and India ink and that they are metallophilic while still in the lymphocytic stage, properties which are characteristic of monocytes and histiocytes but not of lymphocytes. Similarly, Lennert *et al.* [202, 203] observed that Rebuck's lymphocytes are rich in acid phosphatase and unspecific esterases, enzymes which are characteristic of macrophages but not of lymphocytes. For these and other reasons, Rebuck's observations cannot be looked upon as conclusive.

The view that small lymphocytes may differentiate into plasma cells [82] has been supported in recent years especially by Dixon *et al.* [204, 205]. It was observed that lymphoid cells of lymph nodes, following transfer to another host, were rapidly replaced by plasma cells. This was interpreted to mean that lymphocytes changed into plasma cells. However, the transferred lymphoid cells in each experiment included as many as 5 to 15 million plasma cells. If we consider that small lymphocytes are very motile and that after transfer they either disintegrate or rapidly move away [206], Dixon's observations were explainable by the assumption that the plasma cells which later predominated were left behind in the area of injection by the lymphocytes which moved away [140]. Because following stimulation by antigen the plasma cells rapidly incorporated tritiated thymidine, while the small lymphocytes did not, Baney, Vazquez, and Dixon [89] later concluded that the plasma cells arise from mitotic division of a "precursor," not "by direct, nonmitotic differentiation from lymphocytes."

The approach to the problem of the lymphocyte took a new turn when several British workers [71, 174–176, 207] by means of tritiated thymidine and adenosine and by chromosomal studies observed that during the graft-versus-host reaction a "small fraction" of the small thoracic duct lymphocytes entered the lymph sheaths of the spleen and the cortex of lymph nodes and here changed into "large pyroninophilic cells." In the lymph nodes they appeared first around postcapillary veins. They did not enter germinal centers or plasma cell areas.

The appearance of similar cells following single injections of killed staphylococci, typhoid vaccine, sheep erythrocytes, and other antigens had previously been described and illustrated by several investigators (Fig. 18-24) [1, 125, 127, 174]. They were called "large lymphoid cells" by Scothorne and McGregor [178] and "large-type cells" by Langevoort *et al.* [134]. Although they were interpreted as lymphoblasts arising from undifferentiated

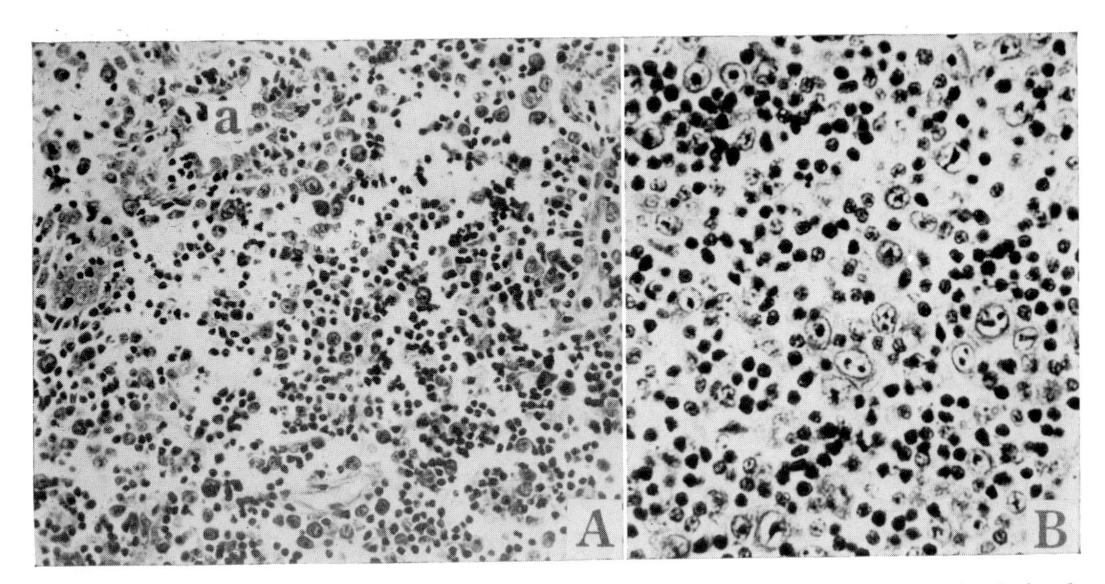

Fig. 18-24. Appearance of large blast forms in the cortex of lymph nodes following stimulation by antigen. In *A,* note their presence around postcapillary veins (*a*). (*B* from Ehrich [124]; courtesy of the publisher.)

mesenchymal cells, we may now state that at least some of them are derivates of small lymphocytes.

The transformation of small lymphocytes into large pyroninophilic cells has been observed also in tissue cultures and Millipore diffusion chambers. In tissue cultures such transformation followed the addition to human blood cells of phytohemagglutinin, an extract of the bean *Phaseolus vulgaris* [54, 145, 208–211] or of pertussis vaccine or other antigens to cultures of blood lymphocytes from human beings sensitive to these antigens [211]. In Millipore diffusion chambers "differentiation" and "modulation" of small lymphocytes into large pyroninophilic cells followed the addition of typhoid bacilli to human lymph node or spleen cells [212] or incubation of specifically sensitized rat ductus thoracicus lymphocytes with sheep erythrocytes [213].

Carstairs [209], who used phytohemagglutinin in tissue cultures, observed replacement during the first 3 days of almost all the small lymphocytes by large cells with deeply basophilic cytoplasm and prominent nucleoli resembling "reticulum cells, plasmablasts, or proerythroblasts." The cells were difficult to identify. They "seemed primitive and of somewhat atypical morphology." This change seemed to occur without mitoses. If the cultures were continued, however, mitoses became frequent. MacKinney *et al.* [210], who described a change of small lymphocytes into "young lymphocytes" and "large mononuclear cells," reported that after 24 hours 25 percent and after 75 hours 85 percent of the lymphocytes had completed this change. After 40 to 50 hours mitoses appeared and thereafter increased rapidly.

Shelton and Rice [214], who were the first to study the fate of lymphoid cells in Millipore diffusion chambers, concluded that the small lymphocytes are pluripotential stem cells. However, because they gathered their lymphoid cells from the peritoneal cavity, and these are widely believed to be monocytes and histiocytes [49, 50, 215, 216], their deductions are not conclusive. Nettesheim [213], who used rat ductus thoracicus lymphocytes, observed the appearance in the chambers of large blasts two days after implantation. On the sixth day, over 40 percent of the cells seemed to be transformed. Studies with tritiated thymidine revealed that the blasts arose via replication of DNA. As no mitoses were seen, they must have arisen through endomitosis, i.e., replication of chromosomes without nuclear division.

The nature of the large pyroninophilic cells is being vigorously studied. Like other blast forms, they are rich in ribosomes, but lack endoplasmic reticulum [178, 217]. Binet and Mathé [217] reported that they are capable of incorporating ferritin, so thought that they were histiocytes. Others, however, concluded that they were undifferentiated blasts which gave rise to plasma cells [134, 161, 211, 213, 218–220] or, again, to small lymphocytes [71, 178, 209]. The transformation of large pyroninophilic cells into plasma cells was proved by Hirschhorn *et al.* [211] through demonstration by the Coons's fluorescent antibody technique of specific antibodies in the cytoplasm of these cells and the observation that in cultures of blood of a patient with agammaglobulinemia lymphocytes developed into blast forms but failed to change into antibody-forming plasma cells. Transformation of the large cells into small lymphocytes was proved by Turk and Stone [221] through labeling of the large cells with tritiated thymidine.

The significance of these observations cannot be overrated. They prove for the first time that the small lymphocytes are not end forms but are capable of changing into blast forms which, through mitotic division, then form new small lymphocytes or differentiate into plasma cells. Whether or not they can turn into other blood or connective tissue cells remains to be seen.

ROLE OF LYMPHOCYTES IN THE IMMUNE RESPONSE

In 1955, Chang *et al.* [7, 8, 222] accidentally found that removal in the neonatal period of the bursa in the chicken depresses or prevents the development of immunological competence. This was soon confirmed by Mueller and associates [223]. In 1961, Miller [152, 157] found (confirmed by Good *et al.* [159, 224, 225]) that early removal of the thymus in mice delays or prevents homologous graft rejection. In the same year, Archer and Pierce [151, 226] demonstrated (soon confirmed [159]) that in rabbits removal of the thymus during the first five days after birth causes reduction in the formation of serum antibodies later in life. Finally, Waksman and his associates [160, 173] showed that delayed hypersensitivity is also impaired by thymectomy early in life. As thymectomy and bursectomy cause a reduction in the number of circulating lymphocytes and the weight of the other lymphoid tissues, these various observations have led to the suggestion that the small lymphocytes of the thymus and bursa are the originators of the immunologically competent cells, that they migrate from the thymus to the lymph nodes, spleen, and other lymphoid organs, and that only here do they unfold their immunological activity [14, 90, 152, 159, 163, 173]. However, recent studies have shown that the thymus and presumably the bursa stimulate the development of the lymphoid apparatus and of immunological competence by means of humoral factors rather than through delivery of lymphocytes (see above, under lymphopoiesis).

Between 1912 and 1926, Murphy presented several papers to show that the small lymphocytes were the cellular sources of transplantation immunity (homograft reaction). This theory was revived recently when Anderson [227] and Billingham [228] and their associates succeeded in causing runt disease by injecting allogenic thoracic duct lymphocytes into newborn rats. In 1952, Wesslen [229] reported that sensitized thoracic duct lymphocytes were capable of transferring delayed hypersensitivity. From this he concluded that the small lymphocytes were the sources of cellular antibodies. Although these views have been widely accepted [90, 179, 194, 230], other observations implicate the reticulum cells or the macrophages rather than the small lymphocytes [231–234].

Gowans *et al.* [110, 161] found that in rats made immunologically unresponsive (tolerant) by various experimental procedures, the capacity to form antibodies can be restored by injection of thoracic duct lymphocytes from normal, nonimmunized rats. As "only a small fraction" of the injected small lymphocytes changed into large pyroninophilic cells, they postulated that there may be two classes of small lymphocytes: those which are immunologically "committed" in that they, or their precursors, have already reacted to antigen, and those which are uncommitted. "The simplest view would be that small lymphocytes interact with antigen—and give rise to a dividing cell line—which generates the cells which eventually synthesize antibody." As an equal number of thoracic duct lymphocytes of immunologically unresponsive rats failed to restore the capacity of such rats to form antibodies, they concluded that the restorative power of small lymphocytes was not a nonspecific effect due to the injection of any cellular material, but a specific function of living cells. Gowans and associates did not

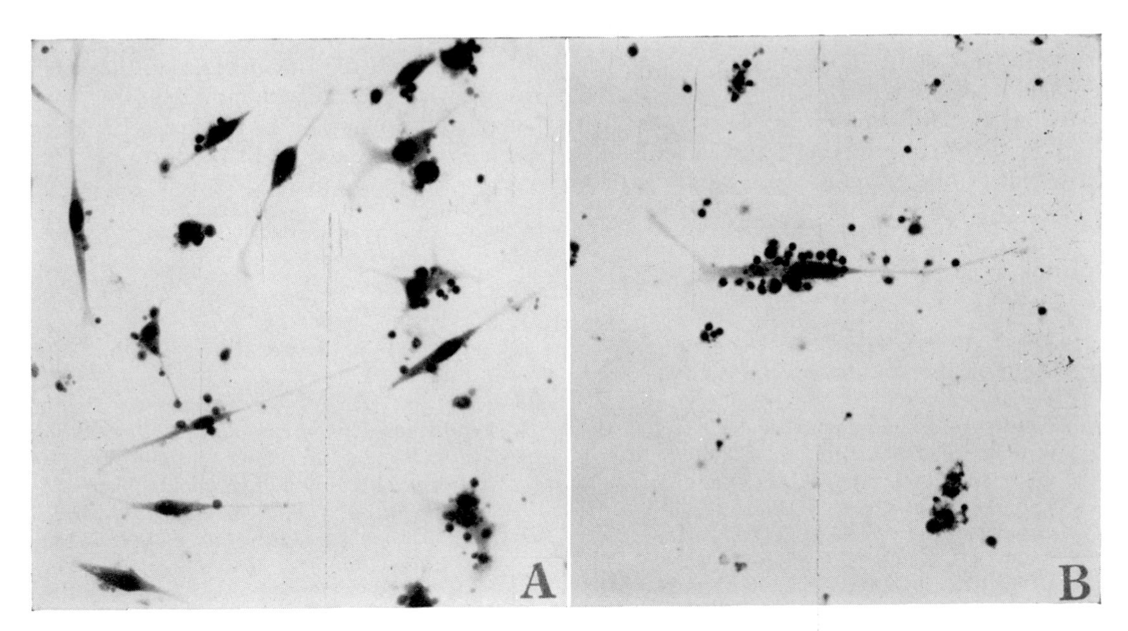

Fig. 18-25. Emperipolesis by small lymphocytes sensitive to L cells. (*A*) Some L cells have partially withdrawn their cell processes. (*B*) One of the L cells has been lysed. (×280.) (From Rosenau [241]; courtesy of the publisher.)

discuss the work of Taliaferro *et al.* [235, 236], who showed quite clearly that antibody formation following irradiation can be partly or completely restored by the administration of yeast autolysates, extracts of Hela cells, spleen extracts, ribonuclease, or specific nuclease digests of nucleic acids implicating nucleic acid derivatives as the active principle.

Recently, it has been postulated that the rejection of homografts [71, 110] and development of delayed hypersensitivity (cellular antibodies) [217] are a function of the large pyroninophilic cells which, during the immune response, derive from small lymphocytes, as discussed earlier (p. 150). It is true that Turk and Stone [221] by means of cyclophosphamide and immunological paralysis were able to show that the development of delayed hypersensitivity depended on the formation of the large cells. But as methotrexate prevented the immunological response without interfering with formation of the blasts or their uptake of tritiated thymidine, and as it caused a marked reduction in formation of small lymphocytes from the large cells, it appears that the development of delayed hypersensitivity and probably also the rejection of homografts are functions of the small lymphocytes rather than of the large pyroninophilic cells.

That this is the proper explanation is apparent also from the curious phenomena known as "peripolesis" [237] and "emperipolesis" [238]. Peripolesis was well described by Berman and Stulberg [145]. "The small lymphocytes wander about and between the macrophages and giant cells, often pausing or stopping when in contact." Emperipolesis, the invasion by lymphocytes of other cells, received considerable attention at a recent symposium on cell-bound antibodies [239–241] and elsewhere [242]. In a study by time lapse cinematography, Rosenau [241] first observed attachment of small lymphocytes to the surface of many but not all of the L cells provided they were sensitive to them. Following the attachment, the L cells withdrew their cell processes and became rounded. After some violent movement, all motility ceased suddenly, and the cells underwent lysis (Fig. 18-25).

In view of these observations it seems safe to conclude that the small lymphocytes play an important role in the immune response. When exposed to antigenic substances or to mediators formed by phagocytes, small lymphocytes change into large pyroninophilic blasts (Fig. 18-15). These then divide and differentiate into plasma cells or again into small lymphocytes. While the plasma cells are retained in the areas where they develop and they dispatch the antibodies which they form through the lymph into the general circulation, the small lymphocytes which contain cellular antibodies are themselves dispatched through lymph and blood to distribute their cellular function throughout the system. It appears, therefore, that the small lymphocytes are the immunologically competent cells proper, the plasma cells being specialized derivates or by-products of these cells.

REFERENCES

1. Ehrich, W. E. The role of the lymphocyte in the circulation of the lymph. *Ann. N.Y. Acad. Sci.* 46:823, 1946.
2. Ehrich, W. E. Studien über das lymphatische Gewebe: V., *Beitr. Path. Anat.* 86:287, 1931.
3. Hellman, T. Lymphgefässe, Lymphknötchen, Lymphknoten. In v. Möllendorff, W. (Ed.), *Handbuch der mikroskopischen Anatomie des Menschen.* Berlin: J. Springer, 1930. Vol. 6/1, p. 233.
4. Hellman, T. Lymphgefässe, Lymphknötchen, Lymphknoten. *Ibid.,* 1943, Vol. 6/4, p. 173.
5. Ehrich, W. E. Die Entzündung. In Büchner, F., Letterer, E., and Roulet, F. (Eds.), *Handbuch der allgemeinen Pathologie.* Berlin: Springer-Verlag, 1956. Vol. 7/1, p. 1.
6. Ackerman, G. A., and Knouff, R. A. Lymphopoiesis in the bursa of Fabricius. *Amer. J. Anat.* 104:163, 1959.
7. Glick, B., Chang, T. S., and Jaap, R. G. The bursa of Fabricius and antibody production. *Poult. Sci.* 35:224, 1956.
8. Chang, T. S., Rheins, M. S., and Winter, A. R. The significance of the bursa of Fabricius in antibody production in chickens. *Poult. Sci.* 36:735, 1957.
9. Hammar, J. A. *Die normal-morphologische Thymusforschung.* Leipzig: J. A. Barth, 1936.
10. Bargmann, W. Der Thymus. Ref. 4, p. 1.
11. Chievitz, J. H. Zur Anatomie einiger Lymphdrüsen im erwachsenen und fetalen Zustande. *Arch. Anat.,* p. 247, 1881. Vol. 5.
12. Ehrich, W. E. Studies of the lymphatic tissue: II. *Amer. J. Anat.* 43:385, 1929.
13. Hellman, T. Studien über das lymphoide Gewebe. *Beitr. Path. Anat.* 68:333, 1921.
14. Papermaster, B. W., and Good, R. A. Relative contributions of the thymus and the bursa of Fabricius to the maturation of the lymphoreticular system and immunological potential in the chicken. *Nature* (London) 196:838, 1962.
15. Ruth, R. F. Ontogeny of the blood cells. *Fed. Proc.* 19:579, 1960 (abst.).
16. Hammar, J. A. Die Menschenthymus. *Z. Mikr. Anat. Forsch.* 6:1, 1926.
17. Löwenthal, K. Thymus. In Hirsch, M. (Ed.), *Handbuch der inneren Sekretion.* Leipzig: Curt Kabitzsch, 1932. Vol. I, p. 709.
18. Boyd, E. The weight of the thymus gland in health and in disease. *Amer. J. Dis. Child.* 43:1162, 1932.
19. Gedda, E. Zur Altersanatomie der Kaninchenthymus. *Upsala Läk. Förh.* 26:9, 1922.
20. Ehrich, W. E., and Seifter, J. The Effect of Corticosteroids upon Lymphoid Tissue. In Shwartzman, G. (Ed.), *The Effect of ACTH and Cortisone upon Infection and Resistance.* New York: Columbia University Press, 1953. P. 25.
21. Hellman, T. J. Ueber die normale Mange des lymphoiden Gewebes bei Kaninchen in verschiedenen postfötalen Altern. *Upsala Läk. Förh.* 19:363, 1914.
22. Hellman, T. J. Die Altersanatomie der menschlichen Milz. *Z. Konst.-Lehre* 12:270, 1926.
23. Berggren, S., and Hellman, T. Die chronische Tonsillitis. *Acta Otolaryng.,* supp. XII, 1930.
24. Aschoff, L. Das retikuloendotheliale System. *Ergebn. Inn. Med.* 26:1, 1924.
25. Aschoff, L. Morphologie des retikuloendothelialen Systems. In Schittenhelm, A. (Ed.), *Handbuch der Krankheiten des Blutes.* Berlin: J. Springer, 1925. P. 473.
26. Metchnikoff, E. *Immunity in Infective Diseases.* Cambridge: Cambridge University Press, 1905.
27. Weidenreich, F. Zur Morphologie und morphologischen Stellung der ungranulierten Leukozyten-Lymphozyten des Blutes und der Lymphe. *Arch. Mikr. Anat.* 73:793, 1909.
28. Downey, H., and Weidenreich, F. Ueber die Bildung der Lymphocyten in Lymphdrüsen und Milz: IX. *Arch. Mikr. Anat.* 80:306, 1912.
29. Downey, H. Histiocytes and macrophages and their relations to the cells of normal blood in animals stained with acid colloidal dyes intra vitam. *Anat. Rec.* 11:350, 1917.
30. Downey, H. The development of histiocytes and macrophages from lymphocytes. *J. Lab. Clin. Med.* 45:499, 1955.
31. Fagraeus, A. Antibody production in relation to the development of plasma cells. *Acta Med. Scand.* 130 (supp. 204): 3, 1948.
32. Unno, G., Hanaoka, M., Iwai, H., Hashimoto, S., and Morita, S. Cytological studies on lymphogonia, *Act. Path. Jap.* 4:75, 1954.
33. Trowell, O. A. Re-utilization of lymphocytes

in lymphopoiesis. *J. Biophys. Biochem. Cytol.* 3:317, 1957.
34. Bargmann, W. *Histologie und mikroskopische Anatomie des Menschen.* Stuttgart: Georg Thieme Verlag, 1959.
35. Letterer, E. *Allgemeine Pathologie,* Stuttgart: Georg Thieme Verlag, 1959.
36. Rebuck, J. W., and LoGrippo, G. A. Characteristics and interrelationships of the various cells in the RE cell, macrophage, lymphocyte and plasma cell series in man. *Lab. Invest.* 10:1068, 1961.
37. Trowell, O. A. The lymphocyte. *Int. Rev. Cytol.* 7:236, 1958.
38. Amano, S. Antibody producing cell series—a review of molecular biology of immunological phenomena. *Ann. Rep. Inst. Virus Res.* (Kyoto University) 5:194, 1962.
39. Tanaka, H. Mesenchymal and epithelial reticulum in lymph nodes and thymus of mice as revealed in the electron microscope. *Ibid.,* p. 146.
40. Maximow, A. Thymus. *Arch. Mikr. Anat.* 74: 525, 1909.
41. Maximow, A. Ueber undifferenzierte Blutzellen und mesenchymale Keimlager im erwachsenen Organismus. *Klin. Wschr.* 5:2193, 1926.
42. Maximow, A. Bindegewebe und blutbildende Gewebe. Ref. 3, 1927, Vol. 2/1:232.
43. Marchand, F. Ueber die bei Entzündungen in der Peritonealhöhle auftretenden Zellformen. *Verh. Deutsch. Ges. Path.* 1:63, 1898.
44. Marchand, F. Die örtlich reaktiven Vorgänge. In Krehl, L., and Marchand, F. (Eds.), *Handbuch der Allgemeinen Pathologie.* Leipzig: Hirzel, 1924, Vol. 4/1, p. 78.
45. Herzog, G. Ueber adventitielle Zellen und über die Entstehung von granulierten Elementen. *Verh. Deutsch. Ges. Path.* 17:562, 1914.
46. Herzog, G. Ueber die Bedeutung der Gefässwandzellen in der Pathologie. *Klin. Wschr.* 2:730, 1923.
47. Herzog, G. Aussprache. *Verh. Deutsch. Ges. Path.* 42:200, 1959.
48. Benacerraf, B., Kivy-Rosenberg, E., Sebestyen, M. M., and Zweifach, B. W. The effect of high doses of x-irradiation on the phagocytic, proliferative, and metabolic properties of the reticulo-endothelial system. *J. Exp. Med.* 110: 49, 1959.
49. Cunningham, R., Sabin, F. R., and Doan, G. A. The development of leucocytes, lymphocytes and monocytes from a specific stem cell in adult tissue. *Contrib. Embryol.* 16:227, 1925.
50. Ehrich, W. E. Die Leukozyten und ihre Entstenhung. *Ergebn. Path.* 29:1, 1934.
51. Gordon, A. S., and Katsh, G. F. The relation of the adrenal cortex to the structure and phagocytic activity of the macrophagic system. *Ann. N.Y. Acad. Sci.* 52:1, 1949.
52. Marshall, A. H. S. *An Outline of the Cytology and Pathology of the Reticular Tissue.* Springfield, Ill.: Charles C Thomas, Publisher, 1956.
53. Yoffey, J. M., and Courtice, F. C. *Lymphatics, Lymph and Lymphoid Tissue.* Cambridge, Mass.: Harvard University Press, 1956.
54. Schrek, R., and Rabinowitz, Y. Effects of phytohemagglutinin on rat and normal and leukemic human blood cells. *Proc. Soc. Exp. Biol. Med.* 113:191, 1963.
55. Paschkis, K. E. Zur Biologie des reticuloendothelialen Apparates. *Z. Exp. Med.* 43:175, 1924.
56. Ehrich, W. E., and Harris, T. N. Site of antibody formation. *Science,* 101:28, 1945.
57. Harris, T. N., and Ehrich, W. E. The fate of injected particulate antigens in relation to the formation of antibodies. *J. Exp. Med.* 84:157, 1946.
58. Ehrich, W. E. Die cellulären Bildungsstätten der Antikörper. *Klin. Wschr.* 33:315, 1955.
59. Fishman, M. Antibody formation in tissue culture. *Nature* (London) 183:1200, 1959.
60. Fishman, M. Antibody formation in vitro. *J. Exp. Med.* 114:837, 1961.
61. Campbell, D. H., and Garvey, J. S. The fate of foreign antigen and speculations as to its role in immune mechanisms. *Lab. Invest.* 10: 1126, 1961.
62. Pernis, B. Personal communication. 1961.
63. Felton, L. D. The significance of antigen in animal tissues. *J. Immun.* 61:107, 1949.
64. McMaster, P. D., and Kruse, H. Persistence in mice of certain foreign proteins and azoprotein tracer antigens derived from them. *J. Exp. Med.* 94:323, 1951.
65. Speirs, R. S. Antigenic material: Persistence in hypersensitive cells. *Science* 140:71, 1963.
66. Lennert, K., and Remmele, W. Karyometrische Untersuchungen an Lymphknotenzellen des Menschen: I. *Acta Haemat.* 19:99, 1958.
67. Yoffey, J. M., Everett, N. B., and Reinhardt, W. O. Labeling of cells in thoracic duct lymph of the guinea pig after tritiated thymidine. *Nature* (London) 182:1608, 1958.
68. Cronkite, E. P., Bond, V. P., Fliedner, T. M., and Rubini, J. R. The use of tritiated thymidine in the study of DNA synthesis and cell turnover in hemopoietic tissues. *Lab. Invest.* 8:263, 1959.
69. Cronkite, E. P., Fliedner, T. M., Bond, V. P., Rubini, J. R., Brecher, G., and Quastler, H. Dynamics of hemopoietic proliferation in man and mice studied by H^3-thymidine incorporation into DNA. *Ann. N.Y. Acad. Sci.* 77:803, 1959.
70. Gowans, J. L. The recirculation of lympho-

cytes from blood to lymph in the rat. *J. Physiol.* (London) 146:54, 1959.

71. Gowans, J. L. The fate of parental strain small lymphocytes in F_1 hybrid rats. *Ann. N.Y. Acad. Sci.* 99:335, 1962.
72. Everett, N. B., Reinhardt, W. O., and Yoffey, J. M. The appearance of labeled cells in the thoracic duct lymph of the guinea pig after the administration of tritiated thymidine. *Blood* 15:82, 1960.
73. Schooley, J. C., and Berman, I. Morphologic and autoradiographic observations of H^3-thymidine-labeled thoracic duct lymphocytes, cultured in vivo. *Blood* 16:1133, 1960.
74. Nossal, G. J. V., and Mäkelä, O. Genetic aspects of antibody formation. *Lab. Invest.* 10:1094, 1961.
75. Fliedner, T. M., Kesse, M., Cronkite, E. P., and Robertson, J. S. Cell proliferation in germinal centers of the rat spleen. *Ann. N.Y. Acad. Sci.* 113:578, 1964.
76. Aschoff, L., and Kiyono, K. Zur Frage der grossen Mononukleären. *Folia Haemat.* 15: 383, 1913.
77. Schilling, V. Der Monocyt in trialistischer Auffassung und seine Bedeutung im Krankheitsbilde. *Med. Klin.* 22:563, 1926.
78. Pappenheim, A. Bemerkungen über örtliche Unterschiede und die gegenseitige genetische Beziehung zwischen den verschiedenen lymphoiden Zellformen. *Folia Haemat.* 9:321, 1910.
79. Ferrata, A. Ueber die Klassifizierung der Leukozyten des Blutes. *Folia Haemat.* 5:655, 1908.
80. Maximow, A. Der Lymphocyt als gemeinsame Stammzelle der verschiedenen Blutelemente in der embryonalen Entwicklung und im postfetalen Leben der Saeugetiere. *Folia Haemat.* 8:125, 1909.
81. Downey, H. The Myeloblast. In Cowdry, E. V. (Ed.), *Special Cytology*. New York: Paul B. Hoeber, Inc., 1932, Vol. 2, p. 653.
82. Marschalko, T. U. Ueber die sogenannten Plasmazellen. *Arch. Dermat.* (Leipzig) 30:3, 1895.
83. Miller, F. R. Induced development and histogenesis of plasma cells. *J. Exp. Med.* 54:333, 1931.
84. Amano, S., Unno, G., and Hanaoka, M. Studies on the discrimination of plasma cells. *Act. Path. Jap.* 1:117, 1951.
85. Vazquez, J. J. Antibody and gamma globulin-forming cells as observed by the fluorescent antibody technique. *Lab. Invest.* 10:1120, 1961.
86. Thorbecke, G. J. *Over de vorming van antilichamen en gamma-globuline "in vitro" in bloedvermende organen.* Groningen: Proefschrift, 1954.
87. Movat, H. Z. Experimentelle Studien uber die allergische Gewebsreaktion. *Beitr. Path. Anat.* 116:238, 1956.
88. Leduc, E. H., Coons, A. H., and Connolly, J. M. Studies on antibody production. *J. Exp. Med.* 102:61, 1955.
89. Baney, R. N., Vazquez, J. J., and Dixon, F. J. Cellular proliferation in relation to antibody synthesis. *Proc. Soc. Exp. Biol. Med.* 109:1, 1962.
90. Nossal, G. J. V. Genetic control of lymphopoiesis, plasma cell formation, and antibody production. *Int. Rev. Exp. Path.* 1:1, 1962.
91. Joannovics, G. Ueber Plasmazellen. *Zbl. Path.* 20:1011, 1909.
92. Braunsteiner, H., Fellinger, K., and Pakesch, F. Ergebnisse und Probleme histologischer Untersuchungen im Elektronenmikroskop. *Klin. Wschr.* 31:357, 1953.
93. Movat, H. Z., and Fernando, N. V. P. The fine structure of connective tissue. *Exp. Mol. Path.* 1:535, 1962.
94. Bing, J., and Plum, P. Serum proteins in leukopenia. *Acta Med. Scand.* 92:415, 1937.
95. Gormsen, H. Investigation of the role of plasma cells as antibody producers. *Sang* 21: 483, 1950.
96. Good, R. A., and Zak, S. J. Disturbances in gamma globulin synthesis as "experiments of nature," *Pediatrics* 18:109, 1956.
97. Carlson, B., and Gyllensten, L. Plasma cells in the growing lymphatic system of young guinea pigs. *Acta Path. Microbiol. Scand.* 43: 365, 1958.
98. Bridges, R. A., Condie, R. M., Zak, S. J., and Good, R. A. The morphological basis of antibody formation development during the neonatal period. *J. Lab. Clin. Med.* 53:331, 1959.
99. Barandun, S., Stampeli, K., Spengler, G. A., and Riva, C. Die Klinik des Antikörpermangelsyndroms. *Helv. Med. Acta* 26:163, 1959.
100. Gitlin, D., Gross, P. A. M., and Janeway, C. A. The gamma globulins and their clinical significance. *New Eng. J. Med.* 260:21, 72, 121, and 170, 1959.
101. Reiss, E., Mertens, E., and Ehrich, W. E. Agglutination of bacteria by lymphoid cells in vitro. *Proc. Soc. Exp. Biol.* 74:732, 1950.
102. Coons, A. H., Leduc, E. H., and Connolly, J. M. Studies on antibody production. *J. Exp. Med.* 102:49, 1955.
103. Coons, A. H. The cytology of antibody formation. *J. Cell. Comp. Physiol.* 52 (supp. 1):55, 1958.
104. Nossal, G. J. V. Antibody production by single cells. *Brit. J. Exp. Path.* 39:544, 1958.
105. Nossal, G. J. V. Antibody production by single cells: II and III. *Brit. J. Exp. Path.* 40:118 and 301, 1959.
106. Nossal, G. J. V. Antibody production by single cells: IV. *Brit. J. Exp. Path.* 41:89, 1960.

107. Ehrich, W. E. Eigenschaften und Bildung humoraler und zellständiger Antikörper. *Arch. Klin. Exp. Dermat.* 213:313, 1961.
108. Burnet, F. M., and Fenner, F. *The Production of Antibodies.* Melbourne: Macmillan & Co. Ltd., 1949.
109. Schultz, J. Antigens and antibodies as cell phenotypes. *Science* 129:937, 1959.
110. Gowans, J. L., McGregor, D. D., Cowen, D. M., and Ford, G. E. Initiation of immune responses by small lymphocytes. *Nature* (London) 196:651, 1962.
111. Mottura, G. On the origin and peripheric function of the lymph system. *Sci. Med. Ital.* 2:534, 1952.
112. Fliedner, T. M., Cronkite, E. P., and Bond, V. P. Potentialities and Limitations of H^3-Thymidine Labelling of Hemopoietic Cell Systems in the Study of Their Dynamics of Proliferation. In *Proceedings of the 8th Congress of the European Society of Haematology.* Basel: Karger AG, 1962. P. 62.
113. Heiberg, K. Das Aussehen und die Function der Keimzentren des adenoiden Gewebes. *Virchow. Arch. Path. Anat.* 240:301, 1923.
114. Cottier, H. *Strahlenbedingte Lebensverkürzung.* Berlin: Springer-Verlag, 1961.
115. Hamilton, L. D. Nucleic acid turnover studies in human leukemic cells and the function of lymphocytes. *Nature* (London) 178: 597, 1956.
116. Medawar, P. B. Transplantation immunity and subcellular particles. *Ann. N.Y. Acad. Sci.* 68:255, 1957.
117. Hamilton, L. D. Control and functions of the lymphocyte. *Ann. N.Y. Acad. Sci.* 73:8, 1958.
118. Hill, M. Re-utilization of lymphocyte remnants by reticular cells. *Nature* (London) 183: 1059, 1959.
119. Lennert, K., and Löffler, H. Ferment-histochemische Untersuchungen der Antikörperbildungsstätten. *Verh. Deutsch. Ges. Path.* 46: 115, 1962.
120. Trowell, O. A. Some properties of lymphocytes in vivo and in vitro. *Ann. N.Y. Acad. Sci.* 73:105, 1958.
121. Yoffey, J. M., Hanks, G. A., and Kelly, L. Some problems of lymphocyte production. *Ibid.*, p. 47.
122. Yoffey, J. M. *Quantitative Cellular Hematology,* Springfield, Ill.: Charles C Thomas, Publisher, 1960.
123. Flemming, W. Studien über Regeneration der Gewebe. *Arch. Mikr. Anat.* 24:355, 1885.
124. Ehrich, W. E. Studies of the lymphatic tissue: I. *Amer. J. Anat.* 43:347, 1929.
125. Ehrich, W. E. Studies of the lymphatic tissue: III. *J. Exp. Med.* 49:347, 1929.
126. Sjoevall, A., and Sjoevall, H. Experimentelle Studien ueber die Sekundaerknoetchen in den Kniekehlenlymphknoten des Kaninchen bei Bacillus pyocyaneous Infektion. *Virchow. Arch. Path. Anat.* 278:258, 1930.
127. Ringertz, N., and Adamson, C. A. The lymph node response to various antigens. *Acta Path. Scand.*, supp. 86, 1950.
128. Ortega, L. G., and Mellors, R. C. Cellular sites of formation of gammaglobulin *J. Exp. Med.* 106:627, 1957.
129. Lang, F. J. Experimentelle Untersuchungen über die Histogenese der extramedullaren Myelopoiese. *Z. Mikr. Anat. Forsch.* 4:417, 1926.
130. Lang, F. J. Die Keimzentren der lymphatischen Organe, *Folia Haemat.* 36:31, 1928.
131. Hughes, W. L., Bond, V. P., Brecher, G., Cronkite, E. P., Painter, R. B., Quastler, H., and Sherman, F. G. Cellular proliferation in the mouse as revealed by autoradiography with tritiated thymidine. *Proc. Nat. Acad. Sci. U.S.A.* 44:476, 1958.
132. Yoffey, J. M., Reinhardt, W. O., and Everett, N. B. The uptake of tritium-labelled thymidine by lymphoid tissue. *J. Anat.* 95:293, 1961.
133. White, R. G. The Relation of the Cellular Responses in Germinal or Lymphocytopoietic Centers of Lymph Nodes to the Production of Antibody. In Holub, M., and Jarošková, L. (Eds.), *Mechanisms of Antibody Formation.* Prague: Publishing House of Czechoslovak Acadamy of Sciences; and New York: Academic Press, Inc., 1960. P. 25.
134. Langevoort, H. L., Keuning, F. J., Meer, J. v.d., Nieuwenhuis, P., and Oudendijk, P. Histogenesis of the plasmacellular reaction in the spleen during the primary antibody response in normal and sublethally x-irradiated rabbits. *Proc. Kon. Ned. Akad. Wet.* [Biol. Med.] 64:397, 1961.
135. Ehrich, W. E., and Harris, T. N. The formation of antibodies in the popliteal lymph node in rabbits. *J. Exp. Med.* 76:335, 1942.
136. Ehrich, W. E., Drabkin, D. L., and Forman, C. Nucleic acids and production of antibody by plasma cells. *J. Exp. Med.* 90:157, 1949.
137. Matsumura, T. Studies on whooping cough. *Acta Sch. Med. Univ. Kioto* 27:103, 1949.
138. Thorbecke, G. J., Asofsky, R. M., Hochwald, G. M., and Siskind, G. W. Gammaglobulin and antibody formation in vitro: III. *J. Exp. Med.* 116:295, 1962.
139. Gyllensten, L., Ringertz, N., and Ringertz, N. R. The uptake of labelled phosphate in lymph nodes during experimental lymphadenitis in relation to the morphological picture. *Acta Path. Microbiol. Scand.* 38:81, 1956.
140. Ehrich, W. E. Morphologie und Physiologie der Antikörperbildung. *Verh. Deutsch. Ges. Path.* 46:9, 1962.

141. Pappenheim, A., and Ferrata, A. Ueber die verschiedenen lymphoiden Zellformen des normalen und pathologischen Blutes. *Folia Haemat.* 10:78, 1910.
142. Bessis, M. C. Ultrastructure of lymphoid and plasma cells in relation to globulin and antibody formation. *Lab. Invest.* 10:1040, 1961.
143. Trowell, O. A. The culture of lymph nodes in vitro. *Exp. Cell Res.* 3:79, 1952.
144. Hulliger, L. Ueber die unterschiedlichen Entwicklungsfähigkeiten der Zellen des Blutes und der Lymphe in vitro. *Virchow. Arch. Path. Anat.* 329:289, 1956.
145. Berman, L., and Stulberg, C. S. Primary cultures of macrophages from normal human peripheral blood. *Lab. Invest.* 11:1322, 1962.
146. Little, J. R., Brecher, G., Bradley, T. R., and Rose, S. Determination of lymphocyte turnover by continuous infusion of H^3-thymidine. *Blood* 19:236, 1962.
147. Ottesen, J. On the age of human white cells in peripheral blood. *Acta Physiol. Scand.* 32: 75, 1954.
148. Cronkite, E. P., Fliedner, T. M., Bond, V. P., Rubini, J. R., Brecher, G., and Quastler, H. Dynamics of Hemopoietic Proliferation in Man and Mice Studied by H^3-Thymidine Incorporation into DNA. In *Progress in Nuclear Energy*, Series VI. London: Pergamon Press, 1959. Vol. 2, p. 92.
149. Kindred, J. E. Quantitative study of hemopoietic organs of young albino rats. *Amer. J. Anat.* 67:99, 1940.
150. Yoffey, J. M. The mammalian lymphocyte. *Biol. Rev.* 25:314, 1950.
151. Archer, O. K., Pierce, J. C., Papermaster, B. W., and Good, R. A. Reduced antibody response in thymectomized rabbits. *Nature* (London) 191:191, 1962.
152. Miller, J. F. A. P. Role of the thymus in transplantation immunity. *Ann. N.Y. Acad. Sci.* 99:340, 1962.
153. Kindred, J. E. Quantitative study of hemopoietic organs of young adult albino rats. *Amer. J. Anat.* 71:207, 1942.
154. Andreasen, E., and Ottesen, J. Studies on lymphocyte production. *Acta Physiol. Scand.* 10:258, 1945.
155. Sainte-Marie, G., and Leblond, C. P. Tentative pattern for renewal of lymphocytes in cortex of the rat thymus. *Proc. Soc. Exp. Biol. Med.* 97:263, 1958.
156. Reinhardt, W. P., and Yoffey, J. M. Thoracic duct lymph and lymphocytes in the guinea pig. *Amer. J. Physiol.* 187:493, 1956.
157. Miller, J. F. A. P. Immunological function of the thymus. *Lancet* 2:748, 1961.
158. Schooley, J. C., and Kelly, L. S. The thymus in lymphocyte production. *Fed. Proc.* 20:71, 1961 (abst.).
159. Good, R. A., Dalmasso, A. P., Martinez, C., Archer, O. K., Pierce, J. C., and Papermaster, B. W. The role of the thymus in development of immunologic capacity in rabbits and mice. *J. Exp. Med.* 116:773, 1962.
160. Arnason, B. G., Jankovic, B. D., Waksman, B. H., and Wennersten, C. Role of the thymus in immune reactions in rats: II. *Ibid.*, p. 177.
161. McGregor, D. D., and Gowans, J. L. The antibody response of rats depleted of lymphocytes by chronic drainage from the thoracic duct. *J. Exp. Med.* 117:303, 1963.
162. Waksman, B. H., Arnason, B. G., and Jankovic, B. D. Role of the thymus in immune reactions in rats: III. *J. Exp. Med.* 116:187, 1963.
163. Dalmasso, A. P., Martinez, B., and Good, R. A. Failure of spleen cells from thymectomized mice to induce graft vs. host reactions. *Proc. Soc. Exp. Biol. Med.* 110:205, 1962.
164. Kelsall, M. A., and Crabb, E. D. *Lymphocytes and Mast Cells.* Baltimore: Williams & Wilkins Company, 1959.
165. Metcalf, D. The effect of thymectomy on the lymphoid tissues of the mouse. *Brit. J. Haemat.* 6:324, 1960.
166. Levey, R. H., Trainin, N., and Law, L. W. Evidence for function of thymic tissue in diffusion chambers implanted in neonatally thymectomized mice. *J. Nat. Canc. Inst.* 31: 199, 1963.
167. Law, L. W., Trainin, N., Levey, R. H. and Barth, W. F. Humoral thymic factor in mice: further evidence. *Science,* 143:1049, 1964.
168. Osoba, D., and Miller, J. F. A. P. Evidence for a humoral thymus factor responsible for the maturation of immunological faculty. *Nature* (London) 199:653, 1963.
169. Nossal, G. J. V. Studies on the rate of seeding of lymphocytes from the intact guinea pig thymus. *Ann. N.Y. Acad. Sci.* (in press).
170. Dantschakoff, W. Untersuchungen über die Entwicklung von Blut und Bindegewebe bei Vögeln. *Arch. Mikr. Anat.* 73:117, 1909.
171. Auerbach, R. Morphogenetic interactions in the development of the mouse thymus gland. *Develop. Biol.* 2:271, 1960.
172. Auerbach, R. Experimental analysis of the origin of cell types in the development of the mouse thymus. *Develop. Biol.* 3.336, 1961.
173. Jankovic, B. D., Waksman, B. H., and Arnason, B. G. Role of the thymus in immune reactions in rats: I. *J. Exp. Med.* 116:159, 1963.
174. Movat, H. Z., van Erkel, G. A., and Fernando, N. V. P. The lymphoid tissue in the spleen and thymus in newborn and fetal rabbits. *Fed. Proc.* 22:600, 1963.
175. Drinker, C. K., and Yoffey, J. M. *Lympha-*

tics, Lymph and Lymphoid Tissue. Cambridge, Mass.: Harvard University Press, 1941.

176. Gowans, J. L. The effect of the continuous re-infusion of lymph and lymphocytes on the output of lymphocytes from the thoracic duct of unanesthetized rats. *Brit. J. Exp. Path.* 38:67, 1957.
177. Sjövall, H. *Experimentelle Untersuchungen ueber das Blut und die blutbildenden Organe.* Lund: Håkan Ohlssons Boktryckeri, 1936.
178. Burwell, R. G. Studies of the primary and the secondary immune response of lymph nodes draining homografts of fresh cancellous bone (with particular reference to mechanisms of lymph node reactivity). *Ann. N.Y. Acad. Sci.* 99:821, 1962.
179. Porter K. A., and Cooper, E. H. Transformation of adult allogeneic small lymphocytes after transfusion into newborn rats. *J. Exp. Med.* 115:997, 1962.
180. Porter, K. A., Chapuisa, G., and Freeman, M. K. Responsibility of small lymphocytes for the killing effect of blood-marrow mixtures on irradiated rabbits. *Ann. N.Y. Acad. Sci.* 99:456, 1962.
181. Jordan, H. E., and Speidel, C. C. The fate of the mammalian lymphocyte, *Anat. Rec.* 26:223, 1923.
182. Kindred, J. E. Quantitative studies on lymphoid tissues. *Ann. N.Y. Acad. Sci.* 59:746, 1955.
183. Cronkite, E. P., Bond, V. P., Fliedner, T. M., and Killmann, S. A. The Use of Tritiated Thymidine in the Study of Hemopoietic Cell Proliferation. In Wolstenholme, G. E. W., and O'Connor, M. (Eds.), *Haemopoiesis.* Boston: Little, Brown, 1960. P. 70.
184. Jacobson, L. O., Marks, E. K., Simmons, L. L., and Gaston, E. O. Immune response in irradiated mice with Peyer's patch shielding. *Proc. Soc. Exp. Biol. Med.* 108:487, 1961.
185. Campbell, I. L., and Ross, M. H. Protectic experiments against radiation injury with lymphocytes. *Oak Ridge Nat. Lab., Biol. Div., Unclass. Rep.,* 1952.
186. Barnes, D. W. H., Ford, C. E., Gray, S. M., and Loutit, J. F. Spontaneous and induced changes in cell populations in heavily irradiated mice. Ref. 148, p. 2.
187. Anderson, D. O., and Whitelaw, D. M. Transfer of homologous thoracic duct lymphocytes to irradiated rats. *Amer. J. Physiol.* 199:824, 1960.
188. Loutit, J. F. Biocycles in the reticuloendothelial system. *Ann. N.Y. Acad. Sci.* 88:122, 1960.
189. Delorme, E. J. Recovery from lethal irradiation in rats after intravenous administration of isogenic lymphocytes. *Lancet* 2:855, 1961.
190. Fliedner, T. M., Thomas, E. D., Meyer, L. M., and Cronkite, E. P. The fate of transfused H^3-thymidine labelled bone marrow cells in irradiated recipients. (In press.)
191. Rebuck, J. W. Cytology of Acute Inflammation in Man as Demonstrated by Two Original Technical Procedures with Particular Reference to the Role of the Lymphocytes. University of Minnesota Ph.D. Thesis, 1947.
192. Sieracki, J. C., and Rebuck, J. W. Role of the Lymphocyte in Inflammation. In Rebuck, J. W. (Ed.), *The Lymphocyte and Lymphocytic Tissue.* New York: Paul B. Hoeber, Inc., 1960. P. 71.
193. Rebuck, J. W., Boyd, C. B., and Riddle, J. M. Skin windows and the action of the reticuloendothelial system in man. *Ann. N.Y. Acad. Sci.* 88:30, 1960.
194. Braunsteiner, H., Paertan, J., and Thumb, N. Studies on lymphocytic function. *Blood* 13:417, 1958.
195. Riis, P. *The Cytology of Inflammatory Exudates.* Copenhagen: Eijnar Munksgaard Forlag, 1959.
196. Perillie, P. E., and Finch, S. C. The local exudative cellular response in leukemia. *J. Clin. Invest.* 39:1353, 1960.
197. Mlczoch, F., and Kohout, J. Das Gewebsbild bei verschiedenen Erkraukungen. *Klin. Wschr.* 40:99, 1962.
198. Volkman. Personal communication.
199. Amano, S. Inflammation, especially the cell-physiological analysis of its fundamental forms. *Acta Sch. Med. Univ. Kioto* 27:188, 1949.
200. Marchesi, V. T. Some electron microscopic observations on interactions between leukocytes, platelets, and endothelial cells in acute inflammation. *Ann. N.Y. Acad. Sci.* 116:774, 1964.
201. Becker, H., Kudo, Y., Argenton, H., and Fischer, H. Cytologische Untersuchungen bei der lokalen Entzuendung. *Folia Haemat.* 5:1, 1961.
202. Lennert, K., Loeffler, H., and Leder, L. D. Fermenthistochemische Untersuchungen am lymphoretikulären Gewebe. In Merker, H. (Ed.), *Zyto-und Histochemie in der Hämatologie,* Berlin: Springer-Verlag, 1963. P. 363.
203. Leder, L. D., and Lennert, K. Diskussionsbeitrag. *Ibid.,* p. 401.
204. Dixon, F. J., Weigle, W. O., and Roberts, J. C. Comparison of antibody responses associated with the transfer of rabbit lymph node, peritoneal and thymus cells. *J. Immun.* 78:56, 1957.
205. Dixon, F. J., Weigle, W. O., and Deichmiller, M. P. The duration of responsiveness of lymph node cells transferred to adult homologous recipients. *J. Immun.* 82:248, 1959.

206. Beckfield, W. J., and Hirata, M. A new approach to the study of the lymphocyte. *Proc. Soc. Exp. Biol. Med.* 106:263, 1961.
207. Porter, K. A., and Cooper, E. H. Recognition of transformed small lymphocytes by combined chromosomal and isotopic labels. *Lancet* 2:317, 1962.
208. Nowell, P. C. Phytohemagglutinin: An initiation of mitosis in cultures of normal human leukocytes. *Cancer Res.* 20:462, 1960.
209. Carstairs, K. The human small lymphocyte: Its possible pluripotential quality. *Lancet* 1:829, 1962.
210. MacKinney, A. A., Stohlman, F., and Brecher, A. G. The kinetics of cell proliferation in cultures of human peripheral blood. *Blood* 19:349, 1962.
211. Hirschhorn, K., Bach, F., Kolodny, R. L., Firschein, I. L., and Hashem, N. Immune response and mitosis of human peripheral blood lymphocytes in vitro. *Science* 142:1185, 1963.
212. Gengozian, N. Heterotransplantation of human antibody-forming cells in diffusion chambers. *Ann. N.Y. Acad. Sci.* (in press).
213. Nettesheim, P. Differentiation of lymphocytes cultured in diffusion chambers. Thesis. University of Pennsylvania Graduate School of Medicine. 1964.
214. Shelton, E., and Rice, M. E. Growth of normal peritoneal cells in diffusion chambers: A study in cell modulation. *Amer. J. Anat.* 105:281, 1959.
215. Cunningham, R. On the origin of the free cells of the serous exudates. *Amer. J. Physiol.* 59:1, 1922.
216. Schilling, V., and Bansi, H. W. Dar verhalten der Exsudatmonozyten zur Oxydasereaktion, ein weiterer Beitrag zur Monozytenfrage. *Z. Klin. Med.* 99:248, 1923.
217. Binet, J. L., and Mathé, G. Optical and electron microscope studies of the immunologically competent cells during the reaction of graft against the host. *Ann. N.Y. Acad. Sci.* 99:426, 1962.
218. Holub, M. Morphology of antibody production by different cell systems in diffusion chambers. *Folia Microbiol.* 5:347, 1960.
219. Holub, M. Potentialities of the small lymphocyte as revealed by homotransplantation and autotransplantation experiments in diffusion chambers. *Ann. N.Y. Acad. Sci.* 99:477, 1962.
220. Fernando, N. V. P., and Movat, H. Z. Fine structural changes in lymphoid tissue after antigenic stimulation. *Fed. Proc.* 22:373, 1963 (abst.).
221. Turk, J. L., and Stone, S. H. Implications of the Cellular Changes in Lymph Nodes during the Development and Inhibition of Delayed Type Hypersensitivity. In Amos, B., and Koprowski, H. (Eds.), *Cell-bound Antibodies.* Philadelphia: Wistar Institute Press, 1963.
222. Chang, T. S., Glick, B., and Winter, A. R. The significance of the bursa of Fabricius of chickens in antibody production. *Poult. Sci.* 34:1187, 1955.
223. Mueller, A. P., Wolfe, H. R., and Meyer, R. K. Precipitin production in chickens: XXI. *J. Immun.* 85:172, 1960.
224. Martinez, B., Dalmasso, A., and Good, R. A. Acceptance of tumor homografts by thymectomized mice. *Nature* (London) 194:1289, 1962.
225. Martinez, C., Kersey, J., Papermaster, B. W., and Good, R. A. Skin homograft survival in thymectomized mice. *Proc. Soc. Exp. Biol. Med.* 109:193, 1962.
226. Archer, O., and Pierce, J. C. Role of thymus in development of the immune response. *Fed. Proc.* 20:26, 1961 (abst.).
227. Anderson, N. F., Delorme, E. J., and Woodruff, M. F. A. Induction of runt disease in rats by injection of thoracic duct lymphocytes at birth. *Transplant. Bull.* 7:93, 1960.
228. Billingham, R. E., Brown, J. B., Defendi, V., Silvers, W. K., and Steinmuller, D. Quantitative studies on the induction of tolerance of homologous tissues and on runt disease in the rat. *Ann. N.Y. Acad. Sci.* 87:457, 1960.
229. Wesslen, T. Passive transfer of tuberculin hypersensitivity by viable lymphocytes from the thoracic duct. *Acta Tuberc. Scand.* 26:38, 1952.
230. Waksman, B. H., Arbouys, S., and Arnason, B. G. The use of specific "lymphocyte" antisera to inhibit hypersensitive reactions of the "delayed" type. *J. Exp. Med.* 114:997, 1961.
231. Cole, L. J., and Garver, R. M. Homograft-reactive large mononuclear leukocytes in peripheral blood and peritoneal exudates. *Amer. J. Physiol.* 200:147, 1961.
232. Eisen, H. N. Delayed-type Hypersensitivity Reactions. In Shaffer, J. H., LoGrippo, G. A., and Chase, M. W. (Eds.), *Mechanisms of Hypersensitivity.* Boston: Little, Brown, 1959. P. 413.
233. Pincus, W. B., and Flick, J. A. Inhibition of the lesions of primary vaccinia and of delayed hypersensitivity by an "antimononuclear" cell serum. *Fed. Proc.* 21:276, 1962 (abst.).
234. Maeir, D. M., and Forschirm, R. Cytochemical effects of a specific antigen on sensitized macrophages in vitro. *Fed. Proc.* 22:197, 1963.
235. Jaroslow, B. N., and Taliaferro, W. H. The restoration of hemolysin-forming capacity in x-irradiated rabbits by tissue and yeast preparations. *J. Infect. Dis.* 98:75, 1956.
236. Taliaferro, W. H., and Jaroslow, B. N. The restoration of hemolysin formation in x-rayed

rabbits by nucleic acid derivates and antagonists of nucleic acid synthesis. *J. Infect. Dis.* 107:341, 1960.

237. Sharp, J. A., and Burwell, R. G. Interaction ("peripolesis") of macrophages and lymphocytes after skin homografting or challenge with soluble antigens, *Nature* (London) 188: 474, 1960.
238. Humble, J. G., Jayne, W. H. W., and Pulvertaft, R. J. V. Biological interaction between lymphocytes and other cells. *Brit. J. Haemat.* 2:283, 1956.
239. Boyden, S. V., Cytophilic Antibody. Ref. 221, p. 7.
240. Rose, N. R., Kite, J. H., Doebbler, T. K., and Brown, R. C. In vitro Reactions of Lymphoid Cells with Thyroid Tissue. Ref. 221, p. 19.
241. Rosenau, W. Interaction of lymphoid cells with target cells in tissue culture. Ref. 221, p. 75.
242. Koprowski, H., and Fernandes, M. V. Autosensitization reaction in vitro. *J. Exp. Med.* 116:467, 1962.
243. Moeschlin, S., Pelaez, J. R. and Hugentobler, F. Experimental investigations of relationship between plasma cells and antibody formation. *Acta Haemat.* 6:321, 1951.

19. The Immunoglobulins

MART MANNIK AND HENRY G. KUNKEL

TISELIUS FIRST PROPOSED THE TERM γ-globulin for serum proteins with the slowest mobility on free electrophoresis. Subsequently, antibody activity of human serum was localized in this serum protein fraction, and therefore the concept of antibody activity became closely associated with γ-globulin. However, the methods for separation, isolation, and identification of serum proteins have advanced. Serum proteins with electrophoretic mobility of γ-globulin have been subdivided according to their molecular size. Serum proteins with β-mobility on electrophoresis have been demonstrated to contain antibody activity. For these reasons, the term immunoglobulins has been applied to the family of serum proteins containing antibody activity, primarily to avoid the ambiguity of the electrophoretic connotation of the term γ-globulin. The family of immunoglobulins is comprised of four classes of distinct proteins: (1) 7S γ-globulins, (2) 19S γ-globulins, (3) β_{2A}-globulins, and (4) low molecular weight γ-globulins or γ_L-globulins. A major reason for grouping them as immunoglobulins is that they all cross-react antigenically and most of them contain antibody activity. Furthermore, the immunoglobulins appear to be products of the plasma cell series.

Contributions to the characterization and description of immunoglobulins have come from many laboratories in the world, and thus several terms have been applied to each of these proteins. Table 19-1 summarizes some properties of the immunoglobulins and lists the commonly encountered synonyms for the terms used in this text.

The normal immunoglobulins are heterogeneous proteins even in a single class of antibodies, rendering their study difficult. In certain diseases of the plasma cell series, notably in multiple myeloma and Waldenström-type macroglobulinemia, large amounts of very homogeneous proteins accumulate in serum apparently due to proliferation of cells from a single clone. The study of these proteins has been of great significance in advancing the knowledge of normal immunoglobulins. For this reason, throughout the discourse to follow, frequent reference will be made to the study of multiple myeloma proteins and Waldenström-type macroglobulins.

Initially, the physical, chemical, and antigenic characteristics and the current concepts of molecular structure of immunoglobulins will be discussed. The genetic factors of the immunoglobulins and the relationships among these proteins will be considered. Finally, the current knowledge of the antibody function and the physiology of the immunoglobulins will be described.

7S γ-GLOBULINS (IgG)

Gamma globulin, by the original definition proposed by Tiselius, is the serum protein with the slowest electrophoretic mobility at pH 8.6. Similarly, in zone electrophoresis on starch, starch gel, and many other media, 7S γ-globulin has the slowest mobility of all serum proteins at neutral or slightly alkaline pH. Immunological analysis of the electrophoretically separated fractions of serum proteins indicates that the 7S γ-globulins extend from serum proteins with the slowest mobility well into the α_2-globulin peak [1]. The broad distribution is also well demonstrated with immunoelectrophoresis [2]. In this technique, human serum is subjected to electrophoresis in agar medium, and subsequently an antiserum is placed in adjacent troughs. Precipitin lines form where a serum protein diffusing through agar encounters the antibodies to this protein diffusing from the opposite direction. On immunoelectrophoresis the 7S γ-globulin precipitin line extends from the slowly migrating proteins on the cathodal side well into the α mobility range. Such broad distribution by a variety of electrophoretic techniques indicates

TABLE 19-1. Summary of Immunoglobulins

Terms used in this text	7S γ-globulin	19S γ-globulin	β_{2A}-globulin	γ_L-globulin
Recommended terms[a]	γG globulin	γM globulin	γA globulin	—
Synonyms	γ_2-globulin IgG	β_{2M}-globulin γ_{1M}-globulin IgM	γ_{1A}-globulin IgA	L chain γ_u-globulin
Sedimentation constant in Svedberg units	7	19	7–15	1.6
Approx. molecular weight	150,000	1,000,000	150,000–500,000	20,000
Carbohydrate content	2.6%	10.0%	7.0%	—
Placental transfer	Yes	No	No	—
Genetic Gm factors	Present	Absent	Absent	Absent
Genetic Inv factors	Present	Present	Present	Present
L chains	Present	Present	Present	Present
Unique antigenicity	Present	Present	Present	Absent

[a] At an international meeting in Prague sponsored by the World Health Organization in May, 1964, recommendations were made for adopting notations for the immunoglobulins that would be uniform throughout the world. These recommendations were made available after this chapter was completed, and therefore the terminology is not adjusted throughout the text. The proposal is comprehensive and includes symbols for immunoglobulins, for polypeptide chains, for 'abnormal' globulins and for fragments obtained by enzymatic digestion. A summary of these recommendations ("Notes on Nomenclature") can be found on page xxi.

that this protein is composed of a continuous range of molecules differing in their isoelectric points. Since the 7S γ-globulin has the slowest electrophoretic mobility of all serum proteins by conventional methods, it has also been termed γ_2-globulin in some laboratories to distinguish it from other related proteins with slightly faster mobility in the zone between γ- and β-globulins of the classic electrophoretic concept.

The most widely quoted ultracentrifugal sedimentation constant for γ-globulin is about 7 Svedberg units. From this determination the term "7S γ-globulin" has been derived to distinguish γ-globulin from other similar proteins with larger molecular size and correspondingly higher sedimentation constant. More precise determinations of the sedimentation constant of γ-globulin disclose heterogeneity, with an average sedimentation constant of 6.56 Svedberg units, standard deviation 0.32 units [3]. The molecular weight of 7S γ-globulin is 150,000 to 160,000, based on the ultracentrifugal analyses. These estimates are in agreement with molecular weight values obtained by light-scattering, low-angle x-ray diffraction, and osmotic pressure calculations discussed in Chapter 3.

Normal 7S γ-globulin and its electrophoretic fractions contain 2.6 percent carbohydrate by weight [4]. In contrast, the other immunoglobulins contain a much higher percentage of carbohydrate (Table 19-1). The 7S γ-globulin contains 1.2 percent hexose and 1.14 percent hexosamine by weight. In moles per mole it contains the following carbohydrates: galactose 3, mannose 5, fucose 2, galactoseamine 8, sialic acid 1. Hexonic acid, uronic acid, pentoses, and other hexoses are not present [5]. Amino acid analyses and terminal amino acid determinations of 7S γ-globulin have been reviewed in Chapter 3. The molecular size of these proteins is too large to permit amino acid sequence studies. However, advances in the understanding of the molecular subunits of 7S γ-globulin and the study of homogeneous proteins of multiple myeloma as models have reopened this field for promising investigations.

Degradation of γ-globulin by proteolytic

enzymes with retention of biological activity was described many years ago [6, 7], but Porter's work on the degradation of rabbit γ-globulin by crystalline papain [8] became the impetus for many studies on the subunits of human immunoglobulins. The details of this and subsequent work on enzymatic degradation of human and animal immunoglobulins are thoroughly discussed also in Chapter 3.

In brief, degradation of human 7S γ-globulin with cysteine-activated papain yields fragments separable on the basis of their electrophoretic mobility [9]. The fragments with relatively slow electrophoretic mobility at pH 8.6 are termed S fragments (A and C fragments by other investigators [10]), and the fragments with relatively faster mobility under the same conditions are termed F fragments (B fragments by other investigators). As discussed in Chapter 3, the S fragments retain the antibody combining site and are functionally univalent antibodies [10, 11]. The F fragments lack antibody-combining activity, but they carry most of the carbohydrate of the parent molecules and also the major antigenic determinants unique to this class of immunoglobulins [12]. The F fragments of human 7S γ-globulin are crystallizable under appropriate conditions [13]. They appear to provide the 7S γ-globulin molecules with many of their functions other than combining with the antigen. These fragments without the antibody combining site play a major role in binding complement [14–17] and are essential for fixation of the 7S γ-globulin to tissue for passive and reverse passive cutaneous anaphylaxis [18]. They also play a role in binding 7S γ-globulin to microsomes during their synthesis [19], and they appear to be important in the transfer of 7S γ-globulin across the placenta.

The digestion of 7S γ-globulin with pepsin in the absence of a reducing agent degrades the F fragments into dialyzable peptides, and the S fragments remain as bivalent precipitating antibodies. These molecules have a sedimentation constant of 5 Svedberg units and are broken into single S fragments upon addition of cysteine. Antigenically, the bivalent 5S fragments as well as the univalent S fragments produced by pepsin in the presence of cysteine are very similar to the S fragments produced by cysteine-activated papain.

The molecules of 7S γ-globulin can be degraded without preceding proteolysis, but the products of cleavage differ from those obtained by enzymatic degradation. Exposure of 7S γ-globulin to 2-mercaptoethanol or other agents capable of cleaving disulfide bonds, followed by alkylation and treatment with 6 to 8 M urea, leads to dissociation of the parent molecules into polypeptide chains [20]. The heavier polypeptide chains, with approximate molecular weight of 60,000 to 103,000 in 6 M urea, are termed H chains, and the lighter chains, with approximate molecular weight of 20,000 in 6 M urea, are L chains [21]. At neutral pH the H chains tend to aggregate and render the determination of their molecular weight difficult. However, studies on horse and rabbit 7S γ-globulin have indicated that the molecular weight of the H chains is 50,000 to 55,000 and that of the L chains, 20,000 to 25,000 [21a, 21b]. The H and L chains differ significantly in their amino acid composition. Antigenically the H and L chains contain all of the antigenic determinants of unaltered 7S γ-globulin, and the isolated H and L chains do not share any antigenic determinants [22]. The L chains correspond antigenically to a part of the S fragment of 7S γ-globulin derived by cysteine-activated papain; the H chains contain all of the F fragments and also a segment of the S fragments [22–24]. The H and L chains of 7S γ-globulin are separable on the basis of their size by gel filtration [25]. By this technique the H chains are eluted first and were termed A chains, and the L chains termed B chains. The H chains contain 95 percent of carbohydrate present on the 7S γ-globulin molecules [26]. In addition, the H and L chains are separable on starch gel electrophoresis in 6 M urea. Reduced and alkylated normal 7S γ-globulins resolve by this technique into slow-moving H chains in a somewhat discrete band and a diffuse spread of L chains with higher mobility, suggesting a spectrum of L chains with differing isoelectric points [27]. Reduced and alkylated γ-type myeloma proteins are separable by the same technique into H chains, similar to those of normal 7S γ-globulin, and into L chains with a very sharply defined band, characteristic of each myeloma protein and in contrast to the diffuse smear of L chains from normal 7S γ-globulin [27].

The L chains from a myeloma protein and the Bence Jones protein from the same patient have precisely the same electrophoretic mobility when subjected to identical conditions [27], are identical antigenically [28], and, furthermore, have identical amino acid composition [29]. These observations and studies of the rate of synthesis of Bence Jones and myeloma proteins [30, 31] have led to the notion that Bence Jones proteins are L chains of the myeloma proteins and are produced asynchronously from the H chains. Strikingly, the L chains of normal 7S γ-globulin have the property of aggregation and precipitation upon heating, reversible by boiling [29], similar to the classic characteristic of Bence Jones proteins [32].

Current evidence strongly suggests that multiple myeloma proteins are normal γ-globulins produced in abundant amounts due to the disease process but lack antibody activity. Further, it has seemed that specific antibodies to a single antigenic determinant should behave like myeloma proteins in that they are separable into H chains and a discrete band of L chains. Indeed, guinea pig antibodies to haptens, isolated from specific precipitates, demonstrate discrete bands of L chains differing from antibody to antibody, in contrast to the diffuse smear of L chains from 7S γ-globulin of the same species [33]. Similarly, isolated specific human antibodies of the 7S class show discrete bands of L chains on electrophoresis. However, the number of bands is variable, and only few antibodies to limited antigenic determinants show single bands. In addition, some isolated antibodies show unique antigenicity like myeloma proteins [34].

19S γ-GLOBULINS (γ_{1M}, IgM)

Antibodies with molecular weight close to 1 million were demonstrated some time ago [35], and their relation to the 7S γ-globulins has since been elucidated. The study of Waldenström-type macroglobulins, the pathological counterparts of normal 19S γ-globulins, has contributed greatly to the understanding of this class of antibodies.

The electrophoretic mobility of 19S γ-globulins at pH 8.6 is faster than that of the major portion of the 7S γ-globulin. In zone electrophoresis, these proteins migrate generally between the peaks of γ- and β-globulins. The distribution of 19S γ-globulins, best observed on immunoelectrophoresis, is broad but less so than that of the 7S γ-globulins. Because of their electrophoretic mobility, the 19S γ-globulins have also been termed γ_{1M}- or β_{2M}-globulins.

The major component of this class of immunoglobulins has a sedimentation constant of 19 Svedberg units, so they have been termed the 19S γ-globulins. Normal 19S γ-globulins and Waldenström-type macroglobulins have a characteristic ultracentrifugal heterogeneity [36, 37]. In addition to the major component, two minor components exist, with sedimentation constants of approximately 29S and 38S. The relative amounts of these heavier components are surprisingly constant from isolated preparations of normal as well as of the pathological proteins. The 29S components comprise roughly 17 percent and the 38S components 5 percent of the total protein in the preparations of 19S γ-globulins. The heavier components may represent polymers of the 19S γ-globulins [38]. The approximate molecular weight of 19S γ-globulins is 1 million as determined from the ultracentrifugal analyses. Normally, the 19S γ-globulins comprise up to 10 percent of total serum γ-globulin.

The total carbohydrate content of normal 19S γ-globulins, Waldenström-type macroglobulins, and isolated rheumatoid factors, which are 19S γ-globulins occurring primarily in patients with rheumatoid arthritis, is approximately 10 percent by weight [37, 39], in contrast to 2.6 percent of carbohydrate by weight in 7S γ-globulins. The hexose content of 19S γ-globulin is 5.2 percent and the hexosamine content 2.9 percent by weight. Fucose, sialic acid, galactose, and mannose are present in smaller quantities. Antigenically, the 19S γ-globulins cross-react with 7S γ-globulin, but in addition they contain antigenic determinants unique to this class of immunoglobulins [40, 41]. Normal 19S γ-globulins and Waldenström-type macroglobulins are dissociated into subunits with sedimentation constants of 6.5 Svedberg units by exposure to mercaptoethanol due to rupture of disulfide bonds. Upon removal of mercaptoethanol by dialysis, the 6.5S subunits reaggregate to form the 19S protein [42]. Stable 6.5S subunits are obtained with mercaptoethanol in the presence of iodoacetamide, since the latter blocks the free sulfhydryl groups and thus prevents reformation of disulfide bonds. The antigenic properties of the 19S γ-globulin are retained on the 6.5S subunits, including the antigenic determinants cross-reacting with 7S γ-globulin and those unique to 19S γ-globulins [43]. However, these 6.5S subunits lose all antibody activity [44–46]. Therefore, this procedure has become a method for distinguishing 19S from 7S γ-globulin antibodies, since, as pointed out, treatment of the latter with mercaptoethanol will not degrade the molecules. This method, however, has pitfalls, since certain polymers of 7S γ- and β_{2A}-globulin also lose their antibody function on exposure to mercaptoethanol, as will be elaborated in the discussion of antibody function.

Although on removal of mercaptoethanol the 6.5S subunits of 19S γ-globulin reaggregate to form a high molecular weight material closely resembling the starting material, antibody activity of the 19S γ-globulins is not usually recovered [46]. On the other hand, return of antibody activity has been demonstrated for a homogeneous macroglobulin with rheumatoid factor activity [47]. Similarly, on reaggregation, 19S γ-globulin antibody activity is regained when isolated antibodies are used as starting material and the dissociation is performed with borohydride [48]. Hybrid 19S γ-globulin antibodies to blood group substances A and B have been reported when equal amounts of purified and dissociated anti-A and anti-B antibodies are mixed prior to reoxidation and formation of 19S antibodies [48]. In view of these findings, the failure to recover antibody activity on reaggregation of the 6.5S subunits of 19S γ-globulin may be explained by random recombination of the subunits and therefore failure to form functioning antibodies. These experiments of dissociation and reassociation of 19S γ-globulin into subunits with loss and subsequent recovery of the antibody activity clearly point to the importance of the large molecular structure of this protein in its function as an antibody.

Just as 7S γ-globulin and myeloma proteins can be dissociated into H and L chains, experiments on Waldenström-type macroglobulins reveal the presence of L chains that have electrophoretic mobilities comparable to the L chains of myeloma proteins. The H chains of the 19S proteins differ from those of 7S γ-globulin on starch gel electrophoresis [49]. The H chains of 19S γ-globulin contain the antigenic characteristics unique to this class of immunoglobulins [24].

β_{2A}-GLOBULINS (γ_{1A}, IgA)

Many of the physical, chemical, and antigenic characteristics of β_{2A}-globulins have been clarified through the study of β_{2A} type multiple myeloma proteins, since the isolation of normal β_{2A}-globulins has been difficult. Some time ago it was observed that about one third of multiple myeloma proteins, particularly those with fast electrophoretic mobility, differ markedly from other myeloma proteins antigenically and are closely related to normal proteins in the γ_1 or β_2 area [50]. These multiple myeloma proteins were called group 3 myeloma proteins by some investigators [51], but subsequently were termed β_{2A} type myeloma proteins because of their antigenic relationship to normal β_{2A}-globulin [52]. Normal β_{2A}-globulins have been considerably purified through the use of buffered zinc sulfate solutions that precipitate 7S γ-globulin but fail to precipitate β_{2A}-globulins [53, 54]. This class of immunoglobulins, like the other classes already discussed, has a broad electrophoretic mobility, reflecting molecular heterogeneity, best observed on immunoelectrophoresis.

The β_{2A} type multiple myeloma proteins frequently show a characteristic ultracentrifugal heterogeneity [55–57]. Some of these are composed primarily of molecules with sedimentation constant of 7 Svedberg units, but the majority have multiple components with sedimentation constants from 7S to 15S. Varying amounts of these proteins may be present, and rarely is the same ultracentrifugal pattern encountered twice (Fig. 19-1). All β_{2A} type multiple myeloma proteins with sedimentation constants above 7S are dissociated with mercaptoethanol into proteins with sedimentation constants of approximately 7S. This effect is illustrated in Figure 19-2. The 9S to 10S peak as well as the larger polymers dissociate in the presence of mercaptoethanol into a major peak of protein with sedimentation constant of 7S along with some heterogeneous very low molecular weight material. This preparation of β_{2A} type myeloma protein contained no 19S γ-globulin on antigenic analysis. On agar gel electrophoresis the β_{2A} type multiple myeloma proteins form multiple bands. The larger polymers thus have slower electrophoretic mobility than the 7S monomers of these proteins [58].

Polymerization of normal β_{2A}-globulins to

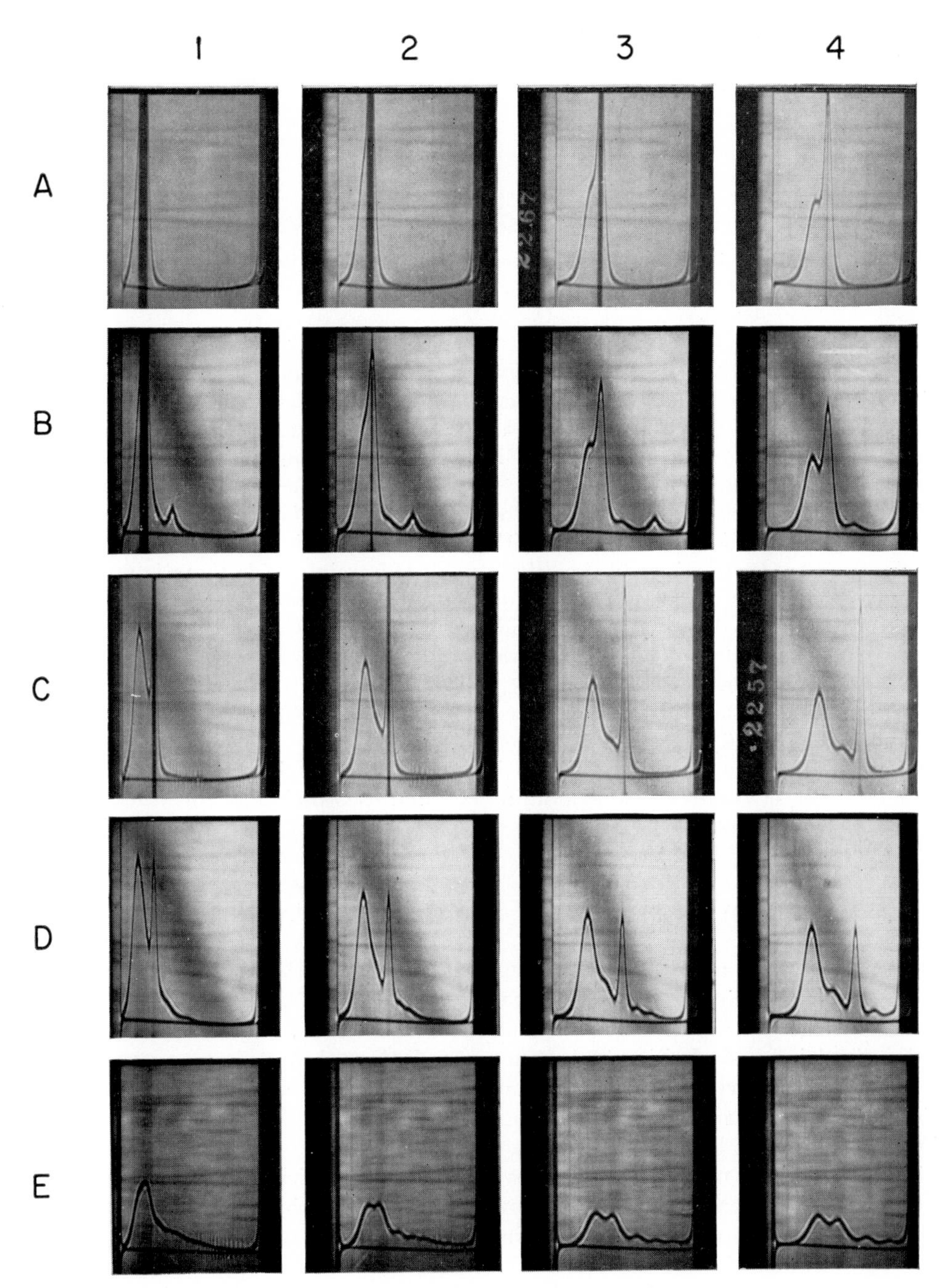

Fig. 19-1. Ultracentrifugal patterns of five sera from patients with β_{2A} type myeloma proteins. Sedimentation proceeds from left to right. Sera *A* and *B* show a predominant 7S peak; serum *B* also illustrates a small heavier component. Sera *C* and *D,* in contrast, show a predominant 9S to 10S peak. Serum *E* illustrates heterogeneity, with several myeloma protein peaks.

proteins with higher molecular weights has not been established, but preliminary evidence exists for this [52]. The β_{2A} type myeloma proteins and normal β_{2A}-globulins with sedimentation constants of 7S have an approximate molecular weight of 150,000 to 160,000, similar to the 7S γ-globulin, but the polymers with higher sedimentation constants have correspondingly higher molecular weights. The carbohydrate content of β_{2A} myeloma proteins is higher than that of 7S γ-globulin but not as high as that of 19S γ-globulins and Walden-

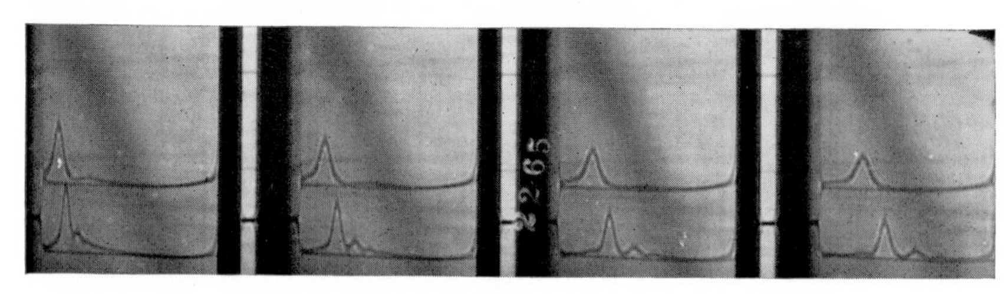

Fig. 19-2. Ultracentrifugal patterns of an isolated β_{2A} type myeloma protein, in 0.1 M mercaptoethanol in the upper pattern and without mercaptoethanol in the lower pattern, showing the dissociation in presence of mercaptoethanol.

ström-type macroglobulins. Hexose and hexosamine acount primarily for the increased carbohydrate content of the β_{2A} type myeloma proteins. Their total carbohydrate content is approximately 7 percent by weight [4].

Antigenically, β_{2A} type myeloma proteins as well as normal β_{2A}-globulins cross-react with 7S γ-globulin [50, 51], but in addition these proteins have antigenic determinants unique to this class of immunoglobulins [12], providing an easy basis for immunological identification [52]. On reduction and alkylation β_{2A} type myeloma proteins are readily dissociated into H and L chains in 6 M urea on starch gel electrophoresis [49]. The H chains differ antigenically from the H chains of 7S γ-globulins and γ type myeloma proteins [24].

γ_L-GLOBULINS

Certain patients with multiple myeloma excrete Bence Jones proteins in their urine that are characterized by precipitation upon heating and redissolving upon boiling [32]. Bence Jones proteins cross-react with normal immunoglobulins, and their molecular weight is approximately 20,000 [59]. Recent studies of proteins in the urine of normal persons have demonstrated, in addition to 7S γ-globulin, low molecular weight γ-globulins, the γ_L-globulins [60–63]. On heating, these behave like the classic Bence Jones proteins. The γ_L-globulins also exist in normal human plasma [64]. Antigenically, γ_L-globulins from plasma and urine are identical to the isolated L chains from normal 7S γ-globulin, and the relative amino acid content of both is nearly identical [65]. Furthermore, the L chains of normal 7S γ-globulin have the thermosolubility characteristics well known for the Bence Jones proteins [29]. The functional significance of γ_L-globulins remains to be determined. They may represent a by-product of immunoglobulin synthesis rather than a breakdown product. The latter notion is supported by the observation that intravenously administered 7S γ-globulin labeled with I^{131} does not lead to excretion of radioactively labeled γ_L-globulins in urine [66]. In addition, on administration of C^{14}-labeled amino acids there is rapid incorporation of the radioactive label into urinary γ_L-globulins [67].

GENETIC CHARACTERS

One area of investigation of the immunoglobulins which has furnished some of the best evidence of their interrelationship is the work on localization of genetic factors to different portions of the γ-globulin molecules. Groups of alleles at two genetic loci involving ordinary 7S γ-globulin are now recognized. The first of these, the Gm locus, includes Gm(a), Gm(b), Gm(x), Gm(r), and probably certain other factors. These have been widely studied, and hereditary patterns have been worked out in various populations. The subject has been thoroughly reviewed by Steinberg [68].

Recent studies on the H chain subgroups of 7S γ-globulins have clarified certain peculiarities in the Gm system [68a]. It is now apparent that Gm(a) and Gm(b) characters occur on different subgroups of γ-globulin and are not determined by allelic genes, as had been thought. Earlier observations with myeloma proteins had demonstrated the rarer occurrence of Gm(b) than of Gm(a). The localization of Gm(b) to a minor subgroup explains this peculiarity and clarifies the unique characteristics of these determinants in Negroes. Each of the H chain subgroups appears to be controlled by genes at separate but closely linked genetic loci. There is also evidence that

TABLE 19-2. Gm and Inv Types of Isolated Myeloma Proteins, Macroglobulins, and Urinary Bence Jones Proteins

	Gm Type				Inv Type			
Class of Protein	a+b−	a+b+	a−b+	a−b−	a+b−	a+b+	a−b+	a−b−
7S γ	15	0	2	30	3	0	17	6
19S γ	0	0	0	6	0	0	2	4
β_{2A}	0	0	0	15	1	0	9	5
Bence Jones	0	0	0	11	1	0	5	5

the Inv(a) and Inv(b) factors too may well occur on different γ-globulin subgroups and therefore that their genetic relationship is not as simple as had been believed.

These factors have been measured primarily through the use of incomplete Rh antibodies as red cell coats which are then agglutinated by a specific anti-γ-globulin reagent. Initially, the latter came from rheumatoid arthritis sera, but in recent years far better reagents have been obtained from certain rare normal sera which possess anti-γ-globulin antibodies. The origin of these antibodies remains a mystery, although some evidence has been obtained that they arise through immunization by placental transfer of maternal 7S γ-globulin [69]. Others may arise through transfusions or injections of γ-globulin. Such antibodies have been demonstrated in high incidence in the sera of children receiving multiple transfusions [70]. Certain sera from monkeys immunized with human γ-globulin also can be used [71].

It has been clearly shown that the genetic factors from the two different loci occur on different portions of the 7S γ-globulin molecules [72–74]. Initially this was done through the localization on different fragments recovered from papain-splitting. The F fragments contain all the Gm factors and the S fragments the Inv factors. Pepsin digestion, which destroys the F fragments, destroyed the Gm factors and left the Inv with the residual S component. Since the Inv factors were localized to Bence Jones proteins, it was clear that they were on the L chains and the Gm factors on the H chains. Direct evidence of this localization was obtained recently through localization on isolated L and H chains [24, 75].

Since it is known that the cross-reactive component of 7S γ-globulin which is also found in the 19S and β_{2A} immunoglobulins occurs on the S fragment and on the L chains, it might be expected that all of the immunoglobulins would possess the Inv factors but that the Gm factors would be restricted to the 7S γ-globulins. This, indeed, proved to be the case. Table 19-2 shows that all of the macroglobulins and β_{2A} proteins are Gm-negative but that many are positive in the Inv system. It seems probable that separate genetic factors will be found for the 19S and β_{2A}-globulins that correspond to the Gm factors of 7S γ-globulin which will be localized to the specific H chains of these proteins.

RELATIONSHIPS AMONG IMMUNOGLOBULINS AND GROUP I AND II IMMUNOGLOBULINS

In the preceding pages the subunits of the four classes of immunoglobulins were discussed. As already stated, the 7S γ-globulins have unique antigenic determinants present on the F fragments and the H chains of the molecules, not present in the other immunoglobulins [12, 22, 24]. The F fragments and the piece of the H chains incorporated into the S fragments are present in all 7S γ-globulin molecules [23, 76]. Furthermore, the γ type myeloma proteins possess similar antigenic determinants unique to the class of 7S γ-globulins.

The β_{2A} type myeloma proteins as well as normal β_{2A}-globulins have antigenic determinants unique to this class of immunoglobulins [12, 52]. The subunits of these proteins carrying the unique antigenic determinants apparently correspond to the H chains of the 7S γ-globulin, but they have not been well defined nor have any genetic factors been defined for these polypeptide chains. Similarly, the Waldenström-type macroglobulins and the normal 19S γ-globulins have antigenic determinants unique to this class of immunoglobulins. Again, the subunits of these proteins that correspond to the H chains of the 7S γ-globulins carry the unique antigenicity. The H chains of 19S γ-globulin have not been well characterized, and genetic factors specific for the 19S γ-globulins have not been described.

The normal immunoglobulins and their pathological counterparts, the γ and β_{2A} type myeloma proteins, Bence Jones proteins, and Waldenström-type macroglobulins, all have common antigenic determinants. Through the study of multiple myeloma proteins, the 7S γ-globulins and other immunoglobulins were further subdivided into two basic types of molecules on the basis of antigenic determinants on their L chains. Some time ago the myeloma proteins were divided into three groups, termed group 1, 2, and 3 on the basis of their degree of cross-reactivity with normal human 7S γ-globulins, by utilizing antisera to the latter [51]. In these studies the group 1 myeloma proteins seemed most closely related to normal 7S γ-globulins, group 2 proteins contained a lesser number of common antigenic determinants with 7S γ-globulins, and group 3 proteins shared only a few antigenic determinants with normal 7S γ-globulin. Subsequent studies demonstrated that the group 3 myeloma proteins are actually β_{2A} type myeloma proteins [52]. By similar analysis, the Bence Jones proteins fall into two groups, initially termed group A and group B on the basis of mutually exclusive antigenic determinants [77]. In another laboratory, these two groups of Bence Jones proteins were termed group 1 and group 2 proteins [78].

Recent evidence demonstrates that the antigenic determinants permitting the grouping of myeloma proteins are identical to those allowing the grouping of Bence Jones proteins [79–81]. Therefore the Bence Jones proteins are also termed group I and group II, rather than group B and A, respectively. Furthermore, the serum myeloma protein group of a patient corresponds to the group of Bence Jones proteins of the same patient; e.g., if the patient has a group I serum myeloma protein, a group I Bence Jones protein also is excreted in the urine [79]. Similarly, the β_{2A} type myeloma proteins and the Waldenström-type macroglobulins fall into two groups on the basis of the same antigenic determinants [79, 80], termed group I and group II proteins. The grouping of all pathological immunoglobulins is best performed with antisera to Bence Jones proteins. An antiserum to a purified group I Bence Jones protein reacts with other group I Bence Jones proteins as well as with group I myeloma proteins and group I Waldenström-type macroglobulins. No reaction occurs with group II Bence Jones proteins, and such antisera contain no antibodies to the H chains of any immunoglobulins, thus rendering the reaction only specific to the group I determinants. Similarly, an antiserum to a purified group II Bence Jones protein reacts only with other group II Bence Jones proteins and all group II immunoglobulins, thus showing specificity to group II determinants.

Since in all instances pathological immunoglobulins belong either to group I or to group II, it was thought that normal immunoglobulins should also consist of two major types of molecules. Indeed, this proved to be the case.

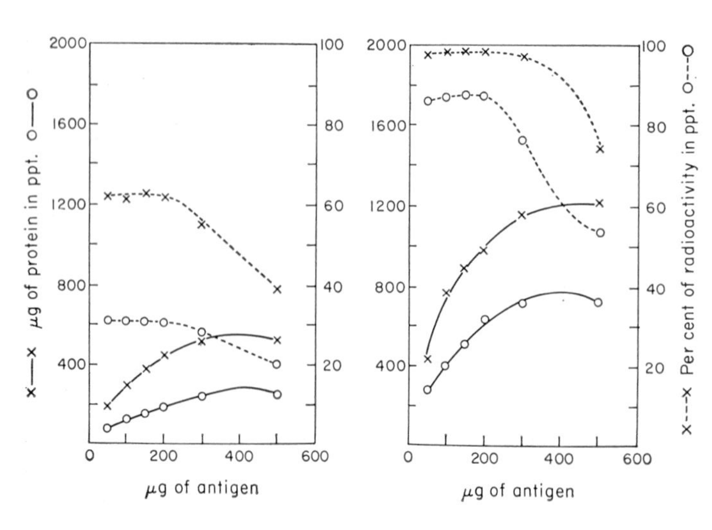

Fig. 19-3. Precipitin curves with I^{131}-labeled normal 7S γ-globulin. On the *left*, x——x indicates protein and x— — —x the percentage of radioactivity precipitated by an antiserum to group I determinants; o——o indicates protein and o— — —o the percentage of radioactivity precipitated by an antiserum to group II determinants. On the *right*, x——x indicates protein and x— — —x, the percentage of radioactivity precipitated by an antiserum to 7S γ-globulin; o——o indicates protein and o— — —o the percentage of radioactivity precipitated by a mixture of equal aliquots of antisera used on the left half of this figure.

Quantitative studies show that approximately 60 percent of the 7S γ-globulin molecules carry group I determinants, therefore termed group I molecules, and approximately 30 percent of molecules carry group II determinants, therefore termed group II molecules [76]. In these studies, again, antisera to isolated Bence Jones proteins of group I and group II are most useful, since they are specific for the group determinants and contain no antibodies to other determinants of normal immunoglobulins. Figure 19-3 illustrates such experiments. An antiserum to group I determinants precipitates 60 percent of I^{131}-labeled 7S γ-globulin, and antiserum to group II determinants precipitates 30 percent of I^{131}-labeled 7S γ-globulin in the antibody excess zone of the precipitin curve. Both antisera simultaneously precipitate nearly 90 percent of the labeled material, indicating that the group I and group II determinants exist on separate molecules. If some molecules would carry both group I and group II determinants, the percentage of radioactive 7S γ-globulin precipitated at antibody excess would be less than the percentage of radioactivity precipitated by both antisera separately. Furthermore, the fact that only 90 percent of 7S γ-globulin is precipitated by the two antisera suggests that a third, but minor, antigenic group of 7S γ-globulin may exist, constituting around 10 percent of molecules [76]. Certain antisera to normal or pathological immunoglobulins demonstrate a double precipitin line of 7S γ-globulin on immunoelectrophoresis. This phenomenon is encountered because of group I and group II molecules and an appropriate ratio of antibodies in the antiserum used [76]. The double precipitin line phenomenon and study of individual electrophoretic fractions of 7S γ-globulin indicate that group I and group II molecules are present in the 60 percent and 30 percent ratio, respectively, throughout the broad distribution of this protein.

The same two antigenic groups of molecules exist in normal β_{2A}-globulins [82], normal 19S γ-globulin [83], and normal γ_L-globulins of plasma and urine [64, 66]. The group-specific antigenic determinants exist only on the L chains of immunoglobulins [28, 80]. Current amino acid sequence studies on Bence Jones proteins in several laboratories show that group I Bence Jones proteins have a number of common peptides that differ from the peptides common among the group II Bence Jones proteins [84, 85]. These studies clearly indicate that certain basic structural features are common to the L chains of group I immunoglobulins and that different basic structural elements are common to the L chains of group II immunoglobulins, as suggested by the antigenic studies of these proteins. The reasons for existence of two types of immunoglobulins, differing in structure of their L chains, are not apparent at this time.

From many of the studies discussed, the concept emerges that each of the three classes of immunoglobulins is composed of two types of polypeptide chains. The H chains of the 7S γ-globulin and corresponding chains of the 19S γ-globulins and the β_{2A}-globulins are unique to each class of immunoglobulins. The L chains are common to all classes of immunoglobulins, and two basic types of L chains exist. This concept is presented schematically in Figure 19-4.

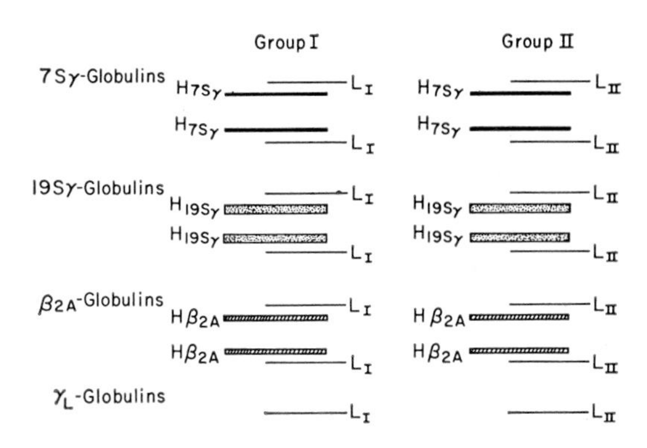

Fig. 19-4. Schematic presentation of the four classes of immunoglobulins and their groups.

The possibility that the H chains of the 7S γ-globulin actually consist of two or more subchains has been raised by several investigators. Recent studies on a group of patients with what has been termed "H chain disease" [86, 87] indicate that in these individuals excessive production of a portion of the H chains occurs. These isolated proteins resemble closely the F fragments produced by cysteine-activated papain and do not seem to represent the entire H chains of 7S γ-globulin. These proteins lack the antigenic determinants that exist on the portion of H chains that becomes part of the S fragment on cleavage of 7S γ-globulin with papain. If an analogy to Bence Jones proteins holds true, these partial H chains may represent a basic subunit of the 7S γ-globulin molecule.

It seems highly probable that some type of subgrouping of L chains within each of the major group I and II categories will be possible [88]. Observations in our laboratory indicate that a very complex system is involved and that many different antisera will be required to delineate it. An alternative to the concept of pure subgroups is that a large number of antigenic determinants detected in various L chains occur in different combinations in individual myeloma and Bence Jones proteins. It has become apparent that the group II type proteins differ much more strikingly from one another than do those of group I.

H CHAIN SUBGROUPS OF 7S γ-GLOBULINS

Recent observations indicate that at least four subgroups of γ-globulins can be distinguished by rabbit antisera to individual myeloma proteins [89]. Some of them are also demonstrated by monkey antisera to fraction II γ-globulin [89a]. Most of the differences have been localized to the F fragment of the H chains, but there is evidence of additional differences involving the portion of the H chains found in the S fragment. These subgroups do not have permanent names; in our laboratory, they have been given the name of the prototype myeloma protein. The major We group consists of 60 to 70 percent of myeloma proteins as well as γ-globulin molecules in fraction II. The Vi group, which contains the Gm(b) character, represents 7 to 10 percent of γ-globulin and myeloma proteins. The Ge group occurs in somewhat lower percentage but is of particular interest because of a unique fast mobility of the F fragments as compared to other myeloma proteins of the 7S type [89]. A fourth group also exists but has not been clearly delineated.

The exact chemical basis for these various subgroups remains to be determined. Their H chains show some cross-reaction antigenically and thus are not as distinct as the H chains of the 19S and β_{2A} immunoglobulins, which fail to cross-react. It is of particular interest that the H chains of the four subgroups, like those of the other immunoglobulins, appear to contain independent genetic determinants [68a]. There is evidence available that similar subgroups also exist for the β_{2A} and 19S immunoglobulins. It is clear that Figure 19-4 will have to be enlarged quite considerably to include all of these H chain subgroups, all of which are apparently combined to both group I and group II L chains.

ANTIBODY FUNCTION

A large body of evidence has accumulated to demonstrate that all three main classes of immunoglobulins possess antibody activity. The β_{2A} class is the subject of intensive study and remains largely undefined. However, certain antibodies clearly have been localized in this fraction. Another subject of current interest involves the localization of antibodies in group I and II immunoglobulins. This work on the group determinants shows that actually six classes of immunoglobulins exist with antibody function, since the 7S, 19S, and β_{2A} types are all divisible into the two groups. Even further subdivision appears likely. The basic principles involved in the formation of antibodies of the six types remain largely unknown. It is clear that they differ strikingly for the group I and group II categories which involve the L chains as opposed to the 7S, 19S, and β_{2A} types which involve H chain differences. Recent work has gone far to elucidate the 7S–19S relationship in terms of stages of antibody production. Just where the β_{2A} class fits into this scheme remains an enigma.

7S–19S RELATIONSHIP

Early work on 19S antibodies was performed primarily with the pneumococcus system and suggested that high molecular weight antibodies were characteristic of horse and related species and were not observed in the rabbit or man. It was already apparent in this work that the 19S antibodies occurred early in immunization, with the 7S antibodies predominating in the later states [35, 90]. Subsequent observations clearly showed that rabbits also produce 19S antibodies to sheep cells [91] and even to pneumococci [92]. Here again the 19S antibodies occurred primarily in the early stages of immunization [91]. Recent work in rabbits and other species has greatly expanded these observations [93–95], and it now is apparent that all antigens, even haptens, can produce 19S antibodies early in immunization [96]. The most interesting finding is that there is little or no secondary 19S response, as in the case of the 7S system [97]. "Immunological memory" appears to be lacking, and a sustained antigenic stimulus is required to preserve 19S antibody levels. It seems likely that different cells are involved in the two responses, although in man, some evidence has been obtained of the production of 7S and 19S antibodies by the same cell [98]. The question of whether these same principles apply in other species, particularly the horse, remains unanswered. The extreme 19S response noted by the earlier workers requires explanation. Such effects have not been noted in the recent rabbit work.

19S ANTIBODIES IN MAN

It is clear that in man, too, the 19S antibody response usually appears early in immunization and declines as the 7S secondary response becomes operative. The similarity to the rabbit system has become most evident in recent work with the bacteriophage system [99]. However, some observations in human beings are difficult to fit into this picture. Certain antigens produce only 19S antibodies and never appear to result in 7S responses [100, 101]. In addition, injection of blood group substance A or B results in different responses in different individuals and appears to be governed by the blood group of the individual [102, 103]. Type O individuals tend to produce 7S antibodies, as is dramatically illustrated by hemolytic disease. However, in some type O mothers single injections of A or B substances produce high titers of 19S antibodies which may persist for many years. This interesting problem requires further investigation. The recent finding that many individuals, following immunization, produce a third type of isoagglutinin, which has an intermediate sedimentation rate [104], must be fitted into the picture. This new type of antibody was formerly considered in part in the 19S group [103].

Observations on the allotypic antibodies produced to foreign genetic types of γ-globulin indicate that the vast majority of them are of the 19S type. Here again it is not clear why more 7S antibodies are not produced; secondary responses would be expected. The question of the development of tolerance needs evaluation with respect to the 19S response in this case, because of exposure to the mother's γ-globulin. That this might be important has become evident from the observations that individuals who possess anti-γ-globulin factors specific for a foreign genetic type of γ-globulin have mothers possessing this type of γ-globulin [69]. These 19S anti-γ-globulins persist for many years.

Extreme levels of 19S anti-γ-globulins are frequently found in individuals with rheumatoid arthritis to such an extent that they can be visualized by direct analysis of whole serum in the analytical ultracentrifuge [105]. They appear to be antibodies to altered γ-globulin, perhaps antigen-antibody complexes. Here it seems possible that a sustained antigenic stimulus gives rise to the high and persistent titers, particularly since similar factors found in the sera of patients with bacterial endocarditis disappear following antibacterial therapy [106].

Other 19S γ-globulins which appear to have antibody activity are found in a variety of human sera in extreme amounts. These include cold agglutinins, certain other red cell agglutinins, and some anti-γ-globulin factors. Current evidence indicates that these are analogous to Waldenström macroglobulins with specific biological activity [107]. They seem to arise from a single cell line and show great homogeneity in physical and antigenic properties [34, 102, 108]. These proteins do not show the heterogeneity characteristic of antibodies formed to antigenic stimulus. It seems likely that they are products of rapidly proliferating mutant cell lines resembling the myeloma proteins and Waldenström macroglobulins but having somewhat less malignant characteristics. The cold agglutinins have been shown to have red cell specificity in the I system [109]. The anti-γ-globulin factors of this type are frequently cryoglobulins, primarily because of their ability to react with the individual's own 7S γ-globulin [110]. A number of such sera have been studied in our laboratory recently. These macroglobulins show some tendency to precipitate in the cold alone, but in the presence of 7S γ-globulin this is strikingly accentuated. These proteins differ from those observed in rheumatoid arthritis sera because of their marked electrophoretic homogeneity. The cold agglutinins and the anti-γ-globulin factors appear to be the most common proteins of this type, but an aged red cell agglutinin [111] and antinuclear factors have also been encountered. There are probably a number of others, and perhaps all Waldenström macroglobulins may have antibody activity. One reason these proteins are of interest now is that they probably represent antibodies to single antigenic determinants and are readily isolated for the many current studies concerning the structure of antibodies.

β_{2A} ANTIBODIES

Observations on the antibody activity of the β_{2A} fraction have been hampered by the paucity of methods for separating this fraction readily from the other immunoglobulins. Actually, the only entirely adequate characteristic delineating the β_{2A} proteins is their specific antigenic activity. A simple method such as density gradient ultracentrifuge analysis, that has proved so useful for 19S antibodies, is not available. The difficulty arises from the fact that 7S γ-globulin has a broad electrophoretic distribution, and the chemical and chromatographic characteristics of fast-migrating 7S γ-globulin are very similar to those of the β_{2A} proteins.

The ultracentrifugal characteristics of β_{2A} antibodies also are not entirely clear. Antigenic analyses of density gradient fractions indicate that the bulk of the β_{2A}-globulins correspond to 7S γ-globulin in their sedimentation rate [104, 112]. However, the fact that many β_{2A} myeloma proteins have higher sedimentation constants, as mentioned earlier, raises the possibility that at least certain antibodies in this group might have similar increased s-rate. The many blood group antibodies with intermediate s-rate also may be related to the β_{2A} fractions, although in the main these appear to be polymers of 7S γ-globulin [113]. Considerable evidence indicates that the skin-sensitizing antibodies which appear to be β_{2A} proteins have an s-rate above 7 [104]. The β_{2A} proteins found in saliva are predominantly of higher s-rate [114]. An anti-B isoagglutinin has been isolated from a high-titer serum in which the specific precipitate with B substance consists predominantly of β_{2A} protein. This isoagglutinin shows intermediate sedimentation in the 9S to 15S range [112]. An anti-γ-globulin useful for genetic typing in the Gm(a) system has been observed. It appears to be β_{2A}-globulin and also shows an intermediate sedimentation rate [115]. These results all remain somewhat confusing, but it is evident that many antibodies in the β_{2A}-globulin class have sedimentation constants above 7S.

These antibodies also appear to be sensitive to sulfhydryl compounds, although this seems to be somewhat less than for 19S antibodies. The skin-sensitizing antibodies clearly show greater sensitivity than control 7S class antibodies [104, 116]. This, of course, may be a function of the delicate *in vivo* test system. However, the isoagglutinins and the anti-γ-globulin antibody described above also show increased sensitivity to mercaptoethanol. This might be expected if these antibodies were of intermediate s-rate, since the higher s-rate myeloma proteins are readily dissociated by these reagents.

Relatively few antibodies have thus far been clearly delineated in the β_{2A} fraction, but the number is increasing rapidly and may include all types. Initial observations [117] on fractions of serum enriched in β_{2A} through zinc precipitation showed evidence of antibody activity. However, these fractions were admittedly contaminated with ordinary 7S γ-globulin. More recent work, utilizing this approach, has furnished further evidence in the same direction [54]. Fractions have been prepared virtually free from 7S γ-globulin which show considerable antibody activity. *Brucella* agglutinins and diphtheria antitoxins have been studied particularly.

In our laboratory [113], a large number of isoagglutinins have been isolated from specific precipitates with A or B substance, and varying amounts of β_{2A}-globulin have been found. One anti-B serum mentioned earlier contained β_{2A}-globulin as the dominant antigen in the isolated antibody. Isolated teichoic acid antibodies in many human sera have been found to contain β_{2A}, but in no instance was this the dominant immunoglobulin. Antinuclear antibodies have also been found of the β_{2A} class by means of specific fluorescent antisera [118] and analysis of eluates prepared with DNAse [119]. Certain rheumatoid factors, particularly those from patients with Sjögren's syndrome [120], and certain anti-γ-globulins useful for genetic typing have been shown to be of the β_{2A} type [115].

Particular success in the localization of antibodies to the β_{2A} fraction has been obtained through the use of the autoradiographic technique of immunoelectrophoresis developed by Morse and Heremans [11]. Here, labeled antigen is added to the trough containing an antiserum to β_{2A}-globulins. The antigen localizes in the β_{2A} line if the serum which was separated contains antibodies of this character. This technique permits the localization of antibodies to all of the immunoglobulins in one simple experiment if an antiserum is used which reacts specifically with the three major immunoglobulins. The method has been applied with particular success to thyroglobulin antibodies in human sera [121]. Antibodies falling into all three classes of immunoglobulins were encountered in many sera. The method has also been applied to insulin antibodies [122] and to ragweed pollen antibodies [123] with similar results.

A question which has intrigued a number of investigators concerning the β_{2A} fraction is whether it contains the skin-sensitizing antibodies. It has long been known that these antibodies must be of a special type, primarily because of their failure to cross the placenta. Initial observations suggested that they might be of the 19S type, but this is definitely ruled out [104]. Skin-sensitizing antibodies are concentrated in a fraction rich in β_{2A}-globulin [124]. Skin sensitization is abolished if the β_{2A}-globulins are precipitated with an antiserum to this protein [125]. These results appear conclusive.* However, some results in our laboratory are not readily interpreted on this basis [126]. One individual, whose serum is completely lacking in β_{2A}-globulins, is under investigation concerning the formation of skin-sensitizing antibodies. Preliminary observations indicate that such antibodies are indeed present. In addition, certain individuals with clear β_{2A} isoagglutinins do not appear to have demonstrable skin-sensitizing antibodies. The problem remains unsettled; the role of the β_{2A}-globulins remains undetermined. No results are available concerning the stage of immunization, as in the case of the 19S antibodies. The problem is hampered by the failure to recognize this fraction clearly in most experimental animals, although β_{2A} myeloma proteins are recognized in mice [127].

ANTIBODIES OF INTERMEDIATE S-RATE

The study of the isoagglutinins in the past has furnished considerable knowledge that later found application to antibodies in general. A more recent development concerns the finding of many isoagglutinins of intermediate s-rate, covering a spectrum readily separable from the classic 7S and 19S groups. Figure 19-5 illustrates the pattern of distribution of a high titer anti-A agglutinin following ultracentrifugation in a sucrose density gradient; a 19S cold agglutinin and a 7S anti-D are shown from the same experiment for comparison. In a study of a large number of individuals of blood group A or B in whom high titers of anti-B or anti-A developed following one injection of B or A substance, the intermediate type antibodies represented a frequent finding and in some sera was the dominant type. These isoagglutinins have also been observed in recent work with Sephadex G-200 [128]. In diethylaminoethyl chromatography they come off the column in later fractions but before the bulk of the 19S antibodies [104]. The antibodies have only been demonstrated clearly for isoagglutinins. However, recent work [129] indicates that certain antibacterial antibodies also appear in this intermediate fraction.

The exact relationship of these intermediate type antibodies to the β_{2A} fraction remains to be determined. Their isolation from specific precipitates has proved feasible, and in each case some β_{2A} is found in the precipitate. However, in most instances antigenic analysis indicates that the bulk of the protein is ordinary 7S γ-globulin even in the intermediately sedimenting peak of density gradient experiments on the isolated antibody. Acid extraction of the specific precipitate from sera containing primarily intermediate antibodies has in most instances resulted in protein showing an s-rate of approximately 7S, suggesting dissociation in the process of acid extraction. Controlled conditions of acetate buffer extraction at pH 3.8 have resulted in isolation of intermediately sedimenting antibodies. One anti-B antibody has been encountered which shows primarily β_{2A} in the isolated antibody. This, too, is of intermediate s-rate indistinguishable from those already described, except in this case relatively little 7S γ-globulin is apparent through antigenic analysis. Most of these antibodies show some sensitivity to sulfhydryl compounds. These assorted observations are difficult to put together into a rational picture at present.

* *Editor's comment:* Further evidence for the association of B_{2A} with reagin was provided by Allansmith and Buell (*J. Allerg.* 35:339, 1964), who examined maternal blood of 26 atopic mothers and corresponding cord blood of their babies. All maternal samples were positive for B_{2A} and reagin both by direct and P.K. testing. One cord sample had both reagin and B_{2A}, but all others were negative. Of 58 normals (nonallergic mothers), all had B_{2A} but no reagin. The corresponding cord blood was negative for both factors.—B. R.

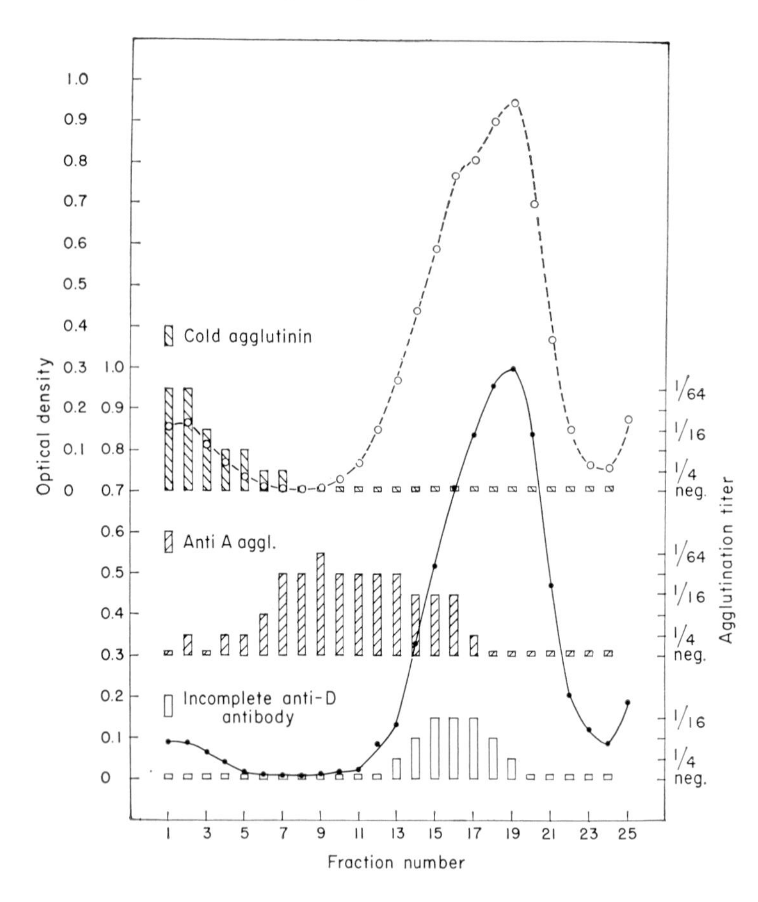

Fig. 19-5. Curves of protein concentration and distribution of agglutination obtained by simultaneous density gradient ultracentrifugation of an intermediate sedimenting anti-A isohemagglutinin, 7S incomplete anti-D antibody, and a 19S cold agglutinin. Base-line values represent negative agglutination at lowest dilution indicated. •——• indicates the protein concentration of a mixture of the sera containing anti-A and anti-D antibodies. o— — —o indicates the protein concentration of a mixture of the sera containing anti-A and cold agglutinins; only the cold agglutinin titer is recorded. (From Kunkel and Rockey [112].)

ANTIBODIES IN GROUP I AND II IMMUNOGLOBULINS

The division of 7S and 19S γ-globulins and β_{2A}-globulins into two basic groups on the basis of their mutually exclusive antigenic determinants on the L chains indicates that antibodies of the different immunoglobulin classes also can be localized into these two groups. Recent work demonstrates this to be the case [130]. Rh antibodies, isoagglutinins, thyroglobulin antibodies, dextran antibodies, and teichoic acid antibodies have been demonstrated in both groups of immunoglobulins.

Three methods have been utilized to demonstrate this distribution. Antisera to either group I or group II Bence Jones proteins can be obtained which show no reaction with proteins of the opposite groups. These antisera serve as Coombs sera for the agglutination of red cells coated with incomplete Rh antibodies. Seven different anti-Rh sera showed Rh antibodies belonging to both groups. A second method, which proved useful for many antibodies, involves the precipitation of group I or group II immunoglobulin molecules with a specific antiserum in the region of antibody excess. Analysis of the antibodies remaining in the supernate after such precipitation indicates the antibodies belonging to the opposite group. This method has been used successfully for Rh antibodies, thyroglobulin antibodies, and isoagglutinins. The third method, which proved most useful, is direct antigenic analysis of isolated antibodies. For this purpose, specific precipitates dissolved in antigen excess have sufficed. Serial dilutions of these antibody preparations on agar slides with the group I antiserum on one side in a trough and the group II antiserum on the other side in a trough furnish semiquantitative results in comparison with normal 7S γ-globulin. Figure 19-6 illustrates one such experiment. The striking finding by this technique is that certain antibodies belong predominantly to one group or the other. In Figure 19-6, one anti-A is predominantly group II and the other shows a stronger reaction with the group I antiserum.

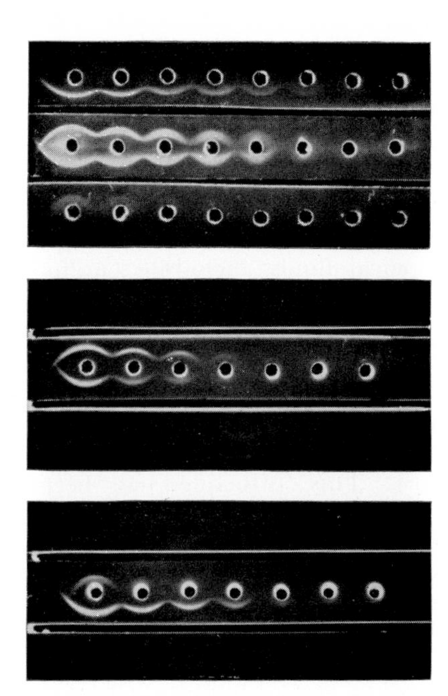

Fig. 19-6. Double diffusion agar slides showing the reaction of serial dilutions of isolated antibodies with group I and group II antisera. The upper trough in each slide contains an antiserum specific to group II determinants, and the lower trough, an antiserum specific to group I determinants. In the upper slide the outer wells contain isolated antibodies to blood group substance A from donor Th., and the inner wells contain similar antibodies from donor 66, adjusted to equal protein concentration. Clearly, the isolated antibodies from Th. react primarily with group II antiserum, in contrast to those from donor 66. In the center and bottom slides the wells contain isolated anti-teichoic acid antibodies from donors Es. and Ga., respectively. The antibodies from Es. (center) show predominance of group II molecules and those from Ga., predominance of group I molecules.

A study of a variety of antibodies indicated that this is a general finding. Labeling of isolated antibodies with I^{131} and selective precipitation with the two antisera confirmed in an accurate quantitative fashion the selective distribution [130].

It appears that antibodies to very limited determinants tend to show predominance of one or the other group. Antibodies known to be heterogeneous with respect to multiplicity of sites on the antigen show a distribution of group I and group II molecules similar to that of 7S γ-globulin. Thus far no reason has become apparent for the distribution of antibodies into one or the other group. The same principles appear to apply for 19S and β_{2A} antibodies, although these have not been studied as closely [131]. The cold agglutinins belong to group I and the homogenous anti-γ-globulins belong to one or the other group but not to both, furnishing further evidence that these are "monoclonal" in type and more closely resemble the Waldenström macroglobulins, which always belong to a single group. The determination of the homogeneity with respect to groups appears to be a very simple way of determining the homogeneity of an antibody.

MEASUREMENT OF IMMUNOGLOBULINS

Physical and chemical methods are not adequate for accurate quantitation of immunoglobulins separately. At present their most accurate quantitation in biological fluids depends on immunochemical methods, utilizing the unique antigenic characteristics of each of these classes of proteins. However, the reagents for these methods must be prepared with great care, so these methods are not used as routine. Other techniques used for quantitation of one or all immunoglobulins include electrophoresis, ultracentrifugation, and salting out or precipitation by chemicals.

Free electrophoresis was widely employed to determine the quantity of γ-globulin in serum. More recently, paper electrophoresis with appropriate staining and scanning devices is frequently used for clinical quantitation of γ-globulins. By such techniques, 11 to 14 percent of the total serum protein consists of γ-globulin, primarily composed of 7S γ-globulin. However, as already pointed out, some normal 7S γ-globulin migrates with the β- and α_2-globulins. Furthermore, electrophoretic methods will not permit the quantitation of other immunoglobulins, and they are rather inaccurate for quantitation of subnormal levels of serum 7S γ-globulin as well as 7S γ-globulin in other body fluids. Nevertheless electrophoretic methods have value in detecting diseases involving the immunoglobulins, as discussed elsewhere in this volume.

Ultracentrifugation can be used to determine the presence of normal or excess 19S γ-globulins [132], but it will not detect 19S γ-globulins in concentrations less than 1 mg. per ml. of serum or other biological fluids. By ultracentrifugal determinations adult normal serum contains 50 to 100 mg. of 19S γ-globulin per 100 ml., compared to 35 to 70 mg. per 100 ml. by immunochemical techniques [132].

For large-scale screening purposes and serial estimation of 7S γ-globulins during the course of a disease, turbidimetric measurements of γ-globulin with precipitation by zinc ions has proved useful [133–135]. Other salting out or precipitation procedures give variable degrees of success. In such methods, not all 7S γ-globulin is precipitated, and other immunoglobulins cannot be estimated.

Immunochemical methods are accurate and the only methods for quantitation of each immunoglobulin individually. The technical aspects of these methods are well reviewed and described elsewhere [136]. In general, the methods utilize specific antisera to each of the classes of immunoglobulins. Specific antisera from rabbit, horse, or chicken may be used to react with the protein under study to form the specific precipitate. The amount of protein in the precipitate is determined, and from standards constructed with known pure samples of the protein in question the quantity of the immunoglobulin under study is calculated. Nephelometry may be used for convenience and speed to quantitate the specific precipitation instead of protein determination [137]. Both methods, however, require a standard curve constructed with the same antiserum and a purified preparation of the protein under study. The latter is easily obtained for 7S γ-globulin, relatively easily for 19S γ-globulin, but with difficulty for β_{2A}-globulin. The possibility of utilizing homogeneous myeloma proteins of the β_{2A} type as a standard needs to be fully evaluated. Immunochemical quantitation of each class of immunoglobulins separately is possible due to the antigenic determinants characteristic of each class (discussed earlier). For accurate quantitation of 7S γ-globulins, an antiserum to the F fragments should be utilized. Quantitation of 19S γ-globulins should be performed with an antiserum specific for this protein, and similarly, a specific antiserum should be utilized for the quantitation of β_{2A}-globulins. The absolute concentrations of normal immunoglobulins in serum or other body fluids have not been determined by these methods in large series. Quantitative immunochemical methods can detect as little as 0.5 μg. of 7S γ-globulin per ml. [138]. Immunochemical determinations of serum 7S γ-globulins usually yield values higher than those obtained by electrophoresis, and the normal values for adults are around 12 mg. per ml. of serum [137, 139].

Various gel diffusion techniques have been employed to quantitate the immunoglobulins in biological fluids, including Oudin tubes, Preer tubes, and Ouchterlony plates [140]. All depend on the principles discussed above. Relative concentrations of proteins are determined accurately, and absolute values can be obtained by comparison with standards constructed with purified individual immunoglobulins. This principle has been well applied to modified immunoelectrophoretic techniques to quantitate 7S and 19S γ-globulins, but adequate standards for the β_{2A}-globulins were not available [141, 142]. Careful measurements in a modified diffusion in agar technique have shown that the average normal serum concentration of 19S γ-globulin is 1.08 mg. per ml. and 1.56 mg. per ml. for β_{2A}-globulin [143].

Inhibition of immune precipitation, whereby the standard antigen is labeled with radioactive isotopes, has been used successfully to quantitate serum immunoglobulins in normal individuals. By such methods the normal values are: 7S γ-globulin, 12.63 mg. per ml.; β_{2A}-globulin 3.94 mg., and 19S γ-globulin 1.16 mg. per ml. [144, 145]. In this study the serum concentration of β_{2A}-globulin is higher than observed in previous studies by different methods. Differences in the standard antigen and in the method of quantitation may account for these discrepancies.

Qualitative demonstration of the three major classes of immunoglobulins, including 7S γ-globulins, 19S γ-globulins, and β_{2A}-globulins, depends on the same considerations outlined for the quantitative determinations. Immunoelectrophoresis is the most useful procedure for identification of each of the immunoglobulins and has gained wide use as a clinical and research tool.

DISTRIBUTION AND TURN-OVER OF IMMUNOGLOBULINS

Once the 7S γ-globulins have been formed by plasma cells in lymph nodes, spleen, and bone marrow, they enter the blood stream directly or via the lymphatics and become distributed primarily in the extracellular space. By immunofluorescent techniques, 7S γ-globulins are noted in lymphatics, interstitial spaces, connective tissue, and a variety of cells [146]. A dynamic equilibrium exists between the intravascular and extravascular 7S γ-globulin [147]. Its concentration varies from tissue to tissue; in muscle, for example, 200 to 250 mg. of 7S γ-globulin exists per 100 ml. of interstitial fluid [148]. Calculations from turn-over studies indicate that about 45 percent of 7S γ-globulins is in the intravascular space at any one time and that 55 percent of these proteins exist in the extravascular spaces [149, 150]. Further calculations indicate that normal adults have approximately 1.22 gm. of γ-globulin per kg. of body weight, i.e., approximately 85 gm. of γ-globulin in a 70-kg. man, whose serum contains about 11 mg. of 7S γ-globulin per ml.

The quantity of 7S γ-globulin in the body at any one time represents an equilibrium between its rate of synthesis and its rate of catabolism. The serum level reflects the level at which such equilibrium has been reached. The pathways and mechanisms of catabolism of 7S γ-globulins and other immunoglobulins are poorly understood, as are the factors that maintain the normal adult 7S γ-globulin serum level rather constant over many years. The turn-over of 7S γ-globulin has been investigated extensively by labeling the protein with I^{131}; internal labels in the form of N^{15} [151] and S^{35} [152] have also been used. By such labeling, the half-life of 7S γ-globulin has been calculated to be 20 to 25 days [150–153]. The daily production of 7S γ-globulins in normal adults is about 0.036 gm. per kg. of body weight [150].

The distribution of 19S γ-globulin is primarily intravascular. Its turn-over is faster than that of 7S γ-globulin, and its half-life has been estimated at about five days [154]. Since the isolation of normal β_{2A}-globulins is difficult, no data are available on their turnover and distribution.

PLACENTAL TRANSFER AND NEONATAL DEVELOPMENT OF IMMUNOGLOBULINS

Placental transfer of immunoglobulins from maternal circulation to the fetus has been the subject of many investigations. In older studies, only 7S γ-globulin was investigated since the other immunoglobulins were not adequately defined. As early as the end of the Nineteenth Century, investigators noted that certain antibodies did not appear in fetal circulation in spite of their presence in the maternal serum, in contrast to other antibodies that appeared in fetal serum in higher concentration than in maternal serum [155]. Salting out procedures as well as paper strip electrophoresis, conducted before development of the immunoglobulin concept, indicate that γ-globulin concentration in the serum of the infant was slightly higher than that of the mother [156–158]. More recent immunochemical analyses show that, at the time of delivery, maternal serum contains about 11.0 mg. of 7S γ-globulins per ml., and the concentration of 7S γ-globulins in the cord serum is 12.5 mg. per ml. [159]. Isolated 7S γ-globulins from cord sera contain 60 percent group I molecules and 30 percent group II molecules, similar to the ratio of both groups of molecules in adult normal sera [160]. Ultracentrifugation does not show the cord serum of infants to contain a 19S γ-globulin peak, indicating that its level in the infant is less than one tenth of that in maternal serum [132]. Thorough immunochemical analyses of the cord sera show minute quantities of 19S γ-globulins as well as β_{2A}-globulins, but their concentration is markedly less than in the maternal circulation [142, 159]. There are abundant data that the 7S γ-globulin antibodies from maternal circulation are transferred across the placenta, whereas the 19S γ-globulin antibodies are not [155, 161–163]. Antibodies among β_{2A}-globulins have not been investigated, but their behavior in regard to placental transfer is probably similar to that of the 19S γ-globulin antibodies.

The exact mechanism of placental transfer of 7S γ-globulins to fetal circulation is not known. However, several observations suggest that this is active transport rather than filtration. As already indicated, the concentration of 7S γ-globulin is higher in the serum of the infant than in that of the mother. Serum proteins of equal or smaller molecular size are not transferred across the placenta [159]. Furthermore, horse diphtheria antitoxin cleaved with pepsin does not cross the placental barrier, in contrast to the unaltered antitoxin [164]. In rabbits, 7S γ-globulin fragments I and II fail to cross the placenta, whereas fragments III, corresponding to F fragments of human 7S γ-globulins, readily cross the placental barrier [165]. In humans S fragments have a very short and variable half-life, but F fragments reach a higher fetal serum concentration relative to maternal serum concentration than S fragments [165a]. However, the placental transfer of immunoglobulins in relation to molecular subunits is not entirely settled. Although 7S γ-globulin antibodies exist in the amniotic fluid, 19S γ-globulins and β_{2A}-globulins have not been detected [166, 167].

Placental transfer of maternal 7S γ-globulin antibodies provides the infant with protection against many viral and bacterial organisms. However, the 19S γ-globulin bactericidal antibodies, e.g., antibodies to *Salmonella typhosa* and *Escherichia coli,* fail to pass the placental barrier and the infant must rely on his own immunological mechanisms to produce antibodies to these organisms [163]. This may be a reason for the high susceptibility of infants to certain bacterial infections.

Maternal 7S γ-globulin in the infant is catabolized, and the serum concentration begins to fall, reaching the lowest level in the second to third month of extrauterine life [157–159]. On immunochemical assay, the 7S γ-globulin level falls to around 5.8 mg. per ml. [159]. During the ensuing months of infancy and childhood, the level gradually rises and approaches 10 mg. per ml. during the second year of life [158]. During the neonatal period, marked paucity of plasma cells is noted in bone marrow and lymphoid tissue [168], accounting for the slow production of immunoglobulins. Both 19S γ-globulin and β_{2A}-globulin are detectable in the neonatal period, and their concentration begins to rise around the third month of extrauterine life [139, 159].

During the neonatal period, the serum level of 7S γ-globulin declines due to catabolism and also to growth of the infant. In spite of these two factors, the decrease is slower than would be expected, assuming a half-life of 25 days. This suggests that the infant is producing his own 7S γ-globulin, even though at a slow rate initially [159]. Full-term as well as premature infants are capable of forming antibodies. This is well demonstrated with typhoid and paratyphoid vaccine [162, 169] and with bacteriophage in newborn premature infants [99]. The infant first forms 19S γ-globulin antibodies to these administered antigens and only subsequently produces 7S γ-globulin antibodies. A study of 19S γ-globulin Wassermann antibodies suggests that the fetus is able to produce antibodies *in utero* as early as the fifth month [170]. All of these observations clearly show that infants are capable of producing antibodies. Furthermore, the same observations coupled with the evidence that germ-free animals have low levels of γ-globulin [171, 172] raise the possibility that the immunoglobulins of the newborn are produced only due to antigenic stimulation.

IMMUNOGLOBULINS IN BODY SECRETIONS

A number of body secretions have been investigated for the presence of each of the immunoglobulins. In spite of progress in this area, the function of immunoglobulins in many secretions remains unknown in health as well as in relation to diseases.

Recent studies on normal human parotid saliva demonstrate that approximately 1.5 mg. of immunoglobulins is present per 100 ml. of saliva. This protein component of saliva consists entirely of β_{2A}-globulins [173]. The 7S γ-globulins are not detectable in parotid saliva by sensitive methods, and only occasionally are minute quantities of 19S γ-globulins encountered. These observations raise the possibility that β_{2A}-globulin is preferentially excreted by the parotid gland, as compared to the other immunoglobulins. In addition, it remains to be seen which subunit of the β_{2A}-globulin confers this function to the molecules. The physiological significance of the relatively high β_{2A}-globulin in saliva is an enigma.

Neutralized and quickly cooled gastric juice from normal subjects contains variable amounts of 7S γ-globulins and up to 300 mg. of this protein may be secreted into gastric juice per day [174]. Intestinal juice from normal individuals also contains 7S γ-globulins [175], but quantitation of 7S γ-globulin in the intestine has not been achieved. The significance of intestinal secretion of immunoglobulins in relation to the total turn-over of these proteins remains to be determined.

The immunoglobulins in human milk and colostrum have been extensively investigated [176, 177]. Colostrum and milk both contain 7S γ-globulin and group I and group II molecules. In addition, 19S γ-globulin and β_{2A}-globulin are elaborated into colostrum and milk, and γ_L-globulins occur in both secretions [178]. Many antibodies of the 7S and 19S γ-globulin class, present in maternal serum, are also demonstrable in colostrum and milk [155]. Their absorption to the circulation of the infant does not seem to occur, but this question is not entirely settled.

SITE OF SYNTHESIS

Mature plasma cells are the site of synthesis of 7S γ-globulins, as established by a variety of techniques. Fluorescein-labeled antibodies to human 7S γ-globulins demonstrate this protein in mature plasma cells [98, 179] and the cytoplasm of germinal center cells of lymph nodes. In patients with agammaglobulinemia, lymph nodes and bone marrow lack plasma cells [180]. Incubation of tissue slices from lymph nodes of immunized animals shows a parallel in the increase of plasma cells and the rise of antibody titer in the incubation medium [181]. Similarly, a suspension of lymph node cells from an animal immunized with bacteria shows agglutination of the bacteria and plasma cells [182].

With fluorescent antibody techniques it has been shown that group I and II immunoglobulins are produced in different mature plasma cells [182a, 182b], whereby about two-thirds of cells produce group I proteins and one-third group II proteins, corresponding to the relative distribution of these proteins in serum. However, both group I and group II antigens exist in single cells in the germinal centers of lymphoid follicles [182a]. This observation suggests that immature and perhaps immunologically uncommitted cells are capable of producing both kinds of molecules. Once antibody production begins, only one kind of molecules is produced, the others being repressed.

The exact cell type involved in 19S γ-globulin synthesis is not established. The cells differ somewhat from those forming 7S γ-globulin and have been given a variety of names. The cells producing Waldenström-type macroglobulins have been called plasmacytoid lymphocytes as well as lymphocytoid plasma cells [183, 184]. Rheumatoid factor production has been demonstrated in cells of the plasma cell series present in the lymph nodes and synovial lesions of patients with rheumatoid arthritis [185, 186]. Patients with absence of 7S γ-globulins, but capable of synthesizing 19S γ-globulins, possess plasmacytoid lymphoctyes, primarily in the spleen [187], as demonstrated with fluorescein-labeled antibodies to 19S γ-globulins.

In vitro incubation of human lymph nodes with radioactive amino acids shows definite incorporation of radioactivity into β_{2A}-globulins as well as into other immunoglobulins, indicating that β_{2A}-globulins are produced in lymph nodes [188]. Immunofluorescent techniques show that β_{2A}-globulins are produced in plasma cells of human lymph nodes, splenic white pulp, and lymphoid tissue elsewhere in the body [98, 189]. The number of cells producing β_{2A}-globulin is less than the number of cells producing 19S γ-globulin.

The current evidence clearly shows that all of the major immunoglobulins are produced in plasma cells and related cells, thus providing another reason for grouping these proteins in one family. However, these observations raise many unanswered questions in regard to the formation of antibodies in the three classes of immunoglobulins. Are the precursors of plasma cells producing 7S γ-globulins, 19S γ-globulins, or β_{2A}-globulins identical? If the precursor cells are identical, what is the stimulus that leads to the formation of antibodies in the three classes of immunoglobulins and what is the stimulus for producing 19S γ-globulin antibodies early in immunization and subsequently only 7S γ-globulin antibodies to the same antigen? Do antibodies to single antigenic determinants, which fall into the three classes of immunoglobulins, have identical combining sites? These represent just a few of the many interesting questions concerning the immunoglobulins which remain unanswered.

REFERENCES

1. Slater, R. J. The serum γ-globulins defined by electrophoretic and immunologic analyses. *Arch. Biochem.* 59:33, 1955.
2. Williams, C. A., and Grabar, P. Immunoelectrophoretic studies on serum proteins: I. The antigens of human serum. *J. Immun.* 74:158, 1955.
3. Cann, J. R. Ultracentrifugal properties of human γ-globulins prepared by electrophoresis convection. *J. Amer. Chem. Soc.* 75:4213, 1953.

4. Müller-Eberhard, J. H., and Kunkel, H. G. The carbohydrate of γ-globulin and myeloma proteins. *J. Exp. Med.* 104:253, 1956.
5. Rosevear, J. W., and Smith, E. L. Glycopeptides: I. Isolation and properties of glycopeptides from a fraction of human γ-globulin. *J. Biol. Chem.* 236:425, 1961.
6. Northrop, J. H. Purification and crystallization of diphtheria antitoxin. *J. Gen. Physiol.* 25:465, 1941–42.
7. Petermann, M. L. The splitting of human γ-globulin antibodies by papain and bromelin. *J. Amer. Chem. Soc.* 68:106, 1946.
8. Porter, R. R. The hydrolysis of rabbit γ-globulin and antibodies with crystalline papain. *Biochem. J.* 73:119, 1959.
9. Edelman, G. M., Heremans, J. F., Heremans, M.-T., and Kunkel, H. G. Immunological studies of human γ-globulin. Relation of the precipitin lines of whole γ-globulin to those of the fragments produced by papain. *J. Exp. Med.* 112:203, 1960.
10. Franklin, E. C. Structural units of human 7S γ-globulin. *J. Clin. Invest.* 39:1933, 1960.
11. Morse, J. H., and Heremans, J. F. Immunoelectrophoretic analysis of human insulin binding antibody and its papain-produced fragments. *J. Lab. Clin. Med.* 59:891, 1962.
12. Franklin, E. C., and Stanworth, D. R. Antigenic relationships between immune globulins and certain related paraproteins in man. *J. Exp. Med.* 114:521, 1961.
13. Hershgold, E. J., Cordoba, F., Charache, P., and Gitlin, D. A crystalline fragment from human γ-globulin. *Nature* (London) 199:284, 1963.
14. Taranta, A., and Franklin, E. C. Complement fixation by antibody fragments. *Science* 134: 1981, 1961.
15. Amiraian, K., and Leikhim, E. J. Interaction of fragment III of rabbit γ-globulin and guinea pig complement. *Proc. Soc. Exp. Biol. Med.* 108:454, 1961.
16. Schur, P. H., and Becker, E. L. Complement-fixing properties of papain-treated rabbit and sheep antibodies. *Science* 141:360, 1963.
17. Reiss, A. M., and Plescia, O. Fixation of complement to fragments of antibody. *Ibid.*, p. 812.
18. Ovary, Z., and Karush, F. Studies on the immunological mechanism of anaphylaxis: II. Sensitizing and combining capacity in vivo of fractions separated from papain digests of antihapten antibody. *J. Immun.* 86:146, 1961.
19. Kern, M. E., Helmreich, E., and Eisen, H. N. The solubilization of microsomal antibody activity by the specific interaction between the crystallizable fraction of γ-globulin and lymphnode microsomes. *Proc. Nat. Acad. Sci. U.S.A.* 47:767, 1961.
20. Edelman, G. M. Dissociation of γ-globulin. *J. Amer. Chem. Soc.* 81:3155, 1959.
21. Edelman, G. M., and Poulik, M. D. Studies on structural units of the γ-globulins. *J. Exp. Med.* 113:861, 1961.
21a. Small, P. A., Kehn, J. E., and Lamm, M. E. Polypeptide chains of gamma globulin. *Science* 142:393, 1963.
21b. Pain, R. H. The molecular weights of the peptide chain of γ-globulin. *Biochem. J.* 88: 234, 1963.
22. Olins, D. E., and Edelman, G. M. The antigenic structure of the polypeptide chains of human γ-globulin. *J. Exp. Med.* 116:635, 1962.
23. Mannik, M., and Kunkel, H. G. Unpublished observations, 1962.
24. Cohen, S. Properties of the separated chains of human γ-globulin. *Nature* (London) 197: 253, 1963.
25. Fleischman, J. B., Pain, R. H., and Porter, R. R. Reduction of γ-globulins. *Arch. Biochem.*, supp. 1, p. 174, 1962.
26. Fleischman, J. B., Porter, R. R., and Press, E. M. The arrangement of the peptide chains in γ-globulin. *Biochem. J.* 88:220, 1963.
27. Poulik, M. D., and Edelman, G. M. Comparison of reduced alkylated derivatives of some myeloma globulins and Bence Jones proteins. *Nature* (London) 191: 1274, 1961.
28. Mannik, M., and Kunkel, H. G. Antigenic specificity of individual "monoclonal" γ-globulins. *Fed. Proc.* 22:264, 1963 (abst.).
29. Edelman, G. M., and Gally, J. A. The nature of Bence Jones proteins: Chemical similarities to polypeptide chains of myeloma globulins and normal γ-globulins. *J. Exp. Med.* 116:207, 1962.
30. Putnam, F. W., and Hardy, S. Proteins in multiple myeloma: III. Origin of Bence Jones proteins. *J. Biol. Chem.* 212:261, 1955.
31. Hardy, S., and Putnam, F. W. Proteins in multiple myeloma: IV. Interaction with metabolic nitrogen. *Ibid.*, p. 371.
32. Jones, H. B. Papers on Chemical Pathology, *Lancet* 2:88, 1847.
33. Edelman, G. M., Benacerraf, B., Ovary, Z., and Poulik, M. D. Structural differences among antibodies of different specificity. *Proc. Nat. Acad. Sci. U.S.A.* 47:1751, 1961.
34. Kunkel, H. G., Mannik, M., and Williams, R. C. Indivivual antigenic specificity of isolated antibodies. *Science* 140:1218, 1963.
35. Heidelberger, M., and Pedersen, K. O. The molecular weight of antibodies. *J. Exp. Med.* 65:393, 1937.
36. Wallenius, G., Trautman, R., Kunkel, H. G., and Franklin, E. C. Ultracentrifugal studies of major non-lipid electrophoretic components of normal human serum. *J. Biol. Chem.* 225:253, 1957.

37. Müller-Eberhard, H. J., and Kunkel, H. G. Ultracentrifugal characteristics and carbohydrate content of macromolecular γ-globulin. *Clin. Chim. Acta* 4:252, 1959.
38. Kunkel, H. G. Macroglobulin and High Molecular Weight Antibodies. In Putnam, F. W. (Ed.), *Plasma Proteins.* New York: Academic Press, Inc., 1960.
39. Müller-Eberhard, H. J., Kunkel, H. G., and Franklin, E. C. Two types of γ-globulin differing in carbohydrate content. *Proc. Soc. Exp. Biol. Med.* 93:146, 1956.
40. Franklin, E. C., and Kunkel, H. G. Immunologic differences between the 19S and 7S components of normal human γ-globulin. *J. Immun.* 78:11, 1957.
41. Korngold, L., and Van Leeuwen, G. Macroglobulinemia: I. The antigenic relationship of pathological macroglobulins to normal γ-globulins. *J. Exp. Med.* 106:467, 1957.
42. Deutsch, H. F., and Morton, J. J. Dissociation of human serum macroglobulins. *Science* 125: 600, 1957.
43. Morton, J. J., and Deutsch, H. F. Human serum macroglobulins and dissociation units. II. Immunochemical properties. *J. Biol. Chem.* 231:1119, 1958.
44. Fudenberg, H. H., and Kunkel, H. G. Physical properties of the red cell agglutinins in acquired hemolytic anemia. *J. Exp. Med.* 106: 689, 1957.
45. Deutsch, H. F., and Chan, P. C. Human serum hemagglutinins. *Fed. Proc.* 17:210, 1958 (abst.).
46. Grubb, R., and Swahn, B. Destruction of some agglutinins but not of others by two sulfhydryl compounds. *Acta Path. Microbiol. Scand.* 43:305, 1958.
47. Kunkel, H. G., Rockey, J. H., and Tomasi, T. B. Methods of Separation and Properties of Antibodies of High Molecular Weight. In Heidelberger, M., and Plescia, O. J. (Eds.), *Immunochemical Approaches to Problems in Microbiology.* New Brunswick, N.J.: Rutgers University Press, 1961.
48. Jacot-Guillarmod, H., and Isliker, H. Scission et réassociation des iso-agglutinines: Préparation d'anticorps "mixtes." *Chimia* 15:405, 1961.
49. Edelman, G. M. Structural relations between normal and pathologic γ-globulins. *Ann. N.Y. Acad. Sci.* 101:246, 1962.
50. Slater, R. J., Ward, S. M., and Kunkel, H. G. Immunological relationships among the myeloma proteins. *J. Exp. Med.* 101:85, 1955.
51. Korngold, L., and Lipari, R. Multiple myeloma proteins: I. Immunological studies. *Cancer* 9:183, 1956.
52. Heremans, J. F. *Les globulines sériques du système gamma.* Brussels: Éditions Arscia, S. A., 1960.
53. Heremans, J. F., Heremans, M.-T., and Schultze, H. E. Isolation and description of a few properties of the β_{2A}-globulin of human serum. *Clin. Chim. Acta* 4:96, 1959.
54. Heremans, J. F., Vaerman, J.-P., and Vaerman, C. Studies on the immune globulins of human serum: II. A study of the distribution of anti-brucella and anti-diphtheria antibody activities among γ_{ss}-, γ_{1M}-, and γ_{1A}-globulin fractions. *J. Immun.* 91:11, 1963.
55. Laurell, A. H. Sera from patients with myeloma, macroglobulinemia and related conditions as studied by ultracentrifugation. *Acta Med. Scand.,* supp. 367, p. 69, 1961.
56. Kunkel, H. G. Unpublished observations, 1960.
57. Fahey, J. L. Heterogeneity of myeloma proteins. *J. Clin. Invest.* 42:111, 1963.
58. Zingale, S. B., Mattiolo, C. A., Bohner, H. D., and Bueno, M. P. Disc electrophoresis study of serum proteins from patients with multiple myeloma and macroglobulinemia. *Blood* 22: 152, 1963.
59. Putnam, F. W. Aberrations of protein metabolism in multiple myeloma: Interrelationships of abnormal serum globulins and Bence Jones proteins. *Physiol. Rev.* 37:512, 1957.
60. Webb, T., Rose, B., and Sehon, A. H. Biocolloids in normal human urine: II. Physicochemical and immunochemical characteristics. *Canad. J. Biochem. Physiol.* 36:1167, 1958.
61. Franklin, E. C. Physicochemical and immunologic studies of γ-globulin of normal human urine. *J. Clin. Invest.* 38:2159, 1959.
62. Stevenson, G. T. Detection in normal urine of protein resembling Bence Jones protein. *J. Clin. Invest.* 39:1192, 1960.
63. Berggård, I. Studies on the plasma proteins in normal human urine. *Clin. Chim. Acta* 6:413, 1961.
64. Berggård, I. On a γ-globulin of low molecular weight in normal human plasma and urine. *Ibid.,* p. 545.
65. Berggård, I., and Edelman, G. M. Normal counterparts to Bence Jones proteins: Free L polypeptide chains of human γ-globulin. *Proc. Nat. Acad. Sci. U.S.A.* 49:330, 1963.
66. Stevenson, G. T. Further studies of the gamma-related proteins of normal urine. *J. Clin. Invest.* 41:1190, 1962.
67. Gordon, D. A., Eisen, A. Z., and Vaughan, J. H. γ-Globulin Metabolism in Rheumatoid Arthritis. Presented at the Annual Meeting of the American Rheumatism Association, Atlantic City, June, 1963.
68. Steinberg, A. G. Progress in the study of genetically determined human γ-globulin types (the Gm and Inv groups). *Progr. Med. Genet.* 2:1, 1962.

68a. Kunkel, H. G., Allen, J. C., Grey, H. M., Mårtensson, L., and Grubb, R. A relationship between the H chain groups of 7S γ-globulin and the Gm system. *Nature* (London) 203: 413, 1964.

69. Steinberg, A. G., and Wilson, J. A. Hereditary globulin factors and immune tolerance in man. *Science* 140:303, 1963.
70. Allen, J. C., and Kunkel, H. G. Antibodies to genetic types of γ-globulin after multiple transfusions. *Science* 139:418, 1963.
71. Hess, M., and Bütler, R. Anti-Gm specificities in sera of rhesus monkeys immunized with human γ-globulin. *Vox Sang.* 7:93, 1962.
72. Harboe, M., Osterland, C. K., and Kunkel, H. G. Localization of two genetic factors to different areas of γ-globulin molecules. *Science* 136:979, 1962.
73. Harboe, M., Osterland, C. K., Mannik, M., and Kunkel, H. G. Genetic characters of human γ-globulins in myleoma proteins. *J. Exp. Med.* 116:719, 1962.
74. Franklin, E. C., Fudenberg, H., Meltzer, M., and Stanworth, D. R. The structural basis for genetic variations of normal human γ-globulins. *Proc. Nat. Acad. Sci. U.S.A.* 48:914, 1962.
75. Allen, J. C., Mannik, M., and Kunkel, H. G. Localization of genetic characters to the L and H chains of human γ-globulin. To be published.
76. Mannik, M., and Kunkel, H. G. Two major types of normal 7S γ-globulin. *J. Exp. Med.* 117:213, 1963.
77. Korngold, L., and Lipari, R. Multiple myeloma proteins: III. The antigenic relationships of Bence Jones proteins to normal γ-globulins and multiple myeloma serum proteins. *Cancer* 9:262, 1956.
78. Burtin, P., Hartmann, L., Fauvert, R., and Grabar, P. Études sur les protéines du myélome: I. Étude critique des techniques d'identification de la protéine de Bence Jones et de leur valeur diagnostique. *Rev. Franc. Etudes Clin. Biol.* 1:17, 1956.
79. Mannik, M., and Kunkel, H. G. Classification of myeloma proteins, Bence Jones proteins, and macroglobulins into two groups on the basis of common antigenic characters. *J. Exp. Med.* 116:859, 1962.
80. Fahey, J. L., and Solomon, A. Two types of γ-myeloma proteins, β_{2A}-myeloma proteins, γ_1-macroglobulins and Bence Jones proteins identified by two groups of common antigenic determinants. *J. Clin. Invest.* 42:811, 1963.
81. Migita, S., and Putnam, F. W. Antigenic relationships of Bence Jones proteins, myeloma globulins, and normal human γ-globulin. *J. Exp. Med.* 117:81, 1963.
82. Franklin, E. C. Two types of γ-globulin in sera from normals and patients with multiple myeloma. *Nature* (London) 195:393, 1962.
83. Fahey, J. L. Two types of 6.6S γ-globulins, β_{2A}-globulins and 18S γ_1-macroglobulins in normal serum and γ-microglobulins in normal urine. *J. Immun.* 91:438, 1963.
84. Hilschman, N. Personal communication, 1963.
85. Putnam, F. W., and Easley, C. W. Peptide maps of normal γ-globulin, myeloma globulins, and Bence Jones proteins. *Fed. Proc.* 22:657, 1963 (abst.).
86. Franklin, E. C., Meltzer, M., Guggenheim, F., and Lowenstein, J. An unusual micro-gammaglobulin in the serum and urine of a patient. *Fed. Proc.* 22:264, 1963 (abst.).
87. Osserman, E. F., and Takatsuki, K. Plasma cell myeloma: Gamma globulin synthesis and structure. *Medicine* 42:357, 1963.
88. Stein, S., Nachman, R. L., and Engle, R. L. Individual and subgroup antigenic specificity of Bence Jones protein. *Nature* (London) 200: 1180, 1963.
89. Grey, H. M., and Kunkel, H. G. H chain subgroups of myeloma proteins and normal 7S γ-globulin. *J. Exp. Med.* 120:253, 1964.

89a. Terry, W. D., and Fahey, J. L. Heterogeneity of H chains of human 7S γ-globulin. *Fed. Proc.* 23:454, 1964 (abst.).

90. Kabat, E. A. Review: Immunochemistry of the proteins. *J. Immun.* 47:513, 1943.
91. Talmage, D. W., Freter, G. G., and Taliaferro, W. H. Two antibodies of related specificity but different hemolytic efficiency separated by centrifugation. *J. Infect. Dis.* 98:300, 1956.
92. Kunkel, H. G., Fudenberg, H., and Ovary, Z. High molecular weight antibodies. *Ann. N.Y. Acad. Sci.* 86:966, 1960.
93. Benedict, A. A., Brown, R. J., and Ayengar, R. Physical properties of antibodies to bovine serum albumin as demonstrated by hemagglutination. *J. Exp. Med.* 115:195, 1962.
94. Bauer, D. C., and Stavitsky, A. B. On the different molecular forms of antibody synthesized by rabbits during the early response to a single injection of protein and cellular antigens. *Proc. Nat. Acad. Sci. U.S.A.* 47:1667, 1961.
95. Uhr, J. W., Finkelstein, M. S., and Baumann, J. B. Antibody formation: III. The primary and secondary antibody response to bacteriophage ØX 174 in guinea pigs. *J. Exp. Med.* 115:655, 1962.
96. LoSpalluto, J. Personal communication, 1963.
97. Uhr, J. W., and Finkelstein, M. S. Antibody formation: IV. Formation of rapidly and slowly sedimenting antibodies and immunological memory to bacteriophage ØX 174. *J. Exp. Med.* 117:457, 1963.
98. Mellors, R. C., and Korngold, L. The cellular origin of human immunoglobulins (γ_2, γ_{1M}, γ_{1A}). *J. Exp. Med.* 118:387, 1963.
99. Uhr, J. W., Dancis, J., Franklin, E. C., Finkel-

stein, M. S. and Lewis, E. W. The antibody response to bacteriophage ØX 174 in newborn premature infants. *J. Clin. Invest.* 41:1406, 1962.

100. Smith, R. T. Immunity in infancy. *Pediat. Clin. N. Amer.* 7:269, 1960.

101. LoSpalluto, J., Miller, W., Jr., Dorward, B., and Fink, C. W. The formation of macroglobulin antibodies: I. Studies on adult humans. *J. Clin. Invest.* 41:1415, 1962.

102. Fudenberg, H., Kunkel, H. G., and Franklin, E. C. High Molecular Weight Antibodies. Presented at 7th International Congress of Blood Transfusion, Rome, 1958.

103. Rawson, A. J., and Abelson, N. M. Studies of blood group antibodies: III. Observations on the physicochemical properties of isohemagglutinins and isohemolysins. *J. Immun.* 85:636, 1960.

104. Rockey, J. H., and Kunkel, H. G. Unusual sedimentation and sulfhydryl sensitivity of certain isohemagglutinins and skin-sensitizing antibody. *Proc. Soc. Exp. Biol. Med.* 110:101, 1962.

105. Franklin, E. C., Holman, H., Müller-Eberhard, H. J., and Kunkel, H. G. An unusual protein component of high molecular weight in the serum of certain patients with rheumatoid arthritis. *J. Exp. Med.* 105:425, 1957.

106. Williams, R. C., and Kunkel, H. G. Rheumatoid factor, complement, and conglutinin aberrations in patients with subacute bacterial endocarditis. *J. Clin. Invest.* 41:66, 1962.

107. Kritzman, J., Kunkel, H. G., McCarthy, J., and Mellors, R. C. Studies of a Waldenström-type macroglobulin with rheumatoid factor properties. *J. Lab. Clin. Med.* 57:905, 1961.

108. Mehrotra, T. N. Individual specific nature of the cold autoantibodies of acquired hemolytic anemia. *Nature* (London) 185:323, 1960.

109. Jenkins, W. J., Marsh, W. L., Noades, J., Tippett, P., Sanger, R., and Race, R. R. The I antigen and antibody. *Vox Sang.* 5:97, 1960.

110. LoSpalluto, J., Dorward, B., Miller, W., and Ziff, M. Cryoglobulinemia based on interaction between a γ-macroglobulin and 7S γ-globulin. *Amer. J. Med.* 32:142, 1962.

111. Ozer, F. L., and Chaplin, H., Jr. Agglutination of stored erythrocytes by a human serum. Characterization of the serum factor and erythrocyte changes. *J. Clin. Invest.* 42:1735, 1963.

112. Kunkel, H. G., and Rockey, J. H. Unpublished observations, 1962.

113. Kunkel, H. G., and Rockey, J. H. β_{2A} and other immunoglobulins in isolated anti-A antibodies. *Proc. Soc. Exp. Biol. Med.* 113:278, 1963.

114. Tomasi, T. B. Personal communication, 1963.

115. Allen, J. C., and Kunkel, H. G. To be published.

116. Leddy, J. P., Freeman, G. L., Luz, A., and Todd, R. Inactivation of the skin-sensitizing antibodies of human allergy. *Proc. Soc. Exp. Biol. Med.* 111:7, 1962.

117. Schultze, H. E. The synthesis of antibodies and proteins. *Clin. Chim. Acta* 4:610, 1959.

118. Barnett, E. V., Condemi, J. J., Leddy, J. P., and Vaughan, J. H. γ_2, γ_{1A}, and γ_{1M} Antinuclear Factors in Human Sera. Ref. 67.

119. Tan, E. M., and Kunkel, H. G. Unpublished observations, 1962.

120. Tomasi, T. B. Personal communication, 1962.

121. Goodman, H., Robbins, J., and Exum, D. Radioimmunoelectrophoretic characterization of antibody globulins in human and rabbit sera. *Arthritis Rheum.* 6:273, 1963.

122. Yagi, Y., Maier, P., and Pressman, D. Two different anti-insulin antibodies in guinea pig antisera. *J. Immun.* 89:442, 1962.

123. Yagi, Y., Maier, P., Pressman, D., Arbesman, C. E., and Reisman, R. E. The presence of the ragweed-binding antibodies in the β_{2A}, β_{2M} and γ-globulins of sensitive individuals. *J. Immun.* 91:83, 1963.

124. Heremans, J. F., and Vaerman, J. P. β_{2A}-globulin as a possible carrier of allergic reagenic activity. *Nature* (London) 193:1091, 1962.

125. Fireman, P., Vannier, W. E., and Goodman, H. C. The association of skin-sensitizing antibody with the β_{2A}-globulins in the sera from ragweed sensitive patients. *J. Exp. Med.* 117:603, 1963.

126. Rockey, J. H., and Loveless, M. To be published.

127. Clausen, J., Heremans, J., Heremans, M. T., and Rask-Nielsen, R. Immunoelectrophoretic studies of serums from mice carrying two transplantable plasma-cell leukemias. *J. Nat. Cancer Inst.* 22:57, 1959.

128. Killander, J. Fractionation of Antibodies of 19S, 7S and "Intermediate" Types by Gel Filtration and Ion Exchange Chromatography or Preparative Electrophoresis. Presented at the 11th Colloquium on Protides of the Biological Fluids, Bruges, Belgium, 1963.

129. Smith, R. T. Personal communication, 1963.

130. Mannik, M., and Kunkel, H. G. Localization of antibodies in group I and group II γ-globulins. *J. Exp. Med.* 118:817, 1963.

131. Fahey, J. L., and Goodman, H. Antibody activity in six classes of human immunoglobulins. *Science* 143:588, 1964.

132. Franklin, E. C., and Kunkel, H. G. Comparative levels of high molecular weight (19S)

γ-globulin in maternal and umbilical cord sera. *J. Lab. Clin. Med.* 52:724, 1958.

133. Kunkel, H. G. Estimation of alterations of serum γ-globulin by a turbidimetric technique. *Proc. Soc. Exp. Biol. Med.* 66:217, 1947.
134. Kunkel, H. G., Ahrens, E. H., Jr., and Eisenmenger, W. J. Application of turbidimetric methods for estimation of γ-globulin and total lipid to the study of patients with liver disease. *Gastroenterology* 11:499, 1948.
135. Fudenberg, H., German, J. L., and Kunkel, H. G. The occurrence of rheumatoid factor and other abnormalities in families of patients with aggammaglobulinemia. *Arthritis Rheum.* 5:565, 1962.
136. Kabat, E. A., and Mayer, M. M. *Experimental Immunochemistry,* (2nd ed.). Springfield, Ill.: Charles C Thomas, Publisher, 1961.
137. Goodman, M., Ramsey, D. S., Simpson, W. L., Remp, D. G., Basinski, D. H., and Brennan, M. J. The use of chicken antiserum for the rapid determination of plasma protein components: I. The assay of human serum albumin and γ-globulin. *J. Lab. Clin. Med.* 49:151, 1957.
138. Schultze, H. E., and Schwick, G. Quantitative immunologische Bestimmung von Plasmaproteinen. *Clin. Chim. Acta* 4:15, 1959.
139. Zak, S. J., and Good, R. A. Immunochemical studies of human serum γ-globulins. *J. Clin. Invest.,* 38:579, 1959.
140. Hitzig, W. H., Scheidegger, J. J., Bütler, R., Gugler, E., and Hässig, A. Zur quantitativen Bestimmung der Immunoglobuline. *Helv. Med. Acta* 26:142, 1959.
141. West, C. D., Hinrichs, V., and Hinkle, N. H. Quantitative determination of the serum globulins β_{2A} and β_{2M} by immunoelectrophoretic analysis. *J. Lab. Clin. Med.* 58:137, 1961.
142. West, C. D., Hong, R., and Holland, N. H. Immunoglobulin levels from the newborn period to adulthood and in immunoglobulin deficiency states. *J. Clin. Invest.* 41:2054, 1962.
143. Tomasi, T. B. Personal communication, 1963.
144. Fahey, J. L., and McLaughlin, C. Preparation of antisera specific for 6.6S γ-globulin, β_{2A}-globulin, γ_1-macroglobulins, and for type I and II common γ-globulin determinants. *J. Immun.* 91:484, 1963.
145. Fahey, J. L., and Lawrence, M. E. Quantitative determination of 6.6S γ-globulins, β_{2A}-globulins and γ_1-macroglobulins in human serum. *Ibid.,* p. 597.
146. Gitlin, D., Landing, B. H., and Whipple, A. The localization of homologous plasma proteins in the tissue of young human beings as demonstrated with fluorescent antibodies. *J. Exp. Med.* 97:163, 1953.
147. Gitlin, D., and Janeway, C. A. Dynamic equilibrium between circulating and extravascular plasma proteins. *Science* 118:301, 1953.
148. Gitlin, D., and Janeway, C. A. Studies on plasma proteins in interstitial fluid of muscle. *Science* 120:461, 1954.
149. Gitlin, D., Janeway, C. A., and Farr, L. E. Studies on metabolism of plasma proteins in nephrotic syndrome: I. Albumin, γ-globulin and iron-binding globulin. *J. Clin. Invest.* 35:44, 1956.
150. Solomon, A., Waldmann, T. A., and Fahey, J. L. Metabolism of normal 6.6S γ-globulin in normal subjects and in patients with macroglobulinemia and multiple myeloma. *J. Lab. Clin. Med.* 62:1, 1963.
151. London, I. M. Studies on Rates of Formation of Serum Proteins in Man. In Youmans, J. B. (Ed.), *Plasma Proteins.* Springfield, Ill.: Charles C Thomas, Publisher, 1950. Vol. 2.
152. Volwiler, W., Goldsworthy, P. D., MacMartin, M. P., Wood, P. A., Mackay, J. R., and Fremont-Smith, K. Biosynthetic determination with radioactive sulfur of turnover rates of various plasma proteins in normal and cirrhotic man. *J. Clin. Invest.* 34:1126, 1955.
153. Dixon, F. J., Talmage, D. W., Maurer, P. H., and Deichmiller, M. Half life of homologous γ-globulin (antibody) in several species. *J. Exp. Med.* 96:313, 1952.
154. Barth, W. F., Wochner, R. D., Waldmann, T. A., and Fahey, J. L. Metabolism of human gamma globulins. *J. Clin. Invest.* 43: 1036, 1964.
155. Valquist, B. Transfer of antibodies from mother to offspring. *Advances Pediat.* 10:305, 1958.
156. Moore, D. H., Martin du Pan, R., and Buxton, C. C. An electrophoretic study of maternal, fetal and infant sera. *Amer. J. Obstet. Gynec.* 57:312, 1949.
157. Orlandini, T. O., Sass-Kortsak, A., and Ebbs, J. H. Serum γ-globulin levels in normal infants. *Pediatrics* 16:575, 1955.
158. Oberman, J. W., Gregory, K. O., Burks, F. G., Ross, S., and Rice, E. C. Electrophoretic analysis of serum proteins in infants and children: I. Normal values from birth to adolescence. *New Eng. J. Med.* 255:743, 1956.
159. Hitzig, W. H. Das Bluteiweissbild beim gesunden Säugling: Spezifische Proteinbestimmungen mit besonderer Beruecksichtigung immunochemischer Methoden. *Helv. Paediat. Acta* 16:46, 1961.
160. Mannik, M., and Kunkel, H. G. Unpublished observations, 1962.

161. Kochwa, S., Rosenfield, R. E., Tallal, L., and Wasserman, C. R. Isoagglutinins associated with AB0 erythroblastosis. *J. Clin. Invest.* 40:874, 1961.
162. Fink, C. W., Miller, W. E., Jr., Dorward, B., and LoSpalluto, J. The formation of macroglobulin antibodies: II. Studies on neonatal infants and older children. *J. Clin. Invest.* 41:1422, 1962.
163. Gitlin, D., Rosen, F. S., and Michael, J. G. Transient 19S γ_1-globulin deficiency in the newborn infant, and its significance. *Pediatrics* 31:197, 1963.
164. Hartley, P. The effect of peptic digestion on the properties of diphtheria antitoxin. *Proc. Roy. Soc.* [Biol.] 138:499, 1951.
165. Brambell, F. W. R., Hemmings, W. A., Oakley, C. L., and Porter, R. R. The relative transmission of the fractions of papain hydrolysed homologous γ-globulin from the uterine cavity to the foetal circulation in the rabbit. *Proc. Roy. Soc.* [Biol.] 151:478, 1960.
165a. Gitlin, D., Kumate, J., Urrusti, J., and Morales, C. The selectivity of the human placenta in the transfer of plasma proteins from mother to fetus. *J. Clin. Invest.* 43: 1938, 1964.
166. Beecham, C. T., Moltham, L., Boutwell, J., and Rohrbeck, C. W. Amniotic fluid studies in Rh-sensitized women. *Amer. J. Obstet. Gynec.* 83:1053, 1962.
167. Auerswald, W., Doleschel, W., Reinhardt, F., and Schüller, E. Zur Frage der Permeation von Plasmaproteinen in den Liquor amnii. *Wien. Klin. Wschr.* 75:129, 1963.
168. Bridges, R. A., Condie, R. M., Zak, S. J., and Good, R. A. The morphological basis of antibody formation development during the neonatal period. *J. Lab. Clin. Med.* 53:331, 1959.
169. Smith, R. T. Response to active immunization of human infants during neonatal period. In Wolstenholme, G. E. W., and O'Connor, M. (Eds.), *Ciba Foundation Symposium on Cellular Aspects of Immunity*. Boston: Little, Brown, 1960.
170. Silverstein, A. M. Congenital syphilis and timing of immunogenesis in human foetus. *Nature* (London) 194:196, 1962.
171. Thorbecke, G. J., Gordon, H. A., Wostman, B., Wagner, M., and Reyniers, J. A. Lymphoid tissue and serum γ-globulin in young germfree chickens. *J. Infect. Dis.* 101:237, 1957.
172. Gustafsson, B. E., and Laurell, C.-B. Gamma globulins in germfree rats. *J. Exp. Med.* 108: 251, 1958.
173. Tomasi, T. B., and Zigelbaum, S. The selective occurrence of γ_{1A}-globulins in certain body fluids. *J. Clin. Invest.* 42:1552, 1963.
174. Cohen, N., Horowitz, M. J., and Hollander, F. Serum albumin and γ-globulin in normal human gastric juice. *Proc. Soc. Exp. Biol. Med.* 109:463, 1962.
175. Holman, H., Nickel, W. F., Jr., and Sleisenger, M. H. Hypoproteinemia antedating intestinal lesions and possibly due to excessive serum protein loss into the intestine. *Amer. J. Med.* 27:963, 1959.
176. Hanson, L. A. The serological relationship between human milk and blood plasma. *Int. Arch. Allerg.* 17:45, 1960.
177. Hanson, L. A. Comparative immunological studies of the immune globulins of human milk and of blood serum. *Int. Arch. Allerg.* 18:241, 1961.
178. Hanson, L. A., and Berggård, I. An immunological comparison of immunoglobulins from human blood serum, urine and milk using diffusion-in-gel methods. *Clin. Chim. Acta* 7:828, 1962.
179. Coons, A. H., Leduc, E. H., and Connolly, J. M. Studies on antibody production: I. Method for histochemical demonstration of specific antibody and its application to study of hyperimmune rabbit. *J. Exp. Med.* 102:49, 1955.
180. Craig, J. M., Gitlin, D., and Jewett, T. C. Response of lymph node of normal and congenitally agammaglobulinemic children to antigenic stimulation. *Amer. J. Dis. Child.* 88:626, 1954.
181. Fagraeus, A. Plasma cellular reaction and its relation to formation of antibodies in vitro. *J. Immun.* 58:1, 1948.
182. Reiss, E., Mertens, E., and Ehrich, W. E. Agglutination of bacteria by lymphoid cells in vitro. *Proc. Soc. Exp. Biol. Med.* 74:732, 1950.
182a. Pernis, B., and Chiappino, G. Identification in human lymphoid tissues of cells that produce group 1 or group 2 gamma-globulins. *Immunology* 7:500, 1964.
182b. Bernier, G. M., and Cebra, J. J. Polypeptide chains of human gamma-globulin: cellular localization by fluorescent antibody. *Science* 144: 1590, 1964.
183. Dutcher, T. F., and Fahey, J. L. Histopathology of macroglobulinemia of Waldenström, *J. Nat. Cancer Inst.* 22:237, 1959.
184. Solomon, A., Fahey, J. L., and Malmgren, R. A. Immunohistologic localization of γ_1-macroglobulins, β_{2A} myeloma proteins, 6.6S γ-myeloma proteins, and Bence Jones proteins. *Blood* 21:403, 1963.
185. Mellors, R. C., Heimer, R., Corcoss, J., and Korngold, L. Cellular origin of rheumatoid factor. *J. Exp. Med.* 110:875, 1959.
186. Mellors, R. C., Nowaslawski, A., Korngold, L., and Sengson, B. L. Rheumatoid factor

and the pathogenesis of rheumatoid arthritis. *J. Exp. Med.* 113:475, 1961.

187. Cruchaud, A., Rosen, F. S., Craig, J. M., Janeway, C. A., and Gitlin, D. The site of synthesis of the 19S γ-globulins in dysgammaglobulinemia. *J. Exp. Med.* 115:1141, 1962.
188. Asofsky, R., and Thorbecke, G. J. Sites of formation of immune globulins and of a component of C′3: II. Production of immunoelectrophoretically identified serum proteins by human and monkey tissue in vitro. *J. Exp. Med.* 114:471, 1961.
189. Carbonara, A. O., Rodhain, J. A., and Heremans, J. F. Localization of γ_{1A}-globulin (β_{2A}-globulin) in tissue cells. *Nature* (London) 198:999, 1963.

20. *Delayed Hypersensitivity in Man**

JONATHAN W. UHR

THE GENERAL PRINCIPLES UNDERlying delayed hypersensitivity reactions are based on a rapidly accumulating body of knowledge derived almost entirely from animal experimentation. These topics are covered in Chapter 11. The purpose here is to review delayed hypersensitivity in man. The paucity of experimental data, however, and the need to place delayed hypersensitivity in human beings in perspective necessitate reference to and occasional discussion of data obtained from studies of animals. We shall review first the characteristics of the hypersensitive state and then the transfer of hypersensitivity with leukocyte extracts, an accomplishment at present unique to man. Several disease states in man that can affect the delayed hypersensitive state as well as homotransplantation and autoimmunity, frequently considered to be expressions of delayed hypersensitivity, are discussed elsewhere in this volume.

CHARACTERISTICS OF THE DELAYED HYPERSENSITIVE STATE

SKIN REACTIVITY

After intradermal injection of specific antigen into sensitized individuals, no macroscopic inflammation is usually visible for 5 to 24 hours [1], although pain may be present at the injection site. After this interval, induration and erythema appear and reach peak intensity at 16 to 72 hours before gradually declining. If the reaction is severe, peak intensity occurs late and the local reaction may be accompanied by regional lymphadenopathy and fever. In such instances, necrosis and scarification may occur at the injection site. Erythema is variable, but *firm induration,* indicative of cellular infiltration, is the hallmark of a positive reaction. The simultaneous presence of large amounts of precipitating antibody may cause the appearance of early inflammation and swelling (Arthus reaction) which complicate interpretation of the delayed reaction.

Histologically, there are initially dilatation of capillaries and exudation of fluid and cells with a predominance of polymorphonuclear leukocytes [1–3]. After several hours the proportion of mononuclear cells increases, and by twenty-four hours the inflammatory response is almost exclusively mononuclear. The cells are distributed throughout the dermis and subcutaneous tissue, frequently concentrated around small venules, and can also be seen surrounding underlying muscle fibers. Hemorrhage and vascular lesions are not seen in an uncomplicated delayed reaction. If necrosis occurs, epithelioid and giant cells may be found several days later [4]. In contact hypersensitivity reactions (another form of delayed hypersensitivity), the cellular exudate is similar to that described above [5]. In addition, the epidermis participates in the inflammatory process and may show spongiosis (edema), microvesicles, and an increase in mitosis.

That sensitivity comes from the circulation and not from the local skin site is shown by transfer studies, to be discussed later, and by the cross-grafting experiment of Haxthausen [6]. Using identical twins, one of whom had been previously sensitized to dinitrochlorobenzene, he showed that skin from the nonsensitive donor was soon able to display sensitivity in the sensitive host, in contrast to skin from the sensitive donor transplanted into the nonsensitive host.

The mechanism by which tissue damage occurs in delayed hypersensitivity reactions is not known; damage does not appear to be due to the release of histamine [7] or to the type of vascular damage responsible in part for the Shwartzman [8] and Arthus reactions [9]. Studies involving the passive transfer of delayed hypersensitivity in guinea pigs by

* This work was supported in part by U.S. Public Health Service Grant No. AI-01821-07, by the Commission on Immunization of the Armed Forces Epidemiological Board, and by the Office of the Surgeon General, Department of the Army, Washington, D.C.

means of lymphocytes labeled with tritiated thymidine [10–13] suggest that the vast majority of cells that participate in delayed hypersensitivity reactions are *not* specifically sensitized cells. It appears, therefore, that interaction between antigen and a small number of specifically sensitized cells *in vivo* [14] can result in the eventual participation of large numbers of previously unsensitized lymphoid cells at the reaction site. This may be analogous to the inhibiting effect of specific antigen on migration of cells obtained from the peritoneal exudate of guinea pigs with delayed hypersensitivity [15]. Specific antigen can affect mixtures of cells from normal and sensitized animals in which the latter population constitutes less than 2.5 percent of the total cells.

SYSTEMIC REACTIVITY

When sufficient amounts of tuberculoprotein are absorbed into the circulation of a tuberculin-hypersensitive individual, systemic reactions follow [16]. Several hours after the injection, fever begins, often accompanied by malaise and, in more severe reactions, by headache, anorexia, backache, and joint pains; in extreme cases, the reaction may progress to prostration and death. In addition, there may be focal reactions in the pre-existing tuberculous lesions which may result in renewal of their activity and extension. In a moderate reaction, however, fever and symptoms disappear in 18 to 36 hours. Typical systemic reactions have occurred in tuberculin-sensitive laboratory workers who have inhaled vapors of heated tuberculin. Fever and joint pains have also been reported in individuals convalescing from brucellosis after intravenous injection of as little as 10 μg. of *Brucella* extract [17].

There is little doubt that the febrile response with its associated symptoms is a specific systemic reaction of the delayed hypersensitive type, because analogous reactions can be induced by specific challenge of guinea pigs with intense delayed hypersensitivity to purified proteins but without circulating antibody [18]. In such animals, however, shock and death do not follow intravenous injection of large amounts of specific protein. These findings suggest that complicating factors may be responsible for tuberculin shock. It is known, for example, that old tuberculin (OT) may be contaminated by endotoxin [19] and that tuberculous guinea pigs are hypersusceptible to the toxic effect of endotoxin [20, 21]. These findings have led Stetson [19] to postulate that endotoxin may be responsible for the vascular collapse observed in tuberculin shock. An additional consideration is the role played by specific serum antibodies, frequently not usually detectable by precipitation present in tuberculin-sensitized animals and tests [22].

The fever observed in specifically challenged tuberculin-sensitive rabbits, like many other experimental fevers, was found to be associated with a circulating endogenous pyrogen (EP) [23]. Johanovsky [24] concludes that the source of EP in hypersensitivity fever is the hypersensitive cell itself, since lymphocytes obtained from hypersensitive guinea pigs release EP after exposure to specific antigen *in vitro*. Acceptance of this conclusion should await confirmation of this work, however, since it is the only report of a cell other than the polymorphonuclear leukocyte [25] producing EP.

INDUCTION OF HYPERSENSITIVITY

The classic means of acquiring delayed hypersensitivity is by infection. Thus delayed skin reactions to microbial antigens have clinical significance as indications of previous contact with the corresponding organism, frequently through asymptomatic infection. Hypersensitivity acquired by this means appears to be long lasting, frequently for decades, possibly abetted by persistence of microorganisms or their products (tuberculosis) or because of recurrent contact with the particular infective agent (streptococci, *Trychophyton*, etc.).

In attempting to understand the role played by infection, one does well to remember that the route of entrance of antigen into the host is an important factor in induction of hypersensitivity. Experiments in animals have shown that the intradermal and subcutaneous routes, in contrast to other parenteral routes, favor the development of this type of hypersensitivity [26–30]. The importance of the intradermal route in inducing delayed hypersensitivity in man is underlined by the work of Mote and Jones [31]. They showed that repeated small intradermal injections of rabbit serum proteins eventually induced in adult "normal" males a delayed type skin reactivity to the antigen(s) in question. There was considerable individual variation in the development of delayed hypersensitivity to a given antigen, but eventually *all individuals could be rendered delayed type hypersensitive.* Such sensitivity could last two years, but if skin testing was continued, it was later accompanied or replaced by immediate wheal and erythema reactivity. In these instances, after cessation of antigenic challenge, there was reversion back to delayed hypersensitivity reactivity. The disappearance of delayed type skin reactivity during the period of wheal and erythema reactivity may reflect not the disappearance of hypersensitivity but simply interference with its expression by the binding of antigen by skin-sensitizing antibody.

Another method of sensitization in man is the injection of protein antigens in the form of antigen-antibody precipitates [30] which can sensitize without stimulating detectable antibody formation. The facility of this method may depend on slow release of antigen from the specific precipitates [32].

Another factor which influences induction of delayed hypersensitivity is the use of adjuvants such as oil. A high proportion of nonallergic patients given injections of ragweed pollen extract emulsified in Arlacel A-Drakeol developed delayed skin reactivity to this antigen [33, 34], confirmed by histological examination of the test site and by transfer of the hypersensitivity with peripheral leukocytes to nonsensitive recipients.

The common denominator of these factors is probably the stimulation of a particular type of immunologically competent cell, formed in the thymus gland [35, 36] or other primary lymphoid organs [37] and later localized in lymph nodes and perhaps at the site of adjuvant-induced inflammation. Competition for such a cell type may explain the interference phenomenon in allergic contact dermatitis in man [38]. The simultaneous application of two contact allergens of unequal sensitizing capacity resulted in a striking inhibition of the expected sensitization to the weaker allergen. This phenomenon appears to be similar to the "competition of antigens" effect on antibody formation [39].

The similarity between sensitization to bland proteins such as was described by Mote and Jones and that to bacterial products following an infection has not been universally accepted [40, 41], however, for several reasons. (1) In animals sensitized to purified proteins and without detectable serum antibody, specific challenge, intradermal or systemic, does not lead to skin necrosis or shock, respectively [18, 30]. (2) Raffel [40] has reported a diminished intensity and duration of this hypersensitivity compared to tuberculin hypersensitivity. (3) In human beings, multiple skin testing with tuberculin [42, 43], coccidiodin [44, 45], and other skin-testing materials does not usually induce the delayed hypersensitivity state unless there is pre-existing low-grade sensitization. In such instances, reactions originally negative to dilute but not concentrated solutions of the specific antigen develop to the dilute antigen solution following multiple skin tests.

The complexities of the tuberculin hypersensitivity system have already been mentioned as possible causes of cytotoxicity phenomena in this system. As to differences in degree of sensitization, the remarkable capacity of mycobacteria to enhance the development of delayed hypersensitivity can be utilized for antigens other than tuberculoprotein; hence it is a *nonspecific* attribute of the tubercle bacillus. Thus intense and long-lasting delayed hypersensitivity to bland proteins is achieved when complete adjuvant is used in the sensitizing injection [30, 46–48]. In the consideration of the significance of differences based on macroscopic appearance of delayed reactions to bland proteins and to bacterial products, the unsatisfactory nature of this criterion for assessing immunological reactivity should be emphasized. Gell and Benacerraf [49] have observed numerous variations within the purified antigen group itself in the quality of the delayed hypersensitivity skin reaction: salmine—small, intensely indurated, occasionally necrotic reactions; γ-globulins—larger, well-defined and indurated reactions; and ovalbumin—widespread and only slightly erythematous and indurated reactions. They suggest that the capacity of each antigen to remain at the injection site may be an important factor in these differences. Finally, the failure of human beings to sensitize routinely after skin testing may be quantitative in nature, relating to the immunogenicity of the antigen (tuberculin, for example, is denatured), the dose, or the immunization schedule. Such operational differences in the development of hypersensitivity are not unexpected and might also be present in a group of human beings following various infections; this has not been studied systematically. It therefore appears to be unnecessary at present to subdivide delayed type hypersensitivity.

ONTOGENY

Studies on the ontogeny of human delayed type hypersensitivity are few. Straus [50] has shown that some human infants can be sensitized to poison ivy within 4 weeks after birth. Uhr *et al.* [51] induced contact hypersensitivity to 2,4-dinitrofluorobenzene (DNFB) in 3 or 4 weeks in 3 of 10 premature infants and in 2 of 5 full-term infants sensitized percutaneously during the first week of life. All of 5 older children were successfully sensitized by the same regimen. One of the premature infants successfully sensitized in 3 weeks weighed only 1,080 gm. at birth. These results show striking similarities to studies of antibody formation to diphtheria toxoid in full-term and premature newborn infants [52–54]. In both studies, the immune response was inconsistently obtained in the newborns, but no difference was observed between the premature and the full-term infants. In contrast, in a similar type of study using a highly antigenic bacteriophage, ØX174, *all* newborns formed antibody within 2 weeks, usually detectable by precipitation [55]. By analogy with these studies of antibody formation, it is probable that all newborn infants can develop delayed hypersensitivity if stimulated sufficiently with the proper antigen, although their capacity to be sensitized or to express hypersensitivity to less antigenic materials is quantitatively deficient as compared to adults. This deficiency may reside at the level of expression of skin inflammation in general [56] or, alternatively, in the development of sensitization. In the latter event, it is possible that the low responsiveness of the newborn immune system may reflect primarily a lack of stimulation of the lymphoreticular system. This possibility is supported by studies of the sheep embryo, which has undeveloped lymphoid tissue (except for the thymus) [57] and is essentially agammaglobulinemic throughout the 150 days of gestation [58]. After stimulation with certain antigens, however, there is rapid maturation of lymphoid tissue and the formation of large amounts of γ-globulin, of which only a small fraction can be demonstrated to be antibody [59, 60].

Another aspect of newborn immunology that has recently received attention is the capacity of newborn infants to be sensitized by transfer of leukocytes from donors sensitive to one or more of the commonly encountered microbial antigens. Warwick *et al.* [61] demonstrated that viable leukocytes from highly sensitized donors failed to transfer delayed skin reactivity to newborn infants, although a similar aliquot transferred intense delayed type skin reactivity to adult recipients. Even exchange transfusion of 500 to 600 ml. of whole blood failed to transfer sensitivity despite the use of donors who showed a high degree of delayed allergy. Either newborns are unable to accept or actively utilize transfer factor, or their quantitative deficiency in expressing delayed hypersensitivity reactions is strikingly exposed by the technique of passive transfer.

DESENSITIZATION

Studies of desensitization of delayed hypersensitivity in man have been concerned primarily with tuberculin hypersensitivity. Older studies documented the loss of skin and systemic reactivity after repeated injections of OT [62, 63], but in view of the severe systemic reactions and general condition of the subjects it was unclear whether or not the desensitization was specific. Evidence that specific desensitization can be accomplished comes from experiments in doubly sensitized animals [64] and in human beings. The latter experiments, of Oliveira-Lima [65], were performed in normal adult male subjects with tuberculin and streptococcal skin reactivity two to three months after institution of a desensitizing regimen of OT. Tuberculin but not streptococcal skin reactivity had disappeared. At this time, transfer of leukocytes from the desensitized donors to normal recipients resulted in transfer of streptococcal hypersensitivity only, demonstrating that specific desensitization had occurred.

It is not known why tuberculin desensitization requires administration of extremely large doses of tuberculin for long periods, sometimes months. In animals with delayed type hypersensitivity to highly purified proteins, a single injection of a relatively small amount of the specific protein (1 mg.) may suffice for complete desensitization [64]. It is possible that the difficulty in desensitizing to tuberculin reflects the antigenic complexity of the tubercle bacillus, or the intensity of sensitization may be an important factor.

The difficulty in desensitization to contact

dermatitis such as *Rhus* dermatitis is well illustrated by the studies of Kligman [66], who showed that repeated intramuscular administrations of the hapten (a total of 2 gm. of *Rhus* allergen oleoresin injected during a five to nine month period) were necessary to decrease significantly the skin reactivity to the *Rhus* antigen. These results are understandable in the light of the recent accumulation of evidence that the specificity of delayed hypersensitivity reactions involves broader areas of the antigen molecule than that required for interaction with serum antibody [67–69]. This conclusion results from experiments showing that the specificity of delayed hypersensitivity reactions in guinea pigs to hapten-protein conjugates involves, to a considerable degree, the protein carrier. For example, in guinea pigs intensely sensitized with picrylated guinea pig albumin, picrylated bovine γ-globulin, in contrast to the homologous antigen, is relatively ineffective in eliciting delayed skin reactions; similar results have been obtained in desensitization studies with hapten-protein conjugates [70, 71]. Desensitization to contact hypersensitivity, therefore, requires sensitizing conjugates made from the carrier proteins to which the hapten allergen is conjugated *in vivo;* unfortunately, these proteins have not been identified.

"Nonspecific" desensitization can also occur in man, as exemplified by temporary loss of tuberculin skin reactivity during certain acute infections such as measles [72] and influenza [73]. This phenomenon may be similar to the one observed in doubly sensitized guinea pigs, in which injection of a large dose of one antigen causes a transitory loss of skin reactivity to the second, unrelated antigen [64]. The hypersensitivity response to the measles virus (which may be responsible for the rash, as von Pirquet first suggested [72]), presumably depletes temporarily a factor(s) necessary for the expression of delayed hypersensitivity skin reactions. It would be helpful to know whether or not the leukocytes of such "nonspecifically" desensitized individuals can still transfer delayed hypersensitivity to tuberculin.

TOLERANCE

Immunological tolerance with respect to contact hypersensitivity has been induced in adult guinea pigs by feeding them hapten in such a way as to avoid contact with skin or buccal mucosa [74]; a similar long-lasting tolerance to protein antigens has been induced by exposing fetal guinea pigs to antigen by way of maternal administration [75].

In human beings, Rollof *et al.* [76] compared tuberculin hypersensitivity responses to BCG vaccination at birth in 50 infants of healthy mothers with those in 98 infants of tuberculous mothers. At 3 months, 86 percent of the control infants were tuberculin-positive, 60 percent of the infants of mothers with inactive tuberculosis, and 28 percent of the infants of mothers with active tuberculosis. The last group were separated from their mothers after birth until protected by BCG vaccination. Revaccination of the unsuccessfully vaccinated infants resulted in 100 percent sensitization of the controls but only 70 percent sensitization of infants of mothers with active tuberculosis. Antibody titrations of infants from mothers with tuberculosis, active or inactive, did not contain detectable anti-tubercle antibody by the Middlebrook-Dubos test. Similar results were obtained by Thurell [77].

These results are consistent with the concept that partial tolerance to tuberculoprotein has resulted from prenatal exposure to antigens presented to the fetus via the maternal circulation. The possibility is not excluded, however, that maternal antibody, transplacentally transmitted but undetected by the assay method used, has inhibited development of tuberculin hypersensitivity.

RELATION TO IMMUNITY

Despite a half-century of study and controversy, the role of delayed hypersensitivity in immunity remains unclear. The extent of this hypothetical role is limited to infections in which the microbes exist intracellularly. Particular attention has been focused on tuberculosis, brucellosis, salmonellosis, systemic mycosis, and viral infections. There is a considerable body of literature on the inhibition of intracellular multiplication of such microorganisms in macrophages from specifically sensitized animals [78] and on the capacity of sensitized macrophages to endow normal animals with increased resistance to the corresponding microorganism [79, 80]. The resistance of immune macrophages appears to be nonspecific, however [81].

Several observations in man bear on this subject.

1. BCG vaccination of tuberculin-negative young adults has been reported to reduce the

subsequent incidence of clinical reinfection [82–84], but this observation is contested [85].

2. Human splenic and lymph node tissues cultivated *in vitro* in the presence of OT showed inhibition of migration of the cells of the explant only when the tissues were obtained from a tuberculin-sensitive donor [86]. This result is similar to those previously described in which cells were obtained from tuberculin-sensitive animals [87]. The specificity of this reaction has been proved by the recent experiments of David *et al.* [15].

3. Enders *et al.* [88] demonstrated that individuals exhibiting delayed hypersensitivity reactions greater than 10 mm. in diameter to inactivated mumps virus were usually resistant to mumps infection whether or not complement-fixing antibody to mumps was detectable. The larger the reaction, the smaller the possibility of reinfection.

4. Viral infections in agammaglobulinemic children cause a typical clinical syndrome, and there are, with rare exceptions, normal recovery from infection and development of the usual long-lasting immunity to reinfection [89, 90]. This finding would be of the greatest significance in demonstrating a role of cellular hypersensitivity in specific resistance to viral infections if these patients were truly *agamma*globulinemic. Unfortunately, all have small amounts of γ-globulin; moreover, some can produce trace amounts of serum antibody detectable only by extremely sensitive methods of antibody assay [91, 92]. If immunity to the small dose of virus presented by a naturally transmitted infection is a more sensitive test for serum antibody than any known *in vitro* titration, viral immunity in agammaglobulinemia may be due entirely to conventional antibody. (Presumably, all serum antibody can be mobilized for interaction with the virus at the local invasion site, in contrast to *in vitro* tests which utilize a minute aliquot of the total serum volume.)

In addition, Friedman *et al.* [93] were unable to demonstrate a role for delayed hypersensitivity in recovery from experimental vaccinia infection. They showed that guinea pigs previously treated with X-ray and methotrexate, and therefore unable to develop demonstrable delayed hypersensitivity to vaccinia virus, nevertheless recover from vaccinia virus infection as rapidly as nontreated control animals. Since a virus-inhibiting substance with the properties of interferon was demonstrated in the skin of recovering animals, whether untreated or treated with methotrexate and X-ray, these authors concluded that interferon was responsible for recovery from the primary infection.

5. A patient with vaccinia gangrenosum studied by Kempe [94] appeared to be unresponsive to administration of hyperimmune vaccinial γ-globulin but began to improve following injections around the lesion of leukocytes from a recently vaccinated donor. It is possible, however, that nonspecific effects of the transferred leukocytes, such as interferon production [95], may have been responsible for the improvement.

It is clear that, at present, there is insufficient evidence to support the view that delayed hypersensitivity is a factor in immunity to certain infectious agents.

RELATION TO ANTIBODY FORMATION

Experimental evidence regarding the earlier time of appearance of delayed skin reactivity than of detectable antibody formation [46–48] and the elicitation of a secondary type of antibody response in sensitized animals [96, 97] have led to the hypothesis that the delayed type of hypersensitivity is an integral part of antibody formation [48, 98]. This hypothesis has been challenged in turn by the inability to demonstrate delayed hypersensitivity to polysaccharides which can stimulate antibody formation [99] and by the effect of neonatal thymectomy on the immunological responsiveness of adult animals in which delayed hypersensitivity reactivity is severely inhibited with considerably less effect on antibody formation [35, 100]. A similar dissociation has been described in man, associated with Hodgkin's disease and sarcoidosis.

In human beings, there is evidence associating delayed skin reactivity to diphtheria toxoid with antitoxin formation. Individuals with delayed skin reactivity to "purified" diphtheria toxoid almost always have detectable serum antitoxin [101, 102]. Such individuals produce unusually large amounts of antitoxin when later immunized with small amounts of toxoid, and there appears to be a general correlation between the intensity of delayed skin reactivity and the magnitude of the subsequent secondary antitoxin response [102].

This finding has practical significance because individuals with delayed skin reactivity to toxoid are routinely immunized by the tiny dose of toxid used for skin testing (0.01 Lf). Skin testing, therefore, eliminates the need for an injection of the large immunizing dose (5–50 Lf) which in many would have caused unpleasant local and systemic reactions. This type of correlative evidence does not, of course, answer basic questions about the relationship of hypersensitivity to antibody formation.*

TRANSFER OF HYPERSENSITIVITY

Patterned after the initial demonstration by Landsteiner and Chase [103] of the cellular transfer system of delayed hypersensitivity in the guinea pig, similar experiments were attempted in human subjects by Lawrence [104] using viable peripheral blood leukocytes. In this study, 0.3 to 0.5 ml. of packed white cells obtained from blood donors with intense delayed type hypersensitivity to tuberculin was injected intradermally or subcutaneously into the tuberculin-negative recipient, who was challenged with the usual skin-testing dose of tuberculin or purified protein derivative (PPD) 1 to 14 days later. Typical tuberculin reactions were obtained in the formerly tuberculin-negative recipients; subsequently, similar successful transfer in man of hypersensitivity to streptococcal products [105] and other antigens [106, 107] was accomplished.

The results of these early experiments in human beings were qualitatively similar in every respect to those previously reported in animals. Several quantitative differences were noted, however. (1) A smaller dose of leukocytes relative to body surface area was required for transfer in man. (2) Transferred hypersensitivity was more intense and of longer duration in man (usually months to years, but usually weeks in animals). (3) Adult donors did not need to be actively sensitized by an antigenic challenge just before transfer of their leukocytes. These operational differences may express a greater intensity of donor sensitization in men than in animals.

Of greater interest was the subsequent finding by Lawrence [108] that *extracts* of hypersensitive leukocytes, prepared by distilled-water lysis or by freeze-thawing for 10 cycles, were equally effective in transferring delayed type hypersensitivity. The important implications of this observation stimulated further experiments by Lawrence [109, 110] and others [111, 112]. It was shown that systemic transfer is effective as early as four to six hours, as evident from the "firing off" of previously negative skin test sites where antigen had been injected days earlier. Sensitivity of the transfer could be increased approximately tenfold if antigen was injected into the site of the transfer (test for "local-transfer) or incubated with the extract before transfer. With this technique as little as 0.01 ml. of leukocytes could be used, in contrast to 0.1 ml. for "systemic" transfer.

In experiments using leukocytes from donors sensitized against two antigens, diphtheria toxoid and PPD, it was shown that incubation of PPD but not of toxoid with aliquots of the cells specifically released the corresponding transfer factor into the supernatant, leaving a "desensitized" cell pellet [110]. This suggests either that specific desensitization can be accomplished *in vitro* by this technique but, for reasons not understood, toxoid was ineffective under the particular experimental conditions employed, or that the observed desensitization with PPD was nonspecific, possibly due to contaminating materials, perhaps endotoxin. In experiments with diphtheria toxoid-sensitive donors [109], it was possible to transfer sensitivity with extracts devoid of any detectable neutralizing diphtheria antitoxin; moreover, toxoid treatment of the extract did not block the transfer. The conclusion that serum antibody was not present in the extract was not proved, however, because with the diphtheria toxoid system it was difficult to exclude rigorously the participation of contaminating antigens [113]. However, further support for the absence of a role by serum antibody was obtained by Maurer [2], who transferred delayed hypersensitivity to ethylene

* *Editor's comment:* Although the relation of circulating antibodies to delayed hypersensitivity is obscure, the findings of Turcotte *et al.* (Turcotte, R., Freedman, S. O., and Sehon, A. H., *Amer. Rev. Resp. Dis.* 88:725, 1963) are of interest. In analyzing hemagglutinating antibody titers by chromatography in the sera of healthy subjects with positive skin tests to PPD, the major activity was found in Fraction XII (14S, macromolecules). In contrast, the sera of patients with active pulmonary tuberculosis and positive skin reactivity had higher titers generally with the major activity in Fraction I (7S, γ_2-globulin). Although these findings appear to be consistent for pulmonary tuberculosis, it is not known if they pertain to other forms as well.—B. R.

oxide-treated human serum in man, using leukocyte extracts. This antigen was incapable of stimulating detectable antibody formation after repeated intradermal immunizations during a one and a half year period; the hypersensitivity of recipients lasted for at least one year.

Another important step in the development of an understanding of the nature of transfer factor was the observation that dialysates of leukocyte extracts were effective in transfer [114]. In contrast to transfer factor, papain-digested rabbit γ-globulin fragments did not leave the dialysis bag, suggesting that transfer factor has a molecular weight of less than 40,000. Moreover, fractionation of the dialysate using Sephadex G-25 suggested a molecular weight of *less than 10,000*. The dialysate did not react on agar diffusion in gel with antibody to human γ-globulin, γ_2-globulin, or albumin, nor was protein detected by precipitation in 5 percent TCA. The soluble factor was resistant to desoxyribonuclease (DNAse), ribonuclease (RNAse), trypsin, and storage at 20° C. for six months or at room temperature for eight hours.

The interpretation of these findings has presented one of the more challenging problems in immunology. The following explanations must be considered.

1. Transfer of antigen. This seems unlikely because (*a*) intense inflammation can develop at previously tested skin sites in the recipient within six hours after transfer, and (*b*) incubation of antigen-normal leukocytes did not endow them with the capacity to transfer hypersensitivity. The possibility that a previous undetected reactivity in the recipient is heightened to detectable levels by the transfer appears to be excluded by the transfer of sensitivity to ethylene oxide-treated human serum, since *new* antigenic determinants are created by this procedure [2].

2. Transfer of effector (antibody-like) material. The apparent low molecular weight of transfer factor suggests a relatively small polypeptide chain. The implication of this possibility is that delayed type hypersensitivity is not due to antibody activity of the recognized intact immunoglobulins but is due to a smaller molecule with stereospecificity for antigen. This hypothesis requires that (*a*) reaction with antigen is not demonstrated by mixing isolated factor together with antigen *in vitro* by the procedures employed to date and (*b*) after transfer, it is not readily catabolized in host (to explain sensitization that lasts for years).

Although the polypeptide theory is unlikely, it has not been excluded. Theoretically, an antibody combining site could be formed from such a small molecule since the relation of the geometry of the combining site to the structure of γ-globulin is not yet known. The failure to detect antigen-antibody-like interactions in a test tube is not unexpected since such reactions are usually not detectable when well-washed leukocytes that can transfer hypersensitivity are mixed with specific antigen. In addition, the long duration of passive sensitization could be explained if the polypeptide chain has an affinity for certain long-lived small lymphocytes or if the polypeptide is passed from cell to cell as suggested by Pappenheimer [110].

3. Transfer of material that contains information for formation of effector (antibody-like) material. A transfer of this type may account for the *in vitro* antibody response to T-2 bacteriophage described by Fishman [115], but the material in his studies was RNAse-sensitive. If transfer factor is an informational molecule, then presumably it is a messenger RNA (mRNA) since the failure of DNAse to affect transfer factor appears to exclude DNA as the factor. If so, to explain the immunological and biochemical observations, this mRNA has at least the following three characteristics: (*a*) resistance to RNAse, (*b*) stability or capacity for self-replication, and (*c*) molecular weight of less than 25,000. None of these characteristics are to be expected from other studies of mammalian protein synthesis [115a]. Thus, in all other studies of mRNA function, mRNA is extremely sensitive to RNAse except for "artificial" messengers having unusual base sequences; mRNA does not appear to replicate in mammalian systems, and only the mRNA in the nonnucleated reticulocyte appears stable; the expected molecular weight of mRNA for the L and H chains of γ-globulin (assuming no repeating monomeric units) would be over 250,000.

It is immediately apparent that a great deal more information is needed before reaching any conclusions concerning the mechanism of transfer, particularly because of the importance of this mechanism to an understanding of the immune response and, indeed, the behavior, in general, of mammalian informational macromolecules.

DISEASES AFFECTING THE DELAYED HYPERSENSITIVE STATE

A number of human diseases are known to affect delayed hypersensitivity. These include Hodgkin's disease, lymphoma, leukemia, multiple myeloma, sarcoidosis, and agammaglobulinemia. During Hodgkin's disease, skin reactions to tuberculin or histoplasmin are rarely positive, even in patients with active tuberculosis and histoplasmosis, respectively; and those with Hodgkin's disease as well as the lymphoma-leukemia group show a diminished capacity to become sensitized to DNFB or to bacterial antigens [116–121]. The immunological abnormalities associated with this particular group of diseases are discussed in detail in the separate chapters devoted to each condition.

REFERENCES

1. Rich, A. R. *The Pathogenesis of Tuberculosis.* Springfield, Ill.: Charles C Thomas, Publisher, 1951. P. 376.
2. Maurer, P. H. Immunologic studies with ethylene oxide-treated human serum. *J. Exp. Med.* 113:1029, 1961.
3. Black, S., Humphrey, J. H., and Niven, J. S. F. Inhibition of Mantoux reaction by direct suggestion under hypnosis. *Brit. Med. J.* 1:1649, 1963.
4. Stewart, F. W., and Rhoads, C. P. The significance of giant cells in the intradermal tuberculin reaction. *Arch. Path.* 2:571, 1926.
5. Allen, A. C. *The Skin.* St. Louis: C. V. Mosby Company, 1954.
6. Haxthausen, H. Allergic dermatitis: Studies in identical twins. *Acta Dermatovener.* 23:438, 1943.
7. Inderbitzin, T. Histamine in Allergic Responses of the Skin. In Shaffer, J. H., Lo-Grippo, G. A., and Chase, M. W. (Eds.), *Mechanisms of Hypersensitivity.* Boston: Little, Brown, 1959.
8. Thomas, L. The physiological disturbances produced by endotoxins. *Ann. Rev. Physiol.* 16:467, 1954.
9. Stetson, C. A. Similarities in the mechanisms determining the Arthus and Shwartzman phenomenon. *J. Exp. Med.* 94:347, 1951.
10. Najarian, J. S., and Feldman, J. D. Passive transfer of tuberculin sensitivity by tritiated thymidine-labeled lymphoid cells. *J. Exp. Med.* 114:779, 1961.
11. Turk, J. L. The passive transfer of delayed hypersensitivity in guinea pigs by the transfusion of isotopically-labelled lymphoid cells. *Immunology* 5:478, 1962.
12. Najarian, J. S., and Feldman, J. D. Passive transfer of contact sensitivity by tritiated thymidine-labeled lymphoid cells. *J. Exp. Med.* 117:775, 1963.
13. McCluskey, R. T., Benacerraf, B., and McCluskey, J. S. Studies on the specificity of the cellular infiltrate in delayed hypersensitivity reactions. *J. Immun.* 90:466, 1963.
14. Najarian, J. S., and Feldman, J. D. Specificity of passively transferred delayed hypersensitivity. *J. Exp. Med.* 118:341, 1963.
15. David, J. R., Al-Askari, S., Lawrence, H. S., and Thomas, L. Studies on delayed hypersensitivity in vitro. *Fed. Proc.* 22:618, 1963.
16. Rich, A. R. Ref. 1, p. 385.
17. Spink, W. W. The significance of endotoxin in brucellosis: Experimental and clinical studies. *Trans. Ass. Amer. Physicians* 67:283, 1954.
18. Uhr, J. W., and Brandriss, M. W. Delayed hypersensitivity: IV. Systemic reactivity of guinea pigs sensitized to protein antigens. *J. Exp. Med.* 108:905, 1958.
19. Stetson, C. A., Schlossman, S., and Benacerraf, B. Endotoxin-like effects of old tuberculin. *Fed. Proc.* 17:536, 1958 (abst.).
20. Freund, J. The effect of heterologous bacterial products upon tuberculous animals. *J. Immun.* 30:241, 1936.
21. Bordet, P. Contribution à l'étude de l'allergie: L'allergie nonspécifique. *Ann. Inst. Pasteur* (Paris) 56:325, 1936.
22. Boyden, S. V. The immunological response to antigens of the tubercle bacillus. *Progr. Allerg.* 5:149, 1958.
23. Hall, C. H., Jr., and Atkins, E. Studies on tuberculin fever: I. The mechanism of fever in tuberculin hypersensitivity. *J. Exp. Med.* 109:339, 1959.
24. Johanovsky, J. Production of pyrogenic substances in the reaction of cells of hypersensitive guinea pigs with antigen in vitro. *Immunology* 3:179, 1960.
25. Atkins, E. Pathogenesis of fever. *Physiol. Rev.* 40:580, 1960.

26. Landsteiner, K., and Chase, M. W. Studies on the sensitization of animals with simple chemical compounds: VII. Skin sensitization by intraperitoneal injection. *J. Exp. Med.* 71:237, 1940.
27. Derick, C. L., and Swift, H. F. Reactions of rabbits to nonhemolytic streptococci: General tuberculin-like hypersensitiveness, allergy, or hyperergy following secondary reaction. *J. Exp. Med.* 49:615, 1929.
28. Julianelle, L. A. Reactions of rabbits to intracutaneous injection of pneumococci and their products: III. Reactions at the site of injection. *J. Exp. Med.* 51:463, 1930.
29. Eisen, H. N., Orris, L., and Belman, S. Elicitation of delayed allergic skin reactions with haptens: The dependence of elicitation on hapten combination with protein. *J. Exp. Med.* 95:473, 1952.
30. Uhr, J. W., Salvin, S. B., and Pappenheimer, A. M., Jr. Delayed hypersensitivity: II. Induction of hypersensitivity in guinea pigs by means of antigen-antibody complexes. *J. Exp. Med.* 105:11, 1957.
31. Mote, J. R., and Jones, T. D. The development of foreign protein sensitization in human beings. *J. Immun.* 30:149, 1936.
32. Uhr, J. W., and Baumann, J. B. Antibody formation: I. The suppression of antibody formation by passively administered antibody. *J. Exp. Med.* 113:935, 1961.
33. Feinberg, S. M., Rabinowitz, H. I., Pruzansky, J. J., Feinberg, A. R., and Kaminker, A. Repository antigen injections: Absorption studies by immunologic and radioactive methods. *J. Allerg.* 31:421, 1960.
34. Becker, R. J., Sparks, D. B., Feinberg, S. M., Patterson, R., Pruzansky, J. J., and Feinberg, A. R. Delayed and immediate skin reactivity in man after injection of antigen in emulsion: Cell transfer of the delayed sensitivity. *J. Allerg.* 32:229, 1961.
35. Warner, N. L., Szenberg, A., and Burnet, F. M. The immunological role of different lymphoid organs in the chicken: I. Dissociation of immunological responsiveness. *Aust. J. Exp. Biol. Med. Sci.* 40:373, 1962.
36. Aspinall, R. L., Meyer, R. K., Graetzer, M. A., and Wolfe, H. R. Effect of thymectomy and bursectomy on the survival of skin homografts in chickens. *J. Immun.* 90:872, 1963.
37. Sutherland, D. E. R., Archer, O. K., and Good, R. A. The role of the appendix in development of immunologic capacity. *Proc. Soc. Exp. Biol. Med.* 115:673, 1964.
38. Epstein, W. L., and Kligman, A. M. The interference phenomenon in allergic contact dermatitis. *J. Invest. Derm.* 31:103, 1958.
39. Adler, F. L. Competition of Antigens. Ref. 7.
40. Raffel, S., and Newel, J. M. The "delayed hypersensitivity" induced by antigen-antibody complexes. *J. Exp. Med.* 108:823, 1958.
41. Rostenberg, A., Jr. Ref. 7, p. 465.
42. Furcolow, M. L., Hewell, B., Nelson, W. E., and Palmer, G. E. Quantitative studies of tuberculin reaction: Titration of tuberculin sensitivity and its relation to tuberculous infection. *Public Health Rep.* 56:1082, 1941.
43. Magnus, K., and Edwards, L. B. The effect of repeated tuberculin testing on post-vaccination allergy. *Lancet* 2:643, 1955.
44. Smith, C. E., Whiting, E. G., Baker, E. E., Rosenberg, H. G., Beard, R. R., and Saito, M. T. The use of coccidioidin. *Amer. Rev. Tuberc.* 57:330, 1948.
45. Rapaport, F. T., Lawrence, H. S., Millar, J. W., Pappagianis, D., and Smith, C. E. The immunologic properties of coccidioidin as a skin test reagent in man. *J. Immun.* 84:368, 1960.
46. Dienes, L. The first manifestation of the developing hypersensitiveness. *Proc. Soc. Exp. Biol. Med.* 28:75, 1930.
47. Dienes, L. The specific immunity response and the healing of infectious diseases. *Arch. Path.* 21:357, 1956.
48. Salvin, S. B. Occurrence of delayed hypersensitivity during the development of Arthus type hypersensitivity. *J. Exp. Med.* 107:109, 1958.
49. Gell, P. G. H., and Benacerraf, B. Delayed hypersensitivity to simple protein antigens. *Advances Immun.* 1:319, 1961.
50. Straus, H. W. Artificial sensitization of infants to poison ivy. *J. Allerg.* 2:137, 1931.
51. Uhr, J. W., Dancis, J., and Neumann, C. G. Delayed-type hypersensitivity in premature neonatal humans. *Nature* (London) 187:1130, 1960.
52. Vahlquist, B., Murray, U., and Persson, N. G. Studies on diphtheria in newborn babies and in infants. *Acta Paediat.* 35:130, 1948.
53. Osborn, J. J., Dancis, J., and Julia, J. F. Studies of the immunology of the newborn infant: I. Age and antibody production. *Pediatrics* 9:736, 1952.
54. Dancis, J., Osborn, J. J., and Kunz, H. W. Studies on the immunology of the newborn infant: IV. Antibody formation in the premature infant. *Pediatrics* 12:151, 1953.
55. Uhr, J. W., Dancis, J., Franklin, E. C., Finkelstein, M. S., and Lewis, E. W. The antibody response to bacteriophage ØX174 in newborn premature infants. *J. Clin. Invest.* 41:1509, 1962.
56. Eitzman, D. V., and Smith, R. T. The nonspecific inflammatory cycle in the neonatal infant. *Amer. J. Dis. Child.* 97:326, 1959.
57. Silverstein, A. M. Unpublished data, 1963.
58. Silverstein, A. M., Thorbecke, G. L., Kraner, K. L., and Lukes, R. J. Fetal response to

antigenic stimulus: III. γ-globulin production in normal and stimulated fetal lambs. *J. Immun.* 91:384, 1963.

59. Silverstein, A. M., Uhr, J. W., Kraner, K. L., and Lukes, R. J. Fetal response to antigenic stimulus: II. Antibody production by the fetal lamb. *J. Exp. Med.* 117:799, 1963.
60. Silverstein, A. M., Prendergast, R. A., and Kraner, K. L. Homograft rejection in the fetal lamb: The role of circulating antibody. *Science,* 142:1172, 1963.
61. Warwick, W. J., Good, R. A., and Smith, R. T. Failure of passive transfer of delayed hypersensitivity in the newborn human infant. *J. Lab. Clin. Med.* 56:139, 1960.
62. Bauer, J. Über Immunitätsvorgänge bei der Tuberkulose. *Beitr. Klin. Tuberk.* 13:383, 1909.
63. Fernbach, H. Über langdauernde, ohne klinische wahrnehmbare Herd- und Allgemeinreaktionen durchegefuhrte Tuberkulinkuren und über den nach ihnen auftretenden Unempfindlichkeitszustand. *Beitr. Klin. Tuberk.* 81:301, 1932.
64. Uhr, J. W., and Pappenheimer, A. M., Jr. Delayed hypersensitivity: III. Specific desensitization of guinea pigs sensitized to protein antigens. *J. Exp. Med.* 108:891, 1958.
65. Oliveira-Lima, A. Passive transfer of the delayed dermal sensitivity to tuberculin by means of blood leukocytes. *Amer. Rev. Tuberc.* 78:346, 1958.
66. Kligman, A. M. Hyposensitization against Rhus dermatitis. *Arch. Derm.* 78:47, 1958.
67. Benacerraf, B., and Gell, P. G. H. Studies on hypersensitivity. III. The relation between delayed reactivity to the picryl group of conjugates and contact sensitivity. *Immunology* 2:219, 1959.
68. Salvin, S. B., and Smith, R. F. Delayed hypersensitivity and the anamnestic response. *J. Immun.* 84:449, 1960.
69. Gell, P. G. H., and Benacerraf, B. Studies on hypersensitivity: IV. The relationship between contact and delayed sensitivity. *J. Exp. Med.* 113:571, 1961.
70. Gell, P. G. H., and Silverstein, A. M. Delayed hypersensitivity to hapten-protein conjugates: I. The effect of carrier protein and site of attachment to hapten. *J. Exp. Med.* 115:1037, 1962.
71. Silverstein, A. M., and Gell, P. G. H. Delayed hypersensitivity to hapten-protein conjugates: II. Anti-hapten specificity and the heterogeneity of the delayed response. *Ibid.,* p. 1053.
72. von Pirquet, C. E. Allergy. *Arch. Intern. Med.* 7:383, 1911.
73. Bloomfield, A. L., and Mateer, J. G. Changes in skin sensitiveness to tuberculin during epidemic influenza. *Amer. Rev. Tuberc.* 3:166, 1919.
74. Chase, M. W. Inhibition of experimental drug allergy by prior feeding of sensitizing agent. *Proc. Soc. Exp. Biol. Med.* 61:257, 1946.
75. Turk, J. L., and Humphrey, J. H. Immunological unresponsiveness in guinea pigs: II. The effect of unresponsiveness on the development of delayed type hypersensitivity to protein antigens. *Immunology* 4:310, 1961.
76. Rollof, S. I., Lagercrantz, R., and Lind, J. Antibodies to tubercle bacilli and tuberculin response after BCG vaccination in infants of mothers with tuberculosis. *Acta Paediat.,* supp. 100, p. 179, 1954.
77. Thurell, I. B. Tidpunkfen for tuberkulinpositivitet hos BCG-vaccinerade spadborn till tuberkulose modrar. *Nord. Med.* 52:1139, 1954.
78. Mitsuhashi, S., Sato, I., and Tanaka, T Experimental salmonellosis: Intracellular growth of *Salmonella enteritidis* ingested in mononuclear phagocytes of mice, and cellular basis of immunity. *J. Bact.* 81:863, 1961.
79. Suter, E. Passive transfer of acquired resistance to infection with *Mycobacterium tuberculosis* by means of cells. *Amer. Rev. Resp. Dis.* 83:535, 1961.
80. Saito, K., Nakano, M., Akiyama, T., and Ushiba, D. Passive transfer of immunity to typhoid by macrophages. *J. Bact.* 84:500, 1962.
81. Holland, J. J., and Pickett, M. J. A cellular basis of immunity in experimental *Brucella* infection. *J. Exp. Med.* 108:343, 1958.
82. Heimbeck, J. Éssais sur le sérothérapie de quelques maladies tuberculeuses. *Tubercle* 18: 97, 1936.
83. Scheel, O. La tuberculose parmi les étudiants en médecine à Oslo et sa prévention par la vaccination au BCG. *Bull. Acad. Med.* 114:149, 1935.
84. Aronson, J. D., and Palmer, C. E. Experience with BCG vaccine in control of tuberculosis among North American Indians. *Public Health Rep.* 61:802, 1946.
85. Blanch, P. C., Blanch, H. C., and Lieutier, H. *Rev. Tuberc. Urug.* 13:1, 1945.
86. Gangarosa, E. J., Inglefield, J. T., Thomas, C. G. A., and Morgan, H. R. Studies of hypersensitivity of human tissues in vitro: I. Tuberculin hypersensitivity. *J. Exp. Med.* 102: 425, 1955.
87. Rich, A. R., and Lewis, M. R. The nature of allergy in tuberculosis, as revealed by tissue culture studies. *Bull. Hopkins Hosp.* 50:115, 1932.
88. Enders, J. F., Kane, L. W., Maris, E. P., Stokes, J. Immunity in mumps: V. The correlation of the presence of dermal hypersensitivity and resistance to mumps. *J. Exp. Med.* 84:341, 1946.
89. Gitlin, D., Janeway, C. A., Apt, L., and Craig,

J. M. Agammaglobulinemia. In Lawrence, H. S. (Ed.), *Cellular and Humoral Aspects of the Hypersensitive States.* New York: Paul B. Hoeber, Inc., 1959.

90. Good, R. A., Zak, S. J., Condie, R. M., and Bridges, R. A. Clinical investigations of patients with agammaglobulinemia and hypogammaglobulinemia. *Pediat. Clin. N. Amer.* 7:397, 1960.
91. Baron, S., Nasou, J. P., Friedman, R. M., Owen, G. M., Levy, H. B., and Barnett, E. V. Antibody production by hypogammaglobulinemic patients. *J. Immun.* 88:443, 1962.
92. Good, R. A., and Gabrielsen, A. E. Agammaglobulinemia and Hypogammaglobulinemia —Relationship to the Mesenchymal Diseases. In Uhr, J. W. (Ed.), *Streptococcus, Rheumatic Fever and Glomerulonephritis.* Baltimore: Williams & Wilkins Company, 1964.
93. Friedman, R. M., Baron, S., Buckler, C. E., and Steinmuller, R. I. The role of antibody, delayed hypersensitivity, and interferon production in recovery of guinea pigs from primary infection with vaccinia virus. *J. Exp. Med.* 116:347, 1962.
94. Kempe, C. H. Studies on smallpox and complications of smallpox vaccination. *Pediatrics* 26:176, 1960.
95. Glasgow, L. A., and Habel, K. Interferon production by mouse leukocytes *in vitro* and *in vivo*. *J. Exp. Med.* 117:149, 1963.
96. Scharff, M., Uhr, J. W., and Pappenheimer, A. M., Jr. Antibody Production and the Delayed Hypersensitive State. In Tunevall, G. (Ed.), *Proceedings of VIIth International Congress of Microbiology.* Stockholm: Almqvist & Wiksells, 1959. P. 257.
97. Sell, S. and Weigle, W. O. The relationship between delayed hypersensitivity and circulating antibody induced by protein antigens in guinea pigs. *J. Immun.* 83:257, 1959.
98. Pappenheimer, A. M., Jr., Scharff, M., and Uhr, J. W. Delayed Hypersensitivity and Its Possible Relation to Antibody Formation. Ref. 7, p. 417.
99. Sabin, F. R., Joyner, A. L., and Smithburn, K. C. Cellular reactions to polysaccharides from tubercle bacilli and from pneumococci. *J. Exp. Med.* 68:563, 1938.
100. Arnason, B. G., Jankovic, B. D., Waksman, B. H., and Wennersten, C. Role of the thymus in immune reactions in rats: II. Suppressive effect of thymectomy at birth on reactions of delayed (cellular) hypersensitivity and the circulating small lymphocytes. *J. Exp. Med.* 116:117, 1962.
101. Pappenheimer, A. M., Jr., and Lawrence, H. S. Immunization of adults with diphtheria toxoid: II. An analysis of the pseudoreactions to the Schick test. *Amer. J. Hyg.* 47:233, 1948.
102. Pappenheimer, A. M., Jr., and Lawrence, H. S. Immunization of adults with diphtheria toxoid: III. Highly purified toxoid as an immunizing agent. *Ibid.*, p. 241.
103. Landsteiner, K., and Chase, M. W. Studies on the sensitization of animals with simple chemical compounds: VII. Skin sensitization by intraperitoneal injections. *J. Exp. Med.* 71:237, 1940.
104. Lawrence, H. S. The cellular transfer of cutaneous hypersensitivity to tuberculin in man. *Proc. Soc. Exp. Biol. Med.* 71:516, 1949.
105. Lawrence, H. S. The cellular transfer in humans of delayed cutaneous reactivity to hemolytic streptococci. *J. Immun.* 68:159, 1952.
106. Warwick, W. J., Page, A., and Good, R. A. Passive transfer with circulating leucocytes of delayed hypersensitivity to cat scratch antigen. *Proc. Soc. Exp. Biol. Med.* 93:253, 1956.
107. Freedman, S. O., and Fish, A. J. The passive cellular transfer of delayed type hypersensitivity to intradermal procaine. *J. Invest. Derm.* 38:363, 1962.
108. Lawrence, H. S. The transfer in humans of delayed skin sensitivity to streptococcal M substance and to tuberculin with disrupted leucocytes. *J. Clin. Invest.* 34:219, 1955.
109. Lawrence, H. S., and Pappenheimer, A. M., Jr. Transfer of delayed hypersensitivity to diphtheria toxin in man. *J. Exp. Med.* 104: 321, 1956.
110. Lawrence, H. S. Some Biological and Immunological Properties of Transfer Factor. In Wolstenholme, G. E. W., and O'Connor, M., (Eds.), *Cellular Aspects of Immunity.* Boston: Little, Brown, 1960. P. 243.
111. Rapaport, F. T., Lawrence, H. S., Millar, J. W., Pappaglanis, D., and Smith, C. E. Transfer of delayed hypersensitivity to coccidioidin in man. *J. Immun.* 84:358, 1960.
112. Baram, P., and Mosko, M. M. Chromatography of the human tuberculin delayed hypersensitivity transfer factor. *J. Allerg.* 33: 498, 1962.
113. Finger, I., and Kabat, E. A. A comparison of human antisera to purified diphtheria toxoid with antisera to other purified antigens by quantitative precipitin and gel diffusion techniques. *J. Exp. Med.* 108:453, 1958.
114. Lawrence, H. S., Al-Askari, S., David, J., Franklin, E. C., and Zweiman, B. Transfer of immunological information in humans with dialysates of leucocyte extracts. *Trans. Ass. Amer. Physicians* 76:84, 1963.
115. Fishman, M. Antibody formation in vitro. *J. Exp. Med.* 114:837, 1961.

115a. Michelson, A. M. *The Chemistry of Nucleosides and Nucleotides.* London and New York: Academic Press, 1963.
116. Bastai, P. Kurze wissenschaftliche Mitteelungen: Ueber die klinische Bedentung der Tuberkulin-anergie bie malignem Lymphogranulom. *Klin. Wschr.* 7:1606, 1928.
117. Parker, F., Jr., Jackson, H., Jr., FitzHugh, G., and Spies, T. D. Studies of diseases of the lymphoid and myeloid tissues: IV. Skin reactions to human and avian tuberculin. *J. Immun.* 22:277, 1932.
118. Bunnell, I. L., and Furcolow, M. L. Variations in histoplasmin sensitivity in certain cities in Eastern Kansas. *Public Health Rep.* 63:1298, 1948.
119. Schier, W. W., Roth, A., Ostroff, G., and Schrift, M. H. Hodgkin's disease and immunity. *Amer. J. Med.* 20:94, 1956.
120. Good, R. A., Kelly, W. D., Rottstein, J., and Vargo, R. L. Immunological deficiency diseases. *Progr. Allerg.* 6:187, 1962.
121. Rostenberg, A., Jr., McCraney, H. C., and Bluefarb, S. M. Immunologic studies in the lymphoblastomas: II. The ability to develop an eczematous sensitization to a simple chemical and the ability to accept passive transfer antibody. *J. Invest. Derm.* 26:209, 1956.

21. Homograft Rejection

JOHN P. MERRILL

GENERAL PHENOMENA ACCOMPANYING HOMOGRAFT REJECTION IN MAN

The general immunological aspects of tissue transplantation have been dealth with in Chapter 13. In large part this information has been obtained from experiments with inbred strains of mice, with rabbits, guinea pigs, and more recently hamsters. The general principles derived from these experiments apply also to man, but there are a number of differences, to be pointed out later. As Medawar [1] has put it, "perhaps the behavior of inbred and homozygous mice is not the best theoretical guide as to what may be expected of animals so obstinately heterozygous as human beings." The data from truly experimental graftings of skin and organs in man are necessarily limited. Nevertheless the fact that most, if not all, nucleated tissues of an individual (and also platelets) share the transplantation antigenic configuration makes it possible to obtain information about the grafting of kidney and liver, for example, by the use of skin grafts and "grafts" of peripheral leukocytes between well-motivated human volunteers. Although the publications of Medawar [2, 3] confirm the significance of immunity as a basis for the rejection of skin homografts in rabbits, it is interesting to note that more than twenty years before his work a clinical surgeon, Holman [4], suggested an immunological basis from the observation of skin grafts in burned patients.

In general, there is similarity in the sequence of events which follows the placing of an autograft or first and second homograft in both man and the experimental animal. Converse and Rapaport and their colleagues [5, 6] and our own group [7, 8] have extensively studied these phenomena in healthy adult human volunteers. The behavior of autografts and first-set homografts followed the general outline described for autografts and homografts of animal tissue. On the first day, both autograft and homograft depend for their nutrition and oxygenation on "plasmatic" circulation from the graft bed. In a full-thickness graft and to a lesser extent in a thin graft, some degree of ischemic change takes place in the autograft. Capillaries in the upper dermis collapse and the nuclei of the endothelial cells degenerate, although the capillary basement membrane remains intact. Some minor changes may take place in the epidermis, and there may be slight degeneration of the dermal appendages. Revascularization of the autograft commences the second or third day and is complete by day 6 or 7. Following this, the ischemic changes regress rapidly. The first-set homograft in man is vascularized in a manner identical to that of the autograft, and the changes are similar for the first few days. The first signs of rejection of the homograft appear in the deeper layers of the graft, where a few lymphocytes are noted around the small venules and the blood vessels supplying the sweat glands. The appearance of these perivascular round cells correlates well in our studies with the first observation of gross edema. Others have noted first changes as dilatation of the capillary bed as seen through the stereoscopic microscope [5]. As the rejection process continues, perivascular infiltration intensifies. Lymphocytes continue to accumulate in the dermis, which becomes edematous. On day 9 or later, the vascular lesion may progress to thrombosis; and once this occurs, rejection is rapid as far as the epidermis is concerned, the latter becoming necrotic with pyknotic nuclei, eosinophilic cytoplasm, and later separation from the dermis. The first day of rejection as estimated grossly from edema may vary between 6 and 8 days. There are, however, specific individual variations in man, some subjects showing rejection completed by day 11 and others slowly deteriorating up to day 14. In one pair of closely related nonidentical twins studied by us [9], the first evidence of rejection was not apparent until day 23 after grafting. In a series of dizygotic twins reported by Rogers [10], skin grafts survived for periods ranging from 19 to 29 days.

When a second homograft from the same human donor is placed after a first has been rejected by the recipient, rejection of the second-set homograft occurs more quickly and in a somewhat different fashion. The period of time of placing the graft influences the course of events. The second graft, if placed three weeks or more after the first, appears for three days to follow a course similar to that of the autograft and the first-set homograft. Vascularization begins on the second day with the appearance of dilated blood vessels in the epidermis. However, the blood supply becomes abruptly "cut off" about the fifth day, and thereafter the epidermis undergoes "infarct" necrosis with eosinophilic cytoplasm, pyknosis, and ghosting of the nuclei. It is of interest that little or no cellular infiltrate is seen in the epidermis or the dermis in these circumstances. Similar observations have been made in animals.

It has been found in man that if the second graft is placed exactly fourteen days after the first homograft, the second graft is rejected as a "white graft." In these circumstances circulation is never re-established; the graft never blanches as do autografts and first-set homografts. The histological changes are nonspecific, with epidermal necrosis, a dermal polymorphonuclear infiltrate, and collapse of the superficial capillaries with loss of endothelial cells. Perhaps a better term, therefore, is "avascular graft." These findings in man, as in the animal, suggest that cellular infiltrate is not necessarily part of the rejection response. Indeed, much other evidence that we have suggests that the first effect of the beginning immune process is on the vasculature. It has been suggested that the characteristic nature of the white graft depends on the fact that the graft is placed at the peak of immunity generated by the first graft and that humoral factors involved will affect the vasculature so that the graft never obtains a blood supply. The histological observations in man suggesting the possible role of humoral factors acting on vasculature independent of host round cells have considerable importance to our understanding of homograft rejection in general, in both man and the experimental animal. In spite of this presumptive evidence of humoral antibodies in man, however, and an occasional report to the contrary [11], there is no conclusive serological evidence that the rejection of homograft in man is accompanied by causally related humoral antibodies.

The "obstinately heterozygous" state of the human being makes possible a wide range of rejection times for skin grafts placed between individuals. This apparently has to do with quantitative similarity or differences between the histocompatibility antigens of man, presumably genetically determined as they are in the inbred mouse. Prolonged survival of skin grafts between dizygotic human twins has been well documented [9, 10]. The long survival of skin grafts between mother and offspring has also been reported, and although this is less common than was once supposed [12], it is a reality. Even though some nonidentical twins might show prolonged survival of grafts, in others survival may be the same as between unrelated donor recipient pairs. Although Medawar [1] pointed out that "evidently the immune reaction does not necessarily extend with equal vigor to the skin from a graft donor other than that which generated the immune state," there has been a general impression that homograft immunity, particularly in man, is individual-specific. Medawar's data from rabbits, however, show that following an immunizing dose of homograft in one rabbit and a second dose from three others, two reacted with a second-set response and the third as a first-set, suggesting in this heterozygous population a cross-reactivity which appears to be the rule rather than the exception in man.

This sharing of histocompatibility antigens in man is exemplified in the pioneer work of Rapaport *et al.* [13], who reported a nine-year study of 147 skin grafts in a group of unrelated normal subjects. Survival time of the first set of grafts ranged from 6 to 21 days, with a median survival time of 8 to 11 days. Second-, third-, and fourth-set homografts applied to recipients from the same donor 10 to 26 days after rejection of the preceding graft had a median survival of 4.7 days. If a second-set graft was applied to the recipient within 1 to 5 days after the first-set rejection, the white graft rejection previously referred to occurred. However, when a longer latent period (10 to 26 days) was allowed between first-set rejection and application of a second-set graft, the accelerated rejection reaction occurred. In one isolated instance, a first-set graft persisted for 21 days. In studies of cross-sensitization, two recipients received two successive grafts from the same donor. Fifteen days after the rejection of the first-set graft, both received a second-set graft from the same donor and showed an accelerated rejection. Twenty-four hours after second-set rejection, the two recipients received (1) a third-set graft from the original test donor and (2) 6 first-set grafts obtained from six unrelated donors. The third-set graft from the original donor underwent accelerated rejection in both recipients. More important, however, is the fact that of the 12 first-set grafts whose survival times were being compared with that of the original donor, 3, or 25 percent, underwent accelerated rejection, paralleling behavior of third-set grafts from the original donor. When this cross-sensitization experiment was conducted so that a white graft reaction had occurred as a result of a second graft from the original donor, 5 of the 8 first-set unrelated donors underwent accelerated rejection instead of the first-set survival time usually accorded the graft from an unrelated individual. It is obvious from these experiments that a considerable sharing of strong histocompatibility antigens occurred as a result of chance distribution in the human population at large. This sharing, however, is exhibited only in relation to the ability of the indifferent recipient to respond to the shared antigen and does not necessarily represent the full complement of antigenic similarity or differences between the donors themselves. For instance, although exposure to a graft from donor A had cross-sensitized recipients to first-set grafts from donor B in two of three subjects, the first-set grafts exchanged between donors A and B did not exhibit any prolongation of survival time.

The sharing of histocompatibility antigens in man has obvious relevance to the problem of organ grafting. It is well established that the vigor of efforts necessary to suppress the immune response to animal tissue grafts is related to the quantitative difference between the histocompatibility antigens of donor and recipient. The search for the ideal human donor-recipient pair therefore should concern itself initially with an effort to quantitate these histocompatibility differences. Unlike the situation in the inbred mouse, however, the locus for histocompatibility on the human gene has not been well established. It is possible that "skin groups" (reflected in other nucleated tissues) do exist in man. However, as Woodruff [14] has pointed out:

> . . . If skin groups do exist there is likely to be a very large number of them. It is conceivable that some skin groups like some red cell groups might be common and others rare, in which case the chance of any two people chosen at random belonging to the same group would be much greater than the reciprocal of the number of groups. Moreover, the probability of obtaining permanent survival of a homograft made in one direction from a randomly chosen donor to a randomly chosen host is likely to be much greater than the probability that two randomly chosen people should belong to the same skin groups. That is to say that grafts could be made successfully from one to the other and vice versa.

The relation of blood group antigens to histocompatibility antigens in man, as determined by skin grafting, shows a correlation only in specific circumstances. In the case of our nonidentical twins [9], although the donor and recipient shared 23 identical blood groups, tissue was rejected between them, though at a slower rate than in the random population. Woodruff and Allen [15] exchanged small full-thickness skin grafts between two volunteers with 11 identical blood groups and found, in spite of the remarkable degree of red cell compatibility, that the homografts were destroyed within three weeks. In discussing this problem, Newth [16] pointed out:

> . . . Blood group correspondence is not a reliable indication of correspondence in other loci in pairs taken at random from a large population. If, therefore, histocompatibility were entirely independent of blood group antigens, blood grouping would be of little value in selecting unrelated donors for a particular recipient. At present it seems likely that many of the histocompatibility loci are independent of the blood group loci though in the mouse at least, this appears not to be true of the very important H-2 locus whose antigens are expressed in circulating cells. Blood group compatibility is likely to prove a necessary but not a sufficient condition of homograft survival. When considering relatives, however, and particularly if called upon to choose a donor from among parents and siblings of the prospective recipient, it should be remembered that while each child should have one-half the total chromosomal equipment of each parent and hence one-half of

all its genes which must be present in either parent, the actual complement going into each child may be very different. Thus for siblings the expectation of compatibility is subject to a variability which does not apply to parent-child pairs. Siblings may be genetically closer to each other than to either of the parents or equally may be genetically more remote. In this situation the blood grouping of siblings could well be helpful. A very high correspondence in blood antigenicity would indicate greater than chance genetic correspondence at other loci.

A detailed review of these problems was written by Rogers [17]. It can be concluded that, in general, there is no correlation between donor and recipient blood groups and the ability to elicit transplantation immunity.

Entirely apart from the correlation of blood group antigens and histocompatibility, blood isoagglutinins may play a role in the acceptance or rejection of vascularized homografts. If, for instance, the transplanted kidney from a donor of blood group A is perfused by recipient blood containing anti-A isoagglutinins, intravascular clumping, agglutination, and hemolysis are apt to cause tissue damage. Szulman [18] has clearly demonstrated that blood group antigens A and B have widespread localization in the cell walls of endothelium of capillaries, veins, and arteries of man. It is quite probable that the perfusion of vessels containing these antigens by plasma containing specific isoagglutinins for them is not helpful. Furthermore, preliminary data on renal homografting in man suggest strongly that the chance of initial success is considerably lessened if donor and recipient are chosen so that the graft must cross the major blood group barriers [19].

Attempts to elicit "tissue types" in man have been made by the use of nucleated tissue. Dausset [20–22], utilizing the serum of patients in whom leukoagglutinins had been produced by multiple transfusions, compared agglutination by donor and recipient leukocytes. On the basis of this comparison he has suggested that, because all nucleated tissues contain the same histocompatibility antigens, agglutination or lack thereof of leukocytes from a panel of human beings to be tested might reveal a similarity between tissue antigens. Such similarity has been proved for monozygotic twins [22]. However, as Dausset himself points out, the leukoagglutinins were produced by transfusions from multiple, presumably heterozygous donors. The correlation between this leukoagglutinin test and the survival of kidney homografts or skin grafts has not been exact.

A somewhat more sophisticated test has been proposed by Van Rood and Van Leeuwen [23]. They screened 66 sera containing leukocyte agglutinins formed during pregnancy, i.e., presumably by exposure to the antigens of a single donor, the fetus. These sera were screened against a panel of 100 random leukocyte samples, and, by taking into account the agglutination-negative, absorption-positive phenomena, they were able to select a number of sera that gave similar agglutination patterns. By cross-absorption it could be shown that some of these sera recognized only one antigen. In this way it was possible to recognize two allelic leukocyte antigens, 4a and 4b. Mathé *et al.* [24], studying mice, and Wilson *et al.* [25], working with human beings, have proposed a system by which histocompatibility between donors A and B might be classified by studying the degree of immunity elicited to one of the donor pair by prior skin grafting to an indifferent recipient by the other donor. Mathé's work showed that one could not distinguish between weak histocompatibility antigens (H-3). In man [25], by use of time sequence referred to earlier for eliciting a white graft, it was possible to show that all identical twins tested in this fashion produced a white graft. Nonidentical twins, however, varied from white graft, accelerated, and first-set reactions, again indicating a spread even in these presumably closely related individuals. The difficulty with such a system, however, is that in man, at least, it indicates only the strong antigens shared by the panel to be tested and not those in which they differ. In addition, the variable imposed by the antigenic configuration of the indifferent recipients is an unknown factor.

Ideally, one would seek a direct answer to the question: "How will the proposed recipient respond when directly confronted with the antigens of the donor?" Unfortunately, direct testing for this answer would sensitize the prospective organ recipient by immunization to the antigens of the prospective donor. Brent and Medawar [26] have recently suggested a method for eliciting the direct answer to this question without endangering the recipient. It has been shown that circulating lymphocytes in the peripheral blood are immunologically competent. If, therefore, one were to harvest such lymphocytes from the peripheral blood of the prospective tissue recipient and inject them into the prospective tissue donor, antibodies produced by these lymphocytes against the tissues of the prospective donor should portray in some degree the reaction of the donor of the lymphocytes when subjected to a graft of tissue from the recipient of the lymphocytes. Brent and Medawar have shown that the degree of skin reaction elicited correlates well with the survival of skin grafts from donor guinea pigs when grafted onto the lymphocyte donor. A report by Gray and Russell [27] suggests that the screening procedure may have some application in man, although the preliminary nature of their communication and the meager data require substantiation. In our own laboratory, rather more extensive work on this subject [28] suggests that the correlation in man between the skin reaction observed and the survival of skin homografts is considerably less exact than in the guinea pig.

The extent to which such animal studies have applicability to man bears some explanation. As pointed out in Chapter 13, guinea pigs sensitized by skin homografts respond to subsequent intradermal challenge with living donor cells or antigenic extracts with a delayed inflammatory response by a classic tuberculin reaction. We [29] have been able to show that the immunity occasioned by the rejection of a skin homograft in man is also manifested by delayed intradermal sensitivity to the injection of donor white cells and to a lesser extent to a noncellular extract of these white cells. The reaction is not specific for donor leukocytes but was elicited by the injection of nondonor leukocytes into a sensitized recipient in 16 of 19 patients studied—a considerably higher percentage than the cross-reactivity for skin homografts themselves found by Rapaport *et al.* [13]. Furthermore, as in the experimental animal, we were able to show that the intradermal inoculation of peripheral leukocytes prior to full-thickness skin grafting induced white grafts and accelerated rejection of first-set homografts in man [30]. Here again, 10 of 14 skin grafts from donors whose leukocytes had not been used to pre-immunize the recipient showed an accelerated rejection or white graft when placed for the first time on the recipient immunized by nondonor leukocytes. The efficacy of immunization with donor cells depends on the route of administration. In both man [30] and the experimental animal [31], the immunizing effect of homologous leukocytes in subsequent skin homografts is considerably more effective when they are given intradermally than when given intravenously. It is of interest that patients with disseminated lupus, one of the typical "autoimmune diseases" in man, showed a similar delayed type of hypersensitivity when given injections of their own leukocytes as well as those obtained from other donors [32]. A normal individual shows no such reaction on injection of autologous leukocytes. Although the similarities of these responses in man and animal are striking, man is a much more complex animal than the guinea pig in characteristics other than his heterozygosity. Our failure to correlate the results in man of histocompatibility tests by the techniques proposed by Brent and Medawar [26] and by direct skin grafting must be viewed in this light. These difficulties can be no better explained than by the fact that it is possible to inhibit completely the skin reaction to tuberculin by hypnotic suggestion in man [33] (although no change in the degree of cellular infiltration is evident on biopsy). A unique difference in skin reactivity between man and the experimental animal has been described by Lawrence *et al.* [34], who pointed out that it is possible to transfer delayed hypersensitivity to skin homografts in man with cell-free leukocyte extracts. This is not possible in the experimental animal.

Other factors which may affect immunity elicited in man by skin homografts, and thus the survival of these grafts, are indicated in the following studies. Our group [35] has demonstrated the long survival of skin grafts in uremic patients. This appears to be true in other patients with serious illnesses such as burns [36], and lymphoma [37], and other forms of cancer. This modification of the immune response to skin grafts in chronically ill patients is exemplified by the fact that in one patient with chronic lymphatic leukemia, a human skin homograft survived for 300 days [38]. He subsequently received a heterograft of pig skin which survived for 33 days! In the patients with lymphoma and leukemia it is possible that abnormalities of the lymphopoietic, and thus the antibody-forming, system may account for prolonged survival, since it has been demonstrated that in patients with congenital aplasia of these tissues, the skin grafts may survive for prolonged periods [39].

MARROW TRANSPLANTATION

In 1951, Jacobson *et al.* [40] pointed out that the intraperitoneal injection of isologous splenic tissue decreased mortality of mice given large doses of radiation. Subsequent work by a number of investigators suggested that this was due to repopulation of marrow by primitive hemopoietic cells originating in the spleen. Later work [41] showed that radiation injury may be modified by bone marrow injection in mice and guinea pigs. By the use of cell markers such as chromosomes, the specific female configuration of polymorphonuclear leukocytes in rabbits, and weak erythrocyte antigens, it has been shown without question that hemopoietic tissue destroyed by large doses of radiation may be repopulated by the donor source, which then continues to proliferate, producing erythrocytes, leukocytes, and platelets of donor origin. Of particular interest was the demonstration by Main and Prehn [42] that once the homologous marrow was successfully established, the marrow recipient would also "tolerate" skin grafts from animals isologous with the marrow donor, thus confirming the evidence from other experiments that once tolerance has been produced to one tissue, such tolerance holds for all tissues. Since, however, the donor tissue is also immunologically competent, it is quite capable of reacting against the host, and the resultant graft-versus-host reaction or homologous disease has been extensively studied [43–45]. Since, as has been mentioned elsewhere, fetal tissue has not yet obtained immunological competence, the use of fetal hemopoietic tissue to prevent deaths in radiation chimera has been tried with some success [46]. With this brief background, we may now discuss the problem of marrow transplantation in man.

Woodruff quotes Migdalska [47] as describing the experiments of Raszek, who attempted to treat lymphatic leukemia and pernicious anemia by transplantation of bone marrow in 1939. The current status of marrow transplantation in man was reviewed by Ferrebee and Thomas [48] in 1960. The infusion of homologous and isologous marrow in man for the treatment of leukemia following large doses of radiation has received much attention. Marrow has been obtained from cadavers, fetuses, ribs removed at surgery and multiple biopsy aspirations of living donors. The tissue may be injected directly after suspension in Hank's medium and filtering, or it may be preserved frozen in glycerol. It has been shown that man can withstand 2,000 r of continuous whole-body exposure to x-rays if the dose is administered slowly enough. This is adequate to destroy completely lymphopoietic and hemopoietic function. The therapeutic efficacy of this technique in man has been extremely limited, although some success has been obtained in dogs. Thomas *et al.* [49] reported on five patients with acute leukemia treated by total body irradiation and bone marrow infusion. As much as 2,000 r was given. Two of the patients received marrow from identical twin donors. In one patient, evidence of marrow repopulation from another's tissue was obtained, but not in two others. In one identical twin, recipient marrow function returned but the patient died of recurrent leukemia after 72 days. In the other identical twin, partial marrow recovery was evident at autopsy, but death from jaundice occurred at 20 days. One of the patients who received fetal hemopoietic tissue showed no evidence of marrow repopulation at autopsy. Infection from gram-negative organisms and fungus were major problems. The authors were impressed by the possibility that failure of the marrow in one instance might have been due to prior sensitization of the recipient to homologous cells as a consequence of previous transfusion. They had some evidence also that immunologically competent lymphocytes contained in fresh blood transfusions after irradiation might lead to a graft-versus-host reaction. These investigators believe that it might be possible to avoid such reactions by exposing fresh blood to large doses of radiation prior to its administration. Such irradiation, in theory, would destroy the capacity of the transfused lymphocytes to react against the host.

Mathé *et al.* [50] had similar experience with bone marrow grafts in infants with leukemia. One patient had the characteristic signs of "the secondary or homologous syndrome" with fever, anorexia, diarrhea, dermatitis, and desquamation. This syndrome has also been seen by Mathé [51] in adults in whom apparently bone marrow was repopulated by homologous marrow. Mathé, too, has suggested the transfusion of bone marrow in individuals exposed accidentally to large doses of irradiation. In a group of subjects studied following accidental exposure to irradiation Mathé [52] found some evidence of temporary survival of bone marrow, but in none of the individuals so treated was there more than temporary survival. However, he concluded that temporary repopulation may be helpful in maintaining the patient until regeneration of his own marrow has occurred. This experience has been true generally until the most recent case reported by Mathé and his colleagues [53] in which a 26-year-old man with lymphoblastic leukemia received bone marrow from multiple donors. In this instance, six donors were used and the patient received both x-ray and chemical immunosuppressive therapy before marrow transplantation. He was alive and well six months after this experience, with evidence of survival of bone marrow obtained from one of the donors. This donor previously had been shown to be the most closely related by the histocompatibility test of Dausset [21]. It was felt that the recipient had "selected" the most compatible donor, and this was confirmed by the fact that skin grafting at a later date showed rejection of all other donors but survival of both the autologous graft and that of the marrow donor. It is of particular interest that the patient underwent a crisis characterized by many of the manifestations of the secondary syndrome and apparently was able to overcome this in spite of the persistence of donor marrow. This phenomenon has also occurred in animals, and the suggestion has been made that while the host lymphocytic cells are destroyed by radiation, the donor's more differentiated lymphocytic cells consume themselves in reactions against tissue antigens, leaving less well differentiated cells which become "tolerant" to the host. It is possible also that the lymphocytic cells of donor origin undergo changes similar to the transformation achievable in bacterial species [54], allowing them to adapt themselves to host antigens.

Transplantation of bone marrow has been attempted in the therapy of hypoplastic anemia [55]. Apparent remissions accompanied by reticulocytosis were obtained in a few instances. X-irradiation and antimetabolites obviously could not be given because of the nature of the underlying disease. The donor marrow was not tagged, and it could not be ascertained with certainty whether the patients who responded did so as a result of transplantation or because of recovery of their own marrow. However, patients who received marrow from closely related donors seemed to respond significantly better than those given marrow from unrelated donors. In three instances, splenectomy two weeks after transplantation led to a sustained, prompt rise in hemoglobin, white cell, and platelet values. It was concluded, however, that "the value of bone marrow infusion in the treatment of hypoplastic anemia is uncertain."

The use of autologous bone marrow collected prior to irradiation of patients with widely disseminated neoplastic diseases and replaced following treatment as an autotransplant was first reported by Kurnick *et al.* [56] and has been studied by a number of workers. Evidence of repopulation of a marrow made hypoplastic by irradiation was obtained in several instances, and this experience has been repeated [57]. However, autologous marrow did not contribute effectively to hemopoietic regeneration in a group of patients given large doses of nitrogen mustard [58].

The mechanism of rejection of skin grafts and bone marrow in man has been dealt with in some detail because much of what we know of graft rejection in animals has been learned from orthotopic skin grafts or by the injection of marrow or spleen cells as suspensions of homologous or isologous tissue. The parallel between graft rejection in man and similar rejection in animals (on which there are abundant data) is therefore more clearly compared. The rejection or retention of homografts other than skin and marrow appear to follow the same basic rules in the human species. Grafts of blood vessels and bone are destroyed, and their usefulness is not as living viable tissue but as a supporting structure or bridge over which the host's own tissue may grow.

CORNEAL TRANSPLANTS

The cornea appears to survive in man as a successful homograft largely because it is not vascularized. In animals, when the cornea is transplanted to the anterior chest wall where it is vascularized, it is destroyed in much the same way as any other homograft, and presumably this fact holds also for man. Although this seems to be the most probable explanation of prolonged survival of the cornea, it has also been suggested that the cells of the graft may have been systematically replaced by host cells [59] or that some form of adaptation may have taken place.

ENDOCRINE AND GONAD HOMOGRAFTS IN MAN

Transplantation of endocrine tissue and gonads in man has received extensive attention. Excellent bibliographies of this work are to be found in Woodruff's book [14] and in the review of Brooks [60].

In all of these tissues, the same general laws relating to histocompatibility appear to apply. It is possible, though not probable, that the human ovary may be less antigenic than skin, as appears to be the case in certain animal strains [61]. The successful results reported with endocrine tissue grafts in man may have been due to regeneration of remnants of the patient's own tissue or to supplies of hormones passively transferred with the graft. In many instances, particularly those involving homografting or heterografting of gonads, improvement might have been purely psychological. Convincing evidence that such homografts function must be based either on histological evidence of homograft survival and proliferation or on the results of stimulating the homografts with trophic hormones. This evidence is almost completely lacking, with extremely rare exceptions. In the case of the parathyroid, the issue is confused by the ability of the organism to adapt after a certain period to total absence of parathyroid tissue, even in the absence of a homograft.

In a few isolated instances, questionable success seems to have been obtained. Goldzieher and Barishaw [62] reported that some functioning cortical tissue was seen at autopsy following an adrenal transplant. Broster and Gardner-Hill [63] described remarkable clinical improvement following transplantation of an adrenal into a patient with Addison's disease. However, clinical improvement is not a reliable criterion of graft survival. These criticisms apply also to grafts of thyroid and of parathyroid tissue. The most impressive series with parathyroid tissue is that of Gaillard [64]. This author, using parathyroid from fetuses and infants dying soon after birth, cultivated the tissue for a time in a medium containing serum from the prospective host. Gaillard reported on 30 patients treated in this way, 7 of whom appeared to be cured and 2 showed some improvement. No biopsy specimens were examined, so the significance of the apparent success is therefore uncertain. Brooks *et al.* [66] employed grafts of ovary and adrenal protected in millipore diffusion chambers. Some temporary evidence of hormone secretion was obtained for short periods, but ultimately all of the grafts failed. Interestingly, the failure here was not a typical rejection of the transplanted tissue by the host; this apparently was prevented by the diffusion chamber. However, the pores of the diffusion chamber became plugged with host tissue cells, preventing adequate oxygenation and nutrition of the graft. Upon removal, millipore chambers frequently contained only a few apparently viable cells and much fibrous tissue. Brooks *et al.* [66] recently placed fragments of an insulin-secreting adenoma of the pancreas in millipore chambers and transplanted them in two diabetics. They observed a significant decrease in the patients' insulin requirements for four months. Eventually, however, none of the grafts was successful, and at the present writing the grafting of endocrine tissue and gonads in man is not a feasible procedure.

TRANSPLANTATION OF THE KIDNEY

Of the vascularized tissue grafted in both man and animal, the kidney has been most extensively studied. A kidney transplanted from one individual to another of the same species, either human or animal, generally fails to survive. There are, however, some differences between the kidney and other tissues which advantageously affect the survival of the former. First, the transplanted kidney represents a large antigenic dosage, and large doses of antigen are known to produce tolerance more effectively than smaller ones, as has been pointed out elsewhere. Second, antigens shed from a transplanted kidney reach the recipient by the intravenous route, i.e., the renal vein. It is known that intravenous administration of the antigen is preferable to subcutaneous or intracutaneous administration in the production of tolerance. The kidney also represents a large dosage of actively metabolizing viable tissue, and cell viability is one of the prerequisites to the production of homograft tolerance. Properly, it is also possible to demonstrate that the kidney is incapable of forming antibodies against the host [67, 68] and thus producing a graft-versus-host reaction, frequently seen with successful grafts of spleen cells or bone marrow. From the point of view of the potential human donor the kidney has a special place also. The normal donor has two kidneys and can live perfectly well with only one. On the other hand, the potential recipient needs only one kidney to live a normal life-span. Furthermore, recipients of transplanted kidneys should be chronically uremic, and it has been pointed out previously that such patients tolerate grafts of skin (and presumably kidney) better than normal healthy individuals [35].

The sequence of events which take place when a kidney is homografted resembles in many respects the changes which follow a skin homograft, always keeping in mind the fact that such studies have not taken into account the chance similarity or disparity of antigenic configuration of donor and recipient and, in man, the effect of uremia. In the dog, the autograft and homograft behave similarly for the first three or four days. Secretion of urine continues in normal quantities for the first few days, the urine containing traces of albumin and occasional casts and red cells. On the third or fourth day, however, a noticeable difference between homograft and autograft appears. The blood urea nitrogen in dogs with the homograft begins to rise. The urine contains more albumin, red cells, and occasionally red cell casts. The urine volume diminishes and the urine becomes isotonic with plasma. The kidney fails to concentrate even on Pitressin stimulation. Finally, the secretion of urine ceases, and the animal dies shortly thereafter of uremia.

Serial biopsies of autografted kidneys show few or no changes or, rarely, degenerative tubular lesions secondary to ischemia induced by narrowing of the renal artery. Occasionally in dog autografts and in grafts between identical twins, one may see odd foci of round cell infiltration. The histological changes of the homograft, however, follow a predictable sequence. Initially, these changes are localized largely to the cortex. Classically focal interstitial infiltrations are seen, localized around the glomeruli and the small vessels. The small arteries and the thin-walled subcapsular veins are particularly affected. The glomeruli themselves appear to be normal. The cellular infiltrate consists largely of mononuclear cells, of which roughly one half are small lymphocytes and the rest larger mononuclear cells with varying forms showing marked pyroninophilia. Clumps of these cells are scattered throughout the interstitium, some having no discernible relation to the glomeruli or blood vessels. At a later stage one may see proliferation of the endothelium of the small arteries sufficient to reduce the size of a lumen. In the small arteries, fibrinoid necrosis may involve the whole of the vessel wall, and the vascular changes may be similar to those seen in malignant hypertension. At this stage, the tubules themselves are widely separated by edema, cellular infiltration, and occasionally hemorrhage. With further necrosis and interstitial hemorrhage, polymorphonuclear leukocytes appear.

When a kidney is transplanted into an animal previously sensitized to the tissue antigens of that animal, an "accelerated rejection" occurs which differs histologically from that occurring in a first-set graft. After four days, the reaction in the "second-set" kidney is one of extensive edema and hemorrhage in the interstitial tissue, with a lesser accumulation of pyroninophilic cells. The tubules are more widely separated by edema and have undergone much more severe degenerative changes, including necrosis. Now one finds that the glomeruli themselves are involved, with the tufts showing swelling and increased cellular pyroninophilia and in some instances even fibrin thrombi. The function of these kidneys is impaired within the first twenty-four hours, and urine secretion virtually ceases at the end of the third day.

In the human recipient of a kidney transplant, the changes are similar but somewhat more variable [69]. In patients in whom no attempt was made to modify the immune response, the histological findings were complicated by infection which obviously modified the cell type found in the renal interstitium. In the chronically uremic human recipient, homograft rejection did not follow a regular pattern. Although cellular infiltration occurred, prolonged periods of renal homograft survival have been observed. In one of our first unmodified human homografts, the kidney functioned well for five and one-half months. This kidney was obtained from a cadaver and the recipient had chronic uremia. The transplant at autopsy showed "round cell infiltration, marked polymorphonuclear infiltration, and marked arteriosclerosis involving both small and large vessels." In the case reported by Michon *et al.* [70], in which donor and recipient were closely related and in which the recipient was acutely, rather than chronically, uremic, the histological picture more closely resembled that in the experimental animal. Human identical twins behave as individuals of an isologous animal strain. Provided the technical procedure is satisfactory, no rejection response occurs and the kidney may survive indefinitely [71]. In spite of this, however, 6 of our 25 identical twins have developed glomerulonephritis (histologically similar to the disease in their own kidneys) in the transplanted kidney.

In the first successful kidney homograft between nonidentical twins [72], advantage was taken of the fact that there was considerable sharing of tissue antigens. The healthy donor twin rejected a skin graft from his sick brother, but only after twenty-three days. He did, however, show accelerated rejection of a second skin homograft. The immune response of the recipient was modified by whole body irradiation (450 r). The kidney homograft functioned well, both of the diseased kidneys of the recipient were removed, and he is alive and well more than five years after the procedure. In this patient was demonstrated for the first time in man an important phenomenon which has been a part of all subsequent homografts between donor and recipient pairs who are not identical twins. At six months the recipient began to reject his kidney at a time when the skin graft was also rejecting. Biopsy at this time showed round cell infiltration of the renal homograft. Further whole body irradiation and large doses of cortisone completely reversed the findings in the urine sediment, and the patient has had normal renal function while receiving small doses of cortisone since that time.

This episode delineated the fact that in man, *partial tolerance* (i.e., retention of a renal homograft for six months) could be obtained between closely related individuals with the aid of immunosuppressive therapy. It demonstrated also that once rejection became apparent, it could be *reversed* by further immunosuppressive therapy. In all subsequent cases in which the homograft has been partially tolerated for more than a few days, these episodes of beginning rejection have occurred and have been "aborted" by the use of steroids or other immunosuppressive agents. More recently, immunosuppressive therapy in the form of antimetabolite drugs has replaced x-irradiation in our hands [73], although the latter seems still to be effective if properly administered. Rejection response has varied from the appearance of proteinuria and red cells or casts, without other phenomena to fever, oliguria, massive hematuria, and necrosis of the graft. In some instances it appears that presensitization of the recipient by the white cell or platelet elements of blood transfusion has resulted in sensitization to these elements which cross-sensitizes them to the vascular endothelium of the renal homograft. In such instances, the homograft may function well for two or three days and then suddenly cease to function. The histological picture in such kidneys is that of diffuse vasculitis with thrombosis of the afferent arterioles of the glomeruli, infarcts of the glomeruli, and diffuse interstitial hemorrhage. It is possible to reproduce such lesions in the dog by prior sensitization of the recipient to platelet transfusions from the kidney donor. Evidence of early rejection of a kidney may be found in the urine by the appearance of large atypical lymphocytes with eccentrically placed nuclei, one or two nucleoli, and a granular cytoplasm. The administration of large doses of corticosteroids results in disappearance of these cells from the urinary sediment and improvement in renal function.

It seems probable from these data, and from the data previously mentioned pertaining to the rejection of skin grafts, that involvement of the vasculature plays a primary role in the rejection process. The role of the cellular infiltrate is unclear and seems to bear little, if any, quantitative relation to the impairment of renal hemodynamics. In the homografts surviving for more than one year, large focal collections of round cell infiltrates are found in individuals with relatively normal kidney function. This observation is particularly true in the dogs in whom homografts have been maintained for more than two years with immunosuppressive therapy. On the other hand, in a series of cases of cadaver transplants reported by Porter [19], diffuse vasculitis with marked narrowing of the vascular lumen has been seen within a period of weeks or months.

In man, recent evidence suggests that the use of immunosuppressive therapy with x-irradiation or with antimetabolites and steroids may result in marked prolongation of a renal homograft. Although thymectomy and splenectomy have both been used to modify the immune response in human renal transplantation [74], there is no real evidence that it prolonged the life of the graft. One of the individuals treated by Hamburger [19] with x-irradiation alone developed lobular glomerulonephritis in the transplant and died of this disease. Whether or not the rejection process or the immune process related to the original disease may slowly and insidiously destroy the transplant after months or years remains to be seen. At the present time, however, it is certainly possible to modify the rejection response in human renal homografts for considerable periods and with adequate renal function. As in the animal experiments, it appears that the more closely related the individuals, the better the tolerance for the graft and the less immunosuppressive therapy is necessary. It thus appears that, with one most recent and important exception, human renal homografting follows the general biological laws for tissue grafting in the mouse; i.e., the closer the antigenic relationship, the longer the period of tolerance and the less immunosuppressive therapy necessary to repress the rejection response. This most recent "exception" is the grafting of two chimpanzee kidneys to a human subject, with good function for more than sixty days but failure shortly thereafter [75]. The lessons to be derived from this fascinating experience with a heterograft are still unclear.

In man, the liver, lung, and spleen have been transplanted as homografts. All appear to have functioned temporarily but not permanently. It is unclear why the liver, which technically can be successfully transplanted, which certainly has no more antigenic potential than the kidney, and which constitutes a large vascularized homograft, should not be at least as successful as a kidney homograft. Preliminary evidence indicates that failure is due to a diffuse but patchy involvement of the hepatic vasculature.

REFERENCES

1. Medawar, P. B. Immunological Tolerance. *Le Prix Nobel en 1960,* Stockholm, 1961.
2. Medawar, P. B. The behavior and fate of skin autografts and skin homografts in rabbits. *J. Anat.* 78:176, 1944.
3. Medawar, P. B. A second study of the behavior and fate of skin homografts in rabbits. *J. Anat.* 79:157, 1945.
4. Holman, E. Protein sensitization in isoskin-grafting: Is the latter of practical value? *Surg. Obstet. Gynec.* 38:100, 1924.
5. Converse, J. M., and Rapaport, F. T. The vascularization of skin autografts and homografts: An experimental study in man. *Ann. Surg.* 143:306, 1956.
6. Rapaport, F. T., Thomas, L., Converse, J. M., and Lawrence, H. S. The specificity of skin homograft rejection in man. *Ann. N.Y. Acad. Sci.* 87:217, 1960.
7. Marshall, D. C., Friedman, E. A., Goldstein, D. P., Henry, L., and Merrill, J. P. The rejection of skin homografts in the normal human subject: I. Clinical observations. *J. Clin. Invest.* 41:411, 1962.
8. Henry, L., Marshall, D. C., Friedman, E. A., Dammin, G. J., and Merrill, J. P. The rejection of skin homografts in the normal human subject: II. Histological findings. *Ibid.,* p. 420.
9. Merrill, J. P., Murray, J. E., Harrison, J. H., Friedman, E. A., Dealy, J. B., Jr., and Dammin, G. J. Successful homotransplantation of the kidney between nonidentical twins. *New Eng. J. Med.* 262:1251, 1960.
10. Rogers, B. O. The genetics of skin homotransplantation in the human. *Ann. N.Y. Acad. Sci.* 64:741, 1957.
11. Gorer, P. A. The antibody response to skin homografts in mice. *Ann. N.Y. Acad. Sci.* 59:365, 1955.
12. Peer, L. A. Behavior of skin grafts exchanged between parents and offspring. *Ann. N.Y. Acad. Sci.* 73:584, 1958.
13. Rapaport, F. T., Lawrence, H. S., Thomas, L., Converse, J. M., Tillett, W. S., and Mulholland, J. H. Cross reactions to skin homografts in man. *J. Clin. Invest.* 41:2166, 1962.
14. Woodruff, M. F. A. *The Transplantation of Tissues and Organs.* Springfield, Ill.: Charles C Thomas, Publisher, 1960.
15. Woodruff, M. F. A., and Allen T. M. Blood groups and the homograft problem. *Brit. J. Plast. Surg.* 5:238, 1953.
16. Newth, D. R. Chance compatibility in homografting. *Transplant. Bull.* 27:452, 1961.
17. Rogers, B. O. Genetics of transplantation in humans. *Dis. Nerv. Syst.* 24:3, 1963.

18. Szulman, A. E. The histological distribution of blood group substances A and B in man. *J. Exp. Med.* 111:785, 1960.
19. *Proceedings of International Conference on Human Renal Homografts.* Washington, D.C.: National Academy of Sciences, 1963.
20. Dausset, J. Iso-leuco-anticorps. *Acta Haemat.* 20:156, 1958.
21. Dausset, J. Iso-anticorps et antigénes de leucocytes et de plaquettes indépendants de ceux des érythrocytes. *Sang* 30:634, 1959.
22. Dausset, J., and Brecy, H. Identical nature of the leucocyte antigens detectable in monozygotic twins by means of immune iso-leucoagglutinins. *Blood* 9:696, 1954.
23. Van Rood, J. J., and Van Leeuwen, A. Leucocyte grouping, a method and its application. *J. Clin. Invest.* 42:1382, 1963.
24. Mathé, G., Amiel, J.-L., and Niemetz, J. Récherche d'un test d'histocompatibilité pour des essais de greffes allogéniques. *Rev. Franc. Etudes Clin. Biol.* 6:684, 1961.
25. Wilson, R. E., Henry, L., and Merrill, J. P. A model system for determining histocompatibility in man. *J. Clin. Invest.* 42:1497, 1963.
26. Brent, L., and Medawar, P. B. Tissue transplantation: A new approach to the "typing" problem. *Brit. Med. J.* 2:269, 1963.
27. Gray, J. G., and Russell, P. S. Donor selection in human organ transplantation. *Lancet* 2:863, 1963.
28. Carpenter, C., Glassock, R., Merrill, J. P., *et al.* Unpublished observations, 1964.
29. Merrill, J. P., Friedman, E. A., Wilson, R. E., and Marshall, D. C. The production of "delayed type" cutaneous hypersensitivity to human donor leucocytes as a result of the rejection of skin homografts. *J. Clin. Invest.* 40:631, 1961.
30. Friedman, E. A., Retan, J. W., Marshall, D. C., Henry, L., and Merrill, J. P. Accelerated skin graft rejection in humans pre-immunized with homologous peripheral leucocytes. *Ibid.,* p. 2162.
31. Medawar, P. B. Immunity to homologous grafted skin: II. The relationship between antigens of blood and skin. *Brit. J. Exp. Path.* 27:15, 1946.
32. Friedman, E. A., Bardawil, W. A., Merrill, J. P., and Hanau, C. "Delayed" cutaneous hypersensitivity to leucocytes in disseminated lupus erythematosus. *New Eng. J. Med.* 262: 486, 1960.
33. Black, S., Humphrey, J. H., and Niven, J. S. F. Inhibition of Mantoux reaction by direct suggestion under hypnosis. *Brit. Med. J.* 1:1649, 1963.
34. Lawrence, H. S., Rapaport, F. T., Converse, J. M., and Tillett, W. S. Transfer of delayed hypersensitivity to skin homografts with leukocyte extracts in man. *J. Clin. Invest.* 39:185, 1960.
35. Dammin, G. J., Couch, N. P., and Murray, J. E. Prolonged survival of skin homografts in uremic patients. *Ann. N.Y. Acad. Sci.* 64: 1967, 1957.
36. Kay, G. D. Prolonged survival of a skin homograft in a patient with very extensive burns. *Ibid.,* p. 767.
37. Green, I., and Corso, P. F. A study of skin homografting in patients with lymphoma. *Blood* 14:235, 1959.
38. Miller, D. G., Lizardo, J. G., and Snyderman, R. K. Homologous and heterologous skin transplantation in patients with lymphomatous disease. *J. Nat. Cancer Inst.* 26:569, 1961.
39. Good, R. A., Varco, R. L., Aust, J. B., and Zak, S. J. Transplant studies in patients with agammaglobulemia. *Ann. N.Y. Acad. Sci.* 64: 882, 1957.
40. Jacobson, L. O., Simmons, E. L., Marks, E. K., Gaston, E. O., Robson, M. J., and Eldredge, J. H. Further studies on recovery from radiation injury. *J. Lab. Clin. Med.* 37: 683, 1951.
41. Lorenz, E., Uphoff, D., Reid, T. R., and Shelton, E. Modification of irradiation injury in mice and guinea pigs by bone marrow injections. *J. Nat. Cancer Inst.* 12:197, 1951.
42. Main, J. M., and Prehn, R. T. Successful skin homografts after administration of high dosage x-radiation and homologous bone marrow. *J. Nat. Cancer Inst.* 15:1023, 1955.
43. Barnes, D. W. H., Ibery, P. L. T., and Loutit, J. F. Avoidance of "secondary disease" in radiation chimeras. *Nature* (London) 181:488, 1958.
44. Trentin, J. J. Induced tolerance and "homologous disease" in x-irradiated mice protected with homologous bone marrow. *Proc. Soc. Exp. Biol. Med.* 96:139, 1957.
45. Trentin, J. J. Tolerance and homologous disease in irradiated mice protected with homologous bone marrow. *Ann. N.Y. Acad. Sci.* 73: 799, 1958.
46. Porter, K. A. Use of foetal haematopoietic tissue to prevent late deaths in rabbit radiation chimeras. *Brit. J. Exp. Path.* 40:273, 1959.
47. Migdalska, Z. Letter cited by Editor. *Blood* 13:300, 1958.
48. Ferrebee, J. W., and Thomas, E. D. Transplantation of marrow in man. *Arch. Intern. Med.* 106:523, 1960.
49. Thomas, E. D., Herman, E. C., Jr., Greenough, W. B., Hager, E. B., Cannon, J. H., Sahler, O. D., and Ferrebee, J. W. Irradiation and marrow infusion in leukemia. *Arch. Intern. Med.* 107:829, 1961.
50. Mathé, G., Bernard, J., DeVries, J., Schwarzenberg, L., Larrieu, M. J., Lalanne, C. M., Dut-

riex, A., Amiel, J.-L., and Surmont, J. Nouveaux essais de greffe de moelle osseuse homologue après irradiation totale chez des enfants: Atteints de leucémie aigue en rémission. *Rev. Hemat.* 15:115, 1960.

51. Mathé, G. Transfusion et greffe de moelle osseuse homologue chez l'homme. *Antibiot. Chemother.* (Basel) 8:395, 1960.
52. Mathé, G. Problèms posés à l'hématologiste par le traitement de sujéts irradiés accidentellement à 'haute dose. *Rev. Hemat.* 15:3, 1960.
53. Mathé, G., Amiel, J.-L., Schwarzenberg, L., Cattan, A., and Schneider, M. Haematopoietic chimera in man after allogenic bone marrow transplantation: Control of the secondary syndrome. Specific tolerance due to the chimerism. *Brit. Med. J.* 2:1633, 1963.
54. Avery, O. T., MacLeod, C. M., and McCarty, M. Studies on the chemical nature of the substance inducing transformation of pneumococcal types. *J. Exp. Med.* 79:137, 1944.
55. McFarland, W., Granville, N., Schwartz, R., Oliner, H., Misra, D. K., and Dameshek, W. Therapy of hypoplastic anemia with bone marrow transplantation. *Arch. Intern. Med.* 108:23, 1961.
56. Kurnick, N. B., Montano, A., Gerdes, J. C., and Feder, B. H. Preliminary observations on the treatment of postirradiation hematopoietic depression in man by the infusion of stored autogenous bone marrow. *Ann. Intern. Med.* 49:973, 1958.
57. Humble, J. C. The application of stored autologous bone marrow in the treatment of advanced malignant disease: (B) Haematological aspects. *Brit. J. Radiol.* 33:393, 1960.
58. Kretchmar, A. L., Andrews, G. A., and Sitterson, B. W. Attempted bone-marrow autografts after large doses of nitrogen mustard. *New Eng. J. Med.* 268:427, 1963.
59. Katzin, H. M. The ultimate fate of the graft. *Am. J. Ophthal.* 33:35, 1950.
60. Brooks, J. R. Greffes de glandes endocrines. In Mathé, G., and Amiel, J.-L. (Eds.). *La Greffe, Aspects Biologiques et Cliniques.* Paris: Masson et Cie., 1962.
61. Krohn, P. L. Ovarian Transplantation in Mice. In Albert, F., and Medawar, P. B. (Eds.), *Biological Problems of Grafting.* Oxford: Blackwell Scientific Publications, 1959.
62. Goldzieher, M. A., and Barishaw, S. B. Transplantation of adrenal tissue in Addison's disease. *Endocrinology* 21:394, 1937.
63. Broster, L. R., and Gardner-Hill, H. A case of Addison's disease successfully treated by a graft. *Brit. Med. J.* 2:570, 1946.
64. Gaillard, P. J. Transplantation of Cultivated Parathyroid Gland Tissue in Man. In Wolstenholme, G. (Ed.), *Preservation and Transplantation of Normal Tissues. Ciba Symp.* Boston: Little, Brown, 1954.
65. Castellanos, H., and Sturgis, S. H. Ovarian homograft survival within millipore filter chambers in the monkey. *Obst. Gynec.* 12:603, 1958.
66. Brooks, J. R., Sturgis, S. H., and Hill, G. J. An evaluation of endocrine tissue homotransplantation in the Millipore chamber with a note on tissue adaptation to the host. *Ann. N.Y. Acad. Sci.* 87:487, 1960.
67. Porter, K. A., and Calne, R. Y. Origin of cells infiltrating skin and kidney homografts. *Transplant. Bull.* 26:2, 1960.
68. Wheeler, H. B., and Corson, J. M. Graft-host interaction after kidney slice transplantation in inbred mice. *Surg. Forum* 11:472, 1960.
69. Hume, D. M., Merrill, J. P., Miller, B. F., and Thorn, G. W. Experiences with renal homotransplantation in the human: Report of 9 cases. *J. Clin. Invest.* 34:327, 1955.
70. Michon, J., Hamburger, J., Oeconomos, N., Delinotte, P., Richet, G., Vaysse, J., and Antoine, B. Une tentative de transplantation rénale chez l'homme: aspects médicaux et biologiques. *Presse Med.* 61:1419, 1953.
71. Merrill, J. P., Murray, J. E., Harrison, J. R., and Guild, W. R. Successful homotransplantation of the human kidney between identical twins. *J.A.M.A.* 160:277, 1956.
72. Merrill, J. P., Murray, J. E., Harrison, J. H., Friedman, E. A., Dealy, J. B., Jr., and Dammin, G. J. Successful homotransplantation of the kidney between nonidentical twins. *New Eng. J. Med.* 262:1251, 1960.
73. Murray, J. E., Merrill, J. P., Harrison, J. H., Dammin, G. J., and Wilson, R. E. Prolonged survival of human kidney homografts by immunosuppressive drug therapy. *New Eng. J. Med.* 268:1315, 1963.
74. Starzl, T. E., Marchioro, T. L., Talmage, D. W., and Waddell, W. R. Splenectomy and thymectomy in human renal homotransplantation. *Proc. Soc. Exp. Biol. Med.* 113:929, 1963.
75. Reemtsma, K., McCracken, B. H., Schlegel, J. U., Pearl, M. A., DeWitt, C. W., and Creech, O., Jr. Reversal of early graft-rejection following renal heterotransplantation. *J.A.M.A.* 187:691, 1964.

22. *Transfusion Reactions*

SCOTT N. SWISHER

BLOOD TRANSFUSION WAS AMONG the earliest attempted heterografting and homografting of tissues to man. The first efforts to transfuse the blood of animals to man now appear irrational and excessively empirical. These crude beginnings led, however, not only to the present highly effective clinical practice of blood transfusion but *also* to important biological concepts concerning the nature of individual differences.

Following prompt recognition of the fact that animal blood could not be transfused to man, the technique of blood transfusion lay essentially dormant until the latter part of the Nineteenth Century. Increasing physiological awareness then accentuated the disastrous effects of severe hypovolemia and anemia and again aroused interest in the possibility of human blood transfusion. Sporadic attempts were undertaken, utilizing a variety of techniques, with donor and recipient paired essentially by chance. The erratic but fairly common clinical disasters following this type of transfusion limited its use. In retrospect, this appears fortunate, since it seems certain that more harm than good would have resulted from unrestricted blood transfusions in the absence of a serological basis for choice of appropriate donors.

Following the monumental discovery by Landsteiner of the major blood groups of man and recognition of their significance for blood transfusion practice, the use of transfusions increased rapidly as improved methods for the technical aspects were developed. The introduction of citrate as an anticoagulant for transfusion and later the development of acidified citrate with added dextrose as a preservative for blood stored *in vitro* are the major technical achievements which led to present-day blood banking and blood transfusion practices.

The discovery of blood grouping systems other than the ABO system, particularly elucidation of the role of the Rh system in so-called intragroup hemolytic reactions and in erythroblastosis fetalis, was a milestone in the development of immunological understanding of blood transfusion. Recognition of the Rh blood grouping system led to development of greatly improved techniques for the detection of isoantibodies. These findings also resulted in vigorous search for still other isoantibody-antigen systems which might be part of known blood groups or evidence of independent blood grouping systems. Out of this research has grown the present concept of the complex antigenic structure of the individual human erythrocyte, reflecting as it does the individual's genetic makeup, now known to be potentially so variegated as to raise the possibility that each individual is, in fact, unique in terms of the constellation of antigenic components present in his erythrocytes.

Broadly defined, a transfusion reaction is any unfavorable effect which follows directly upon the transfusion of donor blood into a recipient. This chapter is restricted to consideration of those transfusion reactions which have an immunological basis. The most important of these immunological incompatibilities are reflected in excessively rapid destruction of the donor's red cells by an immunized recipient. The reverse situation, in which antibodies in the donor's plasma destroy some of the red cells of the recipient, is also encountered. Immune reactions which appear to involve the leukocytes and platelets of the donor or recipient also will be discussed.

CLINICAL ASPECTS OF HEMOLYTIC TRANSFUSION REACTIONS

A hemolytic transfusion reaction may be defined as any situation in which there is abnormally rapid destruction of either donor or recipient erythrocytes following a transfusion. The classic example, which is easily recognizable clinically, involves the rapid destruction of the donor's erythrocytes by the action of an isoantibody in the plasma of the recipient. Slower rates of destruction of donor red cells with little or no associated symptomatology are encountered but may not be recognized unless the *in vivo* life span of the donor erythrocytes is under surveillance. In other circumstances, accelerated destruction of the donor red cells may occur only after a delay of 7 to 10 days, during which primary isoimmunization of the recipient occurs, or after a lag of 3 to 5 days, during which there is anamnestic recall of a prior isoimmunization. The only clinical indications of these delayed and slower processes of red cell destruction may be slight to moderate icterus and the finding that the transfusion has not maintained an increased red cell mass and hematocrit for an appropriate period.

The clinical picture of an acute hemolytic transfusion reaction is well known. Usually there are restlessness, apprehension, and vague general discomfort after only a portion of the donor red cells has been infused. Increasing discomfort, with pain in the extremities and back, air hunger, and a sense of constriction in the chest then develop, followed by tachycardia, falling blood pressure, and clinical shock in severe cases. Hypothermia may occur initially, followed by fever. Transitory suppression of urinary output is common, and in severe cases, particularly when prolonged shock has been encountered, the patient may become rapidly oliguric and then anuric.

The prompt and proper investigation of patients suspected of having hemolytic transfusion reactions is of great practical importance. An attempt to identify with certainty the occurrence of hemoglobinemia as an indication of rapid *in vivo* blood destruction is essential. A sample of blood should be drawn carefully from a vein other than that into which the infusion was given, utilizing a scrupulously dried syringe and needle and a dry test tube. The blood sample may be anticoagulated with appropriate amounts of ethylenediaminetetracetic acid or mixed potassium and ammonium oxalate, in which case the sample should be promptly centrifuged and the plasma examined for the presence of hemoglobin. Significant levels of hemoglobinemia are usually obvious. Identification of free plasma hemoglobin by the use of a hand spectroscope makes the examination more certain, particularly when the plasma is discolored by other pigments. If there is a delay in obtaining the blood sample from the suspected recipient and the recipient has had hemoglobinemia for a relatively prolonged period, the plasma may show brownish discoloration due to the presence of the pigment methemalbumin. Demonstration of this pigment, even in small amounts, by the Schumm test has essentially the same significance in this situation as the direct demonstration of free plasma hemoglobin.

Hemoglobinuria may or may not occur, depending on the level of free plasma hemoglobin that was achieved. Similarly, there may be a variable rise in serum bilirubin. Both of these changes should be searched for, but it should be emphasized that neither constitutes as reliable an indication of acute intravascular hemolysis as the prompt demonstration of free plasma hemoglobin following the suspected hemolytic reaction.

A sample of clotted blood from which serum can be obtained should also be procured promptly from the recipient, and this, with a sample of the red cells and plasma taken directly from the bottle of blood given to the recipient, should be utilized for the serological investigation of donor-recipient incompatibility. It is most important that all specimens be carefully preserved until the immunological basis of the transfusion reaction has been identified.

The management of patients with hemolytic transfusion reactions is directed toward prompt correction of hypovolemic shock with plasma volume expanders and compatible fresh blood if necessary, correction of dehydration, and observation of the patient for development of oliguria and anuria. If anuria supervenes, the problem becomes one of management of fluid, electrolyte, and caloric intake to minimize endogenous protein breakdown and prevent excessive body fluid accumulation which may lead to pulmonary edema and death. With proper management, mortality should be low even in patients in whom complete anuria develops, provided they can be carried long enough to permit tubular regeneration and restoration of renal function [1].

SEROLOGY OF INCOMPATIBLE TRANSFUSION REACTIONS

The blood grouping isoantibodies of man appear either spontaneously or as a result of known immunizing antigenic exposure, such as occurs with blood transfusion or pregnancy. The reason for the regular appearance of anti-A and anti-B in the sera of persons lacking these red cell antigens, and the occasional spontaneous appearance of isoantibodies of other specificities, is unknown. It has been proposed that these isoantibodies are in fact due to immunization and develop because of contact with substances in the environment having essentially the same specificity as the red cell antigen. This hypothesis remains unproved but seems quite tenable, particularly in the case of blood group A and B substances, which seem to appear widely in nature [2].

Blood grouping antibodies exhibit a great deal of diversity in serological behavior. In the past, this led to substantial confusion when it was assumed that at least the major differences in serological behavior were associated with peculiarities of the molecular species of antibody involved. Although certain differences in serological behavior of blood group isoantibodies are now clearly recognized as related to the molecular characteristics of an antibody, major attention is focused on the diversity of antigen sites on the erythrocyte surface in relation to differences in serological characteristics.

Isoantibodies may agglutinate red cells suspended in saline or hemolyze them in the presence of fresh serum which provides complement (C′). Antibodies having either of these properties are termed "complete." By contrast, many isoantibodies require modification of the physicochemical conditions of agglutination tests or the use of antiglobulin sera for their demonstration. These isoantibodies are "incomplete." Although the two terms are ingrained in the literature, they are unfortunate in that they suggest basic differences in the molecular structure of isoantibodies; this does not seem justified in the light of present knowledge. Antibodies which fail to agglutinate in one test system may agglutinate strongly in a modified system. It would seem to be more useful to regard the antigen-antibody interaction as essentially the same in both instances. However, what may be observed following the antigen-antibody interaction, i.e., agglutination, appears to depend primarily on the conditions of the test and possibly secondarily on the physicochemical characteristics of the antibody involved.

Blood grouping antibodies appear as both 19S (γ_{1M}) and 7S (γ_2) immunoglobulins [3]. Isoantibodies have been sought among the γ_{1A} class of serum proteins with equivocal results. In general, the naturally occurring isoantibodies, as in the ABO system, are found largely to be 19S proteins; isoantibodies which appear as the result of deliberate immunization are primarily 7S proteins. The capacity to agglutinate red cells suspended in saline is also usually associated with 19S antibody fractions, although a major exception exists in the case of the ABO system, in which it has been shown that 7S anti-A and anti-B are also capable of agglutinating saline-suspended test red cells.

A detailed discussion of the serological techniques used to demonstrate isoantibodies *in vitro* is beyond the scope of this chapter. Table 22-1 summarizes the essential characteristics of the basic systems employed now and in the past. Numerous variations of these test systems have been developed and are utilized for special purposes. In addition to hemolysis when fresh serum is present in the test system as a source of C′ and agglutination of test red cells suspended in saline, there are three other basic methods of demonstrating isoantibody activity *in vitro;* (1) alteration of the medium of the test by addition of a colloid, (2) alteration of the agglutinability of the test erythrocytes by treating them with a variety of weak proteolytic enzymes, and (3) use of the indirect antiglobulin technique.

An antiglobulin serum reactive with the γ_2 type of human immunoglobulin (anti-γ) is generally employed, and the attachment of the γ_2 isoantibody molecules to the test red cells is demonstrated directly in this way [4]. The antiglobulin technique provides a second useful mechanism for detection of blood grouping isoantibodies [5]. This involves carrying out the reaction between certain isoantibodies and test red cells in the presence of C′. Partial C′ fixation results, and the presence of C′ protein on the test red cell surface is detected by use of a "non-γ" (anti-C′) antiglobulin reagent. Antiglobulin reagents prepared by using fresh whole human serum as the immunizing antigen may be expected to have both anti-γ and anti-non-γ reactivity. By appropriate additions of purified human γ_2 globulin, the anti-γ_2 reactivity of the serum can be neutralized, leaving the anti-non-γ activity behind. It has been shown that this type of anti-non-γ antiglobulin reaction occurs with the first component of C'_3 (C'_{3a}) at-

TABLE 22-1. Blood Group Isoantibody Serological Methods

Method	Serological Principle of Method	Blood Groups for Which Test Is Useful	Comment
Saline agglutination test	Direct agglutinin activity for red cells suspended in saline solution	ABO MN P Lutheran	Certain sera of many specificities react in this test, best done at room temp. or lower
Colloid media tests	Use of colloid red cell suspension medium to enhance agglutination phase after interaction with an antibody weakly or nonreactive in saline test	Rh	Many colloids can be used: human or bovine albumin, gelatin, dextran, PVP solutions, acacia
Anti-γ antiglobulin test	Use of antiglobulin serum to agglutinate cells coated with γ-globulin isoantibody	Rh Duffy Kell	Original Coombs test involved this mechanism
Anti-non-γ globulin antiglobulin test	Antiglobulin serum vs. complement (C′) component (C'_{3a}) attached to red cell by specific antibody interaction in presence of fresh serum	Lewis Kidd Kell Duffy	Antisera which become inactive in this test may have lost C′ activity by deterioration or become anticomplementary; may be reactivated by adding fresh serum after adsorption
Enzyme test	Use of weak proteolytic enzymes to modify RBC surface and render cells agglutinable by antisera previously nonagglutinating	Lewis Rh P	Many enzymes have been used: trypsin, cholera filtrate, papain, ficin, bromelin; many modifications proposed; enzyme destroys MNSs and Duffy antigens
"Blocking" test	Interaction of test RBC with incomplete antibody renders them nonagglutinable by a complete agglutinin of same specificity	Rh-anti-D	First technique for use in Rh system; of historical interest, largely
Hemolysin test	Production of hemolysis by C′-fixing antibody in presence of fresh human or animal sera	ABO	High ratios of serum to cells required to demonstrate weak hemolysins; of limited use in blood typing or cross-match tests, but of interest in antibody characterization
Lectin test	Use of a plant substance which specifically agglutinates red cells carrying a specific blood group antigen	H antigen of ABO system	Many phytohemagglutinins exist; they are *not* antibodies!

tached to the red cells; this protein has been identified as a β_{1c}-globulin in human serum [6]. Antibodies of the Lewis (Le) blood grouping system are particularly well detected by demonstrating the specific attachment of C′ components to test red cells by the use of anti-non-γ antiglobulin sera. Alternatively, the γ_{1M} antibody molecules of the Lewis system may be demonstrated directly on the surface of the red cells by use of an antiglobulin reagent having anti-γ_{1M} specificity [7].

Complement-dependent hemolysis is demonstrable with many antibodies of anti-A, anti-B, and anti-Le^a specificity. It is irregularly associated with antibodies of other specificities and never with antibodies of the human Rh system. Rare individual Rh antisera capable of producing partial C′ fixation have been demonstrated. Sera of some specificities may not hemolyze human test red cells in the presence of human C′ but may become hemolytic when tested with animal sera as a source of C′. The basis of this interesting difference in the behavior of C′ of various species is unknown.

In recent years, convincing evidence has been presented that not all significant incompatibilities between recipient and donor can be demonstrated by *in vitro* serological methods. This type of incompatibility must be demonstrated by showing that the life span of the donor erythrocytes *in vivo* is significantly shortened in the immunized recipient's circulation but normal in other recipients, and that other normal donor erythrocytes, presumably lacking the important antigens, have normal survival in the immunized recipient. The line of evidence is completed by showing that the donor's erythrocytes survive normally in his own circulation or that there is no clinical or laboratory evidence of a hemolytic process in the donor. Although a humoral isoantibody of the usual kind may not be involved in such incompatibilities, presumably an immune process is involved. In some reported cases, prior, and presumably immunizing, transfusions have been administered. In other instances, transitory and weak serological evidence of donor-recipient incompatibility has been noted at some time. It is also apparent that not all reported instances of this phenomenon fulfill rigid criteria; indeed, other data suggest that there are mechanisms, probably nonimmune in type, which lead to the excessively rapid removal of Cr^{51}-labeled donor red cells [1].

Knowledge of human blood grouping systems has accumulated rapidly in the past fifteen years. Only the briefest discussion of them can be included here. Table 22-2 lists the known human blood grouping systems and summarizes some of their more important characteristics.

The clinical importance of the various blood grouping systems and the several antigens contained in a single system depend on the incidence of each antigen in a randomly selected population of donors and recipients, the immunizing potency of the antigens, and the usual serological characteristics of the antibodies which may be evoked. As can be seen in Table 22-2, blood group antigens occur with widely varying frequency in the randomly selected population. Furthermore, certain antigens occur with substantially different frequencies in populations of varying ethnic origin [8, 9]. An antigen which has very low or virtually universal incidence in a population will cause few antigenic challenges when donors and recipients are randomly paired. On the other hand, when the incidence of the antigen approaches 50 percent, antigenic challenges will occur with maximal frequency if the same policy of donor-recipient pairing is followed. Antigens which are potent, in that they will immunize a large proportion of individuals who are challenged, may cause more frequent isosensitization of recipients, even if the occurrence of antigenic challenge is rare, than in the case of more commonly occurring antigenic challenges with antigens which are relatively incapable of inducing isosensitization. If the antibody resulting from isosensitization is capable of causing rapid *in vivo* destruction of incompatible erythrocytes which might be subsequently transfused, a more hazardous situation will result for the recipient than if the induced antibody were capable of only slow destruction of incompatible red cells. The serological characteristics of an isoantibody are also important in terms of the ease with which it can be detected *in vitro* on subsequent transfusion cross-matches.

The present practice in blood transfusion is to type and match donor and recipient for the antigens of the ABO system and the major antigen of the Rh system, $Rh_o(D)$. This is practical only because virtually all other blood grouping antigens either are rarely involved in an antigenic challenge of a recipient or, more importantly, are relatively incapable of sentisizing eligible recipients. It is both somewhat remarkable and very fortunate that this relatively simple strategy is effective. As can be seen from Table 22-2, with the number of different blood grouping systems and blood grouping antigens known and their distributions in the population, some antigenic differences between the erythrocytes of the donor and those of recipient will occur in a large proportion of transfusions, even when donor and recipient are compatible within the ABO system and for the antigen Rh_o. Indeed, if the antigens present in the donor leukocytes, platelets, and plasma proteins are considered,

*TABLE 22-2. Summary of 10 Human Blood Grouping Systems**

Name of System; Date of Discovery	Major Antigens of System	Approx. Incidence of Major Antigens (Caucasians)†	Original Source of Antibody	Estimate of Antigenicity	Characteristics of Usual Isoantibody	Relative Clinical Importance	Comment
ABO 1900	A_1	37	Naturally occurring reciprocal isoantibodies	Antigenic for all normal persons	Agglutinin and weak hemolysin	Most important	Antibody reciprocal to RBC antigens appears in serum; rare weaker variants of A and B exist
	A_2	10.5					
	B	11.5					
	H‡	Nearly universal	Animal sera	Antigenic for all persons lacking H antigen	Agglutinin (serum of Bombay type person)	Excessively rare	Bombay type lacks H antigen because of rare recessive suppressor gene
MNSs 1927	M	78	Heteroimmune rabbit serum	Low	Cold agglutinin	Little	At least 8 other related antigens have been found; M and N alleles closely linked to S and s alleles; anti-s always due to isoimmunization; others commonly spontaneous
	N	72					
	S	55	Heteroimmune rabbit serum	Low	Cold agglutinin or incomplete	Little	
	s	89	HDNB§				
P 1927	P_1	79	Heteroimmune rabbit serum	? low	Weak cold agglutinin	Little	Anti-P_1 common in serum of P_1 negative persons‖
	$P + P_1$ (T_{ja})‖	99.9+	Isoimmunization	High	Incomplete	Little	Rare isosensitization; Donath-Landsteiner antibody has anti-$P + P_1$ specificity
Rh 1939	Rh_o or D	85	Rabbit anti-monkey serum	Very high	Incomplete	Great	Weak reacting variant, D^u, common
	rh′ or C	70	Human sera from HDNB and hemolytic transfusion reactions	Intermediate to low	Incomplete	Much less than D antigen; next most common problem	No antibody defining expected Hr_o or d antigen; at least 20 related antigens in this system
	hr′ or c	80					
	rh″ or E	30					
	hr″ or e	97					

Lutheran 1945	Lu^a Lu^b	7.6 99.9	Isoimmunized transfusion recipient	Low	Saline agglutinin at room temp.	Very little	Anti-Lu^a much more common than anti-Lu^b
Kell 1946	K k	9 99.8	HDNB	High	Incomplete; may fix C′	Next to Rh system	Several other closely associated or allelic antigens in the system
Lewis 1946	Le^a Le^b	22 72	Normal human serum	Moderate (?) (antibody appears spontaneously)	Saline aglutinin at room temp.; incomplete; fixes C′	Little	6% of persons are Le^a—, Le^b—, Le system involves soluble antigens and is related to secretor gene: Le(a— b+) = secretors, Le(a+ b—) = nonsecretors
Duffy 1950	Fy^a Fy^b	66 80	Transfusion recipient and HDNB	Low	Incomplete; may fix C′	Little	About 68% Negroes are (Fy^a— Fy^b—)
Kidd 1951	Jk^a Jk^b	75 75	HDNB	Low	Incomplete; may fix C′	Little	Rare person is Jk^a—Jk^b—; other alleles probably exist
Xg 1962	Xg^a	F, 88.8 M, 61.7	Transfusion recipient	Very low	Incomplete (requires antiglobulin technique)	Virtually none	Gene responsible for Xg is in X chromosome and thus a sex-linked dominant characteristic

* Diego, Auberger, and Sutter blood group systems await demonstration of independence from other established systems. (Race and Sanger's book [8] is a comprehensive and scholarly source of information on human blood groups.)

† Marked differences in incidence of many antigens are found in different ethnic groups. These differences are of value to physical anthropologists in studies of population migrations and relationships.

‡ Normal serum incomplete cold antibody has anti-H specificity. Pathological cold antibodies frequently have specificity for an antigen, "I," which is nearly universally distributed; this antigen is related to another, "i."

§ HDNB = hemolytic disease of the newborn.

|| Antigens of P system are related in a manner analogous to those of A system: anti-P is analogous to anti-A_1, and anti-P + P_1 (anti-T_{Ja}) to anti-A (i.e., α_1 plus common α). Another rare allele is known in the P system. Persons lacking known P system antigens, phenotype "p," are rare in the population, $<1 : 10{,}000$; they commonly form anti-P + P_1.

Note: In addition, a number of very high incidence antigens, termed "public" antigens, and many very low incidence antigens, termed "private" antigens, are known. These may be part of established systems, but excessively high or low incidence prevents critical tests of independence.

it is reasonable to assume that every transfusion is potentially antigenic. Thus the safety of the recipient of a second transfusion depends on the serological cross-matching procedure to detect isosensitization of that recipient to essentially all erythrocyte antigens except A, B, and D.

MECHANISM OF RED CELL DESTRUCTION ACTIVATED IN VIVO BY ANTIBODIES

There are two general *in vivo* mechanisms of red cell destruction by antibodies. These have been called, somewhat unfortunately, "intravascular" hemolysis and "extravascular" red cell destruction. The intravascular mechanism refers to rapid processes of red cell destruction, such as those brought about by complement-fixing hemolysins. In this instance, red cell destruction *in vivo* and *in vitro* appears to be essentially the same. The extravascular mechanism is, in general, slower and occurs primarily in the liver and spleen, where sinusoidal patterns of circulation are present. With this mechanism, erythrocytes which have interacted with antibodies are first sequestered in either or both of these organs; the final process of disruption of the red cell membrane occurs secondarily.

These two general mechanisms of red cell destruction are not sharply separated. Certain isoantibodies, such as anti-Rh, destroy red cells primarily by the extravascular mechanism, yet commonly cause sufficiently rapid red cell destruction to produce hemoglobinemia, the hallmark of the intravascular mechanism. The occurrence of hemoglobinemia after red cell destruction by what is primarily the extravascular mode is probably related to the rate at which the red cells are sequestered and then broken down. Why this varies when antibodies with different specificity, serological characteristics, and concentration are involved is unknown.

Red cells destroyed by the action of a C′-fixing hemolysin release their hemoglobin directly into the circulation. The mechanism of C′-induced injury to the erythrocyte membrane is not understood in biochemical terms. However, it has been shown that heteroantibodies and C′ can interact to produce functional red cell membrane holes which result in loss of electrolytes and other small molecules but retention of the osmotically active hemoglobin. Red cell destruction in this instance then proceeds by an osmotic mechanism, with cellular swelling, rupture of the membrane, and release of the hemoglobin [10]. More recent work has shown that antibodies of human A specificity do not involve a colloid osmotic process in producing hemolysis, since the primary membrane defect created by the antibody and C′ appears to be sufficiently large to permit direct escape of hemoglobin without the necessity of prior cell swelling [11].

Red cell sequestration seems to be the primary process involved in the extravascular mechanism of red cell destruction. Antibody-coated erythrocytes are removed from the circulation, presumably by the sinusoidal reticuloendothelial (RE) cells of the spleen and liver by some process of cell recognition and trapping, the intimate details of which are not understood. In certain circumstances, particularly when the rate of red cell destruction is relatively low, sequestration is carried out primarily by the spleen. With more powerful antibodies and more rapid rates of red cell destruction, the liver usually plays the more prominent role in the sequestration process. Again, the reason for the differential behavior of these two RE organs is unknown, but may be related to the fact that there are substantial differences in the structure of splenic and hepatic sinusoids. Furthermore, the liver receives a much larger fraction of the cardiac output, and when it is active in removing incompatible erythrocytes, it can be expected to remove more red cells on this basis alone.

Erythrophagocytosis by peripheral leukocytes or the fixed macrophages of the RE system is a known mode of red cell destruction, but its significance has been difficult to evaluate. It has been proposed that erythrophagocytosis is only a final and nonspecific mode of removal of red cells that already have been rendered nonviable by other processes. Conversely, erythrophagocytosis may be a significant primary mechanism of red cell destruction; phagocytes may, in fact, have both types of function. Quantitative measurements of erythrophagocytosis *in vivo* in situations involving antibody-induced red cell destruction have seldom been attempted. As a consequence, little is known of the *in vivo* process of erythrophagocytosis, particularly in man.

Erythrophagocytosis can be induced *in vitro*

in peripheral blood leukocytes by both isoimmune and heteroimmune antibodies. Antibodies capable of inducing this phenomenon appear to be capable of fixing C′, including at least the first component of C'_3, which attaches to antibody-sensitized erythrocytes [12]. Thus most of the antibodies capable of inducing this phenomenon *in vitro* are heteroimmune hemolysins or isoantibodies of specificity actually or potentially capable of hemolysis *in vitro,* such as human anti-A, anti-B, and anti-Le^a. Rare examples of human anti-Rh have been encountered which are capable of inducing erythrophagocytosis; these antibodies also fix an incomplete sequence of C′ components and thus do not hemolyze *in vitro.* Recent work has emphasized the importance of energy-producing metabolic processes and physicochemical conditions of the incubation system which affect the capacity of leukocytes to carry out erythrophagocytosis *in vitro* [13].

Detailed physicochemical and biochemical studies of the changes induced in red cells by interaction with antibodies are greatly needed. Information of this type may be crucial to the understanding of all mechanisms of red cell destruction initiated by antibodies. Certainly in the case of hemolysis by C′, a major change is produced in the character of the red cell membrane, involving relatively large membrane defects of macromolecular size. Changes in the glycolytic processes of red cells which have interacted with antibodies *in vivo* have been observed in experiments carried out in dogs and in infants with erythroblastosis fetalis. The significance of the observed changes is difficult to assess. They may be unrelated to the actual process of red cell damage and may only secondarily reflect changes induced in the cell membrane and its function.

The Cr^{51} technique of labeling red cells permits determination of the *in vivo* survival of small doses of incompatible erythrocytes and relative localization of their fate in the spleen and liver. This method has greatly advanced our knowledge of *in vivo* mechanisms of red cell destruction. The work of Mollison [1, 14] and of Jandl *et al.* [15] is particularly important in this regard. Table 22-3 summarizes the principal results of these investi-

TABLE 22-3. Correlation of in Vitro *and* in Vivo* *Characteristics of Human Blood Group Isoantibodies*

In Vitro Characteristics	Example	*In Vivo* Mechanism of Hemolysis	Principal Organ Site of RBC Removal	Comment
In vitro hemolysis	"Immune" anti-A	Intravascular	RE system	Acts by C′ fixation
Nonlytic agglutinins	Usual anti-A or B, moderate or low titer	Intravascular and ? extravascular	Liver	May fix C′ and hemolyze if small numbers of cells are involved
	Anti-Rh agglutinin, high titer	Extravascular	Liver	If cells are destroyed rapidly, hemoglobinemia may result
	Anti-Lu^b, low titer	Extravascular	Spleen	Very low titered anti-A and anti-B also act by splenic sequestration
Agglutinins active 34°C. and below	Anti-P_1	—	—	*In vivo* destruction may be very slow or inactive
Incomplete C′-fixing antibodies	Anti-Fy^a	Extravascular	Liver	Splenic sequestration if antibody is weak
Incomplete antibody incapable of C′ fixation	Anti-Rh_0	Extravascular	Spleen	Hepatic sequestration if antibody is potent

* Most tests of *in vivo* fate of incompatible red cells are carried out with infusion of very small volumes of erythrocytes, i.e., 1–3 ml.

gations which correlate *in vivo* fate of infused incompatible erythrocytes and *in vitro* characteristics of the isoantibody responsible for initiating hemolysis.

The severity of the clinical manifestations accompanying a hemolytic transfusion reaction, such as cardiovascular collapse and renal injury, may not be related in all cases to the rate of blood destruction alone or to the number of incompatible erythrocytes destroyed. In general, the more serious clinical manifestations are associated with rapid intravascular blood destruction, such as commonly occurs with an incompatibility involving the ABO blood group system. Serious or fatal hemolytic transfusion reactions, primarily due to renal damage which may not have been adequately managed, have been encountered with donor-recipient incompatibilities involving virtually all of the commonly encountered isoantibody specificities.

The mechanism of renal injury produced by incompatible hemolytic transfusion reactions is poorly understood. It does not appear to be due solely to renal filtration by free plasma hemoglobin, although this factor may interact with other injurious effects. Coexistent shock increases the incidence and severity of renal injury after transfusion-induced acute hemolysis. It is probable that some change in the pattern of circulatory perfusion of the renal tubules induced by shock, reflex mechanisms, or vascular obstruction by agglutinated red cells, or other yet unidentified mechanisms will be found to be responsible for the primary injury which ultimately results in acute tubular necrosis.

HEMOLYTIC TRANSFUSION REACTIONS DUE TO INFUSION OF ANTIBODIES

It has long been recognized that transfusion of group O donor blood into a recipient of any other ABO blood group involves the infusion of an antibody which will interact with the recipient's own erythrocytes. This can be done safely in the majority of instances, in which only a few transfusions of group O blood are given, primarily because the antibody is diluted in the recipient's plasma and is distributed over a relatively large mass of the recipient's red cells. When large amounts of group O donor blood are infused into A, B, or AB recipients, particularly those who possess the blood group A antigen, a concentration of antibody in the recipient's circulation sufficient to induce destruction of the recipient's own red cells may be produced. Rare persons of blood group O carry anti-A of extremely high titer in their plasma [16, 17]. A single unit of this plasma (250 ml. or less) may be capable of inducing serious hemolysis of a group A or AB recipient's red cells. Such group O donors are referred to as "dangerous universal donors." It should be emphasized, however, that it is fundamentally the quantitative relationship between the amount of infused antibody and the recipient's red cell mass which determines the safety or hazard of such transfusions. The anti-A of group O donors of the hazardous type commonly exhibits many of the so-called immune characteristics; in particular, it is usually difficult to neutralize this type of anti-A by the addition of soluble blood group A substance. For these reasons, routine addition of soluble A and B substances to group O blood is of limited value in avoiding immune injury to the recipient's erythrocytes. Well-operated transfusion services seldom find it necessary to transfuse a recipient with blood of other than his own major ABO blood group, except in times of emergency when bloods of the less common types are in short supply.

A particularly hazardous situation may be encountered when group O blood is transfused to a recipient of group A_2 or A_2B, particularly in emergency. In this situation, the common alpha antibody of the donor's anti-A will be absorbed by the recipient's group A_2 erythrocytes, usually without resulting hemolysis. This fractionation has the effect of leaving the donor's anti-A_1 antibody circulating in the recipient's plasma. If a subsequent unit of blood, now of the recipient's apparent "A or AB" type, is given again in emergency circumstances without cross-match following the unit of group O blood, a donor of group A_1 or A_1B may be unwittingly chosen. As a result, the second donor's A_1 or A_1B erythrocytes interact with the anti-A_1 now circulating in the recipient. Since there will now be a relatively high ratio of antibody to incompatible erythrocytes, a prompt and severe hemolytic reaction commonly occurs. Fatal outcome has been encountered in this situation.

Hemolytic reactions due to infusion of isoantibodies of other specificity are uncommon.

Mohn *et al.* [18, 19] have shown that relatively large amounts of plasma containing anti-Rh in moderate to low titer may be infused into recipients whose red cells react with the antibody without demonstrable evidence that a hemolytic process has been induced. However, these investigators have shown that a severe hemolytic reaction could be induced by the infusion of an unusual Rh isoantibody of anti-C plus anti-D specificity. This antibody was of very high titer. A prolonged hemolytic episode occurred in the recipient. There was evidence that a self-sustaining type of immune hemolytic process may have been established for a period, occurring a relatively long time after the antibody infusion [18, 19]. It should be emphasized that Rh isoantibodies capable of inducing this type of hemolytic reaction are uncommon. Other investigators have demonstrated somewhat equivocal evidence of hemolysis after infusion of relatively large amounts of anti-Rh with the more commonly encountered characteristics.

The mechanism of red cell destruction induced by infusion of antibodies which react with the recipient's own erythrocytes is probably quite like that which operates in the more common situation of infusion of incompatible erythrocytes. Again, the importance of quantitative relationships between the amount of infused antibody and the red cell mass with which it interacts in determining the mechanism of red cell destruction which is activated has been emphasized by the elegant experiments of Jandl and Kaplan [20]. They have shown that when the ratio of infused antibody to incompatible red cells is low, splenic sequestration of the incompatible erythrocytes occurs if any red cell destruction is induced. When higher ratios of antibody to incompatible erythrocytes are reached, hepatic sequestration with red cell destruction is prominent; at still higher ratios, if the antibody is capable of fixing C′ as in the case of the anti-B studied by these workers, intravascular hemolysis is produced.

Immunized donors may be detected in two ways. The minor cross-match, in which the recipient's erythrocytes are tested with the donor's serum, will detect isoantibodies which may be important to that particular recipient. A more general approach to this problem involves the testing of the sera of all donors with a panel of selected erythrocytes known to contain virtually all of the recognized significant blood group antigens. In this way, immunized donors who may reappear as blood donors at a later date may be detected. This approach is gaining favor in blood transfusion practice, and in a number of institutions the minor cross-match has been abandoned.

OTHER TRANSFUSION REACTIONS WHICH HAVE AN IMMUNOLOGICAL BASIS

Febrile reactions are common among blood transfusion recipients, particularly those who have received multiple transfusions. There is evidence that these reactions are often related to isosensitization of the recipient to the leukocyte and platelet cellular fractions of the infused blood. These reactions have been termed "buffy coat" sensitivity [21]. Direct serological demonstration of the presence of platelet and white cell isoantibodies in a recipient's serum is difficult. The buffy coat sensitivity reaction may be avoided by the simple expedient of removing the donor's platelets and white cells by washing or by filtration or sedimentation techniques. It should be pointed out that probably not all febrile reactions are ascribable to buffy coat sensitivity. Furthermore, not all patients, even those who receive large numbers of leukocytes and platelets by deliberate transfusion, will have buffy coat sensitivity febrile reactions. Even in those showing this type of febrile response, occurrence of the reaction is somewhat erratic and unpredictable.

Shulman [22] has also demonstrated a mechanism by which immunothrombocytopenia may be produced in a recipient some time after a transfusion by inducing isosensitization of the recipient to antigens of the donor's platelets. If donor platelets are still circulating in the recipient when the isoantibody appears, they are rapidly destroyed; by some poorly understood mechanism this also results in removal of many of the recipient's own platelets. Destruction of the recipient's platelets may be sufficiently severe to result in thrombocytopenic bleeding.

Isosensitization of blood transfusion recipients to protein components of the donor plasma has also been reported [23]. This appears to involve allotypic differences in the protein structure of donor and recipient. Clinical phenomena involving this type of donor-recipient incompatibility have not been identified.

Allergic reactions, particularly urticaria, may be induced in recipients following transfusion. The basis of this type of transfusion reaction, which is quite common, is not clear. It is thought to result from the infusion either of a soluble antigen present in the donor's plasma into an allergic recipient or of a donor's antibody to a common allergen to which the recipient is exposed but not ordinarily sensitive.

Blood transfusion immunology is obviously closely related to the problems of hemolytic disease of the newborn. The serological problems and techniques, and the mechanism of antibody-induced red cell destruction, are common to both. Hemolytic disease is, in many respects, analogous to the type of hemolytic reaction encountered following infusion of isoantibodies which interact with a recipient's own erythrocyte antigen. Two factors explain the major differences between these conditions. In hemolytic disease of the newborn, the antibody infusion process is slow and continuing; second, the placenta passes only low molecular weight antibodies of the 7S type from maternal to fetal circulation. Quantitative considerations of the red cell mass and amount of antibody involved are again important. It should be noted that, in general, large amounts of antibody are involved in hemolytic disease of the newborn in this relative sense. Maternal isosensitization by the fetus probably occurs by transplacental hemorrhage of fetal red cells into the mother's circulation. Severe erythroblastosis fetalis is commonly associated with isosensitization of the mother by previous blood transfusion.

REFERENCES

1. Mollison, P. L. *Blood Transfusion in Clinical Medicine.* Springfield, Ill.: Charles C Thomas, Publisher, 1961.
2. Springer, G. F., Horton, R. E., and Forbes, M. Origin of anti-human blood group B agglutinins in white Leghorn chicks. *J. Exp. Med.* 110:221, 1959.
3. Fahey, J. L., and Morrison, E. G. Separation of 6.6S and 18S gamma globulin with isohemagglutinating activity. *J. Lab. Clin. Med.* 55: 912, 1960.
4. Coombs, R. R. A., Mourant, A. E., and Race, R. R. A new test for the detection of weak and "incomplete" Rh agglutinins. *Brit. J. Exp. Path.* 26:255, 1945.
5. Polley, M. J., and Mollison, P. L. The role of complement in the detection of blood group antibodies: Special reference to the anti-globulin test. *Transfusion* (Philadelphia) 1:9, 1961.
6. Müller-Eberhard, H. J., and Nilsson, U. Relation of a β_1 glycoprotein of human serum to the complement system. *J. Exp. Med.* 111:217, 1960.
7. Stratton, F. Complement-fixing blood group antibodies with special reference to the nature of anti-Le^a. *Nature* (London) 190:240, 1961.
8. Race, R. R., and Sanger, R. *Blood Groups in Man.* Philadelphia: F. A. Davis Company, 1962.
9. Mourant, A. E. *The Distribution of the Human Blood Groups.* Oxford: Blackwell Scientific Publications, Ltd., 1954.
10. Green, H., and Goldberg, B. The action of antibody and complement on mammalian cells. *Ann. N.Y. Acad. Sci.* 87:352, 1960.
11. Sears, D. A., Weed, R. I., and Swisher, S. N. Characterization of the mechanism of hemolysis of human erythrocytes by antibody and complement. *J. Clin. Invest.* 42:977, 1963.
12. Nelson, R. A., Jr. Complement and body defense. *Transfusion* (Philadelphia) 3:250, 1963.
13. Greendyke, R. M., Brierty, R. E., and Swisher, S. N. *In vitro* studies on erythrophagocytosis. *Blood* 22:295, 1963.
14. Mollison, P. L. Blood-group antibodies and red-cell destruction. *Brit. Med. J.* 2:1035 and 1123, 1959.
15. Jandl, J. H., Richardson-Jones, A., and Castle, W. B. The destruction of red cells by antibodies in man: I. Observations on the sequestration and lysis of red cells altered by immune mechanisms. *J. Clin. Invest.* 36:1428, 1957.
16. Ervin, D. M., and Young, L. E. Dangerous universal donors: I. Observations on destruction of recipient's A cells after transfusion of group O blood containing high titer of A antibodies of immune type not easily neutralizable by soluble A substance. *Blood* 5:61, 1950.
17. Ervin, D. M., Christian, R. M., and Young, L. E. Dangerous universal donors: II. Further observations on the *in vivo* and *in vitro* behaviour of isoantibodies of immune type present in group O blood. *Ibid.*, p. 553.
18. Mohn, J. F., Lambert, R. M., Bowman, H. S., and Brason, F. W. Experimental transfusion of donor plasma containing blood-group anti-

bodies into incompatible normal human recipients: I. Absence of destruction of red-cell mass with anti-Rh, anti-Kell and anti-M. *Brit. J. Haemat.* 7:112, 1961.

19. Bowman, H. S., Brason, F. W., Mohn, J. F., and Lambert, R. M. Experimental transfusion of donor plasma containing blood-group antibodies into incompatible normal human recipients: II. Induction of isoimmune haemolytic anaemia by a transfusion of plasma containing exceptional anti-CD antibodies. *Ibid.*, p. 130.
20. Jandl, J. H., and Kaplan, M. E. The destruction of red cells by antibodies in man: III. Quantitative factors influencing the patterns of hemolysis *in vivo*. *J. Clin. Invest.* 39:1145, 1960.
21. Brittingham, T. E., and Chaplin, H., Jr. Febrile transfusion reactions caused by sensitivity to donor leukocytes and platelets. *J.A.M.A.* 165:819, 1957.
22. Shulman, N. R. Mechanism of blood cell destruction in individuals sensitized to foreign antigens. *Trans. Ass. Amer. Physicians* 76:72, 1963.
23. Blumberg, B. S., and Riddell, N. M. Inherited antigenic differences in human serum beta lipoproteins. *J. Clin. Invest.* 42:867, 1963.

SECTION II. DISEASES WITH ABNORMAL IMMUNE RESPONSES

23. The Thymus and Immunological Deficiency Disease*

ROBERT A. GOOD, RAYMOND D. A. PETERSON,
AND ANN E. GABRIELSEN

DURING THE PAST FEW YEARS THERE has been impressive progress in our understanding of the functions of the mammalian thymus. Although we tend to think of this progress as stemming from observations made in the very recent past, a considerable body of knowledge concerning the thymus had accumulated before the turn of the century, and intensive investigations of this organ were in progress in the early 1900's. Several figures from this era are of particular interest in the light of the recent findings on the immunological function of the thymus and the mechanism of this activity: John Beard [1, 2], for example, who saw the thymus as the original source of the leukocytes which later populate other body tissues, and J. August Hammar [3], who set the thymus apart from what he called "real lymphoid tissue" and later postulated antitoxic functions of the thymus. Some of these concepts are close to current notions of the "peripheralization" of thymic lymphoid cells, the distinction between central and peripheral lymphoid tissues, and the role of the thymus in the development and sustenance of adaptive immunological function.

The original stimulus to reconsideration of the immunological role of the thymus at the University of Minnesota was a 50-year-old patient with acquired agammaglobulinemia [4–6]. During a period of hospitalization for pneumonia, a mediastinal mass was observed on x-ray studies. The tumor was removed without affecting the immunological deficit, and it proved to be a benign growth, weighing 565 gm., largely epithelial and stromal in composition, and generally lacking in lymphoid elements. The immunological status of this patient was studied intensively: he had a circulating γ-globulin level ranging between 40 and 70 mg. per 100 ml., formed little or no detectable circulating antibody to a wide range of antigens, showed persistent failure of plasma cell formation in lymph nodes and bone marrow under conditions of intense antigenic stimulation, and took three months to reject a skin graft from an unrelated donor.

Since primary acquired agammaglobulinemia is a rare disease and thymoma an unusual tumor, it seemed at the time [4, 7] that this was a meaningful association of immunological failure with thymic abnormality. Up to the present, seven other patients with thymoma and acquired agammaglobulinemia have been observed [8–13], perhaps 7 or 8 percent of the total number of cases of acquired agammaglobulinemia. Several of the eight have had other hematological defects as well; most of these were aregenerative anemia or pancytopenia, but isolated eosinopenia and thrombocytopenia also occurred.

As noted elsewhere [14], agammaglobulinemia-hypogammaglobulinemia occurs in several forms in children. Boys with congenital sex-linked recessive agammaglobulinemia tend to have normal-appearing thymus tissue, although their other lymphoid tissues are usually small and of poor structure [4, 15–17].

* Aided by grants from the National Foundation, the U.S. Public Health Service (HE-02085, AI-00798, 5TI-HE-5462), American Heart Association, and American Cancer Society.

The thymus of such a patient often shows depletion of lymphocytes and varying degrees of atrophy, but usually this has not been more extreme than it would be in an immunologically normal child having a similar infectious illness. The thymic tissue seems to have normal structure, Hassall's corpuscles, and lymphoid elements in each instance (Fig. 23-1).

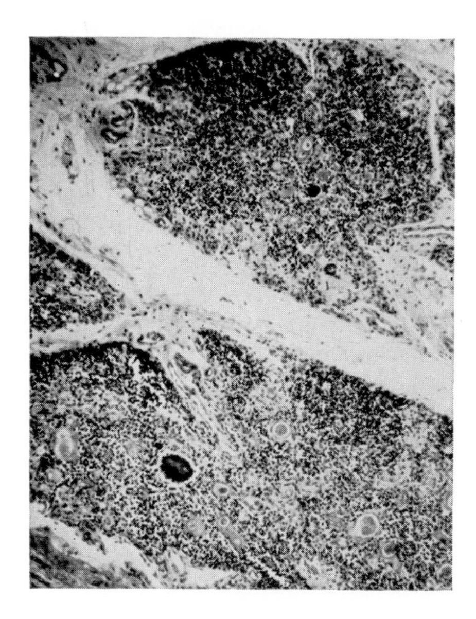

Fig. 23-1. Low-power photomicrograph of thymic tissue from a child with congenital sex-linked recessive agammaglobulinemia. Structure is relatively normal, with Hassall's corpuscles and appreciable number of lymphoid cells. (From Good *et al.* [21].)

Gitlin and Craig [17] recently documented the appearance of the thymic and other lymphoid tissues in their group of children with congenital sex-linked recessive agammaglobulinemia. Although they tend perhaps to emphasize the atrophy and depletion of lymphoid cells, the material they illustrate is quite comparable to ours.

In a second group of immunologically deficient children, those with the Swiss or lymphopenic type of agammaglobulinemia, the thymus has usually been abnormal in both structure and cellular composition and has often, though not always, been a very small organ, weighing less than 1 gm. [18–22]. In one of our patients [21] and in patients studied by Tobler and Cottier [23], the thymus was also in an abnormal location, high in the mediastinum in the thyroid region of the neck. Apparently this represents a failure of descensus, and it suggests that the very abnormal thymus in at least some of these patients is not a result of involution following disease but is a rudimentary tissue that failed to develop.

Although the initial description of this disease, by Glanzmann and Riniker [24] in 1950, came from Switzerland, as have the most definitive studies of the syndrome [18–20, 25] and the characterization of the thymic abnormalities [18–20, 23], patients with this disease have been observed in France [26, 27], in Malmo, Sweden [28], in Canada [29, 30], and in Boston [17, 22] and Minneapolis in the United States. The major threat to patients with sex-linked recessive agammaglobulinemia is bacterial infection with the pyogenic pathogens [14]. The Swiss agammaglobulinemia group, however, is also inordinately susceptible to fungal and virus infections, and these patients have often died of such diseases as *Pseudomonas* pneumonia and overwhelming *Candida* infection [21, 22, 27]. The data available suggest that they have a failure of delayed hypersensitivity and homograft immunity as well [22, 31].

The efforts at replacement therapy in these children have emphasized γ-globulin but generally have not met with success; few of these children have survived to the age of 2 years. Rosen *et al.* [22] undertook the only effort at organ replacement known to us: they grafted thymus tissue from another young child subcutaneously. The period of observation was forty days; as far as could be determined at the time of the recipient child's death, no reconstitution had occurred although the thymic tissue was not rejected. A skin graft remained intact for the same forty days.

We have studied the lymphoid tissues of six lymphopenia-agammaglobulinemia patients, one at the University of Minnesota and five at Children's Hospital, Winnipeg. Figure 23-2 illustrates splenic tissue from one of these patients and Figure 23-3 a lymph node. The spleen has foci of reticulum cell accumulation around the penicillary arteries but lacks true lymphoid development. The lymph nodes are hard to find; when located, they are very small and histologically are almost entirely reticular and stromal in composition, with only a few scattered lymphoid cells. The abnormal thymic tissue of this patient (Fig. 23-4) is very different from the thymus of the

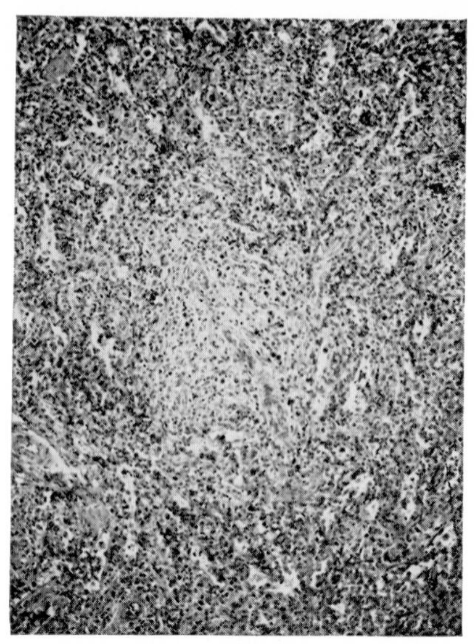

Fig. 23-2. Photomicrograph of splenic tissue from a child with the Swiss or lymphopenic form of agammaglobulinemia. Follicular development is lacking, and lymphoid cells are few.

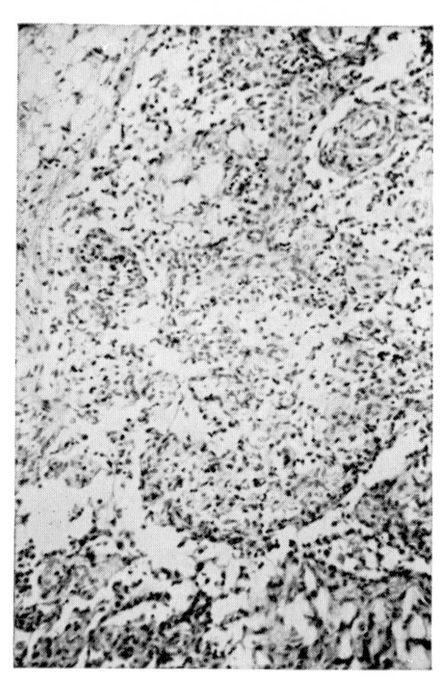

Fig. 23-3. Low-power view of lymph node from a Swiss agammaglobulinemic patient. Lymph nodes in these children are very small and located with difficulty. Microscopic examination reveals a dearth of lymphocytes and absence of characteristic lymphoid structure.

sex-linked recessive agammaglobulinemic patients (Fig. 23-1).

One of the most provocative of the thymus-linked immunological deficiency diseases is the defect associated with ataxia-telangiectasia in children. This rare neurological disease, originally described in 1941 by Madame Louis-Bar [32], has become known in this country largely because of the work of Dr. Elena Boder [33, 34] and her associates in Los Angeles. The disease is characterized by cerebellar ataxia, usually progressive, oculocutaneous telangiectases, and, in 70 to 80 percent of the patients, inordinate susceptibility to respiratory infections. Many of them show striking growth failure as well.

Several other findings suggest that these patients are an extraordinary "experiment of nature" in which thymic abnormality is associated with immunological deficiency, abnormalities of the immunoglobulins, and unusual susceptibility to certain types of lymphoid malignancy [35, 36]. All of these facets of the syndrome have not been observed in all patients; however, one of our patients showed all of them in an extraordinary way. Her ataxia had first become evident at 9 months of age, and her susceptibility to recurrent ear infections and severe pulmonary infections had developed at about 4 and 6 years of age, respectively. Cutaneous telangiectasia was first observed at age 8, at about the time we first saw her. The γ-globulin level was 150 mg. per 100 ml. She formed no antibodies to a variety of bacterial and particulate antigens and did not develop delayed allergy to 2,4-dinitrofluorobenzene despite repeated efforts at sensitization. A skin graft from an unrelated donor survived for an extended period and was thereafter rejected slowly. Eighteen months after our initial evaluation, the child

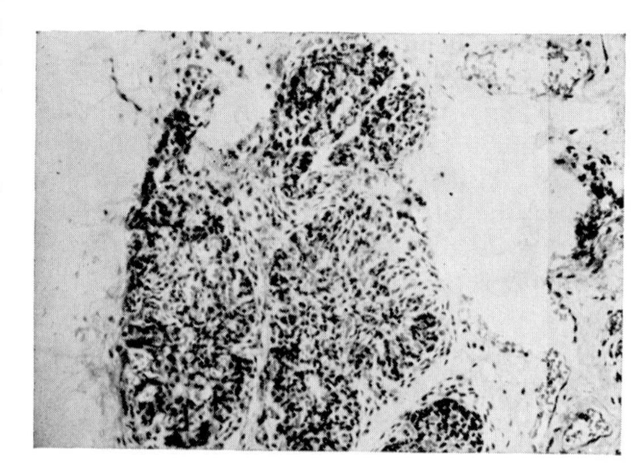

Fig. 23-4. Medium-power view of vestigial thymus tissue from a patient with the lymphopenic form of agammaglobulinemia. The organ, in addition to its very small size, lacked separation of cortex and medulla. Its composition was largely epithelial, with no Hassall's corpuscles and extreme lack of lymphoid elements.

died of lymphosarcoma involving most of the body organs. Although extensive sections of the mediastinal and neck regions were examined, no thymic tissue was found.

In a broad survey of the literature on reported cases of ataxia-telangiectasia, supplemented by a number of personal communications and material from our own laboratories, we have found that 25 to 35 percent of ataxia-telangiectasia patients have definable deficiencies of the immunoglobulins by present criteria [35, 36]. At least 6 have had an epithelial, embryonic type of thymus or no thymus at all, and at least 8 have died of lymphocytic malignancies [36]. Thus, among the estimated 110 reported cases of this syndrome, there is an extraordinary clinical constellation of thymic abnormality, immunological deficiency, and inordinate susceptibility to certain kinds of neoplasia, underscoring the experimentally demonstrated link of thymus and bursa of Fabricius to both the ontogeny of immunity and the development of malignant lymphoma in mice and chickens [37–42]. The relation of these aspects of the ataxia-telangiectasia syndrome to the central nervous system disease and to the cutaneous and visceral vascular ectasia is unknown, but it has been suggested [36] that a faulty mesenchyme may be reflected in abnormal thymic induction, vascular abnormalities, and progressive central nervous system disease. The lymphoma may be a reflection of the presumed failure of thymic induction, but it could also be secondary to the immunological defect: agammaglobulinemic patients without ataxia-telangiectasia also seem to have inordinate susceptibility to neoplasia of the lymphoid system [43–46].

LYMPHOMA AND LEUKEMIA IN AGAMMAGLOBULINEMIC PATIENTS

The relation of the thymus to pathological processes can be extended by consideration of the association of leukemia or lymphoma with the congenital sex-linked recessive form of agammaglobulinemia. Two such cases have been studied in our laboratory. One was a 4½-year-old boy, studied from early infancy because his older brother had sex-linked recessive agammaglobulinemia. He had done well clinically on an antibiotic regimen and had never been given γ-globulin. However, at 3 years and 8 months of age, he received a scalding burn, and treatment included administration of γ-globulin and tetanus antitoxin. Although the burn healed without complication, urticarial episodes began and recurred for several months. At about 4 years of age, he had a sudden onset of fever and lymphadenitis, with evidence of obstruction of venous return from his arms, neck, and head. A large mediastinal mass was seen on chest x-ray films, and hematological studies established a diagnosis of acute lymphatic leukemia. The remissions induced with 6-mercaptopurine and cortisone were brief, and he died of the fulminant leukemic process at 4 years and 4 months of age.

Thus we observed a congenitally agammaglobulinemic child who, following a hypersensitivity type of reaction, developed a leukemic process presenting as a thymic tumor.

The second child also had the typical history of congenital agammaglobulinemia, a succession of recurrent severe respiratory and gastrointestinal infections having their onset at about 6 months of age, following the loss of passively transferred maternal γ-globulin and antibody. At age 2, typical dermatomyositis developed, with edema, muscle weakness, flexion contractures, a heliotrope rash, and atrophic changes at the knuckles, knees, and elbows, and the serious infectious episodes continued. Agammaglobulinemia was definitely diagnosed at age 3, and γ-globulin therapy was begun. The number of infections decreased, but the dermatomyositis progressed. At age 4½, the boy died of an overwhelming infection; at autopsy, characteristic manifestations of lymphoma were found in lymph nodes, liver, and kidneys.

Two instances of this type of malignant development among fewer than 30 patients with congenital agammaglobulinemia suggest a relation between the two conditions. This is supported by two more instances of this type of malignant development in adults with agammaglobulinemia, documented by Fudenberg and Solomon [44], and by a report from Washington University Medical Center [45]. One additional childhood case has also been reported [46], and there are undoubtedly others.

That at least one of these, our first case cited above, should have involved a thymoma again links the thymus with both immunological defect and lymphocytic malignancy, as in ataxia-telangiectasia.

The relation of the mouse thymus to spontaneous and induced lymphomas was first reported in 1944. McEndy *et al.* [37] discovered that removal of the thymus early in life in AK mice, destined by heredity to manifest leukemia in high incidence, reduced markedly the tendency to development of this disease. Others [47–49] have shown a similar effect of early thymectomy on leukemias in mice induced or influenced by radiation, virus, and hormonal manipulation.

About 1950, the thesis of thymic origin of certain human leukemias had some currency, fostered principally by the evidence brought forward by Simmons [50]. Thymectomy in leukemic patients was not clearly of benefit in the investigations of Earle *et al.* [51], and such intervention was unusual until recently. Peterson *et al.* [52] have lately observed a group of leukemic children following thymectomy and, again, have observed no difference in their subsequent course from that of nonthymectomized leukemic children.

In 1955, Thomson [53], who had studied a large series of patients with Hodgkin's disease, suggested that a thymic origin of this disease was usually obscured by the generalized disease process at the time of diagnosis. His conclusion has been disputed [54–56]. Several thymectomies were performed in England on Hodgkin's disease patients, and the results reported in 1963 by Patey [57]. In only two of the five excised thymuses was Hodgkin's disease evident. The question of clinical benefit remained unanswered: all operated patients were alive six years later, but all had been clinically benign prior to surgery.

Many of these observations regarding a possible thymic role in lymphocytic malignancies merit re-examination in the light of the findings in ataxia-telangiectasia and agammaglobulinemia patients as well as the recent experimental extension of the thymus-lymphoma link in mice to another species, the chicken.

THE THYMUS AND AUTOIMMUNE DISEASE

One of the best-known clinical correlates of thymic abnormality is myasthenia gravis. Although the figures vary in different groups of patients, about 15 percent of those with myasthenia gravis have a thymoma, and another 60 to 70 percent have histological abnormalities of the thymus, featuring germinal center formation and plasma cell development. Furthermore, in young women with myasthenia gravis of short duration, thymectomy often results in clinical improvement and at times in cure.

Myasthenia gravis has come to the forefront in the recent consideration of the immunological role of the thymus for several reasons. First, beginning with the work of Strauss *et al.* [58], and continuing with the studies of several other groups of investigators [59–64], it has become evident that myasthenia gravis patients often have antimuscle and antinuclear antibodies. Such authors as Smithers [65] and Simpson [66] have offered other evidence to support the thesis that myasthenia gravis may be an autoimmune disease. (See Chap. 81.) Second, there have been a number of instances of actual symptomatic and pathological overlap of myasthenia gravis and systemic lupus erythematosus (LE) [67–73]. There are reports of several patients with thymoma who appeared to have elements of one or both diseases. Most often they have had myocarditis or myositis or both [74–77]; at least one had a positive reaction to the LE cell test [78]. There have also been some instances of the occurrence of LE and thymoma in the same patient. One of these patients, studied by Larsson [79], had a thymic tumor lacking in germinal center development. Another, observed by Wolf *et al.* [80], had a tumor in which lymphoid constituents were prominent, and configurations of the follicular type were evident. This man was a member of a family group in which immunological abnormalities, blood dyscrasias, and mesenchymal diseases occurred in high frequency. Mackay and deGail [81] described a patient who, in the early stages of LE, had evidence of germinal center formation in thymic tissue removed as a therapeutic measure. The question of the value of thymectomy in these patients is open; in the case reported by Mackay *et al.* [82] and in one observed here [52], there was no clear indication of benefit. There are at least two instances in which systemic LE developed following thymectomy for myasthenia gravis [83].

There are some experimental observations that link the thymus to autoimmune processes. One of these is the regular occurrence of a Coombs-positive hemolytic anemia in strain NZB mice, originally described by Bielchowsky *et al.* [84] and studied further by Burnet and Holmes [85, 86]. A thymic lesion, characterized by germinal center and plasma cell formation, also develops in the course of the illness [85]. Data on a small group of animals completely thymectomized at an early age suggest that the onset of the disease was not much affected by thymectomy; indeed, splenectomy showed greater effects [86].

Helyer and Howie [87] reported extensive studies of thymectomy and thymic replacement in NZB/Bl mice, as well as in the (NZB/Bl $\times$ NZW)F_1 hybrid, which develops positive reactions to LE cell tests and renal glomerulitis in high incidence. Here too, the effect of neonatal thymectomy was negligible. However, neonatally thymectomized CBA animals grafted with thymus from either the NZB/Bl strain or the F_1 hybrid often developed positive reactions to the Coombs and LE cell tests and other characteristics of the thymus donors. On the other hand, grafting of CBA thymus into either of the autoimmune strains did not prevent disease.

THE THYMUS AND OTHER DISEASES

Space does not permit more than mention of certain other diseases associated with thymic abnormality, particularly thymoma. Among these are Cushing's disease [14, 56], nephrotic syndrome [65, 88], and dermatomyositis [89, 90]. The question of specificity has been raised in connection with Cushing's syndrome in particular, since similar tumors in other locations have also been associated with a similar development and since the question of corticosteroid production by the tumors themselves has not been resolved [91–93].

REFERENCES

1. Beard, J. The development and probable function of the thymus. *Anat. Anz.* 9:476, 1894.
2. Beard, J. The source of leucocytes and the true function of the thymus. *Anat. Anz.* 18:550, 1900.
3. Hammar, J. A. The new views as to the morphology of the thymus gland and their bearing on the problem of the function of the thymus. *Endocrinology* 5:543 and 731, 1921.
4. Good, R. A. Agammaglobulinemia—a provocative experiment of nature. *Bull. Univ. Minnesota Hosp.* 26:1, 1954.
5. MacLean, L. D., Zak, S. J., Varco, R. L., and Good, R. A. Thymic tumor and acquired agammaglobulinemia—a clinical and experimental study of the immune response. *Surgery* 40:1010, 1956.
6. Good, R. A., and Page, A. R. Fatal complications of virus hepatitis in two patients with agammaglobulinemia. *Amer. J. Med.* 29:804, 1960.
7. Good, R. A., and Varco, R. L. A clinical and experimental study of agammaglobulinemia. *J. Lancet* 75:245, 1955.
8. Ramos, A. J. Presentation of a case, with discussion by V. Loeb. *J.A.M.A.* 160:1317, 1956.
9. Martin, C. M., Gordon, R. S., and McCullough, N. B. Acquired hypogammaglobulinemia in an adult: Report of a case, with clinical and experimental studies. *New Eng. J. Med.* 254:449, 1956.
10. Lambie, A. T., Burrows, B. A., and Sommers, S. C. Clinicopathologic conference: Refractory anemia, agammaglobulinemia, and mediastinal tumor. *Amer. J. Clin. Path.* 27:444, 1957.
11. Gafni, J., Michaeli, D., and Heller, H. Idiopathic acquired agammaglobulinemia associated with thymoma: Report of two cases and review of the literature. *New Eng. J. Med.* 263: 536, 1960.
12. Rötstein, J., and Good, R. A. Unpublished observations, 1961.
13. Wollheim, F., and Waldenström, J. Personal communication, 1962.
14. Good, R. A., Martinez, C., and Gabrielsen, A. E. Clinical Considerations of the Thymus in Immunobiology. In Good, R. A., and Gabrielsen, A. E. (Eds.), *The Thymus in Immunobiology*. New York: Hoeber Med. Div., Harper & Row, 1964.
15. Good, R. A., and Zak, S. J. Disturbances in gamma globulin synthesis as experiments of nature. *Pediatrics,* 18:109, 1956.
16. Gitlin, D., Janeway, C. A., Apt, L., and Craig, J. M. "Agammaglobulinemia." In Lawrence, H. S. (Ed.), *Cellular and Humoral Aspects of the Hypersensitive States.* New York: Paul B. Hoeber, Inc., 1959.
17. Gitlin, D., and Craig, J. M. The thymus and other lymphoid tissues in congenital agammaglobulinemia. *Pediatrics* 32:517, 1963.
18. Tobler, R., and Cottier, H. Familiäre Lymphopenie mit Agammaglobulinämie und schwerer Moniliasis. *Helv. Paediat. Acta* 13: 313, 1958.

19. Hitzig, W. H., Biró, Z., Bosch, H., and Huser, H. J. Agammaglobulinämie und Alymphocytose mit Schwund des lymphatischen Gewebes. *Ibid.*, p. 551.
20. Hitzig, W. H., and Willi, H. Hereditäre lymphoplasmocytäre Dysgenesie ("Alymphocytose mit Agammaglobulinämie"). *Schweiz. Med. Wschr.* 91:1625, 1961.
21. Good, R. A., Martinez, C., Dalmasso, A. P., Papermaster, B. W., and Gabrielsen, A. E. Studies on the Role of the Thymus in Developmental Biology, with a Consideration of the Association of Thymus Abnormalities and Clinical Disease. In Grabar, P., and Miescher, P. (Eds.), *Immunopathology* (3rd International Symposium). Basel: Benno Schwabe & Co., 1963.
22. Rosen, F. S., Gitlin, D., and Janeway, C. A. Alymphocytosis, agammaglobulinemia, homografts and delayed hypersensitivity: A study of a case. *Lancet* 2:380, 1962.
23. Cottier, H. Discussion. Ref. 14.
24. Glanzmann, E., and Riniker, P. Essentielle Lymphocytophthise: Ein neues Krankheitsbild aus der Säuglingspathologie. *Ann. Paediat.* (Basel) 175:1, 1950.
25. Barandun, S. *Das Antikörpermangelsyndrom.* Basel: Benno Schwabe & Co., 1959.
26. Jeune, M., Larbre, F., Germain, D., and Freycon, F. Lymphocytophtisie, alymphocytose et hypogammaglobulinémie. *Arch. Franc. Pediat.* 16:14, 1959.
27. Sacrez, R., Willard, D., Beauvais, P., and Korn, R. Étude des troubles digestifs et réspiratoires dans un cas de lymphocytophtisie du nourrisson. *Arch. Franc. Pediat.* 20:401, 1963.
28. Waldenström, J. Monoclonal and polyclonal gammopathies and the biological system of gamma globulin. *Progr. Allerg.* 6:320, 1962.
29. Donohue, W. L. Alymphocytosis. *Pediatrics* 11:129, 1953.
30. Medovy, H., Stone, P., and Zipurski, A. Personal communication, 1961–1962.
31. Good, R. A., Peterson, R. D. A., and Gabrielsen, A. E. The thymus; current concepts. *Postgrad. Med.* 36:505, 1964.
32. Louis-Bar. Sur un syndrome progressif comprénant des télangiectasies capillaires, cutanées et conjonctivales symétriques, à disposition naevoïde et des troubles cérébelleux. *Confin. Neurol.* 4:32, 1941.
33. Boder, E., and Sedgwick, R. P. Ataxia-telangiectasia: A familial syndrome of progressive cerebellar ataxia, oculocutaneous telangiectasia, and frequent pulmonary infection. *Pediatrics* 21:526, 1958.
34. Boder, E., and Sedgwick, R. P. Ataxia-telangiectasia. A review of 101 cases. In Walsh, G. (Ed.), *Cerebellum Posture and Cerebral Palsy.* London: William Heinemann, Ltd., 1963.
35. Peterson, R. D. A., Blaw, M. E., and Good, R. A. Ataxia-telangiectasia: A possible clinical counterpart of the animals rendered immunologically incompetent by thymectomy. *J. Pediat.* 63:701, 1963.
36. Peterson, R. D. A., Kelly, W. D., and Good, R. A. Ataxia-telangiectasia: Its association with a defective thymus, immunological deficiency disease and malignancy. *Lancet* 1:1189, 1963.
37. McEndy, D. P., Boon, M. C., and Furth, J. On the role of the thymus, spleen and gonads in the development of leukemia in a high-leukemia stock of mice. *Cancer Res.* 4:377, 1944.
38. Miller, J. F. A. P. The immunological function of the thymus. *Lancet* 2:748, 1961.
39. Martinez, C., Kersey, J., Papermaster, B. W., and Good, R. A. Skin homograft survival in thymectomized mice. *Proc. Soc. Exp. Biol. Med.* 109:193, 1962.
40. Glick, B., Chang, T. S., and Jaap, R. G. The bursa of Fabricius and antibody production. *Poult. Sci.* 35:224, 1956.
41. Peterson, R. D. A., Burmester, B. R., Fredrickson, T. N., and Good, R. A. The prevention of lymphatic leukemia in the chicken by the surgical removal of the bursa of Fabricius. *J. Lab. Clin. Med.* 62:1000, 1963 (abst.).
42. Peterson, R. D. A., Burmester, B. R., Fredrickson, T. N., Purchase, H. G., and Good, R. A. The effect of bursectomy and thymectomy on the development of visceral lymphomatosis in the chicken. *J. Nat. Cancer Inst.* 32:1343, 1964.
43. Page, A. R., Hansen, A. E., and Good, R. A. Occurrence of leukemia and lymphoma in patients with agammaglobulinemia. *Blood* 21:197, 1963.
44. Fudenberg, H., and Solomon, A. Acquired agammaglobulinemia with autoimmune hemolytic disease: Graft-versus-host reaction? *Vox Sang.* 6:68, 1961.
45. Recant, L., and Hartroft, W. S. (Eds.) Clinicopathological conference: Rademacher's disease. *Amer. J. Med.* 32:80, 1962.
46. Reisman, L. E., Mitani, M., and Zuelzer, W. W. Chromosome studies on leukemic children with and without congenital abnormalities. *J. Pediat.* 63:739, 1963.
47. Kaplan, H. S. Influence of thymectomy, splenectomy and gonadectomy on the incidence of radiation induced lymphoid tumors in strain C57B1 mice. *J. Nat. Cancer Inst.* 11:83, 1950.
48. Gross, L. Effect of thymectomy on development of leukemia in C3H mice inoculated with leukemic "passage" virus. *Proc. Soc. Exp. Biol. Med.* 100:325, 1959.

49. Kirschbaum, A., Shapiro, J. R., and Mixer, H. W. Synergistic action of leukemogenic agents. *Cancer Res.* 13:262, 1953.
50. Simmons, V. P. Thymic function and leukemia. *Pediatrics* 5:574, 1950.
51. Earle, A. M., Reilly, W. A., and Dean, G. O. Thymectomy and ACTH in lymphatic leukemia. *J. Pediat.* 38:63, 1951.
52. Peterson, R. D. A., Varco, R. L., and Good, R. A. Unpublished observations, 1962–1964.
53. Thomson, A. D. The thymic origin of Hodgkin's disease. *Brit. J. Cancer* 9:37, 1955.
54. Annotations: Hodgkin's disease. *Lancet* 2:490, 1955.
55. Discussion on the possible significance of the thymic origin of Hodgkin's disease. *Proc. Royal Soc. Med.* 49:97, 1956.
56. Fisher, E. R. Pathology of the Thymus and Its Relationship to Human Disease. Ref. 14.
57. Patey, D. H. A contribution to the study of Hodgkin's disease. *Brit. J. Surg.* 50:389, 1963.
58. Strauss, A. J. L., Seegal, B. C., Hsu, K. C., Burkholder, P. M., Nastuk, W. L., and Osserman, K. E. Immunofluorescence demonstration of a muscle binding, complement-fixing serum globulin fraction in myasthenia gravis. *Proc. Soc. Exp. Biol. Med.* 105:184, 1960.
59. Beutner, E. H., Witebsky, E., Ricken, D., and Adler, R. H. Studies on autoantibodies in myasthenia gravis. *J.A.M.A.* 182:46, 1962.
60. Feltkamp, T. E. W., van der Geld, H., Kruyff, K., and Oosterhuis, H. J. G. H. Antinuclear factor in myasthenia gravis. *Lancet* 1:667, 1963.
61. Hess, E. V., Eliasson, G. S., Grigson, J. P., and Ziff, M. L.E. Cells, Antinuclear and Antimuscle Factor, and Thymus Abnormality in Myasthenic Patients. Ref. 14.
62. van der Geld, H., Feltkamp, T. E. W., van Loghem, J. J., Oosterhuis, H. J. G. H., and Biemond, A. Multiple antibody production in myasthenia gravis. *Lancet* 2:373, 1963.
63. van der Geld, H., and Oosterhuis, H. J. G. H. Muscle and thymus antibodies in myasthenia gravis. *Vox Sang.* 8:196, 1963.
64. Feltkamp, T. E. W., van der Geld, H., and Oosterhuis, H. J. G. H. Studies on sera from cases of myasthenia gravis, using the fluorescent antibody technique. *Ibid.*, p. 317.
65. Smithers, D. W. Tumours of the thyroid gland in relation to some general concepts of neoplasia. *J. Fac. Radiol.* 10:3, 1959.
66. Simpson, J. A. Myasthenia gravis: A new hypothesis. *Scot. Med. J.* 5:419, 1960.
67. Cross, R. J. Combined staff clinics: Systemic lupus erythematosus. *Amer. J. Med.* 28:416, 1960.
68. Denny, D., and Rose, R. L. Myasthenia gravis followed by systemic lupus erythematosus. *Neurology* 11:710, 1961.
69. Harvey, A. M., Schulman, L. E., Tumulty, P. A., Conley, C. L., and Schoenrich, E. H. Systemic lupus erythematosus. *Medicine* 33: 291, 1954.
70. White, R. G., and Marshall, A. H. E. The autoimmune response in myasthenia gravis. *Lancet* 2:120, 1962.
71. Rowland, L. P. Prostigmine-responsiveness and the diagnosis of myasthenia gravis. *Neurology* 5:612, 1955.
72. Goldin, H., and Robbins, W. C. A patient with myasthenia gravis, thymoma and lupus nephritis. *Arthritis Rheum.* 6:272, 1963.
73. Larson, D. L. *Systemic Lupus Erythematosus.* Boston: Little, Brown, 1961.
74. Bignami, A., and Calcara, S. Myocardite e miosite a cellule giganti associate a tumore del timo. *Policlinico* [Prat.] 69:857, 1962.
75. Bonduelle, M., Bordet, F., Bouygues, P., and Charles, F. Un cas de polymyosite avec thymome: Vérification anatomique. *Rev. Neurol.* (Paris) 92:551, 1955.
76. Langston, J. D., Wagman, G. F., and Dickenman, R. C. Granulomatous myocarditis associated with thymoma. *Arch. Path.* 68:367, 1959.
77. Waller, J. V., Shapiro, M., and Paltauf, R. Congestive heart failure in postmenopausal muscular dystrophy: Myositis, myocarditis, thymoma. *Amer. Heart J.* 53:479, 1957.
78. Funkhouser, J. W. Thymoma associated with myocarditis and the LE-cell phenomenon. *New Eng. J. Med.* 264:34, 1961.
79. Larsson, O. Thymoma and systemic lupus erythematosus in the same patient. *Lancet* 2:665, 1963.
80. Wolf, J. K., Gokcen, M., and Good, R. A. Heredo-familial disease of the mesenchymal tissues: Clinical and laboratory study of one family. *J. Lab. Clin. Med.* 61:230, 1963.
81. Mackay, I. R., and deGail, P. Thymic "germinal centers" and plasma cells in systemic lupus erythematosus. *Lancet* 2:667, 1963.
82. Mackay, I. R., Goldstein, G., and McConchie, I. H. Thymectomy in systemic lupus erythematosus. *Brit. Med. J.* 2:792, 1963.
83. Alarcón-Segovia, D., Galbraith, R. F., Maldonado, J. E., and Howard, F. M., Jr. Systemic lupus erythematosus following thymectomy for myasthenia gravis. *Lancet* 2:662, 1963.
84. Bielschowsky, M., Helyer, B. J., and Howie, J. B. Spontaneous haemolytic anaemia in mice of the NZB/BL strain. *Proc. Univ. Otago Med. School* 37:9, 1957.
85. Burnet, F. M., and Holmes, M. C. Thymus lesions in an autoimmune disease of mice. *Nature* (London) 194:146, 1962.
86. Burnet, F. M., and Holmes, M. C. Thymic Lesions Associated with Autoimmune Disease in Mice of Strain NZB. Ref. 14.

87. Helyer, B. J., and Howie, J. B. The thymus and autoimmune disease. *Lancet* II: 1026, 1963.
88. Hallman, N., Hjelt, L., Eklund, J., and Paatela, M. Microcystic disease simulating nephrotic syndrome. *Ann. Paediat.* 199:493, 1962.
89. Hegglin, R., and Siegenthaler, W. Maligne Tumoren bei Dermatomyositis. *Schweiz. Z. Tuberk.* 16:205, 1959.
90. Rundle, L. G., and Sparks, F. P. Thymoma and dermatomyositis. *Arch. Path.* 75:276, 1963.
91. Allott, E. N., and Skelton, M. O. Increased adrenocortical activity associated with malignant disease. *Lancet* 2:278, 1960.
92. Hymes, A. C., and Doe, R. P. Adrenal function in cancer of the lung, with and without Cushing's syndrome. *Amer. J. Med.* 33:398, 1962.
93. Meador, C. K., Liddle, G. W., Island, D. P., Nicholson, W. E., Lucas, C. P., Nuckton, J. G., and Luetscher, J. A. Cause of Cushing's syndrome in patients with tumors arising from "nonendocrine" tissue. *J. Clin. Endocr.* 22:693, 1962.

24. *Multiple Myeloma**

ELLIOTT F. OSSERMAN

MULTIPLE MYELOMA IS CONSIDERED to represent an autonomous neoplastic disease of those plasmacytic lines of the reticuloendothelial system (RES) normally responsible for the synthesis of the 7S γ_2 and the γ_{1A} (β_{2A})-globulins [1]. The neoplastic proliferation of these cells is characteristically associated with the elaboration of large quantities of γ_2 or γ_{1A} type serum globulins or Bence Jones (L-polypeptide) constituents, or both. The extensive physicochemical and immunochemical studies of myeloma proteins carried out in recent years have established the close relationship of these proteins to the normal immunoglobulins and at the same time have helped to elucidate the structure and polypeptide composition of the normal immunoglobulins. The important question of whether the myeloma proteins are truly abnormal constituents or whether they represent great quantitative excesses of proteins which are present in normal serum in minute amounts has not been answered. Although it has not been possible to demonstrate functional (antibody) specificity for any of the myeloma proteins thus far studied, the possibilities remain that these proteins possess antibody specificity for unrecognized antigens or, alternatively, that they represent abnormal antibodies elaborated in response to a particular form of (antigenic) stimulation of the RES.

The well-documented physicochemical homogeneity of individual myeloma serum and urinary proteins is consistent with the hypothesis that these proteins represent the products of single clones of γ-globulin-producing cells. Since it is now recognized that homogeneous, myeloma type γ-globulin abnormalities can also, on occasion, be found in the serum of individuals without clinically evident plasma cell myeloma, the possibility must be considered that "monoclonal proliferations" (Waldenström's [2] term) can occur without development of the destructive skeletal lesions and other clinical manifestations characteristic of plasma cell myeloma, at least for periods of several years or within the life span of a particular individual. Whether the distinction between these cases of so-called "asymptomatic monoclonal gammopathy" or "premyeloma" and overt plasma cell myeloma is qualitative or whether these different clinical patterns are the result of variations in the rate and/or the duration of the plasmacytic clonal proliferation in different subjects remains to be determined.

ETIOLOGY AND PATHOGENESIS OF PLASMA CELL NEOPLASIA

Although the etiological factors responsible for the induction of plasma cell neoplasms in man are undefined, observations on a variety of experimental plasma cell tumors in different inbred strains of mice may offer some leads. As detailed in a recent review of these studies [1], several spontaneous plasma cell tumors have been described in strain C_3H mice and in F_1 hybrids of CBA × DBA/2 strain mice [3–5]. Several of these tumors have subsequently been maintained by serial transplantation and have continued to elaborate myeloma type proteins after many transplant generations. Of further interest is the fact that several of the tumors apparently originated in older animals in the ileocecal lymphoreticular tissues [5], suggesting that prolonged and repetitive stimulation of these tissues by intestinal organisms may have been responsible for their ultimate neoplastic transformation. In another inbred strain of mice (BALB/c), the intraperitoneal introduction of a variety of substances, including Freund's adjuvants, mineral oil, and plastics, induces the formation of plasma cell neoplasms in a high per-

* These studies have been supported by Grant No. CA 02332 of the National Cancer Institute.

centage of animals after latent periods of six to twelve months [6–8]. The initial cellular response to the intraperitoneal introduction of such chronic and apparently nonspecific irritants in these mice is a lymphoreticular proliferation and the formation of aggregates of reticulum cells, lymphocytes, and lipid-laden macrophages. After these lesions have been present for several months, plasmacytic elements increase, followed by the development of multiple plasma cell tumor nodules on the peritoneal surface. These nodules can then be cloned and transplanted to normal BALB/c mice, where they grow as typical plasma cell tumors associated with the elaboration of myeloma type serum or urinary proteins, or both. Furthermore, several functionally distinct plasma cell tumors, as shown by their distinctive protein abnormalities, can be cloned from among multiple tumors which develop in the primary (adjuvant-treated) animal [8].

This experience has now been repeated in several laboratories. The fact that it has not been possible to reproduce this phenomenon in other murine strains indicates that specific genetic factors in the BALB/c mouse apparently predispose this strain to the induction of plasma cell neoplasms. The nature of the genetic factors remains to be elucidated. The common feature of the diverse agents shown to be capable of inducing plasma cell tumors in this mouse strain, e.g., plastics, Freund adjuvant-mineral oil mixtures, and mineral oil alone, appears to be related to their adjuvant properties, i.e., their ability to act as long-term stimulants to the proliferation of lymphoreticular cell populations, and to the fact that these substances are not readily eliminated by the cellular response which they induce, as are soluble antigens. Several attempts to induce functionally specific plasma cell tumors, i.e., plasma cell tumors which would elaborate functional antibody globulin, by the incorporation of specific bacterial or protein antigens in the adjuvant mixtures have been unsuccessful [6].

The relevance of these observations on spontaneous and induced plasma cell tumors in inbred strains of mice to the pathogenesis of human plasma cell neoplasias remains to be determined.

The possibility that viral agents may be involved in the pathogenesis of plasma cell tumors has been suggested by electron microscopic observations of virus-like particles in several of the spontaneous and adjuvant-induced plasma cell tumors in mice [9–13]. The significance of these particles is obscure, since it has not been possible to transmit these tumors by cell-free tumor filtrates. Whether, in the case of the adjuvant-induced tumors, the stimulation of the lymphoreticular tissues by the intraperitoneal irritants activates a latent oncogenic virus or whether these tumors are serving merely as host tissues for nonpathogenic agents is unknown. Although there have been several electron microscopic studies of human myeloma cells [14–17], virus-like particles were observed in only one of eleven cases studied by Sorenson [17]. In this case, round particles 30 to 50 $m\mu$ in diameter, located within doubly membraned cytoplasmic vacuoles, were found in approximately 10 percent of the marrow cells. There was a suggestion that these particles developed from the wall of the vacuoles in a manner similar to that of the virus-like particles in the mouse plasma cell tumors. The fact that similar structures were not observed in the myeloma cells of other cases examined suggests, but does not prove, that these particles are not of etiological significance. Thus it is recognized that the oncogenic viral agents of several experimental tumors may be demonstrable only in the initial stages of tumor development. Further studies of a possible viral etiology of plasma cell neoplasia are needed.

Studies in recent years of the pathogenesis of several experimental neoplasms, including leukemias, lymphomas, and mammary carcinomas, have demonstrated the intimate interaction of genetic factors, oncogenic viruses, and chemical and physical (x-ray) carcinogens. It is not unlikely, therefore, that a similar *combination* of factors may be involved in the genesis of experimental as well as human plasma cell neoplasms.

A possible hereditary factor in the genesis of plasma cell myeloma in man is suggested by the sporadic occurrence of the disease in two or more family members [18, 19], but the possibility of coincidence cannot be excluded. There are only two reports [20, 21] of chromosomal studies in multiple myeloma. In the first [20], the chromosomes of the myeloma cells of three patients were examined, and no specific chromosomal marker abnormalities were detected prior to the administration of a chemotherapeutic agent, L-aminocyclopentanecarboxylic acid (NSC-1023). Examination of marrow buffy coats in one patient, after this drug had been administered, showed an abnormal karyotype. In the other study [21], the cells from one patient (untreated) were examined, and the majority were found to have an aberrant number of chromosomes, 44, and several chromosomal rearrangements. An aberrant, medium-sized metacentric chromosome was found in all cells examined, but it was not established that this was a specific abnormality. Additional chromosomal studies in myeloma are needed.

CYTOLOGICAL CONSIDERATIONS

It has been well documented that the morphology of normal plasma cells changes significantly in the course of cell differentiation and maturation, and it is also recognized that the morphology of the plasma cells in myeloma varies from case to case and within the same case. Part of this variability is related to the changes in the nuclear and cytoplasmic constituents of these cells which occur in the process of synthesis and release of their specific protein products. Thus, as the plasma cell differentiates and develops the capacity for protein synthesis, there is a progressive accumulation of cytoplasmic ribonucleic acid (RNA). This RNA is responsible for the characteristic basophilia and pyroninophilia of the plasma cell cytoplasm. Electron microscopic studies of normal and neoplastic plasma cells have disclosed a highly developed network of endoplasmic reticulum [14–17, 23], and studies of these cells with ferritin-labeled antibody to their specific protein products have confirmed the presence of γ-globulin within the endoplasmic cisternae [13, 23].

Several studies have attempted to establish a correlation between the morphological characteristics of the abnormal plasma cells in individual cases of myeloma and the type of protein being synthesized by these particular cells. In 1949, Olhagen *et al.* [24] carried out cytometric and microspectrophotometric analyses of the distribution and concentration of nucleic acid in the cells of 16 patients with myeloma. Eleven of them had hyperglobulinemia with or without Bence Jones proteinuria, and 5 had Bence Jones proteinuria without hyperproteinemia. In the first group (with hyperglobulinemia and characteristic serum electrophoretic patterns), the predominant cells had the morphological features of mature plasmacytes with abundant cytoplasm, eccentrically placed nuclei, dense chromatin, large nucleoli, and prominent perinuclear clear zones (Golgi region). In these cells, designated A type, the cytoplasmic RNA was peripherally distributed, probably due to the paucity of RNA in the Golgi region. The predominant cell type in the 5 cases with Bence Jones proteinuria *without* hyperglobulinemia appeared to be relatively more primitive, with a larger nucleus (higher nucleocytoplasmic ratio), more sparse and evenly distributed chromatin, and somewhat larger and more conspicuous nucleoli. The cytoplasmic RNA of these Bence Jones protein-secreting (B type) cells was more evenly distributed than in the serum globulin-producing cells. In 3 of the 16 patients, an admixture of A and B type cells was found, and 2 of these patients had both Bence Jones proteinuria and hyperglobulinemia. These observations, which have been confirmed in subsequent studies, indicate that the production of a complete γ-globulin molecule with a molecular weight of the order of 160,000 requires a more highly differentiated cell organization than is required for the production of a lower molecular weight polypeptide of the Bence Jones type.

Attempts to demonstrate a correlation between the electrophoretic mobility of myeloma serum globulins and the morphological characteristics of the cells responsible for their production yielded generally inconclusive results until it was established that there are two major types of myeloma serum globulins, i.e., the γ_2- and γ_{1A}-globulins. Although the majority of γ_{1A} myeloma globulins have an electrophoretic mobility which is relatively greater (i.e., in the fast gamma or beta mobility range) than that of the γ_2 type myeloma globulins, there is considerable overlap. It is, therefore, impossible to distinguish γ_2- from γ_{1A}-globulins on the basis of electrophoretic mobility. The major chemical differences between the γ_2 and γ_{1A} myeloma globulins, however, particularly the significantly higher carbohydrate content of the latter, suggest that there might be discernible differences between their respective cells of origin, and this has been reported [25]. In a cytochemical and cytometric study of the marrow smears of 72 patients with myeloma, macroglobulinemia, and atypical forms of lymphatic or reticulum cell disease with myeloma type serum globulin abnormalities, Paraskevas *et al.* [25] found Undritz type "flame" cells and so-called "thesaurocytes" ("storage cells" with cytoplasm markedly distended by accumulations of protein) exclusively in 13 cases of γ_{1A} type myeloma. Subsequent electron microscopic studies of Bessis and co-workers [15] partially confirmed the findings of Paraskevas *et al.* with the observation of "flame" cells and "thesaurocytes" predominantly in 3 of their 4 cases of γ_{1A} type myeloma. In the electron microscope, these cells were seen to have markedly distended endoplasmic cisternae, filled with amorphous material of intermediate electron density, indicating that a high percentage of γ_{1A} myeloma cells have large intracytoplasmic aggregates of their specific protein products. This intracellular accumulation may be the result of the tendency of these carbohydrate-rich γ_{1A}-globulins to form high molecular weight polymers, with consequent hindrance of the protein-secreting mechanisms. The release of protein from these "flame" cells and "thesaurocytes" may require the dissolution and disintegration of cytoplasm, i.e., the process termed "clasmatosis" [22].

Intracytoplasmic crystals are found in a small percentage of normal and neoplastic plasma cells as well as in the cells comprising the plasmacytic reactions in certain infections. These crystals are usually within the endoplasmic cisternae and have been demonstrated by electron micrography to have a lamellar structure with a periodicity of approximately 100 A [22]. Cytochemical and immunohistochemical studies have shown that these crystals are comprised of γ-globulin, but the precise type (i.e., γ_2, γ_{1A}, γ_{1M}, or low molecular weight γ_L) has not been determined.

Future studies with improved cytochemical and immunocytochemical methods, particularly in association with electron microscopy, will unquestionably establish further correlations between the ultrastructure and the protein-secreting functions of these cells.

MYELOMA PROTEINS

The physicochemical and immunochemical properties of the myeloma γ_2- and γ_{1A}-globulins and of the Bence Jones proteins and their relation to the normal immunoglobulins are considered in detail in Chapter 19 and have been reviewed elsewhere [1]. As noted, the available evidence indicates that the neoplastic plasma cells in any given case of myeloma may produce: (1) an excess of L (light)-polypeptide subunits of the γ-globulins, i.e., the Bence Jones proteins, which can further be classified as either antigenic type I or type II (never I and II); (2) complete γ-globulin molecules with either γ_2 or γ_{1A} type H (heavy) chains combined with either type I or type II L chains, or (3) complete γ_2- or γ_{1A}-globulins plus an excess of free L chains (Bence Jones protein). Recent studies have also demonstrated that there are at least two antigenic (structural) types of γ_2 H chains [26–28] as well as several subtypes of Bence Jones proteins [29], and future studies will unquestionably reveal additional classes and subclasses of these molecules. Of 262 cases of myeloma studied in our clinic in the past ten years, 142 (54 percent) had γ_2 type serum protein abnormalities, and 58 (22 percent) were of the γ_{1A} type. Bence Jones proteinuria was present in 32 percent of the 142 γ_2 cases and 29 percent of the 58 γ_{1A} cases. In 59 cases (23 percent), only Bence Jones protein was produced by the myeloma cells. In 3 of the 262 cases (1 percent), it was not possible to detect an abnormal protein by either electrophoretic or immunoelectrophoretic analyses. By conventional filter paper electrophoretic analysis of the serum in these 262 cases, a characteristic electrophoretically homogeneous protein abnormality was found in 200 (76 percent). Urine protein electrophoresis demonstrated a Bence Jones type peak in 121 (46 percent), and, as noted, this was the only demonstrable protein abnormality in 59 (23 percent). These results provide further confirmation of the diagnostic value of serum and urine protein electrophoresis in myeloma.

Although the serum or urinary proteins, or both, which are elaborated in individual cases of myeloma can be classified into the categories already noted, it must be recognized that each Bence Jones protein and each myeloma serum globulin is apparently unique and distinctive with respect to its primary structure, i.e., its amino acid sequence, and necessarily also unique in its secondary and tertiary structure. A comparable degree of individuality has been demonstrated for the Bence Jones proteins and serum globulins produced by the various mouse plasma cell tumors [30] and applies not only to different tumors in the same inbred mouse strains but to separate transplantable plasma cell tumor lines which were initially isolated or "cloned" from a single adjuvant-treated mouse [8]. In addition to providing an exceptionally fertile field for biochemical exploration, this phenomenon of "paraprotein individuality" has several significant clinical implications, since it is now possible to relate a number of the specific clinical and pathological manifestations in individual patients to the specific physicochemical properties of the paraproteins elaborated [31]. These paraprotein-related clinical manifestations of myeloma are considered later.

CLINICAL ASPECTS OF MULTIPLE MYELOMA

Multiple myeloma is usually defined, for clinical purposes, as a neoplastic disease of plasma cells which is manifested primarily by the development of widespread skeletal lesions resulting from the replacement of bone by plasma cell tumors. Commonly associated with the skeletal symptoms are anemia, hypercalcemia, hyperuricemia, renal functional impairment, coagulation defects, and an increased susceptibility to infections. Proteinaceous tissue infiltrates, so-called "paramyloid" deposits, develop in about 10 percent of cases. The diagnosis of multiple myeloma generally depends on the x-ray demonstration of skeletal destruction (diffuse osteolytic lesions and/or osteoporosis), the documentation of an increased number of plasma cells in the marrow, and the finding of myeloma type serum or urinary (Bence Jones) proteins, or both. The disease usually pursues a relentless course, with average duration of life from the onset of symptoms (usually skeletal pain) of 20 to 24 months [31–34].

Although this clinical pattern is displayed by a significant number of patients, there is great variability in the manifestations and clinical course in individual cases. Thus, in certain patients, the disease may initially present as an apparently solitary plasma cell tumor and be followed by the development of disseminated lesions only after many years. In others, the finding of a myeloma type serum or urinary protein abnormality, or both, may be the first evidence of an abnormal plasma cell population, or plasma cell dyscrasia, and clinically evident signs and symptoms of myeloma may not emerge for several months or years [33, 35–37]. Finally, it is known that there are certain patients whose serum contains an electrophoretically homogeneous, myeloma type γ-globulin for ten years or longer, but in whom the signs and symptoms of multiple myeloma never develop [1, 2, 33]. Because these diverse clinical patterns and associated biochemical abnormalities apparently merge through a continuous spectrum, it may be postulated that they represent varying manifestation of a common pathological process, i.e., the proliferation of a limited population of plasma cells or "plasma cell dyscrasia." This hypothesis further suggests that the observed differences in the rate of disease progression and cell proliferation are due to quantitative rather than qualitative differences among the abnormal plasma cell populations in individual cases or to undefined host factors, or both. Contrariwise, it can be postulated that the pathogenic mechanisms and cell populations involved in the "typical" case of multiple myeloma are different from those involved in the "atypical" and asymptomatic monoclonal gammopathies. Which of these postulates is more nearly correct is not clear. As previously noted, however, the observations on experimental murine plasma cell tumors indicate that several pathogenic factors may induce plasma cell dyscrasias. Thus the diversity of the clinical and biochemical patterns in the human plasma cell dyscrasias may well be the result of different initiating mechanisms acting on related but distinct cell populations, but this remains to be proved.

PATHOLOGICAL EFFECTS OF MYELOMA GLOBULINS AND BENCE JONES PROTEINS

As previously noted, the abnormal serum and Bence Jones proteins elaborated in individual cases of myeloma differ considerably in their specific physicochemical properties due to dissimilarities in their primary structure. These structural dissimilarities result in differences in the solubility characteristics of these proteins with respect to pH, temperature, and ionic concentration, in their tendency to aggregate and form higher molecular weight polymers, in their intrinsic viscosity, and in their propensity to form complexes with other proteins. The fact that certain of these specific physicochemical properties of individual myeloma proteins can be related to specific clinical and pathological manifestations in individual cases of myeloma has become increasingly evident. Thus, certain Bence Jones proteins have the capacity to impair renal function as a direct consequence of their precipitation with renal tubules [38–40]. More recently, the finding that in certain patients with myeloma and Bence Jones proteinuria specific defects develop in renal tubular reabsorption mechanisms [41–43] also suggests that certain of these proteins have the capacity to damage specific tubular transport mechanisms through direct (protein : protein) interaction with specific tubular cytoplasmic constituents. That a nephrotoxic potential is not common to all Bence Jones proteins is apparent from the clinical fact that Bence Jones proteinuria is not invariably associated with impairment of renal function. Also, it is evident that several factors in addition to Bence Jones proteinuria, particularly hypercalciuria and anemia, and in some cases an increase in serum viscosity, can contribute to renal functional impairment in individual cases of myeloma and that a combination of these and other factors may be operative in specific cases. From the standpoint of the clinical management of myeloma, recognition of the several factors which may contribute to renal damage is of obvious importance. In particular, the need to maintain adequate hydration and urine volume cannot be overemphasized. In this regard it is now documented that intravenous pyelography can be extremely hazardous in patients with myeloma and Bence Jones proteinuria [44–46] and can precipitate irreversible renal shutdown, probably owing to the period of water withdrawal and dehydration which routinely precedes these studies.

Another important group of clinical signs and symptoms in patients with myeloma can be directly related to certain of the specific physicochemical properties of individual γ_2 and γ_{1A} serum globulins. Thus it has been recognized for several years that some of the myeloma proteins, particularly of the γ_2 type, have a high intrinsic viscosity which is further increased at lowered temperatures. Their presence in the serum can result in marked circulatory impairment with central nervous system manifestations, retinal vascular complications, and other manifestations of circulatory slowing, including peripheral and central thromboses and hemorrhages [47–50]. This property of high intrinsic and temperature-dependent viscosity is apparently closely related to the property of temperature-dependent solubility which is also displayed by certain of the myeloma γ_2-globulins, and to an even greater extent by the γ_1 macroglobulins [51–53]. Thus, it can be demonstrated that lowering of the temperature of serum containing certain of these proteins results solely in an increase in viscosity without precipitation, whereas in others, cooling causes precipitation of the globulin, either as a floccule (cryoprecipitation) or as a firm gel ("cryogel"). These viscosity and solubility properties are pH- and ionic strength-dependent as well as being dependent on temperature and protein concentration. Recognition of the several factors which influence the physical state of these proteins both *in vitro* and *in vivo* provides at least a partial explanation of the diversity in the clinical signs and symptoms which can be related to these properties [51–53].

Another group of clinical and laboratory manifestations of myeloma which can be related to specific properties of the myeloma globulins are those which apparently result from an interaction between certain of these proteins and one or more of the coagulation factors, including fibrinogen, factors V and VII, prothrombin, and the antihemophilic globulin [54–58]. Although the precise nature of these protein : protein interactions is undefined, it is probable that a variety of intermolecular bonds, including covalent linkages, hydrogen bonds, and possibly disulfide bridges, can be formed between certain of the myeloma globulins and these clotting factors. Because of the complexity of these phenomena and the fact that capillary damage from increased serum viscosity and thrombocytopenia may also contribute to a hemorrhagic diathesis in myeloma, it is often difficult, if not impossible, to pinpoint the precise defect in the clotting mechanism in a particular case. Also, the relating of the laboratory and clinical findings with respect to coagulation reactions in cases of myeloma is frequently unsatisfactory, again unquestionably due to the multiplicity of factors involved and the inherent limitations of available techniques.

TISSUE PROTEINOSIS (PARAMYLOIDOSIS) AND BENCE JONES PROTEINS

Proteinaceous tissue infiltrates, variously designated as amyloid, paramyloid, atypical amyloid, and so on, develop in 8 to 10 percent of cases of overt multiple myeloma. There is considerable evidence [59–65] that a large proportion of cases usually classified as "primary" amyloidosis, in which there is no recognized predisposing chronic infection, rheumatoid arthritis, or other obvious chronic disease, are in fact examples of occult myeloma, i.e., cases in which the abnormal plasma cells are diffusely distributed throughout the bone marrow and skeletal signs and symptoms fail to develop in the course of the illness. The possibility that "primary" amyloidosis and the amyloidosis associated with overt myeloma might have a similar pathogenesis was initially suggested because of the similarity in distribution and staining properties of the tissue infiltrates in these conditions and was substantiated by the demonstration by Apitz [60] of abnormal numbers of plasma cells in the marrow of these subjects irrespective of the presence of osteolytic lesions. It was recognized also that clinical manifestations of amyloidosis (macroglossia, the carpal tunnel syndrome, cardiac failure, gastrointestinal symptoms, etc.) frequently preceded the onset of skeletal signs and symptoms in individuals who ultimately manifested overt myeloma and might indeed cause death from cardiac failure or malnutrition before the development of clinically evident skeletal damage. In these cases, the abnormal plasma cell proliferations would only be documented if specifically sought by repeated bone marrow aspirations or meticulous postmortem examination of multiple skeletal sites.

A specific association between Bence Jones proteins and amyloidosis in both overt and occult myeloma was first suggested by Magnus-Levy [59], and several subsequent studies have provided further evidence of this association. Thus, among 27 cases of amyloidosis studied in our laboratory in the past ten years, Bence Jones proteins were demonstrable in 25 [65]. In 13, amyloidosis was associated with skeletal destruction; in 14, there were no demonstrable skeletal lesions. The clinical and pathological diagnosis in the latter group was usually "primary," atypical, or idiopathic amyloidosis. In 13 of these 14 "primary" cases, an increased number of plasma cells was documented by bone marrow aspiration but, significantly, in several instances only after several specimens had been obtained. By paper electrophoresis or immunoelectrophoresis, or both, Bence Jones type proteins could be demonstrated in all of the 13 cases with skeletal lesions and in 12 of the 14 "primary" cases. It is noteworthy that the routine Bence Jones heating test gave negative results in several samples subsequently shown to contain Bence Jones protein by the more sensitive electrophoretic and immunoelectrophoretic procedures.

Although the precise role of Bence Jones proteins in the pathogenesis of amyloid infiltrates remains to be determined, studies employing fluorescein-labeled Bence Jones proteins have suggested that the Bence Jones proteins from patients with amyloidosis may possess a greater binding affinity for certain normal tissue constituents than those from patients without associated amyloidosis [65]. These observations are consistent with the hypothesis that the amyloid infiltrates in these cases of overt or occult myeloma (or plasma cell dyscrasia) represent insoluble complexes of Bence Jones proteins with normal tissue proteins or polysaccharides, or both.

DEFICIENCY IN ANTIBODY PRODUCTION

An increased susceptibility to bacterial infections in general, and particularly to bacterial pneumonias, is exhibited in many cases of overt or occult myeloma. This is at least partially the result of an impaired capacity to elaborate the normal γ-globulins and functional antibody [66–69]. Immunoelectrophoretic studies have further established that the serum concentrations of all three of the major classes of normal immunoglobulins, i.e., γ_2, γ_{1A}, and γ_1, macroglobulins, are usually diminished in myeloma, irrespective of whether the myeloma protein is of the γ_2, γ_{1A}, or Bence Jones type [70–72]. These γ-globulin deficiencies are apparently similar to the deficiencies observed in lymphosarcoma and chronic lymphatic leukemia [73–75], but there is some evidence that the precise nature of the immunological deficits in myeloma may be qualitatively different from those of the lymphomas [76]. Turn-over studies of labeled 7S γ_2-globulin of myeloma [77, 78] have demonstrated an accelerated rate of catabolism in some cases, but this has not been a consistent finding. Thus the basis for the deficiencies in the normal γ-globulins in myeloma is obscure, but it is likely that deficient production is a more significant factor than enhanced catabolism or excessive loss.

Although the antibody-deficient status of most patients with myeloma would suggest that prophylactic γ-globulin administration might be of value, this has only rarely been found to be indicated. In the majority of cases, the bacterial infections that develop respond readily to appropriate antibiotic therapy.

THERAPY

It is now well established that several therapeutic agents are useful, although obviously not curative, in the management of multiple myeloma. Since spontaneous regressions virtually never occur, the remissions observed in a variable percentage of cases following radiotherapy or administration of chemotherapeutic agents can properly be ascribed to a direct or an indirect suppressive effect of these agents on the neoplastic plasma cells or their precursors. The variability in responsiveness in individual cases is probably the result of qualitative or quantitative differences in the metabolic requirements of different cell populations, to differences in dosage schedules, or to a combination of these and several other undefined tumor and host factors.

The majority of myelomatous tumors are relatively radiosensitive, and irradiation is of established value in the symptomatic management of localized skeletal infiltrates and large tumors. Irradiation frequently facilitates the mobilization of a patient who is incapacitated by a local area of pain. The importance of maintaining ambulation in these patients cannot be overemphasized, since the skeletal demineralization and negative calcium balance of immobilization can compound the effects of myelomatous skeletal destruction. Similarly, the need for maintaining adequate hydration, particularly in the presence of hypercalcemia, hypercalciuria, and Bence Jones proteinuria, is well established. It has further been demonstrated that prednisone is a useful adjunct in the management of hypercalcemia [79], but neither ACTH nor the corticosteroids significantly suppress the over-all progress of the disease.

Of the available chemotherapeutic agents, L-phenylalanine mustard (Melphalan) seems to be the most effective in long-term management of myeloma. The Soviet investigators, Blokhin *et al.* [80], were the first to report the therapeutic usefulness of D,L-phenylalanine mustard (sarcolysin) in a limited number of cases of myeloma. It was subsequently established by Bergel and Galton of the Chester Beatty Institute in London that the L-isomer of phenylalanine mustard (Melphalan) was the more active and less toxic form of this substituted alkylating agent. Although these investigators have not published the results of their own clinical studies with Melphalan, they have been responsible in significant measure for the clinical trials which have been carried out in several institutions in Europe and the United States, including those reported from our clinic [81]. We have had the opportunity to evaluate the effect of Melphalan in 24 patients in the past 3 years [81]. In 17 of them there has been objective evidence of disease suppression (decrease in abnormal serum and/or urinary proteins; hematological improvement; improved functional status) for periods ranging from 6 to 36 months. In 4 cases there has been radiographic evidence of skeletal improvement, and, significantly in 6 cases, there has been an unequivocal increase in the serum concentration of normal γ_2-globulin, coincident with the decrease in level of the myeloma serum or urinary proteins, or both. No evidence of a significant difference in the responsiveness of the different immunological types of myeloma has been noted. These results are essentially in accord with those obtained in other clinics [82–84]. Preliminary evidence suggests that the survival of these patients may be significantly prolonged by the use of this agent, but because of the great variability in the natural history of myeloma in individual cases, further studies will be necessary to confirm this. There is no question, however, that the useful life of many myeloma patients can be extended by this agent when given in combination with proper general management.

REFERENCES

1. Osserman, E. F., and Takatsuki, K. Plasma cell myeloma: Gamma globulin synthesis and structure. *Medicine* 42:357, 1963.
2. Waldenström, J. Studies on conditions associated with disturbed gamma globulin formation (gammopathies). *Harvey Lect.* 56:211, 1961.
3. Potter, M., Fahey, J. L., and Pilgrim, I. H. Abnormal serum protein and bone destruction in transmissible mouse plasma-cell neoplasm. *Proc. Soc. Exp. Biol. Med.* 94:327, 1957.
4. Rask-Nielsen, R., and Gormsen, H. Spontaneous and induced plasma-cell neoplasia in a strain of mice. *Cancer* 4:387, 1951.
5. Dunn, T. B. Plasma-cell neoplasms beginning in the ileocecal area in strain C_3H mice. *J. Nat. Cancer Inst.* 19:371, 1957.
6. Potter, M., and Roberston, C. L. Development of plasma-cell neoplasms in BALB/c mice after intraperitoneal injection of paraffin-oil adjuvant, heat killed staphylococcus mixtures. *J. Nat. Cancer Inst.* 25:847, 1960.
7. Potter, M., and Boyce, C. R. Induction of plasma-cell neoplasms in strain BALB/c mice with mineral oil and mineral-oil adjuvants. *Nature* (London) 193:1086, 1962.
8. Potter, M. Plasma cell neoplasia in a single host: A mosaic of different protein-producing cell types. *J. Exp. Med.* 115:339, 1962.
9. Howatson, A. F., and McCulloch, E. A. Virus-like bodies in transplantable mouse plasma cell tumor. *Nature* (London) 181:1213, 1958.
10. Dalton, A. J., Potter, M., and Merwin, R. M. Some ultrastructural characteristics of a series of primary and transplanted plasma cell tumours of the mouse. *J. Nat. Cancer Inst.* 26:1221, 1961.
11. Parsons, D. F., Darden, E. B., Jr., Lindsley, D. L., and Pratt, G. T. Electron miscroscopy of plasma cell tumors of the mouse: I. MPC-1 and X5563 tumors. *J. Biophys. Biochem. Cytol.* 9:353, 1961.
12. Parsons, D. F., Bender, M. A., Darden, E. B., Jr., Pratt, G. T., and Lindsley, D. L. Electron microscopy of plasma-cell tumors of the mouse. II. Tissue cultures of the X5563 tumor. *Ibid.*, p. 369.
13. Rifkind, R. A., Osserman, E. F., Hsu, K. C., and Morgan, C. The intracellular distribution of gamma globulin in a mouse plasma cell tumor (X5563) as revealed by fluorescence and electron microscopy. *J. Exp. Med.* 116:423, 1962.
14. Bessis, M. Ultrastructure of lymphoid and plasma cells in relation to globulin and antibody formation. *Lab. Invest.* 10:1040, 1961.
15. Bessis, M., Breton-Gorius, J., and Binet, J. L. Étude comparée du plasmocytome et du syndrome de Waldenström. *Nouv. Rev. Franc. Hemat.* 3:159, 1963.
16. Braunsteiner, H., Fellinger, K., and Pakesch, F. Demonstration of a cytoplasmic structure in plasma cells. *Blood* 8:916, 1953.
17. Sorenson, G. D. Electron miscroscopic observations of viral particles within myeloma cells of man. *Exp. Cell Res.* 25:219, 1961.
18. Mandema, E., and Wildervanck, L. S. La maladie de Kohler (myélomes multiples) ches deux soeurs. *J. Génét. Hum.* 3:170, 1954.
19. Nadeau, L. A., Magalini, S. I., and Stefanini, M. Familial multiple myeloma. *Arch. Path.* 61:101, 1956.
20. Richmond, H. G., Ohnuki, Y., Awa, A., and Pomerat, C. M. Multiple myeloma—an *in vitro* study. *Brit. J. Cancer* 15:692, 1961.
21. Castoldi, G. L., Ricci, N., Punturieri, E., and Bosi, L. Chromosomal imbalance in plasmacytoma. *Lancet* 1:829, 1963.
22. Thiery, J. P. Études sur le plasmocyte en contraste de phase et en microscopie électronique: III. Plasmocytes à corps de Russell et à cristaux. *Rev. Hemat.* 13:61, 1958.
23. DePetris, S., Karlsbad, G., and Pernis, B. Localization of antibodies in plasma cells by electron microscopy. *J. Exp. Med.* 117:849, 1963.
24. Olhagen, B., Thorell, B., and Wising, P. The endocellular nucleic acid distribution and plasma protein formation in myelomatosis. *Scand. J. Clin. Lab. Invest.* 1:49, 1949.
25. Paraskevas, F., Heremans, J., and Waldenström, J. Cytology and electrophoretic patterns in γ-1A (β-2A) myeloma. *Acta Med. Scand.* 170:575, 1961.
26. Ballieux, R. E., Bernier, G. M., Tominaga, K., and Putnam, F. W. Gammaglobulin antigenic types defined by Heavy Chain determinants. *Science* 145:168, 1964.
27. Takatsuki, K., and Osserman, E. F. Structural differences between two antigenic types of "heavy ($H\gamma^2$) chain disease" proteins and of gamma-2 myeloma globulins of corresponding antigenic types. *Science* 145:499, 1964.
28. Osserman, E. F., and Takatsuki, K. Clinical and immunochemical studies of four cases of $H\gamma^2$-chain (Franklin's) disease. *Amer. J. Med.* 37:351, 1964.
29. Stein, S., Nachman, R. L., and Engle, R. L. Individual and sub-group antigenic specificity of Bence Jones protein. *Nature* (London) 200: 1180, 1963.
30. Fahey, J. L., and Askonas, B. A. Enzymatically produced sub-units of proteins formed by plasma cells in mice: I. γ-globulin and γ-myeloma proteins. *J. Exp. Med.* 115:623, 1962.
31. Osserman, E. F. Plasma-cell myeloma: II.

Clinical aspects. *New Eng. J. Med.* 261:952, 1006, 1959.

32. Snapper, I., Turner, L. B., and Moscovitz, H. L. *Multiple Myeloma.* New York: Grune & Stratton, Inc., 1953.
33. Adams, W. S., Alling, E. L., and Lawrence, J. S. Multiple myeloma: Its clinical and laboratory diagnosis with emphasis on electrophoretic abnormalities. *Amer. J. Med.* 6:141, 1949.
34. Mandema, E. *Over het Multipel Myeloom, het Solitaire Plasmocytoom en de Macroglobulinaemie.* Groningen: Dijkstra's Drukkerij N.V., 1956.
35. Waldenström, J. Die Frühdiagnose der Myelomatose. *Acta Chir. Scand.* 87:365, 1942.
36. Wallerstein, R. S. Multiple myeloma without demonstrable bone lesions. *Amer. J. Med.* 10:325, 1951.
37. Osserman, E. F. Natural history of multiple myeloma before radiological evidence of disease. *Radiology* 71:157, 1958.
38. Forbes, W. D., Perlzweig, W. A., Parfentjev, I. A., and Burwell, J. C., Jr. Bence-Jones protein excretion and its effect upon kidney. *Bull. Hopkins Hosp.* 57:47, 1935.
39. Oliver, J. New directions in renal morphology: method, its results, and its future. *Harvey Lect.* 40:102, 1944–45.
40. Greenwald, H. P., Bronfin, G. J., and Auerbach, O. Needle biopsy of kidney: Report of five cases of multiple myeloma. *Amer. J. Med.* 15:198, 1953.
41. Sirota, J. H., and Hamerman, D. J. Renal function studies in adult with Fanconi syndrome. *Amer. J. Med.* 16:138, 1954.
42. Engle, R. L., and Wallis, L. A. Multiple myeloma and adult Fanconi syndrome: I. Report of case with crystal-like deposits in tumor cells and in epithelial cells of kidney. *Amer. J. Med.* 22:5, 1957.
43. Dedmon, R. E., West, J. H., and Schwartz, T. B. The adult Fanconi syndrome: Report of two cases, one with multiple myeloma. *Med. Clin. N. Amer.* 47:191, 1963.
44. Bartels, E. D., Brun, G. C., Gammeltoft, A., and Gjørup, P. A. Acute anuria following intravenous pyelography in patient with myelomatosis. *Acta Med. Scand.* 150:297, 1954.
45. Myhre, J. R., Brodwall, E. K., and Knutsen, S. B. Acute renal failure following intravenous pyelography in cases of myelomatosis. *Acta Med. Scand.* 156:263, 1956.
46. Perillie, P. E., and Conn, H. O. Acute renal failure after intravenous pyelography in plasma cell myeloma. *J.A.M.A.* 167:2186, 1958.
47. Shapiro, S., Ross, V., and Moore, D. H. Viscous protein obtained in large amount from serum of patient with multiple myeloma. *J. Clin. Invest.* 22:137, 1943.
48. Bichel, J., Bing, J., and Harboe, N. Another case of hyperglobulinemia and affection of central nervous system. *Acta Med. Scand.* 138:1, 1950.
49. Wuhrmann, F. Über das Coma paraproteinaemicum bei Myelomen und Makroglobulinämien. *Schweiz. Med. Wschr.* 86:623, 1956.
50. Berneaud-Kötz, G., and Jahnke, K. Ueber einen Fall von ungewöhnlicher Dys- und Paraproteinämie mit auffallenden Augenhintergrundveränderungen (Fundus paraproteinaemicus). *Klin. Mbl. Augenheilk.* 125:160, 1954.
51. Lerner, A. B., and Watson, C. J. Studies of cryoglobulins: I. Unusual purpura associated with presence of high concentration of cryoglobulin (cold precipitable serum globulin). *Amer. J. Med. Sci.* 214:410, 1947.
52. Watson, C. J., and Lerner, A. B. Clinical significance of cryoglobulinemia. *Acta Med. Scand.* 196 supp.: 489, 1947.
53. Mackay, I. R., Eriksen, N., Motulsky, A. G., and Volwiler, W. Cryo- and macgroglobulinemia: Electrophoretic, ultracentrifugal and clinical studies. *Amer. J. Med.* 20:564, 1956.
54. Uehlinger, E. Ueber eine Blutgerinnungsstörung bei Dysproteinämie: (Beitrage zur Kenntnis der körpereigenen Antikoagulantia). *Helvet. Med. Acta* 16:508, 1949.
55. Lüscher, E., and Labhart, A. Blutgerinnungsstörung durch $\beta\gamma$-Globuline: zur Kenntnis der Gerinnungsstörungen durch körpereigene Antikoagulantien. *Schweiz. Med. Wschr.* 79:598, 1949.
56. Nilsson, I. M., and Wenckert, A. Hyperglobulinemia as cause of hemophilia-like disease. *Blood* 8:1067, 1953.
57. Ratnoff, O. D. Delayed blood coagulation in multiple myeloma. *J. Clin. Invest.* 32:596, 1953.
58. Craddock, C. G., Jr., Adams, W. S., and Figueroa, W. G. Interference with fibrin formation in multiple myeloma by unusual protein found in blood and urine. *J. Lab. Clin. Med.* 42:847, 1953.
59. Magnus-Levy, A. Multiple Myeloma: VII. Euglobulinämie zur Klinik und Pathologie; Amyloidosis. *Z. Klin. Med.* 126:62, 1933.
60. Apitz, K. Die Paraproteinosen (über die Störung des Eiweisstoffwechsels bei Plasmacytom). *Virchow. Arch. Path. Anat.* 306:631, 1940.
61. Eisen, H. N. Primary systemic amyloidosis. *Amer. J. Med.* 1:144, 1946.
62. Bayrd, E. D., and Bennett, W. A. Amyloidosis complicating myeloma. *Med. Clin. N. Amer.* 34:1151, 1950.
63. Magnus-Levy, A. Amyloidosis in multiple myeloma: Progress noted in 50 years of personal observation. *J. Mount Sinai Hosp.* N.Y. 19:8, 1952.
64. Osserman, E. F. Amyloidosis: Tissue protein-

osis; Gammaloidosis. *Ann. Intern. Med.* 55: 1033, 1961 (editorial).

65. Osserman, E. F., Takatsuki, K., and Talal, N. The pathogenesis of "amyloidosis": Studies on the role of abnormal gamma globulins and gamma globulin fragments of the Bence Jones (L-polypeptide) type in the pathogenesis of "primary" and "secondary amyloidosis," and the "amyloidosis" associated with plasma cell myeloma. *Seminars Hemat.* 1:3, 1964.
66. Larson, D. L., and Tomlinson, L. J. Quantitative antibody studies in man: II. Relation of serum proteins to antibody production. *J. Lab. Clin. Med.* 39:129, 1952.
67. Marks, J. Antibody formation in myelomatosis. *J. Clin. Path.* 6:62, 1953.
68. Zinneman, H. H., and Hall, W. H. Recurrent pneumonia in multiple myeloma and some observations on immunologic response. *Ann. Intern. Med.* 41:1152, 1954.
69. Lawson, H. A., Stuart, C. A., Paull, A. M., Phillips, A. M., and Phillips, R. W. Observations on antibody content of blood in patients with multiple myeloma. *New Eng. J. Med.* 252:13, 1955.
70. Grabar, P., Fauvert, R., Burtin, P., and Hartmann, L. Étude sur les protéines du myélome: II. L'analyse immuno-électrophorétique des sérum de 30 malades. *Rev. Franc. Etud. Clin. Biol.* 1:175, 1956.
71. Heremans, J. F. *Les globulines sériques du système gamma: Leur nature et leur pathologie.* Brussels: *Éditions Arscia, S.A.*, 1960.
72. Osserman, E. F., and Lawlor, D. P. Immunoelectrophoretic characterization of the serum and urinary proteins in plasma cell myeloma and Waldenström's macroglobulinemia. *Ann. N.Y. Acad. Sci.* 94:93, 1961.
73. Grabar, P., Burtin, P., and Seligmann, M. Études immuno-électrophorètiques et immunochimiques des agammaglobulinémies. *Rev. Franc. Etud. Clin. Biol.* 3:1 and 41, 1958.
74. Gitlin, D., Janeway, C. A., Apt, L., and Craig, J. M. Agammaglobulinemia. In Lawrence, H. S. (Ed.), *Cellular and Humoral Aspects of Hypersensitive States.* New York: Paul B. Hoeber, Inc., 1959.
75. Miller, D. G. Patterns of immunological deficiency in lymphomas and leukemias. *Ann. Intern. Med.* 57:5, 703, 1962.
76. Cone, L. A., and Uhr, J. W. Immunological deficiency disorders associated with multiple myeloma and chronic lymphatic leukemia. *J. Clin. Invest.* 42:925, 1963 (abst.).
77. Lippincott, S. W., Korman, S., Forg, C., Stickley, E., Wolins, W., Hughes, W. L. Turnover of labeled normal gamma globulin in multiple myeloma. *J. Clin. Invest.* 39:565, 1960.
78. Solomon, A., Waldmann, T. A., and Fahey, J. L. Metabolism of 6.6S γ-globulin in normal subjects and in patients with macroglobulinemia and multiple myeloma. *J. Lab. Clin. Med.* 62:1, 1963.
79. Adams, W. S., and Skoog, W. A. The management of multiple myeloma. *J. Chron. Dis.* 6:446, 1957.
80. Blokhin, N., Larionov, L. F., Perevodchikova, N. I., Chebotareva, L., and Merkulova, N. Clinical experiences with sarcolysin in neoplastic diseases. *Ann. N.Y. Acad. Sci.* 68:1128, 1958.
81. Osserman, E. F. Therapy of plasma cell myeloma with Melphalan. *Proc. Amer. Assc. Cancer Res.* 2:50, 1963.
82. Bergsagel, D. E., Sprague, C. C., Austin, C., and Griffith, K. M. Evaluation of new chemotherapeutic agents in the treatment of multiple myeloma: IV. L-phenylalanine mustard (NSC-8806). *Cancer Chemother. Rep.* No. 21, p. 87, 1962.
83. Bernard, J., Seligmann, M., and Danon, F. Essai de traitment de 21 malades atteints de myelome ou de macroglobulinémie par le p-di-2-chloro-éthyl-amino-L-phénylalanine (Melphalan). *Nouv. Rev. Franc. Hémat.* 2:611, 1962.
84. Waldenström, J. Personal communication, 1963.

25. *Macroglobulinemia**

JAN WALDENSTRÖM

THE DISEASE

Among the diseases related to the antibody-forming cells, myeloma or plasmacytoma was long regarded as unique. In this condition, the plasma cells show a more or less unlimited proliferation, and the usual result is marked increase in their metabolic product, hypergammaglobulinemia. This is one of the classic symptoms of myeloma, which became one of the diseases important in the study of antibody synthesis.

In the early nineteen-forties, K. O. Pedersen and I became interested in conditions with increased γ-globulins in the serum that could be investigated by electrophoresis and ultracentrifugation. It became evident that the sera of some patients contained a previously unknown type of globulin with a much higher molecular weight than normal γ-globulin. The sedimentation constant was 19 to 20S, whereas normal γ-globulin has the value 7S. This meant that their molecular weight could be calculated to be about 10^{-6}, i.e., six to seven times that of the 7S component. We called these globulins macroglobulins. It was found that they migrated as β- or γ-globulins on free electrophoresis (Tiselius), that they sometimes behaved like cryoglobulins (gel at low temperatures), that their viscosity increased more with lowering temperature than did that of 7S globulins, and that they were euglobulins and therefore often precipitated on dilution of the serum with water (positive Sia test) [1–3].

We were able to collect a number of patients whose sera showed a very marked content of macroglobulins. The condition was therefore called macroglobulinemia. Our first patients were elderly men. Anemia and a very high sedimentation rate are among the first signs noted. Lymph nodes and spleen may be slightly enlarged. In some instances, there is even marked splenomegaly. Subjective complaints are mostly lassitude and headache, but not bone pain. In this respect we found the disease to differ from myeloma. Several patients complained of a bleeding tendency, especially nosebleed, and also diffuse bleeding in the mouth: "I wake up in the morning with my mouth full of blood." Purpura is not common. Nerve involvement in the form of polyneuritis may occur (Bing-Fog-Neel syndrome).

Further investigation showed a very high sedimentation rate, and often normochromic anemia, which may become quite severe and is sometimes, though rarely, hemolytic. Serological findings will be discussed later. The white cell picture is usually lymphocytic, but increased absolute values are rare, whereas leukopenia with a high lymphocyte percentage is quite common. Platelet count is mostly normal but may be lowered. From the findings of palpable lymph nodes and marked lymphocytosis in the blood, it might be inferred that this is really *a lymphatic disease* [3].

Examination of the bone marrow showed a picture that was interpreted as lymphocytic and later, according to the terminology of Rohr, as indicating proliferation of lymphocytoid reticulum cells. These small round cells, with a very scarce cytoplasm that was obviously quite fragile and showed budding and shedding, have ever since been regarded as the cytological basis for the disease. The bone marrow may contain more or less typical plasma cells, but the dominant cell is the lymphocytoid. Tischendorf and Hartmann [4] later noted tissue mast cells, and this combination of the two cell types is at present regarded as the most typical both in the bone marrow and in lymph nodes and other lymphatic tissue. The best published colored pictures of the cells are to be found in Reference 5.

Roentgenological examination of the skeleton showed that these cells, distinct from

* Supported by grants from the Swedish Cancer Fund and the Alfred Österlund Foundation.

plasma cells in most myeloma patients, were not osteoclastic, and this of course accounts for the absence of severe bone pain and bone destruction. Later investigations have disclosed rare patients who may have an increase in macroglobulins and still have a skeletal process resembling myeloma. All of these possible transitions have been discussed elsewhere at some length [6]. It was found that transitions between macroglobulinemia and myeloma, lymphatic leukemia, lymphosarcoma, and reticulum cell sarcoma were by no means rare. It is thus evident that the anatomical basis for the classification of different *tissues* is sometimes not sufficient for a clinical diagnosis. With the advent of modern staining methods on a cytochemical basis and with further development of electron microscopy [7], the *cell* will more often become the basis for diagnostic differentiation. The metabolic products of cell activity will be regarded as an increasingly valuable means of classification. The possible explanation for the many overlappings regarding proliferation of reticulum cells and their descendants—certainly connected with the pluripotentiality of the "stem cell"—will be discussed in another connection.

It seems to be a well-established fact that the plasma cell is involved in formation of 7S γ-globulin and the lymphocytoid cell in formation of macroglobulin (19S–20S) [8].

The course of macroglobulinemia is usually much more protracted than that of myeloma. Our first patients were seen in late stages, and this gave a pessimistic outlook when they died with severe anemia, edema, cachexia or during an acute infection. It seems probable that they also suffer from immunoparesis, just as do patients with myeloma, as their normal γ-globulin level tends to be low. Recent investigations seem to show that antibody titers are, on the whole, low in both diseases [9]. With increasing experience, it has become clear that macroglobulinemia is a disease that may last for ten years without causing much trouble. At this stage it is really an essential hyperglobulinemia, as I stated many years ago (1944). It is not known if this condition may last indefinitely or if the ultimate development is always progressive and malignant.

Many authors have pointed out that there could be a connection between macroglobulinemia and *carcinoma* [10, 11]. I have been rather hesitant to accept this, as the majority of persons with both diseases are quite old and cancer is, of course, so common that it must arise in a number of elderly patients, who live long with any other disease. Our experience with this problem in Malmö, where we have probably seen most patients with macroglobulinemia in this city of 230,000 inhabitants during the past 12 years, may be worth citing. In this period we have seen 4 to 6 patients out of 10 with severe macroglobulinemia who have had or have active carcinoma. The same relation for myeloma would be 3 to 4 out of 65. This problem certainly deserves the interest of immunologists and several possible explanations may be discussed. For instance, there could be reduced resistance against carcinoma, a tendency to develop malignancies other than macroglobulinemia, or, on the contrary, development of antibodies of a macroglobulin nature against carcinoma cells. All of these leads may possibly become important for a better understanding of cancer immunity.

In recent years, knowledge regarding active therapy in myeloma has made great strides. Starting in 1947 with urethane (Alwall), which is not very well tolerated, other cytostatic drugs were tried. The latest is Melphalan (bis-chlorethylaminophenylalanine). We have had experience with this drug in well over fifty patients with myeloma. Our results have been remarkably positive [12]. We have also tried the drug in macroglobulinemia and noted marked reduction of macroglobulins. In our opinion, the drug of choice in this disease is Chlorambucil. It is important to realize, however, that response may come late and that the drug should be given continuously for years. [See Ref. 13, and Figs. 25-1 and 25-2.]

THE MACROGLOBULIN MOLECULE

As may be expected from its name, the molecule is unusually large even though there are other globulin molecules of the same size, e.g., the α macroglobulin. In the electrical field the macroglobulin described by Pedersen migrates as β- or γ-globulin. In free electrophoresis it appears as a narrow spire; on paper it gives a narrow band. A great many arguments favor Burnet's [14] idea that one clone of plasma cells is responsible for the disease we call myeloma. The same holds true in principle for macroglobulinemia. The globulin bands are narrow, they remain the same

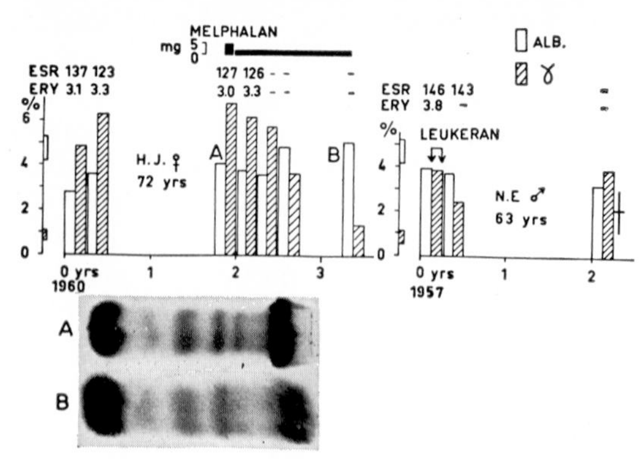

Fig. 25-1. (*A*) H. J. had had anemia for some time. Serum electrophoresis, done because of a very high erythrocyte sedimentation rate, showed pronounced monoclonal hyperglobulinemia consisting of macroglobulins. Treatment with Melphalan produced rapid decrease in macroglobulins and increase in serum albumin as well as considerable improvement in general health. The electrophoretic diagram has become practically normal after treatment for about a year and a half. (*B*) N. E. had typical macroglobulinemia. He was treated for a short time with Leukeran but did not continue his treatment at home, in another part of the country. There was good immediate effect of the short course, but he suffered a relapse and died in cachexia at home.

and the globulin obviously does not change, and they never disappear spontaneously but tend to increase in myeloma and in progressive macroglobulinemia and remain completely unchanged for years in essential benign hypergammaglobulinemia. I have chosen the word monoclonal for this type of γ-globulin increase, whereas the broad type seen in so-called autoimmune and collagen diseases is polyclonal. The monoclonal globulin is often called an M component (for M-yeloma and M-acroglobulinemia, and also for M-onoclonal!).

It is evident that polyclonal hypergammaglobulinemia is really formed by a very large number of monoclonal products. Pedersen and I studied a number of patients with polyclonal hyperglobulinemia, and it was evident that the percentage of macroglobulins was usually not much increased even though the absolute amount was higher than normal. As a rule, a polyclonal hypergammaglobulinemia consists mainly of 7S γ-globulin. These important problems have been studied in great detail by the German investigators Jahnke and Scholtan; the reader is referred to their monograph on ultracentrifugation of serum in a large variety of diseases chiefly with polyclonal type globulins [15].

I shall not enter upon a detailed discussion of different physical constants obtained by ultracentrifugation of macroglobulins. Suffice it to say that equipment newer than the ultracentrifuge first devised by Svedberg in Uppsala has simplified the work—above all, the Spinco centrifuge. The first sedimentation constants of 19S to 20S were found to be too high in many sera, and it is also realized that there are fractions with still larger molecules in most sera from patients with the disease. Constants below 14S are not indicative of real macroglobulins. The term atypical macroglobulins has been coined for these fractions. It was pointed out in 1952 [16] that globulins with sedimentation constants 9S to 12S were not altogether uncommon in clinically typical cases of myeloma. They are not macroglobulins according to our first definitions, but belong to the most recently discovered members of the γ family, the so-called γ_A (β_{2A})-globulins [17]. It is probable that the high molecular weight in this instance is caused by complex formation, as it is common to find both 7S and 11S γ values increased in such cases.

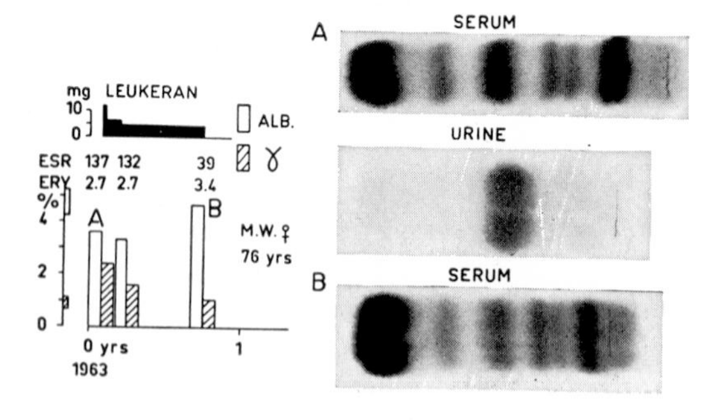

Fig. 25-2. M. W. had a very high erythrocyte sedimentation rate (ESR) and a fever of unknown origin with no physical symptoms. Electrophoresis: white columns indicate serum albumin, and cross-hatched columns, macroglobulin. She was treated with Leukeran in diminishing doses and the fever disappeared after three weeks. There were great improvement in well-being and some increase in the red cell count, as seen on the graph.

SEROLOGY

The serological grouping of the members of the γ-system was first achieved by the technique of immunoelectrophoresis worked out by Grabar [18]. It then became possible to separate γ_{ss}, γ_{1A}, and γ_{1M} (macroglobulin) in a comparatively simple way (see Chapter 19). New terms have been adopted recently, and γ_{ss}, γ_{1A}, and γ_{1M} are now called γ_G, γ_A, and γ_M respectively. Heremans continued this type of work and presented the findings of his group regarding relationships of the proteins of the three groups on a very simple map (their Figs. 9 and 13, Ref. 19). We shall discuss only his findings regarding macroglobulins here. Earlier, Kratochvil and Deutsch [20] had proved that pathologically increased macroglobulins have antigenic characteristics in common with normal serum proteins, and Müller-Eberhard and Kunkel [21] had isolated the normally occurring γ macroglobulin.

Heremans studied a large number of macroglobulinemia sera with cross-absorption of a polyvalent anti-β_{2M} serum and found that there were different degrees of completeness in the absorption of antigenic groupings. This was to be expected when we assume that the M components are monoclonal and the normal γ macroglobulin must be polyclonal. The map drawn by Heremans demonstrates that one part of the macroglobulin is antigenically identical with γ_G, whereas another is "truly" β_2 or specific; γ_G, of course, also has specific sites [19]. This way of looking at the antigenic constituents of the three different types of γ-globulin has been much extended. Two techniques have been particularly important to the clarification of these problems. One is the application of Korngold's two or three groups of Bence Jones protein to the other members of the γ system. The other is the use of genetically determined markers for the identification of different types of subunits of γ-globulins. Korngold and Lipari [22] showed that the Bence Jones proteins in the urine could be grouped either as A or B or as a third group serologically. It was shown later that this third group corresponds to γ_A globulin antigenically. We too have had a patient with a typical γ_A myeloma whose urinary protein was immunologically not a Bence Jones protein but a γ_A. Through the work of Putnam and his group and the group at the Rockefeller Institute it has been shown definitely that not only the Bence Jones protein but also the M components in the serum may be grouped as Bence Jones protein. A and B correspond to γ-globulin types II and I. In one large survey, the urinary and serum proteins were never of different types. Our knowledge regarding macroglobulinemia is still incomplete, but the available information favors the idea that the same division into I and II groups applies also to these globulins [23–25].

There are other markers on the γ-globulin molecules that may be used for studies, above all, of the genetic conditions. Mårtensson [26], working in Grubb's laboratory on 79 M components isolated by Laurell, was able to show that the group Gm $(a+b+)$ was never found, which is a good argument in favor of a monoclonal origin of these M components. This work has been extended by Harboe *et al.* [27]. Neither they nor Mårtensson found Gm characters on macroglobulins or the γ_{1A}-globulins. Another serological grouping, the Inv system, discovered by Ropartz, is expressed on all three γ types.

Papain-splitting of γ-globulin molecules results in two types of fragments, F and S (fast and slow on gel electrophoresis [28]). The F fragments carry the Gm groups, whereas the S contains the Inv. Obviously, F is present only on γ_G molecules. Another type of splitting results in the formation of L (light) and H (heavy) chains. The former resemble Bence Jones protein and may even be identical. They contain the Inv sites, and the H chains the Gm sites. This must mean that these two sites are present on different polypeptide chains. It is of considerable interest that anticomplementary activity occurs only in sera with γ-globulins of the γ_G type. This would mean that the character is present only on the F or H part of the molecule that is absent from γ_A and macroglobulin molecules. The S part of the molecules that is common to all three groups (γ_G, γ_A, and γ_M) is the carrier of the antibody combining sites [29].

Harboe and collaborators have used the determination of Gm and Inv groups to investigate the genetic influence on the structure of γ-globulins. The reader is referred to their stimulating paper that has the following final lines:

> . . . The accumulated evidence obtained in this study strongly suggested that the presence and absence of genetic characters was compatible with the concept that myeloma proteins were closely analogous to individual moieties in the spectrum of normal γ-globulins rather than truly abnormal proteins. Their study offered evidence of a heterogeneity of genetic characters among the normal

γ-globulins in a given individual. It also appears probable that in normal individuals single plasma cells have a restricted capacity to express genetic information in their protein product.

I would not present these data in detail if I did not think that they constitute important evidence that macroglobulinemia is caused by isolated proliferation of one clone of lymphocytoid reticulum cells with resulting monoclonal hyperglobulinemia of only one individual globulin.

CAUSE OF THE DISEASE

It seems to me that the disease is an exact parallel to myeloma, when the lymphocytoid cell proliferates instead of the plasma cell and macroglobulin increases instead of 7S or 9S to 12S γ (γ_G or γ_A). The more or less unlimited proliferation of a cell that forms antibody globulin is common to both diseases.

Many authors take it for granted that these globulin individuals that occur in increased quantities as M components of γ_G, γ_A, or macroglobulins are pathological—are paraproteins. Are there any indications that this is true? Information so far available has indicated that they may be of a normal type and that they are really monoclonal.

Burnet [14] introduced the concept that somatic mutations are responsible for myeloma. *Benign* essential monoclonal hyperglobulinemia could be a proliferation comparable to normal antibody formation in one clone of cells. We might well assume that the clone could be working at maximal capacity; this would explain the remarkable constancy of the γ-globulin level (γ_G, γ_A, γ_M) through the years [30].

Extremely interesting to my mind is the fact that the cold agglutinin which appears, sometimes, in the macroglobulin that develops after infection with Eaton bodies (pleuropneumonia) also occurs in benign macroglobulinemia. In tropical trypanosomiasis with great increase in γ-globulin (partly as macromolecules), cold agglutinin is also present. This was described by Warrington Yorke in 1910 [31]. French workers have studied tropical diseases with increase in macroglobulins. Charmot *et al.* [32] described what they call tropical splenomegalic macroglobulinemia, in which the probably infectious agent is not known. This seems to be a comparatively common condition in many parts of Africa. French colleagues have told me that this type of hypergammaglobulinemia is broad-banded and would therefore be polyclonal. It is difficult from the publications to obtain information about this. Dreyfus *et al.* [33] published an interesting observation regarding a patient with trypanosomiasis. The patient had hyperglobulinemia with a very high erythrocyte sedimentation rate and positive response to the Sia test. Ultracentrifugation showed 22 percent 7S component and 15 percent macroglobulin. It is thus obvious that more than half of his total globulin was of the 7S type. This, of course, means that he had a polyclonal γ-globulin increase. Pictures of the electrophoretic strip were not published. Sternal puncture showed a large number of Mott cells, which I have never seen in essential macroglobulinemia. It is noteworthy that these cells were first described by Mott in trypanosomiasis. Specific treatment led to complete cure and normal macroglobulin content. Apparently, a symptomatic increase in macroglobulins may become quite pronounced. The occurrence of monoclonal macroglobulin increase as a reaction to an infection remains to be proved. To me, this observation is good evidence that monoclonal and polyclonal hyperglobulinemias must be kept distinct.

It is tempting to assume that the template giving the increased synthesis of cold agglutinin after challenge with the "natural" antigen contained in the infectious agent could also be activated in a nonspecific way, leading to benign monoclonal macroglobulinemia with cold agglutinin. The problem has been illustrated by a patient with monoclonal hyperglobulinemia (γ_G) and an extremely high titer of antistreptolysin (1/12,000) [30].

We have seen two more sera (γ_G) with similar extraordinary titers. Another patient with monoclonal γ_G had a remarkably high titer (1/250,000) of antithyroglobulin in spite of the fact that she was euthyroid and had no goiter. We have seen lower titers of the same kind in the serum from a euthyroid myeloma patient. One patient with increase in macroglobulin had a slightly increased antithyroid titer (1/250). We still do not know whether or not this patient's antibody is contained in the M component. One of our patients with macroglobulin increase had a high titer of rheumatoid factor. Her serum was carefully analyzed by Heremans and by Franklin, and it is evident that she has a pseudomacroglobulin that is caused by aggregation of γ-globulin molecules. Interestingly enough, this patient has had a practically complete remission of her pathological globulin, a development that has never been seen in any of our other macroglobulinemia patients. During the past year we have observed two more patients, in whom results of the Rose-Waaler test were strongly positive and the anti-γ titer was increased. These patients had classic macroglobulinemia. Kritzman *et al.* [34] have pointed out that their macroglobulins must be regarded as antibodies. Recently we have seen two more patients probably belonging to this group.

Perhaps it should be pointed out also that several patients with Sjögren's syndrome (sialoadenitis chronica), in which polyclonal hyperglobulinemia is the rule, have had monoclonal increase in macroglobulins. This may mean, of course, that they have an "autoantibody" of macroglobulin character directed against some antigen in the salivary glands.

It seems very probable that we shall be able to find that an increasing number of M components in the benign nonprogressive group have well-defined "antibody" functions, when we have the opportunity to test them against new antigens.

The significance of antibodies of different molecular weight has been analyzed by Kunkel *et al.* [35]. Recent investigations by pediatricians have shown that there is a different timetable for the maturation of the 7S and the 19S to 20S γ antibodies in ontogenesis [36]. R. T. Smith has shown that the first antibody formed on immunization of infants is a macroglobulin; this is later followed by 7S γ-globulin [37].

Are there any further factors that could be thought to be operative in the development of macroglobulinemia? Heredity has been shown to be a possible factor in polyclonal hyperglobulinemia. Leonhardt [38] studied in detail a family of 14 siblings in which 3 sisters had systemic lupus erythematosus, one had discoid lupus, and a fifth had polyclonal essential increase in γ-globulins (4 gm./100 ml.) with no clinical symptoms. In another family, also studied by Leonhardt but first described by Lindholm, there occurred both hypogammaglobulinemia and monoclonal benign and polyclonal hypergammaglobulinemia as well as myeloma. (For a recent review, see Ref. 39.)

In macroglobulinemia very little is known regarding familial occurrence. We have been able to examine sera from a man and his sister's daughter who had considerable increase in macroglobulins and have hoped to establish identity or nonidentity between the globulin molecules. The latter may seem to be easy, the first, and the most important, impossible. These observations have never been published. Seligmann and Badin [40] in Paris have collected a number of instances of increase in macroglobulins in two or three members of the same family: three mothers with four sons, and one brother and sister. It is remarkable that the three mothers, who must have had the disease longer than their sons, had it in much less severe form. Myeloma is definitely more serious in the male, and there is a male preponderance of patients with macroglobulinemia, but one wonders whether it might be transmitted through the female. Twenty years ago, when I first published my observations on this disease, I wrote: "The hypothesis is put forward that a mechanism analogous to the predominant formation of virus protein in a plant infected with, e.g., tobacco mosaic virus may be present in these cases. A large amount of the protein in the blood would then be found after the image of some abnormal 'virus' protein." In 1952, I discussed the analogy with the gene and wrote: "It does not seem improbable that one or possibly several templates for the synthesis of individual proteins may be modified by a virus-like or gene-like influence." It is possible that these ideas may receive confirmation from family studies.

In 1961, Bottura *et al.* [41] published studies on the karyokinetic picture of cells from a patient with macroglobulinemia which seemed to contain an extra very large chromosome. Some confirmatory observations have been published, together with a large number of negative findings. Final conclusions must be deferred, since negative findings might only mean that abnormal cells, while present, have not been studied in the right mitotic phase.

REFERENCES

1. Waldenström, J. Incipient myelomatosis or "essential" hyperglobulinemia with fibrinogenopenia. *Acta Med. Scand.* 117:216, 1944.
2. Pedersen, K. O. *Ultracentrifugal Studies on Serum and Serum Fractions.* Uppsala: Almqvist and Wiksell, 1945.
3. Waldenström, J. Zwei interessante Syndrome mit Hyperglobulinämie (Purpura hyperglobulinaemica und Makroglobulinämie). *Schweiz. Med. Wschr.* 78:927, 1948.
4. Tischendorf, W., and Hartmann, F. Makroglobulinämie (Waldenström) mit gleichzeitiger Hyperplasie der Gewebsmastzellen. *Acta Haemat.* (Basel) 4:374, 1950.
5. Waldenström, J. Macroglobulinaemia. *Triangle* 3:264, 1959.
6. Waldenström, J. Hypergammaglobulinemia as a clinical hematological problem: A study in the gammopathies. *Progr. Hemato.* 3:266, 1962.
7. Bessis, M., Breton-Gorius, J., and Binet, J. L. Étude comparée du plasmocytome et du syndrome de Waldenström. *Nouv. Rev. Franc. Hemat.* 3:159, 1963.
8. Zucker-Franklin, D., Franklin, E. C., and Cooper, N. S. Production of macroglobulins *in vitro* and a study of their cellular origin. *Blood* 20:56, 1962.
9. Waldenström, J., Winblad, S., and Hällén, J. The occurrence of serological "antibody" reagins or similar γ-globulins in conditions with monoclonal hypergammaglobulinemia, such as myeloma, macroglobulinemia etc. *Acta Med. Scand.* 176:619, 1964.
10. Schaub, F. Gleichzeitiges Vorkommen von Makroglobulinämie Waldenström und von malignen Tumoren. *Schweiz. Med. Wschr.* 83: 1256, 1953.
11. Kappeler, R., Krebs, A., and Riva, G. Klinik der Makroglobulinämie Waldenström. *Helv. Med. Acta* 25:54, 1958.
12. Waldenström, J. Melphalan treatment of myeloma. *Trans. Ass. Amer. Physicians* 76:57, 1963.
13. Waldenström, J. Macroglobulinemia. *Advances Metab. Disord.* (in press).
14. Burnet, M. *The Clonal Selection Theory of Antibody Production.* New York: Oxford University Press, 1959.
15. Jahnke, K., and Scholtan, W. *Die Bluteiweisskörper in der Ultrazentrifuge.* Stuttgart: Georg Thieme Verlag, 1960.
16. Waldenström, J. Abnormal proteins in myeloma. *Advances Intern. Med.* 5:398, 1952.
17. Heremans, J. F. *Les globulines sériques du système gamma: Leur nature et leur pathologie.* Brussels: Editions Arscia, S. A., 1960.
18. Grabar, P. *Analyse Immune Électrophorétique.* Paris: Masson et Cie, 1960.
19. Heremans, J. F., Heremans, M.-T., Laurell, H. F., Laurell, C.-B., Mårtensson, L., Sjöquist, J., and Waldenström, J. Studies on "abnormal" serum globulins (M-components) in myeloma, macroglobulinemia and related diseases. *Acta Med. Scand.*, supp. 367, 1961.
20. Kratochvil, C. H., and Deutsch, H. F. A crystalline macroglobulin from human serum. *J. Biol. Chem.* 222:31, 1956.
21. Müller-Eberhard, H. J., and Kunkel, H. G. Ultracentrifugal characteristics and carbohydrate content of macromolecular γ-globulins. *Clin. Chim. Acta* 4:252, 1959.
22. Korngold, L., and Lipari, R. Multiple myeloma proteins: I and III. *Cancer* 9:183 and 262, 1956.
23. Migita, S., and Putnam, F. W. Antigenic relationship of Bence Jones proteins, myeloma globulins and normal human γ-globulin. *J. Exp. Med.* 117:81, 1963.
24. Mannik, M., and Kunkel, H. G. Classification of myeloma proteins, Bence Jones proteins and macroglobulins into two groups on the basis of common antigenic characters. *J. Exp. Med.* 116:859, 1962.
25. Mannik, M., and Kunkel, H. G. Two major types of normal 7S γ-globulin. *J. Exp. Med.* 117:213, 1963.
26. Mårtensson, L. Ref. 19.
27. Harboe, M., Osterland, C. K., Mannik, M., and Kunkel, H. G. Genetic characters of human γ-globulins in myeloma proteins. *J. Exp. Med.* 116:719, 1962.
28. Schwartz, J. H., and Edelman, G. M. Comparisons of Bence Jones proteins and L polypeptide chains of myeloma globulins after hydrolysis with trypsin. *J. Exp. Med.* 118:41, 1963.
29. Franklin, E. C. Structural units of human 7S γ-globulin. *J. Clin. Invest.* 39:1933, 1960.
30. Waldenström, J. Studies on conditions associated with disturbed gamma-globulin formation (gammopathies). *Harvey Lect.* 56:211, 1961.
31. Yorke, W. On the variation of the haemolytic complement in experimental trypanosomiasis. *Ann. Trop. Med.* 3:565, 1909–10.
32. Charmot, G., Demarchi, J., Orio, J., Reynaud, R., and Vargues, P. Le syndrome splénomégalie avec macroglobulinémie. *Presse Med.* 67:11, 1959.

33. Dreyfus, B., Laroche, C., Fritel, D., Nienna, A., and Schneider, J. Trypanosome responsable d'une maladie de Waldenström. *Presse Med.* 68:590, 1960.
34. Kritzman, J., Kunkel, H. G., McCarthy, J., and Mellors, R. C. Studies of a Waldenström-type macroglobulin with rheumatoid factor properties. *J. Lab. Clin. Med.* 57:905, 1961.
35. Kunkel, H. G., Fudenberg, H., and Ovary, Z. High molecular weight antibodies. *Ann. N.Y. Acad. Sci.* 86:966, 1960.
36. West, C., Hong, R. and Holland, N. Immunoglobulin levels from the newborn period to adulthood and in immunoglobulin deficiency states. *J. Clin. Invest.* 41:2054, 1962.
37. Franklin, E. C., and Kunkel, H. G. Immunologic differences between the 19S and 7S components of normal human γ-globulin. *J. Immun.* 78:11, 1957.
38. Leonhardt, T. Familial hypergammaglobulinaemia and systemic lupus erythematosus. *Lancet* 2:1200, 1957.
39. Waldenström, J. Monoclonal and polyclonal gammopathies and the biological system of gamma globulins. *Progr. Allerg.* 6:320, 1962.
40. Seligmann, M., and Badin, J. β_2-macroglobulinémie familiale. *Rev. Franc. Etud. Clin. Biol.* 7:1107, 1962.
41. Bottura, C., Ferrari, I., and Veiga, A. A. Chromosome abnormalities in Waldenström's macroglobulinemia. *Lancet* 1:1170, 1961.

26. Hodgkin's Disease, Lymphosarcoma, and Chronic Lymphocytic Leukemia

DANIEL G. MILLER

IMMUNE ABNORMALITIES IN LYMphomas and leukemias are as inevitable as circulatory disturbances in heart disease. Consideration of the alterations in the immune system resulting from Hodgkin's disease, lymphosarcoma and chronic lymphocytic leukemia should commence with a perspective on these diseases per se. These entities are manifestations of two fundamentally different neoplastic diseases of the lymphatic system—lymphogranulomatous disease and lymphoproliferative disease. The former is represented by Hodgkin's disease and its histological variants—granuloma, paragranuloma, and sarcoma; the latter by lymphocytic leukemia, acute and chronic, lymphosarcoma, follicular and diffuse, and reticulum cell sarcoma. The separation of Hodgkin's disease from lymphoproliferative diseases is more than a question of semantics and has consequences beyond that of pathological classification. There is a tendency to generalize about these diseases, and the myeloproliferative diseases as well, without regard for their distinctive natural histories, complications, therapeutic individualities, and basically different pathological processes.

The lymphoproliferative diseases may coexist or evolve one into the other during the course. However, it is our distinct impression that in its natural history and evolution, Hodgkin's disease remains a discrete entity and does not evolve into leukemia or lymphosarcoma. Nevertheless the aforementioned histological variants of Hodgkin's disease may coexist. This is contrary to the opinion of others [1, 2]. Hodgkin's disease is one of the few diseases considered to be neoplastic which is not characterized by proliferation of a single cell type. The granulomatous process consists not only of cells of lymphatic origin but of eosinophils and mast cells as well as of connective tissue and endothelial cells. The origin of the Reed-Sternberg cell is ill-defined. There may also be inflammatory changes around the involved nodes, a finding not associated with uncomplicated lymphosarcoma. The necrosis, abscess formation, fibrosis, sarcoid changes, and amyloid degeneration which may be seen in Hodgkin's disease are not found in the lymphoproliferative diseases.

There are significant clinical differences between the lymphogranulomatous and lymphoproliferative diseases. The age incidence in Hodgkin's disease differs from that of the lymphoproliferative diseases [3], and a familial predisposition has been described [4]. Certain characteristics of Hodgkin's disease (fever, night sweats, pruritus, and alcohol-induced pain) are not typical of uncomplicated lymphoproliferative diseases, although they may occur with other malignancies. Just as the pathological process of Hodgkin's disease may be more inflammatory and destructive, the clinical manifestations may be more toxic.

The tendency to regard these diseases as variants of a single process stems not only from the common tissue involved but from the similar response to radiation therapy. However, here, too, there is a difference, for the common observation is that chronic lymphocytic leukemia and lymphosarcoma are more radiosensitive than Hodgkin's disease. A dose-response comparison of these diseases, employing an oral alkylating agent, gave similar results [5]. Lymphocytic leukemia and lymphosarcoma frequently respond to adrenal corticosteroids; Hodgkin's disease seldom does. On the other hand, excellent results are obtained in the treatment of Hodgkin's disease with vinblastine, and such response is uncommon in lymphosarcoma and lymphocytic leukemia. Furthermore, lymphosarcoma as a disease stretches across species barriers and is found with great frequency in many animals. Hodgkin's disease has not been demonstrated clearly in any animal other than man. Thus it would not be unexpected to find that the immunological consequences of these two groups of diseases are different. The changes seen in the myeloproliferative diseases are again different, but these will be considered only parenthetically.

SERUM PROTEINS

Investigations into the immune aspects of these diseases were stimulated in the last decade by the introduction of electrophoretic methods of analyzing serum proteins. Our experience with paper and immunoelectrophoretic analyses of the serum of 240 patients with lymphomas and leukemias has been summarized by Leoncini *et al.* [6]. These findings with regard to γ-globulin are summarized in Figure 26-1 and related to disease activity. In general, the findings are consistent with those of other investigators [7–19]. In Hodgkin's disease, hypoalbuminemia is usually found. It is most often noted in patients with active disease and becomes more profound as the disease advances. The incidence is particularly high in patients with Hodgkin's disease of the liver. The most consistent globulin alteration of Hodgkin's disease is elevation of the α_2 fraction, especially with activity of disease. There may also be elevations of the α_1-, β-, and γ-globulins. Less often, the γ-globulin fraction is depressed. A study of the α_2 fraction of serum protein in uncomplicated Hodgkin's disease revealed three components contributing to the elevation seen in abnormal sera: a haptoglobin portion, one containing protein-bound hexose, and a third consisting chiefly of ceruloplasmin [20]. The elevations of α_1-globulin consisted chiefly of orosomucoid. Use of immunoelectrophoresis has permitted further definition of serum protein change in these diseases. By this technique, the γ-globulin fraction of serum has been separated into three components referred to as the immunoglobulins: γ_{1A}-, γ_{1M}- (macroglobulin), and γ_2-globulin [21].* The quantities of γ-globulin on immunoelectrophoresis in general parallel the findings on paper electrophoresis. But the γ-region on paper electrophoresis represents the sum of the three globulins; therefore there may be significant variations in the three fractions which are masked when only paper electrophoresis is performed. Figure 26-2 shows three paper electrophoretic values of the serum γ-globulin in a patient with Hodgkin's disease. All are normal. Immunoelectrophoretic studies done at the same time show a marked fall of the γ_2- and γ_{1A}-globulins and an elevation of γ_1 macroglobulin in the third specimen.

In chronic lymphocytic leukemia and lymphosarcoma, hypoalbuminemia is not common until the advanced stages of the disease, and here, as in Hodgkin's disease, liver involvement favors the development of this deficiency. Alpha- and β-globulin changes are not characteristic of these diseases, but γ-globulin

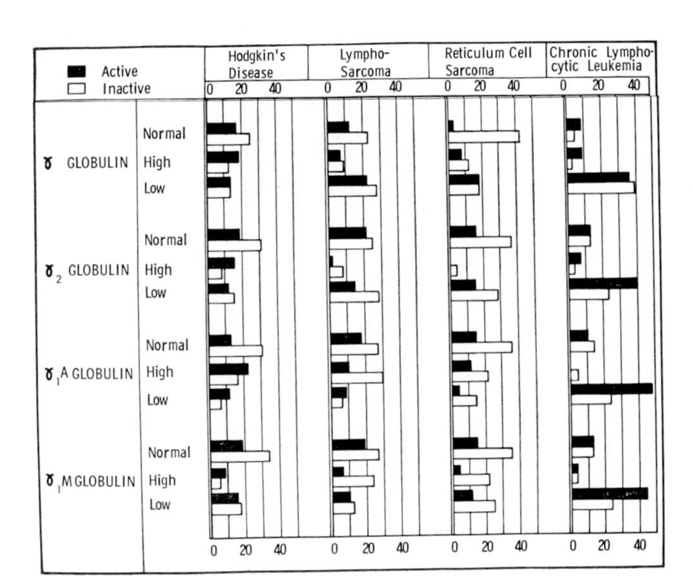

Fig. 26-1. Paper and immune electrophoretic determinations of serum γ-globulin in 240 patients.

* *Editor's comment:* These refer to γ_A, γ_M, and γ_G immunoglobulins; see Chapter 19.—B. R.

TABLE 26-1. Viral Antibody Content of Serum of Patients Compared to Normal Controls[a]

Study Group	Over-all Indices	Antibody Indices of Age Group 20–39	40–59	60–
Control	3.8	4.0	3.8	3.5
HD[b]	3.3	3.7	—	—
LSA	2.9	—	3.3	—
RCS	2.8	—	2.7	—
CLL	2.1	—	—	1.8

[a] Results are summarized for each group as an antibody index $\left(\frac{\text{total no. of antibody reactions}}{\text{no. of individuals tested}}\right)$. Over-all results are presented as well as results for the age groups representing the majority of patients.

[b] HD = Hodgkin's disease; LSA = lymphosarcoma; RCS = reticulum cell sarcoma; CLL = chronic lymphocytic leukemia.

deficiencies are prominent. In Table 26-1, 75 percent of the patients with chronic lymphocytic leukemia had low γ-globulin, and in another study [22], 44 percent of the values were more than 2 standard deviations below the normal mean. Low γ-globulin values are indicative of far-advanced disease and a poor prognosis, little influenced by antileukemic therapy. Ultmann *et al.* [23] found that the survival time of patients with chronic lymphocytic leukemia who did not have low γ-globulin was more than twice that of patients with hypogammaglobulinemia. A low γ-globulin level, when occurring in these diseases, does not remit. Creyssel *et al.* [24] referred to it as a *signe permanent.* Figure 26-3 shows serial determinations of γ-globulin in a patient (R.A.) with chronic lymphocytic leukemia, demonstrating the progression from normal to low values, a feature which remained constant until death. In contrast, the serum γ-globulin levels rose with progression of disease in another patient with chronic lymphocytic leukemia (P.C.); this, too, has remained a constant feature of the disease. Low serum γ-globulin occurs more frequently in chronic lymphocytic leukemia than in lymphosarcoma, but in patients with lymphosarcoma evolving into lymphocytic leukemia, the leukolymphosarcoma group, low γ-globulin levels

	γGlobulin (PEP)	γGlobulin (IEP)
2/20/58	1.12gms%	
5/16/61	1.07gms%	
6/28/61	1.36gms%	

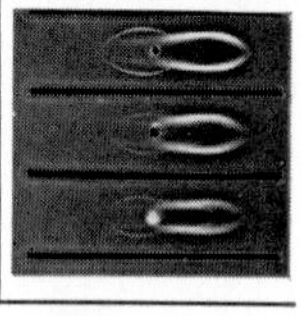

Fig. 26-2. Paper electrophoretic (PEP) and immune electrophoretic (IEP) determinations of γ-globulin in a patient with Hodgkin's disease. All PEP values are within normal limits. However, the IEP of 6/28/61 shows a marked deficiency in γ_2- and γ_{1A}-globulins and an increase in γ_1 macroglobulin. This was just becoming apparent a month earlier and was not present in the first determination. The well contains the patient's serum, and the trough, rabbit antihuman β- and γ-globulin serum.

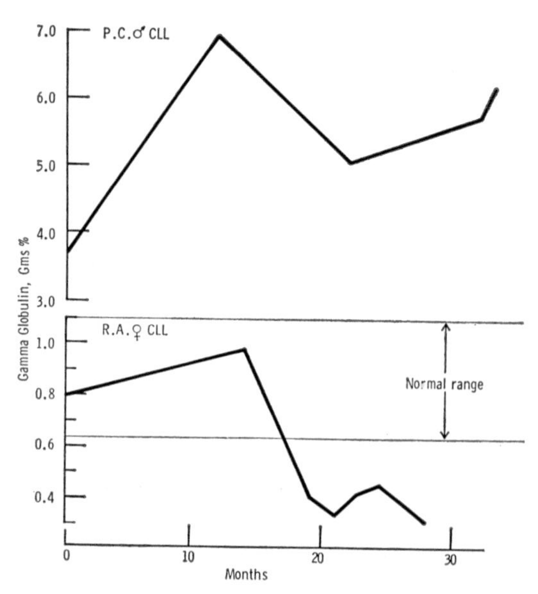

Fig. 26-3. Progressive fall in level of serum γ-globulin in the course of disease in patient R.A., and progressive elevation in patient P.C.

are very common and the degree of hypogammaglobulinemia is likely to be profound. It should be noted that in the less commonly encountered cases of Hodgkin's disease and chronic myelocytic leukemia associated with hypogammaglobulinemia, the depression is seldom as profound as in the aforementioned diseases, nor has this finding been related to susceptibility to infection, as in the lymphoproliferative diseases.

Immunoelectrophoretic studies of the γ-globulins in chronic lymphocytic leukemia and lymphosarcoma have revealed wide variations. Figure 26-4 shows the patterns of the immunoglobulins in a normal control (case 1) and 6 patients with chronic lymphocytic leukemia. Cases 2 and 3 had severe hypogammaglobulinemia. Case 4 had hypo- and case 5, hypermacroglobulinemia. There is a slight increase in macroglobulin in case 6 and an increase in all three γ-globulin fractions in case 7, who also had cryoglobulinemia. The differentiation between γ_{1A}-globulin and γ_1 macroglobulin was made by other means, using specific antisera. The initial finding of normal γ-globulins in many patients with lymphoproliferative disease evolving into various gammopathies with progression of disease suggests that normal lymphatic tissues gradually are replaced by a neoplastic population of lymphocytes rather than that a leukemic or lymphomatous transformation of the entire lymphatic system takes place. The globulin-producing capacity of the proliferating leukemic tissue will become increasingly apparent as this tissue replaces the normal. Thus we may find normal, hyper-, or hypogammaglobulinemia. The hypergammaglobulinemia is usually a broad or diffuse elevation, although sharp monoclonal peaks of macroglobulin and myeloma globulin have been seen in these diseases [25, 26]. In addition, we have encountered cryoglobulinemia in chronic lymphocytic leukemia, lymphosarcoma, and Hodgkin's disease.

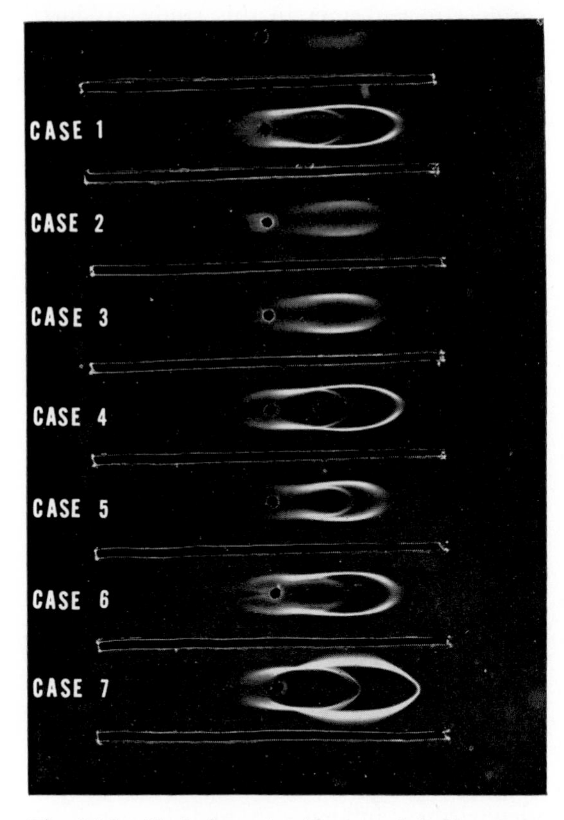

Fig. 26-4. Variations in immunoglobulins in a normal control and six patients with chronic lymphocytic leukemia. The well contains the patient's serum, and the trough, rabbit antihuman γ-globulin serum. (From L. Korngold, *Ann. N.Y. Acad. Sci.* 94:110, 1961; courtesy of author and publisher.)

Haptoglobin and C-reactive protein, which are readily identified by immunoelectrophoresis, generally rise in the serum with diseases characterized by inflammation and tissue damage. Haptoglobin migrates on electrophoresis as an α_2-globulin and C-reactive protein as β-globulin. In Hodgkin's disease; activity and extent of disease can, in general, be correlated with these two factors. In addition, their levels have prognostic significance. In the experience mentioned earlier, all the patients with 2+ to 4+ elevation of haptoglobin, and the majority of those with strong C-reactive protein reactions, died within two years of the study [6]. The same observations could not be made in the patients with chronic lymphocytic leukemia and lymphosarcoma.

The serum protein characteristics described in the foregoing paragraphs apply in general to uncomplicated lymphomas and leukemias. The complications frequently seen with these diseases, such as infection, liver disease, and hemolytic anemia, impose their own characteristics on the serum protein fractions. It is believed that the treatment received by these patients plays a relatively minor role in altering the serum proteins and is not responsible for the changes characteristic of these diseases.

CIRCULATING ANTIBODIES

There have been many studies on the ability to form circulating antibodies in patients having these diseases. The early reports, those in 1914 by Moreschi [27] and Rotky [28] and in 1920 by Howell [29], led to the conclusion that patients with "leukemia" are poor producers of antibodies. Subsequent investigations have substantiated this general conclusion, but it has been qualified, as will be noted.

A poor response to immunization with typhoid-paratyphoid A and B vaccine [17, 30–32] as well as pneumococcal antigen [33–35] has been observed in chronic lymphocytic leukemia and lymphosarcoma. With tularemia vaccine, 8 percent of chronic lymphocytic leukemia and 23.3 percent of lymphosarcoma and reticulum cell sarcoma patients responded, in contrast to 94 percent of normal subjects [36]. Antibodies to mumps, influenza and diphtheria antigens have been found to be deficient in chronic lymphocytic leukemia [17].

Reports on the ability of patients with Hodgkin's disease to produce circulating antibodies differ. Antibody response to mumps vaccine [37] and sheep red cells and isohemagglutinin titers were normal [38, 39]. Typhoid-paratyphoid vaccine produced no measurable antibodies in 8 patients in two studies [29, 38]; in another, 13 patients had antibody titers comparable to those of normal controls, but they did not sustain them as well [40]. In patients with Hodgkin's disease and active brucellosis, antibodies were absent in one study [41]; in another, their presence was demonstrated in some patients [42]. In the aforementioned study with tularemia vaccine, 41 percent of the patients with Hodgkin's disease responded [36]. In two studies, there was a poor antibody response to pneumococcal polysaccharides [33, 35]. In a third [43], significant response was obtained in 15 of 19 patients; however, in this study also, the antibody response in many patients was not sustained as it was in normal subjects. The four patients who did not respond had far-advanced disease. The condition of the patient, extent of disease, and treatment administered all play a role in determining the ability to respond to an antigenic stimulus. However, Geller [33] observed a patient with extensive lymphosarcoma, clinically in the terminal stages and with leukopenia induced by nitrogen mustard, who produced a very high titer of antibody to pneumococcal polysaccharide. It is not unusual to see patients go through the entire course of chronic leukemia or malignant lymphoma without infection or other manifestation of abnormal immunity, despite vigorous therapy and progressive cachexia. In such cases, one must conclude either that sufficient normal lymphatic tissue is present to perform adequately or that the proliferating lymphatic tissue has retained some functional ability.

In 11 untreated patients with acute leukemia, Larson and Tomlinson [35] found that all produced antibodies to pneumococcal polysaccharides, 9 in unusually large amounts. In another group of patients with the same disease but treated with cortisone, antibody production was less, but still greater than in the controls. The 7 patients with chronic myelocytic leukemia in this study produced antibodies in the normal range. In a study of antibody production in 10 patients with acute leukemia, Silver *et al.* [44] found that the response to any one of the antigens used did not differ significantly from that of the controls but that the over-all rise in antibody titer in the leukemic group was poorer than in the controls. However, the authors noted that all the leukemic patients received antimetabolites at some time during the study. There was no correlation between antibody production and the occurrence of infectious complications. In the study using tularemia vaccine, 5 of 10 patients with acute leukemia had a normal antibody response [36].

Millian *et al.* [45] studied the viral antibody content of the serum of 107 patients with Hodgkin's disease, lymphosarcoma, reticulum cell sarcoma, and chronic lymphocytic leukemia. All were ambulatory, and none had received any viral vaccines before the serum specimen was obtained. For control, serum was taken from normal individuals matched with regard to age, sex, and time of bleeding. Sera were studied for antibodies to herpes simplex, mumps, respiratory syncytial and adenoviruses, influenza A and B, parainfluenza 2 and 3, psittacosis-lymphogranuloma venereum virus and rickettsialpox. All groups of patients had relatively high frequency of antibodies to herpes simplex virus, the incidence increasing with age, and of antibodies to parainfluenza 3 and influenza B viruses. A deficiency of influenza A and respiratory syncytial antibodies was seen only in the chronic lymphocytic leukemia patients. The sera of patients with Hodgkin's disease contained mumps antibodies as frequently as did the sera of controls, but progressively fewer patients with reticulum cell sarcoma, lymphosarcoma, and chronic lymphocytic leukemia had mumps antibodies. Antibody to mumps virus represents the ability to maintain antibody production after exposure almost certainly before the onset of Hodgkin's disease, a finding which is in contrast to the experience cited earlier regarding the inability of such patients to maintain antibody production after pneumococcal polysaccharide and typhoid paratyphoid vaccinations. Adenovirus antibodies were not as numerous in any of the disease groups as in the controls; however, the Hodgkin's disease patients again deserve mention, for this deficiency in adenovirus antibodies was an exception in an otherwise normal antibody profile. Such was not the case with the other diseases, in which other antibody deficiencies occurred as well. This may be of interest in view of the oncogenic ability of human adenoviruses in the Syrian hamster and the observation that the onset of disease in the vast majority of patients with Hodgkin's disease is seen in lymph nodes draining respiratory passages. This incidence of antibodies to parainfluenza 3 was very low in both disease and control groups, and none of the sera had antibodies to psittacosis-lymphogranuloma venereum or rickettsialpox. The over-all antibody response to these viruses is summarized in Table 26-1. In keeping with the bacterial experience, Hodgkin's disease patients were close to normal, lymphosarcoma and reticulum cell sarcoma patients poorer, and those with chronic lymphocytic leukemia most deficient in antibody content.

Barr and Fairley [46] have pointed out that some of the contradictory reports on antibody production may be due to failure to distinguish between primary and secondary immunization. In their study, patients with Hodgkin's disease and chronic myelocytic leukemia responded better to secondary than to primary immunization. Those with chronic lymphocytic leukemia and lymphosarcoma were poorest antibody producers on primary and also on secondary immunization.

The incidence of elevated heterophil antibody titers is of interest in differentiating these diseases from infectious mononucleosis. It is not uncommon for the patient to present initially with lymphocytosis, lymphadenopathy, and a history of sore throat [47]. Of 94 patients with acute leukemia, 19 percent had titers of 1 : 112 or higher [48]. Twenty-one percent of 29 patients with Hodgkin's disease had similar elevations, but none of 8 patients with chronic myelocytic leukemia or 10 patients with chronic lymphocytic leukemia, and only 1 of 9 patients with lymphosarcoma, had such a titer. These elevated titers were not diagnostic of infectious mononucleosis, since the antibodies could be absorbed by boiled guinea pig kidney suspension. Use of the guinea pig absorption technique affords a clearcut method of distinguishing the antibody of infectious mononucleosis from the antibody to Forssman antigen. The most likely source of Forssman antigen stimulation is that contained in many species of bacteria. A higher incidence of significant titers in patients with acute leukemia and Hodgkin's disease is in keeping with the finding of relatively intact mechanisms for producing circulating antibodies in these diseases. However, three cases have been reported of infectious mononucleosis occurring simultaneously with Hodgkin's disease [49–51].

DELAYED HYPERSENSITIVITY

Delayed hypersensitivity reactions are believed to be mediated by cell-bound antibodies and do not lend themselves readily to quantitation. Skin testing is a common method of evaluating this type of immune response.

Thirty-one patients with chronic lymphocytic leukemia were given skin tests with tuberculin purified protein derivative, mumps skin test antigen, and *Candida albicans* antigen. Fifteen responded to the tuberculin antigen and 13 to each of the other two antigens. Six of the 31 gave negative responses to all three tests, and 80.6 percent responded to at least one antigen [31, 39]. In the study of Shaw *et al.* [17], most of the patients with chronic lymphocytic leukemia responded normally to skin testing with tuberculin and histoplasmin. Nine of 10 adults with acute leukemia responded to at least one of three antigens [52]. Three of 4 patients with chronic myelocytic leukemia responded to at least one of four skin test antigens [53]. Of 91 patients with carcinoma of various sites, 45 percent responded to at least one of three skin test antigens [54].

Of Dubin's 38 patients with Hodgkin's disease, 1 reacted to tuberculin antigen [55]. Schier *et al.* [37] skin tested 43 patients with Hodgkin's disease, with the following results in comparison with the controls: tuberculin 23 and 71 percent; mumps 14 and 90 percent; *Candida albicans* 19 and 92 percent; and *Trichophyton gypseum* 16 and 68 percent. Kelly *et al.* [56] tested 43 patients with Hodgkin's disease with a battery of five antigens, and 45 percent reacted to at least one antigen. Of 288 controls without Hodgkin's diseases; 98.6 percent reacted to at least one skin test. A correlation has not been made of infectious complications and anergy in Hodgkin's disease.

Sokal and Primikirios [54] studied delayed hypersensitivity reactions in relation to activity of disease. Abnormal reactions were found more frequently in Hodgkin's disease than in lymphosarcoma or chronic lymphocytic leukemia. A high incidence of anergy was found even when the patients were asymptomatic. Of the Hodgkin's disease patients with systemic symptoms, 79 percent were anergic to four skin test antigens, and 60 percent of those with inactive disease were anergic. In asymptomatic patients with lymphosarcoma or chronic lymphocytic leukemia, there was little depression of cutaneous sensitivity: 27 percent of patients were anergic, in contrast to 18 percent of normal controls. None of the patients with active Hodgkin's disease responded to all four test antigens. Three percent of the Hodgkin's disease patients with inactive disease responded to all four test antigens, as did 17 percent of the lymphosarcoma and chronic lymphocytic leukemia patients and 10 percent of the normal controls. In patients who had systemic manifestations of lymphoproliferative disease, 76 percent were anergic, an incidence approaching that of the patients with active Hodgkin's disease. Lamb *et al.* [57] studied the incidence of anergy in patients with Hodgkin's disease, other lymphoma and leukemia (not further classified), and carcinoma. They used seven skin test antigens, five of which caused a positive response in more than 50 percent of 208 male hospital patients in good condition who were used as controls. Of the 192 patients with malignant diseases studied, only those with Hodgkin's disease had a high incidence of anergy while still in good general condition. With progression of disease, there is an increase in the frequency of anergy [57, 58]. Even activity in localized Hodgkin's disease may result in anergy. The converse also appears to be true: anergic patients with active Hodgkin's disease may recover skin sensitivity if remission is achieved, although it may take several months to reappear [54, 58].

The mechanism of anergy in Hodgkin's disease has been studied by passive transfer of delayed hypersensitivity accomplished by injecting leukocytes from a sensitive donor to an anergic recipient. Such transfer has been accomplished in normal individuals and in patients with carcinoma and sarcoid, but not in patients with Hodgkin's disease [59–63]. This is also our experience. The significance of this finding is heightened by the observation that the reaction was negative when tested at the site of injection of the sensitized cells as well as at distant skin sites. This suggests not only a failure to transfer tuberculin sensitivity to the cells of the patient with Hodgkin's disease but an inability of the normal cells to express their sensitivity in the Hodgkin's disease environment. It is known that the tuberculin reaction may be suppressed as a result of debilitation or starvation, in miliary tuberculosis and in febrile viral diseases [62–66], but a common link between the anergy of Hodgkin's disease and these anergic states has not been demonstrated. A tuberculin-neutralizing factor has been found in some normal sera and the sera of patients with sarcoidosis [67–69].*

A group of anergic Hodgkin's disease patients studied by Kelly *et al.* [56] had normal γ-globulin levels, produced plasma cells, and formed circulating agglutinins, antitoxic antibodies, and complement-fixing antibodies on appropriate stimulation. Similar findings were reported by Aisenberg and Leskowitz [43].

Most studies of delayed hypersensitivity have depended on chance prior exposure for immunization. In the case of the tuberculin skin test, the incidence of positive reactors in recent years has fallen off conspicuously, and a negative reaction today would not necessarily

* *Editor's comment:* In contrast, passive transfer of tuberculin sensitivity can be achieved in patients with sarcoid.—B. R.

indicate anergy. Active immunization under standardized conditions is a more reliable and meaningful procedure. Immunization with diphtheria toxoid [56, 70] and BCG [54] has confirmed the association of anergy and Hodgkin's disease. Aisenberg [58] employed skin contact with an acetone solution of dinitrochlorobenzene to sensitize patients with Hodgkin's disease. Twenty-five with active disease remained anergic after being immunized with this antigen; 14 of the 25 were in good general condition and not debilitated in any way. Eight in this group had early and localized disease. Eleven of 12 patients with inactive Hodgkin's disease responded normally. All patients whose disease had been inactive more than two years had normal cutaneous sensitivity.

In patients with chronic lymphocytic leukemia, lymphosarcoma, reticulum cell sarcoma, and Hodgkin's disease who were positive reactors to tuberculin, addition of hydrocortisone to a solution of antigen enhanced skin sensitivity in one study. The same procedure in normal positive controls inhibited the reaction [71]. If this were a replicable phenomenon, it would provide interesting insight into the mechanism of anergy. However, Fairley and Matthias [72] found that the effect of mixing tuberculin and cortisone acetate was to decrease the skin reactivity in patients with these diseases. Five of the 62 tuberculin-negative patients did respond to this procedure, but the frequency (8 percent) was approximately the same as in the controls. Thus the mechanism of anergy is probably different from that seen in sarcoidosis and tuberculosis, for in these diseases the mixture of tuberculin and cortisone converts negative to positive, or enhances skin reactivity in a large percentage of cases, indicating that there is a latent tuberculin sensitivity [73–75].

The abnormality of the immune system in Hodgkin's disease resembles that of another granulomatous disease, sarcoidosis, more than it does that of the lymphoproliferative diseases. Patients with sarcoidosis have a high incidence of skin anergy, and they, too, exhibit the paradox of deficiency of cell-bound antibodies but unimpaired circulating antibody production [76–77]. The significant immunological differences between Hodgkin's disease and sarcoidosis are the latent tuberculin sensitivity in sarcoid, which may be demonstrated by the local injection of cortisone, and the successful passive transfer of tuberculin sensitivity with lymphocytes which has been accomplished in sarcoid but not in Hodgkin's disease.

INFLAMMATORY RESPONSE AND OTHER FACTORS

The inflammatory reaction to the intracutaneous injection of histamine was studied by Schier [53] in 33 patients with Hodgkin's disease and 12 with chronic lymphocytic leukemia, lymphosarcoma, reticulum cell sarcoma, chronic myelocytic leukemia, and sarcoidosis. All were capable of a normal response to histamine. However, this reaction may be altered by thrombocytopenia, and in patients with lymphomas or leukemia and a low platelet count it is not uncommon to find hemorrhagic areas of inflammation. The adrenal corticosteroids find widespread use in this group of diseases and profoundly influence the inflammatory response by reducing vascular permeability. It is likely that this action is as important, if not more important, in altering resistance to infection as its influence on antibody formation [78–80].

The cellular composition of inflammatory exudates studied at autopsy and clinically by the skin window technique has been found to be normal in patients with chronic leukemias and in some patients with Hodgkin's disease [31, 81, 82]. However, Rebuck *et al.* [83], studying nine experimental inflammatory lesions in five patients with Hodgkin's disease, found a striking lymphocytic "hiatus" in the leukocytic cycles of the inflammatory response. Not only was the lesion lacking in lymphocytes but the over-all cellularity was lower than in the control. Four of the five patients had been or were under active treatment at the time of study, but the same deficiency was found in an untreated patient included in this group. This was not the only deficiency noted. The peroxidase activity in the exudate of cells of the inflammatory reaction of two patients with Hodgkin's disease revealed almost complete suppression of this reaction. These observations would be of great importance if they proved to be characteristic of Hodgkin's disease. They would provide cellular and physiological markers for family studies. One would also be interested in knowing whether the abnormalities preceded the onset of the disease and whether the cellular abnormality indicated a transformation of all cells of that series or the presence of two populations of cells.

In acute leukemia, there may be a deficiency in circulating mature granulocytes, and the inflammatory response may be relatively acellular [84]. Cells less mature than metamyelocytes do not migrate to the site of inflammation. The same situation may be seen in other neutropenic states. It should be pointed out that not only is the inflammatory response deficient in the acute stage, in which polymorphonuclear leukocytes predominate, but the cellular deficiencies extend into the period when mononuclear cells would be accumulating in the lesion [82, 85, 86]. Opie [87] suggested that this might be the consequence of the polymorphonuclear leukocyte deficiency, for he found that it was these cells together with the products of tissue injury which acted as the principal stimulant to the accumulation of mononuclear cells. A study of the pharyngeal exudate during infection in acute leukemia failed to reveal a granulocytic response [88]. In the sputum of chronic lymphocytic leukemia patients studied during episodes of pneumonia, the predominant cell was the polymorphonuclear leukocyte. However, the chronic inflammatory response in leukemia may be abnormal; for example, in areas of chronic inflammation such as bronchiectasis, where plasma cells would be found normally, they were absent in an autopsy study of patients with chronic lymphocytic leukemia and infection [89].

The mature granulocytes seen in the peripheral blood in leukemia have been shown to be capable of phagocytosis, although some observers have reported a deficiency in the degree of phagocytosis in the granulocytes of chronic myelocytic leukemia [82, 90–93]. Hoff [94] has indicated a relation between the enzymatic content of phagocytic cells and their function. This may have significance for the manner in which the phagocytized material is subsequently disposed of by the cell. In chronic lymphocytic leukemia, the percentage of mature granulocytes in the peripheral blood is usually reduced but the absolute number frequently remains normal. In Hodgkin's disease there is no deficiency of circulating mature granulocytes; on the contrary, leukocytosis is common. The leukopenia occasionally seen is most often related to treatment or bone marrow involvement.

Biozzi *et al.* [95] measured the phagocytic function of the reticuloendothelial system in man by the use of clearance measurements of denatured human albumin labeled with radioactive iodine. The two patients with Hodgkin's disease had normal clearances.

Serum complement levels in lymphomas and leukemias are usually within normal limits [96]. The properdin levels have been decreased in some patients with chronic lymphocytic leukemia, lymphosarcoma, and Hodgkin's disease, but most patients studied had levels within normal limits [39, 97, 98]. Properdin levels have been low most consistently in acute leukemia. Of 66 patients with acute leukemia, Southam [99] found low titers in 28 and zone phenomena in 8; 49 percent of the determinable titers were low. No correlation was found with ability to accept or reject skin grafts and the properdin titers [39]. We attempted to correlate complement and properdin levels with infectious complications in 19 patients with chronic lymphocytic leukemia [31]. None of those who had been free from infection had deficient complement or properdin titers, nor did they have any abnormality in other aspects of immune function. Two patients were deficient in complement and 6 in properdin titers. All had infections requiring treatment during the course of the disease. In addition, all had deficiencies in γ-globulin, circulating antibodies, or delayed hypersensitivity reactions. One or another of these deficiencies was noted in 7 patients with a history of infections or recurrent infectious complications and normal complement and properdin titers. Properdin is a nonantibody serum protein which is active against gram-negative bacteria [100]. It would be relevant to the known function of properdin to study its role in host resistance against infections with these organisms. In 2 of our patients with Hodgkin's disease and *Salmonella typhimurium* septicemia, properdin was not present.

INFECTION

It is generally recognized that patients with leukemia and lymphoma have poor resistance to infection, but here, too, the fact that these

TABLE 26-2. Infectious Complications in 436 Patients with Lymphomas and Leukemias

Infections	Chronic Lymphocytic Leukemia	Lymphosarcoma	Reticulum Cell Sarcoma	Acute Leukemia	Chronic Myelocytic Leukemia	Hodgkin's Disease
Total no. of admissions	24	87	83	91	7	144
Total no. of bacterial infections	9 (37.2%)	11 (12.6%)	14 (16.9%)	44 (48.5%)	0	18 (12.5%)
Pneumonia, bronchitis, or empyema	8	3	6[a]	5	—	8[b]
Urinary tract infections	—	3	3	8	—	1
Cellulitis, furunculosis, or subcutaneous abscess	—	—	2	7	—	2
Pharyngitis, stomatitis, otitis media, or sinusitis	—	1	—	6	—	1
Septicemia	1	3	3	18	—	5
Unclassified	1	—	—	5	—	1
Other infections	—	—	—	—	—	10[c]

[a] One case associated with local disease.
[b] Three cases associated with local disease.
[c] One retroperitoneal abscess, two cryptococcus meningitis, seven probable viral infection.
SOURCE: Miller [52].

are a heterogeneous group of diseases with characteristic cellular, protein, and immunological abnormalities appears to influence the way in which resistance to infection is impaired. Wintrobe and Hasenbush [101] reported in 1939 that infectious complications were more frequent in chronic lymphocytic than in chronic myelocytic leukemia. They emphasized the frequency with which pneumococcal lobar pneumonia was seen in patients with chronic lymphocytic leukemia, a complication which was not seen among the larger number of chronic myelocytic leukemia patients.

Table 26-2 lists the infectious complications which occurred during 436 hospital admissions of patients with lymphomas and leukemias. This represents all the admissions of patients with these diseases to one institution in a single year. The highest percentage of infectious complications, 48.5, appeared in acute leukemia. These occurred almost invariably during relapse and frequently subsided during remission. There were no infectious complications in chronic myelocytic leukemia. Chronic lymphocytic leukemia had the second highest frequency, 37.2 percent; lymphosarcoma, reticulum cell sarcoma, and Hodgkin's disease had approximately the same incidences. The type of associated infections is also of interest. Pneumonia was seen in all but 1 of the chronic lymphocytic leukemia patients. Septicemia was most common in acute leukemia; next in frequency were infections of the oropharynx and skin. The bacterial complications in Hodgkin's disease were varied. However, the 2 cases of cryptococcal meningitis and the viral infections which occurred in this sampling were in patients with Hodgkin's disease.

Occasionally, infectious complications in the lymphomas and leukemias result from destruction of protective surfaces, production of fistulae, or obstruction of body cavities by the disease. However, these causes are seen more frequently with carcinoma. In the great majority of lymphomas and leukemias, such local factors do not explain the increased sensitivity to infection. However, an indication, if not the complete explanation, is found in the impairments in the immune system characteristic of these diseases. Of 61 patients with chronic lymphocytic leukemia studied by Creyssel *et al.* [24], 21 had complicating hypogammaglobulinemia and numerous infectious complications. Among the 21 were 16 instances of recurrent and chronic pulmonary infections, 8 of skin infections, and 7 of miscellaneous infectious complications. Similar results were reported by Ultmann *et al.* [23] in 60 patients with chronic lymphocytic leukemia and lymphosarcoma. Of our 22 patients with chronic lymphocytic leukemia, 11 had hypogammaglobulinemia and recurrent pulmonary infection. Skin infections were the next most common, and there were a variety of miscellaneous infections. However, the pulmonary infections were the most troublesome clinically, and in most cases responsible for death [31]. No case of tuberculosis was reported in the 143 cases of chronic lymphocytic leukemia mentioned above. Tuberculosis is not common with agammaglobulinemia; pneumonia is. In three patients with prior history of tuberculosis, chronic lymphocytic leukemia did not aggravate the disease [24]. Parkes [102] reviewed evidence that tuberculin sensitivity behaves normally in patients with hypogammaglobulinemia, and in 2 patients observed by him, the natural course of tuberculosis appeared to be affected by the hypogammaglobulinemia. In chronic lymphocytic leukemia, no correlation was found between infectious complications and the absolute number of granulocytes in the peripheral blood [31]. In acute leukemia, bacterial infection frequently was preceded by fall in mature granulocytes in the peripheral blood [88].

Staphylococcus aureus and the *pneumococcus* were the organisms most frequently found in our cases of chronic lymphocytic leukemia and pulmonary infection. In acute leukemia, organisms usually considered nonpathogenic may cause infectious disease [88]. The frequency, variety, and severity of infection in acute leukemia emphasize the primary role of polymorphonuclear leukocytes in host resistance. It should also be emphasized that if the patient with acute leukemia achieves hematological remission, it is usual for resistance to infection to improve. This is concomitant with the appearance of an adequate number of mature granulocytes. However, response to therapy in chronic lymphocytic leukemia is seldom associated with improved host resistance. When these patients reach the stage of disease characterized by hypogammaglobulinemia and recurrent infection, reduction in lymph node size or hematological improvement seldom eliminates the problem of recurrent infection. When hematological remission is achieved in acute leukemia, the bone marrow appears to be normal and hematological functions become normal. In chronic lymphocytic leukemia, hypogammaglobulinemia means that the leukemic process has replaced normal lymphatic tissue to a degree that an adequate amount of γ-globulin cannot be produced. Even if this leukemic tissue is suppressed by irradiation or chemotherapy, lymphoid follicles do not reappear. The lymphatic tissue does not resume its normal architecture nor its normal function.

The situation in Hodgkin's disease is more complex. Recurrent or chronic infection is uncommon except when tissue integrity has been destroyed by local disease or in patients treated to the point of bone marrow depression. That is not to say that there are no infectious complications characteristic of Hodgkin's disease. Jackson and Parker [103] found that 20 percent of their patients with advanced Hodgkin's disease also had active tuberculosis. It was Ewing's [104] opinion that there was a unique association between Hodgkin's disease and tuberculosis. Razis *et al.* [3] found a lower incidence of tuberculosis (5.1 percent), which probably represents diminished opportunity for contact. However, the difference between the incidence of tuberculosis in Hodgkin's disease and that in lymphosarcoma was of high statistical significance.

Another disease which evokes a granulomatous inflammation and results in immunity of the delayed hypersensitivity type is cryptococcosis. Among the 247 cases of cryptococcosis reviewed by Collins *et al.* [105] were 21 cases of lymphoma: 14 of Hodgkin's disease, 4 of lymphosarcoma, and 3 of unspecified types of leukemia. Among the 60 cases of cryptococcosis reported by Zimmerman and Rappaport [106] were 18 lymphoma: 11 of Hodgkin's disease, 2 of reticulum cell sarcoma, 1 of multiple myeloma, and 4 of different types of leukemia. With regard to Hodgkin's disease and cryptococcosis, Gendel *et al.* [107] observed, ". . . the association of these two uncommon diseases occurs much too frequently to be simply a matter of chance." In an area where brucellosis was highly endemic, Wise and Poston [42] found that *Brucella* was isolated frequently from the nodes of Hodgkin's disease but only rarely from nodes of other lymphomatous diseases or in lymphadenopathy due to other causes.

Patients with Hodgkin's disease are particularly susceptible to diseases which normally cause a granulomatous reaction. Whether this susceptibility is a result of Hodgkin's disease, as is generally assumed, or whether it plays a role in the etiology of the disease remains to be determined.

The use of adrenal corticosteroids for long periods in patients with Hodgkin's disease and the lymphoproliferative diseases contributes to their susceptibility to infection. Latent tuberculosis may be reactivated; deep mycotic infections, such as actinomycosis, aspergillosis, nocardiosis, and mucormycosis, may supervene, and cytomegalic inclusion disease may appear. Herpes zoster and simplex are seen with unusual frequency in these diseases, especially in the advanced stages. In some cases the infection may persist over many years, or may be recurrent at the same site. There may be dissemination of herpes zoster to generalized herpetic dermatitis indistinguishable from varicella. We have encountered multiple verrucous infections and condylomata acuminata in these diseases. Fatal vaccinia gangrenosa has been reported in hypogammaglobulinemia [108].

Although it appears that the primary deficiency leading to increased susceptibility to infection in the lymphoproliferative diseases is in the production of γ-globulin and circulating antibodies, and in Hodgkin's disease an abnormal delayed hypersensitivity reaction, one recognizes that the various parameters of host resistance to infection are interrelated. For example, patients with hypogammaglobulinemia may have a normal number of mature granulocytes, but they may not function in an optimal fashion in the absence of opsonins. The relation between polymorphonuclear leukocytes and lymphocytes in the inflammatory response has been mentioned. In addition, there are other aspects of host resistance, such as reticuloendothelial function with regard to phagocytosis and endotoxins and some of the aforementioned nonantibody serological factors which have not been adequately evaluated for clinical significance. Nevertheless clinicopathological patterns are discernible, for pneumonia is the hallmark of hypogammaglobulinemia, congenital or acquired, and pharyngitis or stomatitis is most characteristic of the agranulocytic state, whatever the cause. This is distinctly different from the granulomatous types of infection to which patients with Hodgkin's disease are most susceptible.

IMMUNOPATHIC CONDITIONS IN HODGKIN'S AND LYMPHOPROLIFERATIVE DISEASES

In addition to infection, there are other consequences of these neoplastic diseases of the immune system. Hemolytic anemia is a common complication of chronic lymphocytic leukemia and lymphosarcoma and is seen also in Hodgkin's disease [109]; both warm and cold antibodies have been observed. Paradoxically, Coombs-positive hemolytic anemia has been observed in patients with chronic lymphocytic leukemia who have greatly reduced levels of γ-globulin [89, 110]. Thrombocytopenia may also occur as an autoimmune complication of these diseases [111].

Collagen-vascular diseases are another immunopathic consequence of these disorders. Arthralgia is a common complaint, and bursitis and tenosynovitis may be encountered. This is in contrast to the myeloproliferative diseases, in which arthralgia is usually associated with gout, and acute leukemia, in which joint symptoms are frequently due to leukemic infiltration. In addition to localized joint and soft tissue symptoms, systemic rheumatoid diseases have been recorded in lymphoproliferative disease and Hodgkin's disease. These include rheumatoid arthritis, systemic lupus erythematosus (LE), polyarteritis nodosa, dermatomyositis, scleroderma, rheumatoid spondylitis, and Sjögren's syndrome. Hench *et al.* [112] studied 1,000 patients with a lymphoma diagnosis and found 22 with significant systemic rheumatoid complaints. Cammarata *et al.* [113] reported on 4 patients with such an association.The systemic rheumatoid disease either closely preceded or followed the appearance of lymphoma. In 3 of 58 patients with Sjögren's syndrome observed by Talal and Bunim [114] reticulum cell sarcoma developed, and in a fourth, changes resembling Waldenström's macroglobulinemia. The duration of Sjögren's syndrome before the appearance of lymphoma varied between four and ten years. Blodgett and associates [115] reported on 16 patients with hematological diseases and carpal tunnel syndrome. Three had lymphoma (not further classified) and 1, chronic lymphocytic leukemia. Razis *et al.* [3] found 4 of 1,109 patients with Hodgkin's disease who had polyarteritis, scleroderma, or dermatomyositis. In the same study, Hodgkin's disease was observed in 2 patients who had had idiopathic thrombocytopenic purpura and who had been successfully treated by splenectomy. Similar associations have been reported by others [116–118].

In patients with chronic lymphocytic leukemia, lymphosarcoma, and Hodgkin's disease we have encountered rheumatoid arthritis, systemic LE, discoid LE, cold agglutinin disease, glomerulonephritis, ulcerative colitis, encephalomalacia, cold urticaria, erythema multiforme, generalized exfoliative dermatitis, and Stevens-Johnson syndrome. Hemolytic anemia was frequent in these patients and warm antibodies were common. Other serological abnormalities included macro- and cryoglobulinemia, antinuclear antibodies, positive LE cell preparations, positive latex fixation, and leukocyte and platelet agglutinins (including two patients who had never had a transfusion). In five patients, lymphocytes were stained with fluorescin-labeled antihuman globulin. Cryoglobulinemia associated with Raynaud's syndrome and with hemolytic anemia has been reported in chronic lymphocytic leukemia [119, 120]. Brody and Beizer [121] demonstrated coating of lymphocytes with globulin in patients with chronic lymphocytic leukemia. Positive LE cell preparations have been observed in patients with lymphosarcoma and Hodgkin's disease [122, 123]. Candreviotis [124] described hematoxylin bodies in patients with Hodgkin's disease. Certain neurological disorders seen in lymphomas have been attributed to an autoimmune etiology, e.g., progressive multifocal encephalopathy, cerebral demyelinization, and peripheral neuropathy, motor, sensory, and mixed [125–127]. Careful study has separated such patients from those whose neurological disorder was due to lymphomatous infiltration, hemorrhage, or amyloid disease. Moeschlin [128] postulated that some of the signs and symptoms of Hodgkin's disease, e.g., chills, fever, eosinophilia, are the result of autoimmunization with abnormal proteins produced by the disease. Blood and plasma transfusion reactions and drug allergies are also common in these patients. Dworin *et al.* [129] found the incidence of atopic allergy (asthma, eczema, hay fever, urticaria) in Hodgkin's disease to be the same as in the general population.

A likely link between rheumatoid and lymphomatous disease is an abnormal underlying immune system. Although this cannot be demonstrated in every case at present, supportive evidence is accumulating. Systemic rheumatoid disease and lymphoproliferative disease each occurs more commonly than would be expected by chance in patients with congenital agammaglobulinemia [130, 131]. Page *et al.* [132] observed a child with congenital agammaglobulinemia in whom dermatomyositis developed at age 2 and who died at 4 years of age with malignant lymphoma. Fudenberg and Solomon [133] described lymphoma in an adult with acquired agammaglobulinemia, hemolytic anemia, and a long history of repeated infections. A case referred to as Rademacher's disease has been recorded with the following features: a man aged 20 had frequent infections and thrombocytopenia in childhood; splenectomy (histology normal) relieved the thrombocytopenia, but infectious complications persisted and hypogammaglobulinemia was found and treated; massive lymphadenopathy developed shortly before death, and at autopsy, widespread reticulum cell sarcoma was found [134]. In the NZB/BL strain of inbred mice, hemolytic anemia and hypergammaglobulinemia occur with great regularity, and at death, one third to one half of the animals will have a degree of lymphoproliferation that is classified as either lymphoma or leukemia [135]. In mink carrying the Aleutian gene for light-colored fur, a disease has been described that is characterized by hypergammaglobulinemia, enlargement of the liver, spleen, and kidneys, and marked plasma cell infiltration [136]. Among 24 patients with chronic arthritis, splenomegaly, and leukopenia, Denko and Zumpft [137] described patients with rheumatoid arthritis, systemic LE, Hodgkin's disease, and chronic lymphocytic leukemia.

When the histological appearance of biopsy material is not clear cut, or the clinical course not characteristic, and disturbances of immunity are evident, it may be very difficult to decide whether the patient has malignant lymphoma, autoimmune disease, or both. Such cases suggest that there is a continuous spectrum of immune diseases with autoimmune and rheumatoid processes at one end and malignant lymphomas at the other.

An unusual ability to accept foreign tissue grafts is associated with these diseases [39, 56, 138]. Table 26-3 summarizes the results of three studies of skin homografting in 71 pa-

TABLE 26-3. Results of Skin Homografting in 71 Patients with Lymphomas and Leukemias

References	CLL[a]	LSA	RCS	MM	AL	CML	HD
Miller *et al.* [39]	7/16[b]	2/4	3/4	2/6	0/4	0/2	6/12
Green and Corso [138]	—	0/2	1/1	1/1	0/1	0/1	1/4
Kelly *et al.* [56]	—	—	—	—	—	—	10/13
Totals	7/16	2/6	4/5	3/7	0/5	0/3	17/20
	47%				0%		58.6%

[a] CLL = chronic lymphocytic leukemia; LSA = lymphosarcoma; RCS = reticulum cell sarcoma; MM = multiple myeloma; AL = acute leukemia; CML = chronic myelocytic leukemia; HD = Hodgkin's disease.

[b] Denominator indicates total number of patients; numerator is the number of patients in whom the graft survived 30 days or longer.

SOURCE: Miller [52].

tients with lymphomas and leukemias. None of the grafts in patients with myeloproliferative diseases survived for long. The highest incidence of prolonged survival occurred in the condition most often associated with deficient delayed hypersensitivity reaction, Hodgkin's disease. The lymphoproliferative diseases also had a high incidence of prolonged survival. Despite the suggestive evidence, an association could not be made between graft survival and antibody production, γ-globulin levels, or delayed hypersensitivity reactions. However, this result may reflect the inadequacy of our tests rather than the failure of a concept. The immunological deficiency was sufficiently severe for 2 of 9 patients grafted with skin of suckling pigs to accept these grafts for prolonged periods [39].

An attempt has been made to take advantage of the ability to accept homografts by giving patients with pancytopenia and lymphoma homologous bone marrow transplants [139]. In some cases, such as that illustrated in Figure 26-5, there was temporary growth of the homologous bone marrow. Failure of the graft to take permanently may have resulted from the graft's rejection of the host rather than from the host's reaction against the graft. Beilby *et al.* [140] reported prolonged acceptance of a homologous bone marrow transplant with resulting blood chimerism in a patient with Hodgkin's disease.

It should be emphasized that when a patient with chronic lymphocytic leukemia or lymphosarcoma begins to deteriorate and this cannot be attributed to disease activity or infection, one should look for a second primary malignancy. Hyman *et al.* [141] studied 1,780 patients with carcinoma of the colon and 650 patients with leukemia or lymphoma. In 21 instances, the two malignancies occurred in the same patient. Eighteen patients had chronic lymphocytic leukemia or lymphosarcoma; 2, reticulum cell sarcoma; and 1, acute lymphocytic leukemia. Thirteen of the 20 typed patients had blood group A. Ten percent of the patients with lymphocytic leukemia or lymphosarcoma who had blood

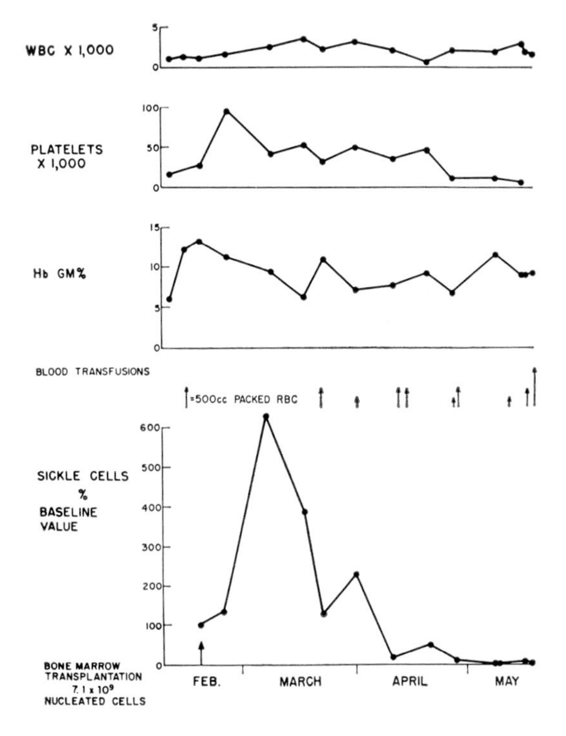

Fig. 26-5. Transitory function of homologous bone marrow in a man, aged 28, with Hodgkin's disease and pancytopenia.

group A or AB had carcinoma of the colon. Warren and Gates [142] reviewed the literature and found a 3.9 percent incidence of multiple primary malignancies at autopsy. In their own series of 8,028 cases, the incidence was 3.7 percent. In chronic lymphocytic leukemia, the incidence of associated malignancies at autopsy has been reported to be 4.3 percent [143], 7.6 percent [144], 16.7 percent [145], 18.9 percent [146], 19 percent [147], and 19.8 percent [148] and appears to be higher than in related diseases [146]. In addition, Gunz [148] found an excess of cancer in the immediate families of patients with chronic lymphocytic leukemia. The incidence was higher than in families of patients with other forms of leukemia, and the difference was significant at the 5 percent level.

We have matched 105 patients for age and sex and studied them for incidence of second primary malignancy. There were three groups of 35 patients having chronic lymphocytic leukemia, chronic myelocytic leukemia, and carcinoma of the colon. The incidence of second primary malignancies in chronic lymphocytic leukemia was 22.9 percent, in carcinoma of the colon 11.4 percent, and in chronic myelocytic leukemia 11.4 percent. The numbers in each group are too small for confidence, but they are in keeping with our experience in frequently finding second primary malignancies at some time in the life of patients with chronic lymphocytic leukemia. However, this conclusion is not shared by all observers [149].

Evidence has been adduced in the preceding discussions that patients with lymphoproliferative diseases and Hodgkin's disease have a disorder which deranges the immune system and results in deficient host resistance. The evidence is good that this impaired host resistance makes the patient susceptible to microbial pathogens. It suggests that the same impairment makes the patient susceptible to allergens and carcinogens. An attempt to unify this concept is presented in Figure 26-6. The suggestion is implicit in this figure that the immune disorders and the neoplasms, as well as the infections which are encountered, are due to environmental pathogens which can penetrate the deficient immune shield. One must also consider the alternate hypothesis, that the lymphomatous tissue represents proliferation of a "forbidden clone" of lymphocytes resulting in immunopathic disorders.

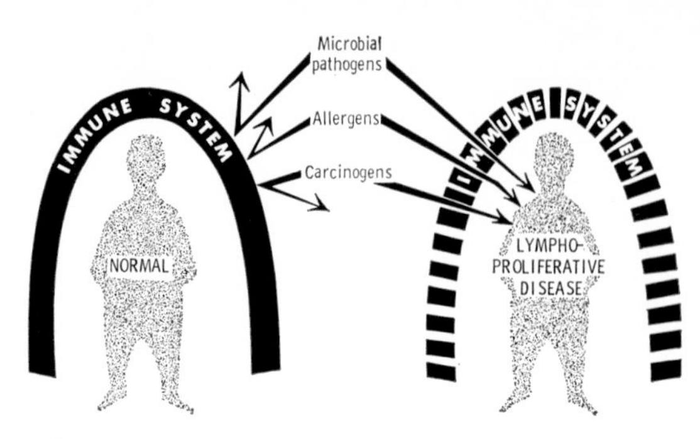

Fig. 26-6. Deficiencies in the immune shield in patients with lymphoproliferative diseases. (See text.)

Unanswered in this diagram is the question of which abnormality came first, the neoplastic process or the deficient host resistance. An intriguing parallel situation exists in the patients with congenital agammaglobulinemia who are susceptible to infection, autoimmune disease, and lymphomas.

THERAPY

Therapy may be considered in terms of: (1) treatment aimed directly at improvement of an immune deficiency; (2) treatment of immunopathic complications, and (3) treatment of the disease and how this may affect immune function and resistance to infection.

IMPROVEMENT OF AN IMMUNE DEFICIENCY

A high incidence of hypogammaglobulinemia in the lymphoproliferative diseases and the concomitant infectious complications have led to the use of γ-globulin for replacement therapy. This is an extension of its use in the treatment of primary agammaglobulinemia in children and is based on that experience [150]. Pooled human γ-globulin is available as a 16 percent solution. When used prophylactically, an initial loading dose of 0.3 ml. per pound of body weight is given intramuscularly. No more than 5 ml. is given in any one site. Since this initial dose for any adult may be in the neighborhood of 50 ml., it is not uncommon to give the loading dose over a two or three day period. Subsequently, one half of the initial dose is given every two to four weeks. If the injections cause great discomfort, 0.5 to 1.0 ml. of 1 percent procaine may be mixed with the serum γ-globulin. Our best results were obtained when antibiotics were given with the γ-globulin. Penicillin V,

125 mg. orally three times a day, was used as the initial antibiotic. Some patients required more than the quantity of γ-globulin recommended above for satisfactory prophylaxis, and some derived no benefit [89]. In this experience, γ-globulin was also used therapeutically in patients with infections which had not responded to conventional management. In these cases, γ-globulin was added to the therapy already employed in doses of 10 to 20 ml. per day. If no improvement was noted after 200 ml., the injections were discontinued.

We have observed three anaphylactic reactions to γ-globulin, two after intramuscular and one after intravenous injection. (They are most common after intravenous injection.) Skin tests and search for precipitins gave negative results. Some patients complained of malaise and severe anxiety and apprehension after receiving γ-globulin, often refusing further injections. In an aforementioned patient with reticulum cell sarcoma and agammaglobulinemia, the injection of γ-globulin was associated with swelling of the lymph nodes [134]. Since the γ-globulin is administered in large quantities and contains antibodies other than antibacterial antibodies, this may be another example of graft-versus-host reaction manifesting itself as reverse anaphylaxis. Patients with hypogammaglobulinemia may have several allergies, and it is possible that the γ-globulin preparation contains allergens that were circulating in the donor's blood. Other considerations for these reactions have been offered [151, 152].

Although γ-globulin may be a helpful adjunct to therapy, it is not a panacea. Occasionally, satisfactory prophylaxis against infection for long periods may be achieved with antibiotics alone, and this should be attempted before therapy with γ-globulin is commenced. We have not found γ-globulin useful against bacterial infections in Hodgkin's disease or myeloproliferative diseases. But our experience suggests, although without adequate controls, that therapeutic doses of γ-globulin may be helpful in the treatment of herpes zoster and herpes simplex associated with lymphomas and leukemias regardless of γ-globulin levels.

IMMUNOPATHIC COMPLICATIONS

The autoimmune hypersensitivity and allergic complications seen in these diseases seldom improve after irradiation or chemotherapy. They usually respond to adrenal corticosteroids or salicylates, as they would if not complicated by lymphomatous disease. However, there is a difference in treating the underlying neoplastic process with adrenal corticosteroids and in treating the immune complications. Lymphoma or leukemia may be treated until improvement is obtained; the remission may persist without therapy for several weeks or months and the drug reutilized as necessary. In hemolytic anemia or autoimmune thrombocytopenia, these hormones must be continued after improvement has occurred and usually must be continued indefinitely, for if the hormones are discontinued, there is a very high risk that the immune complication will recur. The recurrence of hemolytic anemia or thrombocytopenia under these conditions may be rapid and, if it occurs in an outpatient who is not being seen frequently, may be disastrous.

TREATMENT OF THE DISEASE, AND EFFECT ON IMMUNE FUNCTION AND RESISTANCE TO INFECTION

Bacterial and viral infections in Hodgkin's disease usually occur during periods of disease activity, and if treatment leads to remission, infectious complications are unlikely to supervene. Infectious complications in chronic lymphocytic leukemia and the other lymphoproliferative processes have a greater tendency to become chronic and persistent. They may be more troublesome than the leukemic problem per se. Treatment of the disease seldom raises the γ-globulin level to normal. The effect of treatment with prednisone on infections in chronic lymphocytic leukemia has been studied [153]. In the control period, the frequency of infection was 1 in 311 patient days, compared to 1 in 189 patient days during prednisone administration. These results suggest an effect of prednisone on host resistance, although the difference in frequency was not significant at the 5 percent level. While the patients were receiving prednisone, infections were generally more severe and more difficult to control. Tuberculosis was reactivated in two patients, and healing of herpes progenitalis did not occur until prednisone therapy ceased. Paradoxically, we have observed five patients in whom resistance to infection improved while the leukemic process was responding to adrenal corticosteroids [89]. Such improvement did not persist when the leukemia became resistant to these agents.

None of the other patients with infections whose course we analyzed had significant remission of infectious complications after response to alkylating agents or radiation therapy. However, Ultmann *et al.* [23] reported improvement in resistance to infection in a patient whose disease responded to alkylating agents.

There are other factors operative in these diseases which must be considered for their role in causing the immunological deficiencies and susceptibility to infection noted in the foregoing discussion. These are cachexia, debility, and hyperproteinemia, as well as radiation therapy, chemotherapy, and adrenal corticosteroid administration. Except in acute leukemia, the antimetabolites are not ordinarily used in the treatment of these diseases. Keys [154] observed that mass starvation does not invariably lead to infection. Balch [155], Bieler *et al.* [156], and Larson and Tomlinson [157] could not correlate cachexia, anemia, and hyperproteinemia with susceptibility to infection or immune response.

Since it has been shown that ablation of the thymus even in the adult will impair the immune system [158], one can question whether impairment of the thymus by treatment or disease plays a role in the development of immune deficiency. Although we cannot answer this question conclusively, many patients in the studies mentioned had no irradiation to the mediastinum, and in none of our patients with immune impairment was involvement of the thymus found at autopsy.

With regard to the specific parameters of immune function, Barr and Fairley [46], Saslaw *et al.* [36] and Schier [53] could not correlate treatment of these diseases with diminution of antibody production, nor could the ability to accept homografts be correlated with therapy [39]. The conditions which prevail experimentally in the depression of antibody production with alkylating agents and radiation are seldom encountered clinically. In addition, permanent impairment of antibody production is extremely difficult to achieve with these agents in any circumstance. The observations in man using therapeutic levels of the adrenal corticosteroids are not consistent in defining the effects they may have on antibody production [159–162]. At a dose of 1 mg. per kg. of body weight, prednisone did not alter the character of the inflammatory exudate in patients with chronic lymphocytic leukemia [81]. Nevertheless, there may be prominent untoward effects of therapy on host resistance, e.g., the leukopenia induced by alkylating agents or radiation therapy, the pneumonitis, fibrosis, or tissue necrosis that may occasionally be seen with radiation therapy, and the bacterial, mycotic, and viral complications associated with adrenal corticosteroids therapy. However, these are not consistent concomitants of such therapy. These forms of treatment are also used in other neoplastic diseases without inducing antibody deficiency syndromes and do not regularly lead to decreased resistance to infection. Also, their use would not explain the differences in the patterns of immune deficiency seen in Hodgkin's disease and lymphoproliferative diseases. One must conclude that radiation therapy and chemotherapy are at most ancillary factors in the production of immune deficiencies associated with these diseases.

REFERENCES

1. Custer, R. P., and Bernhard, W. G. The interrelationship of Hodgkin's disease and other lymphatic tumors. *Amer. J. Med. Sci.* 216:625, 1948.
2. Warthin, A. S. Genetic neoplastic relationships of Hodgkin's disease, aleukemic and leukemic lymphoblastoma and mycosis fungoides. *Ann. Surg.* 93:153, 1931.
3. Razis, D. V., Diamond, H. D., and Craver, L. F. Hodgkin's disease associated with other malignant tumors and certain non-neoplastic diseases. *Amer. J. Med. Sci.* 327:109, 1959.
4. Razis, D. V., Diamond, H. D., and Craver, L. F. Familial Hodgkin's disease: Its significance and implications. *Ann. Intern. Med.* 51:933, 1959.
5. Miller, D. G., Diamond, H. D., and Craver, L. F. A critical study of the clinical use of chlorambucil. *New Eng. J. Med.* 261:3, 1959.
6. Leoncini, D., Korngold, L., and Miller, D. G. Paper and immunoelectrophoretic studies of the serum proteins of patients with lymphomas and leukemias. (To be published.)
7. Petermann, M. L., Karnofsky, D. A., and Hog-

ness, K. R. Electrophoretic studies on the plasma proteins of patients with neoplastic disease: III. Lymphomas and leukemias. *Cancer* 1:109, 1948.

8. Brown, R. K., Read, J. T., Wiseman, B. K., and France, W. G. The electrophoretic analysis of serum proteins of the blood dyscrasias. *J. Lab. Clin. Med.* 33:1523, 1948.
9. Mider, G. B., Alling, E. L., and Morton, J. J. The effect of neoplastic and allied diseases on the concentrations of the plasma cell proteins. *Cancer* 3:56, 1950.
10. Arends, T., Coonrad, E. V., and Rundles, R. W. Serum proteins in Hodgkin's disease and malignant lymphoma. *Amer. J. Med.* 16: 833, 1954.
11. Sunderman, F. W., Jr., and Sunderman, F. W. Clinical applications of the fractionation of serum proteins by paper electrophoresis. *Amer. J. Clin. Path.* 27:125, 1957.
12. Jim, R. T. S., and Reinhard, E. H. Agammaglobulinemia and chronic lymphocytic leukemia. *Ann. Intern. Med.* 44:790, 1956.
13. Hudson, R., and Wilson, S. J. Hypogammaglobulinemia and chronic lymphatic leukemia. *J. Lab. Clin. Med.* 50:829, 1957.
14. Prasad, A. The association of hypogammaglobulinemia and chronic lymphatic leukemia. *Amer. J. Med. Sci.* 236:610, 1958.
15. Seligmann, M., Alais, L., and Bernard, J. Analyse immunoélectrophorétique du sérum de cent malades atteints de leucoses. *Rev. Franc. Etud. Clin. Biol.* 4:901, 1959.
16. Gross, P. A. M., Gitlin, D., and Janeway, C. A. The gamma globulins and their clinical significance: III. Hypergammaglobulinemia. *New Eng. J. Med.* 260:121, 1959.
17. Shaw, R. K., Szwed, C., Boggs, D. R., Fahey, J. L., Frei, E., III, Morrison, E., and Utz, J. P. Infection and immunity in chronic lymphocytic leukemia. *Arch. Intern. Med.* 106:467, 1960.
18. Rottino, A., Suchoff, D., and Stern, K. G. Electrophoretic study of the blood serum from lymphogranulomatous patients. *J. Lab. Clin. Med.* 33:624, 1948.
19. Grabar, P., and Burtin, P. *Analyse Immuno-Électrophorétique: Applications aux Liquides Biologiques Humains.* Paris: Masson et Cie, 1960.
20. Goulian, M., and Fahey, J. L. Abnormalities in serum proteins and protein-bound hexose in Hodgkin's disease. *J. Lab. Clin. Med.* 57:408, 1961.
21. Heremans, J. F. Immunochemical studies on protein pathology: The immunoglobulin concept. *Clin. Chim. Acta* 4:639, 1959.
22. Boggs, D. R., and Fahey, J. L. Serum-protein changes in malignant disease: II. The chronic leukemias, Hodgkin's disease, and malignant melanoma. *J. Nat. Cancer Inst.* 25:1381, 1960.
23. Ultmann, J. E., Fish, W., Osserman, E., and Gellhorn, A. The clinical implications of hypogammaglobulinemia in patients with chronic lymphocytic leukemia and lymphocytic lymphosarcoma. *Ann. Intern. Med.* 51:501, 1959.
24. Creyssel, R., Morel, P., Pellet, M., Medard, J., Revol, L., and Croizat, P. Déficit en gammaglobulines et complications infectieuses des leucémies lymphoides chroniques. *Sang* 29: 383, 1958.
25. Osserman, E. F. Plasma-cell myeloma: II. Clinical aspects. *New Eng. J. Med.* 261:1006, 1959.
26. Braunsteiner, H., and Sailer, S. Lymphatic leukemia and macroglobulinemia Waldenström. *Acta Haemat.* (Basel) 23:306, 1960.
27. Moreschi, C. Ueber antigene und pyrogene Wirkung des Typhusbacillus bei leukämischen Kranken. *Z. Immunitaetsforsch.* 21:410, 1914.
28. Rotky, H. Ueber die Fähigkeit von leukämikern Antikörper zu erzeugen. *Zbl. Inn. Med.* 35:953, 1914.
29. Howell, K. M. The failure of antibody formation in leukemia. *Arch. Intern. Med.* 26:706, 1920.
30. Evans, R. W. The antibody response in cases of radiation lymphopenia, and in the reticuloses. *J. Path. Bact.* 60:123, 1948.
31. Miller, D. G., and Karnofsky, D. A. Immunologic factors and resistance to infection in chronic lymphocytic leukemia. *Amer. J. Med.* 31:748, 1961.
32. Brem, T. H., and Morton, M. E. Defective serum gamma globulin formation. *Ann. Intern. Med.* 43:465, 1955.
33. Geller, W. A study of antibody formation in patients with malignant lymphomas. *J. Lab. Clin. Med.* 42:232, 1953.
34. Hickling, R. A., and Sutliff, W. D. Pneumonia in a case of chronic lymphatic leukemia. *Amer. J. Med. Sci.* 175:224, 1928.
35. Larson, D. L., and Tomlinson, L. J. Quantitative antibody studies in man: III. Antibody response in leukemia and other malignant lymphomata. *J. Clin. Invest.* 32:317, 1953.
36. Saslaw, S., Carlisle, H. N., and Bouroncle, B. Antibody response in hematologic patients. *Proc. Soc. Exp. Biol. Med.* 106:654, 1961.
37. Schier, W. W., Roth, A., Ostroff, G., and Schrift, M. H. Hodgkin's disease and immunity. *Amer. J. Med.* 20:94, 1956.
38. Davidsohn, I. Discussion of paper by Forbus *et al. Amer. J. Path.* 18:745, 1942.
39. Miller, D. G., Lizardo, J. G., and Snyderman, R. A. Homologous and heterologous skin transplantation in patients with lymphomatous disease. *J. Nat. Cancer Inst.* 26:569, 1961.

40. Hoffman, G. T., and Rottino, A. Studies of immunologic reactions of patients with Hodgkin's disease. Antibody reaction to typhoid immunization. *Arch. Intern. Med.* 86:872, 1950.
41. Forbus, W. D., Goddard, D. W., Margolis, G., Brown, I. W., Jr., and Kerby, G. P. Studies on Hodgkin's disease and its relation to infection by *Brucella. Amer. J. Path.* 18:745, 1942.
42. Wise, N. B., and Poston, M. A. The coexistence of *Brucella* infection and Hodgkin's disease: A clinical, bacteriologic and immunologic study. *J.A.M.A.* 115:1976, 1940.
43. Aisenberg, A. C., and Leskowitz, S. Antibody formation in Hodgkin's disease. *New Eng. J. Med.* 268:1269, 1963.
44. Silver, R. T., Utz, J. P., Fahey, J., and Frei, E., III. Antibody response in patients with acute leukemia. *J. Lab. Clin. Med.* 56:634, 1960.
45. Millian, S. J., Miller, D. G., and Schaeffer, N. Viral complement-fixing antibody in patients with Hodgkin's disease, lymphosarcoma, reticulum cell sarcoma and chronic lymphocytic leukemia. *Cancer* (in press).
46. Barr, M., and Fairley, G. H. Circulating antibodies in the reticuloses. *Lancet,* 1:1305, 1961.
47. Wilson, S. J., Mantz, F. A., and Jackson, H. R. Mononucleosis?—Lymphoma?? Mimicry of infectious mononucleosis and malignant lymphoma. *J. Kans. Med. Soc.* 63:467, 1962.
48. Southam, C. M., Goldsmith, Y., and Burchenal, J. Heterophile antibodies and antigens in neoplastic diseases. *Cancer* 4:1036, 1951.
49. Massey, F. C., Lane, L. L., and Imbriglia, J. E. Acute infectious mononucleosis and Hodgkin's disease occurring simultaneously in same patient. *J.A.M.A.* 151:994, 1953.
50. Kenis, Y., Dustin, P., Jr., and Peltzer, T. Un cas de maladie de Hodgkin avec syndrome hématologique et sérologique de mononucleose infectieuse. *Acta Haemat.* (Basel) 20:329, 1958.
51. Davidsohn, I., and Lee, C. L. The laboratory in the diagnosis of infectious mononucleosis: With additional notes on epidemiology, etiology and pathogenesis. *Med. Clin. N. Amer.* 46:225, 1962.
52. Miller, D. G. Patterns of immunological deficiency in lymphomas and leukemias. *Ann. Intern. Med.* 57:703, 1962.
53. Schier, W. W. Cutaneous anergy and Hodgkin's disease. *New Eng. J. Med.* 250:353, 1954.
54. Sokal, J. E., and Primikirios, N. The delayed skin test in Hodgkin's disease and lymphosarcoma: Effect of disease activity. *Cancer* 14:597, 1961.
55. Dubin, I. N. The poverty of the immunological mechanism in patients with Hodgkin's disease. *Ann. Intern. Med.* 27:898, 1947.
56. Kelly, W. D., Good, R. A., and Varco, R. L. Anergy and skin homograft survival in Hodgkin's disease. *Surg. Gynec. Obstet.* 107:565, 1958.
57. Lamb, D., Pilney, F., Kelly, W. D., and Good, R. A. A comparative study of the incidence of anergy in patients with carcinoma, leukemia, Hodgkin's disease and other lymphomas. *J. Immun.* 89:555, 1962.
58. Aisenberg, A. C. Studies on delayed hypersensitivity in Hodgkin's disease. *J. Clin. Invest.* 41:1964, 1962.
59. Lawrence, H. S. Cellular transfer of cutaneous hypersensitivity to man. *Proc. Soc. Exper. Biol. Med.* 59:134, 1945.
60. Urbach, F., Sones, M., and Israel, H. L. Passive transfer of tuberculin sensitivity to patients with sarcoidosis. *New Eng. J. Med.* 247: 794, 1952.
61. Fazio, M., and Calciati, A. An attempt to transfer tuberculin hypersensitivity in Hodgkin's disease. *Panminerva Med.* 4:164, 1962.
62. Kelly, W. D., Lamb, D. L., Varco, R. L., and Good, R. A. An investigation of Hodgkin's disease with respect to the problem of homotransplantation. *Ann. N.Y. Acad. Sci.* 87:187, 1960.
63. Warwick, W. J., Archer, O., Kelly, W. D., and Page, A. R. Anergy of delayed allergy in Hodgkin's disease patients. *Fed. Proc.* 20:18 1961 (abst.).
64. Long, J. B., and Favour, C. B. The ability of ACTH and cortisone to alter delayed type bacterial hypersensitivity. *Bull. Hopkins Hosp.* 87:186, 1950.
65. Seeberg, G. The tuberculin reaction in hunger cachexia. *Acta Dermatovener.* 31:245, 1951.
66. Mitchell, A. G., Wherry, W. B., Eddy, B., and Stevenson, F. E. Studies in immunity: I. Nonspecific factors influencing the reaction of the skin to tuberculin. *Amer. J. Dis. Child.* 36: 720, 1928.
67. Magnusson, B. The effect of sarcoidosis sera on the tuberculin response. *Acta Dermatovener.,* Vol. 36, supp. 35, 1956.
68. Sterling, K. Erythema nodosum with tuberculin-neutralizing serum: A report of two cases. *Amer. Rev. Tuberc.* 62:112, 1950.
69. Wells, A. Q., and Wylie, J. A. H. A tuberculin-neutralizing factor in the serum of patients with sarcoidosis. *Lancet* 256:439, 1949.
70. Kelly, W. D., Good, R. A., Varco, R. L., and Levitt, M. The altered response to skin homografts and to delayed allergens in Hodgkin's disease. *Surg. Forum* 9:785, 1958.
71. Faulk, A. T., Tellem, M., and Frumin, A. M. Altered tuberculin reaction in lymphoma and leukemia. *Clin. Res.* 7:266, 1959.
72. Fairley, G. H., and Matthias, J. Q. Cortisone and skin sensitivity to tuberculin in reticuloses. *Brit. Med. J.* 2:433, 1960.

73. Pyke, D. A., and Scadding, J. G. Effect of cortisone upon skin sensitivity to tuberculin in sarcoidosis. *Brit. Med. J.* 2:1126, 1952.
74. Citron, K. M., and Scadding, J. G. The effect of cortisone upon the reaction of the skin to tuberculin in tuberculosis and in sarcoidosis. *Quart. J. Med.* 26:277, 1957.
75. James, D. G., and Pepys, J. Tuberculin in aqueous and oily solutions: Skin test reactions in normal subjects and in patients with sarcoidosis. *Lancet* 270:602, 1956.
76. Sones, M., and Israel, H. L. Altered immunologic reactions in sarcoidosis. *Ann. Intern. Med.* 40:260, 1954.
77. Sands, J. H., Palmer, P. P., Maycock, R. L., and Creger, W. P. Evidence for serologic hyper-reactivity in sarcoidosis. *Amer. J. Med.* 19:401, 1955.
78. Germuth, F. G., Jr. The role of adrenocortical steroids in infection, immunity and hypersensitivity. *Pharmacol. Rev.* 8:1, 1956.
79. Kass, E. H., and Finland, M. Corticosteroids and infections. *Advances Intern. Med.* 9:45, 1958.
80. Robinson, H. J. Adrenal cortical hormones and infection. *Pediatrics* 17:770, 1956.
81. Boggs, D. The cellular composition of inflammatory exudates in human leukemias. *Blood* 15:466, 1960.
82. Riis, P. *The Cytology of Inflammatory Exudate: A Study on Normal Subjects and Patients Showing Quantitative or Qualitative Changes in the White Blood Picture.* Copenhagen: Ejnar Munksgaards Verlag, 1959.
83. Rebuck, J. W., Monto, R. W., Monaghan, E. A., and Riddle, J. M. Potentialities of the lymphocyte, with an additional reference to its dysfunction in Hodgkin's disease. *Ann. N.Y. Acad. Sci.* 73:8, 1958.
84. Jaffe, R. H. Morphology of the inflammatory defense reactions in leukemia. *Arch. Path.* 14:177, 1932.
85. Page, A. R., and Good, R. A. Studies on cyclic neutropenia. *Amer. J. Dis. Child.* 94:623, 1957.
86. Page, A. R., and Good, R. A. A clinical and experimental study of the function of neutrophils in the inflammatory response. *Amer. J. Path.* 34:645, 1958.
87. Opie, E. L. Inflammation. *Arch. Intern. Med.* 5:541, 1910.
88. Silver, R. T., Utz, J. P., Frei, E., III, and McCullough, N. B. Fever, infection and host resistance in acute leukemia. *Amer. J. Med.* 24:25, 1958.
89. Miller, D. G., Budinger, J. M., and Karnofsky, D. A. A clinical and pathological study of factors influencing resistance to infection in chronic lymphatic leukemia. *Cancer* 15:307, 1962.
90. Braude, A. I., Feltes, J., and Brooks, M. Differences between the activities of mature granulocytes in leukemic and normal blood. *J. Clin. Invest.* 33:1036, 1954.
91. Hirschberg, N. Phagocytic activity in leukemia. *Amer. J. Med. Sci.* 197:706, 1939.
92. Jersild, M. Phagocytic activities of various types of leucocytes. *Acta Med. Scand.* 213 supp.:238, 1948.
93. Silver, R. T., Beal, G. A., Schneiderman, M. A., and McCullough, N. B. The role of the mature neutrophil in bacterial infections in acute leukemia. *Blood* 12:814, 1957.
94. Hoff, F. Ueber Funktionsänderungen der Leukozyten. *Wien. Klin. Wschr.* 72:495, 1960.
95. Biozzi, G., Benacerraf, B., Halpern, B. N., Stiffel, C., and Hillemand, B. Exploration of the phagocytic function of the reticuloendothelial system with heat denatured human serum albumin labeled with I^{131} and application to the measurement of liver blood flow, in normal man and in some pathologic conditions. *J. Lab. Clin. Med.* 51:230, 1958.
96. Southam, C. M., and Goldsmith, Y. Effect of nitrogen mustard on serum complement in vitro and in patients with neoplastic disease. *Proc. Soc. Exp. Biol. Med.* 76:430, 1951.
97. Rottino, A., and Levy, A. L. Serum-properdin levels in patients with Hodgkin's disease and carcinoma. *Cancer* 10:877, 1957.
98. Baltch, A. L., Osborne, W., Bunn, P. A., Canarile, L., and Hassirdjian, A. Serum complement and bacteriophage neutralization titers in human infections, leukemias and lymphomas. *J. Lab. Clin. Med.* 56:594, 1960.
99. Southam, C. M. Personal communication, 1962.
100. Wardlaw, A. C., and Pillemer, L. The demonstration of the batericidal activity of the properdin system. *Ann. N.Y. Acad. Sci.* 66:244, 1956.
101. Wintrobe, M. M., and Hasenbush, L. L. Chronic leukemia. *Arch. Intern. Med.* 64:701, 1939.
102. Parkes, R. Hypogammaglobulinaemia and tuberculosis: Implications of their association and other observations. *Brit. Med. J.* 1:973, 1958.
103. Jackson, H., Jr., and Parker, F., Jr. *Hodgkin's Disease and Allied Disorders.* New York: Oxford University Press, 1947.
104. Ewing, J. *Neoplastic Diseases.* Philadelphia: W. B. Saunders Company, 1940.
105. Collins, V. P., Gellhorn, A., and Trimble, J. R. The coincidence of cryptococcosis and disease of the reticulo-endothelial and lymphatic systems. *Cancer* 4:883, 1951.
106. Zimmerman, L. E., and Rappaport, H. Occurrence of cryptococcosis in patients with malignant disease of reticuloendothelial system. *Amer. J. Clin. Path.* 24:1050, 1954.

107. Gendel, B. R., Ende, M., and Norman, S. L. Cryptococcosis: A review with special reference to apparent association with Hodgkin's disease. *Amer. J. Med.* 9:343, 1950.
108. White, C. M. Vaccinia gangrenosa due to hypogammaglobulinemia. *Lancet* 1:969, 1963.
109. Rosenthal, M. C., Pisciotta, A. V., Zacharias, D., Komminos, Z. D., Goldenberg, H., and Dameshek, W. The auto-immune hemolytic anemia of malignant lymphocytic disease. *Blood* 10:197, 1955.
110. Pisciotta, A. V., Jermain, L. F., and Hinz, J. E. Chronic lymphocytic leukemia, hypogammaglobulinemia and auto-immune hemolytic anemia—an experiment of nature. *Blood* 15:748, 1960.
111. Ebbe, S., Wittels, B., and Dameshek, W. Autoimmune thrombocytopenic purpura ("ITP" type) with chronic lymphocytic leukemia. *Blood* 19:23, 1962.
112. Hench, P. K., Mayne, J. G., Kiely, J. M., and Dockerty, M. B. Clinical study of the rheumatic manifestations of lymphoma. *Arthritis Rheum.* 5:301, 1962.
113. Cammarata, R. J., Rodnan, G. P., and Jensen, W. N. Systemic rheumatic disease and malignant lymphoma. *Arch. Intern. Med.* 111:330, 1963.
114. Talal, N., and Bunim, J. J. The development of malignant lymphoma in patients with Sjögren's syndrome. *Arthritis Rheum.* 6:302, 1963.
115. Blodgett, R. C., Jr., Lipscomb, P. R., and Hill, R. W. Incidence of hematologic disease in patients with carpal tunnel syndrome. *J.A.M.A.* 182:814, 1962.
116. Christianson, H. B., Brunsting, L. A., and Perry, H. O. Dermatomyositis: Unusual features, complications and treatment. *Arch. Derm.* 74:581, 1956.
117. Beickert, A. Autoimmunologische Komplikationen bei neoplastischen Erkrankungen. *Aerztl. Wschr.* 13:438, 1958.
118. Sigidin, Ia. A. On common elements in collagen and hematological diseases. *Ter. Arkh.* 34:11, 1962.
119. Schwartz, T. B., and Jager, B. V. Cryoglobulinemia and Raynaud's syndrome in a case of chronic lymphocytic leukemia. *Cancer* 2:319, 1949.
120. Craig, A. B., Waterhouse, C., and Young, L. E. Autoimmune hemolytic disease and cryoglobulinemia associated with chronic lymphocytic leukemia. *Amer. J. Med.* 13:793, 1952.
121. Brody, J. I., and Beizer, L. H. Globulin coating of neoplastic lymphocytes in chronic lymphocytic leukemia. *Blood* 22:139, 1963.
122. Howqua, J., and Mackay, I. R. L.E. cells in lymphoma. *Ibid.,* p. 191.
123. Ogryzlo, M. A. The L.E. (lupus erythematosus) cell reaction. *Canad. Med. Ass. J.* 75:980, 1956.
124. Candreviotis, N. Haematoxylin bodies in Hodgkin's disease. *J. Clin. Path.* 15:542, 1962.
125. Aström, E.-E., Mancall, E. L., and Richardson, E. P., Jr. Progressive multifocal leukoencephalopathy: Hitherto unrecognized complication of chronic lymphatic leukemia and Hodgkin's disease. *Brain* 81:93, 1958.
126. Cavanagh, J. B., Greenbaum, D., Marshall, A. H. E., and Rubinstein, L. J. Cerebral demyelination associated with disorders of the reticuloendothelial system. *Lancet* 2:524, 1959.
127. Blanchard, B. M. Peripheral neuropathy (non-invasive) associated with lymphoma. *Ann. Intern. Med.* 56:774, 1962.
128. Moeschlin. S. Malignant Reticulosis: Clinical Symptoms Due to Para-Protein Sensitization ("Autoimmunisation"). *Proceedings of the 8th Congress of the European Society of Haematology*. Basel: S. Karger A. G., 1961. Vol. 1, paper no. 211.
129. Dworin, M., Diamond, H. D., and Craver, L. F. Hodgkin's disease and allergy. *Cancer* 8:128, 1955.
130. Bridges, R. A., and Good, R. A. Connective tissue disease and certain serum protein components in patients with agammaglobulinemia. *Ann. N.Y. Acad. Sci.* 86:1089, 1960.
131. Good, R. A., Page, A. R., Hansen, A., and Fudenberg, H. Occurrence of leukemia and lymphoma in agammaglobulinemia. *Fed. Proc.* 21:30, 1962 (abst.).
132. Page, A. R., Hansen, A. E., and Good, R. A. Occurrence of leukemia and lymphoma in patients with agammaglobulinemia. *Blood* 21:197, 1963.
133. Fudenberg, H., and Solomon, A. "Acquired agammaglobulinemia" with auto-immune hemolytic disease: graft-versus-host reaction? *Vox Sang.* 6:68, 1961.
134. Recant, L., and Hartroft, W. S. Rademacher's disease: Diminished immunity of an unusual form complicated by lymphadenopathy. *Amer. J. Med.* 32:80, 1962.
135. Holmes, M. C., and Burnet, F. M. The natural history of autoimmune disease in NZB mice: A comparison with the pattern of human autoimmune manifestations. *Ann. Intern. Med.* 59:265, 1963.
136. Helmboldt, C. F., and Jungherr, E. L. The pathology of Aleutian disease in mink. *Amer. J. Vet. Res.* 19:212, 1958.
137. Denko, C. W., and Zumpft, C. W. Chronic arthritis with splenomegaly and leukopenia. *Arthritis Rheum.* 5:478, 1962.

138. Green, I., and Corso, P. F. A study of skin homografting in patients with lymphomas. *Blood* 14:235, 1959.
139. Miller, D. G., and Diamond, H. D. The biological basis and clinical application of bone marrow transplantation. *Med. Clin. N. Amer.* 45:711, 1961.
140. Beilby, J. O. W., Cade, I. S., Jelliffe, A. M., Parkin, D. M., and Stewart, J. W. Prolonged survival of a bone-marrow graft resulting in a blood-group chimera. *Brit. Med. J.* 1:96, 1960.
141. Hyman, G. A., Ultmann, J. E., and Slanetz, C. A. Chronic lymphocytic leukemia or lymphoma and carcinoma of the colon. *J.A.M.A.* 186:1053, 1963.
142. Warren, S., and Gates, O. Multiple primary malignant tumors: A survey of the literature and a statistical study. *Amer. J. Cancer* 16:1358, 1932.
143. Osgood, E. E., and Seaman, A. J. Treatment of chronic leukemias. *J.A.M.A.* 150:1372, 1952.
144. Lawrence, J. H., and Donald, W. G., Jr. The incidence of cancer in chronic leukemia and in polycythemia vera. *Amer. J. Med. Sci.* 237:488, 1959.
145. Pisciotta, A. V., and Hirschboeck, J. S. Therapeutic considerations in chronic lymphocytic leukemia. *Arch. Intern. Med.* 99:334, 1957.
146. Moertel, C. G., and Hagedorn, A. B. Leukemia or lymphoma and coexistent primary malignant lesions: A review of the literature and a study of 120 cases. *Blood* 12:788, 1957.
147. Beresford, O. D. Chronic lymphatic leukemia associated with malignant disease. *Brit. J. Cancer* 6:339, 1952.
148. Gunz, F. W. Incidence of some aetiological factors in human leukemia. *Brit. Med. J.* 1:326, 1961.
149. Morrison, M., Feldman, F., and Samwick, A. A. Carcinoma and leukemia: Report of two cases with combined lesions; Review of the literature. *Ann. Intern. Med.* 20:75, 1944.
150. Janeway, C. A., and Gitlin, D. The gamma globulins. *Advances Pediat.* 9:65, 1957.
151. Skvařil, F. Changes in outdated human gamma globulin preparations. *Nature* (London) 185:475, 1960.
152. Glaser, J., and Wyss-Souffront, W. A. Alleged anaphylactic reactions to human gamma-globulin. *Pediatrics* 28:367, 1961.
153. Shaw, R. K., Boggs, D. R., Silberman, H. R., and Frei, E., III. A study of prednisone therapy in chronic lymphocytic leukemia. *Blood* 17:182, 1961.
154. Keys, A. Caloric undernutrition and starvation with notes on protein deficiency. *J.A.M.A.* 138:500, 1948.
155. Balch, H. H. Relation of nutritional deficiency in man to antibody production. *J. Immun.* 64:397, 1950.
156. Bieler, M. M., Ecker, E. E., and Spies, T. D. Serum proteins in hypoproteinemia due to nutritional deficiency. *J. Lab. Clin. Med.* 32:130, 1947.
157. Larson, D. L., and Tomlinson, L. J. Quantitative antibody studies in man: II. The relation of the level of serum proteins to antibody production. *J. Lab. Clin. Med.* 39:129, 1952.
158. Auerbach, R. Thymus: Its role in lymphoid recovery after irradiation. *Science* 139:1061, 1963.
159. McEwen, C., Bunim, J. J., Baldwin, J. S., Kuttner, A. G., Appell, S. B., and Kaltman, A. J. The effect of cortisone and ACTH in rheumatic fever. *Bull. N.Y. Acad. Med.* 26:212, 1950.
160. Havens, W. P., Jr., Shafer, J. M., and Hopke, C. J., Jr. The capacity of patients with chronic hepatic disease to produce antibody and the effect of ACTH and cortisone on this function. *J. Clin. Invest.* 30:647, 1951.
161. Mirick, G. S. The effects of ACTH and cortisone on antibodies in human beings. *Bull. Hopkins Hosp.* 88:332, 1951.
162. Southam, C. M., and Moore, A. E. Antivirus antibody studies following induced infection in man with West Nile, Ilhéus and other viruses. *J. Immun.* 72:446, 1954.

27. *Infectious Mononucleosis*

STUART C. FINCH

INFECTIOUS MONONUCLEOSIS USUally presents a characteristic clinical pattern with relatively few complications. Unfortunately, many common virus illnesses closely resemble this disorder. This has created many misconceptions concerning its clinical and epidemiological features. Until the etiology of infectious mononucleosis is established, many of these misconceptions will persist.

Pfeiffer [1] presented a reasonably accurate description of infectious mononucleosis in 1889. Shortly thereafter, many reports of illnesses and epidemics of uncertain etiology were reported as infectious mononucleosis. Downey and McKinlay's [2] description of the atypical lymphocytes associated with the condition did much to improve diagnosis. It was not until 1932, however, that Paul and Bunnell [3] defined the sheep cell agglutination reaction that has great diagnostic value. Despite improvements in methods of serological testing, it still is not possible to identify with certainty all patients with this illness.

EPIDEMIOLOGY

Infectious mononucleosis probably is a viral illness of relatively low infectivity, with moderate variation in the severity of its clinical manifestations. Some authorities [4–7] think that the characteristic hematological and serological changes must accompany a compatible clinical picture before the diagnosis is established. Others [8, 9] believe that a subclinical form may occur in epidemic proportions, especially in childhood, without significant hematological and serological change. This divergence of opinion has made it exceedingly difficult to define the epidemiological characteristics.

Infectious mononucleosis has a world-wide distribution, but accurate prevalence rates for many countries are not available [10]. Variations in diagnostic criteria and ages surveyed have resulted in wide differences in the rates reported. In England and Wales, rates of 1.6 to $5.9/10^5$ per year have been estimated [11]. The rate in a survey of the general population of Oxford, however, was $56/10^5$ per year [12]. A minimum rate of $9.7/10^5$ per year and an estimated true rate of $68/10^5$ per year for the State of Wisconsin has been reported [13]. Some believe it to be rare in Negroes [5, 14–16]; others have noted little difference between Negroes and whites [17–19]. There is some evidence that the incidence of the illness is increasing [20–22].

Infectious mononucleosis is a disorder primarily of adolescence. Between 70 and 80 percent of all sporadic cases develop in individuals between 15 and 30 years of age [10, 11, 13, 23, 24]. It has been reported in five individuals past 60 and in a 2-month-old child [25, 26]. There is, however, some doubt as to the validity of each of these diagnoses. Certainly, the diagnosis should be seriously questioned in those under 5 and over 35 years.

The sexes are probably affected about equally. Male to female ratios of from 3 : 2 to 1 : 3 have been noted in some of the major clinical reports [10, 13, 21, 24].

There is little evidence of any real seasonal variation in sporadic occurrence in either temperate or tropical regions [23, 27, 28]. Surveys at some colleges have demonstrated increased rates about one month after the opening of school in the autumn and after vacations [8, 29]. Others [10, 13] report the highest incidence in the spring. It should be emphasized, however, that maximal confusion with a variety of virus illnesses occurs during the spring months.

There is no evidence that occupation influences susceptibility to the disease. The impression that it has greatest predilection for students and white-collar workers is due solely to the fact that the best epidemiological studies have been conducted around hospitals and universities [23]. Susceptibility apparently is not related to either the presence or absence of tonsils [8]. Factors of possible importance are recent surgery, transfusions, and contact with individuals harboring subclinical infectious mononucleosis [30].

The bulk of clinical information [6, 8, 31, 32] favors an incubation period of 33 to 44 days. These estimates are based mostly on the experiences of students who have accurately recalled the dates of kissing contacts. Until recent years, the incubation period was thought to be about 11 days, with a range of 1 to 28 days [8].

A number of epidemics of infectious mononucleosis have been reported in children and young adults [1, 9, 18, 33, 34], but the diagnostic criteria in most of these epidemics were probably inadequate [6]. Evans [8, 13] has expressed the opinion that mild, subclinical forms of short duration develop in children and adolescents with little or no antibody production.

Infectious mononucleosis is not highly contagious. A number of family outbreaks were reported before 1930, but all reports lacked serological confirmation, and it is probable that many represented other types of viral illness. More recent investigations indicate that transmission to roommates, fellow hospital patients, and other family members is rare [5, 10, 20, 27, 31]. The only reasonably well-established mode of transmission is through intimate oral kissing [8, 31, 35].

There have been many experimental attempts to transmit infectious mononucleosis from man to man and from man to animal. Before 1947, there were approximately forty attempts, none completely successful [36]. A few investigators produced illnesses which resembled infectious mononucleosis, but most of them have not been reproduced. It seems likely that these human transmission experiments may have been attempted too late in the clinical illness.

ETIOLOGY

A variety of organisms have been suggested as possible etiological agents. Nyfeldt [37] isolated *Listeria monocytogenes* from patients with a disease clinically indistinguishable from infectious mononucleosis. The organisms were capable of producing a generalized infection with monocytosis in dogs, rabbits, guinea pigs, and mice [38, 39]. Others, however, have failed to isolate *L. monocytogenes* from patients with infectious mononucleosis and have found little or no rise in *Listeria* agglutination titers [40, 41]. Injections of these organisms into either animals or man have consistently failed to produce a rise in the heterophil agglutination titer [41, 42]. Reports of cases possibly due to *L. monocytogenes* continue, however, to appear [43, 44]. *Listeria* probably does not cause infectious mononucleosis, but occasionally it is cultured from the throats of patients with pharyngitis, regional adenopathy, and monocytosis [45].

Rickettsia sennetsu has been suggested [46] as the etiological agent. Toxoplasma has produced an infectious mononucleosis-like illness in rabbits and monkeys [47]. Remington *et al.* [48] reported positive results of toxoplasma dye tests in 16 percent and of toxoplasma skin tests in 17 percent of college students with infectious mononucleosis. Only three had a rise in either dye or hemagglutinin titers, however.

Burnet and Anderson [49] reported that serum from patients with infectious mononucleosis will agglutinate human erythrocytes modified with the virus of Newcastle disease of poultry. Evans and Curnen [50] confirmed these results but failed to demonstrate significant hemagglutination inhibition or complement fixation. Swain [51] demonstrated a high incidence of Newcastle virus agglutinin in sera from patients with infectious mononucleosis. He clearly indicated, however, that this is not Newcastle virus antibody, Forssman antibody, heterophil antibody, or antibody to many other bacterial and viral antigens. The agglutination reaction probably involves alteration of the surface antigen structure of the erythrocyte rather than attachment of virus itself [8, 52]. Sendai virus also has been suggested as a possible etiological agent [53]. An increased antibody against Sendai virus was detected in 10 of 116 patients with infectious mononucleosis, but virus was not cultured from throat washings. This virus is a myxovirus of the influenza, mumps, Newcastle group.

Increased *in vitro* uptake of tritium-labeled thymidine by the atypical lymphocytes of infectious mononucleosis suggests that the cells are virus-infected and are producing viral desoxyribonucleic acid [54]. The enzyme content of these aytpical cells is similar to that in the leukocytes of patients with acute and chronic granulocytic leukemia [55].

Infectious mononucleosis has been considered possibly to be a hypersensitivity or autoantibody disorder [8, 9, 51, 56]. It has been suggested [9] that some of the complications may be caused by autoantibody produced by immunologically competent atypical lymphocytes in response to virus-altered tissue. Swain [51] has indicated that the serum agglutinins which react with sheep erythrocytes and Newcastle virus-treated human erythrocytes may be autoantibody produced against damaged red cells.* Evans [8] has searched intensively for hypersensitivity and autoimmune pathways without success. He had negative results of indirect Coombs tests in thirty-nine consecutive heterophil-positive patients with infectious mononucleosis. No evidence of serum antibody to a leukocyte intracellular virus could be demonstrated. Lupus cells were not detected in the blood of patients with active disease, and their sera failed to induce lupus cell change in normal leukocytes. Nor was he able to support the claims that heterophil antibody is related to group A blood substance and that heterophil-negative infectious mononucleosis occurs principally in individuals of blood group A type. Galbraith *et al.* [57] found no evidence of antibody production by the atypical blood lymphocytes. They did believe, however, that they detected immunologically competent primitive cells in the lymph nodes.

There is other evidence suggesting a possible hypersensitivity mechanism. After cardiac surgery, some patients may develop a syndrome which bears close clinical resemblance to infectious mononucleosis, with fever, splenomegaly, lymphocytosis, and eosinophilia [58]. The differential leukocyte count may show 50 to 80 percent lymphocytes, many of which are atypical. Response to the sheep cell agglutination test is negative. Serum of patients with this syndrome may contain antibody to heart muscle [59]. Drug sensitivity reactions to paraaminosalicylic acid (PAS) [60, 61] and aminopyrine have caused illnesses that resembled acute infectious mononucleosis.

* Johnson and Holbrow (*Nature* [London] 198:1316, 1963) recently demonstrated affinity of serum globulin from patients with infectious mononucleosis for vascular endothelium and red cells of calf thyroid tissue. Serum absorption with ox or sheep red cells inhibited the reaction. There was no inhibition of serum reactivity following either the addition of an excess of human Cohn fraction II or absorption with guinea pig kidney emulsion.

PHYSICAL SIGNS AND SYMPTOMS

The clinical course is reasonably uniform [5, 6, 8, 10, 23, 28, 30, 31], with moderate variations in duration and intensity of symptoms and signs (Fig. 27-1). In approximately

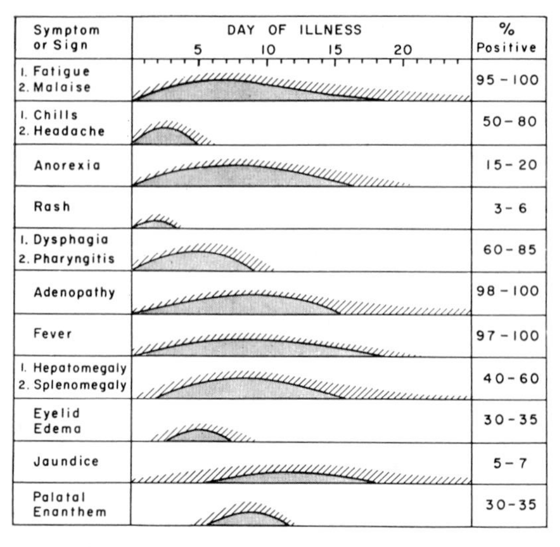

Fig. 27-1. Common symptoms and signs. Heavily shaded areas represent the usual intensity and duration; cross-hatched areas represent the extremes.

80 percent, the illness is primarily pharyngeal. Typhoidal or icteric features will predominate in the rest. Variations may depend on such factors as age, sex, host differences in immune reactivity, and differences in strains of infecting virus.

In many patients it is not possible to date the precise onset of acute symptoms. During the first few days virtually all patients have moderate malaise, easy fatigability, and anorexia. Headaches are common, they have no characteristic features but sometimes are retro-orbital. The temperature gradually rises to levels of 100 to 102° F. by the fifth to seventh day. Temperature above 103° F. is most unusual at any stage of the illness. Sore throat and dysphagia develop in about 50 percent of the patients during the first week. Ultimately 80 to 90 percent complain of soreness of the throat at some stage of the illness. Severity of the pharyngitis usually is proportional to the severity of symptoms, but there are some exceptions. Pharyngeal involvement consists of hyperplasia of lymph follicles, infection and edema of tonsils and pharynx, spotty or generalized membranous pharyngeal exudate, or severe membranous ulceration associated with surrounding inflammation [8].

Palatal enanthem is a relatively late manifestation. It almost always appears between the fifth and twelfth day, but sometimes as late as the seventeenth day [6]. The lesions consist of round, sharply defined petechiae measuring 0.5 to 1 mm. They are symmetrical and appear mostly at the junction of the hard and soft palates. These spots may develop as recurrent crops, at first being red, then turning brownish in 24 to 48 hours. Careful observation may reveal several clusters of new lesions over a 6 to 12 hour period. This enanthem is not specific for infectious mononucleosis, occurring in other viral diseases [5, 6, 31].

Adenopathy is an early sign. The nodes usually begin to enlarge two or three days after the onset of symptoms and are detectable by the end of the first week in 60 to 70 percent of the patients. Sometimes enlargement persists for several weeks and, rarely, for several months after cessation of the acute illness. The nodes are slightly or moderately tender, never exquisitely so or spontaneously painful. Enlargement is mild in 37 percent, moderate in 50 percent, severe in 10 percent, and "bull neck" in 3 percent [6].

A fleeting skin rash develops in 3 to 6 percent of the patients during the first few days. It consists of a faint erythema and generalized maculopapular eruption, mostly on the trunk and proximal portion of the limbs, lasting only for 24 to 48 hours. The skin lesions are very similar to those of rubella. Eruptions of greater intensity or longer duration do not develop.

Tenderness over the liver and spleen appears in 25 to 30 percent of the patients during the first several days of the illness. Moderate hepatomegaly eventually develops in 40 to 50 percent of all patients, with maximal enlargement during the second week. The spleen is enlarged in about 50 percent of the patients, reaching maximum size between the seventh and fourteenth day. In most patients it is barely palpable, soft to moderately firm, and seldom more than 1 to 2 fingerbreadths below the left costal margin, although occasionally it extends down to the iliac crest. Usually the enlargement rapidly recedes during the second and third weeks but, rarely, persists for several weeks or months.

During the first week of the acute illness, jaundice develops in 1 to 3 percent of patients. It appears most frequently during the second week, reaching a peak at the ninth or tenth day and subsiding fairly rapidly on the twelfth to fifteenth day. From 8 to 10 percent of patients with established infectious mononucleosis become visibly jaundiced, but there is only a slight icteric tint of the sclerae and mucous membranes which lasts only a few days. Hepatic enlargement and tenderness are poorly correlated with the degree of icterus. The diagnosis should be seriously questioned if deep jaundice occurs.

Other symptoms and signs have been reported, but most of them are nonspecific and of no diagnostic value.

LABORATORY FINDINGS

The peripheral blood leukocyte changes in most patients with proved infectious mononucleosis are characteristic (Fig. 27-2). They vary somewhat, however, with age, severity of illness, stage of illness, and development of complications. Minimal changes have been re-

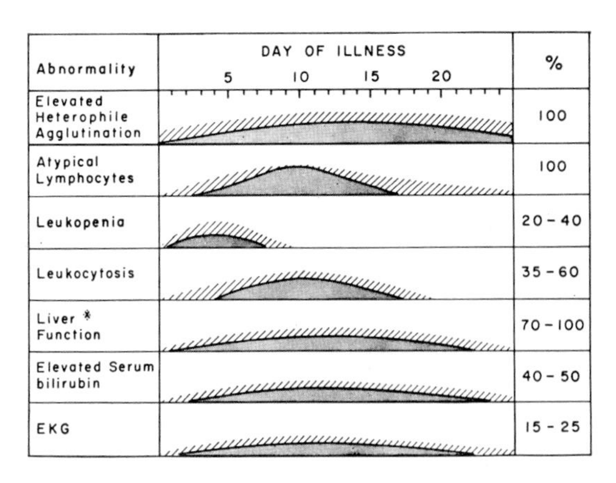

Fig. 27-2. Common laboratory findings. Heavily shaded areas represent the usual intensity and duration of abnormal findings; cross-hatched areas represent the extremes. *Liver function tests include SGOT, SGPT, LDH, alkaline phosphatase, cephalin flocculation, thymol turbidity, and BSP retention.

ported [8], with subclinical infections, during epidemics.

The total leukocyte count usually is normal or moderately reduced during the first week [10, 23, 28, 30, 63, 64]. In 10 to 20 percent, the total leukocyte count is less than 4,000 per mm.^{3}. Occasionally leukopenia is severe, with total counts of 2,000 or less. Moderate leukocytosis with counts ranging from 10,000 to 15,000 persists in some patients throughout the clinical course. Acute onset often is characterized by early polymorphonuclear leukocytosis. Granulocyte immaturity or toxic granulation of the polymorphonuclear leukocytes in patients with early leukocytosis often accompanies a severe clinical course.

Toward the end of the first week or early in the second, mild leukocytosis almost invariably develops. This reaches a maximum during the third week. In 65 to 70 percent, the peak count is between 10,000 and 15,000 per mm.^{3} [10, 66]; in another 10 to 20 percent, the value may exceed 15,000, but rarely exceeds 20,000. Leukocytosis may persist as long as there is fever, but occasionally the white count remains elevated for several months. The total leukocyte count of patients with initial leukopenia rises as the illness progresses, but usually it does not exceed normal values.

More important than the total leukocyte count are the morphological characteristics of the white blood cells. The most consistent finding is relative and absolute increase in atypical lymphocytes. These have been classified as Downey cell types I, II, and III [2]. Unfortunately, none of them is pathognomonic of infectious mononucleosis, being found also in agranulocytosis, toxoplasmosis, rickettsialpox, brucellosis, infectious hepatitis, listeriosis, hypersensitivity reactions, and several other viral illnesses [30]. The frequent association of these cells with virus infections has prompted the suggestion that they be called virocytes [67].

In the first few days or even weeks of illness, only a few atypical lymphocytes may be identified in the peripheral blood smear. Their relative and absolute numbers increase, however, with the rise in total white count. Patients with initial leukocytosis frequently have 30 to 50 percent atypical lymphocytes at the outset. In the second or third week, these cells usually constitute 50 percent or more of the total peripheral leukocytes and may reach levels of 70 to 90 percent. Most of them are Downey types I and II, with only a few type III. In the third and fourth weeks, the atypical lymphocytes disappear rapidly, although in a few patients they may persist for several months to a year or more.

Atypical lymphocytes have been identified both in the cerebrospinal fluid [68] and in stained smears of throat exudate [69]. It has been suggested that cytological study of throat lesion exudate may be of diagnostic value [69].

Most careful studies indicate that the atypical lymphocytes are lymphocytic in origin even though they bear close morphological resemblance to monocytes. Histochemical studies have demonstrated that the atypical lymphocytes are strongly PAS-positive and weakly positive to both methyl green pyronine and Sudan black [57]. They also have been shown to contain acid phosphatase, nonspecific esterase, and reactive sulfhydryl groups [57]. Nuclear fenestration [70] and the development of intersecting intranuclear tunnels [71] have been noted in the atypical lymphocytes following incubation.

Anemia is an extremely rare complication [72–78]. When present, it is an acquired hemolytic type, developing during the second or third week, although it may be present from the outset. It is mild and self-limiting, lasting from a few days to a few weeks. In about one-third, a positive Coombs reaction develops, frequently of the cold antibody type.

Significant thrombocytopenia rarely develops during the acute or convalescent phase. Usually, platelet reduction is slight to moderate, but occasionally severe depression occurs [79–82]. In the later instances, the clinical picture may be indistinguishable from idiopathic thrombocytopenic purpura, with petechiae, purpura, hematuria, and oronasopharyngeal or intestinal bleeding. Usually, the platelet count returns to normal within six weeks, but may remain depressed for six months or longer [82]. Rarely, pancytopenia is associated with the presence of platelet and leukocyte agglutinins [78].

The principal value of bone marrow study is to exclude malignant involvement of the hemopoietic system when the clinical picture is uncertain. Alteration of marrow morphology is found in about 70 percent of patients, but the changes are modest and nonspecific [83, 84]. The most consistent findings are moderate granulocyte hyperplasia, granulocyte immaturity, and increase of mature lymphocytes. Histological bone marrow sections have shown granulomatous lesions with prominent epithelioid cells in about one half of the patients studied [84].

Serum heterophil antibody titers rise during the first 3 to 4 weeks in virtually all patients with the disease. One-half or more have a significant titer during the first week. Usually, the level gradually declines and reaches values close to normal 8 to 10 weeks after the onset. Elevated titers may persist for 3 to 6 months and sometimes for a year or more [30, 85]. Unfortunately, increased titers of sheep erythrocyte antibody alone do not establish the diagnosis of infectious mononucleosis. Elevated levels may be due to naturally occurring Forssman antibody, serum sickness antibody, persistence of heterophil antibody from previous infectious mononucleosis, or an anamnestic response caused by some other infection or possibly other closely related disorders [7, 25, 30, 86–88]. A nonspecific rise in heterophil titer due to other viral illnesses may occur as long as one year after an attack of infectious mononucleosis.

The opinion has been expressed [8, 13, 89] that subclinical or mild infectious mononucleosis of brief duration may develop without rise in heterophil agglutination titer, whereas more protracted infections of greater severity usually cause an increase of serum antibody. About 20 percent of the patients in some of the major reports did not have a significant elevation of the heterophil titer [8, 23, 28, 64].

Variable amounts of antibody that react with sheep cells are present in the serum of healthy individuals. Serum absorption with guinea pig kidney antigen removes heterophil antibody of the Forssman and serum sickness types but has little or no effect on infectious mononucleosis antibody [65, 90]. Serum absorption with beef erythrocytes will not remove Forssman antibody but will remove the heterophil antibodies of infectious mononucleosis and serum sickness. The upper limit for the normal unabsorbed heterophil titer varies widely in different laboratories, ranging from 1 : 20 to 1 : 320 [13, 30]. Usually an unabsorbed titer of 1 : 128 or above in the absence of serum sickness is consistent with the diagnosis of infectious mononucleosis. To minimize false positive reactions, differential absorption tests should be performed on all sera with suspicious elevation of the unabsorbed titer. Guinea pig absorbed titers of 1 : 32 or greater probably are significantly elevated.

Wide variation in the agglutinability of erythrocytes from different sheep [91] suggests that it may be unwise to establish an arbitrary agglutination titer as normal. Probably it is of much greater diagnostic importance to find a rising titer on use of the same sheep cells during the clinical illness. Infectious mononucleosis and other illnesses may elevate serum cold agglutinins for sheep erythrocytes, resulting in a false positive test [92]. Another technical problem is that differences in particle size of guinea pig preparations may cause conspicuous differences in degree of reduction of heterophil titer [93].

Several alternative tests have been developed in an attempt to improve the sensitivity and specificity of serum antibody reactions. Ox cell hemolysis has been reported to be more sensitive and just as specific as the sheep cell test, with serum reactions remaining positive much later in the course of the illness [8, 94]. A satisfactory goat cell agglutination test has been developed [95]. Excellent results also have been reported with tests utilizing either enzyme-treated sheep erythrocytes [93] or guinea pig antigen-absorbed test serum reacted with trypsinized beef erythrocytes [96].

Heterophil antibody has been demonstrated in the cerebrospinal fluid of patients with infectious mononucleosis [97]. The amount of antibody does not bear a linear relationship to the blood level. False positive reactions may occur with tuberculous meningitis, subarachnoid hemorrhage, and trichinosis.

The serum of patients with infectious mononucleosis has been reported to show false positive serological reactions for syphilis, false positive Widal reactions, and agglutinins for *Brucella melitensis* and other microorganisms [10]. Incidence figures for biologically false positive reactions for syphilis vary from 2 to greater than 60 percent [98]. These false positive reactions are stated to be independent of heterophil antibody and to persist for several months after the acute illness has ended [99]. Recently, Hoagland [98] challenged the concept that false positive serological tests for syphilis are a frequent occurrence in infectious mononucleosis, having found an incidence of only 0.66 percent in 300 patients with this disorder. He believes that many of the positive results of serological tests represent either syphilis or false positive reactions in patients with illnesses other than infectious mononucleosis.

Serum protein studies usually disclose moderate hypoalbuminemia and slight increases in α_1-, β-, and γ-globulins [66, 75, 100]. An abnormal protein migrating between α_2- and β-globulin also has been observed [101]. The heterophil antibody is probably a high molecular weight γ-globulin [101a, 101b], but otherwise has not been characterized. The serum lipoproteins are different from those found with hepatitis [102]. In infectious mononucleosis there is significant reduction of both high density lipoprotein fractions and the standard S_f 0 to 12 lipoproteins. The S_f 20 to 100 and S_f 100 to 400 fractions are increased. These changes disappear by the ninth week of illness.

Some of the most consistent laboratory findings in infectious mononucleosis are derangements of liver function. In 85 to 100 percent of patients, some evidence of hepatitis is found on laboratory testing [23, 66, 72, 102–106]. The most sensitive indicators of acute hepatic damage are the lactate dehydrogenase (LDH), serum glutamic pyruvic transaminase (SGPT), serum glutamic oxaloacetic transaminase (SGOT), cephalin flocculation, isocitric dehydrogenase, alkaline phosphatase, phosphohexose isomerase, aldolase, and bromsulphalein tests in about that order [24, 66, 103–106]. Certainly the serum bilirubin is one of the least sensitive indicators of liver involvement. The correlation between elevated serum bilirubin levels and abnormal results of liver function tests, especially the alkaline phosphatase level, is poor [66, 103, 105]. There is some evidence of a direct correlation of the degree of hepatic functional impairment, severity of the general illness, hyperglobulinemia, and possibly the heterophil antibody titer [8, 17, 103]. Demonstration of abnormality of liver function has been useful in the early detection of infectious mononucleosis and in differentiation from acute tonsillitis, certain respiratory infections, and rubella [17, 104, 106]. The SGOT and SPGT levels usually rise during the first week, with maximal values in the second week. Almost invariably they return to normal by the third to fifth week. An occasional instance of persistent abnormality or permanent liver damage has been reported, but there is little evidence that infectious mononucleosis is responsible for chronic liver disease [72, 107].

Elevation of the serum bilirubin to levels in excess of 6 mg. per 100 ml. are rarely encountered [6, 102, 108]. Increasing values usually are found during the first week, with maximal levels on the ninth to eleventh day. Only eleven patients with serum bilirubin levels over 8 mg. have been reported, but seven of them had levels above 17 mg. [108]. Although a high serum bilirubin level is relatively rare, it is likely that it often occurs but has not been reported. On the other hand, it is probable that some of the high levels reported have occurred in patients with infectious hepatitis rather than infectious mononucleosis.

Liver pathology in infectious mononucleosis bears close resemblance to that in infectious hepatitis, but most pathologists agree that there are certain distinctive features of the hepatitis associated with infectious mononucleosis. Focal hepatic cell necrosis, if present at all, is minimal. Sometimes there is extensive portal and perilobular infiltration by swollen reticuloendothelial cells and atypical cells of the mononuclear type [66, 103, 109]. Periportal lymphoid collars may closely resemble the appearance in leukemia. The sinusoids are often dilated, and minor bile duct proliferation may occur [109]. Collections of atypical mononuclear cells sometimes align along the vascular spaces [66]. Correlation is poor between liver pathology and the severity of jaundice [108].

DIAGNOSIS

The diagnosis of infectious mononucleosis requires certain minimal clinical and laboratory findings. These are: a typical clinical course, persistence for ten days or longer of a peripheral blood differential leukocyte count of at least 50 percent lymphocytes of which some are atypical, and a significant serum heterophil titer [6]. It is likely that mild or subclinical infectious mononucleosis occurs with minimal hematological and serological changes [8, 9]. Erroneous identification, however, has greatly clouded the clinical picture. Many bizarre complications have been reported, but rarely in patients with the characteristic clinical and laboratory features. If there are severe nausea, watery diarrhea, painful or extremely tender nodes, chest pain, nasal congestion, paroxysmal or productive cough, joint pains, hematuria, dysuria, or severe abdominal pain, the diagnosis of infectious mononucleosis is unlikely [6].

The importance of individual laboratory features has been overemphasized. Prolonged elevation of heterophil titer following the acute illness has resulted in the reporting of clinical relapse, recurrence, chronic mononucleosis, and a variety of peculiar complications [6, 7, 85, 87]. Clinical relapse is rare, and few well-documented instances of probable recurrence have been reported [6, 30, 31, 85]. Additional difficulty has been encountered due to nonspecific or anamnestic rise in heterophil titer [87, 88]. Most cases of recurrent mononucleosis have been diagnosed on clinical grounds alone, with insignificant rise in heterophil titer.

The differential diagnosis includes a wide variety of neoplastic, bacterial, and viral diseases as well as drug reactions [5, 23, 24, 30, 45, 48, 57, 59, 60, 65–68, 72, 102, 111, 112].

COMPLICATIONS

Most patients with infectious mononucleosis recover completely within a few days after defervescence [5, 10, 18, 31]. The development of complications may slow the recovery period, but, contrary to the general impression, rarely do lethargy and weakness persist for long periods.

Numerous reports of multiple system involvement have created the impression that the disease frequently is associated with various complications, but this opinion probably is the result of poor case documentation and uncritical reporting. In considerably less than 1 percent of patients will unusual problems develop. Table 27-1 summarizes the more common complications.

Cardiac involvement is rare, but minor electrocardiographic abnormalities have been described. Acute pericarditis has been reported in about twenty patients [5, 6, 24, 30, 72, 74, 109, 110].

Neurological difficulties develop in 0.5 percent or less, with a male : female ratio of about 3 : 1. Most of these problems arise during the second and third weeks of the illness [114]. Residual damage in about 15 percent and a mortality of something less than 5 percent in those with serious neurological involvement have been reported [115].

Rupture of the spleen is the single most serious complication. About 40 percent of ruptures are spontaneous [72]. The rest follow trauma, which usually is minor. Rupture most often occurs in the second or third week of the

TABLE 27-1. Reported Complications of Infectious Mononucleosis

General Type of Complication	Specific Problem
Neurological	Meningismus, meningitis, meningoencephalitis, encephalitis, peripheral neuritis, acute polyneuritis, peripheral neuropathy, encephalomyelitis, encephaloneuronitis, primary optic neuritis, transverse myelitis, cerebellar ataxia, hyperesthesia, seizures, mental confusion, psychotic reaction, coma
Hematological	Acquired hemolytic anemia, thrombocytopenia, pancytopenia, splenic rupture
Cardiac	Pericarditis, myocarditis
Ocular	Retro-orbital pain, nystagmus, scotoma, ptosis, diplopia, optic neuritis, hemianopsia, eyelid edema, conjunctivitis, uveitis, lacrimal pericyclitis, retinal edema, retinal hemorrhage
Pulmonary	Pleuritis, virus pneumonia, interstitial pneumonitis, pleural effusion
Other	Orchitis, pancreatitis, thyroiditis, nephritis, hematuria, nephrotic syndrome, vaginitis, porphyrinuria

acute illness [5, 72, 113]; estimated mortality is 30 percent.

Death due to infectious mononucleosis is very unusual, although patients occasionally die of splenic rupture, laryngeal obstruction, or respiratory paralysis. Mortality rates in several of the larger clinical reports have ranged from 0.1 to a little less than 1 percent [5, 30, 117]. Over-all mortality, however, is considerably less than 0.1 percent.

THERAPY

No specific form of therapy is available and treatment is symptomatic. Patients are not isolated.

Medications advocated for uncomplicated infectious mononucleosis have included arsenicals, emetine, γ-globulin, convalescent serum, antibiotics, corticosteroids, and chloroquine phosphate [5, 10, 117–123], but there is little evidence that they are of value. Intrathecal administration of methotrexate has been suggested [120] for central nervous system involvement. BAL (2,3-dimercapto-l-propanol) has been used with good effect for optic neuritis [124].

Most of the severe complications respond to rapid intravenous administration of 400 to 500 mg. of hydrocortisone followed by 60 to 80 mg. of prednisone by mouth daily during the acute phase. Corticosteroid therapy rarely is necessary for more than four to six days [15, 34].

REFERENCES

1. Pfeiffer, E. Drüsenfieber, *Jahrb. Kinderheilk.* 29:257, 1889.
2. Downey, H., and McKinlay, C. A. Acute lymphadenosis compared with acute lymphatic leukemia. *Arch. Intern. Med.* 32:82, 1923.
3. Paul, J. R., and Bunnell, W. W. The presence of heterophile antibodies in infectious mononucleosis. *Amer. J. Med. Sci.* 183:90, 1932.
4. Bender, C. E. Diagnosis of infectious mononucleosis. *J.A.M.A.* 149:7, 1952.
5. Hoagland, R. J. Infectious mononucleosis. *Clin. Sympos.* 10:17, 1958.
6. Hoagland, R. J. The clinical manifestations of infectious mononucleosis: A report of 200 cases. *Amer. J. Med. Sci.* 240:55, 1960.
7. Hoagland, R. J. Diagnosis of infectious mononucleosis. *Blood* 16:1045, 1960.
8. Evans, A. S. Infectious mononucleosis in University of Wisconsin students: Report of a five year investigation. *Amer. J. Hyg.* 71:342, 1960.
9. Editorial. The riddle of infectious mononucleosis. *Brit. Med. J.* 1:111, 1961.
10. Bernstein, A. Infectious mononucleosis. *Medicine* 19:85, 1940.
11. Newell, K. W. The reported incidence of glandular fever: An analysis of a report of the Public Health Laboratory Service. *J. Clin. Path.* 10:20, 1957.
12. Hobson, F. G., Lawson, B., and Wigfield, M. Glandular fever: A field study. *Brit. Med. J.* 1:845, 1958.
13. Evans, A. S. Infectious mononucleosis: Observations from a Public Health Laboratory. *Yale J. Biol. Med.* 34:261, 1962.
14. Rag, E. S., and Cecil, R. C. Infectious mononucleosis in the Negro. *South. Med. J.* 37:543, 1944.
15. Johnson, R. D. Infectious mononucleosis in the Negro. *J.A.M.A.* 124:1254, 1944.
16. Blain, A., 3rd, and Vonder Heide, E. C. Infectious mononucleosis in the Negro. *Amer. J. Med. Sci.* 209:587, 1945.
17. Harley, J. F. Infectious mononucleosis in the Negro: A review of the literature with a report of 9 cases. *J. Pediat.* 39:303, 1951.
18. Wechsler, H. F., Rosenblum, A. H., and Sills, C. T. Infectious mononucleosis: Report of an epidemic in an army camp. *Ann. Intern. Med.* 25:113, 1946.
19. Wintrobe, M. M. *Clinical Hematology* (5th ed.). Philadelphia: Lea & Febiger, 1961.
20. Evans, A. S., and Robinton, E. D. An epidemiologic study of infectious mononucleosis in a New England college. *New Eng. J. Med.* 242:492, 1950.
21. Strom, J. Infectious mononucleosis: Is the incidence increasing? *Acta Med. Scand.* 168:35, 1960.
22. Virtanen, S. Incidence of infectious mononucleosis antibodies in blood donors. *Acta Path. Microbiol. Scand.* 56:53, 1962.
23. Niederman, J. C. Infectious mononucleosis at the Yale–New Haven Medical Center 1946–1955. *Yale J. Biol. Med.* 28:629, 1956.
24. Dunnet, W. N. Infectious mononucleosis. *Brit. Med. J.* 1:1187, 1963.
25. Shapiro, C. M., and Horwitz, H. Infectious mononucleosis in the aged. *Ann. Intern. Med.* 51:1092, 1959.

26. Shibuya, T. Icteric type of infectious mononucleosis in a 2 month old infant. *Tohoku J. Exp. Med.* 78:11, 1962.
27. Contratto, A. W. Infectious mononucleosis. *Arch. Intern. Med.* 73:449, 1944.
28. Keith, T. A., III. Periodicity of mononucleosis-like disease at an army post. *Amer. J. Med. Sci.* 240:340, 1960.
29. Mason, W. R., and Adams, E. Infectious mononucleosis: An analysis of 100 cases with particular attention to diagnosis, liver function tests and treatment of selected cases with prednisone. *Amer. J. Med. Sci.* 236:447, 1958.
30. Leibowitz, S. *Infectious Mononucleosis.* New York: Grune & Stratton, Inc., 1953.
31. Hoagland, R. J. Infectious mononucleosis. *Amer. J. Med.* 13:158, 1952.
32. Hoagland, R. J. The transmission of infectious mononucleosis. *Amer. J. Med. Sci.* 229:262, 1955.
33. Nolan, R. A. Report of so-called epidemic of glandular fever (infectious mononucleosis). *U.S. Nav. Med. Bull.* 33:479, 1935.
34. Hakrow, J. P. A., Owen, L. M., and Rodger, N. Infectious mononucleosis with an account of an epidemic in an E.M.S. Hospital. *Brit. Med. J.* 2:443, 1943.
35. Bender, C. E. Clinical epidemiology of mononucleosis at a state university. *Northwest Med.* 58:697, 1959.
36. Evans, A. S. Experimental attempts to transmit infectious mononucleosis to man. *Yale J. Biol. Med.* 20:19, 1947.
37. Nyfeldt, A. Étiologie de la mononucléose infectieuse. *C. R. Soc. Biol.* (Paris) 101:590, 1929.
38. Nyfeldt, A. Klinische und experimentelle Untersuchungen über die Mononucleosis infectiosa. *Folia Haemat.* 47:1, 1932.
39. Pons, C. A., and Julianelle, L. A. Isolation of *Listerella monocytogenes* from infectious mononucleosis. *Proc. Soc. Exp. Biol. Med.* 40:360, 1939.
40. Janeway, C. A., and Dammin, G. J. Infectious mononucleosis: II. The relationship of the organisms of the genus *Listerella* to the disease. *J. Clin. Invest.* 20:233, 1941.
41. Wising, P. J. A study of infectious mononucleosis (Pfeiffer's Disease) from the etiological point of view. *Acta Med. Scand.* 133 (supp.):5, 1942.
42. Kolmer, J. A. *Listerella monocytogenes* in relation to the Wassermann and flocculation reactions in normal rabbits. *Proc. Soc. Exp. Biol. Med.* 42:183, 1939.
43. Murray, E. G. D. Characterization of listeriosis in man and other animals. *Canad. Med. Ass. J.* 72:99, 1955.
44. Chaiken, B. H., and Michaud, D. T. *Listeria monocytogenes* infection and its relation to infectious mononucleosis. *New Eng. J. Med.* 258:385, 1958.
45. Hoeprich, P. D. Infection due to *Listeria monocytogenes. Medicine* 37:143, 1958.
46. Misao, T., and Kobayashi, Y. Studies on infectious mononucleosis (glandular fever): I. Isolation of etiologic agent from blood, bone marrow and lymph node of a patient with infectious mononucleosis by using mice. *Tokyo Iji Shinshi* 71:683, 1944.
47. Bland, J. O. W. Glandular fever: II. The protozoal nature of the experimental disease. *Brit. J. Exp. Path.* 12:311, 1931.
48. Remington, J. S., Barnett, C. G., Meikel, M., and Lunde, M. D. Toxoplasmosis and infectious mononucleosis. *Arch. Intern. Med.* 110: 744, 1962.
49. Burnet, F. M., and Anderson, S. G. Modification of human red cells by virus action: II. Agglutination of modified human red cells by sera from cases of infectious mononucleosis. *Brit. J. Exp. Path.* 27:236, 1946.
50. Evans, A. S., and Curnen, E. C. Serological studies of infectious mononucleosis. *J. Immun.* 58:323, 1948.
51. Swain, R. H. The nature of the Newcastle agglutinin in infectious mononucleosis and infectious hepatitis. *J. Path. Bact.* 78:67, 1959.
52. Evans, A. S. The interaction of serum with erythrocytes modified by Newcastle disease virus. *J. Immun.* 74:391, 1955.
53. DeMeio, J. L., and Walker, D. L. Sendai virus antibody in acute respiratory infections and infectious mononucleosis. *Proc. Soc. Exp. Biol. Med.* 98:453, 1958.
54. Gavosto, F., Pileri, A., and Mariani, G. Incorporation of thymidine labelled with tritium by circulating cells of infectious mononucleosis. *Nature* (London) 183:1691, 1959.
55. Bertino, J. R., Simmons, B. M., and Donohue, D. M. Increased activity of some folic acid enzyme systems in infectious mononucleosis. *Blood* 19:587, 1962.
56. Hunt, J. S. The pathogenesis of infectious mononucleosis. *Amer. J. Med. Sci.* 228:83, 1954.
57. Galbraith, P., Mitus, W. J., Gallerkeri, M., and Dameshek, W. The "infectious mononucleosis cell": A cytological study. *Blood* 22:630, 1963.
58. Perillie, P. E., and Glenn, W. W. Fever, splenomegaly, lymphocytosis and eosinophilia: A new post-cardiotomy syndrome. *Yale J. Biol. Med.* 34:625, 1962.
59. Robinson, J. F., and Brigden, W. Immunological studies in the post-cardiotomy syndrome. *Brit. Med. J.* 2:706, 1963.
60. Jesiotr, M. A case of severe hypersensitivity to P.A.S. simulating infectious mononucleosis. *Harefuah* 59:267, 1960.

61. Daley, D., and Smith, W. G. Hypersensitivity to P.A.S. simulating glandular fever (infectious mononucleosis). *Tubercle* 41:68, 1960.
62. Paul, J. R. Infectious mononucleosis. *Bull. N.Y. Acad. Med.* 15:43, 1939.
63. Tidy, H. L. Glandular fever and infectious mononucleosis. *Lancet* 2:180, 1934.
64. Gardner, H. T., and Paul, J. R. Infectious mononucleosis at the New Haven Hospital, 1921 to 1946. *Yale J. Biol. Med.* 19:839, 1947.
65. Davidsohn, I. Serologic diagnosis of infectious mononucleosis. *J.A.M.A.* 108:289, 1937.
66. Gelb, D., West, M., and Zimmerman, H. G. Serum enzymes in disease: IX. Analysis of factors responsible for elevated values in infectious mononucleosis. *Amer. J. Med.* 33:249, 1962.
67. Litwins, J., and Leibowitz, S. Abnormal lymphocytes ("virocytes") in virus diseases other than infectious mononucleosis. *Acta Haemat.* 5:223, 1951.
68. Hollister, L. E., Houck, G. H., and Dunlop, W. A. Infectious mononucleosis of the central nervous system. *Amer. J. Med.* 20:643, 1956.
69. Paine, T. F., Jr. Atypical lymphocytes in throat exudate of patients with infectious mononucleosis. *New Eng. J. Med.* 264:240, 1961.
70. Osgood, E. E. Fenestration of nuclei of lymphocytes: A new diagnostic sign in infectious mononucleosis. *Proc. Soc. Exp. Biol. Med.* 33:218, 1935.
71. Ghaemi, A., and Seaman, A. "Swiss cheese" nuclei: An incubation induced lesion of infectious mononucleosis lymphocytes. *Amer. J. Clin. Path.* 39:492, 1963.
72. Erwin, W., Weber, R. W., and Manning, R. T. Complications of infectious mononucleosis. *Amer. J. Med. Sci.* 238:699, 1959.
73. Green, N., and Goldenberg, H. Acute hemolytic anemia and hemoglobinuria complicating infectious mononucleosis. *Arch. Intern. Med.* 105:108, 1960.
74. Editorial. Complications of infectious mononucleosis. *Brit. Med. J.* 1:1553, 1960.
75. Houk, V. N., and McFarland, W. Acute autoimmune hemolytic anemia complicating infectious mononucleosis. *J.A.M.A.* 177:210, 1961.
76. Macpherson, D. J. Hemolytic anemia in infectious mononucleosis. *J. Med. Soc. New Jersey* 60:13, 1963.
77. Denardo, G. L., and Ray, J. P. Hereditary spherocytosis and infectious mononucleosis, with acquired hemolytic anemia: Report of a case and review of the literature. *Amer. J. Clin. Path.* 39:284, 1963.
78. Smith, D. S., Abell, J. D., and Cast, I. P. Autoimmune hemolytic anaemia and thrombocytopenia complicating infectious mononucleosis. *Brit. Med. J.* 1:1210, 1963.
79. Douglas, W. A. Infectious mononucleosis with thrombocytopenic purpura in a child. *Med. J. Aust.* 2:564, 1959.
80. Grossman, L. A., and Wolff, S. M. Acute thrombocytopenic purpura in infectious mononucleosis. *J.A.M.A.* 171:2208, 1959.
81. Lymburner, R. M., and Malcolmson, C. H. Thrombocytopenic purpura complicating infectious mononucleosis. *Canad. Med. Ass. J.* 83:652, 1960.
82. Schumacher, R. H. Infectious mononucleosis complicated by chronic thrombocytopenia. *J.A.M.A.* 177:515, 1961.
83. Limarzi, L. R., Paul, J. T., and Poncher, H. G. Blood and bone marrow in infectious mononucleosis: A review of the literature and a report of 25 cases. *J. Lab. Clin. Med.* 31:1079, 1946.
84. Hovde, R. F., and Sundberg, R. D. Granulomatous lesions in the bone marrow in infectious mononucleosis. *Blood* 5:209, 1950.
85. Bender, C. E. Recurrent mononucleosis. *J.A.M.A.* 182:954, 1962.
86. Davidsohn, I., Stern, K., and Kashiwagi, C. The differential test of infectious mononucleosis. *Amer. J. Clin. Path.* 21:1101, 1951.
87. Bender, C. E. Interpretation of hematologic and serologic findings in the diagnosis of infectious mononucleosis. *Ann. Intern. Med.* 49:852, 1958.
88. Hoagland, R. J. Resurgent heterophil-antibody reaction after mononucleosis. *New Eng. J. Med.* 269:1307, 1963.
89. Evans, A. S. Recurrent mononucleosis. *J.A.M.A.* 184:515, 1963.
90. Virtanen, S. Absorption patterns in the differential absorption test for infectious mononucleosis. *Acta Path. Microbiol. Scand.* 56:57, 1962.
91. Zarafonetis, C. J. D., and Oster, H. L. Heterophile agglutination variability of erythrocytes from different sheep. *J. Lab. Clin. Med.* 36:283, 1950.
92. Zarafonetis, C. J. D., Oster, H. L., and Colville, V. F. Cold agglutination of sheep erythrocytes as a factor in false-positive heterophile agglutination tests. *J. Lab. Clin. Med.* 41:906, 1953.
93. Muschel, L. H., and Piper, D. R. Enzyme-treated red blood cells of sheep in the test for infectious mononucleosis. *Amer. J. Clin. Path.* 32:240, 1959.
94. Ericson, C. Ox cell hemolysin and sheep cell agglutinin in mononucleosis infectiosa. *Acta Path. Microbiol. Scand.* 51 (supp. 144):229, 1961.
95. Wang, S. P., and Grayston, J. T. Goat red

blood cells in agglutination test for infectious mononucleosis. *Proc. Soc. Exp. Biol. Med.* 101: 111, 1959.

96. Tomcsik, J. The serologic diagnosis of infectious mononucleosis. *Triangle* 5:114, 1961.
97. Freedman, M. J., Odland, L. T., and Cleve, E. A. Infectious mononucleosis with diffuse involvement of nervous system. *Arch. Neurol. Psychiat.* 69:49, 1953.
98. Hoagland, R. J. False-positive serology in mononucleosis. *J.A.M.A.* 185:783, 1963.
99. Kahn, R. L. Are there paradoxic serologic reactions in syphilis? *Arch. Derm.* 39:92, 1939.
100. Sterling, K. The serum proteins in infectious mononucleosis: Electrophoretic studies. *J. Clin. Invest.* 28:1057, 1949.
101. Sullivan, B. H., Jr., Irey, N. S., Pileggi, V. J., Crone, R. I., and Gibson, J. R. The liver in infectious mononucleosis. *Amer. J. Dig. Dis.* 2:210, 1957.

101a. Grubb, R., and Swahn, B. Destruction of some agglutinins but not of others by two sulfhydryl compounds. *Acta Path. Microbiol. Scand.* 43:305, 1958.

101b. Kunkel, H. G. Macroglobulins and High Molecular Weight Antibodies. In Putnam, F. W. (Ed.), *The Plasma Proteins.* New York: Academic Press, Inc., 1960. Vol. I.

102. Rubin, L. The serum lipoproteins in infectious mononucleosis. *Amer. J. Med.* 17:521, 1954.
103. Barondess, J. A., and Erle, H. Serum alkaline phosphatase activity in hepatitis of infectious mononucleosis. *Amer. J. Med.* 29:43, 1960.
104. Laursen, T., Faber, V., and Hansen, P. F. Serum glutamic-pyruvic-transaminase in infectious mononucleosis. *Danish Med. Bull.* 8:40, 1961.
105. Futterweit, W. Serum alkaline phosphatase activity in infectious mononucleosis: A clinical study of 55 cases. *Arch. Intern. Med.* 108: 253, 1961.
106. Gold, J. A., O'Connell, F., and Caldwell, F. Serial serum enzymes in infectious mononucleosis. *New York J. Med.* 62:1796, 1962.
107. Davis, T. W., and Bogoch, A. Prolonged hepatitis due to infectious mononucleosis. *Canad. Med. Ass. J.* 82:476, 1960.
108. Corr, W. P., Jr., and Scian, L. F. Deep jaundice in infectious mononucleosis. *J.A.M.A.* 181:52, 1962.
109. Custer, R. P., and Smith, E. B. The pathology of infectious mononucleosis. *Blood* 3:830, 1948.
110. Wilson, D. R., Lenkei, S. C., and Paterson, J. F. Acute constrictive epicarditis following infectious mononucleosis: A case report. *Circulation* 23:257, 1961.
111. Stone, G. E., and Redmond, A. J. Leukopenic infectious monocytosis: Report of a case closely simulating acute monocytic leukemia. *Amer. J. Med.* 34:541, 1963.
112. Dawson, T. A., and Dowling, R. H. Infectious mononucleosis and porphyria. *Ulster Med. J.* 31:82, 1962.
113. Janbon, M., and Bertrand, L. Rupture of spleen in infectious mononucleosis: its physiopathologic mechanism. *Sang* 31:235, 1960.
114. Lawrence, A., Simons, P., and MacGregor, G. A. Glandular fever encephalitis. *Brit. Med. J.* 1:376, 1962.
115. Yarington, C. T., Jr. The neurological complications of infectious mononucleosis. *New Physician* 10:316, 1961.
116. Gardner, C. C. Acute pericarditis as the initial manifestation of infectious mononucleosis. *Amer. J. Med. Sci.* 237:352, 1959.
117. Lassen, H. C. A., and Thomsen, S. Treatment of infectious mononucleosis with specific convalescent serum. *Acta Med. Scand.* 104:498, 1940.
118. Boyer, M. G. Therapeutic trial of gamma globulin in infectious mononucleosis. *Stud. Med.* 8:264, 1960.
119. Chappel, M. R., and Chapman, J. E. A quick ambulatory control for mononucleosis. *Arizona Med.* 18:49, 1961.
120. Schumacher, H. R., Jacobson, W. A., and Bemiller, C. R. Treatment of infectious mononucleosis. *Ann. Intern. Med.* 58:217, 1963.
121. Schultz, A. L., and Hall, W. H. Clinical observations in 100 cases of infectious mononucleosis and the results of treatment with penicillin and aureomycin. *Ann. Intern. Med.* 36:1498, 1952.
122. Gothberg, L. A. Severe infectious mononucleosis treated with chloroquine phosphage. *J.A.M.A.* 173:53, 1960.
123. Cowley, R. G., and Meyers, J. E., Jr. Chloroquine in the treatment of infectious mononucleosis. *Ann. Intern. Med.* 57:937, 1962.
124. Bonyge, T. W., and Von Hagen, K. O. Severe optic neuritis in infectious mononucleosis. *J.A.M.A.* 148:933, 1952.

28. *Sarcoidosis**

HAROLD L. ISRAEL

CLINICAL AND EPIDEMIOLOGICAL FEATURES

Sarcoidosis is a systemic granulomatous disease of unknown etiology. The mediastinal lymph nodes, lungs, peripheral lymph nodes, skin, and eyes are commonly involved, but any organ or tissue may be affected. Since the characteristic epithelioid tubercles with little or no necrosis may be simulated by the granulomas of tuberculosis, beryllium disease, and fungal infections, the diagnosis cannot be established by histological examination alone. Systemic involvement must be demonstrated and other causes of local sarcoid reactions excluded.

Sarcoidosis was once widely considered to be an atypical form of tuberculosis, but this concept has been abandoned by most investigators. Efforts to implicate other infectious agents have been equally unrewarding, and there is growing attention to the possibility that sarcoidosis represents a hypersensitivity disorder.

Sarcoidosis occurs in a remarkable geographic pattern, being fairly common (prevalence of about 4 per 10,000 young adults) in northern Europe, eastern United States, Australia, and New Zealand. It is rare in southern Europe, western United States, South America, and Hawaii and is apparently rare in Asia and Africa. In the United States, most of the patients are Negroes. The disease chiefly affects young adults, with manifestation uncommon before age 18 and after age 50. Symptoms are frequently slight but may be severe. The disease is fatal in almost 10 percent, usually as the result of progressive pulmonary fibrosis. The only therapeutic agents of demonstrated efficacy are the corticosteroids and chloroquine.

Corticosteroids as a rule exert a prompt effect on clinical, radiological, biochemical, and histological manifestations, but most observers believe that steroid therapy does not significantly alter the course. There is no evidence that it averts pulmonary fibrosis, which is the commonest serious development. Generally accepted indications for the administration of adrenal corticosteroids include: active ocular sarcoidosis; progressive pulmonary involvement, on the basis of increasing symptoms, roentgenographic changes, or impaired or deteriorating pulmonary function; persistent hypercalcemia; central nervous system involvement; disfiguring cutaneous lesions; and myocardial sarcoidosis [1]. Dosage is usually in the range of 15 to 20 mg. of prednisone daily for three months. In chronic cases, more prolonged treatment is often required.

DELAYED HYPERSENSITIVITY REACTIONS

TUBERCULIN REACTION

Interest in abnormal immunological responses was aroused by Schaumann's observation in 1917 that most patients with sarcoidosis failed to react to tuberculin. The similarity in tuberculin sensitivity found in patients with sarcoidosis in European and American studies is remarkable (Table 28-1). Less than 10 percent of patients with sarcoidosis react to first- or intermediate strength tuberculin, one-fourth react to second-strength tuberculin, and two-thirds fail to react to second-strength.

In 1917, when tuberculous infection was regarded as almost universal among adults, Schaumann's observation led to ingenious speculation. Jadassohn [8] suggested that pa-

* This work was supported by grants from the American Thoracic Society, Medical Division of the National Tuberculosis Association, and from the Pennsylvania Thoracic Society.

TABLE 28-1. Tuberculin Reaction in Sarcoidosis

Area	% Reacting to 1st-Strength	% Reacting to 2nd-Strength	% Negative to 2nd-Strength	Reference
Boston–Baltimore	12.0	18.3	69.7	[3]
New York	9.0	30.0	61.0	[4]
London	2.0	29.0	69.0	[5]
Scandinavia	5.0	35.0	60.0	[6]
Philadelphia	8.6	21.5	69.9	[7]

tients with sarcoidosis were able to deal with tuberculin so quickly that no reaction, or only a weak reaction, ensued. Martenstein [9] ascribed the anergic state to the production of specific antituberculin antibodies. Pinner [10] and Wells and Wylie [11] reported the demonstration of circulating antibodies which they termed "anticutins," but Pinner *et al.* [12] were subsequently unable to repeat their demonstration of neutralizing antibodies.

Magnusson [13] demonstrated that the influence of serum in enhancing or inhibiting tuberculin reactions was related to the presence or absence of a prompt urticarial response to the injected tuberculin-serum mixture. This effect was similar to that produced by histamine and cortisone. The varied responses reported by early investigators are attributed by Magnusson to differences in the recipients rather than in the serum donors.

The recognition in the middle of this century that tuberculin sensitivity was far from universal in many countries led to the suggestion that the infrequency of reactors among sarcoidosis patients might be merely a reflection of lack of exposure to tuberculosis. Nitter [14], however, documented loss of tuberculin sensitivity as the result of sarcoidosis. Individuals known to be previously tuberculin-positive lost their reactivity on the development of sarcoidosis and were observed to regain sensitivity after regression of the sarcoidosis.

The application of BCG vaccination to patients with sarcoidosis established that an immunological defect was present in this disease. By use of a vaccine which produced tuberculin conversion in 95 percent of normal subjects, it was shown that only one-third of patients with sarcoidosis converted, and in these the sensitivity was not long maintained [15].

The impression that the patients with sarcoidosis were unable to maintain their tuberculin sensitivity because the BCG organisms were being destroyed with extraordinary rapidity was dispelled by subsequent studies. Rostenberg *et al.* [16] administered BCG to patients with sarcoidosis. Biopsy specimens from the vaccination sites were studied bacteriologically, and BCG organisms were found to persist more commonly in sarcoid patients than in a control group. Löfgren, *et al.* [17] used a radioactively labeled BCG vaccine (bacilli grown on medium to which radioactive phosphate had been added) to measure the rapidity with which radioactivity migrated from injection sites. Patients with sarcoidosis had the same rate of migration as controls, and gave no evidence that enhanced immunity was responsible for failure to develop tuberculin sensitivity.

Forgacs *et al.* [18] are the most recent workers to have studied the responses of sarcoidosis patients to BCG. They, too, found that organisms persist in the inoculation site in the same fashion as in controls. Lemming [19], who had been first to study the response to BCG in sarcoidosis, had described a sarcoid type of reaction at the immunization site and proposed this unusual response to BCG as a diagnostic test. However, neither Rostenberg nor Forgacs and their associates nor we have been able to recognize consistent differences between sarcoidosis patients and controls in the gross or histological local reaction to BCG immunization.

Another approach has involved the use of oil emulsions of tuberculin. Seeberg [20] noted that tuberculin in an oily suspension enhanced tuberculin reactions in both tuberculin-positive and tuberculin-negative patients with sarcoidosis. James and Pepys [21] confirmed this observation in a study of 23 patients with sarcoidosis. Four reacted to 100 tuberculin units of ordinary aqueous tuberculin, but 17 reacted to the "depot" tuberculin; 18 tuberculin-negative controls did not react to the depot preparation. Following BCG vaccination of 9 healthy subjects, 2 reacted to depot tuberculin but not to aqueous tuberculin. These authors attribute the phenomenon to localization and persistence of the tuberculin, by reason of the oily vehicle, resulting in detection of a low degree of sensitivity which escapes ordinary tuberculin testing.

Pyke and Scadding [22] found similar enhancement of tuberculin reactivity in patients with sarcoidosis under the influence of locally or systemically administered cortisone. Citron and Scadding [23] injected tuberculin and cortisone mixtures and obtained reactions in 50 percent of sarcoidosis patients who did not react to tuberculin alone.

Recently, tuberculin prepared from unclassified mycobacteria has been tested in sarcoidosis. Israel, *et al.* [7] used Battey purified protein derivative (PPD) derived from a strain of nonphotochromogenic mycobacteria. Reactions to 5 tuberculin units were observed in 9.1 percent of sarcoidosis patients and in 25 percent of nonsarcoid patients. All of the former who reacted to Battey PPD reacted more strongly to human PPD, and the positive reactions to the former antigen presumably represent cross-reactions.

It is curious that the percentage of sarcoidosis patients reacting to tuberculin should be the same in Great Britain as in the United States, since the percentage of reactors in the general British population is considerably greater than that among Americans of the same age. It is also remarkable that the studies in Philadelphia fail to demonstrate a decline in the past two decades of the percentage of reactors among patients with sarcoidosis [7], despite the precipitous drop in incidence of tuberculosis among the general population in recent years.

DELAYED REACTIONS TO OTHER AGENTS

The unusual response to tuberculin has been regarded by some investigators as indicative of a causal relationship between tuberculosis and sarcoidosis [5]. Implicit in such theories was the assumption that the diminished reactivity of sarcoidosis was confined to tuberculin.

That the immunological defect in sarcoidosis was not restricted to the tuberculin reaction was shown by Friou [24] and by Sones and Israel [25], who demonstrated diminished reactivity to a wide spectrum of skin tests, e.g., with histoplasmin, trichophytin, Oidiomycin, mumps virus, and pertussis agglutinogen.

Reactions to histoplasmin (1 : 100) were observed in 8.5 percent of 177 patients with sarcoidosis [7], in contrast to 23.4 percent in nonsarcoid patients. Since the frequency of histoplasmin reactors in the general population varies markedly according to geographic residence, the lower incidence in patients with sarcoidosis is not necessarily the result of immunological depression.

Friou [24] observed reactions to Oidiomycin in 95 percent of tuberculin-negative controls, 93 percent of tuberculin-positive controls, 86 percent of tuberculin-positive sarcoidosis patients, and 53 percent of tuberculin-negative sarcoidosis patients. Sones and Israel [25] found reactions to this extract of *Candida albicans* in 80 percent of controls and 5.9 percent of patients with sarcoidosis. Similar responses were obtained with *Trichophyton gypseum* extract [24]. Reactions to mumps antigen were noted in 29.6 percent and to pertussis agglutinogen in 13.2 percent of patients with sarcoidosis [25]. The percentage of controls reacting was 80.0 and 57.0, respectively. Quinn *et al.* [26] noted negative responses to mumps skin tests in six sarcoidosis patients, all with positive results of mumps complement fixation test. They suggested that, since this combination of adequate circulating antibodies and impaired cutaneous response was rare among normal subjects, such studies might prove useful in diagnosis of sarcoidosis.

RESPONSE TO IMMUNIZATION

Patients who failed to react to pertussis skin tests were immunized with pertussis vaccine [25]. On repetition of the skin tests, positive results were obtained in all controls, whereas only 45 percent of patients with sarcoidosis had reactions, which were frequently transitory.

RESPONSE TO CONTACT SENSITIZERS

Epstein and Mayock [27] studied response of sarcoidosis patients to chemicals which are contact sensitizers: pentadecyl catechol, a highly potent allergen occurring in poison ivy; 2,4-dinitrochorobenzene, a moderately strong sensitizer, and paranitroso dimethyl aniline, a weak one. The incidence of naturally occurring skin sensitivity to the potent poison ivy allergen was the same in sarcoidosis patients and controls, but with the less powerful sensitizers a significantly diminished frequency of sensitization was observed in the sarcoidosis group.

TRANSFER STUDIES

Urbach, Sones, and Israel [28] employed Lawrence's technique in which the centrifuged white blood cells of tuberculin-positive donors were injected into the skin of tuberculin-negative sarcoidosis patients and controls. Tuberculin injected at these sites caused reactions of equal size in both groups, indicating that no neutralizing substance or anticutins were responsible for the diminished tuberculin sensitivity of sarcoidosis patients. Since there was no cutaneous abnormality, the abnormality was thought to be impaired antibody production or transport. Good *et al.* [29] suggested an alternative explanation, a failure of adequate cellular inflammatory response, corrected by the introduction of exogenous cells from a tuberculin-positive donor.

Studies of homograft rejection in sarcoidosis patients have not been reported.

CIRCULATING ANTIBODY RESPONSES

The capacity to form circulating antibody is not affected in sarcoidosis. Carnes and Raffel [30] found complement-fixing antibody titers to multiple antigens prepared from the tubercle bacillus to be as high in tuberculin-negative sarcoidosis patients as in tuberculin-positive controls. Fleming *et al.* [31], employing the Dubos-Middlebrook test, found comparable levels of antituberculosis antibodies in the sera of sarcoidosis patients and normal controls. Sones and Israel [25] measured antibody responses to immunization with pertussis and typhoid vaccines. Titers of 1:1,280 were obtained in both sarcoidosis patients and controls. Quinn *et al.* [26], as has been mentioned, observed a positive response to the mumps complement fixation test in seven patients with sarcoidosis.

The circulating antibody response to tetanus toxoid immunization has been studied in sarcoidosis. Greenwood *et al.* [32] found diminished titers after primary immunization of sarcoidosis patients, but patients with a history of previous immunization showed little impairment of capacity to respond to booster doses. They believe that previous studies of circulating antibodies in sarcoidosis represented measurements of responses in previously immunized patients. Actually, few of our twenty patients had been previously immunized [25]. Another study has shown impaired circulating antibody production; Mankiewicz [33] found that sarcoidosis patients failed to form antibodies against mycobacteriophages (see below).

CLINICAL EVIDENCE OF IMPAIRED RESISTANCE TO INFECTION

The impairment of delayed hypersensitivity mechanisms does not seem to be accompanied by decreased resistance to infection. No increase of frequency of meningeal or urinary infection has been observed in our patients. Pneumonia has been uncommon except in patients with advanced pulmonary fibrosis whose susceptibility to infections appears to be due to lung damage rather than to immunological deficiencies.

Whether there is in sarcoidosis patients an increased susceptibility to tuberculosis and fungal infection is uncertain. Nine of our patients have developed tuberculosis, an incidence in excess of normal expectancy in 325 subjects. Few of them had extensive pulmonary damage from sarcoidosis: in most instances, the sarcoidosis was old and inactive. For this reason we believe that the frequency of tuberculosis is due more to socioeconomic and racial factors than to immunological deficiencies. Sarcoidosis has been associated with two fungal infections in particular, histoplasmosis and cryptococcosis [34,35]. It is uncertain whether these represent instances of fungal infection complicating sarcoidosis or the fungal disease simulated sarcoidosis. Considering the widespread prevalence of histoplasmosis in the United States, instances of its association with sarcoidosis have been few.

NONSPECIFIC IMMUNOLOGICAL ABNORMALITIES

Serological Tests for Syphilis. Moore and Lohr [36] included sarcoidosis among the common causes of biological false positive results of serological tests for syphilis. Buck and McKusick [37] found positive seroreactions in 20.9 percent of 62 patients with sarcoidosis and in 10.4 percent of 115 first-degree relatives of the patients. Mayock *et al.* [38] observed positive seroreactions in 19 percent of 115 patients.

In Norway, on the other hand, Nitter [14] observed a Wassermann reaction in only 1 of 88 patients with sarcoidosis. The high incidence in Negro patients may be due to more syphilis, but there may be a greater likelihood of biological false positive reactions among Negroes, who have been shown to have higher serum levels of globulins than whites [39].

Rheumatoid Factor. Antiglobulin antibodies were found by Kunkel *et al.* [40] in 6 of 61 patients, employing latex particles coated with human globulin. All reactors were females, and no consistent relation with serum protein fractions was demonstrable. Studies in our clinic, also using a latex fixation test, have shown positive results in 24 of 51 patients with sarcoidosis [41]. Sixty percent of females gave positive reactions and 19 percent of males. Serum globulin levels were elevated in 67 percent of females and 80 percent of males.

Serum Proteins. Increased serum proteins and globulins have long been recognized as a feature of sarcoidosis. Paper electrophoresis disclosed serum globulin concentrations greater than 3.5 gm. per 100 ml. in all cases and increased γ-globulin levels in 80 percent [42,43].

These studies were probably performed in patients with advanced chronic disease. A recent study by Norberg [44] included patients in various stages. Patients with early disease, manifested by erythema nodosum, had normal total protein and γ-globulin levels and increased α-globulins. In patients with hilar adenopathy and pulmonary infiltration, the subacute phase, total protein and α_2-globulin levels were slightly increased, and γ-globulin normal. Only in patients with chronic pulmonary sarcoidosis were elevation of total protein and marked increase in γ-globulin values observed.

Properdin. Kallings [45] found serum properdin activity normal in 70 percent of patients with sarcoidosis. None was demonstrable in the rest.

Antinuclear Factor and Thyroid Antibodies. Doniach and Roitt [46] studied 50 patients with sarcoidosis and found none with antinuclear (lupus erythematosus) or thyroid antibodies.

Blood Groups. Lewis and Woods [47] found a difference in ABO blood group distribution in patients with sarcoidosis. The frequency of group O was 40 percent in sarcoidosis and 47 percent in other respiratory diseases, and of group A, 51 and 40 percent respectively.

HYPERSENSITIVITY

In contrast to the familiar impairment of delayed hypersensitivity mechanisms in sarcoidosis is one striking clinical manifestation of sarcoidosis indicative of hypersensitivity. A frequent feature of early sarcoidosis is erythema nodosum. In Great Britain [48] and Sweden [49], sarcoidosis is among the commonest causes of erythema nodosum. It is less often recognized in the United States, for reasons which are uncertain, but has been found frequently in New York City among Puerto Rican patients with sarcoidosis [50].

Two groups of investigators have presented evidence of serological hyperactivity in sarcoidosis. Sands *et al.* [51] measured the agglutinin response to intravenously injected mismatched blood. Patients with sarcoidosis and those with collagen disorders had an 8- to 12-fold increase in titers as against a 2- to 6-fold increase in healthy and tuberculous controls. The increase was inhibited by ACTH.

Pepys *et al.* [52], during a study of precipitins against hay and molds in the sera of patients with farmer's lung (a pulmonary granulomatosis apparently due to hypersensitivity to moldy hay), investigated 50 patients with sarcoidosis. Precipitins to moldy hay were demonstrable in 32 percent of sera from sarcoidosis patients, but in no control sera. Since the sarcoidosis subjects had not had known contact with moldy hay, the authors suggest that the high incidence of precipitins may be due to enhanced ability of granulomata to produce antibodies.

THE KVEIM REACTION

Another "hypersensitivity" phenomenon characteristic of sarcoidosis is the Kveim reaction. Despite disagreement about its diagnostic reliability in its present form [53–55], there can be no doubt about its importance as an immunological phenomenon.

The Kveim reaction is a torpid cutaneous response to certain intracutaneous inoculations, requiring three to four weeks or longer to appear and persisting for long periods. The nodules measure 3 to 10 mm., and biopsy specimens reveal epithelioid granuloma formation.

Numerous intracutaneously injected substances have caused the delayed appearance of a granulomatous nodule in both sarcoidosis patients and other subjects, diseased or healthy. However, these nodules have been most consistently produced in sarcoidosis patients by the injection of coarse extracts of sarcoid lymph nodes. Not all such extracts elicit these reactions; potent extracts may remain so for months or years, but may at any time lose potency and fail to elicit reactions or may lose specificity and elicit reactions in subjects who do not have sarcoidosis [56].

The nature and mechanism of the Kveim reaction are not understood. Rogers and Haserick [57] believe it to be a specific antigen-antibody interaction in which the antigen is the causative agent of sarcoidosis present in the lymph nodes from which the extract was prepared. But since only individuals with "active" sarcoidosis are believed to react to this antigen, they postulated that "active" sarcoidosis results in formation of "sensitizing" antibodies. In support of this hypothesis, they cited experiments in which γ-globulin from the serum of patients with sarcoidosis and Kveim antigen are injected into the skin of healthy subjects. When administered separately, they cause no persistent reaction. When mixed and injected, an indolent papule develops with typical granuloma formation. As Nelson [58] pointed out, however, Rogers and Haserick did not report whether γ-globulin from normal subjects shared this potentiating effect.

Nelson was reluctant to classify the Kveim reaction as an ordinary antigen-antibody process because Kveim antigens can withstand boiling for 30 minutes without great loss of activity. He believed that the Kveim reaction may be but a characteristic reticuloendothelial response of patients with sarcoidosis to one or more chemical complexes.

Fordtran [59] reported a series of studies in which Kveim test material was used as an antigen. After centrifugation, the supernate of an active Kveim preparation and pooled γ-globulin from patients with active sarcoidosis were tested for precipitins. None was demonstrable. The active Kveim material was employed to sensitize guinea pigs and rabbits; the animals were then given Kveim tests, but no differences from controls could be demonstrated. Attempts were made by Fordtran to absorb the postulated serum antibodies with the "antigen" in Kveim material. Paper electrophoretic studies of serum shaken for 48 hours with Kveim material showed no lowering of any serum protein fractions as the result of exposure to the antigen.

If Kveim test material contains an antigen, repeated testing of the same individual might alter the cutaneous reaction. We have retested many patients and observed no intensification of the Kveim reaction nor has such been reported. The Kveim reaction frequently disappears in patients manifesting clinical improvement. It is difficult to believe that antibodies would diminish even earlier than symptoms and radiological changes.

Hurley and Shelley [60] studied the granuloma-producing capacity of 34 patients with sarcoidosis, 6 with zirconium granulomatosis, and 300 normal males. The cutaneous response was measured to a large number of injected substances, including sodium stearate (a soap of high granuloma-producing capacity) and sixty-nine metals and elements such as beryllium, zirconium, bismuth, silicon, silver, and thallium. The 6 patients with zirconium deodorant granulomas manifested, at the site of injection of zirconium, typical delayed sarcoid reactions. In no other instance did a Kveim-like reaction develop; no greater granuloma-producing capacity could be demonstrated in patients with sarcoidosis. The authors therefore believe that a specific unidentified granulomagenic substance is responsible for the Kveim reaction in sarcoidosis.

Kooij and Gerritsen [61] were impressed by the similarity of the Kveim and Mitsuda reactions. The latter is a nodule which develops four weeks after an intracutaneous injection of lepromin in patients with tuberculoid leprosy. They found that Kveim antigen and suspensions of normal liver would also provoke a Mitsuda reaction in patients with tuberculoid leprosy and concluded that these tests do not induce reactions to a specific substance but that reactivity is determined largely by particle size.

In our experience, an important aspect of the conflicting reports regarding the Kveim test is the variability of histological interpretation of granulomas. Although it is commonly thought that epithelioid and other granulomas can be readily differentiated, when histological interpretation is made without clinical data, there is notable variation in reports by different pathologists [54, 81, 86].

Unexpected findings have recently been reported by Hart *et al.* of the Medical Research Council in England [86]. In an attempt to relate tuberculin anergy to the development of sarcoidosis, Kveim tests were made on 64 subjects who had been participants in Medical Research Council trials of tuberculosis vaccines 10 years earlier. Among 10 subjects who had been vaccinated twice without tuberculin conversion, 7 showed Kveim reactions. Positive reactions occurred in 8 of 32 subjects converting after vaccination and in only 1 of 22 subjects not vaccinated. Careful study revealed no evidence of sarcoidosis in the 16 Kveim reactors. These investigators do not believe that these reactors had occult sarcoidosis, and they attribute the results to some novel immunological change produced by BCG vaccination.

Whatever the explanation for these remarkable findings, it should be recognized that Hart *et al.* encountered positive Kveim reactions in many subjects who had no evidence of sarcoidosis. False-positive Kveim tests must still be regarded as a not inconsiderable hazard, even with the best available test materials.

The most reasonable explanation for the conflicting results observed with the Kveim test is provided by Shelley and Hurley's [62] demonstration that cutaneous sarcoid granulomas are of two types. The allergic type is produced in sensitized persons by trace amounts, as in zirconium hypersensitivity. The colloidal type requires a gross amount of particulate material and does not require a sensitized subject; examples are responses to silica and stearate injections. The Kveim test materials in use at present probably induce reactions in some instances by an allergic mechanism and in others by a colloidal mechanism. Confusion is likely to persist until the substance in sarcoid tissues responsible for the allergic production of epithelioid granuloma is isolated.

ETIOLOGICAL INVESTIGATIONS WITH IMMUNOLOGICAL METHODS

Immunological techniques have been used in efforts to support many of the hypotheses advanced concerning the cause of sarcoidosis.

TUBERCULOSIS

Early attempts to interpret the tuberculin hyperergy in sarcoidosis as support for a tuberculous etiology have been vitiated by the demonstration that the impaired delayed hypersensitivity is general rather than confined to tuberculin. Cortisone enhancement of tuberculin reactivity in sarcoidosis is still interpreted as evidence of a causal relationship between tuberculosis and sarcoidosis [5], but an alternative view is that this phenomenon merely demonstrates that sensitivity to tuberculin and other antigens is depressed, not wholly absent, in sarcoidosis.

Mankiewicz [33] isolated mycobacteriophages in the stools of 94 percent of sarcoidosis patients, 36 percent of tuberculosis patients, and 6 percent of a control group. Phage-neutralizing antibodies were demonstrable in the sera of the phage-carrying tuberculosis patients and controls but in none of the patients with sarcoidosis. Mutant forms of tubercle bacilli were isolated from sarcoid lymph nodes on Loewenstein's medium to which phage antiserum had been added. Mankiewicz suggests that the presence of mycobacteriophages and the absence of phage antibodies permit the emergence of lysogenic tubercle bacilli which are responsible for sarcoidosis. Why patients with sarcoidosis fail to produce phage-neutralizing antibodies is unexplained.

Epstein [63] injected zirconium lactate intradermally in 225 patients with arrested tuberculosis and 300 normal subjects. In 8, delayed granulomas developed at the site of infection; 7 were in the arrested tuberculosis group. This important observation suggests that previous mycobacterial infection may contribute to sensitization resulting in granuloma formation. Chase [64] has described the production in guinea pigs of a disease resembling sarcoidosis by injection of killed mycobacteria in oil.

UNCLASSIFIED MYCOBACTERIA

McCuiston and Hudgins [65] noted that serum protein fractionation by paper electrophoresis yielded patterns in chronic pulmonary disease due to unclassified mycobacteria that resemble those observed in sarcoidosis and are unlike those seen in tuberculosis. Chapman [66] reported that gel diffusion studies of sera from sarcoidosis patients showed lines indicative of antibodies against atypical mycobacteria. Similar reactions have been observed by Pepys [67] in control subjects in England; these appear to be confined neither to sarcoidosis nor to infection with atypical mycobacteria.

Chapman *et al.* [68] studied skin reactions to tuberculins derived from unclassified mycobacteria in children in Texas households in which there was a case of sarcoidosis. Reactions in these children to human tuberculin and to tuberculins prepared from group II and group III mycobacteria were rare, but 34 percent (twice the frequency in controls) reacted to group I antigen. This incidence was similar to that in children from households in which there were cases of unclassified mycobacteria disease. However, serological study of the index cases of sarcoidosis did not consistently reveal antibodies against group I mycobacteria.

PINE POLLEN

Support for the ingenious hypothesis that sarcoidosis represents a hypersensitivity to pine pollen antigens has been sought in a variety of immunological procedures. McCuiston *et al.* [69] found 48-hour reactions to a pine pollen antigen to be less common in patients with active sarcoidosis than in other inhabitants of pine-forested counties in Florida. They ascribed this to the impaired immunological mechanisms of sarcoidosis. James [70] injected pine pollen extract intradermally in forty patients with sarcoidosis. A Kveim-like nodule developed in one.

Patnode and Leu [71] prepared pine pollen antigens which on immunization of rabbits produced precipitating antibodies demonstrable by agar diffusion. The same antigens failed to induce precipitating antibodies in the sera of patients with sarcoidosis. The cytotoxicity of pine pollen for peripheral blood leukocytes from sarcoidosis patients did not differ significantly from that of controls.

OTHER INVESTIGATIONS

The results of attempts by Shelley, Hurley and their associates to elicit delayed cutaneous reactions by injection of a variety of possible antigens were mentioned previously. In no instance did a Kveim-like reaction develop [60]. In another study [72], extracts of soil were employed. Eleven patients with sarcoidosis who lived in South Carolina or adjacent Georgia were tested with soil samples from nine counties in South Carolina, representing various soil series of the red-yellow podzolic group. Aqueous, alcohol, chloroform, and acetone extracts were used. No granulomatous reactions were observed.

SIGNIFICANCE OF IMMUNOLOGICAL STUDIES

The cardinal immunological features of sarcoidosis are impairment of delayed hypersensitivity reactions, preservation of circulating antibody formation, and a delayed granulomatous response to the intracutaneous injection of sarcoidosis tissue extracts. Disagreement exists as to whether this immunological pattern is the result of sarcoidosis, a consequence of involvement of the lymphatic system by the disease, or whether a pre-existing immunological peculiarity, possibly genetic in origin, determines the widespread granulomatous reaction. The former hypothesis is consistent with the concept that sarcoidosis is a disease entity caused by exposure to a specific inciting agent. The latter implies the presence of a *terrain sarcoidique* producing sarcoid granulomas in response to a variety of stimuli.

Perhaps the strongest arguments for a single etiological factor are the sharply defined geographic occurrence of sarcoidosis and the similarity of its clinical manifestations and course in northern Europe, North America, and Australia [73]. That involvement of the lymphatic system can lead to the pattern of impaired delayed hypersensitivity with intact circulating antibody formation has been shown in Hodgkin's disease [74]. It is unlikely that the minor differences in antibody response in Hodgkin's disease and sarcoidosis result from different mechanisms of immunological suppression, as Fairley and Matthias [75] have suggested. Suppression of delayed hypersensitivity in guinea pigs has been induced by administration of 6-mercaptopurine, a nucleic acid antimetabolite [76].

Evidence of a primary sarcoidal diathesis, on the other hand, is provided by the variety of substances known to have produced local or systemic sarcoid lesions [61, 77]. A primary immunological peculiarity in persons who have sarcoidosis has been postulated by Burnet [78] and Scadding [79]. Differences in blood group distribution [47], an unusual frequency of hemoglobinopathies [80], and the greater incidence in females than in males [38] suggest constitutional etiological factors. In guinea pigs, Chase [64] found strain differences which influence the granulomatous response to killed mycobacteria and oil injections.

Nevertheless conclusive evidence that a sarcoid diathesis does exist is lacking. Refvem [82] found that sarcoidosis patients and controls alike formed foreign body granulomas after implantation of quartz particles. Hurley and Shelley [60], employing a wide array of test materials, were unable to detect an increased tendency to granuloma formation in patients with sarcoidosis. The epidemiological studies of Buck *et al.* [37] showed that first-degree relatives of sarcoidosis patients exhibit normal immunological responses to tuberculin and fungus skin tests. These conflicting observations are perhaps best reconciled by the reasonable hypothesis that both constitutional and environmental factors are involved in the genesis of sarcoidosis.

Recent investigations [33, 63, 64, 68] have raised anew the possibility that mycobacteria have an etiological role in sarcoidosis. Abundant epidemiological, clinical, and bacteriological studies have failed to show that sarcoidosis results directly from mycobacterial infection [83]. If exposure to mycobacteria contributes to the later development of sarcoidal hypersensitivity, immunological mechanisms hitherto unexplored are involved. Burnet [78] has suggested that an abnormally efficient production of circulating antibody with impaired development of antibody-carrying cells responsible for tuberculin sensitivity might, in the face of an antigenic stimulus by mutant forms of tubercle bacilli, be responsible for sarcoidosis. Mankiewicz [33], on the other hand, proposes that a deficiency of mycobacteriophage antibody production is involved.

Although the impaired immunological mechanisms in sarcoidosis have been emphasized, the hypersensitivity manifestations may be of greater import. Deserving mention are the frequent association of erythema nodosum, increased antibody response to mismatched blood, and the remarkable similarities of sarcoidosis and two disorders which clearly represent uncommon hypersensitivity reactions to widely distributed agents—beryllium and zirconium granulomatoses.

Consideration has recently been given to the possibility that autoimmune mechanisms may be involved in the genesis of sarcoidosis [84]. A clinical feature supporting this hypothesis is that systemic sarcoidosis invariably is first manifested in the mediastinal lymph nodes. Anti-γ-globulin antibody titers are often increased in sarcoidosis, but antinuclear and antithyroid antibodies are not present. Nagaya and Sieker [85] produced lymphocytopenia in rats with an antirat lymph node serum and noted reduction of delayed skin reactions.

One may conclude that immunological investigation offers the most promising approach to discovery of the causative agent and to elucidation of the unusual hypersensitivity mechanisms which seem to be involved in both the etiology and the pathogenesis of this extraordinary disease.

REFERENCES

1. International Conference on Sarcoidosis. *Amer. Rev. Resp. Dis.* 84:172, 1961.
2. Schaumann, J. *Études Bactériologique sur le Lupus Pernio et les Sarcoidoses Cutanées.* Stockholm: P. A. Norstedt et Soner, 1917.
3. Longcope, W. T., and Freiman, D. G. A study of sarcoidosis. *Medicine* 31:1, 1952.
4. Siltzbach, L. E. Pulmonary sarcoidosis. *Amer. J. Surg.* 89:556, 1955.
5. Citron, K. Skin tests in sarcoidosis. *Tubercle* 38:33, 1957.
6. Warfvinge, L. E. Discussion. *Acta Tuberc. Scand.* 45:22, 1959.
7. Israel, H. L., Sones, M., Roy, R. L., and Stein, G. N. The occurrence of intrathoracic calcification in sarcoidosis. *Amer. Rev. Resp. Dis.* 84:1, 1961.
8. Jadassohn, W. L. L'origine tuberculeuse de

la maladie de Boeck. *Bull. Soc. Franc. Derm. et Syph.* 41:1344, 1934.

9. Martenstein, H. Wirkung des Serums von Sarkoid-Boeck und LupuspernioKranken auf Tuberkulin. *Arch. Derm. Syph.* (Berlin) 136: 317, 1921.
10. Pinner, M. Non-caseating tuberculosis. *Amer. Rev. Tuberc.* 37:690, 1938.
11. Wells, A. Q., and Wylie, J. A. H. A tuberculin-neutralizing factor in the serum of patients with sarcoidosis. *Lancet* 1:439, 1949.
12. Pinner, M., Weiss, M., and Cohen, A. C. Procutins and anticutins. *Yale J. Biol. Med.* 15: 459, 1943.
13. Magnusson, B. The effect of sarcoidosis sera on the tuberculin response. *Acta Dermatovener.,* Vol. 36, supp. 35, 1956.
14. Nitter, L. Changes in the chest roentgenogram in Boeck's sarcoid of the lungs. *Acta Radiol.,* supp. 105, 1953.
15. Israel, H. L., Sones, M., Stein, S. C., and Aronson, J. D. BCG vaccination in sarcoidosis. *Amer. Rev. Tuberc.* 62:408, 1950.
16. Rostenberg, A., Jr., Szymanski, F. J., Brebis, G. J., Haeberlin, J. B., and Senear, F. E. Experimental studies on sarcoidosis: Persistence and survival of inoculated microrganisms. *Arch. Derm.* 67:306, 1953.
17. Löfgren, S., Strom, L., and Widstrom, G. Tuberculosis immunity in sarcoidosis studied with the aid of radioactive BCG vaccine. *Acta Paediat.* (Uppsala) 43 (supp. 100):160, 1954.
18. Forgacs, P., McDonald, C. K., and Skelton, M. O. The BCG lesion in sarcoidosis. *Lancet* 1:188, 1957.
19. Lemming, R. An attempt to analyze the tuberculin energy in Schaumann's Disease by means of BCG vaccination. *Acta Med. Scand.* 103:400, 1940.
20. Seeberg, G. Tuberculin sensitivity in lymphogranulomatosis benigna studied with depot tuberculin. *Acta Dermatovener.* 31:426, 1951.
21. James, D. G., and Pepys, J. Tuberculin in aqueous and oily solution: Skin-test reactions in normal subjects and in patients with sarcoidosis. *Lancet* 1:602, 1956.
22. Pyke, D. A., and Scadding, J. G. Effect of cortisone upon skin sensitivity to tuberculin in sarcoidosis. *Brit. Med. J.* 2:1126, 1952.
23. Citron, K., and Scadding, J. G. The effect of cortisone upon the reaction of the skin to tuberculin in tuberculosis and in sarcoidosis. *Quart. J. Med.* 26:277, 1957.
24. Friou, G. J. A study of the cutaneous reactions to oidiomycin, trichophytin, and mumps skin test antigens in patients with sarcoidosis. *Yale J. Biol. Med.* 24:533, 1952.
25. Sones, M., and Israel, H. L. Altered immunologic reactions in sarcoidosis. *Ann. Intern. Med.* 40:260, 1954.
26. Quinn, E. L., Bunch, D. C., and Yagle, E. M. The mumps skin test and complement fixation test as a diagnostic aid in sarcoidosis. *J. Invest. Derm.* 24:595, 1955.
27. Epstein, W. L., and Mayock, R. L. Induction of allergic contact dermatitis in patients with sarcoidosis. *Proc. Soc. Exp. Biol. Med.* 96:786, 1957.
28. Urbach, F., Sones, M., and Israel, H. L. Passive transfer of tuberculin sensitivity to patients with sarcoidosis. *New Eng. J. Med.* 247: 794, 1952.
29. Good, R. A., Kelly, W. D., Rotstein, J., and Varco, R. L. Immunological deficiency diseases. *Progr. Allerg.* 6:187, 1962.
30. Carnes, W. H., and Raffel, S. A. A comparison of sarcoidosis and tuberculosis with respect to complement fixation with antigens derived from the tubercle bacillus. *Bull. J. Hopkins Hosp.* 85:204, 1949.
31. Fleming, J. W., Runyon, E. H., and Cummings, M. M. An evaluation of the hemagglutination test for tuberculosis. *Amer. J. Med.* 10:704, 1951.
32. Greenwood, R., Smellie, H., Barr, M., and Cunliffe, A. C. Circulating antibodies in sarcoidosis. *Brit. Med. J.* 1:1388, 1958.
33. Mankiewicz, E. On the etiology of sarcoidosis. *Canad. Med. Ass. J.* 88:593, 1963.
34. Israel, H. L., DeLamater, E. D., Sones, M., Willis, W. D., and Mirmelstein, A. Chronic disseminated histoplasmosis: An investigation of its relationship to sarcoidosis. *Amer. J. Med.* 12:252, 1952.
35. Shields, L. H. Disseminated cryptococcosis producing a sarcoid type reaction. *Arch. Intern. Med.* 104:763, 1959.
36. Moore, J. E., and Lohr, C. F. The incidence and etiologic background of chronic biologic false-positive reactions in serologic tests for syphilis. *Ann. Intern. Med.* 37:1156, 1952.
37. Buck, A. A., and McKusick, V. Epidemiologic investigations of sarcoidosis: III. Serum proteins; syphilis; association with tuberculosis; familial aggregation. *Amer. J. Hyg.* 74:174, 1961.
38. Mayock, R. L., Bertrand, P., Morrison, C. E., and Scott, J. H. Manifestations of sarcoidosis. *Amer. J. Med.* 35:67, 1963.
39. Rawnsley, H. M., Yonan, V. L., and Reinhold, J. G. Serum protein concentration in North American Negroid. *Science* 123:991, 1956.
40. Kunkel, H. G., Simon, H. J., and Fudenberg, H. Observations concerning positive serologic reactions for rheumatoid factor in certain patients with sarcoidosis and other hyperglobulinemic states. *Arthritis Rheum.* 1:289, 1958.
41. Israel, H. L., Patterson, J. D., and Smukler, N. Latex fixation tests in sarcoidosis. Proceedings

of International Conference on Sarcoidosis. *Acta Med. Scand.* (supp. 425):40, 1964.
42. Sunderman, F. W. W., and Sunderman, F. W. Clinical application of the fractionation of serum proteins by paper electrophoresis. *Amer. J. Clin. Path.* 27:125, 1957.
43. Levitt, N. The clinical application of paper electrophoresis in sarcoidosis. *Dis. Chest.* 36: 243, 1959.
44. Norberg, R. Studies in sarcoidosis. I. Serum proteins. *Acta Med. Scand.* 175:359, 1964.
45. Kallings, L. O. Properdin activity in sarcoidosis. Proceedings of International Conference on Sarcoidosis. *Acta Med. Scand.* (supp. 425):33, 1964.
46. Doniach, D., and Roitt, I. M. Auto-immunity and disease. *What's New,* no. 229, 1962.
47. Lewis, J. G., and Woods, A. C. The ABO and Rhesus blood groups in patients with respiratory disease. *Tubercle* 42:362, 1961.
48. James, D. G. Erythema nodosum. *Brit. Med. J.* 1:853, 1961.
49. Löfgren, S. Primary pulmonary sarcoidosis. *Acta Med. Scand.* 145:424, 1953.
50. Siltzbach, L. E. Ref. 1, p. 166.
51. Sands, J. H., Palmer, P. P., Mayock, R. L., and Creger, W. P. Evidence for serologic hyperreactivity in sarcoidosis. *Amer. J. Med.* 19:401, 1955.
52. Pepys, J., Riddell, R. W., Citron, K. M., and Clayton, Y. M. Precipitins against extracts of hay and moulds in the serum of patients with farmer's lung, aspergillosis, asthma and sarcoidosis. *Thorax* 17:366, 1962.
53. Siltzbach, L. E. Kveim test in sarcoidosis. *J.A.M.A.* 178:476, 1961.
54. Israel, H. L., Sones, M., Beerman, H., and Pastras, T. A further study of the Kveim test in sarcoidosis and tuberculosis. *New Eng. J. Med.* 259:365, 1958.
55. Daniel, T. M., and Schneider, G. W. Positive Kveim tests in patients without sarcoidosis. *Amer. Rev. Resp. Dis.* 86:98, 1962.
56. Nelson, C. T., and Schwimmer, B. The specificity of the Kveim reaction. *J. Invest. Derm.* 28:55, 1957.
57. Rogers, F. J., and Haserick, J. R. Sarcoidosis and the Kveim reaction. *J. Invest. Derm.* 23: 389, 1954.
58. Nelson, C. T. The Kveim reaction in sarcoidosis. *J. Chronic Dis.* 6:158, 1957.
59. Fordtran, J. S. Immunological studies in sarcoidosis. *Bull. Tulane Med. Fac.* 15:143, 1956.
60. Hurley, H. J., and Shelley, W. B. Comparison of the granuloma producing capacity of normals and sarcoid granuloma patients: Experimental analysis of the sarcoid diathesis theory. *Amer. J. Med. Sci.* 237:685, 1959.
61. Kooij, R., and Gerritsen, T. On the nature of the Mitsuda and the Kveim reaction. *Dermatologia* 116:1, 1958.
62. Shelley, W. B., and Hurley, H. J., Jr. Experimental sarcoid reactions in human skin. Ref. 1, p. 45.
63. Epstein, W. L. Induction of allergic zirconium granulomas in normal and tuberculous subjects. *J.A.M.A.* 180:767, 1962.
64. Chase, M. W. Disseminated Granulomata in the Guinea Pig. In Shaffer, J. H., LoGrippo, G. A., and Chase, M. W. (Eds.), *Mechanisms of Hypersensitivity.* Little, Brown and Co., Boston, 1959. P. 673.
65. McCuiston, C. F., and Hudgins, P. C. Serum electrophoresis in sarcoidosis, tuberculosis, and disease due to unclassified mycobacteria. *Amer. Rev. Tuberc.* 82:59, 1960.
66. Chapman, J. S. Mycobacterial and mycotic antibodies in sera of patients with sarcoidosis. *Ann. Intern. Med.* 55:918, 1961.
67. Pepys, J. Discussion. CIBA Foundation Conference on Immune Mechanisms in Sarcoidosis. London, Sept. 7, 1963.
68. Chapman, J. S., Potts, W. E., Speight, M., and Dyerly, M. Cutaneous reactions of household contacts of patients with established diagnosis of sarcoidosis. *Amer. Rev. Tuberc.* 88:95, 1963.
69. McCuiston, C. F., Michael, M., and Hudgins, P. C. Geographic epidemiology of sarcoidosis in Florida. Ref. 1, p. 124.
70. James, D. G. Discussion. Ref. 1, p. 97.
71. Patnode, R. A., and Leu, R. W. Cellular and humoral studies in sarcoidosis. *Amer. Rev. Resp. Dis.* 88:109, 1963.
72. Hurley, H. J., *et al.* Soil extracts as antigens in sarcoidosis. *Amer. Rev. Resp. Dis.* 86:100, 1962.
73. Israel, H. L., and Sones, M. Sarcoidosis. *Advances Tuberc. Res.* 11:214, 1961.
74. Aisenberg, A. C., and Leskowitz, S. Antibody formation in Hodgkin's disease. *New Eng. J. Med.* 268:1269, 1963.
75. Fairley, G. H., and Matthias, J. Q. Cortisone and skin sensitivity to tuberculin in reticuloses. *Brit. Med. J.* 2:433, 1960.
76. Hoyer, J. R., Hoyer, L. W., Good, R. A., and Condie, R. M. The effect of 6-mercaptopurine on delayed hypersensitivity in guinea pigs. *J. Exp. Med.* 116:679, 1962.
77. Michael, M., Jr. Sarcoidosis: Disease or syndrome. *Amer. J. Med. Sci.* 235:148, 1958.
78. Burnet, M. *The Clonal Selection Theory of Acquired Immunity.* Nashville, Tenn.: Vanderbilt University Press, 1959. P. 163.
79. Scadding, J. G.: Calcification in sarcoidosis. *Tubercle* 42:121, 1961.
80. Greenberg, S., Atwater, J., and Israel, H. L. Frequency of hemoglobinopathies in sarcoidosis. *Ann. Intern. Med.* 62:125, 1965.
81. Ringsted, J., and Ferebee, J. B. On the stan-

dardization of the histo-pathologic reading of the Kveim test. *Acta Med. Scand.* (supp. 425): 88, 1964.

82. Refvem, O. The pathogenesis of Boeck's disease (sarcoidosis). *Acta Med. Scand.* 149 (supp. 294), 1954.
83. Israel, H. L. Sarcoidosis and Tuberculosis. In *Excerpta Medical International Congress Series* No. 44, Amsterdam, 1961. Vol. II, p. 565.
84. Waksman, B. H. Autoimmunization and the lesions of autoimmunity. *Medicine* 41:93, 1962.
85. Nagaya, H., and Sieker, H. O. Possible role of lymphoid tissue antibody in immunologic deficiency states. *Clin. Res.* 11:205, 1963.
86. Hart, P. D., Mitchell, D. N., and Sutherland, I. Associations between Kveim test results, previous B.C.G. vaccination, and tuberculin sensitivity in healthy young adults. *Brit. Med. J.* 1:795, 1964.

SECTION III. HYPERSENSITIVITY RESPONSES TO INFECTIOUS AGENTS

29. Poststreptococcal Disease

LEIGHTON E. CLUFF AND JOSEPH E. JOHNSON, III

MANY MICROBIAL DISEASES MAY BE followed by manifestations of illness after subsidence of infection. Group A streptococcal infection, however, is unique in that the late manifestations, such as rheumatic fever and glomerulonephritis, appear after an interval during which the patient has no demonstrable evidence of persistent illness or residual complications of the infection itself. In addition, many of the manifestations of poststreptococcal disease resemble those frequently observed in reactions known to be allergic. These two facts explain the common interpretation that much of the illness following streptococcal infection is attributable to immunological mechanisms. It must be stipulated, however, that none of the poststreptococcal diseases have been proved to be due to hypersensitivity reactions or other immunological processes. This chapter, therefore, will deal with an examination of the immunological responses during and following group A streptococcal infection. The poststreptococcal disease manifestations, possibly immunologically determined, will be described. Unfortunately, completely satisfactory experimental models of the poststreptococcal diseases as seen in man have not been found; the development of such models undoubtedly would further understanding of their pathogenesis.

CHARACTERISTICS OF INFECTION INFLUENCING THE IMMUNOLOGICAL RESPONSE

Streptococcal infection in man may be localized, spreading, or disseminated. These variations can influence the immunological responses developing as a result of infection. For example, streptococcal infections which spread by direct extension or by bacteremia would be expected to elicit a considerably greater antibody response than localized infections, because the bacterial mass undoubtedly would be larger [1]. The probable relationship of antigenic mass to the magnitude of the immunological response in streptococcal infection also is illustrated by the effect of antibiotic therapy. Treatment early in the course is associated with a lower antibody titer than that expected in untreated infection [2]. There is no evidence that antibiotics suppress the immunological response other than by inhibiting bacterial multiplication.

In addition to the antigenic mass, the duration of antigenic stimulation also can influence the immunological response [1]. Therefore persistent infection, even without excessive bacterial replication, may lead to a greater immune response than might otherwise occur. For these reasons, treatment of streptococcal infection with a bacteriostatic antibiotic incapable of eradicating the microorganism would be expected to have less effect on the immunological response than use of a bactericidal antibiotic capable of eliminating the microorganism [2].

Streptococcal infection ordinarily begins in the respiratory tract or integument. It has been suggested from clinical observations that rheumatic fever rarely follows streptococcal infection of the skin, whereas glomerulonephritis may follow either pharyngeal or cutaneous infection. The influence of the site of antigen injection on the nature of the immunological response has been recognized [1]. There is evidence that streptococci and other microorganisms may induce varying degrees of delayed hypersensitivity, as measured by intradermal testing, when the bacteria are injected by different routes [3]. Swift and Derrick [4] and Clawson [5] demonstrated that the intravenous route is less effective in inducing hypersensitivity to streptococci and tubercle bacilli than is injection into skin or subcutaneous tissue. Streptococcal pharyngitis rarely is associated with bacteremia, whereas streptococcal infection of the skin may result in bacteremia even when the skin lesion is inconsequential. It might be anticipated that localization of streptococcal antigens would differ if the streptococcal infection were or were not associated with bacteremia. Obviously the sites of localization of bacteria will be more widespread during bacteremia, and hypersensitivity reactions with microbial antigens may develop wherever the antigens are deposited.

There are over fifty serological types of group A streptococci; however, all types possess common antigens. Since streptococcal infection results in type-specific immunity, reinfection, although common, is usually attributed to a different serological type. For this reason, adverse immunological consequences of group A streptococcal reinfection might be attributable to common antigens elaborated by different bacterial serotypes. On the other hand, adverse immunological reactions following infection by a single serological type would most likely be related to antigens specific for that serotype, or perhaps attributable to some other mechanism.

That tissue proteins subtly altered by streptococcal infection may become antigenic and thus lead to autosensitization is suggested by the appearance of serum antibody which will react with normal, unaltered tissues [6, 7]. Autosensitization induced in this way also may result in delayed hypersensitivity to tissue antigens. In this sense, streptococcal infection could induce an autoimmunological reaction producing late and persistent sequelae. Whether or not this mechanism plays any role in poststreptococcal disease has yet to be conclusively demonstrated. In addition to altered tissue protein inducing autosensitization, certain streptococcal antigens may elicit antibody that has the capacity to cross-react with tissue antigens [8].

Streptococci not shown to produce certain antigens *in vitro* may do so during the course of infection, and some streptococcal antigens not found in culture can be extracted from infected tissues [9]. In addition, streptococci not shown to elaborate certain antigens such as streptokinase, desoxyribonuclease (DNAse) as well as diphosphopyridine nucleotidase (DPNase) *in vitro* have induced specific antibody formation to these enzymes as a result of infection [15]. Repeated passage of some strains of group A streptococci in animals has been associated with appearance of bacterial variants with serologically related but distinguishable group-specific carbohydrate [10, 11]. These phenotypic changes in group A streptococci resulting from infection may be important in relating the adverse immunological sequelae of streptococcal disease to one or more streptococcal antigens.

Bacteriophages specific for streptococci have been identified, and it has been suggested that these phages may induce production of erythrogenic toxin by certain streptococcal strains, similar to the action of specific phage on corynebacteria inducing production of diphtheria toxin [12, 53]. The implication of this phenomenon in the pathogenesis of poststreptococcal disease has not, however, been defined. In addition, L forms or protoplasts of group A streptococci have been produced *in vitro,* devoid of streptococcal cell wall but surrounded by a membrane containing distinct antigens common to all streptococcal types but separable from the antigens of cell wall and cytoplasm [13]. Whether or not these viable forms emerge during infection is not known, but when produced *in vitro* they have not been demonstrated to be pathogenic. Nevertheless their potential role as antigens responsible for immunological responses developing as a result of group A streptococcal infection must be considered.

Group A streptococci have been shown to persist in tissues of experimental animals for long periods, in a relatively dormant state, and may be found on culture in heart, kidney, or liver many days or weeks after intravenous inoculation [14]. The importance of these findings in the pathogenesis of poststreptococcal diseases is obscure but illustrates that streptococcal antigens may be critically localized and persist in certain tissues. Although group A streptococci have been isolated from heart valves of patients dying of acute rheumatic carditis, the infrequency of such observation makes it unlikely that viable streptococci in the heart play a role in this disease.

SPECIFIC IMMUNOLOGICAL RESPONSES TO STREPTOCOCCAL INFECTION

An extraordinary variety of antigens has been isolated from group A streptococci or culture filtrates (Table 29-1). A few have been purified and characterized; others have been obtained only in a crude form. Their variety is impressive, and some have potent toxic effects, but the function of most of these substances in bacterial metabolism, in the pathogenesis of streptococcal infection, and in the poststreptococcal diseases is unknown. For these reasons, each of the streptococcal antigens will not be discussed, but general principles of their immunological function are described.

The M protein of the bacterial cell wall is the antigenic character forming the basis for differentiation of streptococci into serological types. The cell wall polysaccharide is responsible for the antigenic character common to all serological types and is the basis for distinguishing the pathogenic beta hemolytic streptococci from other streptococcal groups. Certain antigens are produced predominantly by

TABLE 29-1. Antigens of Group A Streptococci

Antigens	Substance	Antigenicity	Specificity	Some Properties
Surface	M protein	+	Type specific	Virulence factor
	T protein	+	Not always type specific	—
	R protein	+	Common to 3 types	—
	A polysaccharide	+	Common to all types (rare variants)	—
	Hyaluronic acid	0	Chemically indistinguishable from mammalian hyaluronate	Bacterial capsule
Extracellular	Erythrogenic toxin	+	Produced by most strains	3 serological types; produces rash of scarlet fever
	Streptolysin S	0	Produced by most strains	Hemolytic; formation induced by serum factors
	Streptolysin O	+	Produced by most strains	Hemolytic in reduced form; leukotoxic and cardiotoxic
	DPNase	+	Produced by most strains, but particularly certain types [1, 6, 15]	Probably leukotoxic
	Streptokinase	+	Produced by most strains	Activates plasma protease
	DNAse	+	Produced by all strains	3 serological types (A, B, C); no effect on living cells; lyses dead leukocytes
	RNAse	?	Produced by most strains	?
	Hyaluronidase	+	Produced by most strains of types 4 and 22, less by other types, not type specific	Does not attack chondroitin sulfate
	Proteinase	+(? during infection)	Produced by most types	Released only at pH 5.5–5.6; autocatalytic; pure-form myocardial necrosis
	Amylase	+	Variable formation	—
Intracellular	Cell membrane	+(? during infection)	Group specific	Protein, lipid, CHO complex
	Nucleoproteins	+(? during infection)	Not group specific	—

a few serological types, but others are common to most group A streptococci.

Antigens elaborated by Group A streptococci do not always induce a measurable immunological response in infected individuals. In other words, infection by a single streptococcal serotype may induce a serum antibody response to a particular streptococcal antigen in certain individuals but not in others. This variability in response to bacterial antigens in patients with streptococcal infection illustrates a commonly observed biological phenomenon but has not been explored in the pathogenesis of poststreptococcal disease, although it could provide information about the antigens and immunological reactions possibly involved. The significance of the variability of immunological response in the pathogenesis of experimental glomerulonephritis induced with purified heterologous protein antigens has been shown: only those animals developing antibody at titers permitting antigen excess develop renal lesions [16].

The speed of appearance of serum antibody following group A streptococcal infection is similar to the immunological response to other antigens, whether or not they are of bacterial origin. There are differences, however, in the persistence of serum antibody to streptococcal antigens following infection. For example, the response to M protein, associated with the appearance of specific antibody providing protection against reinfection by type-specific streptococci, may persist for many years after the infection [17]. This may suggest that antigen persists in the tissues, but the mechanism of this protracted immunity is obscure. In contrast to the immunological response to M protein, antibody titers to streptolysin O remain elevated for a very short time (a few weeks). In addition, reinfection by group A streptococci of differing type elaborating an antigenically identical streptolysin O does not appear to induce a booster or secondary response [20].

Administration of specific antibiotics to patients with acute streptococcal infection may suppress the usually expected immunological response to the antigens of the microorganism by preventing bacterial multiplication, as mentioned before. It seems likely that this effect of antibiotics may be related to their ability to reduce the frequency of poststreptococcal disease. However, along with suppression of the immunological response, antibiotic therapy of group A streptococcal infection also interferes with the progression of the infection itself, which could be the means whereby such treatment prevents poststreptococcal disease.

Little is known of the distribution of streptococcal antigens in the host during or following infection. Limited observations of this kind have been made [18], but it is possible that a better understanding of the degradation and localization of these antigens would provide evidence of their implication or insignificance in the manifestations of poststreptococcal disease. It is known, for example, that the group A polysaccharide is rapidly excreted and probably for this reason can be considered of less importance in the pathogenesis of postinfectious complications such as rheumatic fever and glomerulonephritis [18].

In addition to the immunological response characterized by serum antibody production following group A streptococcal infection, it has been shown that delayed hypersensitivity to some streptococcal antigens also develops. Delayed hypersensitivity reactions in human beings to M protein and some extracellular antigens (streptokinase, DNAse) have been detected, and this reactivity has been passively transferred to normal persons with blood leukocytes or leukocyte degradation products [19]. Similar hypersensitivity reactions are probably induced to other streptococcal antigens as a result of streptococcal infection, but this has not been adequately studied. Also, it is likely that immediate hypersensitive reactions to many streptococcal antigens develop, as has been observed in pneumococcal and other infections, but this, too, has not been thoroughly evaluated.

NONSPECIFIC IMMUNOLOGICAL RESPONSES IN STREPTOCOCCAL DISEASE

In addition to the specific immunological responses to streptococcal infection, certain nonspecific changes are of interest. These "acute phase reactions" are nonspecific in that they occur during the active stages of most infections and inflammatory states. The pattern of response, however, may reflect the underlying disease, as, for example, the consistent elevation of C-reactive protein (CRP) in acute rheumatic fever. The acute phase reactions seem particularly pertinent to poststreptococcal disease since it is evident that they express, in part, the host response during acute disease states. The specific immunological host reactions to the microorganism clearly play a central but incompletely understood role in the pathogenesis of the poststreptococcal diseases. In addition, the acute phase reactions may be considered potential keys to pathogenesis.

The poststreptococcal diseases show alterations in *serum proteins* grossly similar to the changes seen in many acute infections. Most often there is an increase in the α-globulin (especially α_2) and γ-globulin fractions and a concomitant decrease in albumin. The rise in the γ-globulin fraction following streptococcal infection rather closely parallels and may be due to the rises in specific streptococcal antibodies [20].

During the active stages of acute rheumatic fever, *C-reactive protein* appears quite regularly in a concentration which roughly reflects the degree of rheumatic activity [21]. This material forms a precipitate when mixed with the somatic C-polysaccharide of the pneumococcus, is not specific for rheumatic activity, and (as with the other acute phase reactants) appears during a variety of acute infections and inflammatory states [22]. CRP is distinct from other serum proteins and can be measured immunochemically [23]. It differs from conventional antibody not only in its nonspecificity but in many of its physical properties. Unlike antibody, it reaches a maximal concentration in serum soon after onset of the acute illness, disappears during convalescence, but is not present in normal serum. It is, of course, this feature which has led to the widespread use of the CRP determination as an index of rheumatic activity. The disappearance of CRP in rheumatic patients treated with corticosteroids seems to indicate a true suppression of the rheumatic process rather than an effect on the synthesis or metabolism of the protein since, during experimental streptococcal infection, corticosteroid treatment is actually associated with an increase in CRP levels [24], and steroid treatment has no influence on levels of specific streptococcal antibodies.

The CRP level is elevated in other poststreptococcal syndromes but without the degree of regularity seen in rheumatic fever. For example, CRP is not present or detectable only with very sensitive techniques in acute glomerulonephritis [24]. In striking contrast to the close correlation between the presence of CRP and the presence of rheumatic activity, CRP disappears from the serum in acute glomerulonephritis early in the disease at a time when other evidence of active disease (urinary abnormalities, hypertension, and blood chemical changes) persists [24]. This observation has led to the suggestion that CRP may reflect a process occurring early in glomerulonephritis and not required for the perpetuation of disease activity. In patients with active chorea, CRP is usually not found unless other manifestations of rheumatic activity are present.

The site of origin of CRP has been of considerable interest. Indirect evidence suggested that it was a product of cells involved in the early response to tissue injury, such as macrophages and polymorphonuclear leukocytes [25]. Recent studies, however, with immunofluorescent techniques have indicated that injured myocardial fibers (at least in rheumatic myocarditis and myocardial infarction) may be a source [26].

Certain serum globulin fractions with relatively high carbohydrate content have particular significance in pathological states, including rheumatic fever. Among them are the serum *glycoproteins* (protein-polysaccharide complexes, including certain hormones, in which the polysaccharides are of the heterosaccharidic and nitrogenous type) and the *mucoproteins* (protein-polysaccharide complexes commonly found in connective tissue ground substance in which the polysaccharide is either chondroitin or mucoitin sulfuric acid). The serum glycoprotein concentration appears to reflect the presence of rheumatic activity [27]. Although elevated in such diverse pathological states as tuberculosis and cancer, there is evidence that the glycoproteins do not respond uniformly in a nonspecific manner in different disease states but show distinct qualitative and quantitative differences [28]. These differences, however, may not be sufficiently distinct to be of diagnostic value in the individual patient. Speculations on the origin of the serum glycoprotein fractions have considered their possible release from injured tissue or their elaboration as part of the host response to injury. A third possibility—that they rise because other low carbohydrate-containing proteins are preferentially metabolized by diseased tissue—seems less likely [29]. Mucoprotein or seromucoid levels in serum also reflect rheumatic activity, perhaps more accurately than other determinations, e.g., CRP, glycoprotein, and erythrocyte sedimentation [30, 31].

Of interest are observations on rheumatic fever patients treated with corticosteroids. The sedimentation rate drops to normal on treatment with cortisone or ACTH, but elevation of serum mucoproteins may persist, often requiring weeks or months to return to normal [24]. Cessation of corticosteroid therapy, while the mucoproteins are elevated, generally results in clinical exacerbation, in contrast to the rarity of exacerbation when therapy is continued until mucoprotein levels have returned to normal.

It now appears substantiated that *complement levels* are elevated in acute rheumatic fever and decline under the influence of corticosteroids or salicylates. This is in striking contrast to the reduction of serum complement levels in the early active stages of acute glomerulonephritis [32]. It has been suggested that complement may contribute to renal damage by increasing the affinity of specific antibody globulin for kidney tissue [33]. The significance of these changes awaits clarification.

In addition to the changes in the acute phase reactants noted above, various other substances which undergo similar changes have been studied. These include *serum hexosamines, hyaluronidase inhibitor, sialic acid,* and *fibrinogen* [24, 34]. Changes in the levels of these substances are either incompletely understood or inconsistent, adding little to our understanding of the pathogenesis of the poststreptococcal states.

POSSIBLE IMMUNOLOGICAL MANIFESTATIONS OF STREPTOCOCCAL INFECTION: THE POSTSTREPTOCOCCAL SYNDROMES

RHEUMATIC FEVER

The etiological importance of group A streptococcal infections as an initial event in the development of rheumatic fever is firmly based on clinical, epidemiological, and immunological grounds. Appreciation of this fact has led to significant success in the prevention of rheumatic fever by appropriate control of streptococcal infection [35]. In addition, repeated streptococcal infections in rabbits have resulted in the induction of myocardial lesions closely resembling those of rheumatic heart disease in man in a small proportion of infected animals [36]. What remains to be demonstrated is the mechanism by which the rheumatic process develops in a relatively small but consistent percentage of infected patients.

Perhaps the most obvious feature suggesting an allergic basis for the development of rheumatic fever is the latent period that regularly follows the acute streptococcal infection and precedes the appearance of rheumatic fever. Furthermore, the latent period coincides roughly with the time required for the appearance of antibodies to streptococcal antigens. The observation that a prior attack of rheumatic fever results in a significant increase in the attack rate per given infection also has suggested that prior sensitization is involved. The fact that the latent period for recurrent attacks of rheumatic fever is not shorter than that of the initial attack may simply indicate that prior sensitization may be required for even the first attack.

There is now also impressive evidence bearing on the question of whether acute rheumatic fever is invariably preceded by streptococcal infection. It appears that when a battery of antibody determinations against different streptococcal antigens is carried out, evidence of preceding streptococcal infection is present in almost every instance of acute rheumatic fever [37]. This observation applies both to the initial attack and to recurrences, but not to recrudescence of activity in the smoldering chronic or polycyclic forms of the disease, which may be triggered by a variety of nonspecific stimuli [38].

Unlike glomerulonephritis which follows certain specific types of streptococcal infection, rheumatic fever may follow infection with any of the more than fifty types of group A streptococci. Also unlike glomerulonephritis, which may reach attack rates of 50 or 60 percent in some epidemics of streptococcal infection, rheumatic fever rather consistently follows 2 to 3 percent of all types of group A streptococcal infection [12] (Table 29-2).

The fact that the occurrence of rheumatic fever is, therefore, actually a rather infrequent sequel of streptococcal infection has led

TABLE 29-2. Comparisons of Rheumatic Fever with Glomerulonephritis

Characteristics	Rheumatic Fever	Glomerulonephritis
Relation to infection by streptococcal type	Follows any of 50+ types	Follows only a few types ("nephritogenic strains")
Attack rate, postinfection	Consistent 2–3%	Varies widely, up to 50–60% in some epidemics
Latent period after infection	Av. 19 days	Av. 10 days
Incidence in 1st 8 days after onset	10%	47%
Frequency in infants (under 2 yr.)	Rare	Relatively frequent
Recurrences	Increased likelihood following any strep. infection	Extremely rare after complete recovery
C-reactive protein	Parallels disease activity	Subsides while evidence of acute disease still present
Serum complement activity	Rises in acute phase	Depressed

to intensive efforts to identify some peculiarity of the host response. In fact, no predisposition to allergic reactions has been shown in rheumatic patients. Monozygotic twins, even when reared together, are discordant for rheumatic fever [39]. Furthermore, rheumatic patients show a normal immunological response to nonstreptococcal antigens [40]. The unique feature of the immunological response to streptococcal infection in individuals with rheumatic fever is a rise in several streptococcal antibodies that is significantly greater than in nonrheumatic but infected patients [20]. This is also true with respect to recurrences. Thus in patients with a history of rheumatic fever, the likelihood that a subsequent streptococcal infection would be followed by rheumatic fever increased progressively from 15 to 78 percent in direct relation to the magnitude of the rise of the antistreptolysin O titer [39]. It also is of interest that older individuals have less of a rise in streptococcal antibodies following infection than do younger ones, corresponding to the reduced rate of rheumatic fever with advancing age. Whether these quantitative differences in immunological response simply reflect a more intense and frequent infectious challenge or whether they indicate differences in host response is not known.

Granted that streptococcal infection is a necessary preliminary event in the development of rheumatic fever, what are the possible ways in which the rheumatic process might occur? Is it the host reaction to the streptococcus or its products which leads to rheumatic fever? We may suppose that streptococcal toxins act directly on the host tissues. Streptolysin O, for example, has been shown to exert a toxic effect on cardiac tissue in animals [41]. Streptokinase is a potent activator of plasminogen, with resultant liberation of the proteolytic enzyme, plasmin [42]. Streptococcal hyaluronidase attacks the connective tissue ground substance [38]. There is, however, no proof that any of these agents are directly involved in the pathogenesis of rheumatic fever. Certainly, rheumatic fever is not manifested at the time of the acute streptococcal infection, when these toxins are produced in maximal quantity.

Hypersensitivity reactions might produce tissue damage in one of several ways. (1) Circulating antigen-antibody complexes might cause tissue injury directly, or (2) streptococcal antigen bound in certain tissues might subsequently participate in an injurious hypersensitivity reaction by combining with circulating antibody. (3) The tissue might be damaged by the infection, with consequent release of modified tissue proteins, and lead to the production of autoantibodies or of autosensitization by a delayed type of cellular hypersensitivity. (4) Finally, streptococcal antigens possessing cross-reactivity with tissue proteins might lead to the production of antibodies reactive to tissue constituents [7].

Attempts to identify an immunopathological mechanism of the sort indicated above have met with little success. In general, it has not been possible to implicate any of the known antistreptococcal antibodies as pathogenic agents. It has been shown, for example, that a delay of nine days in the treatment of the acute streptococcal infection allows antistreptolysin titers to develop significantly but, nevertheless, markedly decreases the incidence of rheumatic fever [12]. Gamma-globulin has been identified in auricular appendages of rheumatic hearts, but such localization may be nonspecific [7]. Perhaps the most promising line of investigation has been the work of Kaplan [8], who has identified a material from streptococcal cell walls associated with, but not identical to, the M protein, which is related antigenically to human cardiac myofibers and the smooth muscle of vessel walls. The presence of such cross-antigenicity, of course, might clarify the unique role of the streptococcus in the etiology of rheumatic fever. It is of interest that the cross-reaction appears to occur with cardiac muscle itself, which is consistent with evidence presented by Murphy [36] that the fibrinoid lesion of the Aschoff body in the rheumatic heart is derived from degenerating myofibers and *not* from collagen.

POSTSTREPTOCOCCAL ACUTE GLOMERULONEPHRITIS

Group A streptococcal infection has been shown to precede the onset of acute glomerulonephritis in at least 90 percent of patients, as determined by bacterial isolation or serological study with several group A streptococcal antigens [43]. The interval between the infection and onset of nephritis averages ten days, which is somewhat shorter than the latent period observed in acute rheumatic fever (Table 29-2). As in acute rheumatic fever, however, there usually is no evidence of disease during the latent period preceding onset of glomerulonephritis, and when the nephritis develops, immunological responses to the preceding streptococcal infection are demonstrable.

Hematuria and proteinuria suggestive of glomerulonephritis commonly are observed *during* the course of many acute infections, including those due to group A streptococci. It must be emphasized that this condition is quite different from poststreptococcal nephritis. For example, in patients with severe infection such as bacterial endocarditis, pneumococcal pneumonia, and meningococcemia, renal abnormalities indistinguishable from glomerulonephritis may develop. In contrast with poststreptococcal nephritis, however, the renal abnormalities of acute infection appear during and do not follow the infection. After infection by group A streptococci, there usually are no urinary abnormalities until the glomerulonephritis supervenes. Although there may be no relation between the renal involvement during infection and poststreptococcal nephritis, it is interesting that patients with the most severe urinary abnormalities during acute streptococcal disease are most likely subsequently to have acute nephritis [12].

Most patients with acute glomerulonephritis recover completely, but a few (10 percent) may have persistent urinary manifestations and develop chronic renal disease [44]. Those who recover completely appear to be insusceptible to recurrent nephritis, in contrast to rheumatic fever, in which recurring streptococcal infection commonly causes reactivation of the disease. Individuals with chronic glomerulonephritis may experience an exacerbation during or following many acute infections, whether or not they are attributable to streptococci. On the other hand, rheumatic fever probably can be reactivated only by infection with group A streptococci, as indicated previously.

In contrast with rheumatic fever, the incidence of acute glomerulonephritis following group A streptococcal infection varies. At times a high percentage and at other times a small or negligible percentage of infected patients will develop nephritis. This variability in occurrence of glomerulonephritis following infection and the infrequency of recurrence in individuals who have recovered from nephritis suggest that not all strains of streptococci induce this poststreptococcal disease. The brilliant epidemiological studies of Rammelkamp and his associates [12] demonstrated that type 12 and occasionally a few other types of group A streptococci were almost exclusively involved in producing nephritis. These observations, now confirmed many times, explain the variability in occurrence of nephritis following infection. In addition, the development of type-specific immunity following streptococcal infection explains why recovery from glomerulonephritis is rarely followed by recurrence with subsequent infection, as reinfection by streptococcal types responsible for nephritis would be unlikely.

The pathogenesis of poststreptococcal glomerulonephritis, however, is not clear. It has been reported that certain strains of group A streptococci may elaborate a nephritogenic toxin capable of producing renal disease in experimental animals [45]. Confirmation of this, however, is lacking. A lower nephron renal disease has been found in rabbits after repeated infection with type 12 streptococci, but such lesions bear only a minor resemblance to poststreptococcal glomerulonephritis in man [46].

The relationship of the development of glomerulonephritis to rising titers of streptococcal antibody, in addition to the interval between the streptococcal infection and onset of nephritis, has long suggested that an altered host reaction may be involved in the pathogenesis of the disease. There is no relationship, however, between the severity of the glomerulonephritis and the height of measured antibody response.

Whether an immunological reaction with streptococcal antigen or induction of autoimmunization is responsible for the development of glomerulonephritis is not known. Group A streptococci have been found to localize partly in the kidney following experimental induction of bacteremia [14]. This localization, however, is not a specific characteristic of type 12 streptococci as many other bacteria (e.g., *Staphylococcus, Escherichia coli* and *Proteus*) behave similarly. Type M protein also has been found to localize in the glomerulus following intravenous injection, and antigens of group A streptococci have been identified by immunological techniques in the kidney of patients with nephritis [7, 18]. The localization of antigens in the kidney, however, is not a peculiarity of type 12 streptococci, being demonstrable with other bacterial antigens and with nonantigenic substances such as polyvinyl alcohol [47]. The localization of foreign substances in the glomeruli appears to be related to molecular weight rather than to a specific affinity for renal tissue. The localization of streptococcal antigens in the kidney, furthermore, is not sufficiently convincing evidence of their implication in the pathogenesis of glomerulonephritis.

Immunoglobulins have been identified in the glomeruli of patients with nephritis, but their presence in the kidney may also have no specific relation to the disease, because γ-globulin also has been found in the renal glomeruli of patients with systemic lupus erythematosus, progressive systemic sclerosis, polyarteritis, amyloidosis, and diabetes mellitus [48]. Immunoglobulin eluted from the kidney of patients with glomerulonephritis does not localize in normal kidney tissue, and it may be present in the diseased kidney for nonimmunological reasons [7].

Serum complement usually decreases in patients with acute glomerulonephritis, suggesting its participation in an immunological reaction. Furthermore, human complement has been detected in the renal glomeruli of patients with nephritis by specific immunofluorescence [7], but this, too, may be a nonspecific phenomenon.

The evidence is compatible with the suggestion that an immunological reaction with streptococcal antigen in the kidney may be an important mechanism in the pathogenesis of glomerulonephritis. In addition, this interpretation is consistent with experimental studies showing that nephritis resembling that following streptococcal infection in man can be produced by immunological reactions in animals involving heterologous foreign protein [16].

The morphological lesions seen in experimental immunological nephritis are similar to the lesions of poststreptococcal glomerulonephritis characterized by (1) an increase in number of cells within the glomerular capillary loops, (2) endothelial proliferation with mitoses, (3) cytoplasmic inclusion in mononuclear cells of material with the same morphological qualities and electron density as glomerular capillary basement membrane, and (4) occasional increase in number of polymorphonuclear leukocytes within the glomeruli, often associated with glomerular necrosis and crescents [44]. Much remains to be done, however, to explain the peculiarities of type 12 group A streptococci in the epidemiology and pathogenesis of the disease. Certainly none of the existing evidence *establishes* an immunological reaction to streptococcal antigen as an important mechanism in the pathogenesis of poststreptococcal glomerulonephritis.

Heterologous antiserum to specific animal kidney can produce nephritis on injection, suggesting the possibility that autoimmunization to renal glomeruli during streptococcal infection may be the mechanism of production of glomerulonephritis in man. However, studies have not demonstrated specific tissue-localizing or complement-fixing antibodies in the serum of patients with nephritis, and skin tests with extracts of normal kidney have not produced positive reactions [6, 7]. There is no evidence at present, therefore, which satisfactorily implicates autosensitization in the pathogenesis of poststreptococcal glomerulonephritis.

It has been speculated that chronic glomerulonephritis may not bear a relationship to poststreptococcal acute nephritis. The studies of Jennings and Earle [44], however, clearly illustrate that a small percentage of patients with acute glomerulonephritis develop morphological lesions typical of chronic nephritis.

ERYTHEMA NODOSUM

Although occasionally seen during rheumatic fever, erythema nodosum most often occurs separately but may be viewed as a poststreptococcal disease since it follows essentially the same pattern of delayed appearance after streptococcal infection and reappearance following reinfection as does rheumatic fever.

It is apparent that a variety of conditions may precede erythema nodosum, including particularly tuberculosis, coccidioidomycosis, and other infectious processes. The apparent "provocative" effect of drugs (especially sulfonamides) in inducing erythema nodosum has suggested hypersensitivity in its pathogenesis [49]. (See also Chap. 28.)

The evidence that streptococcal infection is one of the important preceding events seems well established [49]. Reactions to skin tests with streptococcal antigens in patients with erythema nodosum and streptococcal pharyngitis are consistently positive, and the tests frequently induce systemic reactions, including aggravation of the nodose lesions [50]. The mechanisms involved, however, have been less extensively studied and remain even more obscure than those in rheumatic fever and glomerulonephritis.

OTHER IMMUNOLOGICAL MANIFESTATIONS

Sydenham's Chorea. Convincing evidence now available indicates that this condition, whether occurring with rheumatic fever or as an isolated phenomenon, is a late sequel of streptococcal infection [51]. It is significant that the length of the interval following the streptococcal infection and the onset of chorea occurring without other evidence of rheumatic activity may be quite extended (three to six months). Chorea may, therefore, occur at a time when the usual indices of rheumatic activity (increased sedimentation rate and CRP) are negative and when the titer of specific streptococcal antibodies has fallen to low levels.

Erythema Marginatum. This eruption occurs in up to one-fourth of children with rheumatic fever and may be viewed as the characteristic manifestation of skin involvement in rheumatic fever, although an indistinguishable lesion may occur in nonrheumatic disorders. Like chorea, erythema marginatum occasionally appears late in the rheumatic attack [52], suggesting that a different mechanism may be operative in these disorders.

The changing pattern of acute streptococcal disease which occurs with increasing age has suggested that altered host reactivity to streptococcal products may significantly influence clinical manifestations of infection. The rarity of *scarlet fever* in infants under 3 years (despite Dick test negativity) has suggested that prior sensitization to the erythrogenic toxin may be required for the manifestation of scarlet fever. The tendency of *erysipelas* to recur repeatedly in the same site may indicate altered local tissue reactivity.

REFERENCES*

1. Cluff, L. E., and Allen, J. A. Principles of active immunization for prevention of infection. *J. Chron. Dis.* 15:575, 1962.
2. Denny, F. W., Jr., Perry, W. D., and Wannamaker, F. W. Type-specific streptococcal antibody. *J. Clin. Invest.* 36:1092, 1957.
3. Petroff, S. A., Branch, A., and Jennings, F. B., Jr. Resistance of animals sensitized with heat-killed tubercle bacilli to a measured infecting dose. *J. Immun.* 16:233, 1929.

* Where possible, references have been made to review articles.

4. Swift, H. F., and Derrick, C. L. Reactions of rabbits to nonhemolytic streptococci. *J. Exp. Med.* 49:883, 1929.
5. Clawson, B. J. Experiments relative to vaccination with the Calmette-Guérin bacillus (BCG). *Arch. Path.* 20:343, 1935.
6. Waksman, B. H. Autoimmunization and the lesions of autoimmunity. *Medicine* 41:93, 1962.
7. Cruickshank, B. Nephritis, Nephrosis, Rheumatic Fever and Myocardial Infarction. In Gell, P. G. H., and Coombs, R. R. A. (Eds.), *Clinical Aspects of Immunology.* Oxford: Blackwell Scientific Publications, 1963.
8. Kaplan, M. H. Immunological relation of streptococcal and tissue antigens: I. Properties of an antigen in certain strains of group A streptococci exhibiting an immunologic cross-reaction with human heart tissue. *J. Immun.* 90:595, 1963.
9. Watson, D. W. Host Factors in Experimental Streptococcal Infections. In McCarty, M. (Ed.), *Streptococcal Infections.* New York: Columbia University Press, 1954.
10. McCarty, M. Variations in the group-specific carbohydrate of group A streptococci. I. Immunochemical studies on the carbohydrates of various strains. *J. Exp. Med.* 102:11, 1955.
11. McCarty, M. The Hemolytic Streptococci. In Dubos, R. J. (Ed.), *Bacterial and Mycotic Infections of Man* (3rd ed.). Philadelphia: J. B. Lippincott Company, 1958.
12. Rammelkamp, C. H., Jr. Epidemiology of streptococcal infection. *Harvey Lect.* 51:113, 1955–56.
13. Freimer, E. H. Studies of L forms and protoplasts of group A streptococci. *J. Exp. Med.* 17:377, 1963.
14. Denny, F. W., Jr., and Thomas, L. Persistence of group A streptococci in tissues of rabbits after infection. *Proc. Soc. Exp. Biol. Med.* 88: 260, 1955.
15. Bernhard, G. C., and Stollerman, G. H. Serum inhibition of streptococcal diphosphopyridine nucleotidase in uncomplicated streptococcal pharyngitis and in rheumatic fever. *J. Clin. Invest.* 38:1942, 1959.
16. Dixon, F. J. Tissue Injury Produced by Antigen-Antibody Complexes. In Grabar, P., and Miescher, P. (Eds.), *Mechanisms of Cell and Tissue Damage Produced by Immune Reactions* (II International Symposium on Immunopathology). New York: Grune & Stratton, Inc., 1962.
17. Lancefield, R. C. Current knowledge of type specific M antigens of group A streptococci. *J. Immun.* 89:307, 1962.
18. Schmidt, W. C. The Cellular Localization of Injected Streptococcal Antigens. Ref. 9.
19. Lawrence, H. S. The cellular transfer in humans of delayed cutaneous reactivity to hemolytic streptococci. *J. Immun.* 68:159, 1952.
20. McCarty, M. The Antibody Response to Streptococcal Infections. Ref. 9.
21. Wood, H. F., and McCarty, M. Laboratory aids in the diagnosis of rheumatic fever and in evaluation of disease activity. *Amer. J. Med.* 17:768, 1954.
22. Tillett, W. S., and Francis, T. Serological reactions in pneumonia with a non-protein somatic fraction of pneumococcus. *J. Exp. Med.* 52:561, 1930.
23. Anderson, H. C., and McCarty, M. Determination of C-reactive protein in the blood as a measure of the activity of the disease process in acute rheumatic fever. *Amer. J. Med.* 8:445, 1950.
24. Good, R. A. Acute-Phase Reactions in Rheumatic Fever. In Thomas, L. (Ed.), *Rheumatic Fever: A Symposium.* Minneapolis: University of Minnesota Press, 1952.
25. Rapport, M. M., Schwartz, A. E., and Graf, L. C-reactive protein in patients following operations. *Ann. Surg.* 145:321, 1957.
26. Kushner, J., Rakita, L., and Kaplan, M. H. Studies of acute-phase protein: II. Localization of Cx-reactive protein in heart in induced myocardial infarction in rabbits. *J. Clin. Invest.* 42:286, 1963.
27. Shetlar, M. R., Payne, R. W., Strenge, H. B., and Faulkner, J. B. Objective evaluation of patients with rheumatic diseases: III. Comparison of serum glycoprotein, seromucoid, and C-reactive protein determinations as methods for evaluation of patients with rheumatic fever. *J. Pediat.* 51:510, 1957.
28. Heiskell, C. L., Carpenter, C. M., Weimer, H. E., and Nakagawa, S. Serum glycoproteins in infectious and inflammatory diseases. *Ann. N.Y. Acad. Sci.* 94:183, 1961.
29. Shetlar, M. R. Serum glycoproteins: Their origin and significance. *Ibid.*, p. 44.
30. Kelly, V. C., Adams, F. H., and Good, R. A. Serum mucoproteins in patients with rheumatic fever. *Pediatrics* 12:607, 1952.
31. Singer, J. M. The latex fixation test in rheumatic diseases. *Amer. J. Med.* 31:766, 1961.
32. Osler, A. G. Functions of the complement system. *Advances Immun.* 1:132, 1961.
33. Freedman, P., and Markowitz, A. Immunological studies in nephritis. *Lancet* 2:45, 1959.
34. Payne, R. W. Serum glycoproteins in the rheumatic diseases. *Ann. N.Y. Acad. Sci.* 94: 284, 1961.
35. Stollerman, G. H. A scarlatinal "Nachkrankeheit" of Schick: Rheumatic fever 50 years later. *Int. Arch. Allerg.* 12:287, 1958.
36. Murphy, G. E. Nature of rheumatic heart disease. *Medicine* 39:289, 1960.
37. Stollerman, G. H., Lewis, A. J., Schultz, K.,

and Taranta, A. Relationship of immune response to group A streptococci in the course of acute, chronic, and recurrent rheumatic fever. *Amer. J. Med.* 20:163, 1956.

38. McCarty, M. Present state of knowledge concerning pathogenesis and treatment of rheumatic fever. *Bull. N.Y. Acad. Med.* 28:307, 1952.
39. Taranta, A. Factors associated with the rheumatic fever attack rate following streptococcal infections. *Arthritis Rheum.* 4:303, 1961.
40. Kuhns, W. J., and McCarty, M. Studies of diphtheria antitoxin in rheumatic fever subjects: Analysis of reactions to the Schick test and of antibody responses following hyperimmunization with diphtheria toxoid. *J. Clin. Invest.* 33:759, 1954.
41. Bernheimer, A. W., and Cantoni, G. L. The cardiotoxic action of preparations containing the oxygen-labile hemolysin of streptococcus pyogenes. *J. Exp. Med.* 81:295, 1945.
42. Tillett, W. S., and Garner, R. L. The fibrinolytic activity of hemolytic streptococci. *J. Exp. Med.* 58:485, 1933.
43. Kushner, D. S., Armstrong, S. H. Jr., Dubin, A., Szanto, P. B., Markowitz, A., Maduros, B. P., Levine, J. M., River, G. L., Gynn, T. N., and Pendras, J. P. Acute glomerulonephritis in the adult: Longitudinal, clinical, functional and morphologic studies of rates of healing and progression to chronicity. *Medicine* 40:203, 1961.
44. Jennings, R. B., and Earle, D. P. Poststreptococcal glomerulonephritis: Histopathological and clinical studies of the acute, subsiding acute and early chronic latent phases. *J. Clin. Invest.* 40:1525, 1961.
45. Reed, R. W., and Matheson, B. H. Experimental nephritis due to type-specific streptococci: I. The effect of a single exposure to type 12 streptococci. *J. Infect. Dis.* 95:191, 1954.
46. Reed, R. W., and Matheson, B. H. Experimental nephritis due to type-specific streptococci: II. The effect of repeated exposure to type 12 streptococci. *Ibid.*, p. 202.
47. Hall, C. E., and Hall, O. Polyvinyl alcohol nephrosis: Relationship of degree of polymerization to pathophysiologic effects. *Proc. Soc. Exp. Biol. Med.* 112:86, 1963.
48. Freedman, P., Peters, J. H., and Kark, R. M. Localization of gamma globulin in the diseased kidney. *Arch. Intern. Med.* 105:524, 1960.
49. Beerman, H. Erythema nodosum: A survey of some recent literature. *Amer. J. Med. Sci.* 223:433, 1952.
50. Favour, C. B., and Sosman, M. C. Erythema nodosum. *Arch. Intern. Med.* 80:435, 1947.
51. Taranta, A. Relation of isolated recurrences of Sydenham's chorea to preceding streptococcal infection. *New Eng. J. Med.* 260:1204, 1959.
52. Feinstein, A. R., and Spagnulo, M. The clinical patterns of acute rheumatic fever: A reappraisal. *Medicine* 41:279, 1962.
53. Zabriskie, J. B. The role of temperate bacteriophage in the production of erythrogenic toxin by Group A streptococci. *J. Exp. Med.* 119:761, 1964.

30. Tuberculosis

SIDNEY RAFFEL

TUBERCULOSIS IS A CLASSIC AMONG the infectious diseases of man. It figures largely in the early history of human disease, it was the subject of dramatic disputes concerned with etiology and therapy in the latter part of the last century, it has for years been a center of contention concerning the merits of vaccination, and it is currently the stubborn but slowly yielding object of efforts aimed at its eradication through the prophylactic and therapeutic use of antimicrobial drugs. This interest and activity have built up a massive literary monument to the disease, in textbooks, monographs, and clinical and investigative reports, so that it would be redundant to do more here than to restate the briefest of descriptions of its general features, especially as these relate to immunological aspects.

This infection is a chronic one which causes overt signs and symptoms in only a fraction of individuals who harbor *Mycobacterium tuberculosis.* A quarter-century ago in the large cities of the United States about 80 percent of the population was infected, as indicated by reactivity to skin tests with soluble bacterial constituents (tuberculin). Now the number of infected individuals is at the 20 percent level, i.e., 30 million people in this country show evidence of harboring the bacillus. Of these, 1 in 15 has or has had active disease (about 2 million existing cases), and in one year (1960), the mortality in the United States was 5.9 per 100,000 of the total population, or 1 of 3,400 infected individuals and 1 of 188 of those with active disease. This represents a sharp decrement from the rate of mortality of earlier years. The decline of morbidity has been less steep but very significant, and the total picture reflects the application of antimicrobial drugs [1].

The pattern of incidence of active disease and mortality is also undergoing striking alterations. Historically, the young adult age group was most affected by active disease, but in the past decade there has been a shift to an increased proportion of cases and deaths in the population group above age 50, especially in males. This development has nothing to do with any basic change in host-parasite relationship. It is a result of the recent sharp fall in numbers of total infections in the population. Young adults are still highly susceptible to infection, but there are fewer sources of bacilli open to them. The older group is suffering the effects of implantation of bacteria in their early years and now coming to fruition. As has been pointed out [2], the present older generation in *its* youth suffered a higher tuberculous mortality than it does now. When the present young have attained their seniority, there should be far fewer cases of disease among them than in the current older generations. These considerations indicate that active disease is frequently based on infections acquired earlier, even years in the past. Interesting features of changes in disease pattern related to sex, race, and other factors are also available for study [1].

Another aspect of mycobacterial disease which warrants mention here is the increasingly revealed incidence of infections, both subclinical and overt, caused by a group of acid-fast bacilli variously termed "atypical," "anonymous," or "unclassified" [1]. The last adjective, the one most used now, is becoming rapidly outdated by accumulating information. These bacteria are antigenically related to *M. tuberculosis* and are at present assigned to four groups on the basis of various cultural characteristics, chief among them the production of pigments and rapidity of multiplication. Some of them are etiologically associated with pulmonary disease which is clinically and pathologically indistinguishable from that caused by the tubercle bacillus [3]. The two main organisms so implicated are *Mycobacterium kansasii* (a member of group I which is photochromogenic; i.e., it produces pigment only if exposed to light during incubation), and the Battey bacillus (group III, nonchromogenic). These organisms in the "wild" state are relatively insusceptible to the antimicrobial drugs which act on *M. tuberculosis;* for this reason, the individual fates of diseased patients differ from those of people with conventional tuberculosis. There is an important epidemiological distinction between these diseases also; contacts of patients with unclassified mycobacterial disease rarely develop overt infections, whereas in the same circumstances active tuberculosis is apt to spread readily. Yet skin testing and cultural surveys have made it apparent that many individuals in certain geographic areas are infected by these bacteria at a subclinical level [4, 5]. Presumably some unknown kind of defect of individual capacity to cope with these microbes must account for the development of clinically apparent disease.

PATHOGENESIS

Excellent discussions of pathogenesis have been provided by Rich [6] and Canetti [7], among others. It seems probable that the major concepts derived from investigations of the tubercle bacillus and its disease are entirely applicable to the unclassified mycobacteria and the infections established by them.

The infection begins with a microscopic accumulation of leukocytes and macrophages in which a few bacilli may be found. The macrophages become so altered in appearance as to resemble epithelial cells and are termed epithelioid. Some of these may be multinucleated (Langhans cells). This initial cellular tubercle is called a granuloma, a term reserved for an inflammatory process in which epithelioid cells are a component. During this early phase of infection, the bacteria spread readily via lymphatics to regional lymph nodes to set up similar inflammatory foci. In primary infection of the lung, the combined features of initial parenchymal focus, lymphangitis, and lymphadenitis is known as a Ghon complex.

During the period of these developments, immunological responses to the bacillus become established, so that in three or four weeks the body has acquired three measurable reactive states: humoral antibodies, delayed hypersensitivity, and a degree of acquired resistance to the bacterium. Antibodies are demonstrable by a variety of serological tests. Delayed reactivity may be revealed by the intracutaneous or percutaneous application of tuberculin, and acquired immunity in human beings can be inferred from the ability of infected subjects to contain the process in the sites mentioned, and from a pronounced tendency of such individuals to localize a succeeding infection to the area in which it begins, without lymphatic involvement. In experimental animals this last facet can, of course, be demonstrated directly by deliberate rechallenge with known numbers of bacilli.

An important aspect of the pathogenesis is the pronounced tendency of the cellular lesion, at the time of appearance of the immunological responses, to undergo necrosis. Coincident with this, the number of bacilli in the lesion is apt to drop considerably; whether this is a result of the acquisition of immunity or owing to physical and chemical changes in the local environment inimical to bacillary life is not clear [7]. The dead tissue is usually not attacked by tissue enzymes, so that it remains solid in consistency and appearance and is described as being caseous. Such lesions most often heal, with fibrosis and deposition of calcium and eventual contraction to a scar. However, there may occur a liquefaction of the caseum, accompanied by a spurt of bacillary growth. Any of a number of events may follow this, including discharge of the debris to the outside through the bronchi, or spillage into other uninvolved parts of the lung via the same channels or into blood vessels or lymphatics with resulting systemic spread of disease.

RELATION OF PATHOGENESIS TO CONSTITUENTS OF MYCOBACTERIA

Lipids. The tubercle bacillus differs chemically from most other bacterial cells in possessing a high content of lipids; about one third of its mass consists of fats, which exist mostly in the cell wall [8]. These substances, which have been subjects of intensive study [9, 10], are separable into a number of distinguishable groups, of which some have especial interest for their biological activities. One class consists of a mixture of beta-hydroxy fatty acids about 88 carbon atoms in length, termed mycolic acids. These occur free in the cell or esterified with sugars, either simple, such as trehalose, or nitrogen- and phosphorus-containing polysaccharides [10–12, 22, 25].

The main direct activity of lipids in the pathogenic process in tuberculosis lies in the induction of the typical inflammatory picture of the *granuloma*. The lipopolysaccharides have the property of inducing proliferation of reticuloendothelial cells (RE) in the animal body, and along with certain phosphatides [13], are implicated in the conversion of macrophages to epithelioid cells.

The mycolic acid-trehalose ester has been indicted as an important factor in relation to the *virulence* of the tubercle bacillus [14]. This relationship is suggested by the concomitance of several factors: virulent bacilli grow in serpentine or corded fashion, and the chemical entity associated with this kind of growth is the ester; furthermore, the isolated substance has certain properties of toxicity. It is not yet firmly established that the conclusion suggested by these considerations is valid.

Whether any of the lipids are antigenic is open to question in face of reports implicating them as suitable antigens in tests for antibodies with the sera of infected subjects, as noted later. This class of organic substances in general is only tenuously associated with the molecular endowments required for such activity, perhaps because their limited range of structural possibilities does not provide the almost infinite variety characteristic of proteins and polysaccharides. Therefore, the lipids may not possess the quality of foreignness to tissues which would evoke an immunological response. But certain of these substances participate in immunological activities in a less direct way. Thus whole mycobacteria suspended in water-in-oil emulsion have an appreciable adjuvant effect in antibody production; i.e., the mixture causes an enhanced response to antigens of any kind incorporated in it for injection [15, 16], and the lipopolysaccharides can substitute for the bacteria in this mixture. In analogous fashion, mycobacteria or their lipopolysaccharides participate in the induction of delayed hypersensitive reactivity to proteins of the bacillus. This is indicated by the finding that extraction of these lipids from bacilli largely deprives them of the capacity to induce this state, while readdition of the waxy fat restores it [17]. This activity may depend on the cell-proliferative stimulus supplied by the lipid. Among such cells may be potentially responsive ones, or the lipids may in some other unknown fashion induce cells to respond to antigen with delayed reactivity.

Proteins and Delayed Hypersensitivity. Delayed hypersensitivity represents a response to the proteins of the bacterial cell. A number of these have been studied in considerable detail [18]. All are antigenic, and their unquestionable implication in this response to the bacillus has been shown by the use of fractions for the skin testing of sensitive subjects [19] and by the efficacy of an isolated basic peptide in this respect [20].

The hypersensitive state in this disease is apt to be striking and durable; persons who have attained it as a result of subclinical infection often remain persistently reactive throughout their lives, presumably because they retain a focus of dormant bacilli or perhaps because of occasional restimulation by freshly acquired bacilli from the outside world or even by other antigenically related organisms such as certain of the unclassified mycobacteria. But reversions to nonreactivity can occur spontaneously, and more frequently than was thought to be the case some years ago. This may well relate to diminished opportunities for exposure to overtly infected subjects in the population at this time [21].

The mechanistic aspect of the delayed hypersensitive reaction is discussed elsewhere in this volume. The basis for this appears to be a specific capacity of lymphoid cells, probably small lymphocytes, to interact directly with soluble or cell-borne antigens. The nature of this reactive property has not been defined; it may depend on humoral antibodies with special propensity to adhere to cell surfaces, or the implicated cells may themselves synthesize a reactive factor which is not released into the body fluids [22, 23].

The death of cells which occurs in the cellular tubercle early in its pathogenesis is attributed in large part to the delayed hypersensitive reaction, since a counterpart can be established in the reactive subject by the injection of tuberculin into the skin or, in animals, by the injection of tubercle bacilli themselves. In the latter instance, the resultant local breakdown of tissue in two or three days is referred to as the Koch phenomenon.

One aspect of this necrotizing reaction which requires explanation is the occurrence of general tissue destruction when only specialized cells of the inflammatory infiltrate are vulnerable to antigen. It is apparent that the injury of other cells and tissues must be secondary to the initial specific interaction, but whether this is caused directly by histotoxic derivatives of the primary reaction, by ischemia consequent on vascular injury, or by a damaging action of sensitive cells on parenchymal elements which have adsorbed bacillary antigen is not known (see Chaps. 11 and 20).

ACQUIRED IMMUNITY

This feature of tuberculous infection cannot with certainty be related to any of the known immunological responses to bacillary constituents, although some deductions are permissible. The current status of this subject is best discussed in terms of whether antibodies or cells are the responsible agents of immunity.

Antibodies. These are elaborated against proteins and polysaccharides of the bacterium and perhaps certain of its lipids, as mentioned before. It seems highly doubtful that any of these humoral substances are related to acquired immunity to the disease, if judgment is based on the failure to transfer immunity from vaccinated to normal subjects by repeated injections of serum, or to find evidence of a special activity of the fluids of immune animals on the viability of bacilli in semipermeable chambers installed in the peritoneal cavities for prolonged periods [24]. It is interesting in this connection also that tuberculosis has rarely been encountered in patients with hypogammaglobulinemia despite their relative inability to synthesize antibodies.

It has been suggested that antipolysaccharide antibodies may enter into the immune process indirectly by combining with sugars released from bacilli and thus preventing this substrate from diverting nonantibody antibacterial constituents of the blood, possibly lysozyme, from acting on the organisms [25]. Antibacterial substances of nonantibody nature are present in the blood of normal man and of variously treated animals [26], but the kind of relationship proposed has not been satisfactorily established.

Cells. The cells generally considered to be the alternatives for antibodies as instruments of acquired immunity in tuberculosis are macrophages. In part this idea derives from their well-known propensity to engulf mycobacteria, but more directly it stems from observations that such cells obtained from immune animals and placed in culture have a greater inhibitory effect on multiplication of added microbes than do cells obtained from nonimmune subjects. Although a number of such observations have been recorded, this result has not been found universally, particularly when virulent bacteria have been employed [16]. Efforts have also been made to transfer immunity by means of cells, again with some, but not uniform, success. In one of the more striking of such studies, immunity was conferred on several recipients serially, not only by whole macrophages but by lysates of these cells [27].

Accumulating evidence derived from work in animals suggests that the immunity acquired to tuberculosis may not be entirely specific and, obversely, that subjects made resistant to other bacteria may show heightened protection against the tubercle bacillus. Such findings, with *Brucella* and the staphylococcus among other bacteria [28–30], have raised the question whether immunity may be a nonspecific result of "activation" of cells of the RE system, such as can be brought about by injections of gram-negative bacillary endotoxins [31], histamine [32], and other substances [33]. Perhaps related to this concept are recent observations [34] that the ability of macrophages obtained from appropriately vaccinated animals (with *Listeria* in this case) to suppress bacterial growth parallels a morphological change in these cells coincident with the delayed hypersensitive reaction. That is, such cells appear at a time after vaccination when delayed reactivity sets in and can be found for a time thereafter. With each subsequent antigenic stimulus which reactivates the hypersensitive state, these unusual macrophages reappear. Their capacities to inhibit bacteria are not specific; they may act against microbes other than those providing the stimulus for the hypersensitive response. For example, cells obtained from *Listeria*-sensitive animals act on *Brucella,* and those from tuberculin-sensitive animals on *Brucella* and *Listeria.* Thus the stimulus required to evoke these cells is a specific one, but the antibacterial capacities of the cells are not specific [35]. It may be of interest in this connection that

Myrvik *et al.* [36] have found macrophages of unusual appearance and with extraordinary tuberculostatic properties to accumulate in masses in the lungs of vaccinated animals following subsequent intravenous injections of attenuated tubercle bacilli, and that a "macrophage disappearance" reaction has been described as occurring in the peritoneal cavities of sensitized guinea pigs given small doses of tuberculin [37].

What the precise relationship of these unusual macrophages may be to the delayed hypersensitive state or reaction is not clear. The cells directly implicated in delayed hypersensitivity by most workers are lymphocytes [38–40], but the possibility exists that there are developmental relations between these two cell types (Chap. 11).

If acquired immunity in tuberculosis should prove to be an integral part of the delayed hypersensitive response rather than a concomitant event, the implication is that the protein antigens of the bacillus are the important stimuli for immunity. This view is difficult to reconcile with failures of various investigators to induce immunity by the administration of proteins isolated from the organism, either alone or with lipids which participate in the induction of delayed hypersensitivity [16]. Reconciliation must also be made with older experiments which demonstrated that vaccinated animals may be desensitized without loss of acquired immunity [41].

VACCINATION AGAINST TUBERCULOSIS

Repeated efforts have been made over the years to prepare an effective vaccine consisting of single or multiple constituents of the tubercle bacillus. The results have been variably successful; only rarely have they been described as comparable to those obtainable with the attenuated viable vaccines described below [42–44]. Vaccines composed of killed organisms can unquestionably be effective, but they have found little use in human vaccination, probably because the attenuated vaccine proved its worth early in the quest and was difficult to displace.

The vaccine most widely used in man and animals for induction of resistance to tuberculosis is composed of attenuated but viable organisms derived from a bovine variant of the bacillus, and called BCG (*Bacille Calmette-Guérin*). This mutant was selected early in this century [45], and various strains of it have been propagated throughout the world. Its effectiveness in retarding the course of challenge infections in laboratory animals is easily demonstrated. In man, many millions of vaccinations have been made, but controlled studies for effectiveness are relatively few. However, some such trials have been carefully contrived and followed, and with few exceptions these have shown good results, to the extent of about an 80 percent reduction in the occurrence of active infections in vaccinated populations. This modifying influence has, surprisingly, been found to extend over a period of some years after initial vaccinations [45, 46].

A second viable vaccine is composed of organisms originally isolated from a field mouse (vole) and referred to as *Mycobacterium murius.* In a controlled study in human beings, this vaccine revealed effectiveness about comparable to that of BCG [46].

The rationale for use of vaccine against tuberculosis, aside from its empirically established value, represents an interesting philosophical issue. It is well known that most cases of active tuberculosis are of the "reinfection" type; i.e., they appear in people who some months or years earlier had given evidence of a primary subclinical infection. The fact that the primary infection should be an immunizing one makes the later occurrence of overt disease in such presumably protected individuals a puzzling paradox. One can assume that the affected individual has suffered some lapse in his immune status which permits bacilli to multiply in his tissues; but then why should disease occur so preponderantly in these people in contrast to the unimmunized (i.e., previously uninfected) segment of the population? One explanation for this paradox proposes that it occurs because many or most cases of reinfection disease are caused by bacilli which are already resident in the body as a quiescent residue of the old primary infection, and that when an abrogation of immunity occurs, this is readily taken advantage of by such persisting organisms. If this is the case, the function of a viable vaccine is to evoke immunity in the same fashion as does a spontaneous primary infection, without, however, providing the seed of a possible later reinfection from within ("endogenous reinfection").

ANTIMICROBIAL DRUGS AND IMMUNITY

The therapeutic effectiveness of antimycobacterial drugs has helped to break the chain of tuberculous infection and has resulted in precipitous declines in morbidity and mortality, as discussed earlier. In areas of the world where the drugs are readily available, this fact has had an influence on the use of vaccine; in the United States, for example, BCG was never exploited on more than a restricted scale, and its use now is even more limited.

There is another aspect in which drugs more directly impinge on the issue of biological prophylaxis. This is in the use of isoniazid (isonicotinic acid hydrazide) in subjects with early subclinical primary infection in an effort to take advantage of the immunizing capacity of such an infection while simultaneously destroying the offending bacterium [47]. Further, isoniazid is being used in truly prophylactic fashion in populations with high incidence of disease [48] and in contacts of active disease in households. The administration is begun before known exposure to bacilli has taken place with the purpose of preventing the establishment of the primary infection for at least as long as administration of the drug continues. In a recently conducted experiment of this kind, protection was afforded to the extent of about 75 percent during a one-year period of drug administration [49]. The question as to what may happen after cessation of administration of the agent remains to be answered.

Theoretical as well as practical facets of the rationale for this kind of prophylaxis are promising in this particular situation, although drug prophylaxis as a generalization is not so supported. In this instance the favorable factors are these: isoniazid is relatively nontoxic and may be administered orally for long periods; it acts only on mycobacteria, so that the flora of the body is not disturbed; the treated subject is in normal physiological state and thus not open to "predestined" infection by some other intruder [50]; and it has been found that if infection takes place during drug administration, selection of drug-resistant bacterial mutants does not occur.

IMMUNOLOGICAL DIAGNOSTIC TESTS

SEROLOGICAL TESTS

The mycobacteria causing tuberculosis in man are of the so-called human (hominis) or bovine (bovis) variants. These organisms are distinguishable by differences in certain metabolic activities (e.g., growth on solid medium, production of niacin in culture) and by the range of their pathogenicity for laboratory animals. Antigenically, they are similar [51], and the disease which they produce in human beings cannot be differentiated either on the basis of clinical course or by use of the diagnostic tests to be described. Most of the "unclassified" mycobacteria are related to the tubercle bacilli antigenically, although a few of them appear to fall into distinct groups [51]. This subject is in its early stages of exploration.

The sera of most individuals with active, inactive, or subclinical infection show evidence of exposure to the bacillus through the presence of antibodies detectable by the usual methods, including complement fixation, precipitation in agar, and agglutination of erythrocytes coated with constituents of tuberculin [52]. These antibodies are directed against proteins and polysaccharides; one hemagglutination test is designed to reveal antibodies of the latter kind [53, 54]. As mentioned before, tests in which bacterial lipids serve as antigen have also been described; work is in progress with phosphatides adsorbed to kaolin particles [55].

The usefulness of such tests to the clinician is dubious. Their potential value lies not in the detection of infection per se but rather in the distinction, on the basis of quantitation of the antibody response, between active disease and subclinical infection or inactive disease (the latter consists of previously clinically apparent disease which has left residual deformities revealed by x-ray examination). Several of the tests studied in the past decade have been thought to accomplish this distinction; among them are the Middlebrook-Dubos hemagglutination reaction [54], an agar diffusion test employing concentrated bacillary culture filtrates [56], and a phosphatide-kaolin agglutination test [55]. In all cases, there is doubt that the desired end has been attained, a tentative conclusion which is not surprising in view of the questionable validity of the expectation that antibody responses may be so well attuned quantitatively to extent of disease as to provide such information.*

SKIN TESTS

The classic test for the detection of delayed hypersensitivity in tuberculosis is carried out either with Old Tuberculin (OT), a heat-concentrated filtrate of a fluid culture of the bacillus, or with purified protein derivative (PPD), a less heated product of the precipitation of protein from culture filtrates by salts or trichloroacetic acid [57]. The former is used on the basis of dilutions; 0.10 ml. of 1 : 10,000 dilution of concentrated OT is generally employed as an initial test in order to avoid severe reactions in highly hypersensitive subjects. The concentration may be increased to 1 : 100, if required, without evoking troublesome nonspecific irritation. PPD is supplied as tablets of standardized amounts which are dissolved in buffer for use. It thus possesses the virtue of convenience of storage and quantitation, although OT also is durable and, when standardized on a biological basis, provides results in the same range of quantitation. It should be noted that PPD is a purified but not a pure protein preparation. It contains nucleic acids and some carbohydrate as well. These test substances are injected intracutaneously, and readings are usually made at seventy-two hours.

Patch tests have been used for children, but they have not attained the popularity of the intracutaneous tests. They consist of a gauze dressing containing dried OT and are applied to the skin, usually for forty-eight hours. These detect high levels of sensitivity, such as are revealed by the smallest test quantities of OT or PPD. Negative reactions should therefore be investigated further by application of the intradermal test.

There was recently introduced a multiple puncture method called the "tine test" [58]. This makes use of a four-pronged disposable instrument with concentrated dried OT deposited on the tines. These are punched into the epidermis and the plastic apparatus is discarded. The method is a most convenient one, and a recent comparison of its reliability with that of the intradermal PPD test indicates that it is a worthy substitute [58, 59].

As was suggested by previous discussions of antigenicity among the mycobacteria, cross-reactions in skin testing may be occasioned by subclinical infection with the unclassified mycobacteria, which may be widespread in their occurrence in some geographical areas [60]. "Tuberculins" made from filtrates of these organisms are being investigated for their usefulness in epidemiological studies.

* *Editor's comment:* See footnote p. 311, Chapter 20, which describes the findings of Turcotte *et al.* Since the 14S (macromolecular) antibodies which are predominant in PPD-positive healthy subjects can be depolymerized by mercaptoethanol, a high hemagglutination titer, which is unaltered by mercaptoethanol treatment, is strongly suggestive of active pulmonary disease.—B. R.

REFERENCES

1. Grunberg, E. (ed.) Current status of tuberculosis: 5. The significance of tuberculosis in public health. *Ann. N.Y. Acad. Sci.* 106:1 and 5, 1963.
2. Springett, V. H. Pulmonary tuberculosis in persons aged more than 50 years. *Bull. Int. Un. Tuberc.* 32:215, 1962.
3. Corpe, R. F., and Stergus, I. Is the histopathology of nonphotochromogenic mycobacterial infections distinguishable from that caused by *Mycobacterium tuberculosis? Amer. Rev. Resp. Dis.* 87:289, 1963.
4. Edwards, L. B., and Palmer, C. E. Isolation of "atypical" mycobacteria from healthy persons. *Amer. Rev. Resp. Dis.* 80:747, 1959.
5. Palmer, C. E., and Edwards, L. B. Geographic variations in the prevalence of sensitivity to tuberculin (PPD-S) and to the Battey antigen (PPD-B) throughout the United States. *Bull. Int. Un. Tuberc.* 32:373, 1962.
6. Rich, A. R. *The Pathogenesis of Tuberculosis* (2nd ed.). Springfield, Ill.: Charles C Thomas, Publisher, 1951.
7. Canetti, G. *The Tubercle Bacillus in the Pulmonary Lesion of Man.* New York: Springer Publishing Co., 1955.

8. Kotani, S., Kitaura, T., Hirano, T., and Tanaka, S. Isolation and chemical composition of the cell walls of BCG. *Biken J.*, 2:129, 1959.
9. Anderson, R. J. The chemistry of the lipids of the tubercle bacillus. *Yale J. Biol. Med.* 15: 311, 1943.
10. Asselineau, J. *Les Lipides Bacteriens.* Paris: Hermann et Cie, 1962.
11. Asselineau, J., Choucroun, N., and Lederer, E. Sur la constitution chimique d'un lipopolysaccharide antigénique extrait de *Mycobacterium tuberculosis* var. hominis. *Biochim. Biophys. Acta* 5:197, 1950.
12. Asselineau, J., Buc, H., Jollès, P., and Lederer, E. Sur la structure chimique d'une fraction peptido-glycolipidique (Cire D) isolée de *Mycobacterium tuberculosis* var. hominis. *Bull. Soc. Chim. Biol.* (Paris) 40:1953, 1958.
13. Sabin, F. R. Cellular reactions to fractions from tubercle bacilli. *Amer. Rev. Tuberc.* 44: 415, 1941.
14. Noll, H., Block, H., Asselineau, J., and Lederer, E. The chemical structure of the cord factor of *Mycobacterium tuberculosis. Biochim. Biophys. Acta* 20:299, 1956.
15. Landsteiner, K., and Chase, M. W. Experiments on transfer of cutaneous sensitivity to simple compounds. *Proc. Soc. Exp. Biol. Med.* 49:688, 1942.
16. Raffel, S. *Immunity* (2nd ed.). New York: Appleton-Century-Crofts, Inc., 1961.
17. Raffel, S. Chemical factors involved in the induction of infectious allergy. *Experientia* 6:410, 1950.
18. Seibert, F. B., and Soto-Figueroa, E. Study of tuberculin protein and polysaccharide antigens by gel-diffusion technique. *Amer. Rev. Tuberc.* 75:601, 1957.
19. Seibert, F. B., Figueroa, E. S., and DuFour, E. H. Isolation, identification, and classification of proteins of tuberculin and the tubercle bacillus. *Amer. Rev. Tuberc.* 71:704, 1955.
20. Morisawa, S., Tanaka, A., Shojima, K., and Yamamura, Y. Studies on tuberculin active peptide: I. The isolation, crystallization and properties of tuberculin active peptide from tubercle bacillus. *Biochim. Biophys. Acta* 38: 252, 1960.
21. Blum, H. L., Hesse, F. E., Kent, G. W., and Lichtenstiger, D. S. A tuberculin-testing survey of a school age population in eleven areas in California. *Amer. Rev. Resp. Dis.* 87:181, 1963.
22. Boyden, S. V., Sorkin, E., and Spärck, J. V. Observations on the Antibodies Associated with Spleen Cells at Different Stages of Immunization. In Holub, M., and Jarošková, L. (Eds.), *Mechanisms of Antibody Formation.* Prague: Publishing House of Czechoslovak Academy of Sciences; and New York: Academic Press, Inc., 1960. P. 237.
23. Freedman, S. O., Turcotte, R., Fish, H. A., and Sehon, A. H. The *in vitro* detection of "cell-fixed" hemagglutinating antibodies to tuberculin purified protein derivative (PPD) in humans. *J. Immun.* 90:52, 1963.
24. Raffel, S. The Mechanism Involved in Acquired Immunity to Tuberculosis. In Wolstenholme, G. E. W., Cameron, M. P., and O'Connor, C. M. (Eds.), *Ciba Foundation Symposium on Experimental Tuberculosis.* London: J. & A. Churchill, Ltd., 1955. P. 261.
25. Seibert, F. B. The interplay of an immune substance (possibly lysozyme) with tuberculopolysaccharide and its antibody in tuberculosis. *Amer. Rev. Tuberc.* 78:301, 1958.
26. Kochan, I., Patton, C., and Ishak, K. Tuberculostatic activity of normal human sera. *J. Immun.* 90:711, 1963.
27. Fong, J., Chin, D., and Elberg, S. S. Studies on tubercle bacillus-histiocyte relationships: V. Passive transfer of cellular resistance. *J. Exp. Med.* 115:475, 1962.
28. Nyka, W. Enhancement of resistance to tuberculosis in mice experimentally infected with *Brucella abortus. Amer. Rev. Tuberc.* 73:251, 1956.
29. Elberg, S. S., Schneider, P., and Fong, J. Cross immunity between *Brucella melitensis* and *Mycobacterium tuberculosis:* Intracellular behavior of *Brucella melitensis* in monocytes from vaccinated animals. *J. Exp. Med.* 106: 545, 1957.
30. Boehme, D., and Dubos, R. J. The effect of bacterial constituents on the resistance of mice to heterologous infection and on the activity of their reticulo-endothelial system. *J. Exp. Med.* 107:523, 1958.
31. Shilo, M. Nonspecific resistance to infections. *Ann. Rev. Microbiol.* 13:255, 1959.
32. Gözsy, B., and Kato, L. Studies on the effects of phagocytic stimulation on microbial disease: I. Action of some derivatives of the bicyclo [0.3.5] decapentaene skeleton on endothelial cells of skin vessels. *Canad. J. Microbiol.* 1:455, 1955.
33. Rees, R. J. W. The chemotherapeutic activity of Triton WR 1339 and Macrocyclon in murine leprosy. *Amer. Rev. Tuberc.* 76:915, 1957.
34. Mackaness, G. B. Cellular resistance to infection. *J. Exp. Med.* 116:381, 1962.
35. Mackaness, G. D. The behavior of microbial parasites in relation to phagocytic cells *in vitro* and *in vivo. Sympos. Soc. Gen. Microbiol.* 14:213, 1964.
36. Myrvik, Q. N., Leake, E. S., and Oshima, S. A study of macrophages and epitheloid-like cells from granulomatous (BCG-induced) lungs of rabbits. *J. Immun.* 89:745, 1962.

37. Nelson, D. S., and Boyden, S. V. The loss of macrophages from peritoneal exudates following the injection of antigens into guinea-pigs with delayed-type hypersensitivity. *Immunology* 6:264, 1963.
38. Martins, A. B., Moore, W. D., Dickinson, J. D., and Raffel, S. Cellular activities in hypersensitive reactions. III. Specifically reactive cells in delayed hypersensitivity: tuberculin hypersensitivity. *J. Immun.* 93:953, 1964.
39. Gowans, J. L. The fate of parental strain small lymphocytes in F_1 hybrid rats. *Ann. N.Y. Acad. Sci.* 99:432, 1962.
40. Porter, K. A., and Cooper, E. H. Transformation of adult allogeneic small lymphocytes after transfusion into newborn rats. *J. Exp. Med.* 115:997, 1962.
41. Rothschild, H., Friedenwald, J. S., and Bernstein, C. The relation of allergy to immunity in tuberculosis. *Bull. Hopkins Hosp.* 54:232, 1934.
42. Crowle, A. J. Immunizing constituents of the tubercle bacillus. *Bact. Rev.* 22:183, 1958.
43. Weiss, D. W. Vaccination against tuberculosis with nonliving vaccines. *Amer. Rev. Resp. Dis.* 80:340, 495, and 676, 1959.
44. Crowle, A. J. Tubercle bacillary extracts immunogenic for mice: 5. Specificity of tuberculoimmunity induced by trypsin extracts of tubercle bacilli. *Tubercle* 44:241, 1963.
45. Rosenthal, S. R. *BCG Vaccination against Tuberculosis.* Boston: Little, Brown, 1957.
46. Second Report to the Medical Research Council by the Tuberculosis Vaccines Clinical Trials Committee. BCG and vole bacillus vaccines in the prevention of tuberculosis in adolescents. *Brit. Med. J.* 2:379, 1959.
47. Mount, F. W., and Ferebee, S. H. Preventive effects of isoniazid in the treatment of primary tuberculosis in children. *New Eng. J. Med.* 265:713, 1961.
48. Comstock, G. W. Isoniazid prophylaxis in an undeveloped area. *Amer. Rev. Resp. Dis.* 86:810, 1962.
49. Ferebee, S. H., and Mount, F. W. Tuberculosis morbidity in a controlled trial of the prophylactic use of isoniazid among household contacts. *Amer. Rev. Resp. Dis.* 85:490, 1962.
50. Cassell, E. J. If you can't lick them, join them—or, the tactics of chemoprophylaxis and chemotherapy. *Amer. Rev. Resp. Dis.* 86:726, 1962. (Editorial.)
51. Parlett, R. C., and Youmans, G. P. Antigenic relationships between ninety-eight strains of mycobacteria using gel-diffusion precipitation techniques. *Amer. Rev. Tuberc.* 77:450, 1958.
52. Boyden, S. V. The immunological response to antigens of the tubercle bacillus: Some experimental aspects. *Progr. Allerg.* 5:149, 1958.
53. Meynell, G. G. The antigenic structure of *Mycobacterium tuberculosis* var. hominis. *J. Path. Bact.* 67:137, 1954.
54. Middlebrook, G. Laboratory aids to diagnosis and therapy. *Ann. Rev. Med.* 5:339, 1954.
55. Takahashi, Y. Specific serum agglutination of kaolin particles sensitized with tubercle phosphatide and its clinical evaluation as a serodiagnostic test for tuberculosis. *Amer. Rev. Resp. Dis.* 85:708, 1962.
56. Parlett, R. C., Youmans, G. P., Rehr, C., and Lester, W. The detection of antibodies in the serum of tuberculosis patients by an agar double-diffusion precipitation technique. *Amer. Rev. Tuberc.* 77:462, 1958.
57. Seibert, F. B., and Glenn, J. T. Tuberculin purified protein derivative: Preparation and analyses of a large quantity for standard. *Amer. Rev. Tuberc.* 44:9, 1941.
58. Rosenthal, S. R. The disk-tine tuberculin test (dried tuberculin-disposable unit). *J.A.M.A.* 177:452, 1961.
59. Badger, T. L., Breitwieser, E. R., and Muench, H. Tuberculin tine test: Multiple-puncture intradermal technique compared with PPD-S, intermediate strength (5TU). *Amer. Rev. Resp. Dis.* 87:338, 1963.
60. Edwards, L. B., Hopwood, L., Affronti, L. F., and Palmer, C. E. Sensitivity profiles of mycobacterial infection. *Bull. Int. Uni. Tuberc.* 32:384, 1962.

31. Coccidioidomycosis

CHARLES E. SMITH

COCCIDIOIDOMYCOSIS HAS A BROAD infection spectrum or biological gradient as the parasitic manifestation of the fungus *Coccidioides immitis* [1, 2]. Intrenched in nature, though with restricted geographic distribution, as a saprophyte in the soil [3], *Coccidioides* mainly infects man and other susceptible mammals when its minute arthrospores are inhaled and retained in the deep pulmonary spaces. Occasionally there may be a cutaneous portal of entry [4].

About three fifths of all human infections are asymptomatic [1], detectable only by "conversion" of dermal sensitivity to coccidioidin. At the other extreme are fulminating fatal disseminated infections, fortunately rare, in individuals completely anergic to coccidioidin [5]. Various clinical classifications have been suggested, but a merging spectrum is more descriptive. The manifestations have associated immunological indexes which, although imperfectly understood, assist in comprehension of the pathogenesis, diagnosis, and prognosis.

CLINICAL MANIFESTATIONS

PRIMARY SYMPTOMATIC INFECTIONS

Primary symptomatic infections may cause any or all of the following signs and symptoms in varying degrees of severity: pleural pain, fever, malaise, cough (generally nonproductive), headache, backache, nightsweats, anorexia, rash (a "toxic erythema," not to be confused with erythema multiforme), and nonexudative pharyngitis. Even though extensive pneumonitis may be revealed roentgenographically, physical signs are seldom present unless there is pleural effusion.

The pneumonitis may resolve completely or may leave pulmonary residua ranging from linear fibrosis ("scars") to solid "coin" lesions (coccidioidomas) and cavities. The last frequently develop early or later may shell out of coccidioidomas. Analogy with tuberculous cavitation has tempted some clinicians to assume that patients with these coccidioidal cavities are in grave risk of progressive disease. However, the lesion seldom spreads to new pulmonary sites (the cavity may increase locally in size), and rarely do subsequent extrapulmonary lesions develop [6, 7]. Characteristically, the complement-fixing titers of serum are low in patients with coccidioidal cavities and, indeed, in two fifths of them the serological evidence is not diagnostic [6]. Thus nearly all coccidioidal cavities are manifestations of *in situ* complicating sequelae of the primary infection. Less frequently, they represent progressing "active" infection [7]. Since the cavity often causes no symptoms, it may not be detected until some time after the primary infection. Then waning dermal sensitivity may be confused with the diminished skin sensitivity of disseminated disease. However, the contrasting high complement fixation (CF) titer in the latter assists in differentiation [8]. Occasionally, pulmonic cavities do occur in disseminating disease, but the walls usually are irregular ("moth-eaten") and frequently are thick, in contrast to the cystlike appearance of the "classic" coccidioidal cavities. Even though the cavitary residua never have been implicated in infection of other persons, rarely serve as foci for extrapulmonary disseminations, and seldom cause complicating infectious spread in the patient, they can pose serious problems because of hemorrhage, giant cavity formation (local increase in size), rupture into the pleural space with spontaneous hydropneumothorax, or invalidism due to repeated secondary bacterial infection.

Bronchiectasis, endobronchial disease, and spontaneous pneumothorax also occur occasionally as sequelae of primary coccidioidal infection. They are difficult to diagnose serologically, usually requiring recovery of the fungus.

As has been mentioned, infrequently there is a traumatic cutaneous [4] portal of entry of the primary infection. As with the tuberculous "chancre," the resultant local coccidioidal lesion and secondary lymphatic involvement may be confused with disseminated infection, but more often a single extrapulmonary cutaneous coccidioidal lesion is thought to be primary. Here again, the dermal sensitivity and serological tests assist in differentiation. Experimental infections in mice [9] and monkeys [10] suggest that these rare percutaneous infections are associated with even slighter risk of dissemination [2] than are infections acquired by the usual respiratory route.

Hypersensitivity may evoke erythema nodosum with or without erythema multiforme, phlyctenular conjunctivitis and arthritis, the classic "valley fever," "San Joaquin Valley fever," or "desert rheumatism" [11]. This symptom complex may be precipitated or exacerbated by a coccidioidin skin test. Occasionally, the allergic dermal or joint lesions are confused clinically with the extrapulmonary lesions of progressive primary or disseminated infections, but the exquisite sensitivity to coccidioidin in the former contrasts with the poor dermal sensitivity characteristic of the latter [5].

PROGRESSIVE PRIMARY OR DISSEMINATED COCCIDIOIDOMYCOSIS (COCCIDIOIDAL GRANULOMA)

Progressive primary or disseminated coccidioidomycosis is a complication of the primary infection when the individual's inadequate immune mechanism permits lesions to develop beyond the lungs. The extrapulmonary spread usually occurs during the course of the primary infection, and rarely years later. Occasionally, the extrapulmonary lesions develop after asymptomatic primary infections. We have records of a few patients in whom these lesions developed at the site of trauma experienced some time after they had left coccidioidal endemic areas. Thus one patient had coccidioidal peritonitis in Oregon after the branch of a tree struck his abdomen with sufficient violence to fell him. Another patient, in Idaho, wrenched his shoulder, and this was the site of an extrapulmonary coccidioidal lesion. Neither had had a known clinical primary infection, though they had resided in endemic areas one to two years before. However, these are rare exceptions. Very rarely, too, steroid therapy has been associated with development of late extrapulmonary lesions [12]. There has been some relation of steroids with disseminations during the primary infection, as when a patient in an endemic area is on heavy maintenance steroid therapy for sarcoidosis or leukemia and then acquires a primary coccidioidal infection. Characteristically, these patients develop precipitins and rising CF titers similar to those of other patients with disseminating disease. Their poor dermal sensitivity may be due either to the steroids or to the previously mentioned diminished sensitivity of dissemination. One notes that adrenocortical steroids do not interfere with the development of diagnostic humoral antibodies. Moreover, patients with steroid-associated disseminations usually respond well to amphotericin. Steroids have been used in treating patients given amphotericin to reduce reactions and, hopefully, to assist in its effectiveness. Corticosteroid therapy for cutaneous manifestations of coccidioidal primary infections [13] has not been reported to cause disseminations, but the numbers so treated are few, the dosages of steroids are relatively small, and such patients appear to have especially effective immunity mechanisms.

Table 31-1 contrasts erythema nodosum (classic valley fever [11]) and disseminated coccidioidomycosis as the immunological extremes of clinically manifest primary coccidioidomycosis.

The clinical manifestations depend on the sites and extent of the extrapulmonary lesions. Thus a single cutaneous lesion may evoke no symptoms. Miliary spread or many suppurating lesions with psoas and other cold abscesses usually are accompanied by septic fever and extreme toxicity. Lesions may occur in lymph nodes, bones (especially cancellous), joints, meninges, brain, peritoneal cavity, liver, genitalia, thyroid gland, pericardium, and occasionally myocardium, in fact, in any site involved by extrapulmonary tuberculosis, with the possible exception of the renal calyx or of the mucosal surfaces of the intestines.* The most dreaded extrapulmonary involvement is of the meninges. The clinical pic-

* During the writing of this chapter, I did learn of a patient with coccidioidal nephritis, but, to date, coccidioidal enteritis has not been observed.—C. E. S.

TABLE 31-1. Comparison of Valley Fever and Disseminated Coccidioidomycosis

Characteristics	Erythema Nodosum Valley Fever Complex	Disseminated Disease
Association with primary infection	Absolute	Generally close
Sex	Dominantly female	Dominantly male
Race	Dominantly white	Dominantly Negro-Filipino
Prognosis	Excellent	Grave
Immunological indexes		
Dermal sensitivity to coccidioidin	Very marked	Poor
CF Titer	Variable; generally low	Generally high

ture, cells, and chemistry of the cerebrospinal fluid are similar to those of tuberculous meningitis except that in three fourths of the patients the cerebrospinal fluid will fix complement, and complete CF is virtually diagnostic of coccidioidal meningitis. In a very few patients with extradural coccidioidal abscesses, there is increased protein in the cerebrospinal fluid which also fixes complement but with slight or no increase in cells and with normal glucose levels. Such patients respond satisfactorily to amphotericin intravenously without recourse to the intrathecal route. Because amphotericin does not cross the blood-brain barrier, intrathecal administration is necessary almost invariably for patients with true coccidioidal meningitis [14, 16]. Even with such vigorous combined treatment, the meningitis of only a few patients appears to have been arrested, although one patient apparently survived on intravenous therapy alone [17].

BIOLOGICALLY ACTIVE CONSTITUENTS AND METABOLIC PRODUCTS OF C. IMMITIS

In liquid media, *C. immitis* autolyzes and produces a mixture of antigen-haptens. These react with antibodies produced by *C. immitis* but also in varying degrees with those caused by *Histoplasma capsulatum* and *Blastomyces dermatitidis*. Given intradermally as coccidioidin, they evoke the delayed type of reaction comparable to that of tuberculin [5]. Similarly prepared materials are useful as antigens in serological tests [8, 18, 19]. Coccidioidin also may be prepared by autolysis of young mycelia [20].

The chemical composition of coccidioidin is poorly defined. The immunologically active nondialyzable portion consists of polysaccharides, mainly mannose with some galactose and another reducing sugar, and with 3 to 4 percent nitrogen [21]. The extent to which the nitrogenous material is discrete or combined in the polysaccharide complex is uncertain. However, it is not antigenic [5, 22] in that it rarely if ever sensitizes, nor does it evoke diagnostic humoral antibodies, even anamnestically, as does histoplasmin [23]. Coccidioidin occasionally enhances dermal sensitivity anamnestically [22], and nonviable mycelial suspensions can also evoke it [5]. The immunizing component of sporangial (spherule) vaccines [24, 25] is contained in the particulate components of the disrupted sporangia [26, 27]. Spherule vaccine also sensitizes animals [24, 26] and man and in one instance caused the appearance of CF antibodies (no precipitins) in the serum of an individual known to have been infected over twenty-five years before and in whom hundreds of coccidioidin tests subsequently had never evoked positive serological reactions.

IMMUNOLOGICAL INDEXES OF COCCIDIOIDAL INFECTION

DELAYED CUTANEOUS HYPERSENSITIVITY

Delayed cutaneous hypersensitivity to coccidioidin is a cornerstone in the diagnosis of coccidioidomycosis. However, both technique and interpretation can lead the unwary astray. The transfer of delayed sensitivity to coccidioidin by desoxyribonuclease (DNASE)-treated leukocytes from sensitive donors emphasizes the comparability of coccidioidin with tuberculin and other bacterial hypersensitivities [28].

The coccidioidin available generally is the filtrate of multiple strains of *C. immitis* grown for one to three months at 37°C. on chemically defined liquid asparagin synthetic medium. As already indicated, concomitant autolysis releases a variety of antigen-haptens. Commercial coccidioidin is standardized against Lot 29-31, which in turn was standardized against Lot 9 used throughout the Army-Air Force Studies of 1940–45 [5]. The selection of this coccidioidin is not by omniscience, as many seem to assume, but is based on a deliberate compromise between potency and tolerability coupled with specificity. The routinely dispensed commercial coccidioidin in 1 : 100 dilution may evoke occasional 4-plus reactions (using the same criteria as for reactions to tuberculin). Thus, for patients with erythema nodosum in whom the disease is suspected, a further tenfold dilution is preferable as the initial test. If this is properly performed as a *true* intradermal test and read at 24 *and* 48 hours, patients undergoing primary symptomatic nondisseminating coccidioidomycosis will almost always react. On the other hand, during the investigation of patients with coccidioidal pulmonary residua with or without cavitation, many will require 1 : 10 coccidioidin [6], and, indeed, some will not react even to this strength. In "routine" testing of considerable numbers of long-term asymptomatic residents of the San Joaquin Valley, with simultaneous tests with 1 : 100 and 1 : 1000 Lot 9 coccidioidin, the 1 : 100 coccidioidin elicited 11 percent more reactors than did the 1 : 1000 [5]. A similar comparison has not been made with 1 : 10 and 1 : 100 coccidioidin, but a few small series repeating 1 : 10 coccidioidin in those negative to 1 : 100 strength have detected approximately one-tenth more reactors. Investigation of the successful transfer of delayed hypersensitivity to coccidioidin by DNAse-treated leukocytes from San Joaquin Valley residents negative to 1 : 10 coccidioidin revealed that these donors reacted to *undiluted* coccidioidin [22, 28]. Thus, although dermal sensitivity may be of long duration and appears to be independent of exogenous re-exposure [5], it is subject to irregular and unpredictable waning which at times may be confused with the diminished sensitivity of disseminating disease.

Interpretations also must consider cross-reactions with histoplasmosis and blastomycosis and their respective dermal antigens [29–31]. Indeed, it was recognition of this cross-reactivity of coccidioidin which initiated the hypothesis that pulmonary calcifications in nonreactors to tuberculin might be due to histoplasmosis [29, 30]. Lots of coccidioidin vary in content of such cross-reacting substances produced by autolysis. Without specific means of chemically quantitating these antigen-haptens, we have attempted to screen out "excessive" cross-reactivity in human subjects. This procedure is, however, inexact, for there certainly is considerable individual variation in the cutaneous responses of recipients. Indeed, the variability in content of "specific" and "cross-reacting" antigen-haptens in the skin-testing material appears to be matched by variation in retention of the corresponding dermal sensitivities. Thus the coccidioidins commercially available and which we have used are, like our old Lots 9 and 29-31, of relative low cross-reactivity and have proved reasonably reliable in diagnosis of acute nondisseminating primary coccidioidal infections. However, the apparently greater cross-reactivity of histoplasmin coupled with possibly longer retention of this "group" dermal sensitivity may explain reactions evoked by histoplasmin in "natives" of coccidioidal endemic areas who do not react to 1 : 100 coccidioidin. Moreover, from time to time individual investigators have reported to us that "coccidioidins" which they have prepared have caused reactions in 1 : 100 dilution when our 1 : 100 coccidioidin evoked no reaction in the same individual. Admittedly, the variations in immunological antigenic "coverage" by the strains used are a possibility [31], but more probably there are variations in absolute amounts of the "specific" and especially the "cross-reacting" antigen-haptens. Imperfect as our attempts at standardization of "potency" and "specificity" have been, those individually produced coccidioidins have had no such scrutiny.

Although these complex immunological variations may obscure interpretation of coccidioidin skin tests, the more usual pitfalls are faulty technique and variations relative to the infection spectrum previously mentioned and to be discussed [31]. Attempts to administer coccidioidin by "scratch," "patch," "tine," and "heaf" techniques have been unsuccessful, and only intradermal administration of 0.1 ml. of the appropriate concentration of coccidioidin should be used. Special attention must be given to *true* intradermal administration, careful reading at 24 *and* 48 hours, noting induration with merely faint erythema which is easily overlooked. Moreover, meticulous attention must be paid to the use of Luer's syringes and diluting equipment, for coccidioidin and other adsorbed biologicals are not inactivated by autoclaving [5]. The *stability* both of undiluted and even of the diluted coccidioidin and its virtual lack of "antigenicity" are qualities previously mentioned but warrant emphasis. Moreover, there is absolute freedom from the possibility of "activating" or "exacerbating" a coccidioidal infectious process [5]. One-to-ten or occasionally even 1 : 100 coccidioidin may cause local necrosis ("4-plus" reactions) and even systemic malaise and fever in hypersensitive individuals. Very rarely, giant urticaria has followed. Occasionally, the hypersensitivity manifestations, erythema nodosum and erythema multiforme, may be precipitated or exacerbated by coccidioidin skin tests during the course of "active" primary infection. These lesions may be uncomfortable but have no known serious sequelae.

The association of vigorous dermal reactivity with favorable prognosis of primary coccidioidal infection has been emphasized already. The time sequence in the development of dermal sensitivity must always be kept in mind. While one sixth of those with symptomatic primary nondisseminating coccidioidomycosis do not react to 1 : 100 coccidioidin within the first week of illness, virtually all will react by the fourth week [5]. This "conversion" of dermal sensitivity is the most delicate of diagnostic procedures, although in view of the occasional anamnestic reaction to 1 : 10 coccidioidin [22], such conversion must be scrutinized carefully. If sensitivity to coccidioidin fails to develop or if it is lost during a primary infection, this anergy is ominous. Again, one must be aware of the possibility that intercurrent, unrelated severe illness may interfere with all types of bacterial type delayed hypersensitivity. Conversely, establishment or re-establishment of dermal sensitivity has been shown to be prognostically favorable in coccidioidal dissemination. However, the degree to which the dermal sensitivity *without infection* confers immunity is unknown. Thus far the crucial tests comparing the susceptibility of "normal" nonreacting men and those passively "sensitized" by DNAse-treated leukocytes and these, in turn, to those "sensitized" by spherule vaccine have not been conducted. Such studies will be very difficult, for only the incidence of clinically manifest coccidioidal infections can be compared, since the already induced dermal sensitivity of the second and third groups will make impossible the inclusion of the asymptomatic "converters" who account for 60 percent of the "naturally acquired" infections [1].

We recognize the "relative" immunity to exogenous reinfection of those known to have been infected in the past [2]. Here the positive reaction to coccidioidin indicates prior infection and thus immunity. True, at least one individual had this immunity "broken through" by very heavy respiratory superinfection, as did two others by percutaneous inoculation. However, these were very unusual situations. Even though dermal sensitivity temporally declines to levels no higher than those seen in patients with disseminating disease, those with such reduced levels are at minimal risk of endogenous spread even though viable fungi still may be present. Patients with coccidioidal pulmonary cavities who fail to react even to 1 : 10 coccidioidin do not develop extrapulmonary spread. Still, we must recall that the actual concentration of coccidioidin which we use is arbitrary.

FIXATION OF COMPLEMENT

Complement fixation is the most widely used serological test for coccidioidomycosis. Various types of coccidioidin autolysates are used as antigens [18–20]. The tests are especially valuable because they correlate with the severity of the coccidioidal infection, probably some quantitation of the interreaction of the multiplying fungus with the bodily tissues. Understandably, then, negative results are frequent when the infective process is minimal as in patients with asymptomatic pulmonary infections. Failure to fix complement is also frequent in patients with primary symptomatic infection and is diagnostic only in slightly more than one-half who have coccidioidal cavities [6, 8]. With few exceptions, complement is fixed by serum of patients having a single extrapulmonary lesion, whether in the skin, bone, or meninges, but the titer characteristically is low [8]. In serum of patients with fulminating extensive dissemination, the CF titer is high. Occasionally prezoning or incomplete fixations of complement are noted in serum of patients with extensive disease, but no one has observed terminal disappearance of CF.

The "cross-reactions" noted in skin tests with coccidioidomycosis, histoplasmosis, and blastomycosis also are seen in CF tests [8, 31, 32]. No cross-reactions have been noted with viral, rickettsial, bacterial, or other mycotic infection.

Variations in techniques and antigens make comparisons of titers obtained by different laboratories very risky. Comparison of the results of five techniques in four laboratories led us to predict overoptimistically [33] that each laboratory could use its own favorite technique so that a "standard-titered" control serum might indicate the critical titer below which risk of dissemination was unlikely and above which the possibility became more grave. However, when we extended the collaborative laboratories to eleven, the fluctuations became so great and unpredictable that we could not recommend a satisfactory CF antigen and "control" serum. Possibly "purified" antigens may be more consistent, but the apparent multiplicity of antigens in *C. immitis* and of corresponding humoral antibodies makes one apprehensive that the battery of antigen-antibody tests might be so extensive as to be impractical.

Serial tests on the same patient provide the most aid in prognosis [8, 31]. To minimize variations of technique in the hemolytic system, we always repeat simultaneously the previous positive serum with the new sample. Of course, variations of less than one or two serial dilutions are undependable, but if titers rise over several months there is increasing concern, and, conversely, successive reductions are cause for optimism. Unless these simultaneous comparisons are made, comparative prognostic interpretations are treacherous. Over the years we have become convinced that even though frozen, the titers of some (but not all) older sera have risen slightly, usually only as a "couple of plusses," reinforcing the importance of drawing no major deductions from less than one or preferably two full serial dilutions of changing titers.

The prognostic significance of CF tests is illustrated in Table 31-2. The patients were followed over the years in our coccidioidal studies for the Commission of Acute Respiratory Diseases of the Armed Forces Epidemiological Board. Amphotericin B is fungistatic and not fungicidal, so one strives to restrain the fungus until the individual's immunological mechanism takes over. The CF titer is one of the few indexes of this mechanism. About one-fourth (16/68) of those with initial CF titers exceeding 1 : 32 did not improve or relapsed. In contrast, only one twelfth (2/24) with initial titers *no* higher than 1 : 32 (and thus with less severe disease) experienced failure. During treatment with amphotericin, if a fourfold fall in titer occurred *and was maintained,* all patients ultimately had favorable results. However, this statement must be made cautiously, for occasionally some patients who had fourfold reductions did relapse. Their CF titers invariably *rose concomitantly*. Thus the mere fact of a fourfold fall in CF titer cannot magically transform the patient with disseminated progressive coccidioidomycosis into an individual "immunologically effective" with respect to coccidioidomycosis. We have long maintained that patients who smoothly localize their primary coccidioidal infections almost never "disseminate" years later. On the other hand, patients who disseminate may spontaneously "arrest" their disease. Occa-

TABLE 31-2. Association of Complement-Fixing Titers in Patients with Nonmeningitic Coccidioidal Disseminations Treated with Amphotericin B Intravenously

CF Titers	Good	Poor	Total
Initial CF>1:32	52	16	68
With 4-fold reduction	(43)	(0)	
No 4-fold reduction	(9)	(16)	
Initial CF<1:64	22	2	24
With 4-fold reduction	(19)	(0)	
No 4-fold reduction	(3)	(2)	
Total	74	18	92

sionally some of these patients relapse after ten or even fifteen years. Amphotericin B appears to afford a temporally compressed immunological "model." The CF titer, admittedly imperfect, is one mirror of this immunological model.

We previously mentioned the significance of fixation of complement by cerebrospinal fluid in the diagnosis of coccidioidal meningitis. Under vigorous intravenous and intrathecal treatment with amphotericin B abnormal findings (cells, chemistry, and fixation of complement) sometimes revert to normal, with *no* cells or fixation of complement and with normal ranges of protein and glucose. However, long observation of such patients is necessary to be sure these are "cures" and not just "arrests." But who can say when a patient with "arrested" coccidioidal dissemination is ever truly "cured"? Certainly continued surveillance with periodic cerebrospinal fluid examinations of patients with "arrested" meningitis and CF tests of serum of patients with "arrested" nonmeningitic disseminated disease should be maintained to appraise their immunological status.

PRECIPITINS

Precipitin tests will be mentioned only briefly. As we have reported [8, 18], the mixture of appropriate dilutions of coccidioidin antigens with serum of patients with acute symptomatic primary infections usually results in the formation of a carbohydrate "button." The time sequence is important [8], and the usual pattern is establishment first of dermal sensitivity, then of precipitins, and finally of CF. Although the dermal sensitivity always can be detected in primary nondisseminating disease, neither precipitins nor CF antibodies are detected in serum of *all* patients with symptomatic primary infections. The precipitins disappear first, and dermal sensitivity usually is the most persistent. However, sometimes complement continues to be fixed even after the patient no longer reacts to 1 : 10 coccidioidin. Frequently, precipitins are the sole serological proof of coccidioidomycosis in the relatively mild case.

A recent report [34] concludes that these precipitin tests are relatively valueless, but the technique used was not as we have described. Furthermore, the conclusions were based on examination of two small series, one of 65 "primary" sera and another of 5 sera "in the early stage," without a statement of *any* time relationship to date of onset. They are in contrast to our report [8] of sera from 5,579 *patients* with primary infections (most with multiple sera) to which the authors did not refer.

Admittedly, precipitin tests are crude, show frequent prezoning, and certainly cross-react with histoplasma infections. They probably compare in significance to Campbell's agglutination of sensitized collodion particles in histoplasmosis. Both have established diagnoses which otherwise would have been missed. Moreover, the coccidioidin precipitin tests frequently indicate the recentness of the infection [8]. They are of inconsequential value in the diagnosis of long-standing infections ("pulmonary residual"), nor are they worth performing on cerebrospinal fluid. In literally thousands of precipitin tests on cerebrospinal fluid specimens of hundreds of patients with coccidioidal meningitis, specimens from only two patients ever showed a positive result. Both patients had extensive involvement of the spinal dura with *very* high CF of cerebrospinal fluid. Precipitin titer has no significant prognostic implication. As we have mentioned, precipitins seem to persist longer in patients with progressive disseminating disease. However, they often disappear even in the face of the rising titer of CF concomitant with the manifestations of extrapulmonary lesions. Thus they appear to represent antigen-antibody systems different from CF and with more obscure relationship to pathogenesis. However, like gel diffusion techniques, precipitins may well have important application in the study of "purified" antigens and antibodies.

REFERENCES

For an extensive review of coccidioidomycosis with bibliographic coverage complete to 1958, see the admirably written monograph of the late Marshall Fiese (Fiese, M. J. *Coccidioidomycosis.* Springfield, Ill.: Charles C Thomas, Publisher, 1958). Indeed, a frequent pattern of many authors now is to cite the section in Fiese's monograph rather than the article of the original investigator.

1. Smith, C. E., Beard, R. R., Whiting, E. G., and Rosenberger, H. G. Varieties of coccidioidal infection in relation to the epidemiology and control of the diseases. *Amer. J. Public Health* 36:1394, 1946.
2. Smith, C. E., Pappagianis, D., Levine, H. B., and Saito, M. Human coccidioidomycosis. *Bact. Rev.* 25:310, 1961.
3. Meyer, K. F. Discussion of E. C. Dickson, Valley fever of the San Joaquin Valley and fungus *Coccidioides. Calif. West. Med.* 47:151, 1937.
4. Wilson, J. W., Smith, C. E., and Plunkett, O. A. Primary cutaneous coccidioidomycosis. *Calif. Med.* 79:233, 1953.
5. Smith, C. E., Whiting, E. G., Baker, E. E., Rosenberger, H. G., Beard, R. R., and Saito, M. T. The use of coccidioidin. *Amer. Rev. Tuberc.* 57:330, 1948.
6. Smith, C. E., Beard, R. R., and Saito, M. T. Pathogenesis of coccidioidomycosis with special reference to pulmonary cavitation. *Ann. Intern. Med.* 29:623, 1948.
7. Winn, W. A. Coccidioidomycosis: The need for careful evaluation in clinical pattern and anatomical lesions. *Arch. Intern. Med.* 106:463, 1960.
8. Smith, C. E., Saito, M. T., and Simmons, S. A. Pattern of 39,500 serologic tests in coccidioidomycosis. *J.A.M.A.* 160:546, 1956.
9. Pappagianis, D., Smith, C. E., Berman, R. J., and Kobayashi, G. S. Experimental subcutaneous coccidioidal infection in the mouse. *J. Invest. Derm.* 32:589, 1959.
10. Pappagianis, D., Miller, R. L., Smith, C. E., Kobayashi, G. Response of monkeys to respiratory challenge following subcutaneous inoculation with *Coccidioides immitis. Amer. Rev. Resp. Dis.* 82:244, 1960.
11. Dickson, E. C., and Gifford, M. A. *Coccidioides* infection (coccidioidomycosis): II. The primary type. *Arch. Intern. Med.* 62:853, 1938.
12. Castellot, J. J., Creveling, R. L., and Pitts, F. W. Fatal miliary coccidioidomycosis complicating prolonged prednisone therapy in a patient with myelofibrosis. *Ann. Intern. Med.* 52:254, 1960.
13. Levan, N. E., and Ernstein, H. E. Cortisone in coccidioidomycosis. *Calif. Med.* 84:193, 1956.
14. Winn, W. A. The use of amphotericin B in the treatment of coccidioidal disease. *Amer. J. Med.* 27:617, 1959.
15. Einstein, H., Holeman, C. W., Jr., Sandidge, L. L., and Holden, M. D. Coccidioidal meningitis: The use of amphotericin B in treatment. *Calif. Med.* 94:334, 1961.
16. Winn, W. A. Coccidioidomycosis and amphotericin B. *Med. Clin. N. Amer.* 47:1131, 1963.
17. Castellot, J. J., Pitts, F. W., and Mowrey, F. H. A case of coccidioidal meningitis arrested by prolonged therapy with intravenous amphotericin B. *Antibio. Med. Clin. Ther.* 6:480, 1959.
18. Smith, C. E., Saito, M. T., Beard, R. R., Kepp, R. M., Clark, R. W., and Eddie, B. V. Serologic tests in the diagnosis and prognosis of coccidioidomycosis. *Amer. J. Hyg.* 52:1, 1950.
19. Ajello, L., Walls, K., Moore, J. C., and Falcone, R. Rapid production of complement fixation antigens for systemic mycotic diseases: I. Coccidioidin; Influence of media and mechanical agitation in its development. *J. Bact.* 77:753, 1959.
20. Pappagianis, D., Smith, C. E., Kobayashi, G. S., and Saito, M. Studies of antigens from young mycelia of *Coccidioides immitis. J. Infect. Dis.* 108:35, 1961.
21. Pappagianis, D., Putnam, E. W., and Kobayashi, G. S. Polysaccharide of *Coccidioides immitis. J. Bact.* 82:648, 1961.
22. Rapaport, F. T., Lawrence, H. S., Millar, J. W., Pappagianis, D., and Smith, C. E. The immunogenic properties of coccidioidin as a skin test reagent in man. *J. Immun.* 84:368, 1960.
23. Saslaw, S., and Campbell, C. C. Effect of histoplasmin skin testing on serologic results. *Proc. Soc. Exper. Biol. Med.* 82:689, 1953.
24. Vogel, R. A., Fetter, B. F., Conant, H. F., and Lowe, E. P. Preliminary studies of guinea pigs against respiratory challenge with *Coccidioides immitis. Amer. Rev. Tuberc.* 70:498, 1954.
25. Levine, H. B., Cobb, J. M., and Smith, C. E. Immunogenicity of spherule endospore vaccines of *Coccidioides immitis* in mice. *J. Immun.* 87:218, 1961.
26. Levine, H. B., Miller, R. L., and Smith, C. E. Influence of vaccination on respiratory coccidioidal disease in cynamolgous monkeys. *J. Immun.* 89:242, 1962.
27. Kong, Y.-C.M., Levine, H. B., and Smith, C. E. Immunogenic properties of nondisrupted and disrupted spherules of *Coccidioides immitis* in mice. *Sabouraudia* 2:131, 1963.
28. Rapaport, F. T., Lawrence, H. S., Millar, J. W.,

Pappagianis, D., and Smith, C. E. Transfer of delayed hypersensitivity to coccidioidin in man. *J. Immun.* 84:358, 1960.
29. Smith, C. E. Coccidioidomycosis. *Med. Clin. N. Amer.* 27:790, 1943.
30. Smith, C. E., Saito, M. T., and Beard, R. R. Histoplasmin sensitivity and coccidioidal infection: I. The occurrence of cross-reactions. *Amer. J. Public Health* 39:722, 1949.
31. Smith, C. E., and Campbell, C. C. Question and Answer period on the serology of coccidioidomycosis: Proceedings of the Symposium on Coccidioidomycosis. *U.S. Pub. Health Serv. Pub.* No. 575, p. 53, 1957.
32. Campbell, C. C., and Binkley, G. E. Serologic diagnosis with respect to histoplasmosis, coccidioidomycosis and blastomycosis and the problem of cross-reactions. *J. Lab. Clin. Med.* 42:896, 1953.
33. Smith, C. E., Saito, M. T., Campbell, C. C., Hill, G. B., Saslaw, S., Salvin, S. B., Fenton, J. E., and Krupp, M. A. Comparison of complement fixation tests for coccidioidomycosis. *Public Health Rep.* 72:888, 1957.
34. Schubert, J. H., and Hampson, C. R. An appraisal of serologic tests for coccidioidomycosis. *Amer. J. Hyg.* 76:144, 1962.

32. *Histoplasmosis**

MICHAEL L. FURCOLOW

THE CLINICAL DISEASE

Histoplasmosis is properly classed in the group of hypersensitivity diseases for a variety of reasons. Although the fungus is inhaled into the lungs, as are many bacterial and viral agents, the response is related to the development of hypersensitivity to the organism rather than to spread of the actual infection in most cases. The incubation period is, in general, about two weeks, whereas most bacterial diseases have a much shorter incubation period and hypersensitivity per se seems to play a small part in their natural history, which is determined primarily by multiplication of the organisms and development of specific antibodies. In contrast, in the diseases of hypersensitivity such as tuberculosis, histoplasmosis, and coccidioidomycosis; the subsequent course seems to be much more related to the hypersensitivity phenomenon than to the multiplication of the organisms.

In these more or less chronic diseases, the organism inhaled into the lungs multiplies rather slowly and is carried to the regional lymph nodes from which in many, if not most, cases a few organisms spill over into the lymphatic system and blood stream. This is evident from the presence of calcified lesions in the spleen in a considerable proportion of patients [1]. However, it appears that at about the time when the organisms have multiplied sufficiently to spill over into the blood stream, there is coincident development of hypersensitivity which limits further spread of the organisms. In the very young or very old, or in patients whose immunity is apparently low for unknown reasons, the primary infection may progress fairly promptly to a disseminated systemic infection. This is characterized by multiplication of the fungus in the blood and a clinical picture known as disseminated histoplasmosis, in which the disease is found throughout the body. Clinical characteristics of this type of histoplasmosis are high temperature, large liver and spleen, and usually a rapidly fulminating course. Among older persons, a form of chronic dissemination is recognized which is slower in development and may first be recognized by biopsy of an ulcer in the mouth, pharynx, or larynx. The ultimate prognosis for the chronic disseminated type, however, is as poor as for the acute disseminated type [2].

In the average patient, however, the hypersensitivity develops usually within fourteen days after the initial infection, i.e., approximately simultaneously with the expected onset of symptoms. The acute disease then is localized to the sites in the lung in most cases and pursues a benign course. The acute disease is an influenza-like illness of varying severity, although perhaps one half to two thirds of the patients have no symptoms whatever. With more extensive pulmonary involvement, the influenza-like symptoms may be severe, confining the patient to bed for as long as one month to six weeks. Occasional cough, occasional chest pain, and severe prostration are prominent. The sedimentation rate is elevated. Complement-fixing antibodies begin to develop about two weeks after initial infection and are present in most cases within four to five weeks after the exposure. This would be two to three weeks after onset of illness and development of the skin test reaction. In about one third of the infected patients the lung lesions are sufficiently severe to cause subsequent calcification detectable on chest x-ray films [3].

The infection is widespread throughout the river valleys of the temperate zone, including the central and eastern river valleys of the United States, southern Canada, Central America, the three major river valleys of South America, and much of the central area of Africa. The major river valleys of India and Pakistan appear to be infected, as well as

* From the Communicable Disease Center, Public Health Service, U.S. Department of Health, Education and Welfare.

those of Burma and Thailand and other countries of Southeast Asia. The disease is thus of world-wide significance [4].

In this disease, as in tuberculosis, the primary infection, although localized and successfully resisted by the patient in a great majority of the cases, may become reactivated later on. For some reason, after the age of 50 there appears to be a decline in the resistance of the individual which is, as in tuberculosis, exemplified by flare-up of his previously apparently well-controlled *Histoplasma* infection. The symptoms in such instances are identical to those of chronic cavitary tuberculosis, i.e., low temperature, profuse sputum, sometimes blood-streaked, progressive loss of weight, and slow progression of disease accompanied by extension of the infiltrations in the lungs. Just as in tuberculosis, later reactivations of histoplasmosis occur in the form of apical, usually bilateral, fibrotic and cavitary infiltrations which are indistinguishable from tuberculosis. The prevalence of this type of disease throughout the endemic area is difficult to determine, but estimates have been made that at least 2,000 to 3,000 individuals a year with active histoplasmosis are admitted to sanatoria in the United States alone. This is based on a provable disease rate of 2 to 4 percent of admissions to certain tuberculosis hospitals in which satisfactory studies have been carried out and on widespread serological testing [5]. The untreated chronic pulmonary disease tends to progress, and recognition and treatment are of the utmost importance [6].

It is thus seen that although sensitization to the infectious agent undoubtedly plays a large part in the localization of the disease during the primary stage, hypersensitization or a failure of immunity results in the reinfection type of disease which develops in later life. Thus one is confronted with the problem of whether sensitization per se is helpful or harmful.

TOOLS FOR TESTING SENSITIVITY

Both skin tests and serological tests are employed in the clinical testing of sensitivity in histoplasmosis.

The only antigen widely used for skin testing is the mycelial phase antigen called histoplasmin, similar in general preparation to tuberculin and coccidioidin. This material is, in essence, the metabolic products of the growth of the fungus for four to five months in synthetic media at room temperature. After filtration and sterility tests, the material is titrated on sensitized human beings or guinea pigs and compared with a histoplasmin of known potency. The intradermal test is given and the reaction read in the same manner as in the tuberculin test. It appears from studies of histoplasmin that the active substance is a combination of protein and carbohydrate [7].

Three types of basic serological tests have been used in histoplasmosis: complement fixation, precipitin, and agglutination. It is not known whether these measure the same or different antibody responses. Since the fungus grows in either a mycelial or a yeast phase, depending on temperature, the mycelial phase antigen used in skin tests may be employed or the yeast phase antigen is grown at 37°C. Salvin [8] was the first to employ both the yeast phase and the mycelial phase antigens on the sera of animals in complement fixation tests. The first tests in human beings were performed in our laboratory in 1948 [9]. Ground yeast cells have also been employed in the complement fixation test as antigen, but have not given as satisfactory results as whole yeast cells [7].

Precipitin tests have been performed, both in agar and in capillary tubes, with histoplasmin or concentrates of histoplasmin. The precipitin test in agar does not appear to be as sensitive as the complement fixation test [10]. The capillary tube precipitin test has not been extensively applied [11]. Agglutination tests employing adsorption of histoplasmin on colloidion particles, latex particles, or erythrocytes have been used on a limited scale, as have agglutination tests with whole or disintegrated yeast cells. None of them, however, seems to have any advantage over the complement fixation test employing the histoplasmin and whole yeast phase antigens without modification. All of these tests have been reviewed by Salvin [7].

CLINICAL APPLICATION OF SENSITIVITY TESTS

SKIN TEST AS INDICATOR OF IMMUNITY OR SUSCEPTIBILITY

Skin reactivity in histoplasmosis appears to develop about two weeks after exposure [12]. Once positive, it tends to remain so. As seen in Figure 32-1, the prevalence of sensitivity

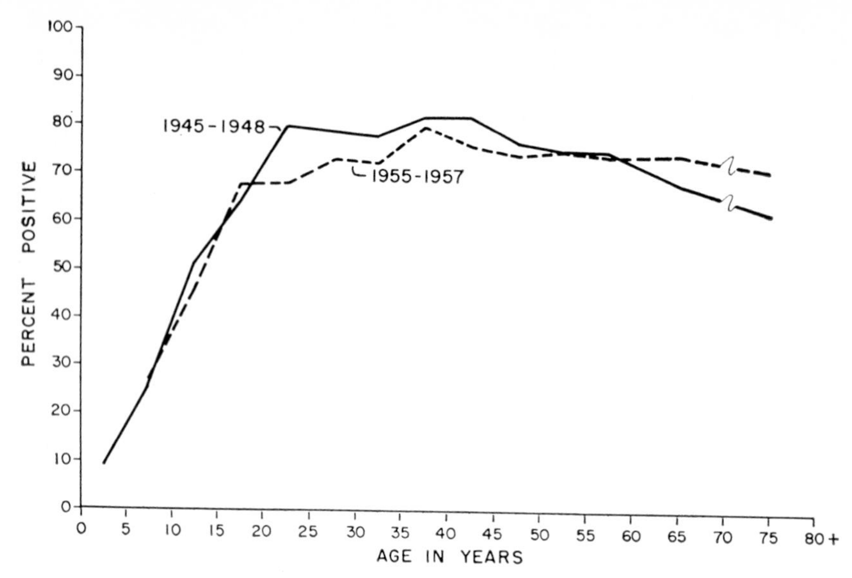

Fig. 32-1. Percentage of Kansas City, Mo., population with positive reactions to histoplasmin by age, 1945–48 and 1955–57.

among large numbers of persons in Kansas City was essentially the same in 1945 and in 1955. Sensitivity tends to decline somewhat in older age groups.

Nearly all patients with acute histoplasmosis as well as most patients with chronic pulmonary histoplasmosis appear to react positively to the skin test. Among 108 patients reviewed in our office, 83 percent had positive skin reactions [2]. However, if critical illness or disseminated disease is present, the reactivity of the skin may be abolished. Thus only 13 of 24 persons with disseminated histoplasmosis showed a positive reaction [2].

In considering skin reactivity as evidence of susceptibility or immunity, one is faced with the same problem as in tuberculosis. Although it seems clear that a positive skin reaction does indicate some resistance to the recurrence of primary disease on subsequent exogenous reinfection, it should be borne in mind that hypersensitization to the fungus must play an important part in the later development of cavitation and fibrosis due to endogenous reinfection. Thus the acquisition of the positive skin reaction is both a protection and a liability to disease in later life.

SEROLOGICAL TESTS AS EVIDENCE OF IMMUNE STATUS

Circulating antibody is demonstrable by serological tests. It does not, as far as we know, indicate immunity in histoplasmosis. Indeed, it appears that it indicates the activity of the infection rather than the degree of the immune response of the individual.

The complement-fixing antibodies develop more slowly than the skin test reaction in histoplasmosis and are only occasionally present two weeks after exposure, when illness occurs and the skin reaction becomes positive [12]. By three weeks, about two thirds of infected persons and at four or more weeks essentially all persons infected develop a positive serological reaction. It remains positive for varying intervals, the yeast phase longer than the mycelial phase, and gradually returns to negative with subsidence of the active disease, unless complications develop. If the disease is disseminated or poorly handled by the host's immune mechanisms, the serological titers tend to remain high and thus the test has some prognostic significance. The advantage of the complement fixation tests in histoplasmosis is that they serve as indicators of active disease and so have diagnostic as well as prognostic value. The question of whether the serological tests can indicate immunity or susceptibility in histoplasmosis is difficult to answer. As shown in Table 32-1, there is no clear relationship between survival and the serological reactions in disseminated histoplasmosis. Indeed, it appears that those who gave negative reactions to serological tests did somewhat better than those who had positive reactions.

The serological tests in chronic pulmonary

TABLE 32-1. Relation of Serological Reactions to Mortality in 36 Cases of Disseminated Histoplasmosis

Mortality	Serological Test: Positive (1:8 or greater)	Serological Test: Negative
Patients	20	16
Deaths	12	7
% Deaths	60	44

TABLE 32-2. Initial Serological Titers in 183 Culturally Proved Cases of Histoplasmosis, 1957–60

Yeast Phase Titer	Mycelial Phase Titer: 0	1:8	1:16	≧1:32	Totals
0	25	1	4	6	36
1:8	9	1	1	2	13
1:16	6	3	8	4	21
≧1:32	25	9	21	58	113
Totals	65	14	34	70	183

TABLE 32-3. Mortality and Reactivity[a] to Histoplasmin Skin Test among Patients with Strongly Positive and with Negative Serological Tests

Patients	Serological Tests: Strongly Pos. ≧1:32	Serological Tests: Neg.
Mortality		
Total patients	58	25
Deaths	16	4
% Deaths	28	16
Skin tests[a]		
Total tested	24	24
Positive	20	18
% Positive	83	75

[a] Skin test records were not available on all patients.

histoplasmosis show similar results. Table 32-2 illustrates the serological results in 183 culturally proved cases observed at the Kansas City Field Station, Communicable Disease Center, between 1957 and 1960 as part of the Communicable Disease Center Cooperative Mycoses Trials. As is quite evident, a large percentage of the patients had high titers in the serological test; indeed, 70 percent of the 183 had a titer of 1 : 32 or greater on one or both antigens and 58 had this titer on both antigens. In contrast to the latter are the 25 patients who had negative titers on both serological tests. One might well consider the significance of the serological tests by contrasting these two very different groups. Table 32-3 shows a comparison of the mortality and reactivity to the histoplasmin skin test of the 58 patients with a titer of 1 : 32 or greater to both antigens and the 25 individuals with negative results on both serological tests. It is seen that 16 of the 58 (28 percent) with strongly positive reactions died, in contrast to 16 percent of those with negative serological reactions. In other words, it certainly looks from this point of view that a negative serologic status was rather more in keeping with a low mortality than with a high one. This resembled the phenomenon in disseminated cases in Table 32-1. Also shown is the reactivity to the histoplasmin skin test among these two contrasting serological groups. It is seen that 20 of 24 (83 percent) of the strongly positive serological reactors had positive reactions to the histoplasmin skin tests in contrast to 18 of 24 (75 percent) of the negative reactors to the serological test. While this suggests perhaps a slight depression of the skin test reactivity among those who had negative serological responses, it does not seem statistically significant. One is forced to conclude, therefore, that the serological test is an indicator of susceptibility rather than of immunity, since patients with strongly positive reactions have greater liability to a fatal outcome than those with negative serological reactions.

FACTORS THAT INFLUENCE THE DISEASE

INFLUENCE OF SEX AND RACE ON IMMUNITY

The reaction rate to the histoplasmin skin test among large numbers of persons is essentially the same in males and females (Fig. 32-2).

When one considers symptomatic forms, however, the sex rates are quite different. Among 145 cases of acute symptomatic disease [12], only 40, or less than one-third, were in females. Among 22 of acute disseminated disease, only 8 were in females, and among 46 disseminated cases, only 10 were in females. Similarly, among 263 treated and untreated individuals with proved chronic pulmonary histoplasmosis included in the Therapy Trials

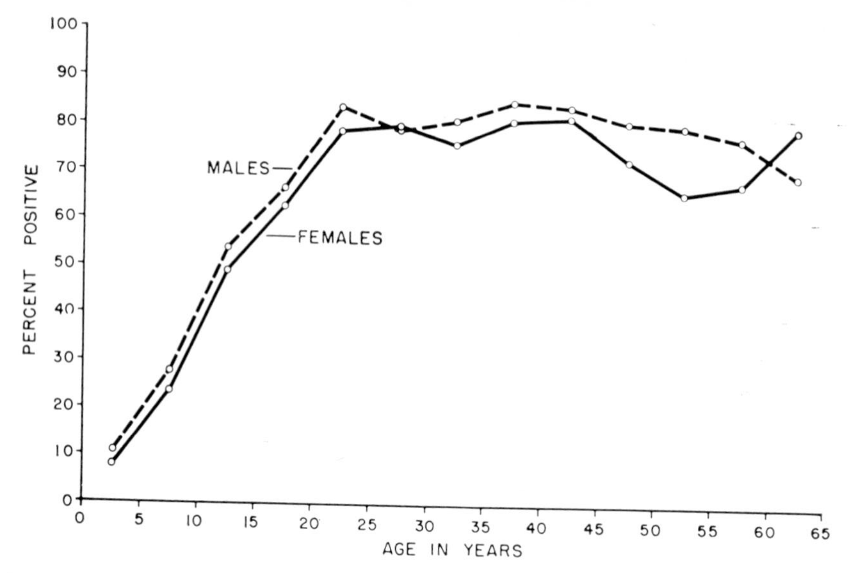

Fig. 32-2. Percentage of Kansas City, Mo., white population with positive reactions to histoplasmin by age and sex, 1945–47.

of the Communicable Disease Center Cooperative Mycoses Study, only 21, or less than 10 percent, were females [6]. It is quite clear, then, that while sex is not important in the incidence of infection, it is in manifest disease, since the acute pulmonary, disseminated, and chronic pulmonary forms are much less frequent in females than in males.

A somewhat similar observation may be made in regard to race. Figure 32-3 shows that the white and Negro rates of infection in Arkansas are essentially alike; similar figures have been gathered elsewhere. Again, when one comes to active disease, the figures are quite different. Only 7 of 145 patients with acute symptomatic disease seen at our Field Station were Negroes [12]. Only 2 of 46 with the disseminated form were Negroes, and there were only 4 Negroes among 263 individuals with treated and untreated chronic pulmonary disease reported to the Therapy Trials [6]. Again, as with sex, although race is not significant in incidence of infection, it does have a striking role in the incidence of disease. Indeed, in histoplasmosis, in contrast to tuberculosis and coccidioidomycosis, the disease is less common among Negroes than among whites.

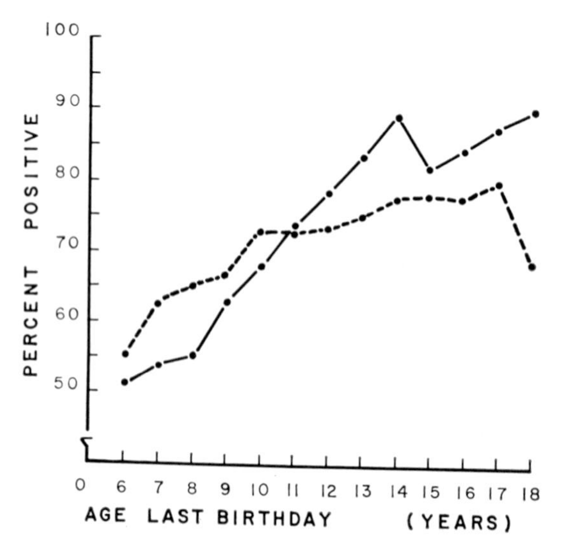

Fig. 32-3. Age-specific histoplasmin sensitivity rates in Crittenden County, Arkansas, March, 1960. *Solid line,* white population; *dashed line,* Negro.

INFLUENCE OF PRIOR INFECTION

The protection offered by primary infection against subsequent secondary or reinfection appears to be definite. No illnesses have been reported among our laboratory personnel, most of whom have positive skin reactions despite repeated exposure to the fungus. On the other hand, it does appear that this immunity is only relative. For example, one of our epidemiologists with a positive skin reaction had an illness shortly after exposure in a cave in New Mexico from which *Histoplasma capsulatum* was recovered. The illness was milder than usual and briefer, although accompanied by a rise in serological antibodies. That this relative immunity can be overcome is also illustrated by the epidemics in Mexico, in which Gonzales-Ochoa [13] has reported nearly 70 percent mortality among almost 200 guano workers who entered caves infected with *H. capsulatum* and acquired acute pulmonary disease. Since they had previously lived in the area of the caves and many had worked in them, it is probable that these cases represent reinfections, rather than primary infections. Also, they probably represent massive reinfections which result in an acute allergic death due to hypersensitization to the fungus rather than to the actual primary infection with the disease.

When one considers the chronic pulmonary or chronic cavitary type of disease, primary infection is certainly a liability rather than the reverse. Many such patients show evidence of what appears to be a well-healed calcified primary complex despite progression and exacerbation of the chronic pulmonary disease with sputum positive for *H. capsulatum*. Many of them are tuberculin-negative. In other words, as in tuberculosis, a primary infection, although reducing the possibility of later primary reinfections, does carry with it the risk of subsequent breakdown, resulting in the apical chronic cavitary "reinfection" type of disease. That this is more likely to occur after the age of 50 again resembles the pattern of tuberculosis.

INFLUENCE OF COINCIDENT DISEASE

The possibility that coincident disease may diminish the immunity to histoplasmosis has not been adequately studied statistically. However, it does not appear from a review of the literature that coincident illness, including neoplastic disease, except that of the blood-forming organs, plays any important part in increasing the susceptibility to histoplasmosis. With neoplasia of the blood-forming organs, such as the leukemia-lymphoma group and Hodgkin's disease, there is clearly an increase in the frequency of severe histoplasmosis. In this group, the disease tends to disseminate and pursue a rapid, progressive, downhill course. Occasionally other fungus diseases predispose to development of the secondary fungus disease which has been reported occasionally [14–16].

In view of the frequency with which chronic pulmonary histoplasmosis is found in tuberculosis sanatoriums and the similarity of chest x-ray appearance of the two diseases, one might question whether the occurrence of one predisposes to the other. Although 20 percent of our patients with proved histoplasmosis have both diseases, it appears from other evidence that this is a chance phenomenon rather than a cause-and-effect relation. In other words, the patient with cavitary histoplasmosis may be sent to a tuberculosis sanatorium because of the similarity of lesions, and occasionally he may also contract tuberculosis in the sanatorium because of inadequate isolation techniques. Some, of course, have both diseases on admission.

A review of the serological records from a large number of sanatoriums in the United States and Canada in which the admissions were surveyed for a five-year period indicates that the frequency of positive serological reactions correlates very well with the frequency of positive skin reactions throughout the general area. That is, the sanatoriums in areas with the largest percentage of skin reactors to histoplasmin also have the largest percentage of individuals with positive serological reactions and proved cases of histoplasmosis [5]. As in other diseases, therefore, it appears that patients with tuberculosis do not, per se, have an increased susceptibility to histoplasmosis.

INFLUENCE OF THERAPEUTIC AGENTS ON IMMUNE STATUS

There has been much discussion recently about the possible aggravation of diseases, particularly fungus diseases, by widespread use of antibiotics. Indeed, there seems no doubt about an increase in incidence of fungus infections in general associated with the use of some drugs or therapeutic agents. On the other hand, as was well brought out in the Symposium on Opportunistic Fungi [17], it seems clear that most of the increase in infections associated with therapy is due to invasions by the so-called "opportunistic" fungi, i.e., fungi which of themselves do not possess much pathogenicity. In this group, *Candida* is especially prominent. On the other hand, there is no evidence that the primary pathogenic fungi, such as *H. capsulatum* and *Coccidioides immitis,* have increased due to the use of therapeutic agents, with the exception of the adrenal corticosteroids. A similar generalization applies to the use of anticancer agents, again except for the adrenal corticosteroids. It is true that patients with leukemia have an increased incidence of systemic fungus infections, but the use of antileukemic agents does not seem to aggravate this situation. However, it has been established that pre-existing histoplasmosis may become disseminated when adrenal corticosteroids are used in the treatment of concomitant disease, including leukemia and sarcoidosis. In these conditions, therefore, corticosteroids are contraindicated in the presence of positive skin reactions or other evidence for histoplasmosis.

THERAPY

The only antifungal agent of value in the treatment of histoplasmosis is amphotericin B. This antibiotic must be given in a total dose of at least 2 gm. and only in severe cases. It is given by slow intravenous infusion and is often accompanied by chills and fever, which can be controlled by adequate premedication. A maximal dose of 50 mg. is recommended, usually given three times a week. A concurrent rise in the blood urea nitrogen level is not uncommon and may necessitate a temporary decrease in dosage. Results with use of this antibiotic have been promising in severe cases of acute pulmonary, disseminated, and chronic pulmonary varieties [6].

REFERENCES

1. Okudaira, M., Straub, M., and Schwarz, J. The etiology of discrete splenic and hepatic calcifications in an endemic area of histoplasmosis. *Amer. J. Path.* 39:599, 1961.
2. Course and Prognosis of Untreated Histoplasmosis: A United States Public Health Service Cooperative Mycoses Study. *J.A.M.A.* 177:292, 1961.
3. Furcolow, M. L. Clinical Types of Histoplasmosis. In Sweany, H. C. (Ed.), *Histoplasmosis.* Springfield, Ill.: Charles C Thomas, Publisher, 1960. P. 382.
4. Furcolow, M. L. Epidemiology of Histoplasmosis. *Ibid.*, p. 113.
5. Furcolow, M. L., Schubert, J., Tosh, F. E., Doto, Irene L., and Lynch, H. J., Jr. Serologic evidence of histoplasmosis in sanatoriums in the U.S. *J.A.M.A.* 180:109, 1962.
6. Comparison of treated and untreated severe histoplasmosis: A Communicable Disease Center Cooperative Mycoses Study. *J.A.M.A.* 183:823, 1963.
7. Salvin, S. B. Immunologic aspects of the mycoses. *Progr. Allerg.* 7:213, 1963.
8. Salvin, S. B. Complement fixation studies in experimental histoplasmosis. *Proc. Soc. Exper. Biol. Med.* 66:342, 1947.
9. Furcolow, M. L., Bunnell, I. L., and Tenenberg, D. J. A complement fixation test for histoplasmosis: II. Preliminary results with human sera. *Public Health Rep.* 63:169, 1948.
10. Schubert, J. H., Lynch, H. J., Jr., and Ajello, L. Evaluation of the agar-plate precipitin test for histoplasmosis. *Amer. Rev. Resp. Dis.* 84:845, 1961.
11. Salvin, S. B., and Furcolow, M. L. Precipitins in human histoplasmosis. *J. Lab. Clin. Med.* 43:259, 1954.
12. Tosh, F. E., Evans, J. C., Varga, D. T., and Furcolow, M. L. Acute pulmonary histoplasmosis: Clinical picture and follow up of over 200 cases. Transactions of the 21st Research Conference on Pulmonary Diseases (VA–Armed Forces), Jan. 22–25, 1962, St. Louis.
13. Gonzalez-Ochoa, A. Peculiaridades de la Histoplasmosis. Pulmonar Primaria Grave en el Pais. *Gac. Med. Mex.* 91:5, 1961.
14. Brandsberg, J., and Furcolow, M. L. Concurrent infection with *Histoplasma capsulatum* and *Blastomyces dermatitidis:* A report of five human cases. *New Eng. J. Med.* 270:874, 1964.
15. Allison, F., Jr., Lancaster, M. G., Whitehead, A. E., and Woodbridge, H. B., Jr. Simultaneous infection in man by *Histoplasma capsulatum* and *Blastomyces dermatitidis. Amer. J. Med.* 32:476, 1962.
16. Layton, J. M., McKee, A. P., and Stamler, F. W. Dual infection with *Blastomyces dermatitidis* and *Histoplasma capsulatum. Amer. J. Clin. Path.* 23:904, 1953.
17. Furcolow, M. L. Fungus diseases. *Arizona Med.* 20:75, 1963.

33. Brucellosis

WESLEY WILLIAM SPINK

THE PATHOGENESIS OF BRUCELLOSIS simulates that of tuberculosis. After invasion of the tissues, brucellae localize within monocytes, granulomatous lesions evolve, and hypersensitivity of the delayed type develops. Brucellosis is characterized by fever, chills, sweats, weakness, headaches, and somatic pains and aches. The illness usually lasts not more than three to six months, although, occasionally, prolonged disease with complications may continue for years with episodes of intermittent chills and fever. There is evidence that some of the manifestations of the acute, and also of the more chronic, stages are related to acquired *Brucella* hypersensitivity.

ETIOLOGY

Although atypical *Brucella* strains are responsible for animal and human disease, three species are usually involved (Table 33-1). *Brucella abortus* causes the less serious disease, although severe illness with complications can occur. This species is responsible for most of the cases in the United States. *Br. melitensis* results in more serious and prolonged illness than that due to *Br. abortus*. Spondylitis and neurological disturbances are common complications. *Br. suis* causes a severe and prolonged illness, often complicated by suppuration of the bones and other tissues. *Br. abortus* strain 19 has also been included as a cause of human illness. This is a stable strain with attenuated virulence and is widely used as a living vaccine for bovine immunization. Veterinarians have become accidentally infected while handling strain 19 vaccine, and in this group of patients *Brucella* hypersensitivity has been observed as a participating factor in their illness [1]. This strain does not cause chronic infection in animals.

TABLE 33-1. Species of Brucella Responsible for Animal and Human Brucellosis

Species	Reservoir
Br. abortus	Cattle
Br. melitensis	Sheep and goats; occasionally swine; rarely cattle
Br. suis	Swine; rarely cattle
Br. abortus strain 19	None

PATHOLOGY

The tissue reactions following the introduction of brucellae into animals have been detailed elsewhere [2]. Briefly, the organisms quickly localize in tissues having an abundance of reticuloendothelial cells, e.g., liver, spleen, bone marrow, and lymph nodes. The key cells of the host in the defense against brucellae are macrophages. Within a week or two after invasion of the host, giant cells consisting of epithelioid cells are seen in the aforementioned tissues. With the appearance of epithelioid cells, which probably evolve from macrophages or monocytes, brucellae disappear from the tissues. Caseation occurs only in very chronic cases usually due to *Br. suis*. The evolution of the noncaseating granuloma reflects a good defense mechanism. The appearance of granuloma does not seem to be dependent on acquired *Brucella* hypersensitivity. If viable brucellae persist, polymorphonuclear leukocytes are noted among necrotic cells, and suppuration may take place. This tissue response denotes an unfavorable defense mechanism.

Coincident with the appearance of the granuloma, *Brucella* agglutinins are found in the blood, and dermal *Brucella* hypersensitivity of the delayed type can be demonstrated. All of these features commonly occur during the incubation period, which is usually one to three weeks. Observations in human subjects have not shown a clear-cut relationship between the appearance of agglutinins and skin hypersensitivity to *Brucella* antigen. The interrelationship of residuum of brucellae in the tissues and acquired hypersensitivity to the genesis of symptoms is discussed below.

SOME IMMUNOLOGICAL FACTORS

Following the introduction of brucellae into experimental animals, e.g., guinea pigs and rabbits, a series of immunological events occurs during the incubation period. *Brucella* agglutinins, precipitins, and complement-fixing antibodies appear in the serum, and a delayed type of skin hypersensitivity can be elicited. The same pattern has been observed in man following infection. It is of interest that there is usually an interval of 1 to 3 weeks following human infections before the onset of symptoms. Agglutinating antibodies have been detected in the γ- and β-globulins of man [3]. At a later period, antibodies that block the agglutination reaction appear first in the γ-globulins and later in the β-globulins. These blocking antibodies often persist in the serum after the agglutinating antibodies disappear. The prozone phenomenon in the agglutination reaction is probably related to the blocking phenomenon.

RELATION OF HYPERSENSITIVITY TO ILLNESS

The contribution of acquired *Brucella* hypersensitivity to the symptoms and signs of active brucellosis has been studied in groups of individuals whose occupations bring them into contact with *Brucella* organisms or antigens, including veterinarians. The relation between hypersensitivity and illness has been most significant in veterinarians known to have had brucellosis in the past and who have accidentally infected themselves with the vaccine, *Br. abortus* strain 19, while immunizing cattle. In these circumstances, following introduction of brucellae into the skin of a finger or hand with a needle, severe local swelling and redness have occurred within 4 to 6 hours, associated with chills and fever. After appropriate antibiotic therapy, the localized swelling and systemic manifestations have usually subsided within 24 to 48 hours. However, if a similar mishap occurs in a veterinarian who has not had a previous *Brucella* infection, i.e., in an individual without *Brucella* agglutinins in the serum and no dermal reaction to *Brucella* antigen, there will be no immediate local reaction following the accident. After a week or more, such an individual may complain of an illness that suggests the "flu" to him. At this time, agglutinins in the serum can be demonstrated, and the skin reaction is usually positive. In addition, *Br. abortus* strain 19 organisms have been isolated from the blood.

Other groups of individuals have been encountered in whom illness was related to acquired *Brucella* hypersensitivity. Laboratory workers, who have had brucellosis in the past, have experienced all of the manifestations of acute brucellosis on inhaling air-borne particles of nonviable *Brucella* antigen. Within a few hours after such exposure they have had chills, fever, sweats, headache, and somatic aches and pains for 24 to 48 hours. A similar pattern of reaction has been observed in laboratory personnel who have been sensitized to *Ascaris lumbricoides* and who are then exposed to *Ascaris* antigen. More limited evidence has been acquired from employees in meat-packing plants who have recovered from brucellosis and then, in a state of good health, have come in contact with the tissues of infected animals. Such individuals have had a temporary illness of only a few days that has been compatible with acute brucellosis but did not reveal serological or bacteriological evidence of reinfection.

One of the most difficult problems in a significant group of patients involves those individuals who have had brucellosis and have recovered, but who have complained subsequently of symptoms consistent with a recurrence of the disease. No definite history of reexposure to the disease could be obtained. However, the possibility did exist that foci of intracellular brucellae remained in the tissues and that, periodically, viable cells or antigen was liberated into the circulation of these highly sensitized individuals, resulting in temporary illness. The persistence of brucellae in the tissues of experimentally infected animals has been demonstrated months after intensive antibiotic therapy [4]. Suppurative *Brucella* foci in man with accompanying illness that endured for several years have been occasionally encountered [5].

The role of *Brucella* antigen in the pathogenesis of brucellosis on the basis of hypersensitivity has been further explored with *Brucella* endotoxin. The injection of endotoxin into patients who had recovered from brucellosis caused fever, chills, sweating, myalgia, headache, and malaise [6]. The severity of the reaction was directly related to the local intensity of the *Brucella* skin reaction. These systemic manifestations could be suppressed or greatly ameliorated by pretreatment with ACTH or adrenal corticosteroids. Furthermore, patients with severe acute brucellosis occurring under natural conditions promptly improved following treatment with ACTH or corticosteroids [7]. These experimental and clinical observations suggested that the action of *Brucella* endotoxin involves an antigen-antibody interaction of the delayed type. Further studies have supported the concept that the action of endotoxin is mediated through complement resulting in the liberation of histamine and probably other amines [8, 9].

The relation of hypersensitivity to inflammation in brucellosis was demonstrated by Dr. A. I. Braude in a patient at the University of Minnesota Hospitals convalescing from acute brucellosis due to *Br. abortus.* Intradermal tests with *Brucella* antigens were followed by chills and fever, and forty-eight hours later icterus was apparent. Liver biopsy revealed numerous granulomas. Sixteen days later the jaundice had subsided and another hepatic biopsy showed only an occasional granuloma. Although jaundice is rare in acute brucellosis, hepatic granulomas with lymphocytic infiltration are common. In the present case, a state of *Brucella* hypersensitivity accentuated the hepatic inflammation because of the intradermal introduction of antigen, and liver function was altered to such an extent that jaundice appeared.

THERAPY IN RELATION TO HYPERSENSITIVITY

Two approaches have been employed in the management of brucellosis, with the common objective of subduing the undesirable effects of hypersensitivity and inflammation. The first procedure is used in patients with presumed chronic brucellosis, the diagnosis of which has been substantiated by correlating nonspecific symptomatology with a positive intradermal *Brucella* reaction. The basic thesis has been that in a persistent low-grade infection, a source of *Brucella* antigen is present in a sensitized patient. Since the chronic illness is due to *Brucella* hypersensitivity, it should be reasonable to desensitize such patients with injections of *Brucella* antigen. Many clinicians have used this method, but the over-all evidence that such therapy is effective remains unconvincing. Desensitization programs have not been used for several years at the University of Minnesota Hospitals.

A second approach has been directed to a more nonspecific control of inflammation and toxemia and has been used most often in patients with severe acute disease. ACTH, cortisol, or prednisone has been successfully administered to such patients along with a tetracycline drug. When an antibiotic has been used alone, improvement has been slow. When combined with a steroid, striking improvement has occurred within 24 hours. Steroid therapy is continued for 48 to 72 hours, and the antibiotic is given for 21 days. This combination is now recommended for seriously ill patients by the Expert Committee on Brucellosis of the World Health Organization [10].

The prevailing opinion in the Minnesota group has been that therapy should be directed at eliminating brucellae from the tissues with appropriate chemotherapy, and rehabilitation of the patient with rest and graduated physical activity.

IMMUNOLOGICAL FACTORS IN RECOVERY

The appearance of *Brucella* agglutinins, precipitins, complement-fixing antibodies, and opsonins in the serum of subjects recovering from brucellosis reflects the humoral aspects of anti-*Brucella* immunity. The titer of agglutinins cannot be correlated with the antibacterial activity of serum. Hall [11] found in *in vitro* studies that undiluted fresh serum possessed considerable bactericidal activity, indicating that a specific inhibitor of anti-*Brucella* activity was present. The clinical significance of this paradox is not understood. Convalescent serum protects animals from the lethal action of *Brucella* endotoxin.

The defense mechanism of the host against brucellae is also dependent on cellular tissue factors, and these may have more significance than the humoral antibodies. The monocyte appears to be the major cell in tissue immunity [12]. Contrasted with mononuclear cells from normal animals, monocytes from infected animals dispose of intracellular brucellae more readily. This anti-*Brucella* action is enhanced by immune serum.

REFERENCES

1. Spink, W. W. The significance of bacterial hypersensitivity in human brucellosis: Studies on infection due to strain 19 *Brucella abortus*. *Ann. Intern. Med.* 47:861, 1957.
2. Spink, W. W. *The Nature of Brucellosis*. Minneapolis: University of Minnesota Press, 1956.
3. Zinneman, H. H., Glenchur, H., and Hall, W. H. The nature of blocking antibodies in human brucellosis. *J. Immun.* 83:206, 1959.
4. Spink, W. W., and Bradley, G. M. Persistent parasitism in experimental brucellosis: Attempts to eliminate brucellae with long-term tetracycline therapy. *J. Lab. Clin. Med.* 55:535, 1960.
5. Spink, W. W. Host-parasite relationship in human brucellosis with prolonged illness due to suppuration of the liver and spleen. *Amer. J. Med. Sci.* 247:129, 1964.
6. Abernathy, R. S., and Spink, W. W. Studies with *Brucella* endotoxin in humans: The significance of susceptibility to endotoxin in the pathogenesis of brucellosis. *J. Clin. Invest.* 37:219, 1958.
7. Spink, W. W., and Hall, W. H. The influence of cortisone and adrenocorticotrophic hormone (ACTH) in acute and chronic human brucellosis. *J. Clin. Invest.* 31:958, 1952.
8. Weil, M. H., and Spink, W. W. A comparison of shock due to endotoxin with anaphylactic shock. *J. Lab. Clin. Med.* 50:501, 1957.
9. Spink, W. W., Davis, R. B., Potter, R., and Chartrand, S. The initial stage of canine endotoxin shock as an expression of anaphylactic shock: Studies on complement titers and plasma histamine concentrations. *J. Clin. Invest.* 43:696, 1964.
10. Joint FAO/WHO Expert Committee on Brucellosis. *Third Report*. Geneva: World Health Organization, 1958.
11. Hall, W. H. The Bactericidal Action of Human Blood Against Brucella and Its Specific Inhibition. In *Third Inter-American Congress on Brucellosis*. Washington, D.C.: Pan American Sanitary Bureau, WHO, 1950. P. 87.
12. Pomales-Lebron, A., and Stinebring, W. R. Intracellular multiplication of *Brucella abortus* in normal and immune mononuclear phagocytes. *Proc. Soc. Exp. Biol. Med.* 94:78, 1957.

34. Candidiasis (Moniliasis) and Aspergillosis

LORRAINE FRIEDMAN

CANDIDIASIS (MONILIASIS)

Candidiasis (Moniliasis) is an acute or chronic infection that usually involves the skin or mucous membranes, but not infrequently the lungs or bronchi, and occasionally disseminates through the blood stream. The infection is caused chiefly by the yeast *Candida albicans,* but other species, e.g., *C. tropicalis, C. krusei, C. parakrusei,* and *C. guilliermondi,* may be responsible [1]. Ordinarily, these agents are part of the saprophytic flora, and man apparently is infected endogenously, although it is not clear why only certain individuals contract the disease. Obviously, there must be predisposing factors, for it has been shown experimentally that contact of human skin even with massive numbers of organisms applied daily to a single area does not result in infection [2]. Debilitating disease has long been thought to predispose to candidiasis, but the increase, of systemic disease in particular, which paralleled the introduction of antibiotics, steroids, roentgen irradiation, and bone marrow depressants leaves little doubt that modern modes of therapy also alter susceptibility to *Candida.* It has been shown that cortisone enhances experimental candidal infections in mice [3], correlating well with clinical experience, and with this as well as antineoplastic therapy it seems probable infection in large part is in some way related to suppression of immune mechanisms [4, 5]. However, a survey of patients with disseminated neoplasia, either leukemia or lymphoma, with or without antineoplastic therapy, revealed that *Candida*-reacting serum antibody was not affected either by the therapy or by the progression of neoplastic growth; the titers were of the same level as in normal populations [6].

In the case of infant infections, it is generally thought that the major source is passage of the newborn through the birth canal [7, 8], although some evidence to the contrary has been presented [9]. The factors predisposing to such infections are not at all clear. Some observers [9] feel that premature or debilitated infants are particularly prone to infection, but this view has not been entirely accepted. In at least one study, these factors were not found operative, nor did preceding antibiotic therapy raise the incidence of disease [10].

The diagnosis of *Candida* infections has been difficult inasmuch as species of *Candida,* especially *C. albicans,* are very common on the mucous membranes and in the feces of a considerable percentage of normal individuals [11, 12], and therefore isolations in culture from sources other than closed systems of the body have little meaning. Nor has detection of antibodies in the sera of patients proved of practical value [2, 13], for antibodies are often present in normal individuals [14–16] and patients with severe infections may have none [17]. There seems to be some correlation, however, between the appearance of complement-fixing antibodies and the anogenital pruritus which often follows tetracycline therapy [18]. Also, a *Candida* polysaccharide was reported [19, 20] to precipitate with the sera of 12 of 13 patients with deep-seated infections but with sera of only 6 of 23 superficially infected individuals; among 16 patients with tuberculosis, only 4 had precipitins, and sera of only 1 of 121 normal adults and of 5 of 59 normal children were positive. Recently, British workers [21] have reported a clear-cut relationship between serum agglutinins and the presence of *Candida,* saprophytic or otherwise, and it was stated that titers higher than 1 : 8 in patients with skin lesions containing *C. albicans* are good evidence of infection by *C. albicans.* They confirmed, however, the general observation that the absence of antibodies does not rule out *Candida* infection.

As in diagnosis, there is little to encourage the use of serology in prognosis, for there is little evidence that a pronounced rise in titer occurs during an infection [13, 16]. In exception, it has been stated that the antibody titer to the polysaccharide described above correlates well with the severity of the disease, with the titer dropping as clinical improvement becomes noticeable [20]. These conclusions, however, are based on experience with only three cases.

Hypersensitivity reactions in the skin also have generally been considered unreliable for diagnostic purposes [13, 21, 22]. In one study, 43 percent of individuals with cutaneous candidiasis failed to react to oidiomycin, an aqueous extract of *C. albicans,** while 46 percent of 192 noninfected individuals gave positive reactions [23]. The antigens prepared by various Japanese workers, however, appear more promising. With soluble substances from disrupted cells, skin hypersensitivity was observed in 19 of 26 patients with candidiasis but none in 56 controls [24], and the polysaccharide antigen described previously [20] had a specificity in skin testing similar to that noted in the serological investigations, i.e., positive reactions occurred primarily among infected individuals. It is claimed also that this antigen is useful in following the progress of a patient because positive reactions seemed correlated with the severity of the disease, converting to negative with clinical improvement. Others [17] have stated that a skin test is useful in the management of a patient. The possibility has been suggested, however, that positive cutaneous reactions to tests with *Candida* materials are not even related to hypersensitivity; rather, they are due to toxic substances of the organism [2]. This property of *Candida* is discussed later.

The sensitizing properties of *Candida* have been demonstrated in experimental candidiasis. Long ago it was shown that the water-soluble fraction, essentially polysaccharide, of several yeasts can elicit anaphylactic shock in sensitized animals [25, 26], and eye hypersensitivity also was demonstrated [27]. These observations have been confirmed in recent years [28], and some suggestive evidence has been presented that a host immunized with *C. albicans* may also develop tuberculin hypersensitivity [29].

There is only scant experimental evidence that hypersensitivity plays a role in the pathogenesis of candidiasis. In one study [30], sensitized rabbits were considered more susceptible to challenge, and later experiments [31], in which immunized rabbits died earlier than nonimmunized rabbits following challenge with *C. albicans,* seem confirmatory. It has also been suggested the occasional lesions with cellular necrosis and inflammatory exudate seen in experimentally infected guinea pigs could be caused by hypersensitivity, although a toxin was equally considered the possible cause [32]. Investigations clearly defining the role of hypersensitivity in *Candida* infections are lacking.

Despite the lack of laboratory data, however, it is rather obvious that hypersensitivity can be an important feature in infection with *Candida,* for patients not infrequently experience secondary eruptions of an allergic nature. Such lesions, termed "ids," are sterile, commonly occurring as a series of vesicles, and the patient usually has a strongly positive skin-test reaction. A number of cases have been reported in which the "candidia" was facial [33]. In recent years, hypersensitivity has also been thought responsible for clinical respiratory allergy to the organism. In one study, 7 patients for whom no other cause of the asthmatic symptoms could be found were hyposensitized beneficially [34], and in another study [35], 129 of 1,131 patients were reported to have respiratory allergy to *C. albicans* and 55 of these responded to hyposensitization. A rather unusual allergy that has been reported is the seasonal mass occurrence in certain areas of Asia of gastrointestinal upsets caused by eating pineapples contaminated with *C. tropicalis* and in which the allergic reaction was to the yeast [36].

The question of whether or not there is an immune response in candidiasis has not been resolved. The lack of resistance of the newborn infant to *C. albicans* infections has been attributed to defects in immunity as yet not understood [10]. In experimental candidiasis, one investigator [37] has repeatedly noted a lack of cellular response with only normal activity of the reticuloendothelial system, and in another instance [32], agglutinating antibodies failed to protect rabbits against the lethal effects of *C. albicans.* Nevertheless there is some evidence that an immune mechanism may be operative, as exemplified by the interesting case of a patient who recovered from pulmonary candidiasis following serum ther-

* Available from commercial sources specializing in the preparation of skin-testing allergens.

apy [38]. Prior to the therapy, the patient seemed to be in antigen excess because reaction to a skin test with autogenous vaccine was negative and agglutinins could not be found in her serum. Injection of 0.1 ml. of anti-*C. albicans* rabbit serum, however, resulted in an immediate wheal and flare while a control skin test with normal rabbit serum caused no response. She was given the immune serum daily for approximately three weeks, during which time there was dramatic clinical improvement, agglutinins appeared, and she lost the dermal reactivity to the immune serum. Another observation [39] suggestive of an immune response is the report that a rabbit immunized against *C. albicans* during the preparation of an antiserum was unaffected by an intravenous inoculation of living *C. albicans* such as had previously caused the death of an unimmunized rabbit. Also, it has been reported that mice vaccinated with *C. albicans* survive longer than nonimmunized mice [40].

Although immunological investigations have yielded relatively little information to explain the pathogenesis of candidiasis or to aid in diagnosis of the human disease, there is abundant literature regarding the antigenic nature of the organisms. The serological classification of the genus has been investigated perhaps most extensively by Tsuchiya *et al.* [41], who "mapped" the agglutinogens of various species, much as the antigenic formulae of *Salmonella* have evolved. Other investigators [42] have shown that *C. albicans* falls into two distinct antigenic groups, and five groups have been established for the entire genus [43]. Many other investigators [19, 44–51] have proved the antigenic heterogeneity of *Candida* species, and an antigenic relationship has even been demonstrated between *C. albicans* and *Blastomyces dermatitidis,* a taxonomically distant organism [52]. Immunology as a taxonomic tool is further exemplified by the report that *C. stellatoidea,* a species of dubious validity, is antigenically identical with *C. albicans* [53].

French workers [54, 55] have studied the antigens of *Candida* by electrophoresis and immunoelectrophoresis and concluded that the major portion of the antigens is protein. Others [56], however, have reported that most of the antibodies to *Candida* are directed toward polysaccharide, and these studies also have been extended by use of electrophoretic methods [43, 57]. There are still other reports of polysaccharide antigens in *Candida,* some mentioned previously [44, 51, 58], and a hemagglutinating antigen also has been prepared from cell washings [59]. On paper chromatography and in other chemical methods, the protein hydrolysates of various species seem to be much the same and the sugars vary only in quantity [60].

Most of the usual antigen-antibody interactions [41, 61–63], including fluorescent antibody [64], have been employed either to detect antibodies to *Candida* or to identify the organisms rapidly in culture, a problem of considerable magnitude in the diagnostic laboratory. Although probably not due to antibody, serum rapidly causes *C. albicans* to become filamentous, and this effect has been employed to differentiate cultures of this species from others [65]. Another curious effect of serum on *Candida* is the marked capacity of normal adult serum to inhibit the *in vitro* growth of *C. albicans* [66]. The mechanism of this action is not known, but it does not seem to conform to the classic conception of antibody. It is interesting, however, that sera of patients with acute blood dyscrasias have a striking reduction in anti-*Candida* capacity.

There is accumulating rather good evidence of a toxin in *C. albicans.* Such a substance was first reported in 1952 [67], but its action could be demonstrated clearly only when mycobacteria were added; and a later group [68], who also thought that *C. albicans* possesses a toxin, could evoke a reaction only in animals pretreated with antibiotics. Subsequently, both intact cells and cytoplasmic extracts were found to be toxic in mice [69], although other work [70] suggests that the pathological changes, at least those induced by the cytoplasm, could have resulted from metabolic disturbances other than those produced by endotoxin. There is much, however, that relates the toxic substances of *Candida* to classic bacterial endotoxin: intact cells are pyrogenic, producing a biphasic fever curve and immediate leukopenia, followed by slight leukocytosis [71]; tolerance to the toxic manifestations of *C. albicans* is induced by previous injection of endotoxin of gram-negative bacilli or of *C. albicans* [72, 73]; necrosis of human skin can be produced with acetone-extracted cells [2]; an acetone extract is lethal in mice [8], and recently a substance which possessed some of the properties of classic bacterial endotoxin was extracted with phenol from *C. albicans* [74, 75]. It is also of interest that a zymosan-like substance has been isolated from *C. albicans* [76], inasmuch as zymosan from other yeasts has proved pyrogenic [77]. None of the toxic substances mentioned has been defined chemically or immunologically, so no comparison with classic bacterial endotoxin is possible. It is interesting, however, that *C. albicans* possesses antigenic relationships with *Salmonella,* a gram-negative bacillus [78], and had an erythrocyte-sensitizing antigen that is lipopolysaccharide [79], as is bacterial endotoxin, thus establishing still other similarities with gram-negative bacilli.

Further information concerning the immunology of *Candida* can be found in the review by Salvin [80].

ASPERGILLOSIS

Aspergillosis is a mycotic disease frequently seen in animals, especially birds, but uncommonly in man. It is usually caused by *Aspergillus fumigatus* or *A. flavus,* although other species have also been reported. All aspergilli are widely distributed in nature, but most often they inhabit soil containing appreciable amounts of organic material where they play a part in the decomposition process. Most species are known to grow at the temperatures of the human body, and at least one, *A. fumigatus,* thrives at temperatures as high as 49° C. [81]. They frequently occur as laboratory contaminants and often are saprophytic in the upper respiratory tract of man, rendering isolation in culture from clinical specimens virtually meaningless. Despite difficulties in diagnosis, however, aspergilli have been associated with chronic infections of the external auditory canal [82] and occasionally invade fingernails, causing "green nails" [83], but most frequently they cause infections of the respiratory tract. Lung infections are usually superficial and localized as nodules (aspergilloma, mycetoma, fungus balls, coin lesions) or abscesses [84], but there may be diffuse pneumonitis. In the case of bronchopulmonary disease, an accompanying pulmonary eosinophilia has been described, presumably a result of sensitization of the host to the fungus [85, 86], and occasionally a lung infection may disseminate, resulting in widespread involvement of various tissues, including brain and endocardium [87]. Aspergilli have long been considered to be possible causes of symptoms in patients with contact and inhalant allergy, and there also have been efforts to relate the genus to "farmer's lung," an allergic syndrome of unknown etiology [88, 89].

The factors which predispose to aspergillic infections are not clear. In the case of pulmonary infections, aspergilli are nearly always secondary invaders and are seen most frequently complicating such chronic debilitating conditions as carcinoma. Experimentally, it has been shown that chickens with induced myelogenous leukemia are more susceptible to aspergillosis than are normal chickens [90]. A factor which has further increased susceptibility to aspergillosis is intensive antimicrobial and adrenal corticosteroid therapy. To support this concept, there is convincing clinical evidence that an actual increase in the incidence of this disease followed the introduction of these modes of therapy [91, 92]. This concept is further supported by the experimental observation that mice so treated die quickly of an ordinarily benign dose of *Aspergillus* spores [93]. Trauma also seems to predispose, for aspergillosis sometimes follows injury, e.g., to the eye, as in keratomycosis, or to the lung, as in pneumoconiosis. And certain occupations predispose, e.g., those which involve prolonged and intimate contact with grains or birds such as is experienced by farmers, threshers, pigeon handlers, and any who work with feeds [94]. The pathogenesis in these occupational cases, however, has been thought to be related to dosage and repetition of exposures rather than to debilitation of the host or other factors.

The immunological aspects of aspergillic disease were first investigated in regard to asthma and other forms of allergy. In 1936, passively transferable antibodies to saprophytic fungi, including *A. fumigatus,* were detected in patients with skin disease [95], and a few years later the same technique demonstrated reagins in asthmatic and hay fever patients who were skin-sensitive to various molds, including species of aspergilli [96]. In the latter study, because some individuals had skin hypersensitivity to molds in the absence of clinical allergy, an attempt was made to provoke the symptoms of asthma and hay fever by applying mold spores or extracts directly to the mucous membranes of the nose and throat. By this technique, 22 of 61 skin-test positive patients had respiratory reactions which correlated with their clinical allergy.

In most geographic areas, the dematiaceous fungi (so-called "black" molds) are the predominant causes of mold allergy and species of *Aspergillus* account for only a small percentage of the cases, perhaps because of their relatively lower incidence in the atmosphere. Aspergilli are more numerous, however, in inside environments, in particular as a constituent of house dust. In one recent study, aspergilli were found even in house dust in far lesser numbers than other genera; nevertheless they seemed to be as often responsible for clinical allergy as were the more commonly occurring molds [97].

In reviewing the problem of selecting the species with which the patient should be desensitized, one investigator [98] has emphasized that a positive skin reaction alone is without meaning but that a positive reaction coupled with cultural evidence of the presence of the mold in great quantity in the patient's environment is strong evidence of the identity of the responsible allergen. For unequivocal evidence, the heroic measure of a sniff test was suggested, although not recommended, for regular use. Yet another group [99] recommended the use of an intranasal provocative test in all patients suspected of having allergic rhinitis due to molds, for they found that eight of eleven patients with dermal sensitivity to *Aspergillus* reacted negatively to the provocative test. Despite these recommendations, cutaneous tests would seem of some help in diagnosis, because the clinically allergic patient would be expected to have an immediate wheal to at least the responsible allergen [100], and, conversely, a negative reaction would make it unlikely that the testing material could be the causative agent [101].

Perhaps the most comprehensive studies concerning *Aspergillus* and allergic diseases are those of Pepys and his associates [101–103], who attempted to determine the clinical and immunological significance of *A. fumigatus* in 145 (7 percent) of 2,080 hospitalized patients with various chest disorders. *A. fumigatus* was present more frequently in the sputum of asthmatics than of nonasthmatics perhaps, the investigators postulated, because the allergic reaction may have caused retention of the spores. Detailed investigation of 27 patients with *A. fumigatus* in the sputum showed two groups, one in which 16 were hypersensitive to both bronchial and skin tests with *Aspergillus* antigens and had episodes of pulmonary eosinophilia; and a second group of 11 who did not react to bronchial tests, gave infrequent reactions to skin tests, and did not have episodes of pulmonary eosinophilia. Among the patients without bronchial sensitivity were those with pulmonary mycetoma and some in whom the fungus appeared merely to be a saprophyte. A few of the allergic patients had "late" reactions following the immediate wheal (discussed later) which at 48 hours showed intense infiltration by eosinophils, in contrast to the typical mononucleated cells of a tuberculin reaction.

Serological tests were also carried out in 60 of these patients. Precipitating antibodies were found in the sera of 13, all of whom had *A. fumigatus* in their sputa and 10 of whom also showed hypersensitivity on both skin and bronchial tests. No precipitins were found in 14 similar patients or in 32 with and without fungus in the sputum and with or without hypersensitivity. As a result of these investigations, it was suggested that there are at least two types of antibody against *Aspergillus*, one, a nonprecipitating, skin-sensitizing antibody of the type found in allergies (reagin), and another which mediates the "late" (Arthus) skin reaction and plays a role in pulmonary eosinophilia. It was further suggested that allergic hypersensitivity to aspergilli can cause respiratory disturbances in two ways: (1) by asthma, rhinitis, and in other ways, as in patients sensitive to allergens such as pollen, and (2) by the appearance of transient infiltrations in the lungs by eosinophils.

Serological tests on patients with "farmer's lung" have revealed antibodies against *Aspergillus*. Earlier studies [104] suggested that these antibodies were present in significantly higher titer than in control sera. The results of more recent investigations, however, indicate that this condition is due to an allergy to hay undergoing decomposition by *Aspergillus* rather than to the mold itself [105]. Although such patients have precipitins to *A. fumigatus*, moldy hay, and good hay, they have bronchial hypersensitivity only to moldy hay [106]. Immunological investigations since then greatly strengthen these conclusions [107, 108].*

The multiplicity of antigenic components in aspergilli has been demonstrated repeatedly. By immunoelectrophoretic analysis, 16 antigens have been found in *A. fumigatus* [109], and similar observations have been made by sensitizing guinea pigs anaphylactically [110]. By agar-gel diffusion and electrophoresis, the extracts of *A. fumigatus* show at least 2 main antigens with at least 1 in common with other aspergilli, and in some instances antigenic relationships with *Cladosporium* and *Penicillium* also have been demonstrated [100].

A species-specific antigen is claimed to have been extracted from the mycelia of *A. fumigatus,* although it was not tested with antisera prepared against other species [111]. In the skin of infected rabbits this antigen produced delayed (tuberculin type) reactions, which seems in contradiction to the observations of Pepys *et al.* [101], who noted only immediate and "late" (Arthus) skin reactions in human beings. This divergence could be explained, however, by the innate differences in reactive capacities of the hosts and in the nature of the infections, for when yet another mycelial antigen [112] was used in a skin-test survey of zoo birds, the reactions observed were of a delayed type also.

The serological response to *A. fumigatus* has been followed also in experimentally infected chickens, using latex and collodion agglutination and agar-gel precipitation, but cross-reactivity was not included in the study [113].

Whether or not any of the previously described antigens can induce protective antibodies has not been reported. At least one antigenic polysaccharide, isolated from *A. fumigatus,* has been tested, but it was incapable of protecting animals against large doses of spores [114]. In this study, the observation was made, however, that the lipid of this fungus has adjuvant properties and can incite tubercle formation. Aspergilli possess yet another property which is not immunological per se but is of interest because it bears a superficial relation to antigen-antibody interactions and could be confused with them. This is the ability of their positively charged polysaccharides to precipitate negatively charged polysaccharides, and when mixed with cells of *Cryptococcus neoformans* in the absence of antibody, a "capsular reaction" and even agglutination occur [115].

Although the role in human infections has not been established, certain species of *Aspergillus* form toxins. In 1939, Henrici [116] isolated a substance from *A. fumigatus* with toxic and chemical properties similar to those of the poisonous mushroom, *Amanita phalloides.* The fungal toxin, however, was thermolabile. This substance was also antigenic, but much difficulty was encountered in active immunization, in part because of the toxicity but also because of a pronounced tendency to hypersensitization. Nevertheless precipitating antibodies were induced in rabbits, and animals so immunized acquired resistance to the toxin. In 1961, investigations of these toxins were reopened in the hope of developing an immunization procedure to protect animals, especially birds, but Henrici's observation of protection was not confirmed [117].

There has recently been a revival of interest in *Aspergillus* toxicosis as a result of a newly observed disease which killed more than 100,000 turkeys in England within a few months and which was associated with diet. Moldy groundnuts (peanuts) were incriminated, and the toxic fraction was identified as a product of *A. flavus* [118]. Perhaps more alarming than the toxicity were the observations that the moldy groundnuts were carcinogenic [119] and that cows fed experimental rations of toxic groundnut meal excreted a toxic factor into their milk [120]. The formula of this toxin, now referred to as aflatoxin, is thought probably to be $C_{17}H_{12}O_6$ or $C_{17}H_{12}O_7$, but little else is known regarding its chemical nature and virtually nothing is known of its immunological properties. The toxin of *A. fumigatus,* however, has been purified, but only to the extent that its hemolytic and other toxic fractions have been separated [121].

There have since been speculations regard-

* *Editor's comment:* According to Pepys *et al.* (*Lancet* 2:607, 1963) the prime antigen in hay which causes farmer's lung is a thermophilic actinomycete, *Thermopolyspora polyspora.* An extract of this species when inhaled produces many features of the disease, and when reacted with the serum of patients with farmer's lung by immunoelectrophoresis has improved discrimination between antigens involved in the etiology of farmer's lung and other fungal antigens.—B. R.

ing a possible causal relationship between *Aspergillus* toxins and malignant hepatomas, especially among certain races in Africa [122], where groundnuts constitute a major source of protein and where an environmental carcinogen has long been postulated. For example, among Bantu males, liver cancer is the commonest form of malignancy, whereas among Europeans it is the rarest.

The problem of mold toxicosis in human beings in Russia has been reviewed by Mayer [123], and still other references to mycotoxins can be found in the veterinary literature [124–127].

REFERENCES

1. Haley, L. D. Yeasts of medical importance. *Amer. J. Clin. Path.* 36:227, 1961.
2. Maibach, H. I., and Kligman, A. M. The biology of experimental human cutaneous moniliasis (*Candida albicans*). *Arch. Derm.* 85:233, 1962.
3. Louria, D. B., and Browne, H. G. The effects of cortisone on experimental fungus infections. *Ann. N.Y. Acad. Sci.* 89:39, 1960.
4. Torack, R. M. Fungus infections associated with antibiotic and steroid therapy. *Amer. J. Med.* 22:872, 1957.
5. Frenkel, J. K. Role of corticosteroids as predisposing factors in fungal disease: International symposium on opportunistic fungus infections. *Lab. Invest.* 11:1192, 1962.
6. Brody, J. I., and Finch, S. C. Candida-reacting antibody in the serum of patients with lymphomas and related disorders. *Blood* 15:830, 1960.
7. Kozinn, P. J., Wiener, H., Taschdjian, C. L., and Burchall, J. J. Is isolation of infants with thrush necessary? *J.A.M.A.* 170:1172, 1959.
8. Dobias, B. Moniliasis in pediatrics. *Amer. J. Dis. Child.* 94:234, 1957.
9. Csillag, A., Vince, I., and Simon, G. Occurrence of "*Candida albicans*" in the throat-mucus of healthy and diseased infants. *Ann. Paediat.* (Basel) 190:352, 1958.
10. Kozinn, P. J., Taschdjian, C. L., and Wiener, H. Incidence and pathogenesis of neonatal candidiasis. *Pediatrics* 21:420, 1958.
11. Skinner, C. E., and Fletcher, D. W. A review of the genus *Candida. Bact. Rev.* 24:397, 1960.
12. Stenderup, A., and Pedersen, G. T. Yeasts of human origin. *Acta Path. Microbiol. Scand.* 54:462, 1962.
13. Riddell, R. W. Precipitins in the diagnosis of fungous infections. *Brit. J. Derm.* 73:323, 1961.
14. Todd, R. L. Studies on yeast-like organisms isolated from the mouths and throats of normal persons. *Amer. J. Hyg.* 25:212, 1937.
15. Norris, R. F., and Rawson, A. J. Occurrence of serum agglutinins for *Candida albicans* and *Saccharomyces cerevisiae* in a hospital population. *Amer. J. Clin. Path.* 17:813, 1947.
16. Winner, H. I. A study of *Candida albicans* agglutinins in human sera. *J. Hyg.* (Camb.) 53:509, 1955.
17. Conant, N. F., Smith, D. T., Baker, R. D., Callaway, J. L., and Martin, D. L. *Manual of Clinical Mycology* (2nd ed.). Philadelphia: W. B. Saunders Company, 1954. P. 456.
18. Peck, S. M., Bergamini, R., Kelcec, L. C., and Rein, C. R. The serodiagnosis of moniliasis. *J. Invest. Derm.* 25:301, 1955.
19. Akiba, T., Iwata, K., and Inouye, S. Studies on the serologic diagnosis of the deep-seated candidiasis. *Jap. J. Microbiol.* 1:11, 1957.
20. Akiba, T., Iwata, K., and Inouye, S. Studies on the Serological Diagnosis of Candidiasis. In *Studies on Candidiasis in Japan.* Tokyo: Research Committee of Candidiasis, Education Ministry of Japan, February, 1961.
21. Comaish, J. S., Gibson, B., and Green, C. A. Candidiasis—serology and diagnosis. *J. Invest. Derm.* 40:139, 1963.
22. Kligman, A. M., and DeLamater, E. A. The immunology of the human mycoses. *Ann. Rev. Microbiol.* 4:283, 1950.
23. Lewis, G. M., Hopper, M. E., and Montgomery, R. M. Infections of the skin due to *Monilia albicans:* I. Diagnostic value of intradermal testing with a commercial extract of *Monilia albicans. New York J. Med.* 37:878, 1937.
24. Kitamura, S. Study on the Preparation of the Antigen for Diagnostic Intradermal Reactions, obtained from *Candida albicans* on Electric Dissolution. Ref. 20.
25. Kesten, H. D., and Mott, E. Hypersensitiveness to soluble specific substances from yeast-like fungi: I. Anaphylaxis. *J. Exp. Med.* 53:803, 1931.
26. Kurotchkin, T. J., and Lim, C. E. Anaphylaxis with water soluble specific substance from yeast-like fungi. *Proc. Soc. Exp. Biol. Med.* 28:223, 1930.
27. Mott, E., and Kesten, H. D. Hypersensitiveness to soluble specific substances from yeast-like fungi: II. Eye hypersensitivity. *J. Exp. Med.* 53:815, 1931.
28. Vogel, R. A., and Krehl, W. Experimental sensitization of guinea pigs with *Candida albicans* and adjuvants. *Amer. Rev. Pulm. Dis.* 76:692, 1957.
29. Vogel, R. A., Koger, M., Johnson, M., and Hunter, M. Tuberculin hypersensitivity as-

sociated with immunization of guinea pigs with *Candida albicans* and the presence of this organism in normal guinea pigs. *Mycopathologia* 16:117, 1961.

30. Kurotchkin, T. J., and Lim, C. E. Experimental bronchomoniliasis in sensitized rabbits. *Proc. Soc. Exp. Biol. Med.* 31:332, 1933.
31. Hurd, R. C., and Drake, C. H. *Candida albicans* infections in actively and passively immunized animals. *Mycopathologia* 6:290, 1953.
32. Winner, H. I. An experimental approach to the study of infections by yeast-like organisms. *Proc. Roy. Soc. Med.* 51:496, 1958.
33. Moreno, G. R. Candide alergica facial, en Sesiones Dermatologicas en Homenaje al Profesor Luis E. Pierini, Nov. 11, 1949.
34. Liebeskind, A. *Candida albicans* as an allergenic factor. *Ann. Allerg.* 20:394, 1962.
35. Charpin, J., Zafiropoulo, A., Aubert, J., and Blanc, M. Allergie gegen *Candida albicans*. *Allerg. Asthma* (Leipzig) 4:189, 1958.
36. Cernik, V. L., Ho Tan-Phi, Doan Hong-Hoa, Sery, V., and Pham Van-Nong. Allergic shock in mycotic hypersensitivity. *Allerg. Asthma* (Leipzig) 6:14, 1960.
37. Winner, H. I. Experimental moniliasis in the guinea-pig. *J. Path. Bact.* 79:420, 1960.
38. Hiatt, H. S., and Martin, D. S. Recovery from pulmonary moniliasis following serum therapy. *J.A.M.A.* 130:205, 1946.
39. Christie, R., and Morton, M. M. The detection of *Candida albicans*. *Aust. J. Derm.* 2:88, 1953.
40. Mourad, S., and Friedman, L. Pathogenicity of *Candida*. *J. Bact.* 81:550, 1961.
41. Tsuchiya, T., Fukazawa, Y., and Kawakita, S. Serological Classification of the Genus *Candida*. Ref. 20.
42. Hasenclever, H. F., and Mitchell, W. O. Antigenic studies of *Candida:* I. Observation of two antigenic groups in *Candida albicans*. *J. Bact.* 82:570, 1961.
43. Jonsen, J., Rasch, S., and Strand, A. Specific polysaccharides in genus *Candida:* I. Preparation and properties of water soluble fractions. *Acta Path. Microbiol. Scand.* 37:449, 1955.
44. Bombara, G., and Morabito, D. Attivita edemizzante nel ratto albino di polisaccaridi estratti da *C. albicans* e da *S. cerevisiae*. *Boll. Soc. Ital. Biol. Sper.* 37:372, 1961.
45. Hasenclever, H. F., and Mitchell, W. O. Antigenic relationships of *Torulopsis glabrata* and seven species of the genus *Candida*. *J. Bact.* 79:677, 1960.
46. Hasenclever, H. F., and Mitchell, W. O. Antigenic studies of *Candida:* III. Comparative pathogenicity of *Candida albicans* Group A, Group B, and *Candida stellatoidea*. *J. Bact.* 82:578, 1961.
47. Seelinger, H. P. R. Advances in mycological serodiagnosis. *German Med. Monthly* 4:272, 1961.
48. Pospisil, L. Chromatografie polysacharidových a protein-ových komplexů některých druhu rodu *Candida*. *Cesk. Derm.* 34:158, 1959.
49. Rawson, A. J., and Norris, R. F. Occurrence of a common group antigen among *Candida albicans, Saccharomyces cerevisiae* and *Hansenula Anomala*. *Amer. J. Clin. Path.* 17:807, 1947.
50. Martin, D. S. Studies on the immunologic relationships among various species of the genus *Candida* (*Monilia*). *Amer. J. Trop. Med.* 22:295, 1942.
51. Kesten, H. D., and Mott, E. Soluble specific substances from yeastlike fungi. *J. Infect. Dis.* 50:459, 1932.
52. Salvin, S. B. The serologic relationship of fungus antigens. *J. Lab. Clin. Med.* 34:1096, 1949.
53. Jonsen, J., Thjøtta, T., and Rasch, S. Quantitative agglutination studies in fungi: 2. Serological relationship between *C. albicans* and *C. stellatoidea*. *Acta Path. Microbiol. Scand.* 33:86, 1953.
54. Biquet, J., Tran Van Ky, P., and Andrieu, S. L'étude immunoélectrophorétique de la structure antigènique des levures permet-elle de rattacher les formes anascosporées aux formes ascosporées correspondantes? *Bull. Soc. Pharm. Lille* 2:75, 1962.
55. Tran Van Ky, P., Biquet, J., and Andrieu, S. Étude par l'électrophorése et la double diffusion en gélose des substances antigèniques excrétées dans le milieu de culture de *Candida albicans*. *Sabouraudia* 2:164, 1963.
56. Jonsen, J. Serological studies in fungi: Comparison of agglutinins and precipitins in anti-*Candida* sera. *Acta Path. Microbiol. Scand.* 37:79, 1955.
57. Jonsen, J., Thjøtta, T., and Rasch, S. Electrophoretic studies of yeast-antisera. *Acta Path. Microbiol. Scand.* 33:271, 1953.
58. Vogel, R. A. The polysaccharides of *Candida albicans*. *Proc. Soc. Exp. Biol. Med.* 86:373, 1954.
59. Vogel, R. A., and Collins, M. E. Hemagglutination test for detection of *Candida albicans* antibodies in rabbit antiserum. *Proc. Soc. Exp. Biol. Med.* 89:138, 1955.
60. Pospisil, V. L. Agglutinations-, Komplementbindungs- und Hämagglutinationsreaktion bei der Bestimmung von Candida-Arten. *Dermatologica* 118:65, 1959.
61. Rosenthal, S. A., and Furnari, D. Slide agglutination as a presumptive test in the laboratory diagnosis of *Candida albicans*. *J. Invest. Derm.* 31:251, 1958.
62. Trimble, J. R. The use of a precipitin test to differentiate *Candida albicans* from *Candida stellatoidea*. *J. Invest. Derm.* 28:349, 1957.
63. Gordon, M. A. Rapid serological differentiation of *Candida albicans* from *Candida stellatoidea*. *J. Invest. Derm.* 31:123, 1958.

64. Kemp, G., and Solotorovsky, M. Fluorescent antibody studies of pathogenesis in experimental *Candida albicans* infections of mice. *J. Immun.* 88:777, 1962.
65. Taschdjian, C. L., Burchall, J. J., and Kozinn, P. J. Rapid identification of *Candida albicans* by filamentation on serum and serum substitutes. *Amer. J. Dis. Child.* 99:212, 1960.
66. Roth, F. J., and Goldstein, M. I. Inhibition of growth of pathogenic yeasts by human serum. *J. Invest. Derm.* 36:383, 1961.
67. Salvin, S. B. Endotoxin in pathogenic fungi. *J. Immun.* 69:89, 1952.
68. Roth, F. J., and Murphy, W. H. Lethality of cell-free extract of *Candida albicans* for chlortetracycline-treated mice. *Proc. Soc. Exp. Biol. Med.* 94:530, 1957.
69. Mourad, S., and Friedman, L. Active immunization of mice against *Candida albicans*. *Proc. Soc. Exp. Biol. Med.* 106:570, 1961.
70. Mankowski, Z. T. The pathological activity of metabolic products of *Candida albicans* on newborn mice. *Mycopathologia* 17:165, 1962.
71. Braude, A. K., McConnell, J., and Douglas, H. Fever from pathogenic fungi. *J. Clin. Invest.* 39:1266, 1960.
72. Hasenclever, H. F., and Mitchell, W. O. Production in mice of tolerance to the toxic manifestations of *Candida albicans*. *J. Bact.* 84:402, 1962.
73. Hasenclever, H. F., and Mitchell, W. O. Endotoxin-induced tolerance to toxic manifestations of *Candida albicans*. *J. Bact.* 85:1088, 1963.
74. Isenberg, H. D., Allerhand, J., and Berkman, J. I. An endotoxin-like fraction extracted from the cells of *Candida albicans*. *Nature* (London) 197:516, 1963.
75. Kobayashi, G. S., and Friedman, L. Characterization of the pyrogenicity of *Candida albicans, Saccharoymyces cerevisiae,* and *Cryptococcus neoformans*. *J. Bact.* 88:660, 1964.
76. Yamabayashi, H. A zymosan-like substance extracted from *Candida albicans*. *Med. J. Osaka Univ.* 9:11, 1958.
77. Freedman, H. H., and Sultzer, B. M. Modification of lethality of endotoxin in mice by zymosan. *Proc. Soc. Exp. Biol. Med.* 106:495, 1961.
78. Aksoycan, N., and Le Minor, S. Antigènes communs entre les *Candida* et les *Salmonella*-Arizona. *Ann. Inst. Pasteur* (Paris) 99:723, 1960.
79. Vogel, R. A. Role of lipid in hemagglutination by *Candida albicans* and *Saccharomyces cerevisae*. *Proc. Soc. Exp. Biol. Med.* 94:279, 1957.
80. Salvin, S. B. Immunologic aspects of the mycoses. *Progr. Allerg.* 7:214, 1963.
81. Thom, C., and Raper, K. B. *Manual of the Aspergilli,* Baltimore: Williams & Wilkins Company, 1945.
82. Sharp, W. B., and John, M. B. Pathogenicity of the aspergilli of otomycosis. *Texas Rep. Biol. Med.* 4:353, 1946.
83. Moore, M., and Marcus, M. D. Green nails. *Arch. Derm. Syph.* 64:499, 1951.
84. Riley, E. A., and Tennebaum, J. Pulmonary aspergilloma or intracavitary fungus ball. *Ann. Intern. Med.* 56:896, 1962.
85. Hinson, K. F. W., Moon, A. J., and Plummer, N. S. Bronchopulmonary aspergillosis: A review and a report of eight new cases. *Thorax* 7:317, 1952.
86. Minetto, E., Fazio, M., Galli, E., and Prinotti, C. La varietà allergica dell'aspergillosi polmonare. *Minerva Med.* 152:98, 1961.
87. Wahner, H. W., Hepper, N. G. G., Andersen, H. A., and Weed, L. A. Pulmonary aspergillosis. *Ann. Intern. Med.* 58:472, 1963.
88. Hořejší, M., Šach, J., Tomšíková, A., and Mecl, A. A syndrome resembling farmer's lung in workers inhaling spores of *Aspergillus* and penicillia molds. *Thorax* 15:212, 1960.
89. Page, M. I., and Hawn, C. V. Z. Farmer's lung. *Amer. Rev. Resp. Dis.* 87:575, 1963.
90. Chick, E. W. Enhancement of aspergillosis in leukemic chicken. *Arch. Path.* 75:81, 1963.
91. Louria, D. B. Experiences with and diagnosis of diseases due to opportunistic fungi. *Ann. N.Y. Acad. Sci.* 98:617, 1962.
92. Gruhn, J. G., and Sanson, J. Mycotic infections in leukemic patients at autopsy. *Cancer* 16:61, 1963.
93. Sidransky, H., and Friedman, L. The effect of cortisone and antibiotic agents on experimental pulmonary aspergillosis. *Amer. J. Path.* 35:169, 1959.
94. Coe, G. C. Primary bronchopulmonary aspergillosis, an occupational disease. *Ann. Intern. Med.* 23:423, 1945.
95. Persons, E. L., and Martin, D. S. Passive transfer antibodies for six saprophytic fungi in a patient with a superficial scaling dermatosis. *J. Clin. Invest.* 15:429, 1936.
96. Penington, E. S. A study of clinical sensitivity to air-borne molds. *J. Allerg.* 12:388, 1941.
97. Frey, D., Cross, D. O., and Durie, E. B. Investigation of a series of samples of house dust for the presence of fungi: Correlation with previous investigations of airborne fungi and sensitivity tests on patients. *Mycopathologia* 19:83, 1963.
98. Schaffer, N. Mold allergy during the winter months. *New York J. Med.* 60:49, 1960.
99. Halpern, S. R., Holman, J., and Whittaker, C. The correlation between skin and respiratory mucous membrane tests with molds in allergic rhinitis. *Ann. Allerg.* 19:1407, 1961.
100. Pepys, J. Allergic hypersensitivity to fungi. *Postgrad. Med. J.* 35:436, 1959.
101. Pepys, J., Riddell, R. W., Citron, K. M., Clayton, Y. M., and Short, E. I. Clinical and immunological significance of *Aspergillus fumi-*

gatus in the sputum. *Amer. Rev. Resp. Dis.* 80:167, 1959.

102. Pepys, J., Riddell, R. W., and Clayton, Y. M. Human precipitins against common pathogenic and non-pathogenic fungi. *Nature* (London) 184:1328, 1959.
103. Pepys, J. The role of human precipitins to common fungal antigens in allergic reactions. *Acta Allerg.*, supp. 7, p. 108, 1960.
104. Tomšíková, A., Šach, J., Hořejší, M., Malý, V., Novackova, D. Antikörper gegen Penicillia und Aspergilli. *Z. Immunitaetsforsch.* 120:40, 1960.
105. Pepys, J., Riddell, R. W., Citron, K. M., and Clayton, Y. M. Precipitins against extracts of hay and fungi in the serum of patients with farmer's lung. *Acta Allerg.* 16:76, 1961.
106. Williams, J. J. Inhalation tests with hay and fungi in patients with farmer's lung. *Ibid.*, p. 77.
107. Kobayashi, M., Stahmann, M. A., Rankin, J. R., and Dickie, H. A. Antigens in moldy hay as the cause of farmer's lung. *Proc. Soc. Exp. Biol. Med.* 113:472, 1963.
108. Parish, W. E. Farmer's lung: Part I. An immunological study of some antigenic components of mouldy foodstuffs. *Thorax* 18:83, 1963.
109. Biquet, J., Tran Van Ky, P., Capron, A., and Fruit, J. Analyse immunochimique des fractions antigèniques solubles d'*Aspergillus fumigatus*. *C. R. Acad. Sci.* (Paris) 254:3768, 1962.
110. Landi, S., and Fitzgerald, J. D. L. Sensitization and anaphylactic shock induced in guinea pigs by using fungus extracts. *Mycopathologia* 12:257, 1960.
111. Fukui, M., and Yasuda, J. Serological studies on *Aspergillus fumigatus*. *Mycopathologia* 14:39, 1961.
112. Asakura, S., Nakagawa, S., Masiu, M., and Yasuda, J. Immunological studies of aspergillosis in birds. *Mycopathologia* 18:249, 1962.
113. Schneider, J. Der Nachweis von Antikörpern bei der Aspergillose der Hühner mit Hilfe der Kollodiumagglutination, der Latexagglutination sowie der Agargelpräzipitation. Veterinärhygienischen und Tierseuchen-Institut der Justus Liebig-Universität zu Gieszen, Doktoral Dissertation, 1962.
114. Stanley, N. V. Biological properties of polysaccharide and lipoid fractions from a pathogenic strain of *Aspergillus fumigatus*. *Aust. J. Exp. Biol. Med. Sci.* 28:99, 1958.
115. Evans, E. E. Reaction of an *Aspergillus* polysaccharide with *Cryptococcus* capsules and various acidic polysaccharides. *Proc. Soc. Exp. Biol. Med.* 101:760, 1959.
116. Henrici, A. T. An endotoxin from *Aspergillus fumigatus*. *J. Immun.* 36:319, 1939.
117. Tilden, E. B., Hatton, E. H., Freeman, S., Williamson, W. M., and Koenig, V. L. Preparation and properties of the endotoxins of *Aspergillus fumigatus* and *Aspergillus flavus*. *Mycopathologia* 14:347, 1961.
118. Toxicity Associated with Certain Batches of Groundnuts. Report of the Interdepartmental Working Party on Groundnut Toxicity Research (British Agricultural Research Council, Department of Scientific and Industrial Research Council, Ministry of Agriculture, Fisheries and Food, June, 1962). London: Her Majesty's Stationery Office, 1962.
119. Lancaster, M. D., Jenkins, F. D., and Philip, J. M. Toxicity associated with certain samples of groundnuts. *Nature* (London) 192:1095, 1961.
120. Allcroft, R., and Carnaghan, R. B. A. Groundnut toxicity: An examination for toxin in human food products from animals fed toxic groundnut meal. *Vet. Rec.* 75:259, 1963.
121. Rau, E. M., Tilden, E. B., and Koenig, V. L. Partial purification and characterization of the endotoxin from *Aspergillus fumigatus*. *Mycopathologia* 14:347, 1961.
122. Editorial: Mouldy peanuts and liver cancer. *J.A.M.A.* 184:57, 1963.
123. Mayer, C. F. Endemic panmyelotoxicosis in the Russian grain belt: I. The clinical aspects of alimentary toxic aleukia (ATA); A comprehensive review. *Milit. Surg.* 113:173, 1953.
124. Forgacs, J., Joch, H., Carll, W. T., and White-Stevens, R. H. Additional studies on the relationship of mycotoxicosis to the poultry hemorrhagic syndrome. *Amer. J. Vet. Res.* 19:744, 1958.
125. Schumaier, G., Panda, B., DeVolt, H. M., Laffer, N. C., and Creek, R. D. Hemorrhagic lesions in chickens resembling naturally occurring "hemorrhagic syndrome" produced experimentally by mycotoxins. *Poult. Sci.* 40: 1132, 1961.
126. Zinchenko, A. V. Disease in pigs caused by toxic fungi. *Veterinariia* 36:37, 1959.
127. Kulik, Y.I. *Aspergillus flavus* link (A study of the properties of mouldy peas infected by *A. flavus*). *J. Microbiol.* (Kiev) 19:36, 1957.

35. *Trichinosis, Hydatid Disease, Schistosomiasis, and Ascariasis*

ELVIO H. SADUN

OUR KNOWLEDGE OF HOST RESISTANCE to animal parasites is in its infancy when compared with what we know about host resistance to viral and bacterial infections. The existing evidence suggests a varying amount of natural and acquired resistance of man to several parasitic infections.

Animal parasites often follow a complex route to reach the site within the host where they eventually develop to maturity. The invasiveness of parasitic organisms and their migration within the host are the results of numerous factors, including specialized structures and specific biochemical entities produced by the parasite, on one hand, and host responses on the other. In general, the greater the invasiveness and tissue migration of the parasites, the greater the host response which they elicit.

At first, immunological studies on parasitic infections were limited to the development of immunological and serological tests that could be used as diagnostic aids. Subsequently, however, numerous observations and experimental studies indicated that the extent of infection is often related to the immunological status of the host and that recovery from an infection frequently results in an increased degree of resistance to subsequent infections.

Basically, the mechanisms of natural and acquired immunity against parasitic infections are identical with those against infections by other microorganisms. The most important obstacle to a speedy and rational development of immunological studies in parasitic infections is the inability to cultivate parasites in defined media *in vitro*. Consequently, it has been difficult to collect sufficient amounts of parasites or their metabolic products totally free from host tissues for accurate biochemical assay. Parasites are complex organisms. Complex and large organisms such as helminths do not possess a high degree of immunological specificity; they consist of many cells and tissues, i.e., many different antigens and antigenic determinants.

Parasites, however, have some significant and unique advantages for the study of immunological phenomena. Perhaps the most outstanding is their relatively large size. Large quantities of material available for purification, physical and chemical fractionation, biochemical analyses, and artificial immunizations make up in part, at least, for the lack of *in vitro* cultivation. Furthermore, the size of parasites frequently permits observation of the host response to the parasite directly under an ordinary microscope. As far as helminths are concerned, another great advantage is the fact that most of them do not multiply in the final host. Therefore, since each adult represents one exposure to one embryonated egg, cercaria, or infective larva, quantitative comparison of the host responses is possible. In autopsy studies of experimental animals, one can therefore estimate the worm burden, relative growth of parasites, relative development of various organs or systems within each parasite, and some of the micropathological results of host response. In protozoan infections, quantitative studies are possible but not easy, since multiplication occurs within the host. In malaria, for instance, one can follow the parasitemias at hourly or daily intervals and compare the parasite development curves in different hosts.

Diseases due to animal parasites cause various manifestations of hypersensitivity. One striking feature of these infections, especially those caused by helminths, is eosinophilia. Large numbers of eosinophil granulocytes appear both in the invaded tissue and in the peripheral blood. Eosinophilia may be of diagnostic importance, since it is often the first indication that a helminthic infection is present.

Helminths which enter the host by the percutaneous route induce a dermatitis which, particularly on reinfection, appears to be due to hypersensitivity. Similar reactions may occur when parasites invade abnormal hosts, previously unexposed. Thus skin lesions in normal "immune" and in abnormal "nonimmune" hosts might be indistinguishable. For instance, schistosome dermatitis or "swimmer's itch" occurs after exposure of bathers to the cercariae of nonhuman schistosomes. A similar type of dermatitis is observed in persons exposed repeatedly to human schistosomes.

It is not unlikely that the visceral pathology of many parasitic diseases is linked to hypersensitivity. The host responses to schistosomiasis and to tuberculosis, for example, are very similar, probably because the granulomatous lesions are a result of delayed hypersensitivity.

For brevity, only four helminthic infections will be discussed. These have been chosen both because of their common occurrence in the Western Hemisphere and because they have been the object of intensive immunological studies in recent years.

TRICHINOSIS*

Human infection with the nematode *Trichinella spiralis* constitutes an important clinical and public health problem in Europe, North America, and, to a lesser extent, in Central and South America. *T. spiralis* larvae are encysted in the muscles of several mammalian hosts. After digestion of the muscle in the stomach of man, the freed larvae pass into the intestine, where they develop to maturity in a few days. After mating, the gravid females begin depositing larvae which penetrate the intestinal mucosa, reach the blood stream, and are distributed throughout the body. They encyst primarily in striated muscles, where eventually they become calcified.

NATURAL IMMUNITY

The biology and immunology of *T. spiralis* have been reviewed elsewhere [1, 2]. Very little host specificity is observed with this parasite. Most mammals can serve as natural or experimental hosts. Birds can be experimentally infected, although with some difficulty [3–5]. Cold-blooded animals are resistant to infection with this parasite [5]. However, Matoff [6] was able to infect frogs and other cold-blooded vertebrates by raising their body temperature. Some of the factors that influence the susceptibility of various hosts to this parasite have been studied. Adrenalectomy in mice lowered their natural resistance [7]. On the other hand, addition of milk to the diet [8], abnormal increase in body weight [9], water deprivation before or after infection [10], and intercurrent infection with *Ancylostoma caninum* [11] appeared to increase the natural resistance of experimental animals. Natural resistance was diminished in mice, guinea pigs, and hamsters by concurrent infection with tuberculosis [12], administration of ACTH or cortisone [13–15], and body irradiation [16]. The age of the host also influences resistance to *T. spiralis* infection, resistance with advancing age being observed in dogs [17], pigeons [4], and other animals [18].

ACQUIRED IMMUNITY

Acquired immunity to *T. spiralis* was reported by Ducas [19], and his work was confirmed and extended by several investigators [20–24]. McCoy [25] succeeded in producing artificial immunization by repeated intraperitoneal injections in experimental animals of living *trichinella* larvae, heat-killed larvae, and dried and powdered larvae. In all instances, the resistance was manifested by rapid elimination of adult worms with resultant diminished muscle invasion. Spindler [26] reported the production of a mild degree of re-

* *Editor's comment:* There are three cardinal signs associated with trichinosis in man. These are, first of all, the muscle pain and discomfort which begin about the seventh day and can be associated with fever and skin rashes. The next most common finding is edema, occurring most frequently as a puffiness around the eyes. Central nervous system involvement, such as visual disturbances or headache, is usually transitory. The third is eosinophilia, which may attain from 10 to 70 percent of the total white count, the latter rising to 20,000 or 30,000 per cu. mm. The eosinophilia precedes the development of serological reactions or positive skin reactions and may persist for years. Although the symptoms may be related simply to irritation as a consequence of invasion by the larvae of the roundworm, the presence of eosinophils in the initial invasion of striated muscle fibers and particularly in the muscle walls of arterioles in reinfections, with inflammatory changes resembling those seen in periarteritis nodosa or serum sickness, all suggest an allergic or immune reaction. —B. R.

sistance in rats, rabbits, and guinea pigs after feeding them filtrates from the digested flesh of infected animals. There is some evidence that passive transfer of immunity is possible in human trichinosis. Salzer [27] reported that convalescent serum from patients recovering from trichinosis had both prophylactic and therapeutic activity, but this observation could not be confirmed by others [28–30]. In experimental animals, Travinsky [31] reported that subcutaneous injections of serum from heavily infected rabbits protected rats from lethal doses of larvae. Culbertson and Kaplan [32] found that serum from infected rabbits passively protected mice and reduced considerably the number of larvae developing from a challenging infection.

Mechanisms of Immunity. Acquired immunity in trichinosis is probably mediated primarily through the action of antibodies developed as a result of the infection. The relative role of humoral and cellular factors is unresolved. Oliver-Gonzalez [33] found that in rabbits, two types of antibodies appear that act specifically on the adults and on the larvae. The antiadult antibody appeared about fifteen days after infection, whereas the antilarvae antibody appeared about the thirtieth day. There seems little question, however, that the acquired resistance is directed primarily against the intestinal phase of the parasite. This is evident from the fact that when infective larvae are fed to an immune animal, most of them are promptly eliminated without obvious development [24]. These larvae are, however, still infective for normal animals to which they may be subsequently fed. The importance of humoral factors in the resistance of the small intestine of the mouse has been demonstrated. However, it is also evident that the body cells play a role in acquired immunity to trichinosis. Coker [34, 35] demonstrated that the cellular response in infected mice could be suppressed by the injection of cortisone and that its administration also suppressed the action of acquired immunity. Markell and Lewis [36] extended these observations by showing that after cortisone treatment, antibody titers could be demonstrated in the infected rat in the absence of a demonstrable immune response.

IMMUNOLOGICAL DIAGNOSIS

An unequivocal diagnosis of trichinosis is difficult to obtain since the clinical picture is not well defined and the organisms cannot be recovered by the usual methods. Consequently there is a need for reliable immunological procedures which can provide the basis for an adequate diagnosis of this infection especially in its early phases. The most commonly employed laboratory procedures have been reviewed recently [37, 38, 2]. The intradermal reaction is a valuable aid in diagnosis but is not very specific [39–41]. Negative reactions may occur in the early stages of the disease at the time when the female worms liberate broods of larvae. Furthermore, since in many areas of the world the prevalence of trichinosis is very high and since dermal sensitivity persists for several years, a positive intradermal reaction is by no means proof of recent infection. For these reasons, increasing reliance has been placed in recent years on serological tests. Precipitin tests have been used extensively. However, as a rule they elicit false positive reactions during the use of some chemotherapeutic agents, in infectious mononucleosis, and in the presence of some chronic degenerative diseases, especially those which alter the albumin-globulin ratio [42–44]. Uroprecipitin and microprecipitin tests have been used with varying degrees of success [45–49]. A hemagglutination test which detects antibodies from experimentally infected rabbits and rats was described [50]. Sadun and Allain [51] developed a rapid slide hemagglutination test which could be read in 15 minutes by placing and rotating sensitized cells and the serum on a flocculation slide. These tests have not yet found an important place in the routine diagnosis of trichinosis. Conversely, the complement fixation test has been in use since 1911 and is being employed routinely by several laboratories. In the opinion of many investigators it is greatly superior to various precipitin tests in providing much greater reliability [52–54]. In an outbreak of trichinosis, it was possible to determine that complement-fixing antibodies appear as early as 2 to 3 weeks after infection and persist for periods varying from 10 to 13 months [42].

Flocculation tests are among the simplest procedures for the serodiagnosis of infection. It is not surprising, therefore, that a number of them have been developed for the diagnosis of trichinosis. The flocculation test in which an alkaline extract of powdered *Trichinella* larvae is coated onto cholesterol crystals was developed by Sussenguth and Kline [55]. It was reported to be more sensitive than the complement fixation test [56] but perhaps somewhat less specific. Agglutination tests employing collodion particles [57, 58] and carmine particles [59] have been utilized with some degree of success. To increase the stability of the antigen for flocculation tests, Bozicevich [42] and his co-workers adsorbed it onto bentonite particles. This test appeared to have as great or greater specificity than the complement fixation test [60–62] and was thus regarded as the test of choice by several investigators [63, 2]. A latex agglutination test [64] has given satisfactory results comparable to those previously reported for the bentonite flocculation and the complement fixation tests. Cholesterol-lecithin crystals have also been used in the flocculation test for trichinosis [52]. Sensitivity was improved by coating a buffered saline extract of ether-treated *Trichinella* larvae onto cholesterol-lecithin particles and subsequently washing this complex to remove the excess antigen [65, 66]. A similar antigen was employed in a solution containing charcoal. The tests were performed on printed cards without the need of a microscope, thus greatly facilitating observations under field conditions [66].

A fluorescent antibody test employing *T. spiralis* larvae as antigen [67] appeared to possess a high degree of sensitivity and specificity. Reliable quantitative results were obtained either with fresh sera or with dried blood specimens on absorbent paper.

HYDATID DISEASE*

The incidence of human hydatid disease is unknown for most countries. Although this disease might be regarded as one having no great over-all significance in tropical public health, it causes concern in certain areas. Hydatid disease is highly endemic along the Mediterranean coast, in the Middle East, in Africa, and in Southwest Asia. It is of some public health importance in South and Central Asia but of only limited prevalence in Southeast Asia. It might be important in Alaska and Canada. There are several species of the genus *Echinococcus,* of which at least two have been proved to be responsible for hydatid disease in man. The adult worm (*E. granulosus* and *E. multilocularis*) is a minute cestode living in the small intestine of dogs, wolves, coyotes, jackals and foxes. The egg, being swallowed by man or other intermediate host, passes into the duodenum, where the embryo is liberated from its shell, penetrates the wall of the intestine, and reaches capillaries or mesenteric venules, from where it is carried passively in the blood stream until it lodges in the liver, lungs, or other organs. The surviving embryos increase rapidly in size, begin to vacuolate, and produce tumor masses.

NATURAL RESISTANCE

Few of the factors which influence natural resistance to *Echinococcus* infections have been established. This is due partly, at least, to the fact that experimental studies are complicated by the relative difficulty of creating sufficient safeguards against infection among laboratory workers. The adult worms possess a great degree of host specificity. The larval stage invades many different kinds of animals, including most of the herbivores, a few carnivores, and man. Attempts to establish *E. granulosus* in mice, rats, hamsters, rabbits, guinea pigs, and gerbils have met with no success. In an unsuccessful effort to depress the natural resistance to this parasite, pigeons were kept on a vitamin-free diet for a considerable period [68].

ACQUIRED IMMUNITY

There is no adequate evidence whether or not infection with hydatid disease confers any immunity to reinfection. However, reinfection has been reported frequently in individuals following surgery and in those in whom an initial cyst has been ruptured. Whether or not resistance to hydatid disease can be passively transferred with serum is also unknown. Turner *et al.* [69] reported that sheep could be protected from infection by previous vaccination with killed antigens prepared from

* *Editor's comment:* The allergic manifestations of hydatid cyst are limited by and large to a shocklike anaphylactic state—associated with itching, generalized erythema and urticaria—which occurs with rupture of a cyst or from an exploratory puncture made for diagnostic purposes. Because of the possible danger of an acute and fatal anaphylactic reaction, exploratory puncture is not recommended. In general, eosinophilia is not a feature of hydatid disease. One possible explanation for the anaphylaxis-like syndrome which occurs on rupture of a cyst is the sudden massive release of antigen in an individual who has become sensitized to the organisms. Another, which has apparently not been explored, is that the cyst fluid may actually contain a histamine-liberating component.—B. R.

the hydatid cyst fluid and membranes. Similarly, dogs were rendered partially resistant to infection with the intestinal stage after vaccination with hydatid cyst material [70].

DIAGNOSIS

The laboratory diagnosis of hydatid disease has been widely employed with varying degrees of success. The intradermal test appears to be the most sensitive and the most often used [71]. Both immediate and delayed skin reactions have been reported [72]. Conflicting reports as to the reliability of such a test can possibly be explained by qualitative and quantitative differences in the antigens employed. In general, however, the skin test has proved useful in the hands of most investigators [73, 74]. No demonstrable dermal sensitivity is developed in animals harboring the intestinal stage of the parasite [75]. The main disadvantage of the intradermal test for this as well as for other parasitic infections is that the fixed antibodies persist after removal of the cyst. Serological techniques have been employed since 1906, when the hydatid fluid from a human cyst was used as antigen in the complement fixation test [76]. An excellent review of the early studies on the immunological diagnosis of hydatid disease was prepared by Fairley [77]. Opinion on the relative merits of complement fixation and precipitation tests has been controversial. This may be due primarily to the facts that many sources of antigens have been used and that the reagents employed have frequently been inadequately standardized. An excellent review of the current and potential value of immunodiagnostic tests with various soluble antigens was published by Kent [78]. An analysis of hydatid antigens utilizing agar-gel methods has provided qualitative data on the minimal number of antigen-antibody systems present in antigens and antisera commonly employed [79]. Some of the reasons for nonspecific reactions reported in serologic tests for hydatid diseases have been reviewed [80].

In addition to the complement fixation and precipitation tests, other serological tests have been employed for diagnosis. Among these, the indirect hemagglutination test [81, 82] and the bentonite flocculation test [83] have shown great promise. An evaluation of these techniques [84] indicates that they may be more sensitive than the complement fixation test.

SCHISTOSOMIASIS*

Approximately 150 million people throughout the world are infected with schistosomes. Infection with *Schistosoma mansoni, S. haematobium,* and *S. japonicum* is widely distributed through Africa, the eastern Mediterranean, some countries of Latin America, and the western Pacific. Because of its wide distribution and the large number of people affected, schistosomiasis is being recognized as second only to malaria in importance as a parasitic disease. What may be even more significant is the fact that whereas most communicable diseases are yielding to modern means of control, schistosomiasis is increasing in distribution and prevalence in many parts of the world. This is due primarily to the fact that its spread is closely related to the development of irrigation systems. Man is infected by contact with fresh water in which schistosome cercariae swim freely. The cercariae penetrate the skin and reach the blood circulation, where they mature, copulate, and proceed to the mesenteric veins or the venous plexus around the bladder (*S. haematobium*), where the females begin to lay eggs. The eggs reach the free environment in the feces or urine, and, on contact with fresh water, the ciliated embryos within the egg shell (miracidia) hatch. The miracidia enter various species of snails, where they undergo asexual development and emerge as free-swimming cercariae.

NATURAL RESISTANCE

The three species of schistosomes that involve man differ widely among themselves in their host ranges. In nature, *S. mansoni* and *S. haematobium* are found primarily in man and only occasionally in other mammals, especially rodents. In contrast, *S. japonicum* is found naturally in human beings, most farm animals, and also rodents. This comparatively

* *Editor's comment:* Allergic manifestations in man occur primarily in the intestinal form of schistosomiasis. During the incubation period, when invasion takes place there may be urticaria, asthmatic attacks, subcutaneous edema, leukocytosis, and eosinophilia. Other symptoms such as anorexia, fever, headache, weight loss, and a hypochromic macrocytic anemia may be seen. In vesical schistosomiasis, commonly due to *S. haematobium,* in which the symptoms consist of hematuria and other vesical complaints, the presence of the organisms in the urine may be associated with leukocytosis and eosinophilia.—B. R.

broad host range is observed also among most of the nonhuman mammalian schistosomes. In the intermediate molluscan host, all of the human schistosomes have a strict host specificity. Our information on natural resistance is based chiefly on infections in experimental animals. In different hosts, the degree of natural resistance can be determined by the percentage survival and relative development of worms, their ability to produce eggs, the sex ratio and location of the worms in the host, the viability of eggs and infectivity of miracidia, and the pathological manifestations of infection.

A complete understanding of factors which influence the natural resistance of human schistosomes in the mammalian host is lacking. There is circumstantial evidence that age is probably significant, since schistosomiasis is most severe in children. In experiments with *S. mansoni,* the number of worms developing in animals on a deficient diet is usually greater than in animals on a normal diet. Rats on a vitamin A–free diet are known to have diminished resistance to experimental infections with *S. mansoni* [85]. The host's diet may have a marked effect on the schistosomes as well as on the pathological changes produced by them. A diet deficient in cystine, selenium, and vitamin E was found to have a profound effect on the course of *S. mansoni* infections in mice [86, 87]. The relative susceptibility of various animals to infection by *S. mansoni* has been noted by various investigators [88–95].

ACQUIRED IMMUNITY

The ability of man to resist reinfection after experiencing an initial infection with schistosomes has not been proved. However, there is a large body of circumstantial evidence that, as a result of a primary infection, man develops an immunity to subsequent exposures. Clinical and epidemiological data from human infections and extensive studies in experimental animals provide the bulk of evidence regarding active immunity. The development of acquired immunity following infection by *S. japonicum* has been reported in mice, rabbits, and monkeys [96–98]. However, no immunity to reinfection was observed in mice, hamsters, and rabbits [99]. Attempts to induce resistance against *S. mansoni* following a primary infection have been unsuccessful in mice [100, 101], hamsters, guinea pigs, and rats [102, 103]. Some evidence of a weak degree of acquired resistance was obtained in monkeys by Meleney and Moore [104], and stronger evidence has been reported by others [105–107, 95].

There is some indication that immunity can be acquired in various experimental animals by previous exposure to heterologous schistosomes. After a series of unsuccessful attempts in monkeys, rabbits, and mice [108, 109, 104, 99], concrete evidence of protection was reported by different groups of investigators with different systems [103, 110, 111, 95].

Inoculation with dead parasite material or the media on which parasites have been cultured has also been shown to induce light protective response in experimental animals. Almost always, however, dead vaccines induced a milder degree of resistance than living vaccines. Ozawa [112] protected dogs to a small degree by injection of suspensions of *S. japonicum* worms. Similar results were reported by Kawamura [113]. Lin *et al.* [97] reported some resistance in mice, and experiments by Sadun and Lin [98] provided further evidence of resistance induced by artificial immunization to this parasite. Unsuccessful results were reported in monkeys [96, 114], mice, hamsters, and rabbits [99].

Failure of attempts at passive transfer of resistance to either *S. japonicum* or *S. mansoni* from immunized to nonimmunized hosts has been reported by several groups [96, 115–117, 94]. Conversely, a very mild degree of resistance to *S. japonicum* was passively transferred by Kawamura [113] and by Sadun and Lin [98].

Artificial immunizations against *S. mansoni* have had very limited success. Watts [118] reported that mice given injections of a cercaria antigen of *S. mansoni* had fewer worms. Kagan [119] observed that injections of *S. mansoni* excretory and secretory products delayed the time of death in mice challenged with lethal doses. These results were confirmed by Levine and Kagan [120]. Protection was also reported in rats immunized with worm homogenates [95]. On the other hand, Thompson [102] was unable to obtain protection by inoculation with dead cercariae. Failure to induce resistance in mice against *S. mansoni* was also reported by Ritchie *et al.* [121] following injections of cercariae, adult worms, and egg homogenates and by Sadun and Bruce [122] after injection of eggs.

Acquired immunity to *S. mansoni* and *S. japonicum* has been observed in mice and monkeys following previous exposure to irradiated cercariae [123–127, 95]. Parasitological and histopathological observations reveal that exposure to irradiation interferes with the ability of schistosomes to reach maturity in mice. Since the death and disintegration of schistosome cercariae stimulate a considerable degree of inflammation, different dosage levels provide contrasting pathological situations [128]. Investigations in mice by Szumlewicz and Olivier [129] seem to indicate that the acquired resistance which developed following exposure to irradiated cercariae may be transitory, resulting only in a delay in development of the second infection. However, this was not true in monkeys [95].

The basis of immunity in schistosomiasis is obscure. Although the stage in the life cycle of the parasite which is mainly responsible for stimulating resistance is debatable, there is no doubt that some immunity can be produced in the absence of sexually mature worms and eggs. The main immunogenic stimulus appears to be related to the metabolic activity and the survival time of the living worms within the host. This suggests that resistance is produced by an antigen which is excreted or secreted by the worms or, alternatively, an unstable antigen which is present only in living schistosome cells [130]. Although the immunity seems to depend primarily on the action of serum antibodies, the role of the body defensive cells in this immunity is unknown. There is ample evidence that the cells respond to the presence of the schistosomes and their eggs, and that this response is greater and more rapid in immunized than in unimmunized hosts [98, 131].

IMMUNODIAGNOSTIC TESTS

Reliable intradermal and serological tests for the immunological diagnosis of schistosomiasis have been developed. Several critical reviews of various techniques have been published [132, 78, 133].

The intradermal tests are relatively simple to perform. The reaction obtained is of the immediate type and can be read fifteen minutes after introduction of the antigen. Saline extracts of adult worms provide relatively crude antigens and have been used for many years [134]. Experimentally infected rabbits also give a positive skin reaction [135]. Other mammalian schistosomes have also been used as the source of the skin-testing antigen [136]. The preparation of more purified antigens has greatly increased the specificity of the test, as has standardization in performance of the test and the reading of results [137, 138, 132]. However, the sensitivity and specificity of the intradermal tests in *S. mansoni* infections are somewhat lower than those of serological tests [139, 140].

Serological tests for schistosomiasis have been in existence for more than fifty years. Yoshimoto [141] first described the complement fixation procedure for this infection in 1910. Since the development of a satisfactory technique utilizing an improved lipid-free antigen [142], many other investigators have used the test successfully, and this reaction is still the most widely used and highly regarded. No species specificity has been reported, and usually any one species of schistosomes is employed for diagnosis of any of the human schistosome infections. Numerous other serological procedures have been described. The most notable are the precipitin test [135, 143, 144], the circumoval precipitation test [145], the cercarianhuellen reaction [146], the cercarial agglutination test [147], the miracidial immobilization test [148], the slide flocculation test [149, 150], and the hemagglutination test [151]. Although some of them must still be regarded as being in the experimental stage, others have been evaluated extensively and show great promise. Excellent results were obtained with the slide flocculation test [150] in recent evaluations [139, 152]. A recently developed indirect fluorescent antibody technique for the diagnosis of schistosomiasis employs formalin-fixed cercariae as the source of antigen [153]. This technique was improved and rendered more practical by the introduction of rhodamine bovine albumin as counter stain [154] and by obviating the need of venipuncture [155, 156]. The test now carried out with blood obtained by finger puncture and dried on filter paper is one of the simplest and most practical serological methods for the diagnosis of schistosomiasis. The technique has been evaluated by several investigators in different parts of the world with excellent results [157–159].

Despite these recent advances, the need still existed for an efficient field-testing procedure which would permit the prompt collection of data without the interval required to mail specimens to a central laboratory and to receive the results. This need might be obviated by the development of a plasma card test [160] to be used in conjunction with a plasma collection slide [161], performed by mixing a drop of plasma obtained from finger blood in a rapid and simple manner with a stable antigen suspension containing charcoal. The results are read on a specially designed plastic-coated card surface a few minutes after rotation. Preliminary evaluations in Africa [160] and in Brazil [152] have shown that this procedure may be particularly useful as a screening procedure for field epidemiological investigations.

ASCARIASIS*

Infection produced in man by *Ascaris lumbricoides* is one of the most ubiquitous of all parasitic conditions. Promiscuous defecation by young children, the discharge of feces from houses onto the immediately adjacent soil, and the use of human night soil as fertilizer are often sufficient to maintain a high level of endemicity. The importance of ascariasis as a cause of disease and of death, especially among children, has been emphasized in numerous reports [162]. It can also be a major cause of pulmonary disease and death among people of all ages [163–165].

Man is infected with *A. lumbricoides* by ingesting embryonated eggs from the soil. The eggs in the feces are deposited on the soil and, under suitable conditions of temperature and humidity, develop at a rate depending on prevailing conditions. Eventually, they are mixed with the soil, blown away as dust, and deposited on various objects with which they come in contact. Thus in an endemic area *Ascaris* eggs can be found on most all objects, from where they are transferred to the mouth. The larvae hatch in the small intestine, penetrate the wall of the lumen, reach the blood circulation, and migrate through the lungs, from where they are coughed out with sputum and frequently swallowed, to reach adulthood in the small intestine.

NATURAL RESISTANCE

Complete understanding of factors which influence the natural resistance of human beings to *Ascaris* is lacking. This is due primarily to the fact that there is insufficient knowledge of how human physiological and anatomical endowments may work to the advantage or detriment of this parasite. When embryonated eggs are fed to abnormal hosts, they reach only the larval stage in the lung and do not attain maturity as adult intestinal worms. There is little, if any, racial difference in susceptibility that can be attributed to a purely physiological specificity. However, different modes of behavior and dietary habits of different races frequently play an important role in incidence.

Since prevalence rates are often greater in males than in females, a sex difference in susceptibility has been suggested. However, little is known about the mechanism of such a sex difference or how gonadal hormones influence natural resistance [166]. Other factors such as diet and physiological requirements for hatching of *Ascaris* eggs in the intestine have been found to influence the natural resistance to this infection. Epidemiological observations and experimental infections in laboratory animals have shown that susceptibility to *Ascaris* declines with advancing age, up to the onset of sexual maturity. Although individuals can be infected with *Ascaris* at any age, young people are more frequently and more intensely infected than older individuals. Attention is called to the fact, however, that under human natural conditions the observed differences in incidence and intensity of infection at different ages are probably due, in part at least, to such other factors as the development of acquired resistance and differences in behavior and occupational activities between children and adults.

ACQUIRED IMMUNITY

Human beings acquire only a partial immunity to reinfection with *Ascaris* [167] as

* *Editor's comment:* Of all the metazoan infections of man, ascariasis is, perhaps, the best known to allergists, since all of the usual allergic manifestations, including urticaria, angioedema, asthmatic attacks, nontropical pulmonary eosinophilia (Loeffler's syndrome), and tropical eosinophilia, may be associated with the migration of larvae. Clinical and experimental studies have disclosed the startling increase in eosinophils of blood and tissues which is associated with *Ascaris* infestation (see Chap. 17) or with the injection of *Ascaris* components (Campbell, D. H. *J. Infect. Dis.* 72:42, 1943). Kailin *et al.* (*J. Allerg.* 18:369 and 373, 1947; 21:225, 1950) demonstrated that *Ascaris* induces the formation of reagins in man and carefully analyzed the factors which, like race, sex, concurrent infection, and time, influence their titer.—B. R.

evident from the fact that if the parasites are eliminated by treatment, reinfection can occur [168]. Most of the evidence of acquired resistance to this parasite is obtained from experimental infections in laboratory animals. It has been shown experimentally that the larvae hatching from embryonated eggs are impeded in their progress through the tissues and frequently are either eliminated through the intestinal tract or encapsulated by various cellular components [169]. Even those that survive and succeed in completing their cycle in the experimental animals frequently produce fewer eggs, are stunted, delayed in their development, and eliminated more readily than in nonimmune animals.

Antibodies probably influence the immunity acquired against infections with *Ascaris*. Artificial immunization of guinea pigs by injection of pulverized eggs, introduction of viable eggs under the skin, injection of saline extracts of disintegrated eggs or larval excretions, and intravenous inoculations of third-stage larvae from lungs have been reported [170, 171]. Furthermore, passive transfer of immunity has been achieved in guinea pigs. The demonstration of precipitates when larvae are placed in immune serum [172, 173] gives additional indications that circulating antibodies affect larvae *in vitro* and may affect them *in vivo*. Sadun [172] and Soulsby [173] found that third-stage larvae were primarily involved in the formation of precipitates in immune serum. Furthermore, in immune animals, larvae of a challenge infection were affected by the host resistance in obvious ways only when they approached the moulting period [174], which confirmed our earlier observations [172]. Such work has suggested that the various developmental stages in the host vary in their ability to release antigens which stimulate "protective" antibodies and in their susceptibility to the host response. Excretory and secretory antigens, obtained by *in vitro* cultivation of third-stage *Ascaris* larvae, induced in guinea pigs a significant protection against a challenge dose. These antigens were very labile and were destroyed by freezing. This suggested "that they are macromolecular in character and possibly comparable to the antigens responsible for the graft rejection in transplantation immunity" [175].

Larvicidal activities of serum were not induced by immunization with *Ascaris* cuticle [176], thus indicating that this organ is not primarily involved in inducing "protective" antibodies. However, immune adhesion of red cells occurred on the cuticle of *Ascaris* larvae in the presence of guinea pig complement. White cells also became firmly adherent to the cuticle in the presence of antibody. This reaction, however, is totally independent of complement [175]. It also seems probable than antibodies behave as opsonins and act in conjunction with the defensive body cells.

The cellular activity in immune animals is considerably greater than in those exposed to a primary infection. The cells surround the migrating larvae of the superimposed infection, check their progress, and finally destroy them [169]. The cells primarily involved in the defense mechanism are predominately those of the reticuloendothelial system, lymphoid macrophage system, the plasma cells, and granular leukocytes. A purified polysaccharide from *Ascaris* injected into mice caused liver infiltration by primitive hemopoietic elements of the erythrocyte and leukocyte series [177]. Eosinophilia is a conspicuous feature of infections with *A. lumbricoides*. When *Ascaris* larvae were placed on a mixture of cells from sensitized rabbits, only eosinophils and cells with marked pyroninophil staining were attracted. Other cells such as neutrophils, lymphocytes, and mast cells were not. This observation led Soulsby [175] to suggest that the role of the eosinophil "is likely to be akin to that of similar cells found in other immunological systems, particularly the immunological rejection of skin and other tissue transplants."

IMMUNODIAGNOSTIC TESTS

Despite extensive research conducted over a long period by many investigators, no satisfactory immunodiagnostic tests have been developed for the routine laboratory diagnosis of ascariasis. This is particularly disturbing since the need for a reliable immunodiagnostic method has been increased by the recognition of visceral larval migrans produced by infection with the dog or cat species [178, 179].

Intradermal tests using extracts of *A. lumbricoides* were found to be of limited practical value for the diagnosis of infections in man. Antibodies resulting from infection with *Ascaris* have been detected in human subjects by use of complement fixation, ring precipitation, hemagglutination, bentonite flocculation, and agar-gel diffusion tests. However, lack of strict species specificity is the predominant observation. This is not surprising, since organisms as large and as complex as *A. lumbricoides* are mosaics of an enormous number of antigens. Additional evidence of the multiplicity of antigens in the parasite is provided by the fact that infection of animals with *Ascaris* produces a pronounced elevation of heterophil antibodies [180, 181], thus confirming previous observations [170] that high levels of A antibodies in rabbits could be stimulated by infection with this parasite. Subsequent investigations [182] demonstrated that pigs infected with *Ascaris* showed a marked elevation of the A antibodies and that antigens from this parasite neutralized human A and B antibodies.

Reliable results with serological reactions will be obtainable only after successful fractionation of various components of this nematode parasite. Soulsby [171–173] conducted an antigenic analysis of the parasite by the double diffusion precipitin test. He found large numbers of components and observed that eight of fourteen agar diffusion bands were removed by absorption of anti-*Ascaris* intestine serum with sheep erythrocytes. Kagan [179], using different physicochemical methods of fractionating whole worm homogenates, found that the number of double diffusion bands varied with the fractionation procedure and concluded that the antigens are closely bound protein-carbohydrate complexes. Kent [183] found that glycoprotein complexes isolated from the water-soluble portion of *A. lumbricoides* could be differentiated into five major components by paper and agar-gel electrophoresis. Four of them could be precipitated by corresponding antibodies. An interesting aspect of these fractions is that they appeared to be specific. Most sera from suspected cases of visceral larva migrans failed to react with these antigens, and no cross-reactions were reported with sera from *Echinococcus, Trichinella,* and *Schistosoma* infections.

As emphasized by Goodchild and Kagan [184] and by Soulsby [175], cross-reactions observed among different parasites may be due to the host proteins in the antigenic preparations. The chances of this occurring with *Ascaris* are considerably greater when the antigen preparation is obtained from the whole parasite, thus including in it the contents of helminth gut.

REFERENCES

1. Gould, S. E. *Trichinosis.* Springfield, Ill.: Charles C Thomas, Publisher. 1945.
2. Kagan, I. G. Trichinosis: A review of biologic, serologic and immunologic aspects. *J. Infect. Dis.* 107:65, 1960.
3. Augustine, D. L. Experimental trichinosis in chicks. *Science* 78:608, 1933.
4. Matoff, K. Bei Tauben auf enteralem Wege erzeugte Muskeltrichinellose. *Tieraerztl. Rundsch.* 42:401, 1936.
5. Pavlov, P. Recherches expérimentales sur la trichinose des volailles. *Ann. Parasit.* 15:434, 1937.
6. Matoff, K. Ueber die Möglichkeit der Entwicklung von *Trichinella spiralis* bei Kaltblütern. *Z. Parasitenk.* 13:156, 1944.
7. Baughn, C. O., Jr. The effect of adrenalectomy on natural and acquired resistance of mice to *Trichinella spiralis. J. Elisha Mitchell Sci. Soc.* 68:207, 1952.
8. Riedel, B. B. Milk as a source of some protection against the acquisition of *Trichinella spiralis* in mice. *J. Parasit.* 35:27, 1949.
9. Hendricks, J. R. The effect of body weight on the natural resistance of mice to *Trichinella spiralis. J. Parasit.* 36(supp.):31, 1950.
10. Campbell, C. H. The effect of water starvation on the natural resistance of mice to *Trichinella spiralis. J. Parasit.* 39(supp.):41, 1953.
11. Cox, H. W. The effect of concurrent infection with the dog hookworm, *Ancylostoma caninum,* on the natural and acquired resistance of mice to *Trichinella spiralis. J. Parasit.* 28:197, 1952.
12. Davis, O. T., Harrell, G. T., and King, E. S. The effect of simultaneous tuberculosis infection on experimental *Trichinella* infestations in guinea pigs. *Amer. J. Med. Sci.* 209:758, 1945.
13. Stoner, R. D., and Godwin, J. T. The effects of ACTH and cortisone upon susceptibility to trichinosis in mice. *Amer. J. Path.* 29:943, 1953.
14. Coker, C. M. Effects of cortisone on cellular inflammation in the musculature of mice given one infection with *Trichinella spiralis. J. Parasit.* 42:479, 1956.
15. Ritterson, A. L. Innate resistance of species of hamsters to *Trichinella spiralis* and its reverse by cortisone. *J. Infect. Dis.* 105:253, 1959.
16. Stoner, R. D., and Hale, W. M. The effect of cobalt-60 gamma radiation on susceptibility

and immunity of trichinosis. *Proc. Soc. Exp. Biol. Med.* 80:510, 1952.

17. Matoff, K. Der Mechanismus der Altersimmunität des Hundes gegen die Trichinelleninfektion. *Tieraerztl. Rundsch.* 43:369, 1937.
18. Hendricks, J. R. Comparing the immune response of young and old mice to infections with 50 and 300 larvae of *Trichinella spiralis. J. Parasit.* 34(supp.):31, 1948.
19. Ducas, R. L'immunité dans la Trichinose. Paris: Jouve et Cie, 1921. (Thesis.)
20. McCoy, O. R. Immunity of rats to reinfection with *Trichinella spiralis. Amer. J. Hyg.* 14:484, 1931.
21. McCoy, O. R. Experimental trichiniasis infections in monkeys. *Proc. Soc. Exp. Biol. Med.* 30:85, 1932.
22. Bachman, G. W., and Rodriguez-Molina, R. Resistance to infestation with *Trichinella spiralis* in hogs: The eosinophilic and precipitin response. *Amer. J. Hyg.* 18:266, 1933.
23. Bachman, G. W., and Oliver-Gonzalez, J. Immunization in rats against *Trichinella spiralis. Proc. Soc. Exp. Biol. Med.* 35:215, 1936.
24. Roth, H. Experimental studies on the course of Trichina infection in guinea pigs: III. The immunity of guinea pigs to re-infection with *Trichinella spiralis. Amer. J. Hyg.* 30:(sect. D) 35, 1939.
25. McCoy, O. R. Artificial immunization of rats against *Trichinella spiralis. Amer. J. Hyg.* 21:200, 1935.
26. Spindler, L. A. Resistance to intestinal trichinosis in experimental animals induced by feeding metabolic products of encysted trichinae. *J. Washington Acad. Sci.* 27:36, 1937.
27. Salzer, B. F. A study of an epidemic of fourteen cases of trichinosis with cures by serum therapy. *J.A.M.A.* 67:579, 1916.
28. Schwartz, B. Serum therapy for trichinosis. *J.A.M.A.* 69:884, 1917.
29. Hall, M. C., and Wigdor, M. An experimental study of serum therapy in trichinosis. *Arch. Intern. Med.* 22:601, 1918.
30. Alexander, M. E. Trichiniasis, endemic and sporadic, with a review of the present status of the treatment of the disease. *Amer. J. Med. Sci.* 165:567, 1923.
31. Travinsky, A. Studien ueber Immunität bei Trichinose. *Zbl. Bakt.* (Naturwiss.) 134:145, 1935.
32. Culbertson, J. T., and Kaplan, S. S. A study upon passive immunity in experimental trichiniasis. *J. Parasit.* 30:156, 1938.
33. Oliver-Gonzalez, J. The dual antibody basis of acquired immunity in trichinosis. *J. Infect. Dis.* 69:254, 1941.
34. Coker, C. M. Cellular factors in acquired immunity to *Trichinella spiralis,* as indicated by cortisone treatment of mice. *J. Infect. Dis.* 98:187, 1956.
35. Coker, C. M. Some effects of cortisone in mice with acquired immunity to *Trichinella spiralis. Ibid.,* p. 39.
36. Markell, E. K., and Lewis, W. P. Effect of cortisone treatment on immunity to subsequent reinfection with *Trichinella* in the rat. *Amer. J. Trop. Med. Hyg.* 6:553, 1957.
37. Sadun, E. H., and Norman, L. A practical flocculation test for the serodiagnosis of trichinosis by the state laboratories. *Public Health Lab.* 13:147, 1955.
38. Sadun, E. H. Recent advances in the serological diagnosis of trichinosis. *Wiad. Parazyt.* 6:344, 1960.
39. Theiler, H., and Augustine, D. L. Zur Frage der immunbiologischen Diagnose der Trichinose. *Zbl. Bakt.* (*Naturwiss.*) 135:299, 1935.
40. Harrell, G. T., and Horne, S. F. *Trichinella* skin tests in tuberculosis sanitariums, hospitals for mental diseases, and general hospitals. *Amer J. Trop. Med.* 25:51, 1945.
41. Arbesman, C. E., Witebsky, E., and Osgood, H. Results of intradermal skin tests with Trichina antigen in allergic and normal individuals. *J. Allerg.* 13:583, 1942.
42. Bozicevich, J. Immunological Diagnosis of Parasitic Diseases. In Most, H. (Ed.), *Parasitic Infections in Man.* New York: Columbia University Press, 1951.
43. Bassen, F. A., Thomason, A. E., and Silver, A. The occurrence of false positive Trichina precipitin tests in infectious mononucleosis. *J. Lab. Clin. Med.* 34:543, 1949.
44. Southam, C. M., Thomason, A. E., and Burchenal, J. H. False positive Trichina precipitin reactions in neoplastic disease. *Proc. Soc. Exp. Biol. Med* 72:354, 1949.
45. Barciszewski, M., Janecki, J., and Jezioranska, J. Clinical and serological evaluation of trichinosis. *J. Hyg. Epidem.* (Prague) 3:317, 1959.
46. Oliver-Gonzalez, J. The *in vitro* action of immune serum on the larvae and adults of *Trichinella spiralis. J. Infect. Dis.* 67:292, 1940.
47. Mauss, E. A. The *in vitro* effect of immune serum upon *Trichinella spiralis* larvae. *Amer. J. Hyg.* 32:(sect. D)80, 1940.
48. Roth, H. The *in vitro* action of Trichina larvae in immune serum: A new precipitin test in trichinosis. *Acta Path. Microbiol. Scand.* 18:160, 1941.
49. Jezioranska, A. Investigations on serodiagnosis of experimental and chemical trichinosis: 1. Precipitin and complement-fixation reactions. *Przegl. Epidem.* 9:211, 1959.
50. Kagan, I. G., and Bargai, U. Studies on the serology of trichinosis with hemagglutination, agar diffusion tests and precipitin ring tests. *J. Parasit.* 42:237, 1956.
51. Sadun, E. H., and Allain, D. S. A rapid slide hemagglutination test for the detection of anti-

bodies to *Trichinella spiralis. J. Parasit.* 43: 383, 1957.

52. Vogel, H., Widelock, D., and Fuerst, H. T. A microflocculation test for trichinosis. *J. Infect. Dis.* 100:40, 1957.
53. Witebsky, E., Wels, P., and Heide, A. Serodiagnosis of trichinosis by means of complement-fixation. *New York J. Med.* 42:431, 1942.
54. Jezioranska, A., and Kicuiska, H. Immunological tests during a trichinosis epidemic in Bydogoszcz in 1957. *Wiad. Parazyt.* 6:389, 1958.
55. Sussenguth, H., and Kline, B. S. A simple rapid flocculation slide test for trichinosis in man and in swine. *Amer. J. Clin. Path.* 14:471, 1944.
56. Sussenguth, H., Bauer, A. H., and Greenlee, A. M. Evaluation of the Sussenguth-Kline test for trichinosis. *Public Health Rep.* 72:939, 1957.
57. Campbell, C. H. The use of the collodion particle agglutination test for detecting antibodies formed in response to *Trichinella spiralis* infection. *J. Parasit.* 39(supp.):41, 1953.
58. Coudert, J., and Coly, M. Éssai d'application de la réaction d'agglutination des particules de collodion à quelques parasitoses. *Ann. Parasit. Hum. Comp.* 31:489, 1956.
59. Leikina, E. S., and Poliakova, O. I. Simplified method of immunodiagnovsis of helminthiasis: I. Agglutination reaction with adsorption of the antigen in diagnosis of experimental ascariasis and trichinosis in animals. *Med. Parazit.* (Moscow) 25:131, 1956.
60. Thomas, E. H., Bozicevich, J., and Hoymen, H. M. Flocculation reactions in rabbits experimentally infected with *Trichinella spiralis. J. Infect. Dis.* 92:89, 1953.
61. Sadun, E. H., and Norman, L. The use of an acid soluble protein fraction in the flocculation test for the diagnosis of trichinosis. *J. Parasit.* 41:476, 1955.
62. Norman, L., and Sadun, E. H. The use of metabolic antigens in the flocculation test for the serologic diagnosis for trichinosis. *J. Parasit.* 45:485, 1959.
63. Norman, L., Donaldson, A. W., and Sadun, E. H. The flocculation test with purified antigen in the diagnosis of trichinosis in humans. *J. Infect. Dis.* 98:172, 1956.
64. Innella, R., and Redner, W. J. Latex-agglutination serologic test for trichinosis. *J.A.M.A.* 171:885, 1959.
65. Sadun, E. H., Anderson, R. I., and Schoenbechler, M. J. A new slide flocculation test for trichinosis. *J. Parasit.* 48:(supp.)17, 1962.
66. Anderson, R. I., Sadun, E. H., and Schoenbechler, M. J. Cholesterol-lecithin slide (TsSF) and charcoal card (TsCC) flocculation tests using an acid soluble fraction of *Trichinella spiralis* larvae. *J. Parasit.* 49:642, 1963.
67. Sadun, E. H., Anderson, R. I., and Williams, J. S. Fluorescent antibody test for the serological diagnosis of trichinosis. *Exp. Parasit.* 12:423, 1962.
68. Pavlov, P. Le role de l'avitaminose dans l'inféstation du pigéon par le *Taenia echinococcus. Bull. Soc. Path. Exot.* 33:93, 1940.
69. Turner, E. L., Dennis, E. W., and Berberian, D. A. The production of artificial immunity against hydatid disease in sheep. *J. Parasit.* 23:43, 1937.
70. Turner, E. L., Berberian, D. A., and Dennis, E. W. The production of artificial immunity in dogs against *Echinococcus granulosus. J. Parasit.* 22:14, 1936.
71. Casoni, T. La diagnosi biologica dell' echinococcosi umana mediante l' intradermoreazione. *Folia Clin. Chim. Micros.* 4:5, 1912.
72. Botteri, J. H. Echinokokkenantigen. *Klin. Wschr.* 8:836, 1929.
73. Fairley, N. H. The intradermal test in hydatid disease: A critical analysis of its results. *Med. J. Aust.* 1:472, 1929.
74. Chung, H.-L., and T'ung, T. The non-specificity of the so-called specific biological tests for hydatid disease. *Trans. Roy. Soc. Trop. Med.* 32:697, 1939.
75. Turner, E. L., Dennis, E. W., and Berberian, D. A. The value of the Casoni test in dogs. *J. Parasit.* 21:180, 1935.
76. Ghedini, G. Ricerche sul sierre del sangue. *Gaz. Osped. Med.* (Milano) 27:1616, 1906.
77. Fairley, N. H. Researches on the complement fixation reaction in hydatid disease. *Quart. J. Med.* 15:244, 1921.
78. Kent, J. F. Current and potential value of immunodiagnostic tests employing soluble antigens. *Amer. J. Hyg.* 22:68, 1963.
79. Kagan, I. G., and Norman, L. Antigenic analysis of Echinococcus antigens by agar diffusion techniques. *Amer. J. Trop. Med.* 10: 727, 1961.
80. Kagan, I. G. Seminar on immunity to parasitic helminths: VI. Hydatid disease. *Exp. Parasit.* 13:57, 1963.
81. Garabedian, G. A., Matossian, R. M., and Djanian, A. Y. An indirect hemagglutination test for hydatid disease. *J. Immun.* 78:269, 1957.
82. Garabedian, G. A., Matossian, R. M., and Suidan, F. G. Correlative study of immunological tests for the diagnosis of hydatid disease. *Amer. J. Trop. Med.* 8:67, 1959.
83. Norman, L., Sadun, E. H., and Allain, D. S. A bentonite flocculation test for the diagnosis of hydatid disease in man and animals. *Ibid.,* p. 46.
84. Kagan, I. G., Allain, D. S., and Norman, L. An evaluation of the hemagglutination and flocculation tests in the diagnosis of *Echinococcus* disease. *Ibid.,* p. 51.

85. Krakower, C., Hoffman, W. A., and Axtmayer, J. H. The fate of schistosomes (*S. mansoni*) in experimental infections of normal and vitamin A deficient white rats. *Puerto Rico J. Public Health* 16:269, 1940.
86. DeWitt, W. B. Experimental schistosomiasis mansoni in mice maintained on nutritionally deficient diets: I. Effects of a *Torula* yeast ration deficient in factor 3, vitamin E, and cystine. *J. Parasit.* 43:119, 1957.
87. DeWitt, W. B. Experimental schistosomiasis mansoni in mice maintained on nutritionally deficient diets: II. Survival and development of *Schistosoma mansoni* in mice maintained on a *Torula* yeast diet deficient in factor 3, vitamin E, and cystine. *Ibid.*, p. 129.
88. Barbosa, F. S., Coelho, M. V., and Coutinho-Abath, E. Infestacao natural e experimental de algums mamiferous de Pernambuco por *Schistosoma mansoni. Rev. Brasil. Malar.* [*Publ. Avuls.*] 10:137, 1958.
89. Kuntz, R. E., and Malakatis, G. M. Susceptibility studies in schistosomiasis: II. Susceptibility of wild mammals to infection by *Schistosoma mansoni* in Egypt, with emphasis on rodents. *Amer. J. Trop. Med.* 4:75, 1955.
90. Price, D. L. Laboratory infection of the agouti, *Dasyorocta aguti,* with *Schistosoma mansoni. Amer. J. Trop. Med.* 2:926, 1953.
91. Martins, A. V. Non-human vertebrate hosts of *Schistosoma haematobium* and *Schistosoma mansoni. Bull. WHO* 18:931, 1958.
92. Bruce, J. I., Llewellyn, L. M., and Sadun, E. H. Susceptibility of wild mammals to infection by *Schistosoma mansoni. J. Parasit.* 47:693, 1961.
93. von Lichtenberg, F., Sadun, E. H., and Bruce, J. I. Tissue responses and mechanisms of resistance in schistosomiasis mansoni in abnormal hosts. *Amer. J. Trop. Med.* 11:347, 1962.
94. Stirewalt, M. A. Seminar on immunity to parasitic infections: IV. Schistosoma infections. *Exp. Parasit.* 13:18, 1963.
95. Sadun, E. H. Immunization in schistosomiasis by previous exposure to homologous and heterologous cercariae by inoculation of preparations from schistosomes and by exposure to irradiated cercariae. *Ann. N.Y. Acad. Sci.* 113: 418, 1963.
96. Vogel, H., and Minning, W. Ueber die erworbene Resistanz von macacus Thesus gegenuber *Schistosoma japonicum. Z. Tropenmed. Parasit.* 4:418, 1953.
97. Lin, S. S., Ritchie, L. S., and Hunter, G. W. Acquired immunologic resistance against *Schistosoma japonicum. J. Parasit.* 40:42, 1954 (abst.).
98. Sadun, E. H., and Lin, S. S. Studies on the host parasite relationship to *Schistosoma japonicum:* IV. Resistance acquired by infection, by vaccination and by the injection of immune serum. *J. Parasit.* 45:543, 1959.
99. Hunter, G. W., III, Ritchie, L. S., Lin, S. S., Pan, C., and Tanabe, H. Immunological studies: II. Experiments with bird and human schistosomes in small mammals. *Exp. Parasit.* 5:551, 1956.
100. Olivier, L., and Schneidermann, J. Acquired resistance to *Schistosoma mansoni* infection in laboratory animals. *Amer. J. Trop. Med.* 2:298, 1953.
101. Stirewalt, M. A. The influence of previous infection of mice with *Schistosoma mansoni* on a challenging infection with the homologous parasite. *Ibid.*, p. 867.
102. Thompson, J. H. Host-parasite relationships of *Schistosoma mansoni. Exp. Parasit.* 3:140, 1954.
103. Hunter, G. W., Weinmann, C. J., and Hoffman, R. G. Studies on schistosomiasis: XVII. Non-reciprocal acquired resistance between *Schistosoma mansoni* and *Schistosomatium douthitti* in mice. *Exp. Parasit.* 11:133, 1961.
104. Meleney, H. E., and Moore, D. V. Observations on immunity to superinfection with *Schistosoma mansoni* and *S. haematobium* in monkeys. *Exp. Parasit.* 3:128, 1954.
105. Standen, O. D., and Fuller, K. A. Ultraviolet irradiation of the cercariae of *Schistosoma mansoni:* Inhibition of development to the adult stage. *Trans. Roy. Soc. Trop. Med.* 53:373, 1959.
106. Cram, E. B., and Files, V. S. Experimental mammalian infection with the schistosomes of man: I. Laboratory animals as source of supply of adult schistosomes and their ova. *Nat. Inst. Health Bull.* 189:101, 1947.
107. Naimark, D. H., Benenson, A. S., Oliver-Gonzalez, J., McMullen, D. B., and Ritchie, L. S. Studies on schistosomiasis in primates: Observations on acquired resistance (progress report). *Amer. J. Trop. Med.* 9:430, 1960.
108. Liu, C., and Bang, F. B. The natural course of a light experimental infection of schistosomiasis japonica in monkeys. *Bull. Hopkins Hosp.* 86:215, 1950.
109. Kagan, I. G. Experimental infections of rhesus monkeys with *Schistosomatium douthitti* (Cort 1914). *J. Infect. Dis.* 93:200, 1953.
110. Hsu, S. Y. L., and Hsu, H. F. A new approach to immunization against *Schistosoma japonicum. Science* 133:766, 1961.
111. Sadun, E. H., Yamaki, A., Burke, J. C., and Lin, S. S. Studies on the host parasite relationships to *Schistosoma japonicum:* VI. Acquired resistance in mice and monkeys infected with the Formosan and Japanese strains. *J. Parasit.* 47:891, 1961.
112. Ozawa, M. Experimental study on acquired immunity to schistosomiasis japonica. *Jap. J. Exp. Med.* 8:79, 1930.
113. Kawamura, R. The recent researches on

schistosomiasis in Japan. *C. R. Cong. Int. Med. Trop. Hyg.* 4:311, 1932.
114. Vogel, H. Immunologie der Helminthiasen. *Zbl. Bakt.* 154:118, 1949.
115. Stirewalt, M. A., and Evans, A. S. An unsuccessful attempt to protect mice against *Schistosoma mansoni* by transfer of immune serum. *Proc. Helminth. Soc. Washington* 20: 15, 1953.
116. Meisenhelder, J. E., Olsewski, B., and Thompson, P. E. Observations on therapeutic and prophylactic effects by homologous immune blood against *Schistosoma mansoni* in rhesus monkeys. *J. Parasit.* 3:128, 1960.
117. Weinmann, C. J., and Hunter, G. W. Studies on schistosomiasis: XV. The effect of immune serum upon egg production by *Schistosoma mansoni* in mice. *Exp. Parasit.* 11:56, 1961.
118. Watts, N. P. Prophylactic use of schistosomal antigen. *J. Immun.* 62:183, 1949.
119. Kagan, I. G. Contributions to the immunology and serology of schistosomiasis. *Rice Inst. Pamph.* 45:151, 1958.
120. Levine, D. M., and Kagan, I. G. Studies on the immunology of schistosomiasis by vaccination and passive transfer. *J. Parasit.* 46: 787, 1960.
121. Ritchie, L. S., Frick, L. P., Knight, W. B., and Berrios-Duran, L. A. Effect of the duration of *Schistosoma mansoni* infections on the degree of protection against subsequent exposures. *J. Parasit.* 48:(sect. 2)18, 1962.
122. Sadun, E. H., and Bruce, J. I. Resistance induced in rats by vaccination with fresh homogenates of adult *Schistosoma mansoni* worms. *Exp. Parasit.* 15:32, 1964.
123. Villella, J. B., Bomberg, H. J., and Gould, S. E. Immunization to *Schistosoma mansoni* in mice inoculated with radiated cercariae. *Science* 134:1073, 1961.
124. Villella, J. B., Bomberg, H. J., and Gould, S. E. Immune response in mice to irradiated cercariae of *Schistosoma mansoni. J. Parasit.* 48:(sect. 2)19, 1962.
125. Erickson, D. G., and Caldwell, W. L. Increased resistance of rats to *Schistosoma mansoni* after exposure to gamma irradiated cercariae. *Ibid.,* p. 19.
126. Hsu, H. F., Hsu, S. Y. L., and Osborne, J. W. Immunization against *Schistosoma japonicum* in rhesus monkeys produced by irradiated cercariae. *Nature* (London) 194:98, 1962.
127. Radke, M. G., and Sadun, E. H. Resistance produced in mice by exposure to irradiated *Schistosoma mansoni* cercariae. *Exp. Parasit.* 13:134, 1963.
128. von Lichtenberg, F., and Sadun, E. H. The parasite migration and host reaction in mice exposed to irradiated cercariae of *Schistosoma mansoni. Exp. Parasit.* 13:256, 1963.
129. Szumlewicz, A. P., and Olivier, L. J. *Schistosoma mansoni:* Development of challenge infections in mice exposed to irradiated cercariae. *Science* 140:411, 1963.
130. Smithers, S. R. Acquired Resistance to Bilharziasis. In Wolstenholme, G. E. W., and O'Connor, M. (Eds.), *Bilharziasis.* Boston: Little, Brown, 1962. P. 239.
131. von Lichtenberg, F., and Ritchie, L. S. Cellular response against schistosomula of *Schistosoma mansoni* in *Macaca mulatta* monkeys following prolonged infections. *Amer. J. Trop. Med.* 10:859, 1961.
132. Kagan, I. G., and Pellegrino, J. A critical review of immunological methods for the diagnosis of bilharziasis. *Bull. WHO* 25:611, 1961.
133. Anderson, R. I. Current and potential value of immunodiagnostic tests employing whole organisms. *Amer. J. Hyg.* 22:97, 1963.
134. Fairley, N. H., and Williams, F. E. A preliminary report on an intradermal reaction in schistosomiasis. *Med. J. Aust.* 2:811, 1927.
135. Taliaferro, W. H., Hoffman, W. A., and Cook, D. H. A precipitin test in intestinal schistosomiasis (*S. mansoni*). *J. Prevent. Med.* 2:395, 1928.
136. Khalil, M., and Hassan, A. J. A preliminary note on a new skin reaction in human schistosomiasis. *J. Egypt. Med. Ass.* 15:129, 1932.
137. Pellegrino, J., Brener, Z., and Memoria, J. M. P. A comparative study of intradermal tests and stool examination in epidemiological surveys on schistosomiasis mansoni. *Amer. J. Trop. Med.* 8:307, 1959.
138. Sadun, E. H., Lin, S. S., and Walton, B. C. Studies on the host parasite relationships to *Schistosoma japonicum:* III. The use of purified antigens in the diagnosis of infections in human and experimental animals. *Milit. Med.* 124:428, 1959.
139. Jachowski, L. A., and Anderson, R. I. Evaluation of some laboratory procedures in diagnosing infections with *Schistosoma mansoni. Bull. WHO* 25:675, 1961.
140. Anderson, R. I., and Sadun, E. H. Some recent advances in the diagnosis of schistosomiasis. *Med. Ann. Dist. Columbia* 31:211, 1962.
141. Yoshimoto, M. Ueber die Komplementbindungsreaktion bei der Schistosomum-Krankheit in Japan. *Z. Immunitaetsforsch.* 5:438, 1910.
142. Chaffee, E. F., Bauman, P. M., and Shapilo, J. J. Diagnosis of schistosomiasis by complement-fixation. *Amer. J. Trop. Med.* 3:905, 1954.
143. Oliver-Gonzalez, J., and Pratt, C. K. Skin and precipitin reactions to antigens from the cercariae and adults of *Schistosoma mansoni. Puerto Rico J. Public Health* 20:242, 1944.
144. Okabe, K., Koga, Y., Shibue, H., and Matsuse,

M. Immunological studies on schistosomiasis japonica: 3. Intradermal and precipitin tests for schistosomiasis japonica. *Kurume Med. J.* 1:85, 1954.

145. Oliver-Gonzalez, J. Anti-egg precipitins in the serum of humans infected with *Schistosoma mansoni. J. Infect. Dis.* 95:86, 1954.
146. Vogel, H., and Minning, W. Hullenbildung bei bilharzia-cercarien im Serum bilharzia-infizierter Tiere und Menschen. *Zbl. Bakt.* 153:91, 1949.
147. Liu, C., and Bang, F. B. Agglutination of cercariae of *Schistosoma mansoni* by immune sera. *Proc. Soc. Exp. Biol. Med.* 74:68, 1950.
148. Senterfit, L. B. Immobilization of *Schistosoma mansoni* miracidia by immune serum. *Proc. Soc. Exp. Biol. Med.* 84:5, 1953.
149. Brandt, J. L., and Finch, E. P. A simple flocculation slide test for the diagnosis of schistosomiasis. *Amer. J. Clin. Path.* 16:141, 1946.
150. Anderson, R. I. Serologic diagnosis of *Schistosoma mansoni* infections: I. Development of a cercarial antigen slide flocculation test. *Amer. J. Trop. Med.* 9:299, 1960.
151. Kagan, I. G. Hemagglutination after immunization with schistosome antigens. *Science* 122:376, 1955.
152. Pellegrino, J. Immunological methods for the diagnosis of schistosomiasis mansoni. *Proc. 7th Int. Cong. Trop. Med. & Malar.*, p. 21, 1963 (abst.).
153. Sadun, E. H., Williams, J. S., and Anderson, R. I. Fluorescent antibody technic for serodiagnosis of schistosomiasis in humans. *Proc. Soc. Exp. Biol. Med.* 105:289, 1960.
154. Anderson, R. I., Sadun, E. H., and Williams, J. S. Preserved cercariae in the fluorescent antibody (FA) test for schistosomiasis. *Exp. Parasit.* 11:226, 1961.
155. Anderson, R. I., Sadun, E. H., and Williams, J. S. A technique for the use of minute amounts of dried blood in the fluorescent antibody test for schistosomiasis. *Ibid.*, p. 111.
156. Sadun, E. H., Anderson, R. I., and Williams, J. S. Fluorescent antibody test for the laboratory diagnosis of schistosomiasis in humans by using dried blood smears on filter paper. *Ibid.*, p. 117.
157. Clarke, V. Personal communication, 1963.
158. Kagan, I. G. Personal communication, 1963.
159. Lewert, R. M. Personal communication, 1963.
160. Sadun, E. H., Anderson, R. I., and Schoenbechler, M. J. A plasma card test for rapid serodiagnosis of schistosomiasis (SPC). *Proc. Soc. Exp. Biol. Med.* 112:280, 1963.
161. Brewer, J. H., and Harris, A. Presented at meetings of the Maryland Branch, American Society of Microbiologists, 1962.
162. Beaver, P. C. Control of soil-transmitted helminths. *WHO Public Health Papers,* 1961.
163. Vogel, H., and Minning, W. Beitrage zur Klinik der Lungen-Ascariasis und zur Frage der fluchtigen eosinophilen Lungeninfiltrate. *Beitr. Klin. Tuberk.* 98:620, 1942.
164. Hemming, G. R. Respiratory complications of *Ascaris* infestation in Fiji. *Med. J. Aust.* 1:501, 1956.
165. Beaver, P. C., and Danaraj, T. J. Pulmonary ascariasis resembling eosinophilic lung: Autopsy report with description of larvae in the bronchioles. *Amer. J. Trop. Med.* 7:100, 1958.
166. Sadun, E. H., Bradin, J. L., and Faust, E. C. The effect of ascorbic acid deficiency on the resistance of guinea pigs to infection with *Endamoeba histolytica* of human origin. *Amer. J. Trop. Med.* 31:426, 1951.
167. Roman, E. Biologie d'*Ascaris lumbricoides* jeune: Infestation pulmonaire de rongeurs; réinfestation de l'homme parasite. *C. R. Soc. Biol.* (Paris) 130:1168, 1939.
168. Cort, W. W., Schapiro, L., and Stoll, N. R. A study of reinfection after treatment with hookworm and ascariasis in two villages in Panama. *Amer. J. Hyg.* 10:614, 1929.
169. Kerr, K. B. The cellular response in acquired resistance in guinea pigs to an infection with pig *Ascaris. Amer. J. Hyg.* 27:28, 1938.
170. Oliver-Gonzalez, J. Functional antigens in helminths. *J. Infect. Dis.* 78:232, 1946.
171. Soulsby, E. J. L. Immunization against *Ascaris lumbricoides* in the pig. *Nature* (London) 179:783, 1957.
172. Sadun, E. H. The antibody basis of immunity in chickens to the nematode, *Ascaridia galli. Amer. J. Hyg.* 49:101, 1949.
173. Soulsby, E. J. L. Some immunological phenomena in parasitic infections. *Vet. Rec.* 69: 1129, 1957.
174. Soulsby, E. J. L. Some aspects of the mechanism of immunity to helminths. *J. Amer. Vet. Med. Ass.* 138:355, 1961.
175. Soulsby, E. J. L. The nature and origin of the functional antigens in helminth infections. *Ann. N.Y. Acad. Sci.* 113:492, 1963.
176. Oliver-Gonzalez, J. Antigenic analysis of isolated tissues and body fluids of roundworm *Ascaris lumbricoides* var. suum. *J. Infect. Dis.* 72:202, 1943.
177. Oliver-Gonzalez, J. Histopathological and immunological observations after inoculation of substances isolated from the muscle and cuticle of *Ascaris lumbricoides. J. Infect. Dis.* 107:94, 1960.
178. Kent, J. F. Current and potential value of immunodiagnostic tests employing soluble antigens. *Amer. J. Hyg.* 22:68, 1963.
179. Kagan, I. G. Hemagglutination tests with *Ascaris* antigens. *J. Immun.* 80:396, 1958.
180. Soulsby, E. J. L. Studies on the heterophile antibodies associated with helminth infec-

tions: I. Heterophile antibodies in *Ascaris lumbricoides* infection in rabbits. *J. Comp. Path.* 68:71, 1958.

181. Soulsby, E. J. L. Studies on the heterophile antibodies associated with helminth infection: II. Heterophile antibodies in *Ascaris lumbricoides* infection in pigs. *Ibid.*, p. 345.
182. Soulsby, E. J. L., and Coombs, R. R. A. Studies on blood group substances associated with *Ascaris lumbricoides. Parasitology* 49: 505, 1960.
183. Kent, H. N. Isolation of specific antigens from *Ascaris lumbricoides* var. suum. *Exp. Parasit.* 10:313, 1960.
184. Goodchild, C. G., and Kagan, I. G. Comparison of proteins in hydatid fluid and serum by means of electrophoresis. *J. Parasit.* 47: 175, 1961.

36. Viruses

A. J. RHODES AND K. R. ROZEE

BIOLOGY AND STRUCTURE

It has long been known that a hypersensitivity reaction may occur when heated preparations of viruses, such as vaccinia, mumps, and lymphogranuloma are introduced into the skin. Such skin tests are used in the diagnosis of certain virus infections, but much less attention has been paid to hypersensitivity developing during a natural virus infection and manifesting itself by "allergic" symptoms and signs.

At the outset of this discussion it may be useful to define the term "virus." According to a popular definition originated by Lwoff, a virus is an infectious, potentially pathogenic agent, composed of protein and ribonucleic acid (RNA) or desoxyribonucleic acid (DNA), but not both nucleic acids, multiplying in the intracellular environment, and being devoid of metabolic enzymes. By a strict definition of this type, most of the agents known as viruses are designated as the "true" viruses, while the basophilic viruses and rickettsiae are excluded from the group because they contain both nucleic acids and exhibit some metabolic activity. However, the true viruses, the basophilic viruses, and the rickettsiae all grow in the intracellular position and will not grow in lifeless media. Accordingly, we shall use the term "virus" to include the true viruses, the basophilic viruses of the psittacosis group, and the rickettsiae of typhus and typhus-like infections. We believe there is abundant precedent as well as biological justification for this approach, especially in a study of microbial allergy, which is essentially a response to the protein components of bacteria and viruses.

It is now customary to divide viruses into various taxonomic groups designated with the suffix "virus," e.g., *herpesvirus, adenovirus,* and *enterovirus.* Viruses are assigned to one of fifteen or more major groups on the basis of common properties. The most important property is probably the type of nucleic acid, and viruses are classified into RNA-viruses, DNA-viruses, and the basophilic viruses and rickettsiae, which probably contain both. The next most important property is morphology. Viruses range in diameter from about 500 mμ to about 20 mμ. Another important characteristic is the presence or absence of essential lipid, as shown by sensitivity or resistance to the killing effect of ether.

Modern techniques of staining viruses prior to examination with a high resolution electron microscope have led to the introduction of an elegant form of classification based on shape and internal structure. Briefly, the genetic material in a virus particle, which is nucleic acid, is situated in the center of a surrounding "overcoat" or capsid of protein or lipoprotein. In an increasing number of viruses the nucleic acid has been demonstrated in the form of elongated helical threads, the dimensions of which can be determined. In many viruses, the protein or protective coat is composed of subunits or capsomeres arranged in a regular interlocking structure. Finally, a number of viruses have lipid material, probably deriving from the wall of the host cell, included in their outer envelope.

The precise differentiation between the individual members in any group of viruses is made not on structure but on the characteristics of the protein or lipoprotein capsid. For it is this envelope that determines the antigenic characteristics of the virus and induces the production of antibody and resistance to reinfection. In the case of most viruses the use of the term "protein antigen" is an oversimplification, because several antigenically distinct antigens can be recognized by various technics, such as gradient centrifugation and gel diffusion by the Oudin or Ouchterlony techniques. Because hypersensitivity is essentially a response to protein or protein complexes, it is evident that viruses which incorporate a limited number of antigens separable by various techniques afford interesting models for study. It is a pity that the intriguing possibilities of such models have been little exploited.

Increasing interest is being taken in substances isolated from several viruses that behave like toxins [1], although their role in hypersensitivity is not yet clear. We shall now give a brief description of some of the virus groups of interest to students of hypersensitivity.

PROPERTIES OF VIRUSES

DNA-CONTAINING VIRUSES

The most interesting DNA-containing viruses from the standpoint of hypersensitivity reactions are the herpesviruses and the poxviruses.

Herpesvirus Group. This group comprises the viruses of herpes simplex, virus B of monkeys, and the varicella-zoster (V-Z) virus. The particles measure about 100 mμ and contain 162 capsomeres in the capsid. Lipid is present in an outer coat. There is probably only one antigenic type of herpes simplex, one type of virus B, and one type of V-Z virus. Soluble complement-fixing antigens that readily dissociate from the virus particles are characteristic of the individual members of this group.

Poxvirus Group. This group comprises the viruses of vaccinia, variola, cowpox, contagious pustular dermatitis (CPD or "orf"), and molluscum contagiosum as well as several which infect only animals (myxoma, fibroma, monkeypox, rabbitpox, etc.). These viruses are described as having complex symmetry. The particles are rectangular or oblong and measure 200 to 300 mμ depending on the species. Capsomeres have not been described, but a double membrane encloses a helical core of nucleoprotein which seems to be wound almost like a ball of knitting wool. Most of the poxviruses are sensitive to ether, indicating the presence of essential lipid.

Vaccinia virus is of particular interest to the student of hypersensitivity, because at least six major antigens can be demonstrated in suitable preparations. (1) *LS antigen* is incorporated in the virus particle but dissociates readily from it. LS is a complex of the L (labile) component destroyed at 70° C. and the S (stable) component, resisting even 90° C. (2) *Nucleoprotein (NP) antigen,* extractable with alkali, constitutes about one half of the virus substance and contains 6 percent of DNA. NP antigen is thought to be shared by most members of the poxvirus group. (3, 4) *Hemagglutinins* are of two types. The soluble hemagglutinin is heat-labile and probably a lipoprotein. A second hemagglutinating fraction is heat-stable. (5) *X antigen* is thought to be separate from the above. (6) *The infectivity factor.*

No detailed studies of the role of these fractions in inducing vaccinial hypersensitivity have been made. However, as heated vaccinia virus elicits a dermal reaction in previously infected individuals, it is probable that the various labile fractions play an unimportant role.

RNA-CONTAINING VIRUSES

RNA-containing viruses of interest in a study of allergy include the relatively large myxoviruses and the smaller picornaviruses. Picornaviruses include the enteroviruses (poliomyelitis, Coxsackie, Echo) and the rhinoviruses of "common colds."

The myxovirus group includes the viruses of influenza (A, B, and C), mumps, the several types of parainfluenza virus (six or more), and Newcastle disease virus. Electron microscope studies strongly suggest that the viruses of measles and rabies should be included in this group.

Myxoviruses range from 90 to 200 mμ in size, although some strains appear larger. The individual particles have a complex structure. The central portion is occupied by the RNA in the form of a long helical thread; this material is identical with the S or soluble complement-fixing antigen of earlier workers. Surrounding the core is a limiting membrane, probably comprising the mucoprotein hemagglutinin and the V (viral) complement-fixing antigen. The outermost layer contains lipoprotein derived from the outer layers of the host cell cytoplasm, where myxovirus particles mature.

BASOPHILIC VIRUSES

The basophilic viruses measure from 250 to 500 mμ, and the particles appear to be spherical and cocco-bacillary. Unlike the true viruses, these agents multiply by binary fission. They contain a common complement-fixing antigen which is heat-stable, released by ether, and composed of polysaccharide, lecithin, and nucleoprotein. This antigen is destroyed by periodate and lecithinase but resists pepsin. There is also a type-specific complement-fixing antigen which is a lecithin-nucleoprotein complex. Both antigens are tightly incorporated in the virus particle but can be differentiated by the fact that the specific antigen is destroyed at 60° C. and resists ether but is inactivated by pepsin. Basophilic viruses elaborate a heat-stable hemagglutinin which can be separated from the particles and is probably a lecithin-nucleoprotein complex.

HYPERSENSITIVITY REACTIONS

REACTIONS TO DNA-CONTAINING VIRUSES

Hypersensitivity may develop following injection of or infection with herpesviruses and poxviruses.

Herpesvirus Group. An important observation was made by Nagler [2], who showed that a heat-inactivated antigen prepared from chick amniotic fluid infected with herpes simplex caused a positive reaction of the delayed type when injected into the skin of immune persons. This state of immunity was indicated by the presence of serum antibody. It has also been reported that antigen prepared from infected tissue culture fluid and inactivated by ultraviolet light induces a positive skin reaction in persons whose serum contains neutralizing antibody [3].

Clearly, therefore, a component of herpes virus, which is not the infectivity factor, elicits a hypersensitivity reaction of the delayed type in persons previously naturally infected with the virus. The work of Kilbourne and Anderson [3] suggests that a soluble antigen which readily dissociates from the virus particle is more actively allergenic than the particulate or viral antigen. This active fraction is presumably of small size and could be the soluble complement-fixing antigen, but further work to identify the two is required.

Herpes simplex virus usually causes a primary infection in childhood. This infection may be of the mouth, mucous membranes, skin, meninges, or central nervous system. The virus probably remains latent for life, after the patient has recovered from the acute stage. Virus-neutralizing antibody circulates in the serum and causes a dermal reaction on injection of inactivated virus. From time to time the latent infection may "flare up" into a recurrent infection of mouth, mucous membrane, or skin. There is no clear evidence of a hypersensitivity component in the clinical picture of recurrent herpes simplex virus infection.

Another member of the herpesvirus group is the virus of varicella-zoster. Strains of this virus isolated from children infected with chickenpox cannot be distinguished from strains isolated from adults with shingles (herpes zoster). It has been known since the early observations of Bokay that herpes zoster in adults may give rise to chickenpox in child contacts. The epidemiological studies of Hope-Simpson show that outbreaks of chickenpox initiated by exposure to a case of chickenpox behave exactly like outbreaks initiated by a case of zoster.

Many students of this fascinating "twin manifestation" disease would accept the stimulating hypothesis of Stokes. According to this hypothesis, the primary infection with V-Z virus usually occurs in childhood and is manifested as chickenpox. After recovery from the infection, the virus may persist in the tissues, but later in life may become active and produce the syndrome of zoster. On the rare occasions when zoster in adults does seem to be a direct result of infection contracted from a child with varicella, the illness may show one of the "accelerated" characteristics of a hypersensitivity reaction, for the incubation is said to be only 3 to 7 days instead of the usual 13 to 17 days.

Poxvirus Group. The so-called immediate reaction* on revaccination with vaccinia virus has long been regarded as a classic example of delayed hypersensitivity. The immediate reaction develops between eight hours and three days after inoculation of a person previously vaccinated against or recovered from smallpox. The reaction consists of a papule and areola. There is no vesiculation, and pre-existing blood antibody level is not raised. The immediate reaction is elicited by living as well as heated vaccinia, either in the form of the usual "lymph" or as washed and concentrated virus particles. It is commonly regarded as due to hypersensitivity to vaccinial "protein." Unfortunately, despite all the knowledge of the various antigens present in vaccinia (as pointed out earlier), the hypersensitivity-in-

* *Editor's comment:* Not to be confused with the "immediate" wheal and flare reaction of atopic individuals.—B. R.

ducing component cannot be specifically identified, except that it must be one or more of the heat-stable components.

There does not appear to be any constant relationship between the presence of circulating blood antibody to vaccinia and the development of the immediate reaction on revaccination [4, 5]. One must, of course, consider the possibility that the responsible antibody is bound to the tissues.

In modified smallpox occurring in resistant individuals, the rash is scanty and the systemic reaction slight or absent. This is no definite evidence that there is a hypersensitivity component in this clinical picture of modified smallpox. However, it is probable that the so-called "contact fever" occurring in individuals in contact with smallpox, and who have a moderate degree of resistance, may be explained on such a basis. The transient symptoms include fever, headache, myalgia, and catarrh.

REACTIONS TO RNA-CONTAINING VIRUSES

Influenza Virus. It has been known for some time that skin hypersensitivity can be demonstrated in individuals previously infected with influenza virus by the injection of antigen prepared from allantoic fluid in which the virus has been destroyed by heat [6]. Many of those who react to the injection of virus have circulating virus-neutralizing antibody.

All three types of influenza virus can elicit dermal sensitivity reactions in persons previously infected with the appropriate virus. The factor that elicits the dermal reaction is quite resistant to heat and even withstands boiling for ten minutes. This raises the suspicion that a toxin may be concerned in the phenomenon.

As dermal sensitivity to influenza viruses can be established, it is of interest that children with an allergic history, when infected with a respiratory virus, have an increased tendency to "wheeze" [7]. These symptoms may be explained on the basis of an allergic response to infection with a respiratory virus. Because several strains of influenza virus may contain the same allergenic antigen, it is theoretically possible that allergic manifestations could occur in an individual infected with a strain to which he had never before been exposed. In the acute phase of illness in such a subject, there would be no specific neutralizing antibodies in the serum to the strain eliciting the hypersensitive state.

These speculations may have some bearing on the etiology of virus croup, which is caused by the parainfluenza and sometimes influenza viruses. The parainfluenza viruses belong to the myxovirus group and are distantly related to the influenza viruses. Perhaps some of the recurrent attacks of croup experienced by certain children may be due to infection with a respiratory virus to which they are hypersensitive as a result of a previous infection with an antigenically related virus.

Early in the modern history of influenza it was observed that when type B virus was inoculated in volunteers three to six months after a primary infection, the second infection had a much shorter incubation period, and the severer symptoms were experienced by those with higher serum neutralizing antibody levels [8]. In addition, the symptoms appeared to be allergic in nature. Virus could be isolated readily during the primary illness but seldom in the second bouts of illness. These facts raise the possibility that the symptomatology of influenza virus infections does indeed have an allergic component.

The thermostable property of the hypersensitivity-initiating component of influenza virus is especially interesting when recent work on toxins is considered, for it has been shown that there are at least two toxic factors, and perhaps more, in preparations of influenza virus.

A necrotoxin responsible for intestinal hemorrhages in mice when injected intraperitoneally is present in strains of both A and B types of influenza virus [9]. Toxic reactions develop in mice, rats, and guinea pigs when virus preparations are injected intracerebrally, intravenously, or intraperitoneally. Death occurs in 16 to 72 hours. In the case of intracerebral inoculations, the major site of lesions is the ependymal lining of the ventricles. Intraperitoneal injections cause extreme engorgement of the vessels of the small intestine, and also edema and hemorrhage.

If a toxic preparation is instilled into the eye of rabbits, a corneal opacity will develop in about three days with no evidence of virus multiplication. In this animal, nasal instillation of toxin results in lung lesions with associated pleural edema, as seen in natural infection of man [10]. This toxin seems to be less sensitive to heat than is the property of infectivity, but it is destroyed when exposed to 56° C. for thirty minutes.

It seems that this toxin is not associated with delayed dermal hypersensitivity, but Kato *et al.* [11] have shown that it contains both the preparatory and the provocative factor of the Shwartzman-Sanarelli phenomenon. This toxin is separable from the infectious and hemagglutinating properties as well as from the S nucleoprotein antigen. It is very closely associated with the hemagglutinin but is not essential for its activity. Ether extraction abolishes toxicity but has only a moderate effect on the hemagglutinin.

Another toxic factor, which is thermostable and requires 16 hours at 56° C. for inactivation, causes a marked fall in blood pressure when given to rats intravenously. This hypotensive toxin acts directly on the myocardium and is neutralized by specific immune serum [12]. It may play a part in cardiac irregularities seen in a number of human influenza infections as well as being associated with dermal hypersensitivity.

Mumps and Measles. These viruses also belong to the myxovirus group. A test for skin reactivity to mumps virus was developed in 1945 by Enders *et al.* [13], who employed antigen extracted from the parotid glands of infected monkeys. Later, amniotic and allantoic fluids of infected embryonated chick eggs were used with equal success.

In earlier studies on convalescents, hypersensitivity was demonstrated by the development of a local inflammatory reaction twenty-four to forty-eight hours after intracutaneous injection of antigen. The reaction occurred in virtually all persons with a history of mumps parotitis and in about one half of those who denied having had the disease.

In tests correlating morbidity and dermal hypersensitivity, it was observed that only 2 percent of those who exhibited a reaction between 15 and 25 mm. in average diameter later had mumps. No individual, among over 300 persons in whom the diameter was greater than 25 mm., later had the disease. When the diameter of the reaction was less than 16 mm., the subsequent attack rate varied from 8 to 35 percent, in proportion to the size of the reaction.

From the foregoing, we see that it is possible to estimate within limits, on the basis of the diameter of the hypersensitivity reaction to mumps antigen, whether or not an immune state exists [14]. Reactions that measure less than 10 to 15 mm. in diameter should be taken to indicate a lack of immunity. We can assume that, as with other viruses, dermal reactivity does develop in a high percentage of immune individuals but that some nonimmune subjects may be equally reactive. This is especially true if skin test antigens have been prepared in the embryonated egg. Many individuals will react to the egg protein in the preparation rather than to the specific virus antigen, thereby giving a false positive result. Friedman *et al.* [15] give this as one possible explanation for the poor correlation of skin reactivity and immunity they observed in one series of sixty children in which they used a commercially produced skin test antigen from the embryonated egg. If reliable results are to be obtained, it would seem that the choice of antigen, bearing in mind its potency and method of production, is as important as the demarcation of what constitutes a positive skin reaction as measured by its diameter.

The administration of a skin-test dose of killed antigen is associated with a striking rise in complement-fixing antibodies in a small percentage of individuals. These observations should be borne in mind in any epidemiological studies in which both serological and skin test methods are contemplated.

The immunology of mumps infection is relatively straightforward. Antibodies are produced in convalescence which fix complement with the virus particle and S antigens, prevent virus hemadsorption and hemagglutination and which neutralize virus infectivity.

Two antigens are elaborated during the replication of mumps virus in host cells. The S, or soluble, antigen is first to appear, and, correspondingly, complement-fixing antibodies to S antigen may be present alone early in infection. Later, antibodies to the V, or viral, antigen develop. Which of the various antigenic components is responsible for dermal sensitization is not known.

Since early in this century, measles infection has been known to reduce or eliminate the tuberculin reaction in individuals previously observed to be positive in this respect. Measles virus has a profound effect on lymphoid tissues throughout the body. These tissues become hyperplastic, with large numbers of multinucleate cells in lymph nodes, tonsils, and other sites. Since the lymphocyte appears to have a major role in the development of delayed hypersensitivity, it may be that infection of lymphocytic tissue with measles virus interferes with the proper functioning of the lymphocytes.

Vaccine measles, as well as natural measles, may depress the tuberculin reaction. During natural measles, the tuberculin reaction is depressed in many individuals during the late incubation period and is negative throughout the period of rash and for an average of eighteen days afterward. Vaccine measles does not cause as great a depression of reactivity nor so long a period of negativity as does natural measles [16]. The observation that live measles vaccine does depress the tuberculin reaction and the known dangers of natural measles to tuberculous children suggest that vaccination of these individuals be carefully controlled.

REACTIONS TO BASOPHILIC VIRUSES

In 1925 Frei developed one of the classic hypersensitivity tests for a virus infection, lymphogranuloma venereum (LGV), which in a modified form is still in routine use [18]. The original antigen was heat-inactivated pus obtained from discharging buboes, but since then several other preparations have been used successfully. The antigen most generally used today is obtained from infected yolk sacs. This preparation, called Lygranum, is purified by centrifugation and is phenol-inactivated.

Infection with LGV virus and other members of the basophilic virus group renders the individual reactive to the intradermal injection of Lygranum antigen. A positive reaction consists of an inflammatory area greater than 7 mm. in diameter, with a central papule. Skin reactions which measure between 4 and 7 mm. should be considered of doubtful significance.

An individual becomes reactive between two and six weeks after infection and usually remains so for life. The injection of Frei or Lygranum antigen is attended by a certain element of risk, for in a small proportion of patients it may cause an exacerbation of a quiescent infection.

Children of Frei-positive mothers circulate complement-fixing antibodies for the virus for two to three months after birth [16]. Such children do not, however, all have a positive Frei reaction [19].

In an acute infection, complement-fixing antibodies appear before the reaction to the Frei test becomes positive. After skin reactivity has developed, there is a correlation with the presence of complement-fixing antibodies for some time, but eventually the complement fixation may disappear, while dermal hypersensitivity persists.

These studies can be interpreted on the basis that the common group antigen responsible for the stimulation of basophilic virus complement-fixing antibodies does not also cause skin hypersensitivity. In further support of this conclusion is the demonstration that antigen eliciting a skin reaction may be separated from the virus particle by filtration [20]. In the case of the basophilic viruses we can therefore suggest that the dermal allergen is not related to the components of the virus which determine infectivity or fix complement.

It has been known for some time that clinical cure in LGV does not mean that the individual has necessarily become free from the organism. It appears that the infection becomes dormant and is subject to recall by a sufficiently specific immunological stimulus. This is illustrated by the numerous cases on record in which injection of Frei antigen has provoked an exacerbation of the disease. There is one case on record of death attributable to encephalitis with resulting flaccid paralysis closely following an injection of Frei antigen.

The fact that the great majority of Frei-positive individuals show only the dermal hypersensitivity reaction and no systemic reaction probably means that nondermal manifestations of allergy are relatively uncommon. However, individuals infected with LGV not infrequently have periodic febrile disturbances similar to those seen on intravenous injection of antigen in Frei-positive patients. In addition, lymphogranuloma has been suspect as a cause of erythema nodosum and polyarthritis, both of which may be manifestations of an allergic condition.*

In tests for psittacosis or ornithosis in birds, an antigen prepared by detergent extraction of meningopneumonitis virus, another mem-

* *Editor's comment:* Both conjunctivitis and iritis may occur as well. Injection of antigen (Lygranum) may induce not only a marked skin reaction but a concomitant flare-up in the eye. Although the mechanism of this reaction is not clear, it is probably related to the tuberculin reaction as a manifestation of delayed hypersensitivity. Curiously, not all antigens used for skin-testing as a diagnostic procedure have the capacity to stir up existing disease, such as histoplasmin, for example (see Chap. 32).—B. R.

ber of the basophilic virus group, has proved useful [21]. The range of reactivity of this antigen is indicative of the group sharing of antigens responsible for the induction of dermal hypersensitivity.

REACTIONS TO RICKETTSIAE

Antigenic fractions can be extracted from *Rickettsia burnetii* which cause skin reactions when injected intradermally in individuals recovered from Q fever. The cell wall portions of the organism contain both the immunogenic and the allergenic property; the protoplasmic fraction is inactive in both respects [22]. The cell wall fraction is as potent as killed whole organisms for the initiation of skin reactions in immune animals. It is not known, however, whether the immunogen and allergen are identical or are separable components of the cell wall.

This intradermal test is not in general use for diagnostic purposes, despite the fact that some investigators have employed it with good results [23]. It is probable that Q fever is more prevalent than is generally realized, and a skin test would provide a simple and effective measure of its incidence.

POSTINFECTIOUS AND POSTVACCINATION DEMYELINATING ENCEPHALOMYELITIS

Postinfectious encephalitis occurs as a complication of several virus diseases, particularly measles, varicella, rubella, variola, influenza, mumps, and infectious mononucleosis. An apparently similar complication has been reported to follow mild respiratory infections, scarlet fever, and pertussis. The illness usually begins five to fourteen days after the primary infection and takes the form of acute disseminated encephalomyelitis.

The complications of natural infection with measles, rubella, variola, varicella, and the "accidents" following vaccinia, yellow fever, and rabies vaccinations are clinically and histologically similar. The essential histological change is necrosis of the vessels, followed by hemorrhage and exudation, the demyelination being a secondary phenomenon. These illnesses are now often designated as acute hemorrhagic leukoencephalitis. Unlike the other viruses, mumps only rarely causes demyelination.

Acute hemorrhagic leukoencephalitis occurring spontaneously with no obvious "trigger" is an illness which is fatal within a week of onset. The histological appearance of the brain is similar to that in postinfectious, postvaccination, or post-therapy disseminated encephalomyelitis, and it has been suggested that these conditions are variants of the same basic process and that hypersensitivity is a fundamental feature [24].

It is the currently held opinion that there is an underlying allergic basis in the etiology of postinfectious and postvaccination encephalomyelitis. The primary stimulus is thought to trigger a nonspecific allergic reaction which has the cells of the central nervous system as its target. Experimentally, it is possible to simulate this disease by the injection into animals of animal nervous tissue incorporated with adjuvants [25]. The immunological basis of this reaction has been investigated by Paterson and Beisaw [26], who inactivated the antibody-producing mechanisms of rats by total body irradiation and showed that the allergic encephalomyelitis reaction was much suppressed, whereas tuberculin-delayed hypersensitivity was not affected.

Bornstein and Appel [27] have shown that rabbits exhibiting this reaction have a cytotoxic antibody in their sera, which would seem to associate this type of reaction with the production of antibody rather than with delayed hypersensitivity. However, Field [28] has reported that in the guinea pig, irradiation has no effect on allergic encephalomyelitis, which in this species would thus seem to be related to the delayed hypersensitivity response.

Whether these apparently contradictory reports reflect a genuine difference in causal mechanism in different animal species is not known. It has been observed, however, that brain antigen may elicit dermal hypersensitivity reactions in rabbits, but not in guinea pigs, after the injection of brain antigen to simulate the allergic encephalomyelitis syndrome [29]. Nevertheless some attention should be paid to the possibility that dissimilar experimental irradiation techniques may explain the different reports.

Of interest in this respect are observations that corticosteroids are sometimes of benefit in the treatment of postinfectious or postvaccination encephalomyelitis.

Information gathered recently [30] strengthens a long-held belief that host factors are of vital importance in the etiology of one of the most frequent forms of encephalomyelitis, postvaccinal encephalitis following vaccination with live vaccinia virus. In this study, three different vaccines were used in Germany, of German, Swiss, and Turkish origin. There was no reduction in the customary incidence of postvaccinal encephalitis following the use of Swiss or Turkish vaccines, despite the fact that neurological complications rarely followed use of these vaccines in their countries of origin. In addition, it is reported that the use of different techniques of vaccination caused no reduction in the incidence of these complications.

These facts suggest that possibly environmental, physiological, and probably racial factors may form part of the underlying basis of the development of postvaccinal encephalomyelitis.*

There have been attempts to reduce the incidence of encephalitis by primary vaccination with killed vaccinia. It has been suggested that the incidence of complications is reduced when such persons are revaccinated with live vaccinia [30]. This suggests that the immune status, age, and other host of factors are important. However, the intimate relationships of these factors to the allergic state in acute hemorrhagic leukoencephalitis remain to be elucidated.

The present period of renewed interest in hypersensitivity has stimulated virologists to seek examples of such phenomena in their own field of specialization. Not all viruses appear to be allergenic, but those with this characteristic seem to be relatively large viruses or to belong to the basophilic virus group; the biology of this latter group places it taxonomically between the true viruses and the bacteria.

All of the known viral skin reactions are of the delayed type. The viruses which cause dermal sensitization contain structural lipid, although not all lipid-containing viruses have yet been investigated in this respect. A classification of lipid-containing viruses has been devised by Franklin [31]. In addition, many of the allergenic viruses produce hemagglutinins. What part, if any, the lipid and hemagglutinin of these viruses play in the induction of a hypersensitive state is pure surmise, but experiments could be easily devised to investigate the question. A lipopolysaccharide found in *Mycobacterium tuberculosis* has been shown to be essential for the induction of skin reactions with this organism [32] (see Chap. 30).

In infections with viruses there is no exact correlation between the results of dermal hypersensitivity tests and the state of resistance to reinfection. This illustrates that the two mechanisms are essentially different, although initiated by the same primary event, that of infection. Resistance may wane with the passage of time more rapidly than does skin reactivity. In virus diseases in which resistance is of long duration, such as mumps, a good correlation exists between resistance to reinfection and dermal hypersensitivity. On the other hand, in virus diseases in which resistance is of short duration, such as influenza, the skin test gives only a poor indication of resistance.

It is evident that very little is known about the allergens contained in virus particles. Methods are available for the separation and characterization of these antigens, and one can hope that the present lack of precise knowledge will soon be remedied by use of the techniques of modern immunology and virology.

Acknowledgments: The authors would like to thank Dr. A. C. Wardlaw of the Connaught Medical Research Laboratories for his generous assistance and suggestions.

* *Editor's comment:* The observations of Hotchin and Weigand (*J. Immun.* 86:392, 1961) and of Wagner and Snyder (*Nature* [London] 196:393, 1962) are of considerable interest in this respect. Thus, if mice are made tolerant prenatally or neonatally to the virus of lymphocytic choriomeningitis (LCM), subsequent exposure results in multiplication of the virus but without manifestations of the disease. Despite the fact that such animals fail to form detectable antibody, they may withstand challenge with homologous virus in a dose that would readily kill uninfected adult mice. It has been postulated that both the failure to develop disease and the resistance to superinfection are related to lack of an allergic tissue response to LCM virus in the immunologically unresponsive host. The nature and variety of lesions which may occur in man following postinfectious or postvaccinal encephalomyelitis are similar to those resulting from rabies vaccination. It is most probable that the latter is "autoallergic," since patients receive repeated injections of nervous tissue in a fashion similar to the induction of experimental allergic encephalomyelitis in animals. An explanation for the postinfectious or postvaccinal types in man is lacking, although an antigen common to myelin and viruses has been postulated.—B. R.

REFERENCES

1. Cooke, P. M. Rickettsial and viral toxins. *Amer. J. Med. Sci.* 241:383, 1961.
2. Nagler, F. P. O. Specific cutaneous reaction in persons infected with the virus of herpes simplex. *J. Immun.* 48:213, 1944.
3. Kilbourne, E. D., and Anderson, W. A. Herpes simplex skin test diagnostic antigen of low protein content from cell culture fluid. *J. Invest. Derm.* 37:25, 1961.
4. Ehrengut, W. Über den Nachweis der vakzinalen Allergie mit Formalinaktiviertem Vakzinevirus bei narbenlosen Wiedenimphlingen. *Deutsch. Med. Wschr.* 86:264, 1961.
5. Kaplan, C., McClean, D., and Vallet, L. A. A note on the immunogenicity of ultra-violet irradiated vaccinia virus in man. *J. Hyg.* (Camb.) 60:79, 1962.
6. Beveridge, W. I. B., and Burnet, F. M. Cutaneous reaction to influenza viruses. *Med. J. Aust.* 1:85, 1944.
7. Freeman, G. L., and Todd, R. H. Role of allergy in viral respiratory tract infections. *Amer. J. Dis. Child.* 104:330, 1962.
8. Bull, R., and Burnet, F. M. Experimental immunization of volunteers against influenza virus. *Med. J. Aust.* 1:389, 1943.
9. Henle, G., and Henle, W. Neurological signs in mice following intracerebral inoculation of influenza viruses. *Science* 100:410, 1944.
10. Kato, N., and Hara, H. The toxic effect of influenza virus given intravenously. *Brit. J. Exp. Path.* 42:145, 1961.
11. Kato, N., Shimizu, K., and Hara, H. Local skin reactivity to influenza virus. *Ibid.*, p. 445.
12. Chang, H.-T., and Kempf, J. E. Hypotensive action of influenza virus on rats. *J. Immun.* 65:75, 1950.
13. Enders, J. F., Cohen, S., and Kane, L. W. Immunity in mumps: II. The development of complement-fixing antibody and dermal hypersensitivity in human beings following mumps. *J. Exp. Med.* 81:119, 1945.
14. Angle, R. M. The use of mumps skin test in adults. *J.A.M.A.* 177:650, 1961.
15. Friedman, R. M., Holtz, A. I., Baron, S., Silbergeld, S., and Buckler, C. E. Studies on rapid immunization with mumps vaccine. *Am. J. Hyg.* 78:269, 1963.
16. Starr, S., and Berkovick, S. Effects of measles, gamma-globulin, modified measles and vaccine measles on the tuberculin test. *New Eng. J. Med.* 270:386, 1964.
17. Frei, W. Eine neue Hautreaktion bei Lymphogranuloma Inguinale. *Klin. Wschr.* 4:2148, 1925.
18. Beeson, P. B., and Miller, E. S. Epidemiological study of lymphogranuloma venereum, employing the complement-fixation test. *Amer. J. Public Health* 37:1076, 1944.
19. Axelrod, S. J. Diagnosis of lymphogranuloma venereum: Evaluation of virus antigen (lygranum) prepared from culture on chick embryo. *Amer. J. Syph.* 26:474, 1942.
20. Rake, G., Morris, F., Shaffer, H., Jones, P., and McKee, C. K. Soluble antigen in lymphogranuloma venereum. *Proc. Soc. Exp. Biol. Med.* 46:300, 1941.
21. Benedict, A. A. Intradermal test for epidemiologic studies of turkey ornithosis. *Amer. J. Hyg.* 66:245, 1957.
22. Anacker, R. L., Lackman, D. B., Pickens, E. G., and Ribi, E. Antigenic and skin-reactive properties of fractions of *Coxiella burnetii*. *J. Immun.* 89:145, 1962.
23. Lackman, D. B., Bell, J., Bell, J. F., and Pickens, E. G. Intradermal sensitivity testing in man with a purified vaccine for Q fever. *Amer. J. Public Health* 52:87, 1962.
24. Russell, D. S. Nosological unity of acute haemorrhagic leucoencephalitis and acute disseminated encephalomyelitis. *Brain* 78:369, 1955.
25. Paterson, P. Y. Nature of the Paralytogenic Factor in Nervous Tissue. In Lawrence, H. S. (Ed.), *Cellular and Humoral Aspects of the Hypersensitive States*. New York: Paul B. Hoeber, Inc., 1959. P. 478.
26. Paterson, P. Y., and Beisaw, N. E. Effect of whole body x-irradiation on induction of allergic encephalomyelitis in rats. *J. Immun.* 90:532, 1963.
27. Bornstein, M. B., and Appel, S. H. The application of tissue culture to the study of experimental "allergic" encephalomyelitis: I. Patterns of demyelination. *J. Neuropath. Exp. Neurol.* 20:141, 1961.
28. Field, E. J. Effect of x-irradiation upon development of experimental allergic encephalomyelitis in guinea pigs. *Brit. J. Exp. Med.* 42:303, 1961.
29. Waksman, B. J. In Kies, M. W., and Alvord, E. C. (Eds.), *Allergic Encephalomyelitis*. Springfield, Ill.: Charles C Thomas, Publisher, 1959. P. 419.
30. Dostal, V. Advances in the production of smallpox vaccine. *Progr. Med. Virol.* 4:259, 1962.
31. Franklin, R. M. Significance of lipids in animal viruses: An essay on virus multiplication. *Ibid.*, p. 1.
32. Crowder, J. A., Stodola, F. H., Pangborn, M. C. and Anderson, R. J. The chemistry of lipids and tubercle bacilli: XLIV. Comparative study of the lipids of the human tubercle bacillus. *J. Amer. Chem. Soc.* 58:636, 1936.

37. *Syphilis*

SIDNEY OLANSKY

NATURAL HISTORY

The causative organism of syphilis is *Treponema pallidum.* It is highly parasitic and occurs naturally only in man and therefore requires intimate contact for its transmission. When an individual is exposed to and infected with syphilis, the fact is not immediately apparent. About three weeks after exposure, a lesion appears at the site of contact from which *T. pallidum* may be demonstrated. This is the chancre or primary lesion of syphilis. Because of the nature of the disease, most chancres appear in the anogenital region, but may occur in areas not easily visible, such as the cervix uteri or rectum, and so may be overlooked. At the first appearance of the chancre, reaction to the serological tests for syphilis (STS) may be negative, but within a week or so it becomes positive. The chancre is usually a solitary lesion but occasionally is multiple. It is associated with an enlarged, discrete, rubbery lymph node in the area of drainage of the lesion. The presence of a so-called satellite bubo is very helpful in diagnosis. However, it may not be detectable if the lesion is in an area where the satellite bubo may not be accessible, e.g., the uterine cervix or anus.

In most instances, the chancre heals spontaneously and is followed by secondary lesions of syphilis in six to twelve weeks. Sometimes the chancre persists, and the secondary lesions appear more quickly. Secondary syphilis may be accompanied by signs and symptoms of systemic disease, such as sore throat, malaise, fever, lymphadenopathy, and an eruption. The eruption is the most common diagnostic feature. It may be very extensive or very limited, but it usually does not itch. The basic lesion is papulosquamous, of varying shapes and sizes, and characteristically involves the palms and soles. In moist intertriginous areas, flat papules that are called condylomata appear, most commonly in the anogenital region, and from these *T. pallidum* can be readily demonstrated. The serological reactions are always positive in secondary syphilis. The secondary stage, too, may heal spontaneously, and the disease then becomes latent. Latent syphilis means serological reactivity with no clinical evidence. It is divided for epidemiological purposes into early and late. Early latent syphilis is latent syphilis of two years or less, and late latent syphilis is of two years or more duration.

LATE COMPLICATIONS

The major systemic damage resulting from syphilis is in the central nervous and cardiovascular systems. The former may be damaged early, leading to paresis or meningovascular syphilis, or very late, taking the form of tabes dorsalis. Tabes may have some immunological implications and is discussed below. Damage to the cardiovascular system becomes apparent after many years. Late benign syphilis (gumma) may occur very early or very late in the disease. The relation to allergy is discussed below.

Not all untreated individuals with syphilis have the late complications; it is estimated that 10 to 15 percent do so. Symptoms in others may remain latent for life. However, carefully conducted statistical studies have shown that individuals with syphilis die younger than those who do not have the disease, all other things being equal.

CONGENITAL SYPHILIS

Congenital syphilis is transmitted from the mother to the child in utero. This may be very severe or very mild, depending on the stage of the maternal syphilis during the pregnancy. Presumably, the developing embryo has no means of producing its own antibodies and must depend on its mother's for protection. It is believed that infection from mother to child occurs after four and one-half months of gestation. If the mother becomes pregnant and syphilitic at the same time or at a reasonably close interval, the child will receive a large number of *T. pallidum* with few antibodies and can have an overwhelming infection that is incompatible with life and results in stillbirth. If the mother becomes pregnant when she has latent syphilis, the child may be very mildly involved, if at all, and may show only a reactive STS as its manifestation of syphilis. Certain stigmata may appear later, namely, abnormalities of the permanent teeth (e.g., Hutchinson's incisors and mulberry molars), saddle nose, interstitial keratitis, and eighth nerve deafness. Interstitial keratitis is very interesting in that it usually appears at or after puberty and does not respond to antisyphilitic therapy but is relieved by topical applications of cortisone. Eighth nerve deafness has recently been shown to be benefited by corticosteroid therapy, but it has never responded to antisyphilitic therapy. These complications, like tabes dorsalis, may represent an autoimmune state in which *T. pallidum* merely acts as a trigger mechanism.

THERAPY

All stages of syphilis are treated with penicillin; in the event of penicillin allergy, widespectrum antibiotics may be used. The best results can be expected in the primary and secondary stages, paresis and meningovascular neurosyphilis, and late benign syphilis. In tabes dorsalis and cardiovascular syphilis, the injury is too extensive and irreversible for much response to therapy. It has often been said that the proper time to treat these complications is when the syphilis is in the primary or secondary stage.

Treatment of mothers with penicillin during pregnancy has made congenital syphilis a very rare disease. It is best to treat early in pregnancy, but treatment at any stage is preferable to treating a child after birth. Therapy before the fourteenth week of gestation is believed to prevent syphilis in the infant, whereas treatment thereafter is really treatment of syphilis in utero, and the child may show some evidence of healing syphilis at birth. This can be exceedingly confusing at times. These patients usually do not need further therapy if they have been adequately treated in utero [1].

IMMUNITY

The study of immunity in syphilis has been seriously hampered by the inability to grow *T. pallidum*. Many competent workers have tried to culture it, but with no confirmed evidence of success. During the great epidemic of syphilis in Europe early in the Sixteenth Century, it was recognized that one attack of the disease induced a degree of immunity to a second attack. About one hundred years ago, reinoculation and autoinoculation experiments in human beings provided clear evidence that syphilis gives rise to partial immunity and that the degree of immunity, at least in the early stages of the disease, bears a direct relationship to the duration of infection. Discovery of the causative agent of syphilis and the ability to transmit it to laboratory animals led to the brilliant investigations of immunity, notably by Neisser [2], Kolle [3], and Chesney [4] and their associates. From the earliest studies came the notion that immunity in syphilis is a unique phenomenon and that it is linked closely to the presence of the infecting agent. Neisser believed that cure led to disappearance of immunity. Chesney and his group, using rabbits, showed the importance of the time element in the development of immunity and clearly demonstrated that immunity, once well established in rabbits, persists long after elimination of the infective organism. This basic concept has been confirmed by a number of investigators, including Magnuson and Rosenau [5] and Turner and Hollander [6]. In 1962, Collart *et al.* [7–9], by using a silver stain, demonstrated the presence of presumed spirochetes in the lymph nodes of animals that had been treated for latent syphilis about one year previously. When these nodes were transferred to other rabbits, no lesions ensued. This group also examined lymph nodes from nine patients with the following diagnoses: two, latent but adequately treated syphilis; one, tabes inadequately treated; five, tabes adequately treated, and one, taboparesis adequately treated. In all patients, they found organisms similar to those found in rabbits—typical spirochetes in five and atypical in four. Since these spirochetes were only demonstrable by staining techniques, they have not been proved to be *T. pallidum*. However, if subsequent more specific staining methods confirm the Collart group's hypothesis that these are *T. pallidum* which have not been destroyed by therapy, Neisser's and Kolle's concepts may again be popular, i.e., that immunity disappears when the organism does, or vice versa.

IMMUNITY IN EXPERIMENTAL ANIMALS

Chesney and Kemp [10] in 1926 first presented experimental evidence that immunity persists after curative therapy, demonstrating that negative node transfers to fresh rabbits did not produce infections. There was some criticism of Chesney's work because he used arsenicals to treat his rabbits, and there was some question of whether these studies were made while the arsenicals were still in the tissues and thus acting as a suppressant to the transfer of siprochetes. Using penicillin as a curative drug, Magnuson [11] and Turner and Hollander [6] in 1948–50 confirmed and extended the findings of Chesney. These investigators established the generally accepted concept of acquired immunity in experimental syphilis, namely, that rabbits infected intratesticularly or intradermally with *T. pallidum* begin to develop relative immunity within three weeks after the so-called immunizing infection. This resistance to challenge reaches a maximum within three months after initial infection and remains high for the rest of the untreated animal's life. If the immunizing infection is terminated with curative doses of penicillin less than three months after infection, at a time when resistance is not fully developed, animals can be constantly reinfected on challenge. However, if treatment is initiated after the immunizing infection has persisted three months or longer, when the immune response is at its maximum, a high degree of immunity results and can be demonstrated on challenge months or even years after therapy. Investigators have also shown that resistance develops against challenge with heterologous strains of *T. pallidum* under the foregoing conditions, although not to the same degree as that obtained when homologous strains are used for challenge. The extent of this acquired immunity is relative, not absolute. It depends on the duration of the original immunizing infection, the size of the infecting dose, the host reaction to infection on challenge, and a number of unknown factors.

The degree of immunity in experimental syphilis is measured by the presence or absence of dark-field positive lesions at the site of challenge or the presence or absence of organisms in the inguinal or popliteal lymph nodes as demonstrated by transfer to normal rabbits, or both. Thus rabbits given a relatively small immunizing infection and treated after the three-month period required for the development of maximal resistance may acquire dark-field positive lymph nodes on challenge despite the failure of clinical lesions to develop. This partial immunity of latency whereby the host defenses restrain the challenging organisms but cannot destroy them is not understood. These studies suggest that acquired immunity in experimental syphilis is similar to immunity in other infectious diseases.

It is clear that rabbits acquire a degree of immunity during syphilitic infection. It is also clear that this immunity is not necessarily complete. As for the treponemes introduced in the original infection, animals develop a capability of holding them in check to the extent that clinical lesions rarely become manifest after the third month except in the eye, which is known to participate less actively in the immune process than most other parts of the animal body. But almost without exception, the animal is incapable of eliminating the infection. Lymph nodes are regularly found to be infectious, and intermittent spirochetemia has been demonstrated in some rabbits for at least three years after infection. Rabbits at this stage of infection likewise have limited capabilities of dealing with treponemes introduced from outside. Previously cited studies demonstrated that after the first infection was eliminated by treatment, in some animals a new infection was established by challenge, but this reinfection nearly always remained latent, while in others it was not possible to induce another infection. Although this seems to be a phenomenon of immunity, the precise mechanism is not clear.

Why is it that treponemes remain viable, virulent for other animals, and presumably multiply, and yet induce virtually no tissue reaction in the host? Is there a continued interplay between host antibody and the treponeme? Is the treponemal population maintained at a fairly constant level? There are no data to answer these questions. Reynolds [12] reported a study in which pieces of rabbit syphiloma were implanted under the skin of the lower hindlegs of normal and immune animals. The fate of the implanted treponemes was followed by dark-field microscopy and infectivity tests of the implants and of the popliteal lymph nodes draining the area. In the normal animals, motile treponemes increased in the transplants, and the regional lymph nodes were infected forty-eight hours after implantation. In the immune animals, motile treponemes could be observed in the transplants and infectivity demonstrated as long as four days after introduction, but the regional lymph nodes were never proved to be infected. Evidently, treponemes were by some mechanism held in situ, although they were still viable over a period of several days. A similar study by Waring and Fleming [13] demonstrated that in partially immune rabbits, lymph nodes may remain uninfected even though local lesions containing motile treponemes may occur after challenge inoculation. It seems reasonable to assume that specific antibodies play a role in this situation. Numerous attempts have been made over the years to induce immunity in laboratory animals with killed treponemes of both pathogenic and nonvirulent cultivatable varieties. In all instances, the results have been disappointing. However, most investigators used rather crude emulsions of spirochetes, and it is conceivable that if the organisms were ultimately grown on artificial media, this method might still have merit.

IMMUNITY IN MAN

There are numerous reports of small or large series of human inoculations with syphilis, but none are careful studies with measured doses of identically prepared inocula given in a manner that permits comparison between animal and human strains. However, the following facts can be gleaned from all of these studies: (1) The nonsyphilitic individual is susceptible to infection with *T. pallidum* if the material is introduced below the skin. (2) Strains of *T. pallidum* passed through rabbits and anthropoids are infectious for man. (3) As the duration of the untreated disease increases, the development of lesions following challenge with homologous or heterologous material occurs with diminished frequency. Shortly after development of the chancre, extending through the secondary stage and also in active paresis, the body has been found to be rather highly refractory to challenge. This refractory state seems to depend in part on the size of the inoculum, the method of inoculation, and unknown host factors. (4) The lesion of challenge tends to conform to the state of syphilis reached by the original infection. (5) Nodules and gummatous lesions most commonly follow challenge in the individuals who have had previous late syphilis. (6) Patients with paresis rarely show reaction to challenge. Those with latent syphilis, congenital syphilis, gummatous syphilis, and tabes frequently show a reaction to challenge which seems to represent reinfection or superinfection.

It was necessary to undertake experiments on man in order to reconcile all of the differing views on immunity in syphilis and to set up conditions which would yield unequivocal results. This was accomplished in 1953 and published under the title, "Inoculation of Syphilis in Human Volunteers" [14]. Before the volunteers were inoculated with virulent *T. pallidum,* they were given injections of heat-killed organisms in order to observe the serological response to such inoculations. The STS (nontreponemal test) showed no rise in titer following injection of killed organisms. The *T. pallidum* immobilization test (TPI) response was negative in the nonsyphilitic controls given heat-killed *T. pallidum,* but there was an anamnestic response as measured by the TPI in those previously treated for syphilis.

The volunteers inoculated with virulent *T. pallidum* of the Nichols strain were in the following diagnostic categories: (1) 8, controls; (2) 5, untreated latent syphilis; (3) 11, previously treated for proved or presumed early syphilis; (4) 3, previously treated for proved or presumed reinfection; (5) 26, previously treated for proved or presumed late latent syphilis; (6) 5, previously treated for proved or presumed congenital syphilis; (7) 2, previously treated for asymptomatic central nervous system syphilis. In all controls, dark-field positive lesions developed at the site of inoculation. None of the subjects with untreated latent syphilis were infected; i.e., there were no local lesions and no serological response. All of the 11 previously treated for proved or presumed early syphilis were reinfected, 9 with dark-field positive lesions associated with an increased STS titer, 2 with dark-field negative lesions with an increased STS titer. Of the 3 previously treated for proved or presumed reinfection, 1 had a dark-field positive lesion and increased STS titer, 1 had a dark-field negative lesion with increased STS titer, and 1 was considered not infected. Of the 26 previously treated for proved or presumed late latent syphilis, 1 had a dark-field positive lesion with increased STS titer, 3 had dark-field negative lesions with no increased serological titer, 9 had dark-field negative lesions with increased STS titer, and 13 were not infected. Of those previously treated for proved or presumed congenital syphilis, 1 had a dark-field positive lesion with increased STS titer, 3 had dark-field negative lesions with increased STS titer, and 1 was not infected. Of the 2 previously treated for asymptomatic central nervous system syphilis, neither was considered to be infected. Two patients had a gumma at the site of inoculation, 1 in the late latent category previously treated and 1 in the congenital group.

The results of this study tended to confirm much of the information already obtained from animals and from human inoculation studies but that remained to be proved under adequately controlled conditions. The Nichols strain of *T. pallidum,* although passed through rabbits for many years, is still infectious for man and produces a disease quite similar to that of acquired syphilis. The injection of heat-killed *T. pallidum* produced an anamnestic rise in TPI antibodies in some patients previously treated for early syphilis but failed to induce significant increases in reagin titers. No changes in circulating antibodies were demonstrated in nonsyphilitic controls given the same antigen. Five patients with untreated latent syphilis showed no clinical or serological response to challenge and were assumed to be resistant to superinfection. Of the eleven patients previously treated for proved or presumed early syphilis, all were reinfected and all responded with increased STS and TPI titers more rapidly than did the nonsyphilitic controls. Of those previously treated for proved or presumed late syphilis, many could not be infected at all, and those who were tended to have dark-field negative lesions, suggesting considerable residual immunity to challenge. One of these patients had a gumma, as did one treated for proved or presumed congenital syphilis. The patients who had previously had syphilis differed from nonsyphilitic controls in their reaction to infection. In a general way, this reaction was influenced by the duration of the original infection before treatment, but there was definite difference among individuals. Some of the evidence suggested that the administration of heat-killed *T. pallidum* may have had a booster effect on the immunity of patients previously treated for syphilis, but because of the possible relationship of other variables this finding requires further confirmation.

SEROLOGY

The study on inoculation syphilis in human volunteers, just discussed, provided an opportunity for observing and comparing the behavior of reagin tests and the treponemal tests in known syphilis. The serological tests used today are divided into three basic types [15]: (1) Tests employing crude lipoidal antigens, represented by the Kahn test. This test is a flocculation procedure employing an antigen prepared from beef heart by simple extraction methods. The test measures reagin. This type of testing procedure is generally being abandoned because of the difficulty of standardizing the antigen. (2) The cardiolipin-lecithin tests, illustrated by the VDRL slide test. This test employs a purified cardiolipin and lecithin antigen obtained from beef heart which chemically and serologically can be standarized. The test is performed on the slide and is read under the microscope. This type of test is being used increasingly as a standard procedure. It also measures reagin, but its chief advantage is that it can be standardized in such a manner that uniform results can be expected if the exact procedure is followed. (3) The treponemal tests. These tests use *T. pallidum,* Nichols strain, as the antigen in either viable or killed form or as an extract of the organism. Numerous procedures have come to the fore since development of the TPI test by Nelson, but only three are being used widely: (a) The TPI, which employs live spirochetes obtained from rabbit orchitis as the antigen. It is essentially a complement fixation test, and reactivity is measured by the ability of the unknown serum to immobilize the spirochetes. (b) The fluorescent treponemal antibody (FTA) test, which uses as antigen, dead spirochetes obtained from rabbit orchitis. The organisms are exposed to serum globulins tagged with fluorescein-isothiocyanate and the unknown serum, and the test is read under the fluorescent microscope. Fluorescence of the spirochetes denotes reactivity. (c) The Reiter protein complement fixation (RPCF) test, which employs as the antigen, extracts from the Reiter spirochete, a nonpathogenic strain which can be cultured. The technique is similar to that of the Kolmer complement fixation test with cardiolipin-lecithin antigen.

Presumably the TPI and FTA tests measure the same antibody, which is different from reagin. The antibody measured by the RPCF test was assumed to be similar, until recently questioned by Deacon [16]. He believes that all spirochetes have a common antibody which can be absorbed by use of proper antigens and that by a series of absorptions thereby he can identify the specific antibody to *T. Pallidum*. From the discussion of the study on human volunteers inoculated with virulent *T. pallidum* one can conclude that certainly reagin and the antibodies measured by the TPI and FTA tests are quite different. The subjects who were inoculated with killed *T. pallidum* did not react in the reagin tests, but those previously treated for syphilis did show an anamnestic response in the TPI tests. Presumably this means that the TPI tests measure antibodies to the surface of the spirochete or to the whole spirochete. On the other hand, when live spirochetes were inoculated, the reagin tests showed marked rises in titer in infected subjects, both controls and those previously adequately treated for syphilis. This suggests that reagin is the result of spirochetes combining with tissue and that probably reagin is a response to a hapten. This conceivably might explain some of the false reactions that occur in diseases that produce tissue destruction, such as lupus erythematosus, some of the virus diseases, and leprosy. Attempts to correlate serological titers and positive reactions to the TPI or TFA tests with immunity have not been completely successful. As previously indicated, immunity seems to be related to the size of the inoculum, duration of the disease, time of therapy, plus many other unknown factors. In general, individuals with positive serological reactions have some immunity to challenge, but this is not a direct measure of immunity. It would be most interesting if it were.

BIOLOGICAL FALSE POSITIVE REACTIONS

So-called biological false positive reactions to STS have had wide interest in the past ten or fifteen years. It is well known that reactions to the standard STS do occur in such diseases as lupus erythematosus, leprosy, and certain virus diseases when there is no evidence of syphilis. The meaning of these reactions is not clear, particularly since they occur only in a very small proportion of the patients with these diseases. For example, in systemic lupus erythematosus, 5 percent or less of patients have biological false positive reactions. In leprosy, the percentage is much higher, and probably in the range of 25 to 50 percent. It is in this area that the treponemal tests are most useful. As was previously mentioned, the treponemal tests, particularly TPI and FTA, measure antibodies to the spirochete, and, in general, those infected with syphilis will have a positive reaction to the TPI test. Indeed, this has become the standard "verification test." If the reaction to the TPI test is positive, the reagin STS reaction is not a biological false positive one. If the TPI reaction is negative, the reagin STS reaction is usually considered to be a biological false positive. There are some exceptions to both of these statements, but they are so rare that discussion of them might confuse the issue. Every reaction to the STS must be investigated completely with syphilis in mind, since most of them will turn out to be associated with this disease. However, the mere fact of a positive serological reaction does not mean that the patient has active disease or is in need of therapy.

EFFECT OF ANTISYPHILITIC THERAPY ON SEROLOGICAL TESTS

Treatment of any stage of syphilis may alter the serological reaction. The alteration is greater when the patient is treated during early syphilis than when treated later, but at either end of the time scale, therapy may have an effect. If a patient with seronegative primary syphilis is treated, he will have consistent negative reactions to STS and, indeed, will have no immunity and may be readily reinfected on re-exposure. If the patient has seropositive primary syphilis, the serological titer will become negative in a reasonably short time in the vast majority of cases, i.e., 2 to 3 months. If he is treated during the secondary stage, the serological response will be slower, but in 80 to 90 percent of cases, seronegativity will be achieved ultimately following adequate treatment, although it may take 12 to 18 months to accomplish this. If the patient is treated during latency or for the late complications of syphilis, regardless of the amount of therapy given, the serological reaction may never become negative, although careful follow-up with quantitative serological tests will indicate that the titer gradually goes down. It is this fact that has been most disturbing to clinicians, since a positive seroreaction is associated in their minds with active disease. Careful and prolonged follow-up of patients who remain seropositive after therapy indicates that there is no cause for alarm as long as the titer goes in the direction of negativity or remains static. If there should be a sudden sustained rise in titer, it is possible that the disease is once again active, and this activity may reflect asymptomatic reinfection.

REFERENCES

1. *Syphilis—Modern Diagnosis and Management.* Public Health Service Pub. No. 743. Washington, D.C.: Government Printing Office, 1960.
2. Neisser, A. Immunisierung Versuche. *Arb. Kais. Gesund.* 37:201, 1911.
3. Kolle, W., and Frigge, R. Gibt es eine aktive Immunität bei Syphilis? *Med. Klin.* 30:46, 1934.
4. Chesney, A. M. *Immunity in Syphilis.* Baltimore: Williams & Wilkins Company, 1927.
5. Magnuson, H. J., and Rosenau, B. J. The rate of development and degree of acquired immunity in experimental syphilis. *Amer. J. Syph.* 32:418, 1948.
6. Turner, T. B., and Hollander, D. H. *Biology of the Treponematoses.* Geneva: World Health Organization, 1957.
7. Collart, P., Burel, L. J., and Burel, P. Étude de l'action de la pénicilline dans la syphilis tardive: Persistance du *Tréponeme pale* après traitement. *Ann. Inst. Pasteur* (Paris) 102:693, 1962.
8. Collart, P., *et al. Ibid.,* p. 313.
9. Collart, P., *et al. Ibid.,* vol. 103, p. 953.
10. Chesney, A. M., and Kemp, J. E. Studies in experimental syphilis: Variations in response of treated rabbits to reinoculations; and cryptogenic reinfection with syphilis. *J. Exp. Med.* 44:589, 1926.
11. Cited in Ref. 6.
12. Reynolds, F. W. The fate of *Treponema pallidum* inoculated subcutaneously into immune rabbits. *Bull. Hopkins Hosp.* 69:53, 1941.
13. Waring, G. W., Jr., and Fleming, W. L. The effect of partial immunity on the dissemination of infection in experimental syphilis. *Amer. J. Syph.* 36:368, 1941.
14. Magnuson, H. J., Thomas, E. V., Olansky, S., Kaplan, B. I., De Mello, L., and Cutler, J. C. Inoculation of syphilis in human volunteers. *Medicine* 35:33, 1953.
15. *Serologic Tests for Syphilis.* Public Health Service Manual No. 411. Washington, D.C.: Government Printing Office, 1959.
16. Deacon, W. E. Unpublished work, 1964.

PART THREE: ATOPY AND RELATED DISORDERS

William B. Sherman, Editor

38. The Atopic Diseases

WILLIAM B. SHERMAN

THE FREQUENT OCCURRENCE OF hay fever and asthma in the same individual has long been recognized. It was noted that acute urticaria and gastrointestinal manifestations of idiosyncracy to a specific food were more common in patients with these diseases than in the general population, and a relation to infantile eczema was also observed. Eczema was found to occur more frequently in the children of patients with hay fever or asthma, and individuals who had had eczema in infancy showed an unusual incidence of hay fever and asthma in later life. Some authors have attempted to relate migraine to the same type of constitution, but the findings in this regard are questionable.

Cooke and Vander Veer [1] in 1916 established the relationship of hay fever, asthma, and certain obvious food allergies to a common hereditary factor. They showed that susceptibility to allergy was inherited, but neither the specific disease manifestation nor allergy to a specific antigen.

A large proportion of patients with these diseases was shown to have immediate urticarial reactions to the introduction of antigen into the skin by scratch, prick, or intracutaneous injection. The urticarial nature of the skin reaction and its appearance within 10 to 20 minutes after the introduction of the antigen resembled the skin reactions noted in serum sickness but differed conspicuously from the inflammatory reaction to tuberculin which developed after 12 to 48 hours.

It was apparent that these conditions, particularly bronchial asthma, bore a striking resemblance to the manifestations of anaphylactic shock in experimental animals. However, they developed spontaneously in individuals rendered susceptible by heredity after the normal contacts with pollens, dust, and foods which did not produce sensitization in other persons. The intense artificial exposure to antigen (usually by injection) which induced anaphylactic sensitization in essentially all animals of suitable species was not necessary. Injections into normal individuals of substances which were most prominent as causative factors in spontaneous human allergies did not produce sensitization. In fact, some of these substances, such as the pollens of ragweed and grass, proved relatively inactive as antigens producing anaphylaxis in animals. Hereditary susceptibility rather than the degree of exposure to antigen appeared to be the determining factor in the development of sensitization.

The sera of these allergic human beings did not contain the antibodies which were typical of the anaphylactically sensitized animal or of the human patient recovering from serum sickness. Specifically, they did not form precipitates with the antigen, and they did not passively sensitize guinea pigs.

Ramirez [2] in 1919 reported the passive sensitization of a previously nonallergic man by transfusion of blood from an individual naturally sensitive to horses. The recipient, who had a transfusion because of pernicious anemia, had asthma when next exposed to horses. Prausnitz and Küstner [3] in 1921 showed that the injection of serum from allergic patients into the skin of normal individuals produced local passive sensitization which could be demonstrated by specific reactions to skin tests. The substance in the serum causing this sensitization was early designated by Coca as a reagin, but it has since been shown to satisfy most of the criteria of an antibody and is now more frequently referred to as skin-sensitizing antibody.

Coca and Cooke [4] in 1923 applied the

term "atopy" (or the atopic diseases) to the type of human sensitization which depended on hereditary predisposition rather than unusual exposure to antigen and which was characterized by the immediate urticarial skin reaction to antigen, by the Prausnitz-Küstner reaction, and by the absence of other demonstrable antibodies. The term atopy has been criticized by many writers and discarded by some as new information has modified the concept of these diseases. The usefulness of the term is not lessened by the subsequent demonstration that the condition, originally thought to be limited to man, might also occur in dogs, cattle, and other species or by the observation that skin-sensitizing antibodies producing the Prausnitz-Küstner reaction can be artificially induced in normal human subjects and animals by suitable sensitizing procedures with certain antigens.

More serious difficulty arises from the observation that the hereditary factor and the immunological mechanism of urticarial skin reactions and skin-sensitizing antibodies cannot be demonstrated in all cases of the conditions grouped together as atopic diseases. Seasonal hay fever, which by definition is related to a specific pollen, rarely presents a problem. On the other hand, patients with nonseasonal rhinitis or bronchial asthma, which are clinically similar in symptoms, physical manifestations, and laboratory findings, may or may not have urticarial reactions to skin tests and skin-sensitizing antibodies. Many of these latter nonreactors appear to have infection and some evidence has been offered that they represent instances of allergic reactions to bacteria [5]. However, the typical skin reactions and immunological phenomena of atopy cannot be demonstrated with any available bacterial antigens. Similar problems are encountered in the study of urticaria. A considerable proportion of cases of acute urticaria fulfill all the criteria of atopy, but such a mechanism is less often demonstrable in chronic urticaria. Some cases of angioedema are demonstrably due to atopy, others to a familial tendency apparently unrelated to the atopic factor, and in many cases the cause cannot be determined.

These limitations and problems must be kept in mind when speaking of the atopic diseases. They will be discussed in detail in the chapters on the various disease entities. With these qualifications, the term atopy is used, since it embodies the important concept of a familial tendency to sensitization which may become manifest in successive generations, or at different ages in the same individual, by various diseases and by allergy to various substances. It is also the most convenient term for designating the type of immunological mechanism characterized by immediate urticarial reactions to skin tests, by skin-sensitizing antibody, and by the absence of other antibody activity.

Many surveys of the incidence of atopic diseases have been reported. The figures given vary widely, and, as pointed out by Dublin and Marks [6] in 1946, the variations in the basis of reporting cases, in diagnostic standards, and in many other factors make it difficult to compare the results of different studies. Cooke and Vander Veer [1] in 1916, using criteria similar to those already described, reported that 7 percent of a small unselected group of individuals questioned reported a personal history of atopic disease. Vaughan [7], in a larger survey, including the same diseases and also migraine, reported 10 percent of the population to be affected by allergies. However, the inclusion of his less clearly defined category of "minor allergies" increased the incidence to 60 percent. Results of many similar surveys are summarized by Vaughan and Black [8]. Without attempting to resolve the discrepancies, but allowing some weight to many higher figures, it is reasonable to estimate that 10 percent of the population in the parts of the United States where ragweed is common is affected at some period of life by definite atopic diseases. Since about one half of the cases are due to allergy to ragweed pollen, the incidence is much lower in Europe and other areas where ragweed does not grow.

REFERENCES

1. Cooke, R. A., and Vander Veer, A. Human sensitization. *J. Immun.* 1:201, 1916.
2. Ramirez, M. A. Horse asthma following blood transfusion. *J.A.M.A.* 73:984, 1919.
3. Prausnitz, C., and Küstner, H. Studien über die Ueberempfindlichkeit. *Zbl. Bakt.* [Orig.] 86: 160, 1921.
4. Coca, A. F., and Cooke, R. A. On the classifi-

cation of the phenomena of hypersensitiveness. *J. Immun.* 8:163, 1923.

5. Cooke, R. A.: Infective Asthma: Indication of Its Allergic Nature. *Amer. J. Med. Sci.* 183:309, 1932.
6. Dublin, L. L., and Marks, H. H. In Derbes, V., and Engelhardt, H. T. (Eds.), *Treatment of Bronchial Asthma.* Philadelphia: J. B. Lippincott Company, 1946.
7. Vaughan, W. T. Minor allergy: Its distribution, clinical aspects and significance. *J. Allerg.* 5:184, 1934.
8. Vaughan, W. T., and Black, J. H. *Practice of Allergy* (3rd ed.). St. Louis: C. V. Mosby Company, 1954. P. 55.

39. *Heredity and Antigen Exposure in Development of Atopic Diseases*

WILLIAM B. SHERMAN

HEREDITY

Many of the earliest writings on bronchial asthma mention its tendency to occur in successive generations of certain families. A similar tendency was noted in regard to hay fever, angioedema, and various other diseases now classed as atopic. The familial nature of allergic diseases was carefully studied by Cooke and Vander Veer [1] in 1916. They found that 244 (48 percent) of 504 patients with allergic disease had a family history of diseases of the group. Of 139 nonallergic individuals, only 17 (12 percent) had a similar family history. They also noted that patients with a bilateral family history of allergy tended to have allergic diseases in childhood usually before the age of 10, those with a unilateral family history at about the age of puberty, and those with a negative family history most often in the third and fourth decades. Of 70 subjects with a bilateral family history of allergy (not necessarily affecting the actual parent), 39 (55 percent) showed evidence of allergic disease when they were studied at an average age of 23 years. Of 150 individuals with a unilateral family history of allergy, 77 (51.3 percent) were allergic when seen at an average age of 27.5 years, and of 631 with a negative family history, 205 (32.4 percent) had allergic disease when seen at an average age of 35 years. On the basis of their figures concerning the age of onset of allergy in these various groups, Cooke and Vander Veer calculated that 67.5 percent of individuals with bilateral inheritance would ultimately become allergic, 60 percent of those with unilateral inheritance, and 38.6 percent of those with negative family histories.

These investigators noted that infants were not born allergic, and inherited the tendency equally from the father and mother, indicating that the familial tendency was due to genetic factors rather than to placental transmission of sensitivity. In this respect, human allergy differed strikingly from anaphylaxis in the guinea pig, in which the progeny of anaphylactically sensitized females were born sensitive to the same antigen which affected the mother, whereas sensitization of the father had no effect. The child did not necessarily show sensitivity to the same antigen as the parent or the same disease manifestations. The factor which was inherited was a tendency to develop allergies which was not evident at birth, might not be manifested for years, and might lead to any of the diseases of the group.

This report was followed in 1920 by a study of Adkinson [2] which further stressed the inherited nature of bronchial asthma and its relation to hay fever, eczema, and urticaria. A similar study by Spain and Cooke [3] in 1924 confirmed and expanded these findings.

The evidence presented in these early papers has been subject to some criticism. The information was collected chiefly by questioning the patients about the diseases of their parents and more remote relatives, most of whom were never examined by the investigators. Since the study of allergic diseases was still new, the validity of these retrospective diagnoses was open to question. However, the general principles set forth by Cooke and Vander Veer have been universally accepted. The recognition of hereditary factor has proved useful in the diagnosis of allergic diseases and is one of the bases of the concept of atopy.

Numerous later surveys (summarized by Vaughan and Black [4]) showed evidence of a familial incidence of allergic diseases, with 40 to 70 percent of asthmatic children, 40 to 60 percent of adult asthmatics, and 35 to 80 percent of patients with hay fever giving family histories of allergic diseases.

Most of the authors have considered the allergic diseases as a group, and the results have varied because not all have included the same diseases in the group. Schwartz [5] avoided the problem of deciding in advance which diseases should be classed as allergic by studying only the families of patients with bronchial asthma and of a normal control group. By recording the incidence in each group of families of various diseases which might be considered atopic, he developed statistical evidence that vasomotor rhinitis, hay fever, and atopic dermatitis were genetically related to asthma. He found no genetic relationship between asthma and migraine, epilepsy, contact dermatitis, psoriasis, ichthyosis, and (surprisingly) gastrointestinal allergy. The evidence with regard to urticaria and angioedema was equivocal. When the cases of asthma were divided into those with and those without skin reactions to various antigens, the genetic background of both groups was found to be identical, suggesting that asthma is a genetic entity, regardless of specific causes.

Clarke *et al.* [6], and more recently Schwartz [5], suggested that in addition to the familial tendency to allergy there is an inherited localization factor which makes an individual more liable to the specific disease affecting the parent than to other allergic diseases. The evidence of such a localization factor is less conclusive than that of the genetic tendency to atopy.

The view expressed by Tips [7] that the heredity of hay fever, asthma, and atopic dermatitis is determined by three separate pairs of genes has not been confirmed.

ALLERGY IN IDENTICAL TWINS

Many authors have reported instances in which identical twins have developed identical manifestations of allergy, often at approximately the same period of life. However, studies of groups of twins show that such identical allergies are by no means always present. It should be noted that most of the reports do not give in detail the evidence for considering the twins identical. Cooke and Vander Veer [1] reported on 6 pairs of twins, in each of which 1 twin showed definite allergic tendencies. In 3 of the pairs, the other twin showed similar manifestations, whereas 3 of the twins were entirely normal. Spaich and Ostertag [8] studied 59 sets of twins in which 1 of the pair was affected by allergic disease. Forty-four of these sets were considered to be identical twins. The second twin showed similar allergic manifestations in 20 pairs and did not in 14. In 10 of the 14 pairs not showing similar allergies, there was evidence of another allergic disease in the second twin. In contrast, among 25 sets of twins which were not considered identical, 6 showed concordance of allergic diseases and 19 discordance. Of the 19, 14 showed evidence of other allergic diseases. Thus the similarity between the 2 twins was strikingly greater in the identical than in the fraternal group. Bowen [9] reported on 59 sets of identical twins in which 1 twin had allergic disease of sufficient severity to require medical attention. In only 7 instances did the second twin have identical allergic disease; the remaining 52 were not considered ill. In 3 of these instances skin tests were done on both twins, with positive results in 1 and negative results in the other.

If all of the twins classed as identical were truly homozygous, it would appear that heredity is only one of many factors involved in the development of atopic diseases.

GENETIC MECHANISMS

Cooke and Vander Veer [1] considered that the allergic factor was a Mendelian dominant but were unable to explain on this basis the fact that almost one half of the allergic patients have no family history of allergy. Adkinson [2] suggested that allergy was a recessive factor, but some of the pedigrees published in her article make it appear to be a dominant. Weiner *et al.* [10] assumed that heredity of allergy was determined by a single pair of genes and that the allergic factor was an incomplete recessive. Individuals homozygous for the normal gene were normal and did not transmit the allergic factor. Individuals homozygous for the allergic gene tended to develop allergic diseases before the age of 10. Heterozygous individuals with one normal and one allergic gene were believed to develop allergy later in approximately 18 percent of cases. Thus a majority would be apparently normal throughout life but might transmit the factor to their children.

Most subsequent writers on the subject [5, 11, 12] have considered their results to accord with the concept that susceptibility to atopy is determined by a single pair of genes and is manifested by both homozygous and a certain percentage of heterozygous individuals. They have differed in their estimates of the percentage of homozygous atopic subjects, and of the degree of penetrance of the atopic factor in heterozygous individuals. Schwartz [5] considered the degree of penetrance to be 40 percent; Van Arsdel and Motuesky [11] placed it between 20 and 45 percent.

Penrose [13] has suggested that the figures are equally consistent with a mechanism in which the heredity of atopic disease is determined by a number of pairs of genes. Available data do not permit proof whether one or more pairs of genes are involved.

EXPOSURE TO ANTIGENS

It has been noted that atopy differs from anaphylaxis in that sensitization appears to develop spontaneously after the ordinary contacts of normal life without the necessity of the intense exposure to antigen required for experimental anaphylaxis. On the other hand, it is axiomatic that immunological reactions and antibodies develop only as a result of contact with antigen. The effect of exposure to antigen on the development of atopic sensitization is most clearly demonstrated in the case of pollen antigens of known and limited geographic distribution. The distribution of the pollen together with the past and present places of residence of the patient determine the possibility of exposure more certainly than is possible with most other allergens. Coca and Grove [14] tested 35 patients with hay fever in Berlin with ragweed pollen, which is a causative factor in three fourths of hay fever patients in the United States but does not grow in Europe. The one patient who showed a positive reaction was the only one who had spent time in America and been exposed to ragweed. The same workers tested hay fever patients in New York with *Algeroba* pollen, which is the principal cause of hay fever in Hawaii but is unknown in New York. None of the New York hay fever patients reacted to this pollen. Phillips [15] tested a large number of patients allergic to other substances with sugar beet pollen when the sugar beet was first introduced as an agricultural crop in his area. Initially, all gave negative reactions, but within three to five years a large proportion showed evidence of having an allergy to this pollen. The period of three to five years is in accordance with the usual time at which persons who have arrived in the United States from Europe may develop allergy to ragweed pollen.

Sensitization in the adult may persist for many years without another exposure to the antigen. Cooke [16] cited the case of a patient with hay fever who remained sensitive to ragweed pollen after spending sixteen consecutive years in Europe, where he was not exposed. On the other hand, many food allergies of children are lost by the age of 5.

Allergy to some of the less common but active antigens, such as castor bean, is rather obviously related to exposure. Groups of cases of asthma due to this substance have been reported from North and South America, Europe, and Africa, always from the vicinity of mills producing castor oil. The cases have usually included both employees and residents of the neighborhood exposed to the dust of the dry residue remaining after expression of the oil. Figley and Elrod [17] reported 30 cases from the vicinity of a mill in Toledo, Ohio. Symptoms occurred six to eighteen months after exposure began; 11 (37 percent) of the patients gave a family history of allergy. Modern methods of controlling the dust have greatly reduced the hazard to both employees of such mills and their neighbors.

Intense occupational exposure to some of the common allergens may also cause an unusual incidence of sensitization. Various authors (summarized by Schwartz [5]) have estimated that 10 to 20 percent of bakers eventually become allergic to wheat flour. Schwartz reported that 46 percent of those affected had a family history of allergy.

REACTION TO FIRST KNOWN CONTACT

The relationship of exposure to antigen to the development of atopic sensitization is difficult to demonstrate in the case of food antigens. The first addition of egg to the diet of an infant often evokes an immediate allergic reaction, suggesting that sensitization existed before the contact. It is usually thought that such allergy may be developed as a result of an exposure to antigen which passes through the placenta from mother to child during intrauterine life. Since newborn infants are, in general, unable to produce antibodies, it must also be assumed that the antigen is stored in the infant until the antibody-producing mechanism has become active. That the child is not born sensitive has been shown by examination of the cord blood of 50 infants with atopic mothers which failed to reveal antibodies for egg or other common food allergens in any case [18]. In breast-fed infants, antigens of foods eaten by the mother may be transmitted to the infant through the breast milk. It is also possible that such sensitization may result from the inhalation of antigen when eggs are cooked, handled, or eaten by other members of the household.

NONSPECIFIC FACTORS

There is no satisfactory explanation of why an individual who is rendered susceptible by heredity develops allergy to certain of the antigens to which he is exposed but not to others to which he has apparently equal exposure. This has led to the hypothesis that atopic sensitization might occur during times when the membranes are inflamed by infection or nonspecific irritants and antigens are readily absorbed. Anderson and Schloss [19] suggested that marasmus in infancy favored sensitization by permitting greater absorption of unaltered milk and egg antigens. However, their own subsequent studies indicated that antibodies to these antigens were equally common in normal babies. The studies of Walzer *et al.* [20] by means of the Prausnitz-Küstner phenomenon also showed that active antigen may be readily absorbed through the gastrointestinal tract of normal adults. The symptoms of asthma are frequently apparent for the first time after an acute respiratory infection such as pertussis or pneumonia. However, it seems probable that the infection in such cases precipitates symptoms of a previously latent sensitization rather than facilitating the acquisition of new sensitizations.

INTERRELATIONS OF HEREDITY AND ENVIRONMENTAL FACTORS

In general, it appears that heredity plays a major part in the susceptibility of an individual to atopic sensitization but that the particular allergies developed depend chiefly on the antigens to which the individual is exposed. If one accepts the hypothesis of Weiner *et al.* [10] that only 18 percent of the individuals with a heterozygous genetic makeup will develop allergy during their lives, it seems probable that the intensity of exposure to antigens may be a determining factor in some cases. Although sensitization does not follow exposure with any regularity, many authorities have recommended that children with a known tendency to atopy or a strong family history be kept from contact with potential antigens, to lessen the likelihood of sensitization.

REFERENCES

1. Cooke, R. A., and Vander Veer, A. Human sensitization. *J. Immun.* 1:201, 1916.
2. Adkinson, J. The behavior of bronchial asthma as an inherited characteristic. *Genetics* 5:363, 1920.
3. Spain, W. C., and Cooke, R. A. Studies in specific hypersensitivity: II. The familial incidence of hay fever and bronchial asthma. *J. Immun.* 9:521, 1924.
4. Vaughan, W. T., and Black, J. H. *Practice of Allergy* (3rd Ed.). St. Louis: C. V. Mosby Company, 1954.
5. Schwartz, M. *Heredity in Bronchial Asthma.* Copenhagen: Ejnar Munkzgaards Forlag, 1952.
6. Clarke, J. A., Donnally, H. H., and Coca, A. F. Studies in specific hypersensitiveness: XXXII. On the influence of heredity in atopy. *J. Immun.* 15:9, 1928.
7. Tips, R. C. A study of the inheritance of atopic hypersensitivity in man. *Amer. J. Hum. Genet.* 6:328, 1954.
8. Spaich, D., and Ostertag, M. Study of allergic disease in twins. *Z. Mensl. Vererb. Konstitutionsl.* 19:731, 1936.
9. Bowen, R. Allergy in identical twins. *J. Allerg.* 24:236, 1953.
10. Weiner, A. S., Zieve, J., and Fries, J. H. The inheritance of allergic disease. *Ann. Eugen.* 7:141, 1936.
11. Van Arsdel, P. P., Jr., and Motuesky, H. G. Frequency and hereditability of asthma and allergic rhinitis in college students. *Acta Genet.* (Basel) 9:101, 1959.
12. Schnyder, U. W. Neurodermatitis, Asthma, Rhinitis: Eine genetische-allergologische Studie. *Acta Genet.* (Basel) Vol. 10, supp., 1960.

13. Penrose, L. S. The genetical background of common disease. *Acta Genet.* (Basel) 4:257, 1953.
14. Coca, A. F., and Grove, E. F. In Coca, A. F., Walzer, M., and Thommen, A. A. (Eds.), *Asthma and Hay Fever in Theory and Practice.* Springfield, Ill.: Charles C Thomas, Publisher, 1931. P. 50.
15. Phillips, E. W. Pollen incidence in central Arizona. *J. Allerg.* 3:489, 1932.
16. Cooke, R. A. *Allergy in Theory and Practice.* Philadelphia: W. B. Saunders Company, 1947. P. 12.
17. Figley, K. D., and Elrod, R. H. Endemic asthma due to castor bean dust. *J.A.M.A.* 90: 79, 1928.
18. Sherman, W. B. Unpublished data, 1948.
19. Anderson, A. F., and Schloss, O. M. Allergy to cow's milk in infants with nutritional diseases. *Amer. J. Dis. Child.* 26:451, 1923.
20. Walzer, M. Studies in absorption of undigested proteins in human beings: Simple direct method of studying absorption of undigested proteins. *J. Immun.* 14:143, 1927.

SECTION I. IMMUNOLOGY OF ATOPIC DISEASES

40. Antigens That Cause Atopic Disease*

PHILIP S. NORMAN

ANTIGENS WHICH ARE INNOCUOUS to most of the population may cause disease when an atopic individual is exposed to them by inhalation or ingestion. Atopic individuals, however, often are not sensitive to some antigens to which they are exposed heavily, even though the same antigen causes severe trouble in other atopic people. The factors which cause atopic individuals to develop sensitivity on exposure to some antigens and not to others are quite unknown (see Chapter 38). Furthermore, some protein materials common in the environment are demonstrably antigenic on parenteral injection in animals but almost never cause atopic disease. Therefore the term *allergen* is applied specifically to those antigens which can cause allergic symptoms. Study of the chemical configuration of allergens provides some insight into their peculiar ability to cause disease in atopic individuals. For this reason, much attention has been paid to the isolation of the allergenic principles of the crude plant and animal materials which cause disease when inhaled or ingested. When isolated, such antigens are usually protein in nature, commonly contain some carbohydrate, and are of medium molecular weight, between 3,000 and 40,000. Chlorogenic acid, the active principle of castor bean and coffee bean dust, is the only known exception to this rule, being a simple organic compound.† Because inhalant and ingestion allergy present somewhat different problems, the antigens involved will be considered separately.

INHALED ALLERGENS

Certain wind-borne plant pollens, mold spores, and insect parts are spread in sufficient quantities over large areas to cause a portion of the susceptible population to develop hay fever or asthma. In addition, there may be sufficient local contamination at home or work by animal danders, house dust, plant dusts, or other inhalant materials to cause respiratory symptoms in exposed allergic individuals.

Of these, plant pollens are the principal offenders, and some plants release enough pollen to produce nationwide seasonal epidemics of respiratory disease affecting as much as 5 percent of the population. Most plants depend on insect pollination and produce pollen suitable for spread by temporary attachment to insect bodies. The more perfectly adapted a plant is to insect pollination, the less pollen produced and spread uselessly by wind. On the other hand, a small number of species (referred to as anemophilous) depend on wind for cross-pollination and produce large amounts of light dry pollen easily borne long distances by air currents. The essential features for establishment of an etiological relationship between a pollen and respiratory allergy were listed by Thommen [1] and are referred to as Thommen's postulates. Slightly modified, they are: (1) pollen must be windborne; (2) pollen must occur in large quantities; (3) plant must be widespread; (4) pollen must contain an excitant of hay fever.

* Work supported by Grant No. AI-04866 from the National Institute of Allergy and Infectious Diseases.

† *Editor's comment:* Other simple compounds reported as allergens causing typical atopic reactions include tannic acid, phthalic anhydride, sulfadiazine, and various sulfone-chloramides.—W. B. S.

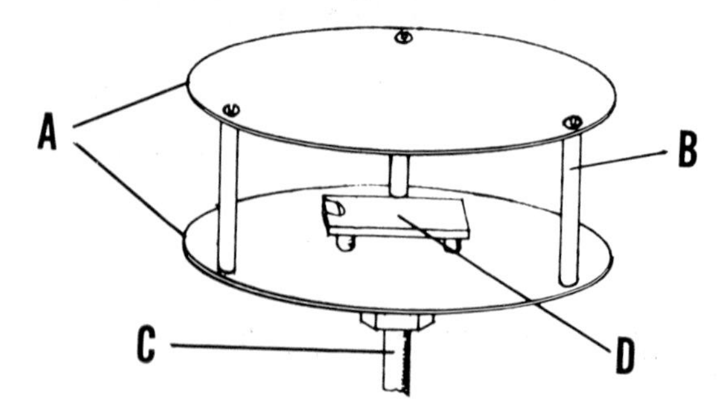

Fig. 40-1. Durham pollen sampler. (*A*) Stainless steel plates, 9-in. diameter; (*B*) separating pillars, 3 in. high; (*C*) support 30 in. high; (*D*) 1 × 3 in. glass slide placed in holder 1 in. above bottom plate.

The small number of species of air-borne plant pollens which are significant in hay fever are produced in definite seasons characteristic for each plant. The dates of pollination of a species may vary by only a week or two from year to year in any one locale, but may be quite different in another climate. Only direct sampling of the air in a locality will define the time of occurrence of pollens and fungi significant in human allergy.

The American Academy of Allergy recommends the Durham sampler (Fig. 40-1), in which a greased microscope slide is exposed for 24 hours in a small shelter designed to protect the slide against rain, snow, and large particles [2]. The slide is removed and stained and the number of pollen grains counted per square centimeter of slide, individual plant pollens being identified by their characteristic morphology. The Durham sampler does not give direct measurements of the concentration of pollens in air because variations of wind velocity influence the number of grains falling on the slide independently of the number of pollen grains per unit volume of air. Various devices to sample measured volumes of air have been developed to obtain more accurate data. A simple quantitative sampler developed by Ogden [3] which catches pollen on the leading edges of two rotating glass slides is shown in Figure 40-2.

Air sampling by the slide method has been performed in thousands of localities in the United States and Canada [4]. The data are reviewed in textbooks of allergy and in handbooks such as *Regional Allergy* [5]. On other continents, different plants are implicated in respiratory allergy [6].

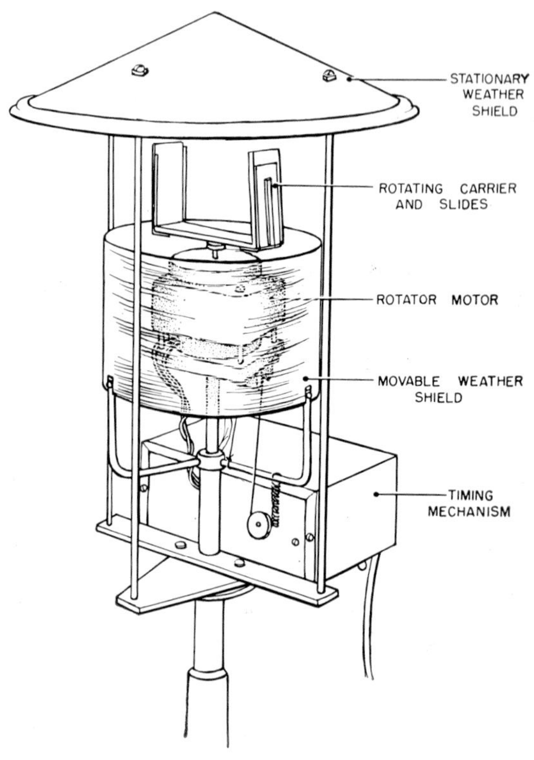

Fig. 40-2. Ogden quantitative pollen sampler.

Air-borne pollens vary in diameter from 10 to 100 μ; particles that are smaller or larger are unsuitable for dispersion from plants by air currents. Particles of 10 to 100 μ are removed by impingement on the moist surfaces of the nasal membranes. In mouth-breathers, such particles land in the pharynx, larynx, and trachea but are too large to be inhaled deeply into the lungs.

Ragweed, widespread and a prolific producer of pollen which contains a potent antigen, is the most common cause of hay fever in North America. There is sufficient cross-reaction between the allergens of the species of ragweed that they may be considered together. Depending on locality and climate, the plant usually matures from late July to early September and begins to shed pollen. It is estimated that a single plant produces 1 billion grains of pollen, or that 1 square mile of ragweed plants produces 16 tons of pollen. The grains are about 25 μ in diameter and are covered by a tough impervious wall which is, however, readily dissolved by the lysozyme of nasal secretions. They are dry and light, easily carried about by air currents, and settle in still air at a rate of 3 ft. per minute. On dry days, ragweed plants shed pollen from about 6:00 to 9:00 A.M. However, air-sampling usually shows the maximal concentration of pollen grains to occur around 3:00 P.M., during the daily maximal wind velocity. On rainy or damp days the plants may not pollinate, which, with the washing effect of rain, lowers the pollen count considerably. The average daily concentration ranges up to several thousand pollen grains per cubic meter of air. Pollen can be blown tremendous distances, and has been found at 14,000 ft. and 400 miles out to sea.

There has been much controversy about the number and biochemical characteristics of the allergens in ragweed pollen. Extracts of ragweed pollen have been shown to contain at least thirteen antigens capable of exciting precipitins in the rabbit. Goldfarb *et al.* [7], however, prepared a highly active protein fraction of giant ragweed which caused skin reactions at 3×10^{-6} gm. per ml. A similar fraction prepared from low ragweed gave a reaction of partial identity on gel diffusion with the fraction from giant ragweed, leading to the hypothesis that the same antigenic specificity is responsible for the allergenicity of both species [8]. The isolation of a nonallergenic antigen from giant ragweed gives further credence to the idea that a single antigenic specificity is responsible for the allergenic activity of ragweed pollen [9]. Recent analyses of the antigens of low ragweed (*Ambrosia elatior*) pollen have identified a single antigen responsible for 90 percent or more of the skin test activity of whole pollen extracts in most hay fever patients [10]. This antigen occurs in several closely related chemical congeners which differ in electrical charge but are immunologically indistinguishable [11]. Other less important allergens are present but are less well characterized. The large quantity of carbohydrate in the pollen, mostly polyarabinose, is not allergenic.

An almost homogeneous preparation of the major allergen has a molecular weight of about 37,800 and is a protein. It represents about 0.005 of the extractable solids of pollen and about 0.05 of the protein. Its biological activity is such that 1 μμg. (10^{-12} gm.) or less causes a positive intracutaneous wheal and erythema reactions in most sensitive human beings. Concentrations of 10^{-8} gm. per ml. cause positive reactions on mucous membranes, and 10^{-10} to 10^{-12} gm. per ml. releases histamine from leukocytes of sensitive individuals [12]. What characteristics make this antigen the most active in ragweed pollen is not known.

Grasses, pollinating in late spring or early summer, are the second most common cause of hay fever in North America and are the most common cause in Europe, where ragweed does not occur. There is a high degree of skin test cross-reaction among extracts of grass pollens causing hay fever, so they are commonly considered together by the allergist. Although most grasses are wind-pollinated, a number are self-pollinated and produce small amounts of pollen, and others are not sufficiently widespread to give high pollen counts. As a result, a small number of species account for practically all grass hay fever. Like ragweed pollen, grass pollens are antigenically complex, both timothy and orchard grass containing at least fifteen antigens. As shown by gel diffusion, the pollens of the five common hay fever grasses, timothy, redtop, June grass, sweet vernal grass, and orchard grass, have a major cross-reacting antigen in common. This antigen is thought to represent the major allergen of these grasses [13]. Although grass pollen allergen has not been prepared in a chemically homogeneous state, highly purified but inhomogeneous allergenic preparations from both timothy and orchard grass have been estimated to have a molecular weight of 14,000 [14]. The allergenic fraction of timothy pollen, however, has been reported by others to have a molecular weight of more than 40,000 [15]. Such preparations are highly active, 10^{-13} or 10^{-14} gm. being sufficient for a positive reaction to an intracutaneous test. Furthermore, one such preparation has been reported in controlled trial to give the same result in desensitization therapy for summer hay fever as whole mixed grass extract [16].

Tree pollens are relatively less frequent causes of hay fever than weed or grass pollens. Most species of trees have a short season of pollination of a few days to a few weeks and do not cause prolonged symptoms. Although oak pollen is produced in very large amounts, it is a less frequent cause of hay fever than ragweed and grass pollens [4].

Some trees are not only widespread but also prolific producers of pollen which is not allergenic. Pine trees, for instance, produce immense quantities of light wind-blown pollen but extremely rarely cause hay fever [4]. The reason that the antigens of some pollens commonly cause hay fever whereas the antigens of other pollens rarely do is unknown.

Little information is available as to the nature of the allergens of tree pollens. The skin test activity of alder (*Alnus glutinosa*) pollen resides in a fraction almost free from carbohydrate which is nondialyzable (more than 10,000 molecular weight) and probably peptide in nature [17].

The place of molds as allergens has been less completely evaluated than that of plant pollens. Nevertheless the spores of a number of molds and fungi seem to fulfill the requirements of Thommen's postulates. These are molds which are widespread in nature, occur in soil or decaying organic matter, and propagate by microscopic spores blown about by wind. The factor of local exposure is important in mold allergy, and some molds grow in houses, particularly in damp cellars, or where the climate is humid. Smuts are obligate parasites of grains which propagate by producing wind-blown spores and have been implicated in allergy to spores. Extracts of the following mold spores are commonly used in diagnosis and treatment of respiratory allergy: *Alternaria, Hormodendrum, Aspergillus, Penicillium, Mucor, Chatomium, Candida, Fusarium,* and smuts [18]. Mold spores may be identified by their microscopic appearance on exposed glass slides or by the colonies appearing on plates of Sabouraud culture medium which have been exposed for a time and then incubated. Some mold spores have definite seasons, particularly *Alternaria* and *Hormodendrum,* which are found from May to December in the eastern United States. *Alternaria* has a definite peak in late September or October, whereas *Hormodendrum* incidence is highest in July. These spores seem to account for the symptoms of hay fever which some people have in July or early August in the gap between the grass and ragweed seasons. Little is known of the chemical nature of the allergens of molds; however, the allergens of *Aspergillus niger, Botrytis cinera,* and *Penicillium frequentans* each appear in a fraction of molecular weight greater than 40,000 [19].

Allergenic parts of insects may be inhaled in sufficient quantities to cause symptoms of hay fever if the insects occur in large enough number. As an example, the sandfly (caddis fly) of the Great Lakes region of the United States swarms from late June to September. The wings have a loose, scaly epithelium and detachable hairs which are easily air-borne [20]. A highly purified preparation active by skin test in sensitive individuals has been prepared from caddis fly extracts. It has two main electrophoretic components, both of which have a sedimentation coefficient of 0.72 S and an estimated molecular weight of about 3,000 [21].

Some very potent allergens pollute the air not over large areas but only in a circumscribed locale such as a house, barn, or factory. The variety in this respect is large, and remarks will be confined to a few common examples. Mold spores in cellars have been mentioned. Animal danders also cause atopic rhinitis and asthma, since domesticated animals shed desquamated skin epithelium which is a potent allergen. Horse dander antigens have been fractionated, and a highly purified but not homogeneous allergen has been obtained of about 34,000 molecular weight. This fraction is a mucoprotein and has been shown not to be horse serum albumin or globulin, although these potent antigens occur in horse dander extracts in small amounts [22].

Industrial exposure to "dusts" arising from a variety of plant materials can cause rhinitis, asthma, or urticaria. Refining of oil from cottonseeds leaves a highly allergenic meal of cottonseed which may cause asthma or rhinitis among workers in plants handling cottonseeds or among farm workers who use the meal as a fertilizer. Spies *et al.* [23] prepared an allergenic fraction of cottonseed meal, referred to as CS-1, which produced passive transfer reactions at concentrations of 10^{-8} gm. per ml. It is precipitable by trichloroacetic acid and therefore thought to be a protein but also contains carbohydrate. It is still highly active after being converted to the picrate. This fraction does not cause skin reactions in every individual who reacts to whole cottonseed and has been useful in differentiating patients with true clinical sensitivity from those with positive reactions but no sensitivity [24]. Further purification leads to removal of nearly all the carbohydrate and a mild enhancement of skin reactivity [25]. The allergen is readily dialyzable and therefore of low molecular weight. Edible cottonseed oil is free from this allergen and probably is only extremely rarely a cause of food allergy.

Two other common examples are green

coffee beans and castor beans, both of which occasionally cause severe trouble in those who handle them in an unrefined state. Castor bean allergen is extremely potent and may be isolated from castor bean meal in a partially purified state by the same methods used for cottonseed allergen [26]. It is also readily dialyzable and quite active when freed from carbohydrate [27] and appears to be a low molecular weight protein. This allergen is to be distinguished from the potent toxin of castor beans, ricin, which is not implicated in respiratory allergy. Castor oil for medicinal purposes is free from the toxin and the allergen. A recent advance is the identification of chlorogenic acid (Fig. 40-3) as the allergen,

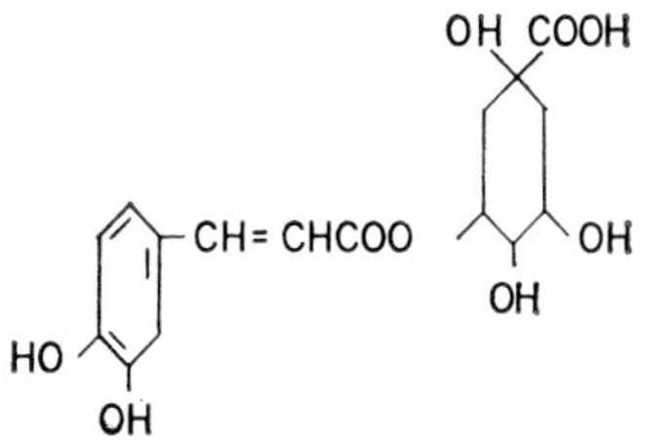

Fig. 40-3. Chlorogenic acid (3-caffeoylquinic acid).

or at least the allergenic determinant, in both green coffee beans and castor beans. Chlorogenic acid in amounts of 2×10^{-11} gm. causes wheal and erythema reactions in patients sensitive to either bean and also neutralizes reagins to whole extracts of either. The identification of chlorogenic acid as a constituent in both coffee and castor beans explains the previously noted cross-reactivity. The relation between chlorogenic acid and previous partially purified preparations of castor bean allergen is unknown.

Roasting of coffee beans destroys chlorogenic acid, and individuals allergic to the green beans can drink coffee without difficulty. Chlorogenic acid has also been identified as the allergen in urticaria caused by ingestion of oranges. Further work of this type may show a biochemical basis for the many known cross-reactions between plant species [28]. Chlorogenic acid is an exception to the general rule that allergens are proteins. Presumably it is a hapten which has the property of spontaneously combining with body protein rapidly in order to become a complete antigen.

House dust extracts commonly cause wheal and erythema reactions among atopic individuals with perennial rhinitis or asthma or with episodic symptoms on exposure to unusual concentrations of dust. House dust is a mixture of epidermal products of man and animals, bacteria, molds, degeneration products of fibrous material, remains of food, plants, and insects. There is evidence, however, that reactions to dust extract cannot be explained by the presence of molds or other known products in dust. An active but heterogeneous house dust allergen fraction has been isolated with a sedimentation coefficient of 2.6 S. It is roughly 5 percent peptide and 95 percent acidic polysaccharide. It remains to be determined if the allergenic activity resides in the peptide or polysaccharide moieties or a combination of the two [29]. The polysaccharide and peptide of crude extracts remain together on electrophoresis at low pH, suggesting that they are linked by covalent bonds [30].

INGESTED ALLERGENS

The antigens responsible for allergic symptoms after ingestion have not been subjected to as much biochemical study as inhalant allergens. The rather dubious place of food allergy as a cause of disease is partly responsible for this. "Gastrointestinal allergy is a diagnosis frequently entertained, occasionally evaluated, and rarely established," according to Ingelfinger *et al.* [31]. Even when history and provocation tests suggest food allergy, reactions to skin tests with the food are often negative. On the other hand, as with pollen antigens, skin tests to food often cause positive reactions in atopic individuals when ingestion of such foods causes no trouble. Nor has the frequent appearance of precipitating antibodies to food antigens in the serum been diagnostically helpful, as they are also frequently present in individuals who are not food-sensitive [32]. These facts have led to the suggestion that the antigen which is absorbed from the intestine has been partially digested and therefore altered to a new antigenic specificity [33]. Cooke, for instance, reported a patient clinically sensitive to milk who had a negative reaction to a skin test to whole milk but a positive one to partially digested milk protein (proteose), but this experience has rarely been duplicated. On the other hand, it has been shown repeatedly that proteins can be absorbed from the intestine in the native state. When passive transfer sites of serum donated by food-sensitive patients who have positive skin reactions are placed on normal recipients, the sites will usually respond with a wheal and erythema when the recipient eats the offending food [34, 35].* Even more convincing is the finding of a protein in the blood a short time after oral administration in a state capable of precipitating with specific rabbit antiserum. Using quantitative precipitin techniques, Gruskay and Cooke [36] estimated that about 0.02 percent of a test dose of egg albumin is absorbed unchanged by normal children and about 0.1 percent is absorbed unchanged by children with diarrhea. It is not essential, therefore, that all of a protein be partially digested before intestinal absorption.

Allergy to cow's milk is the most frequently suspected food allergy, particularly in children. Milk is a complex liquid containing at least sixteen antigens identifiable on immunoelectrophoresis with rabbit antiserum to milk [37]. These antigens include appreciable amounts of serum protein, both globulin and albumin, which are known to be highly antigenic on parenteral injection. Despite some claims that heat-treated milk causes fewer symptoms than unheated milk in milk-allergic individuals, the usual observation is that heated milk is quite capable of provoking symptoms in milk-allergic children [38]. Therefore the heat-resistant antigens, α-lactalbumin, β-lactoglobulin, and casein, are of greatest interest. Alpha-lactalbumin and β-lactoglobulin have molecular weights of 17,600 and 35,000, respectively; casein is a mixture of α-, β-, and γ-caseins in a close molecular association of molecular weight between 75,000 and 100,000 [39]. Assessment of the importance of these antigens and bovine serum albumin was performed in milk-sensitive children by Goldman *et al.* [38]. Forty-five children were studied who had been shown to have symptoms on three different occasions after ingestion of 100 ml. of skim milk. Each child was then given provocative tests at different sittings with purified preparations of each of the four antigens. All 45 reacted positively to one or more of them. Thirteen of the 45 reacted to one antigen, the rest to two, three, or all four of the antigens. The frequency of reaction to the antigens in the children was: α-lactalbumin, 53 percent; β-lactoglobulin, 62 percent; casein, 60 percent; and bovine serum albumin, 52 percent. There is none of the simplicity that is repeatedly suggested by study of inhaled allergens, where it appears that a single allergen is responsible for symptoms of most individuals sensitive to inhalant material. In milk allergy, four different allergens are implicated about equally, and the pattern varies from person to person.

Careful evaluation of individual antigens by provocative test has not been done in other food allergies. Egg-sensitive individuals are usually sensitive only to the egg white and skin reactions can usually be elicited with purified egg albumin as well as whole egg white. The other well-characterized proteins of egg white have not been studied for allergenicity in man.

Urticaria following the eating of fish, shellfish, nuts, or fruit seems to be the food allergy most closely related to atopic disease due to inhaled antigens. Positive skin reactions and presence of passive transfer antibodies are more common than in food allergy associated with other symptoms. The allergens involved have not been identified except in urticaria due to oranges, in which chlorogenic acid, as already mentioned, seems to be the allergenic determinant.

* *Editor's comment:* It is puzzling, indeed, that nonatopic individuals absorb native food and, after absorption, may produce precipitating antibodies, but not reagins. Numerous studies have failed to demonstrate gross differences in the digestion of food by atopic and nonatopic persons. It is conceivable, of course, that the gastrointestinal tract of atopic individuals contributes subtle molecular changes, "labels" which transform food—to use the terminology of the chapter's introduction—from an antigen into an allergen or that the macrophages and the lymphatic system of the atopic person might respond to the ingestion of *any* food with the formation of reagins. These are, at present, unanswered questions.—M. S.

REFERENCES

1. Thommen, A. A. In Coca, A. F., Walzer, M., and Thommen, A. A. (Eds.), *Asthma and Hay Fever in Theory and Practice*. Springfield, Ill.: Charles C Thomas, Publisher, 1931.
2. Durham, O. C. Volumetric incidence of atmospheric allergens: Proposed standard method of gravity, sampling, counting, and volumetric interpolation of results. *J. Allerg.* 17:79, 1946.
3. Ogden, E. C. Unpublished data, 1963.
4. Wodehouse, R. P. *Hay Fever Plants*. Waltham, Mass.: Chronica Botanica Co., 1945.
5. Samter, M., and Durham, O. C. (Eds.), *Regional Allergy of the United States, Canada, Mexico and Cuba*. Springfield, Ill.: Charles C Thomas, Publisher, 1955.
6. Dua, K. L., and Shivpuri, D. N. Atmospheric pollen studies in Delhi area in 1958–1959. *J. Allerg.* 33:507, 1962.
7. Goldfarb, A. R., Bhattacharya, A. K., and Kaemer, S. K. Preparation and immunologic properties of trifidin A, and antigen from giant ragweed pollen. *J. Immun.* 81:302, 1958.
8. Goldfarb, A. R., and Callaghan, O. H. Antigenic relations between fractions from giant and dwarf ragweed. *Int. Arch. Allerg.* 19:86, 1961.
9. Goldfarb, A. R., Bhattacharya, A. K., and Kaplan, M. A. Fractionation of giant ragweed antigens with separation of non-skin reactive antigen. *Int. Arch. Allerg.* 15:165, 1959.
10. King, T. P., Norman, P. S., and Connell, J. T. Isolation and characterization of allergens from ragweed pollen: II. *Biochemistry* 3:458, 1964.
11. King, T. P., and Norman, P. S. Isolation studies of allergens from ragweed pollen. *Biochemistry* 1:709, 1962.
12. Lichtenstein, L. M., and Osler, A. G. *In vitro* studies of histamine release from human leucocytes by ragweed antigen. *Fed. Proc.* 22:560, 1963 (abst.).
13. Wodehouse, R. P. Antigenic analysis by gel diffusion: 2. Grass pollen. *Int. Arch. Allerg.* 6:65, 1955.
14. Augustin, R., and Hayward, B. J. Grass pollen allergens: IV. The isolation of some of the principle allergens of *Phleum pratense* and *Dactylis glomerata* and their sensitivity spectra in patients. *Immunology* 5:424, 1962.
15. Palmstierna, H. On the purification of allergens: I. *Phleum pratense* allergen. *Sci. Tools* 7:29, 1960.
16. Frankland, A. W., and Augustin, R. Prophylaxis of summer hayfever and asthma: Controlled trial comparing crude grass-pollen extracts with isolated main protein component. *Lancet* 1:1055, 1954.
17. Herbertson, S., Porath, J., and Colldahl, H. Studies of allergens from alder pollen (*Alnus glutinosa*). *Acta Chim. Scand.* 12:737, 1958.
18. Feinberg, S. M. Seasonal hay fever and asthma due to molds. *J.A.M.A.* 107:1861, 1936.
19. Palmstierna, H., Ende, H. A., and Ripe, E. On the purification of allergens: II. Allergens from airborne moulds (a preliminary account). *Sci. Tools* 9:25, 1962.
20. Parlato, S. J. The sandfly (caddis fly) as an exciting cause of allergic coryza and asthma: II. Its relative frequency. *J. Allerg.* 1:307, 1930.
21. Shulman, S., Bronson, P., and Arbesman, C. E. Immunologic studies of caddis fly: III. Physical and chemical characterization of the major antigen. *J. Allerg.* 34:1, 1963.
22. Stanworth, D. R. The use of gel-precipitation technique in the identification of horse dandruff allergen, and in the study of the serological relationship between horse dandruff and horse serum protein. *Int. Arch. Allerg.* 11:170, 1957.
23. Spies, J. R., Coulson, E. J., Bernton, H. S., and Stevens, H. The chemistry of allergens: II. Isolation and properties of an active protein component of cottonseed. *J. Amer. Chem. Soc.* 62:1420, 1940.
24. Bernton, H. S., Spies, J. R., and Stevens, H. Significance of cottonseed sensitiveness. *J. Allerg.* 11:1381, 1940.
25. Spies, J. R. The chemistry of allergens: VI. Chemical composition and properties of an active carbohydrate-free protein from cottonseed. *J. Amer. Chem. Soc.* 64:1889, 1942.
26. Spies, J. R., and Coulson, E. J. The chemistry of allergens: VIII. Isolation and properties of an active protein-polysaccharidic fraction, CB-1A, from castor beans. *J. Amer. Chem. Soc.* 65:1720, 1943.
27. Spies, J. R., Coulson, E. J., Chambers, D. C., Bernton, H. S., and Stevens, H. The chemistry of allergens: IX. Isolation and properties of an active, carbohydrate-free protein from castor beans. *J. Amer. Chem. Soc.* 66:748, 1944.
28. Freedman, S. O., Siddiqi, A. I., Krupey, J. H., and Sehon, A. H. Identification of a simple chemical compound (chlorogenic acid) as an allergen in plant materials causing human atopic disease. *Amer. J. Med. Sci.* 244:548, 1962.
29. Vannier, W. E., and Campbell, D. H. The isolation and characaterization of a purified house dust allergen fraction. *J. Allerg.* 30:198, 1959.
30. Vannier, W. E., and Campbell, D. H. A starch block electrophoresis study of aqueous house dust extracts, *J. Allerg.* 32:36, 1961.

31. Ingelfinger, F. J., Lowell, F. C., and Franklin, W. Gastrointestinal allergy. *New Eng. J. Med.* 241:303, 1949.
32. Saperstein, S., Anderson, D. W., Jr., Goldman, M. S., and Knilsen, W. T. Milk allergy: III. Immunological studies with sera from allergic and normal children. *Pediatrics* 32:580, 1963.
33. Cooke, R. A. Protein derivatives as factors in allergy. *Arch. Intern. Med.* 16:71, 1942.
34. Ratner, B., and Gruehl, H. L. Passage of native proteins through the normal gastrointestinal wall. *J. Clin. Invest.* 13:517, 1934.
35. Brunner, M., and Walzer, M. Absorption of undigested proteins in human beings: The absorption of unaltered fish proteins in adults. *Arch. Intern. Med.* 42:173, 1928.
36. Gruskay, F. L., and Cooke, R. E. The gastrointestinal absorption of unaltered protein in normal infants and infants recovering from diarrhea. *Pediatrics* 16:76, 1955.
37. Hanson, L. A., and Mausson, I. Immune electrophoretic studies of bovine milk and milk products. *Acta Paediat.* (Stockholm) 50:484, 1961.
38. Goldman, A. S., Anderson, D. W., Jr., Sellers, W. A., Saperstein, S., Kniker, W. T., Halpern, S. R., *et al.* Milk allergy: I. Oral challenge with milk and isolated milk proteins in allergic children. *Pediatrics* 32:425, 1963.
39. McMeekin, T. L. Milk Proteins. In Neurath, H., and Bailey, K. (Eds.), *The Proteins: Chemistry, Biological Activity and Methods.* New York: Academic Press, Inc., 1954. Vol. II, p. 389.

*41. Antibodies in Nontreated Patients and Antibodies Developed During Treatment**

A. H. SEHON AND L. GYENES

AS IN ACQUIRED IMMUNITY, THE characteristic feature of allergic reactions of both the immediate and the delayed type in man is their specificity with respect to the particular allergen. Since the experiments of Prausnitz and Küstner [1] in 1921, it has been generally accepted that hypersensitivity states of the immediate type, such as hay fever, asthma, and food allergies, are associated with the presence of humoral skin-sensitizing antibodies, produced "spontaneously" by the allergic individual in response to the casual exposure of a given allergen by either inhalation or ingestion. Moreover, since 1935, it has been recognized that treatment of allergic individuals with a series of injections of the offending allergen leads to the formation of an additional humoral antibody, termed blocking antibody, capable of neutralizing the allergen [2]. In the past decade, the presence of agglutinating antibodies has been regularly demonstrated in the sera of both nontreated and treated allergic individuals by passive hemagglutination methods [3, 4].

In contrast, no humoral antibodies have been demonstrated in hypersensitive states of the delayed type, e.g., in tuberculin and contact hypersensitivity, and since these reactions can be passively transferred with the sensitized donor's lymphoid cells, it has been postulated that these states are mediated by a cellular antibody-like factor, referred to as the transfer factor [5].

This discussion will be confined primarily to a consideration of the properties of antibodies present in sera of grass- and ragweed-sensitive individuals†, prior to and after injection therapy, since few systematic studies have been conducted with sera of individuals allergic to other allergens. As will become apparent, despite the many painstaking efforts in numerous laboratories, the exact nature of antibodies in allergic sera and the mechanisms of their interactions *in vivo* and *in vitro* with the appropriate allergens remain unknown. Their elucidation has been hindered partly by the failure to isolate the antibodies from sera of allergic individuals in a pure state, and partly because of the unavailability of pure allergens. Moreover, it will be shown that the differentiation of sera of nontreated allergic individuals from sera of treated patients is arbitrary, since these two types of sera differ mainly in the relative amounts of the various antibodies present rather than in the quality of the antibodies produced.

SKIN-SENSITIZING ANTIBODY (REAGIN)

BIOLOGICAL PROPERTIES

Intradermal injection of the specific allergenic extract into allergic individuals leads to a characteristic reaction which consists of a wheal surrounded by erythema. Prausnitz and Küstner [1] showed that a similar reaction can be obtained by injecting the allergic patient's serum into the skin of a nonallergic individual and challenging the sensitized site, usually 24 or 48 hours later, with the allergen. This has become the recognized test for demonstration of skin-sensitizing antibodies (designated also as reagins) in sera of allergic in-

* The work done in the authors' laboratory and referred to here was supported by grants from the National Institute of Allergy and Infectious Diseases, National Institutes of Health, Bethesda, Md., the Medical Research Council of Canada, and the National Research Council of Canada, Ottawa, Ontario.

† Allergic individuals who have received at least one series of injections of the allergen are denoted as treated individuals; prior to such treatment the allergic patients will be referred to as nontreated individuals. For the sake of brevity, sera of allergic individuals will be designated allergic sera.

dividuals, and the procedure is referred to as the passive transfer (P-K) test. The skin-sensitizing antibody remains attached to the skin for periods of weeks [9]. The P-K test has been also used routinely for the titration of skin-sensitizing antibodies, the P-K titer being equivalent to the reciprocal of the highest dilution of the allergic serum which is still capable of causing a detectable reaction.

It has been repeatedly shown that when blood of an allergic donor is transfused into a nonallergic recipient, skin-sensitizing antibody disappears rapidly from the circulation and becomes fixed in the skin, conjunctivae and mucosae [9, 10]. Exposure of such a passively sensitized recipient to the specific allergen to which the donor was sensitive results in clinical symptoms typical of the allergy of the donor. This transient state of sensitization may persist for several weeks.*

The localization of skin-sensitizing antibody in the skin and in the mucous membranes of the eyes, nose, and respiratory tract of the allergic patient has been exploited in various tests, such as the scratch test, interdermal skin test, conjunctival test, and the insufflation tests used for identification of specific allergens to which the patient is sensitive [12]. Although they have value as diagnostic tools, they are not suited for the quantitation of skin-sensitizing antibodies in serum [13].

In view of the complexity of the mechanism of the local inflammatory reaction, it would be expected that the intensity of the allergic skin reaction will depend not only on the concentration of skin-sensitizing antibodies but on the concentration of the biochemical mediators, which may differ from one allergic individual to another and which determines the over-all response. The P-K titer obtained with a given allergic serum is not an absolutely constant value, since different end points are obtained in different nonallergic recipients and also in different regions of the skin of a given individual [14]. Because of these inherent limitations of the P-K test, a comparison of the reaginic titers of different allergic sera or of serum fractions possessing skin-sensitizing activity may not be meaningful unless these titers are obtained in the skin of the same recipient and with an identical allergenic preparation. For these reasons, the size of a P-K reaction cannot be taken as a measure of the concentration of reagins, and therefore the P-K titer can be determined more objectively in terms of the highest dilution of the reaginic serum or serum fractions which still causes a minimal skin reaction. However, when the number of serum fractions to be tested is too large to titrate all of the fractions in the skin of the same recipient, the P-K titer of each fraction can be expressed in relation to the dilution of the whole serum [15].

Recently it was demonstrated that cutaneous sensitization with sera of allergic individuals could also be achieved in the monkey, *Macaca irus* [16, 17], but attempts to evoke similar reactions in the guinea pig by the passive cutaneous anaphylaxis (PCA) method were usually unsuccessful [18]. It is conceivable that the success of skin sensitization in other species depends on how closely the chemical, anatomical, and physiological makeup of the skin of the animal resembles that of human skin. In this connection it may be mentioned that the skin of young children and of elderly individuals is not suitable for passive transfer test [19]. Since the P-K test in nonallergic volunteers is associated with the unavoidable hazard of transferring homologous serum hepatitis to the test subject, it would be advisable that further investigations be conducted to establish that PCA reactions in monkeys can indeed be used for the demonstration and quantitation of skin-sensitizing antibodies.

Among the other unusual biological properties of skin-sensitizing antibodies are their failure to pass the placenta from maternal to fetal circulation [20, 21] and their retention by the choroid plexus [22]. Although other antibodies to various antigens have been demonstrated in both cord blood and cerebrospinal fluid, no skin-sensitizing antibodies were detected in these two biological fluids. The implications of these findings will be discussed in connection with the physicochemical properties of skin-sensitizing antibody.

CHEMICAL BEHAVIOR

Our knowledge concerning the chemical nature of skin-sensitizing antibody is frag-

* The "spontaneous" production of skin-sensitizing antibody was long believed to be limited to human beings predisposed to hypersensitivity. However, it was recently observed that dogs can also develop spontaneous pollen sensitivity, and their cutaneous, respiratory, and anaphylactic sensitivity could be passively transferred to normal dogs [11].

mentary. Nevertheless all observations made to date indicate that it is much more labile than "conventional" antibodies produced on immunization. Moreover, in conformity with the current concept of diversity of antibodies, skin-sensitizing antibodies have been shown to be heterogeneous with respect to their chemical properties with reference both to sera of different allergic individuals and to the serum of the same individual.

The ability of skin-sensitizing antibody to sensitize human skin is lost on heating at 56° C., the minimal time required for their heat-inactivation varying from serum to serum and ranging from one to ten hours. Moreover, the different skin-sensitizing antibodies present in the same serum and directed against various allergenic fractions of ragweed pollen extract were shown to differ in their thermolability [13]. Heat-inactivation of skin-sensitizing antibody was also found to destroy its eosinophilotactic activity [23].

Sera of allergic individuals stored at 4° C. under sterile conditions for periods up to six months usually show negligible decrease of their skin-sensitizing activity;* prolonged storage, however, was often found to lead to a considerable loss of activity. On the other hand, skin-sensitizing antibodies in serum fractions of relatively low total protein content lost their activity on storage at 4° C. even for short periods. Freezing and thawing of whole sera or of serum fractions were also accompanied by serious loss of skin-sensitizing ability [15].

Dialysis of allergic sera against 0.01 M phosphate buffer at pH 7.5, which is a step used in the chromatographic fractionation of sera on diethylaminoethyl (DEAE) cellulose, was associated with serious loss of skin-sensitizing activity of the order of 50 percent; a further inactivation occurred on chromatographic fractionation of these sera, the final recovered activity in the isolated serum fractions being only 25 to 30 percent of the activity of the sera prior to dialysis† [26]. Similar losses of skin-sensitizing activity were observed on fractionation of allergic sera by starch electrophoresis [15]. However, in both procedures the recovery of serum proteins was almost quantitative. The loss of skin-sensitizing activity reflects thus the lability of reagins when exposed to conditions different from those present in whole serum; the irreversible adsorption of skin-sensitizing antibodies on the supporting material in these procedures cannot be excluded. It is worth mentioning that even a seemingly harmless procedure, such as dilution and reconcentration by ultrafiltration or by pervaporation combined with dialysis, leads to loss of skin-sensitizing activity of the order of 30 to 50 percent [28]. The chemical heterogeneity of skin-sensitizing antibodies is further illustrated by their behavior on exposure to acids. For example, the skin-sensitizing activity of certain allergic sera was partially or completely destroyed on incubation at pH 3 for two hours, whereas other sera were not affected by this treatment [29].

The procedures so far mentioned, i.e., heating, storage, freezing and thawing, dialysis, fractionation procedures on supporting media, and acidification, have no detectable effect on antibodies produced on immunization. Therefore the foregoing observations suggest that skin-sensitizing antibody is not a single, indivisible molecular species but is present in allergic sera in the form of labile complexes and that these complexes may dissociate under certain experimental conditions into smaller fragments with properties different from those of the intact skin-sensitizing antibody molecule.

Like immune antibodies, skin-sensitizing antibodies are degraded with papain, but whereas immune antibodies are split very rapidly, i.e., within the first 30 minutes of digestion 99 percent of the antibodies are destroyed, the skin-sensitizing activity remained practically unchanged within the first 30 to 60 minutes of digestion and decreased gradually over the 24-hour period. Complete inactivation of skin-sensitizing antibodies required about 24 hours of digestion [30].

Unlike immune antibodies, skin-sensitizing antibodies are inactivated by treatment with 0.1 M mercaptoethylamine, in the absence of papain [30–32]. This inactivation may be attributed to the reductive cleavage of these antibodies, since treatment of allergic sera with lower concentrations of the reducing agent or with iodoacetate alone (which is used

* Since the virus responsible for homologous serum hepatitis is inactivated on storage of sera for about six months at 32° C. [24], it has been recommended to use allergic sera for P-K testing after storage for this period [25]. Storage of allergic sera under these conditions does not result in serious loss of reaginic activity.

† This loss of skin-sensitizing activity was minimized in the presence of sucrose [27].

for stabilization of the SH groups liberated during the reductive cleavage) did not lead to a measurable decrease of skin-sensitizing activity. The results obtained in the studies on enzymatic and chemical degradation indicate that during these reactions the portion of the skin-sensitizing antibody molecule responsible for its attachment to the skin becomes destroyed or dissociated from the rest of the molecule.

The weight of all of this evidence supports the view that skin-sensitizing antibodies differ radically from immune antibodies, a conclusion which will be further substantiated in the following discussions.

PHYSICOCHEMICAL PROPERTIES

Salting-out Procedures. The following two examples clearly illustrate that the solubility properties of skin-sensitizing antibodies differ from those of immune antibodies and that they are not 7S γ-globulins.*

At 30 percent saturation with ammonium sulfate, immune antibodies begin to precipitate, and precipitation is complete at about 35 percent saturation. In contrast, skin-sensitizing antibodies do not precipitate at 30 percent saturation with ammonium sulfate, and precipitation is far from being complete at 35 percent saturation; at the intermediate concentration of 33 percent saturation, the skin-sensitizing activity of the supernatants is five to ten times higher than that of the precipitates [33, 34]. Similarly, fractional precipitation with sodium sulfate revealed the different solubility behavior of skin-sensitizing antibodies [35]: skin-sensitizing activity was about equally distributed between the supernatant and the precipitates obtained at 15 and 18 percent salt concentrations; under the same conditions, immune antibodies are quantitatively recovered in the precipitates.

The addition of rivanol (2-ethoxy-6, 9-diaminoacridine lactate) to serum leads to the precipitation of albumin and of α- and β-globulins, leaving γ-globulins (including immune antibodies) in solution. Fractionation of allergic sera by this method resulted in recovery of 60 percent of the original skin-sensitizing activity in the soluble fraction, which was shown to contain 12 percent of the total serum proteins consisting of γ-globulins (75 percent) contaminated with β-globulins [36]. In addition, 22 percent of the original skin-sensitizing activity was associated with the precipitate, which contained most of the other serum proteins and was composed mainly of albumin (75 percent) and contained less than 5 percent γ-globulins.†

Electrophoresis. The electrophoretic behavior of skin-sensitizing antibodies was investigated in a great number of studies. Sera of allergic individuals were fractionated by various electrophoretic procedures, such as Tiselius electrophoresis [37], electrophoresis-convection [38, 39], zone electrophoresis on starch [15, 40], and continuous paper electrophoresis [33], and the isolated fractions were assessed for their skin-sensitizing activity. In another group of studies, serum fractions isolated by other fractionation procedures (i.e., by salting-out, chromatography) and possessing skin-sensitizing activity were further analyzed by electrophoresis [41] or by immunoelectrophoresis [28, 35]. By the latter technique, about thirty distinct components have been revealed in normal human serum on the basis of their electrophoretic mobility and of their specific reactions with homologous antibodies produced in experimental animals [42]. The results of studies identifying skin-sensitizing antibodies with well-defined serum components using this technique are discussed later.

There is general agreement among investigators that the electrophoretic mobility of skin-sensitizing antibody is higher than that of immune antibodies [15, 35, 38–40, 43, 44]. Thus, whereas the bulk of the latter were shown to have an electrophoretic mobility (at pH 8.6, ionic strength 0.1) ranging from -0.5 to -1.3×10^{-5} cm.^{2} per volt per second, corresponding to that of the slow γ-globulins, skin-sensitizing activity was invariably associated with faster moving globulins, having an electrophoretic mobility up to about -2.2×10^{-5} cm.^{2} per volt per second and corresponding to that of γ_1 (or β_2)-globulins.

In a study of the localization of skin-sensitizing antibody by zone electrophoresis on starch, no correlation could be found between the protein concentration of the isolated γ_1-

* Recent recommendations for uniform designations of immunoglobulins—outlined in the beginning of this textbook—suggest that immunoglobulins referred to in this chapter as 7Sγ-, γ_{1A} or β_{2A}, and γ_{1M}- or 19S globulins might be called γG, γA and γM, or alternatively as IgG, IgA, and IgM.

† For a detailed account of this work see Menzel and Sherman [36a].

and γ_2-globulin fractions and the skin-sensitizing activity of the fractions [15]. In some instances, electrophoretic subfractions in the γ_1-globulin region having a protein concentration as low as 800 μg. per ml. caused skin reactions approximating those of the whole unfractionated sera. This indicates that skin-sensitizing antibody is present in sera of allergic individuals in exceedingly low concentration and must possess a high biological activity.

Ultracentrifugation. In a preliminary study [4, 33, 45] using partition cells, it was found that migration of the 19S components into the bottom compartment resulted in the depletion of skin-sensitizing activity from the top compartment and in a concomitant increase of activity in the bottom compartment. (Under the same conditions of centrifugation, immune antibodies were found in both top and bottom compartments.) These results were interpreted to indicate that skin-sensitizing activity was associated not with the 7S globulins but with heavier serum components.

The sedimentation coefficients of skin-sensitizing antibodies were determined in a subsequent study by the more direct solute transport method, which enables one to calculate the sedimentation coefficient of a biologically active substance in terms of the distribution of its activity in the two compartments of the partition cell after centrifugation under precisely established conditions [46]. In practice, the skin-sensitizing activity remaining in the top compartment after different intervals of centrifugation was determined and was related to the skin-sensitizing activity of the serum prior to centrifugation. In this study, the sedimentation coefficients of skin-sensitizing antibodies were invariably found to be larger than 7S, the three calculated values being 12.4, 14.1, and 22.5S. In view of the inherent inaccuracies of the P-K titration used for quantitative estimation of skin-sensitizing antibodies, a narrower range for their sedimentation coefficients could not be established. Nevertheless these results clearly indicate that the sedimentation coefficient(s) of skin-sensitizing antibodies was definitely higher than 7S [47].

These conclusions were subsequently challenged by a number of investigators. By use of a preparative ultracentrifugal method, it was found that serum fractions devoid of 19S components as well as the heavy serum components, isolated in the form of a pellet, had skin-sensitizing activity [48]. However, the activity of each of these fractions was almost equal to that of the original unfractionated serum. Ultracentrifugal analysis of serum fractions, which were isolated by chromatographic or ultracentrifugal fractionation procedures, or both, and were shown to contain skin-sensitizing activity, indicated that these fractions were devoid of 19S components [28]. Furthermore, the results of electrophoretic and immunochemical analyses demonstrated the presence of γ_1-globulins (apparently of the 7S type) in these fractions. However, as was pointed out earlier and as will be further discussed, since the amount of material responsible for the skin-sensitizing activity of allergic sera is exceedingly low, the absence of a detectable amount of faster sedimenting component(s) cannot be considered sufficient evidence that skin-sensitizing antibody is associated exclusively with the 7S globulins. In a similar study [35], it was concluded from the immunoelectrophoretic and gel diffusion analyses of chromatographic and ultracentrifugal fractions of sera of grass- and mold-sensitive individuals that skin-sensitizing antibodies were not macroglogulins but "medium fast γ-globulins of normal molecular weight" [49]; however, the possibility was not excluded that some skin-sensitizing antibodies might be complexed with α_{2M}-globulins [35]. In view of the extreme lability of skin-sensitizing antibodies, it is conceivable that the fractionation procedures used before ultracentrifugal analysis as well as the formation of gummy pellets on prolonged ultracentrifugation of allergic sera or of reaginic fractions may have resulted in the modification of the molecular properties of skin-sensitizing antibodies. Moreover, since in all the latter studies [28, 35, 48] the skin-sensitizing activity of the fractions was recorded in terms of the size of the P-K reactions rather than by the more accurate end point titration procedure, the estimates obtained for the distribution of skin-sensitizing activity between the light and heavy serum globulins cannot be considered to be accurate.

Another explanation for the diverging conclusions of the results presented so far might be that skin-sensitizing activity is associated with neither the 7S nor the 19S serum component, but with other moieties having sedimentation coefficient(s) intermediate between these values [50]; such components would be detected either with the light or with the heavy serum components, depending on the experimental conditions used. Indeed, by means of an improved method of density gradient ultracentrifugation, skin-sensitizing antibodies to glucagon were found to sediment with serum components having sedimentation coefficients of the order of 8 to 11S [32]. At present, however, the question is still open as to whether skin-sensitizing antibodies to other allergens would also belong to this new class of antibodies with intermediate sedimentation coefficients. In this connection it is interesting to note that very recently, in two independent studies, it was demonstrated that skin-sensitizing antibodies of ragweed-sensitive patients sedimented faster than γ-globulins [50a, 50b], their average sedimentation coefficient being 7.7S [50a]. The recent suggestion [51] that they may be associated "essentially and perhaps quantitatively" with the γ_{1A}-globulins (designated also β_{2A}-globulins) will be examined later.

Chromatography. Serum fractions enriched in skin-sensitizing activity were isolated by chromatography of allergic sera on the anion exchange resin, DEAE cellulose [26, 28, 35, 52, 53], and by gel filtration [44] on the cross-linked dextran, Sephadex G-200. The latter technique is essentially a molecular sieving process: i.e., substances with molecular weights higher than about 200,000 do not penetrate this particular gel matrix and are therefore excluded from entering the gel, whereas smaller molecules enter the gel particles and are subsequently displaced in order of decreasing molecular size.

Chromatography of allergic sera on DEAE cellulose demonstrated further that the behavior of skin-sensitizing antibodies was different from that of immune antibodies. Thus, whereas the latter were almost quantitatively recovered in the first chromatographic fraction (eluted with 0.01 M phosphate buffer at pH 7.5), skin-sensitizing antibodies were eluted in later fractions with buffers of higher molarity (0.02 and 0.05) and of lower pH (6.2 and 4.5) [26, 35]. Furthermore, electrophoretic [28], ultracentrifugal [28], and immunochemical [28, 35] analyses revealed that the fractions possessing skin-sensitizing activity were heterogeneous mixtures of proteins. In contrast, the first chromatographic fraction, which contains the bulk of immune antibodies, consists practically of pure 7S γ-globulins [54]. As mentioned earlier, the recovery of skin-sensitizing activity after chromatography on DEAE cellulose was only about 25 to 30 percent of the activity of the original serum [26]. Moreover, skin-sensitizing activity was distributed among three to five distinct chromatographic fractions, usually separated from each other by fractions devoid of such activity [26, 35]. These results suggested that skin-sensitizing antibodies were physicochemically heterogeneous. However, on the assumption that they are labile complexes, it is conceivable that chromatography on DEAE cellulose results in their being broken down into a spectrum of molecules still possessing skin-sensitizing activity but with different physicochemical properties and affinities for the supporting medium.

Fractionation of sera on Sephadex G-200 yields three fractions which are not resolved completely from one another and which are composed of (1) macroglobulins (γ_{1M}- and α_{2M}-globulins), (2) other globulins γ_2-, γ_1-, β-, and α-globulins) of lower molecular weight, and (3) albumin. By use of this method for the fractionation of three sera of treated ragweed-allergic individuals, skin-sensitizing activity was found primarily in the early eluates of the second fraction, i.e., in the eluates corresponding to the region of overlap between the first and second chromatographic fractions, and the bulk of activity emerged before the peak concentration of the second fraction [44]. By immunochemical analysis, the eluates containing skin-sensitizing activity were found to be composed mainly of γ_{1A}-globulins, 7S γ-globulins, a small amount of γ_{1M}-globulins, and possibly also of other components. These results were interpreted to indicate that the distribution of skin-sensitizing activity paralleled best that of γ_{1A}-globulins [44].

ANTIGENIC RELATIONS OF REAGINS AND OTHER GLOBULINS

Reference has been made to the fact that skin-sensitizing activity may be associated with γ_{1A} (β_{2A})-globulins. This conclusion was based not on the direct identification of skin-sensitizing antibodies as γ_{1A}-globulins but on circumstantial evidence. Thus immunoelectrophoretic analysis of serum fractions, isolated by various fractionation procedures and containing skin-sensitizing activity, revealed γ_{1A}-globulins in addition to one or more of other serum proteins, such as 7S and 19S γ-globulins, siderophilin, transferrin, haptoglobin and α_1-glycoprotein [28, 35, 44, 51]. Here will be described the antigenic relationships of skin-sensitizing antibodies to other serum proteins as determined by direct immunochemical procedures with specific antisera.

Specific precipitation of serum components, present in a chromatographic fraction possessing skin-sensitizing activity, with a rabbit antiserum to human γ-globulins resulted in the removal of all skin-sensitizing antibodies; in addition, the specific precipitate was shown to display some skin-sensitizing activity [49]. However, since γ_{1A}-globulins, as well as 7S and 19S γ-globulins, share common antigenic determinants, these results simply indicate that skin-sensitizing antibodies belong to the general class of immunoglobulins but do not specify more precisely their antigenic nature. In contrast, it was demonstrated recently that removal of 7S γ-globulins from a skin-reactive serum fraction by precipitation with an antiserum, rendered specific to 7S γ-globulins by prior absorption with γ_{1A}-globulins, did not diminish its skin-sensitizing titer [44]. However, complete removal of skin-sensitizing activity from the three allergic sera used in this study was achieved by absorption with a specific antiserum to γ_{1A}-globulins [44]; this antiserum had been rendered specific for γ_{1A}-globulins by the precipitation of antibodies directed to the determinants of 7S γ-globulins. These results clearly demonstrated that at least some of the antigenic groups of skin-sensitizing antibodies in these three sera were identical to those of γ_{1A}-globulins. However, since γ_{1A}-globulins tend to complex with other proteins [53a], and since recently three sera of ragweed-sensitive individuals with high P-K titers were found to be devoid of γ_{1A}-globulins [55], it is felt that additional evidence is needed to identify unequivocally skin-sensitizing antibodies with γ_{1A}-globulins. It is conceivable that these antibodies are complex molecular species, one of their building blocks being γ_{1A}-globulin; this latter component might be responsible for the fixation of skin-sensitizing antibodies to tissues* and for their retention by the placenta and choroid plexus. Moreover, although γ_{1A}-globulins are immunochemically homogeneous, i.e., they give a single precipitin band with a homologous antiserum, they display ultracentrifugal heterogeneity; i.e., 85 percent of γ_{1A}-globulins have a sedimentation coefficient of 7S and the remaining 15 percent sediments with rates corresponding to 10S to 15S. The properties of the latter components of γ_{1A}-globulins are practically unknown, and in the light of the experimental results derived from ultracentrifugal, chemical, and chromatographic studies of skin-sensitizing antibodies, it is not unlikely that reagins may belong to the group of γ_{1A}-globulins with higher sedimentation coefficients.

* In this connection it is noteworthy that passive sensitization of normal human skin with reagins was blocked with normal human γ_{1A}-globulins [56] and also with chain A of these globulins [56a].

By use of radio-immunoelectrophoresis, a technique based on immunochemical principles, it was demonstrated that ragweed-binding capacity of allergic sera was not limited to a single serum protein [57]. In this study, allergic sera were separated first by electrophoresis in agar-gel and the various serum components subsequently immobilized as precipitin arcs by reaction with a specific antiserum to human serum proteins. (The procedure described so far is the standard immunoelectrophoresis technique.) After development of the precipitin arcs, I^{131}-labeled ragweed pollen antigens were allowed to diffuse into the gel, and the precipitin arcs corresponding to the γ-, γ_{1A}-, and γ_{1M}- globulins were found, by radioautography, to bind the labeled antigen. The ragweed-binding ability was associated with the γ-globulins of all of the eight sera tested and, in addition, with the γ_{1A}- or γ_{1M}-globulins, or both. However, these results by themselves do not prove that skin-sensitizing antibodies are directly implicated in this reaction since, as will be shown later, sera of nontreated allergic individuals possess, besides reagins, a spectrum of antibodies devoid of skin-sensitizing activity but with a binding capacity for the allergen(s). Nevertheless these results demonstrate strikingly that there exist multiple antibodies in sera of allergic individuals capable of combining with the allergenic constituents of ragweed pollen.

IMMUNOLOGICAL PROPERTIES

Numerous attempts have been made to demonstrate that *in vitro* combination occurs between antibodies in sera of nontreated allergic individuals and the homologous allergens (antigens). All of the classic immunological techniques, such as precipitation, agglutination, complement fixation and/or lysis, as well as the various forms of anaphylaxis, have been used for this purpose. Some of these tests failed altogether to give positive reactions, but other methods were more successful and gave some promising results. However, these tests usually gave more consistent results with sera of treated allergic individuals. Therefore, it is possible that any positive reaction obtained with sera of nontreated allergic subjects could have been attributed to blocking antibodies rather than to skin-sensitizing ones.

It has been repeatedly shown that sera of nontreated allergic individuals fail to give a visible precipitate on incubation with the allergen. The inability of skin-sensitizing antibodies to do this with homologous allergens was ascribed [45, 58] to any of the following three possibilities: (1) the skin-sensitizing antibodies were univalent, (2) the affinity of skin-sensitizing antibodies for the allergen(s) was very small, or (3) these antibodies could be divalent and have a high affinity for the allergen but their concentration was too low to be detected by the standard precipitin test. As will be seen, the experimental data obtained to date strongly favor the third possibility.

If skin-sensitizing antibodies were univalent, the addition of allergic serum to a system consisting of the antigen and of homologous precipitating antibodies produced in another species would be expected to result in a decrease of the amount of specific precipitate.* Theoretically, however, it is also conceivable that, depending on the antibody : antigen ratio and on the relative affinities of the different antibodies for the common antigen, coprecipitation of univalent antibodies would lead to an increase in the amount of specific precipitate. By means of this experimental approach, it was demonstrated in a number of studies [60–63] that the change in the amount of specific precipitate (either increase or decrease) was too small to be considered significant and that therefore no conclusion could be derived regarding the valency and the combining capacity of skin-sensitizing antibodies.

* Inhibition of precipitin reactions were indeed obtained with model systems in which univalent antibody fragments prepared by enzymatic and chemical degradation of divalent antibodies were used [59].

The *in vitro* interaction of antibodies in allergic sera with ragweed allergens has been demonstrated by precipitation of the appropriate soluble complexes either with a potent rabbit antiserum to human γ-globulins [64], or with ammonium sulfate at 40 percent saturation [65]. In view of the recent findings concerning the common antigenic determinants possessed by immunoglobulins [8, 66], it is likely that both blocking and skin-sensitizing antibodies were precipitated with the rabbit antiserum used in the first procedure [64] (see also p. 525). In the second procedure [65], I^{131}-labeled ragweed allergens were used, and although the method was shown to be quantitative and reproducible, about 40 percent of the I^{131}-tagged allergenic constituents was precipitated nonspecifically in the presence of normal serum. In view of this complication and since reagins are probably present in allergic sera in concentrations much lower than those of blocking antibodies, produced during hyposensitization or even "spontaneously" [3, 26, 67], no conclusion could be reached as to whether this method measured reagins, blocking antibodies, or both.

Evidence of the *in vitro* combination between skin-sensitizing antibodies and the homologous allergens was obtained by the use of immunologically specific adsorbents (immunosorbents). Ragweed or grass pollen constituents, or both, were attached by covalent azo bonds to various supporting media, such as polystyrene [29, 68], erythrocytes [69–71], cellulose [72, 73], or cowhide powder [49], and these immunosorbents were shown to remove specifically and completely skin-sensitizing antibodies from allergic sera. Attempts to elute these antibodies from the immunosorbents by the conventional procedure of lowering the pH to about 3 did not lead to their recovery in significant yields [29, 49, 73]. However, in preliminary experiments, elution of substantial amounts of skin-sensitizing antibodies was achieved in the presence of normal serum at pH 3 or with 6 M urea [73]. Moreover, in another series of experiments [71], reagins were displaced off specific immunosorbents with serum fractions containing only blocking antibodies to ragweed. It is to be pointed out that the complete removal of skin-sensitizing antibodies by absorption with immunosorbents was not accompanied by a measurable decrease in the protein concentration or by a change of the protein distribution of allergic sera as determined from comparative electrophoretic and ultracentrifugal analyses [29]. These results indicated further that skin-sensitizing activity of allergic sera was associated with serum components present in concentrations lower than are detectable by the Schlieren optical system or by the Rayleigh interferometric method, i.e., lower than 100 μg. per ml. [74]. Therefore it is not surprising that the classic precipitin test or its variations, such as coprecipitation or inhibition of precipitation, have failed to detect skin-sensitizing antibodies.

The various forms of agglutination techniques, utilizing collodion particles [75] in the earlier studies and erythrocytes [3, 76, 77] more recently, were also applied to the detection of antibodies in sera of allergic individuals. Coating of the surface of these particles with antigens (or allergens) has been achieved by adsorption (as in the collodion or in the tanned red cell techniques [75, 78]), by specific interactions* (as in the red cell linked antigen test [79]), or by coupling of the antigen to erythrocytes by stable covalent bonds using bifunctional reagents (such as bisdiazotized benzidine [69, 80, 81], tolylene-2,4-diisocyanate [82], or 1,3-difluoro-4,6-dinitrobenzene [83]. The last technique has the advantage over the other methods that it is specific and highly sensitive, gives reproducible results, and eliminates the possibility of the antigen's becoming desorbed from the sensitized erythrocytes [84].

Hemagglutination techniques have been adapted for the demonstration of antibodies in sera of individuals allergic to ragweed [69, 85] and grass pollens [68, 86], protein hormones [81], penicillin [87, 88], coffee bean [89], horse serum [90], milk [91], and egg white proteins [92, 93]. The detection of hemagglutinins in sera of both nontreated and treated allergic individuals raises a number of questions concerning their relationship to skin-sensitizing and blocking antibodies.

The complement fixation technique also revealed the presence of antibodies in sera of nontreated allergic individuals, although consistently positive results were obtained primarily with sera of treated patients [94–96]. However, no simple relationship was found between the amount of complement fixed and the amount of skin-sensitizing or blocking antibodies present. Therefore it is difficult to draw any conclusion as to whether skin-sensitizing or blocking antibodies are involved in these reactions or whether complement was fixed by antibodies directed against ragweed components, which bear no relation to skin-sensitizing or blocking antibodies, or both.

The various forms of anaphylaxis, such as passive sensitization of animals with allergic serum [97], the Schultz-Dale technique [98], and PCA in the guinea pig [18], generally failed to detect antibodies in sera of nontreated allergic individuals. (The few positive PCA reactions in guinea pigs should probably be attributed to blocking antibodies, discussed later.) However, as already stated, sera of nontreated allergic individuals regularly caused PCA reactions in the monkey† *Macaca irus* [16, 17].

In addition to these classic immunological techniques, a number of methods based on reactions involving the cellular elements of the blood have been explored in an attempt to develop an *in vitro* method for the detection of skin-sensitizing antibodies. Thus incubation of the blood of allergic individuals with the homologous allergen resulted in the release of histamine from leukocytes [99, 100]. This reaction has been shown to be specific: it could be produced only with the blood of allergic individuals and only with the allergen to which they were sensitive. Moreover, maximal histamine release occurred at an optimal concentration of allergen which seemed to be related to the skin-sensitivity. A similar reaction was also obtained with the leukocytes of

* Recently a double-layer agglutination procedure has been developed (Ridges, A. P., and Augustin, R., *Nature* 202:668, 1964) for the detection of antibodies in allergic sera. In this method, human leukocytes are first incubated with the test serum, then treated with excess antigen and finally exposed to an antiserum containing precipitating antibodies to the antigen. Agglutination of leukocytes results if the test serum contains antibodies against the homologous antigen. Positive results were obtained with sera of nontreated hay fever patients, as well as with precipitating antibodies to pollens which were devoid of reagins. However, from the results with sera devoid of precipitins, it was inferred that this technique showed great promise of being capable of measuring reagins *in vitro*.

† Recently an important discovery was reported: that passive sensitization of monkey ileum with sera of nontreated allergic patients could be reproducibly achieved, and that the modified Schultz-Dale technique was more sensitive than the P-K reaction for the detection of skin-sensitizing antibodies. (Arbesman, C. E., Girard, P., and Rose, N. *J. Allerg.* 35:535, 1964.)

normal individuals (or rabbits) provided the leukocytes were incubated with the allergic serum before addition of the allergen [101]. These findings suggest that skin-sensitizing antibodies also have affinity for leukocytes, and this would explain the success of the transfer of hypersensitive reactions of the immediate type with viable leukocytes or their extracts [102].

It was claimed that leukocytes of allergic individuals show peculiar reactions when exposed to the specific allergen. For example, the number of leukocytes was found to diminish in the blood of ragweed-sensitive individuals on addition of ragweed pollen extract due to lysis of the cells [103, 104]. In another study, it was found that the leukocytes undergo morphological changes associated with their immobilization or lysis, or both [105]. It was reported that this leukocytolytic effect depended on the nature of the allergen: more consistent results were obtained with leukocytes from individuals allergic to house dust or timothy pollen, than with leukocytes from ragweed-sensitive individuals. In other studies, however, no change was observed either in the number of leukocytes or in their morphological aspect [106, 107]. Recently, degranulation of rabbit basophils, incubated with allergic serum, was noted on exposure to the specific allergen [108]. These results, however, have not been consistently reproduced [109]. Due to these contradictory results and to the lack of reproducibility, none of these tests seems to be satisfactory and suitable for the unequivocal demonstration of allergic reactions. The same consideration holds for two other observations, namely, for the agglutination of thrombocytes suspended in allergic serum, which was claimed to occur on addition of the specific allergen [110, 111], and for the increase in the light scattered on addition of the allergen to the allergic serum [112, 113].

BLOCKING ANTIBODY

BIOLOGICAL PROPERTIES

The existence of blocking antibody in sera of allergic individuals who had received hyposensitization treatment was recognized in 1935 [2]. The test for blocking antibody is based on its ability to "neutralize" the allergen(s) and thus prevent the latter from reacting with skin-sensitizing antibodies in the P-K reaction. For the quantitative determination of blocking antibodies, two variations of the test have been adapted [114, 115]. In both procedures, the demonstration of blocking antibodies requires the presence of a reaginic serum, which is used as an indicator. In one method the blocking activity is expressed in terms of the amount of allergen(s) inactivated by blocking antibodies [26]; in the other, the titer of blocking antibodies is expressed in terms of the highest dilution of the serum (or serum fraction) which is still capable of giving a detectable blocking reaction [116].

Although the development of blocking antibody seems to be the major immunological response during hyposensitization treatment, at least in the early stages of immunization of allergic individuals, the appearance of blocking antibody is accompanied by an increase of reagins [117, 118]. The ability of allergic patients to tolerate progressively increasing doses of the allergen during hyposensitization has been, therefore, attributed to the protective capacity of blocking antibodies [2, 117, 119]. However, no simple relation between clinical improvement and the titer of blocking antibodies has been established. In some studies, no correlation was found between clinical symptoms and the titer of blocking or skin-sensitizing antibodies, or both [117, 118, 120–122]; in other studies, the patients' well-being seemed to parallel fairly well their blocking antibody titers [115, 119, 123, 124]. The therapeutic value of blocking antibodies has been demonstrated by passive immunization of a group of allergic individuals with globulin preparations containing large amounts of blocking antibodies which had been produced in nonallergic individuals [125].

In contrast to reagin, blocking antibody appears to have no affinity for human skin or mucous membranes [9]; it passes through the placenta [21, 126] and is capable of neutralizing the allergen [2, 64, 115, 116]. This neutralization was shown to occur *in vitro,* and because of the apparent therapeutic effect of blocking antibody, it is plausible to assume that this reaction occurs also *in vivo* [125].

Formation of blocking antibodies can be induced in both allergic individuals and nonallergic volunteers, and, as shown later, the various properties of blocking antibodies elicited in these two types of inviduals are identical. Blocking ability is not confined to antibodies produced in man but is also possessed by those formed by rabbit, goat, and dog on immunization with the appropriate allergen [30, 33, 127]. From these observations, one may infer that antibodies are produced in all of these species against the same antigenic determinants or against different determinants situated on the same antigenic molecule(s).

CHEMICAL BEHAVIOR

The chemical nature of blocking antibodies resembles that of precipitating antibodies and differs significantly from that of skin-sensitizing antibodies. Thus they are not inactivated by heating at 56° C. [115], are stable under various conditions of storage and handling [26, 30, 116] and are not degraded by reduction with 0.1 M mercaptoethylamine [30]. Moreover, digestion of blocking antibodies with pepsin, papain, or pepsin followed by reduction with mercaptoethylamine—reactions known to lead to the breakdown of precipitating rabbit antibodies to smaller divalent [128] or univalent antibody fragments [128, 129]—resulted in the degradation of blocking antibodies to fragments which were shown to retain the ability of combining with the allergen(s) and thus to block the P-K reaction to the same extent as intact blocking antibodies [30]. Fragments prepared from precipitating rabbit antiragweed antibodies behaved in the same way; i.e., the blocking titers of the fragments were identical to those of the intact antibodies [30].

PHYSICOCHEMICAL PROPERTIES

Salting-out Procedures. The solubility properties of blocking antibodies differ from those of skin-sensitizing antibodies and are similar to those of "conventional" antibodies produced on immunization. Fractional precipitation methods with ammonium sulfate or ethanol demonstrated that the bulk of blocking antibodies was associated with γ-globulins [33, 34, 40, 125]. Like conventional precipitating antibodies, the precipitation of blocking antibodies from whole serum begins at about 30 percent saturation with ammonium sulfate and is almost complete at 35 percent saturation. Under these conditions, most of the skin-sensitizing antibodies remain in solution, as discussed earlier. This method was adopted for the gross separation of blocking antibodies from reagins; i.e., at 33 percent saturation with ammonium sulfate the precipitated globulins contained the bulk of the blocking antibodies (and only 10 to 20 percent of the skin-sensitizing antibodies), and the globulins precipitated subsequently on increase of the ammonium sulfate concentration contained the bulk of skin-sensitizing antibodies [33, 34].

Electrophoresis. With various electrophoretic methods, the bulk of blocking activity was invariably associated with the slowest migrating serum components, namely, with γ_2-globulins [41, 116, 130]. Occasionally, particularly with sera containing large amounts of blocking antibodies, a small portion of the blocking activity was detected also in the faster migrating γ_1-globulin fractions. This behavior is not altogether unique for blocking antibodies; it has been repeatedly shown that conventional precipitating antibodies, particularly those produced on hyperimmunization, are physicochemically heterogeneous, and electrophoretically they extend from the region of the slowest γ-globulins to that of α_2-globulins [131]. In the light of these findings, it seems reasonable to ascribe the ragweed-binding activity of γ_2-globulins, as demonstrated by radio-immunoelectrophoresis [57], to blocking antibodies. Moreover, the binding of I^{131}-labeled ragweed pollen constituents by γ_{1M}- and γ_{1A}-globulins [57] might reflect simply the electrophoretic heterogeneity of blocking antibodies and therefore cannot be considered unequivocal proof for the identification of skin-sensitizing antibodies with these globulins.

Ultracentrifugation. By use of partition cells and calculation of specific activities of globulins in top and bottom compartments for the ultracentrifugal characterization of blocking antibodies, the specific activity of blocking antibodies produced on immunization of nonallergic volunteers was less than unity,* when calculated with respect to the concentration of 7S globulins; the actual value determined in one experiment was 0.4 [34, 47]. In view of the limited accuracy of the

* If the increase of blocking activity of the bottom compartment paralleled the increase in concentration of the 7S components, the specific activity would be unity with respect to 7S globulins. On the other hand, if the accumulation of blocking antibodies in the bottom compartment were greater than the increase in concentration of the 7S components, this specific activity would be larger than unity and would suggest that blocking activity is associated with a component having a sedimentation coefficient higher than 7S.

in vivo method used for titration of blocking antibodies, and because of the technical difficulties involved in the titration of these antibodies with the small volumes of serum which can be recovered from the partition cell, this procedure was not further pursued. Nevertheless, since values significantly higher than unity were obtained for the specific activity of skin-sensitizing antibodies by this method, the results of this experiment were interpreted as indicating that blocking antibodies sedimented in all probability as γ-globulins of the 7S type. In anticipation of the later discussion of the relation of hemagglutinins to skin-sensitizing and/or blocking antibodies, the more accurate passive hemagglutination technique will be considered here to measure blocking antibodies in sera of nonallergic individuals immunized with ragweed pollen extract. On the basis of this assumption, the specific activity of blocking antibodies, measured in terms of the hemagglutination titer and calculated with respect to the concentration of 7S globulins, was 1.1, indicating that indeed the sedimentation coefficient of the hemagglutinins in these sera was close to 7S [33, 47]. In an extension of this study, the sedimentation coefficient of blocking antibodies (again assumed to be measurable in terms of the hemagglutination titer) was determined by the more direct solute transport method and was found to be of the order of 7S for antiragweed antibodies produced on immunization of nonallergic volunteers and rabbits [47].

Chromatography. The chromatographic behavior of blocking antibodies on DEAE cellulose was found to be similar to that of precipitating rabbit antibodies: the bulk of both types was eluted in the first fraction with 0.01 M phosphate buffer at pH 7.5 [26]. However, the protein distribution in this fraction was not symmetrical, and therefore the fraction was subdivided into two subfractions, 1A and 1B. Blocking antibodies, as well as precipitating rabbit antiragweed antibodies, were confined primarily to subfraction 1A, although minute amounts were also found in subfraction 1B and in subsequent chromatographic fractions eluted with buffers of higher concentration and of lower pH. It should be pointed out that, generally, neither blocking antibodies nor precipitins could be demonstrated in these other fractions unless they were first concentrated. Because of the insensitivity of the tests, it is difficult to give an accurate estimate of the extent of recovery of blocking antibodies by chromatography; nevertheless there is no doubt that the bulk of the blocking activity was located in fraction 1A.

Essentially identical results were obtained with sera of nonallergic volunteers and rabbits, immunized with ragweed pollen extract, and of nontreated and treated allergic individuals, except that fraction 1A of sera of nontreated individuals had to be first concentrated before the presence of blocking antibodies could be demonstrated [26]. In addition to the similarity of the chromatographic properties of antibodies to ragweed eluted in fraction 1A, irrespective of the serum used (i.e., sera of immunized nonallergic volunteers or rabbits, or of nontreated and treated allergic individuals), all fractions 1A were shown to contain antibodies demonstrable by the hemagglutination test. Moreover, after appropriate concentration of subfractions 1A of all sera, blocking and precipitating antibodies were readily demonstrable when the hemagglutination titers of the concentrated fractions were at least 2,500 and 40,000, respectively [127, 132]. On the basis of this evidence, it was inferred that these various immunological manifestations could probably be attributed to the same type of antibodies, and consequently it was proposed that blocking antibodies had the properties of normal, immune antibodies [29, 77, 127, 132]. Hence it must be concluded that even nontreated allergic individuals form blocking antibodies and, therefore, that the older classification of sera of allergic individuals into two categories, depending on whether they were obtained from patients before or after hyposensitization treatment, can be regarded as purely arbitrary. However, it should be stressed that during hyposensitization, the patient may produce also antibodies to antigenic constituents in ragweed which may have no relation to the allergenic determinant groups. These antibodies would then escape detection by the *in vivo* procedure for the demonstration of blocking antibodies, although their presence could be verified by *in vitro* methods, i.e., by hemagglutination and precipitation. Similar considerations apply also to blocking antibodies produced "spontaneously" by the nontreated allergic individual, as well as by nonallergic volunteers and rabbits on immunization.

ANTIGENIC RELATIONS OF BLOCKING ANTIBODIES AND OTHER SERUM PROTEINS

As already indicated, the bulk of blocking antibodies is recovered in the first serum fraction isolated by chromatography on DEAE cellulose. This fraction was shown to consist of 7S γ-globulins by a combination of electrophoretic, ultracentrifugal, and immunoelectrophoretic procedures [54]. Furthermore, it was reported that blocking antibodies in sera of treated allergic individuals were precipitated with rabbit antisera produced to human γ-globulins [64]. The specific precipitates were capable of combining *in vitro* with the homologous allergens, indicating that the allergen-binding capacity of blocking antibodies had not been impaired after their incorporation into the precipitate. However, since the purity of the γ-globulin fraction used for immunization of rabbits was not established, and in view of more recent evidence that different immunoglobulins possess common antigenic determinants, it is conceivable that the antiserum used for the precipitation of blocking antibodies was not directed exclusively against 7S γ-globulins (see also earlier discussion under Immunological Properties of skin-sensitizing antibody). Moreover, as previously stated, in all likelihood the immune precipitates would have contained also skin-sensitizing antibodies. On similar grounds, the ragweed-binding activity of allergic sera in the region of slow γ-globulins, as detected by radio-immunoelectrophoresis [57], cannot be considered by itself to be definite proof for the identification of blocking antibodies as γ-globulins. Nevertheless the weight of all of this circumstantial evidence, viewed in the light of our knowledge of the properties of immunoglobulins [53a], strongly suggests that blocking antibodies have the properties of conventional 7S γ-globulins.

IMMUNOLOGICAL PROPERTIES

Absorption of sera containing blocking antibodies with specific immunosorbents resulted in the complete and specific removal of these antibodies [29, 69, 71]; moreover, their concentration in the sera used was shown to be below the limit of detectability by the Schlieren procedure, i.e., below 0.1 mg. per ml. [29]. These results thus provide proof that blocking antibodies combine *in vitro* with the constituents of the appropriate allergenic extract. However, the elution of these antibodies from the immunosorbent by acidification to pH 3, which is the standard procedure for dissociation of the antibody-immunosorbent complexes, was rather poor.

On concentration of sera or serum fractions containing blocking antibodies to a hemagglutination titer of about 40,000, precipitins could be readily demonstrated by the micro-Ouchterlony procedure [132].* Moreover, at least partial, if not complete, reactions of identity were obtained by this procedure with antibodies, isolated by chromatography on DEAE cellulose, in fractions 1A of the sera of nontreated and treated allergic individuals as well as of sera of immunized nonallergic volunteers and rabbits [132]. Also, different ragweed pollen preparations, i.e., the whole water-soluble extract, the nondialyzable and the dialyzable constituents of this extract, and the purified fraction δ [133], gave common precipitin bands with the antibodies of these four types of sera [132]. These results indicate, therefore, that common antigenic constituents are present in the various ragweed pollen preparations and that antibodies in fraction 1A of each of the four types of sera are directed against the same antigenic determinants or against different determinants which are nonetheless situated on the same molecule(s).

It was recently demonstrated that blocking antibodies can sensitize the skin of guinea pigs for PCA [30, 135]. Such positive reactions were readily obtained with blocking antibodies in sera of both treated allergic individuals and nonallergic volunteers immunized with ragweed pollen extracts. In view of the higher concentration of blocking antibodies in the latter group of sera, it is not surprising that their PCA titers were higher, i.e., of the order of 1 : 100 [30], than those of sera of treated allergic individuals, i.e., 1 : 10 to 1 : 40 [135].

RELATION OF HEMAGGLUTININS TO SKIN-SENSITIZING AND BLOCKING ANTIBODIES

From an analysis of the hemagglutination and P-K titers of sera of nontreated allgeric in-

* Similar results were recently reported for two sera of treated patients with hemagglutination titers of the order of 40,000; precipitin bands were readily obtained by immunoelectrophoresis with these unfractionated sera [134].

dividuals, it appears that although all sera tested were never devoid of hemagglutinins, there exists no simple relationship between these two titers; i.e., sera with high P-K titers may have low or high hemagglutination titers, and sera with low P-K titers may have high or low hemagglutination titers. This lack of correlation seems to suggest that the hemagglutinating ability of sera of nontreated allergic individuals is due to multiple factors, the proportion of which differs from one serum to another and represents the individual variation in antibody response [71]. The possibility that multiple hemagglutinins may be present in allergic sera is also supported by the findings that the titers obtained with erythrocytes sensitized via tolylene-2,4-diisocyanate were substantially lower than the bisdiazotized benzidine titers and that there was no obvious relationship between these two sets of titers [82].

The similarity between the physicochemical and chemical properties of blocking antibodies and of hemagglutinins strongly suggests that most of the hemagglutinins of sera of treated allergic individuals may be identified with blocking antibodies. On similar grounds and also in view of the reactions of identity given by antibodies of sera of treated and nontreated individuals in agar-gel diffusion experiments [132], one may postulate that blocking antibodies produced "spontaneously" by the nontreated allergic individual are indistinguishable from those produced on hyposensitization treatment. On the other hand, the lack of correlation between the hemagglutination and P-K titers of sera of nontreated and treated allergic individuals and, more important, the findings that the hemagglutination titers of chromatographic fractions containing the bulk of skin-sensitizing activity were only a small fraction of the hemagglutination titer of the whole serum [26], indicate that even if skin-sensitizing antibodies had hemagglutinating capacity, their contribution to the over-all hemagglutination titers would be minimal [71]. Obviously, to establish whether or not these two different immunological reactions are due to the same serum factor(s), it is necessary to isolate the corresponding antibodies in a pure state or, at least, to separate them from other antibodies reacting with the same antigen. With a view to separating the different types of antibodies from each other by various physicochemical and immunochemical methods, a number of studies have been conducted and the results obtained are summarized below.

By fractional precipitation of allergic sera with salts, partial or complete separation of skin-sensitizing and blocking antibodies was achieved, but none of the fractions containing either type of antibody was devoid of hemagglutinating activity [33, 34]. The hemagglutination titers of fractions containing blocking antibodies were considerably higher than those of fractions containing skin-sensitizing antibodies. All reaginic fractions, isolated under conditions under which blocking antibodies would have been removed prior to the precipitation of skin-sensitizing antibodies, had a low but definite hemagglutination titer. Similar results were obtained by zone electrophoresis on starch or by continuous paper electrophoresis; i.e., skin-sensitizing antibodies were associated with the faster moving γ-globulins [15], blocking antibodies were localized in the slower moving ones [116], and hemagglutinating capacity was associated with fractions containing skin-sensitizing or blocking antibodies, or both, but not with other fractions devoid of either of these antibodies [33, 34].

As stated previously, there is no unanimous agreement among investigators as to the ultracentrifugal properties of skin-sensitizing antibodies [28, 32, 35, 47, 48, 50]. However, it seems fair to state that the weight of experimental evidence strongly supports the belief that reagins have sedimentation coefficients larger than 7S. In this connection, it is to be pointed out that the sedimentation coefficients of hemagglutinins in sera of nontreated allergic individuals were also found to be higher than 7S, the actual values calculated by application of the solute transport method [46] ranging from 9.1S to 20.7S [47]. Moreover, the sedimentation coefficients of these hemagglutinins were found to be time-dependent; i.e., the computed values decreased with increasing periods of centrifugation [47]. This was attributed to the participation of at least two physicochemically distinct hemagglutinins with sedimentation coefficients of the order of 19S and 7S, respectively. From a consideration of the mechanism of sedimentation, it is obvious that the relative contribution of the slower sedimenting hemagglutinins to the over-all titer of the solution in the top compartment of the partition cell becomes more significant with increasing periods of centrifugation and that consequently the sedimentation coefficient becomes weighted in favor of the slower sedimenting factor. Although the coefficients were considered to be accurate only within about 2.5 Svedberg units, it was suggested at the time that the faster sedimenting hemagglutinins may have sedimentation coefficient(s) of the order of 19S, by analogy with the fastest sedimenting components of human sera detectable by Schlieren optics. On the basis of the similarity of the sedimenting properties of these hemagglutinins and of skin-sensitizing antibodies, it was suggested that sera of nontreated allergic individuals might contain two types of antibodies, i.e., antibodies with sedimentation coefficients higher than 7S which possess both skin-sensitizing and hemagglutinating abilities, and antibodies of the conventional 7S type possessing only hemagglutinating activity [47]. The latter hemagglutinins may be thus identifiable with the majority of the blocking antibodies.

Chromatographic fractionation of sera of nontreated allergic individuals on DEAE cellulose led to partial or complete separation of reagins from blocking antibodies [26, 28, 35, 53]. However, hemagglutinating activity was always associated with all chromatographic fractions which had skin-sensitizing or blocking activity, or both.* These findings could be taken as further circumstantial evidence that both skin-sensitizing and blocking antibodies have the capacity of agglutinating erythrocytes coated with ragweed pollen constituents. Obviously one cannot rule out the alternate interpretation, that the hemagglutinins detected in allergic sera are different moieties from skin-sensitizing and blocking antibodies and that the similarity in the physicochemical properties of some of the hemagglutinins and of skin-sensitizing antibodies, or of some of the other hemagglutinins and blocking antibodies, is purely fortuitous.

The experimental data so far presented strongly suggest that most of the hemagglutinating activity of sera of nontreated and treated allergic individuals is due to antibodies which also possess blocking and precipitating ability. This type of antibody may be subdivided into two classes on the basis of their immunochemical properties: (1) antibodies directed against allergenic constitutents of ragweed pollen (theoretically, they may be directed against the allergenic determinants themselves or against some antigenic determinants on the same molecules in the vicinity of the allergenic determinants), and (2) antibodies directed against antigenic constituents of ragweed pollen which are unrelated to the allergens, i.e., against antigenic determinants not situated on the same molecules as the allergenic determinants. Obviously, only antibodies of the first class would be expected to participate in the *in vivo* blocking reaction, although both classes would be detected by the hemagglutination reaction,† provided the homologous allergens or antigens are present on the sensitized erythrocytes. Because of the latter possibility, one could not expect a simple relationship between the hemagglutination and blocking titers of whole sera or of concentrated serum fractions.

On the basis of the foregoing discussion, it is evident that the contribution of skin-sensitizing antibodies to the hemagglutination titer of allergic sera would be only minimal. Nevertheless the result of the physicochemical studies reviewed (fractional precipitation, electrophoresis, ultracentrifugation, chromatography) suggest that skin-sensitizing antibodies may also possess hemagglutinating ability.

The nature of skin-sensitizing, blocking and hemagglutinating antibodies of sera of allergic individuals has as yet not been unequivocally elucidated and no simple relationships have been established among these factors. The solution of these problems is rendered difficult because these antibodies are present in allergic sera in exceedingly low concentrations and because none of these factors has so far been isolated in a pure form in sufficient amount. Consequently, no dose-response relation has been established for any of the different immunological reactions. However, it is obvious that the antibodies in allergic sera are heterogeneous with respect to their size, shape, composition, charge and their affinity for the antigen(s). Moreover, on the basis of the evidence reviewed, it seems plausible to conclude that blocking antibodies are electrophoretically slow γ-globulins with a sedimentation coefficient of 7S, that they have the properties of "conventional" antibodies and can, therefore,

* As mentioned previously, these fractions showed blocking activity provided their hemagglutination titer was at least 2,500 [127].

† As stated previously, hemagglutinating antibodies are by necessity divalent [59].

be detected by classic immunological techniques. On the other hand, skin-sensitizing antibodies are electrophoretically faster-moving globulins belonging possibly to the class of γ_{1A}- and/or γ_{1M}-globulins, they have sedimentation coefficient(s) higher than 7S, and may contribute to a small extent to the overall hemagglutination titer of allergic sera.

REFERENCES*

1. Prausnitz, C., and Küstner, H. Studien über die Ueberempfindlichkeit. *Zbl. Bakt.* [Orig.] 86:160, 1921.
2. Cooke, R. A., Barnard, J. H., Hebald, S., and Stull, A. Serological evidence of immunity with co-existing sensitization in a type of human allergy (hay fever). *J. Exp. Med.* 62: 733, 1935.
3. Boyden, S. V. Approaches to the Problem of Detecting Antibodies. In Shaffer, J. H., Lo-Grippo, G. A., and Chase, M. W. (Eds.), *Mechanisms of Hypersensitivity.* Boston: Little, Brown, 1959. P. 95.
4. Sehon, A. H. The Detection and Nature of Nonprecipitating Antibodies in Allergic Sera. *Ibid.,* p. 61.
5. Lawrence, H. S. The Transfer of Hypersensitivity of the Delayed Type in Man. In Lawrence, H. S. (Ed.), *Cellular and Humoral Aspects of the Hypersensitive States.* New York: Paul B. Hoeber, Inc., 1959. P. 279.
6. Williams, C. A., Jr., and Grabar, P. Immunoelectrophoretic studies on serum proteins: I. The antigens of human serum. *J. Immun.* 74: 158, 1955.
7. Onoue, K., Yagi, Y., and Pressman, D. Multiplicity of antibody proteins in rabbit anti-p-azobenzenearsonate sera. *J. Immun.* 92:173, 1964.
8. Heremans, J. *Les Globulines Sériques du Système Gamma, Leur Nature et Leur Pathologie.* Paris: Masson et Cie, 1960.
9. Loveless, M. H. Immunological studies of pollinosis: II. Passive sensitization of man through transfusion. *J. Immun.* 41:15, 1941.
10. Ramirez, M. A. Horse asthma following blood transfusion: Report of a case. *J.A.M.A.* 73:984, 1919.
11. Patterson, R., and Sparks, D. B. The passive transfer to normal dogs of skin reactivity, asthma and anaphylaxis from a dog with spontaneous ragweed pollen hypersensitivity. *J. Immun.* 88:262, 1962.
12. Criep, L. H. *Clinical Immunology and Allergy.* New York: Grune & Stratton, Inc., 1962.
13. Richter, M., Harter, J. G., Sehon, A. H., and Rose, B. Studies on ragweed pollen: III. Estimation of the minimum number of allergens in the water soluble extract of ragweed pollen and a critical evaluation of the neutralization technique; The demonstration of two different reagins in sera of ragweed sensitive individuals. *J. Immun.* 79:13, 1956.
14. Stanworth, D. R., and Kuhns, W. J. Unpublished work, cited by Stanworth, D. R. Reagins. *Brit. Med. Bull.* 19:235, 1963.
15. Sehon, A. H., Harter, J. G., and Rose, B. The localization of skin-sensitizing antibody in the sera of ragweed-sensitive individuals by electrophoresis. *J. Exp. Med.* 103:679, 1956.
16. Layton, L. L., and Yamanaka, E. Demonstration of human reagins to food, cat dander, an insect, and ragweed and grass pollens. *J. Allerg.* 33:271, 1962.
17. Rose, N., Kent, J. H., Reisman, R.E., and Arbesman, C. E. Passive sensitization of monkey skin with sera of ragweed-sensitive patients. *J. Allerg.* 35:520, 1964.
18. Ovary, Z., and Biozzi, G. Passive sensitization of skin of guinea pig with human antibody. *Int. Arch. Allerg.* 5:241, 1954.
19. Samsoe-Jensen, T., and Kristensen, K. H. On the ability of the skin of infants and young children to fix skin sensitizing antibodies: Passive transfer by the method of Prausnitz-Küstner. *Acta Allerg.* 11:28, 1957.
20. Bell, S. D., and Eriksson, Z. Studies in the transmission of sensitization from mother to child in human beings: I. Transfer of skin sensitizing antibodies. *J. Immun.* 20:447, 1931.
21. Sherman, W. B., Hampton, S. F., and Cooke, R. A. The placental transmission of antibodies in the skin sensitive type of human allergy. *J. Exp. Med.* 72:611, 1940.
22. London, M. Study on reagin content of spinal fluid. *J. Allerg.* 12:244, 1940.
23. Eidinger, D., Raff, M., and Rose, B. Tissue eosinophilia in hypersensitivity reactions as revealed by the human skin window. *Nature* (London) 196:683, 1962.
24. Sayman, W. A., Gauld, R. L., Star, S. A., and Allen, J. G. Safety of liquid plasma: A statistical appraisal. *J.A.M.A.* 168:1735, 1958.
25. Harter, J. G. The effect of storage on human skin-sensitizing antibody (reagin). *Fed. Proc.* 20:259, 1961 (abst.).
26. Perelmutter, L., Freedman, S. O., and Sehon,

* For more recent reviews of this topic refer to the symposia published in the Proceedings of the 5th International Conference of Allergology (Madrid, Oct. 1964) by Editorial Paz Montalvo, Madrid 12.

A. H. Chromatographic fractionation of sera from ragweed-sensitive individuals. *Int. Arch. Allerg.* 19:129, 1961.

27. Perelmutter, L. Characterization of Antibodies in Sera of Allergic Individuals. McGill University, Ph.D. Thesis, 1962.
28. Stanworth, D. R. Studies on the physicochemical properties of reagin to horse dandruff, *Immunology* 2:384, 1959.
29. Gyenes, L., and Sehon, A. H. The use of polystyrene-allergen conjugates for the removal of antibodies from sera of allergic individuals. *Canad. J. Biochem. Physiol.* 38:1249, 1960.
30. Gyenes, L., Sehon, A. H., Freedman, S. O., and Ovary, Z. The properties of fragments of skin-sensitizing and blocking antibodies as revealed by the Prausnitz-Küstner, passive cutaneous anaphylaxis and hemagglutination reactions. *Int. Arch. Allerg.* 24:106, 1964.
31. Leddy, J. P., Freeman, G. L., Luz, A., and Todd, R. H. Inactivation of the skin-sensitizing antibodies of human allergy by thiols. *Proc. Soc. Exp. Biol. Med.* 111:7, 1962.
32. Rockey, J. H., and Kunkel, H. G. Unusual sedimentation and sulfhydryl sensitivity of certain isohemagglutinins and skin-sensitizing antibody, *Proc. Soc. Exp. Biol. Med.* 110:101, 1962.
33. Gordon, J. Antibody-antigen Reactions in Allergy. McGill University, Ph.D. Thesis, 1958.
34. Sehon, A. H. Different Types of Antibodies Produced by Allergic Individuals Depending on Route of Immunization. In Holub, M., and Jarošková, L. (Eds.), *Mechanisms of Antibody Formation*. Prague: Publishing House of Czechslovak Academy of Sciences; and New York: Academic Press, Inc., 1960. P. 79.
35. Augustin, R., and Hayward, B. J. Human reagins to grass pollens and molds: Their purification and physico-chemical characterization. *Immunology* 3:45, 1960.
36. Menzel, A. E. O., Cooke, R. A., and Sherman, W. B. The fractionation of reaginic serums with rivanol. *Excerpta Med.* [Int. Congr. Ser.] 42:108, 1961.

36a. Menzel, A. E. O., and Sherman, W. B. The antibody mechanism of ragweed allergy. Electrophoretic and chemical studies. *Int. Arch. Allerg.* 24:127, 1964.

37. Newell, J. M., Sterling, A., Oxman, M. F., Burden, S. S., and Krejci, L. E. Electrophoretic separation of the antibody from human allergic serum. *J. Allerg.* 10:513, 1938–39.
38. Campbell, D. H., Cann, J. R., Friedman, T. B., and Brown, R. The relation of allergy reagins to electrophoretic components of serum, *Science* 119:289, 1954.
39. Cann, J. R., and Loveless, M. H. Distribution of sensitizing antibody in human serum proteins fractionated by electrophoresis convection. *J. Immun.* 72:270, 1954.
40. Brattsten, I., Colldahl, H., and Laurell, A. H. F. The distribution of reagins in the serum protein fractions obtained by continuous zone electrophoresis. *Acta Allerg.* 8:339, 1955.
41. Cooke, R. A., Menzel, A. E. O., Kessler, W. R., and Myers, P. A. The antibody mechanisms of ragweed allergy; electrophoretic and chemical studies: I. The blocking antibody. *J. Exp. Med.* 101:177, 1955.
42. Grabar, P., and Burtin, P. *Analyse Immuno-Électrophorétique*. Paris: Masson et Cie, 1960.
43. Sehon, A. H., Fyles, W., and Rose, B. Electrophoretic separation of skin-sensitizing antibody from sera of ragweed-sensitive patients. *J. Allerg.* 26:379, 1955.
44. Fireman, P., Vannier, W. E., and Goodman, H. C. The association of skin-sensitizing antibody with the β_{2A} globulins in sera from ragweed sensitive patients. *J. Exp. Med.* 117:603, 1963.

44a. Terr, A. I., and Bentz, J. D. Gel filtration of human skin sensitizing antibody and β_{2A}-globulin. *J. Allerg.* 35:206, 1964.

45. Sehon, A. H. Biophysical and Immunochemical Problems in Allergy. In Halpern, B. N., and Holtzer, A. (Eds.), *Proceedings of the Third Congress of Allergology*. Paris: Éditions Médicales Flammarion, 1958. P. 209.
46. Yphantis, D. A., and Waugh, D. F. Ultracentrifugal characterization by direct measurement of activity: I. Theoretical; II. Experimental. *J. Physiol. Chem.* 60:623 and 630, 1956.
47. Gyenes, L., Gordon, J., and Sehon, A. H. Ultracentrifugal characterization of antibodies in sera of ragweed-sensitive individuals. *Immunology* 4:177, 1961.
48. Heimlich, E. M., Vannier, W. E., and Campbell, D. H. Sedimentation studies of skin-sensitizing antibody. *J. Allerg.* 31:364, 1960.
49. Augustin, R. Precipitins, reagins and blocking antibodies. *Acta Allerg.* 16:473, 1961.
50. Campbell, D. H., and Sehon, A. H. Ref. 3, p. 120.

50a. Anderson, B. R., and Vannier, W. E. The sedimentation properties of the skin-sensitizing antibodies of ragweed-sensitive patients. *J. Exp. Med.* 120:31, 1964.

50b. Terr, A. I., and Bentz, J. D. Density-gradient sedimentation of skin-sensitizing antibody and β_{2A}-globulin in serum of allergic individuals. *Proc. Soc. Exp. Biol. Med.* 115:721, 1964.

51. Heremans, J. F., and Vaerman, J.-P. β_{2A}-globulin as a possible carrier of allergic reaginic activity. *Nature* (London) 193:1091, 1962.
52. Porter, R. R. The reagin content of human gamma-globulin fractions. *Int. Arch. Allerg.* 11:61, 1957.
53. Brown, E. G., and Friedman, H. Chromato-

graphic separation of hemagglutination and reaginic activities of ragweed-sensitive serum. *Ann. Allerg.* 21:17, 1963.

54. Fahey, J. L., McCoy, P. F., and Goulian, M. Chromatography of serum proteins in normal and pathological sera: The distribution of protein-bound carbohydrate and cholesterol, siderophilin, thyroxin-binding protein, B_{12}-binding protein, alkaline and acid phosphatases, radioiodinated albumin and myeloma proteins. *J. Clin. Invest.* 37:272, 1958.

54a. Heremans, J. Ref. 8.

55. Arbesman, C. E., and Rockey, J. H. (Personal communications, 1963).

56. Ishizaka, K., Ishizaka, T., and Hornbrook, M. M. Blocking of Prausnitz-Küstner sensitization with reagin by normal human β_{2A}-globulin. *J. Allerg.* 34:395, 1963.

56a. Ishizaka, K., Ishizaka, T., and Hathorn, E. M. Blocking of Prausnitz-Küstner sensitization with reagin by 'A' chain of human γ_{1A}-globulin. *Immunochem.*, 1:197, 1964.

57. Yagi, Y., Maier, P., Pressman, D., Arbesman, C. E., and Reisman, R. E. The presence of ragweed-binding antibodies in the β_{2A}-, β_{2M}- and γ-globulins of the sensitive individuals. *J. Immun.* 91:83, 1963.

58. Campbell, D. H. The immunochemical aspects of allergy. *J. Allerg.* 19:151, 1948.

59. Gyenes, L., and Sehon, A. H. The mechanism of the hemagglutination reaction. *J. Immun.* 89:483, 1962.

60. Miller, H., and Campbell, D. H. Reagins: Preliminary report on experimental evidence in support of a new theory of their nature. *Ann. Allerg.* 5:236, 1947.

61. Bukantz, S. C., Johnson, M. C., and Hampton, S. Quantitative immunologic studies with allergens. *J. Allerg.* 20:1, 1949.

62. Hampton, S., Johnson, M. C., Alexander, H. L., and Wilson, K. S. Detection of the "thermostable" antibody by means of the precipitin reaction. *J. Allerg.* 14:227, 1943.

63. Orlans, E. S., Rubinstein, L. J., and Marrack, J. R. Detection of antibodies in the serum of patients suffering from hay fever. *Acta Allerg.* 6:33, 1953.

64. Follensby, E. M., and Lowell, F. C. Removal of a skin-reactive component in ragweed pollen extract by human serum protein present as an immunologic precipitate. *J. Allerg.* 28:307, 1957.

65. Lidd, D., and Farr, R. S. Primary interaction between I^{131}-labelled ragweed pollen and antibodies in the sera of humans and rabbits. *J. Allerg.* 33:45, 1962.

66. Fahey, J. L. Heterogeneity of γ-globulins. *Advances Immun.* 2:41, 1962.

67. Gyenes, L., and Sehon, A. H. The nature and properties of antibodies in sera of allergic individuals: A review. *Int. Arch. Allerg.* 18:330, 1961.

68. Frick, O. L., Gyenes, L., and Sehon, A. H. Demonstration of antibodies in sera of grass-sensitive individuals by the bisdiazotized-benzidine hemagglutination technique. *J. Allerg.* 31:216, 1960.

69. Gordon, J., Rose, B., and Sehon, A. H. Detection of "non-precipitating" antibodies in sera of individuals allergic to ragweed pollen by an *in vitro* method. *J. Exp. Med.* 108:37, 1958.

70. Mathews, K. P., and Spear, H. J. A comparative study of the hemagglutinating and skin sensitizing activities of ragweed sensitive human sera. *J. Immun.* 87:274, 1961.

71. Perelmutter, L., Freedman, S. O., and Sehon, A. H. Demonstration of multiple hemagglutinating factors in sera of ragweed-allergic individuals with the help of immunosorbents. *J. Immun.* 89:623, 1962.

72. Malley, A., and Campbell, D. H. Isolation of antibody by means of an immunological specific adsorbent. *J. Amer. Chem. Soc.* 85:487, 1963.

73. Reiner, A., and Sehon, A. H. Unpublished results, 1963.

74. Antweiler, H. J. *Die quantitative Elektrophorese in der Medizin.* Berlin: Springer-Verlag, 1952. P. 17.

75. Jones, F. S. Agglutination by precipitin. *J. Exp. Med.* 48:183, 1928.

76. Stavitsky, A. B., and Arquilla, E. R. Studies of proteins and antibodies by specific hemagglutination and hemolysis of protein-conjugated erythrocytes. *Int. Arch. Allerg.* 13:1, 1958.

77. Sehon, A. H. Hemagglutinating Factors in Allergic Sera. In Brown, E. A. (Ed.), *Allergology.* London: Pergamon Press, 1962. P. 300.

78. Boyden, S. V. The adsorption of proteins on erythrocytes treated with tannic acid and subsequent hemagglutination by antiprotein sera, *J. Exp. Med.* 93:107, 1951.

79. Coombs, R. R. A., Howard, A. N., and Mynors, L. S. A serological procedure theoretically capable of detecting incomplete or non-precipitating antibodies to soluble protein antigens. *Brit. J. Exp. Path.* 34:525, 1953.

80. Pressman, D., Campbell, D. H., and Pauling, L. The agglutination of intact azo-erythrocytes by antisera homologous to the attached groups. *J. Immun.* 44:101, 1942.

81. Stavitsky, A. B., and Arquilla, E. R. Micromethods for the study of proteins and antibodies: III. Procedure and applications of hemagglutination and hemagglutination-inhibition reactions with bis-diazotized benzidine and protein conjugated red blood cells. *J. Immun.* 74:306, 1955.

82. Gyenes, L., and Sehon, A. H. The use of tolylene-2, 4-diisocyanate as a coupling reagent

in the passive hemagglutination reaction, *J. Immunochem.* 1:43, 1964.
83. Ling, N. R. The coupling of protein antigens to erythrocytes with difluorodinitrobenzene. *Immunology* 4:49, 1961.
84. Feinberg, R. J., and Flick, J. A. Elution of pollen antigens from tannic acid treated erythrocytes. *Proc. Soc. Exp. Biol. Med.* 96:71, 1957.
85. (*a*) Arbesman, C. E., Rose, N. R., Kantor, S. Z., and Beede, R. B. Immunologic studies of ragweed-sensitive patients: I. Specificity and sensitivity of hemagglutination reactions. *J. Allerg.* 31:317, 1960. (*b*) Arbesman, C. E., Rose, N. R., and Kantor, S. Z. II. Effect of specific hyposensitization therapy on hemagglutinating antibody titers. *Ibid.,* p. 333.
86. Augustin, R. On the Nature of the Antibody Response to Allergens. Ref. 31, p. 94.
87. Watson, K. C., Joubert, S. M., and Bennett, M. A. E. The occurrence of haemagglutinating antibody to penicillin. *Immunology* 3:1, 1960; Some factors influencing the haemagglutination of penicillin-sensitized erythrocytes. *Immunology* 4:193, 1961.
88. Schwartz, R. H., and Vaughan, J. H. Immunological responsiveness of man to penicillin. *J.A.M.A.,* 186:1151, 1963.
89. Freedman, S. O., Krupey, J., and Sehon, A. H. Chlorogenic acid: An allergen in coffee bean. *Nature* (London) 192:241, 1961.
90. Arbesman, C. E., Kantor, S. Z., Rose, N. R., and Witebsky, E. Serum sickness. *J. Allerg.* 31:257, 1960.
91. Gunther, M., Aschaffenburg, R., Matthews, R. H., Parish, W. E., and Coombs, R. R. A. The level of antibodies to the proteins of cow's milk in the serum of normal human infants. *Immunology* 3:296, 1960.
92. Borduas, A. G., and Grabar, P. L'hémagglutination passive dans la récherche des anticorps antiprotéiques. *Ann. Inst. Pasteur* (Paris) 84:903, 1953.
93. Frick, O. L. Hemagglutination in sera from egg-sensitive individuals. *Ann. Allerg.* 20:794, 1962.
94. Hensel, M. E., and Sheldon, J. M. Complement fixation with specific allergens in hay fever: I. Problem, procedure, diagnostic value. *J. Lab. Clin. Med.* 26:1586, 1941.
95. Cavelti, P. A. Complement fixation studies in allergy. *J. Allerg.* 21:532, 1950.
96. Portnoy, J., and Sherman, W. B. Complement fixation studies in ragweed allergy. *J. Allerg.* 25:229, 1954.
97. Vallery-Radot, L. P., and Hugo, A. Essai de transfert au lapin de l'hypersensibilité pollinique de l'homme. *C. R. Soc. Biol.* (Paris) 101:893, 1929.
98. Adelsberger, L. Anaphylaxie und Atopie: III. Anaphylaxieversuche mit Atopenen. *Z. Hyg. Infektionskr.* 111:577, 1930.
99. Noah, J. W., and Brand, A. Release of histamine in the blood of ragweed-sensitive individuals. *J. Allerg.* 25:210, 1954.
100. (*a*) VanArsdel, P. P., Middleton, E., Sherman, W. B., and Buchwald, H. A quantitative study on the in vitro release of histamine from leukocytes of atopic persons. *J. Allerg.* 29:429, 1958. (*b*) VanArsdel, P. P., and Sells, C. J. Antigenic histamine release from passively sensitized human leukocytes. *Science* 141:1190, 1963.
101. Spain, W. C., Strauss, M. B., and Newman, E. *In vitro* release of histamine by hypersensitive (allergic) serum in contrast to immune (treated) allergic serum in antigen and normal rabbit blood mixtures. *J. Allerg.* 21:318, 1950.
102. Walzer, M., Bowman, K. L., and Stroyman, S. Leukocytic transfer of the immediate types of allergic reaction in man: I. Techniques for the local passive transfer of atopic hypersensitiveness through the use of leukocytes and their derivatives. *J. Allerg.* 28:206, 1957.
103. Pettit, H., Sullivan, H. E., and Hart, E. D. *In vitro* leukocytolysis in presence of pollen and house dust antigens. *J. Allerg.* 32:30, 1961.
104. Audia, M., and Noah, J. Supravital staining of leukocytes from ragweed-sensitive individuals. *Ibid.,* p. 223.
105. Black, A. P. A new diagnostic method in allergic disease. *Pediatrics* 17:716, 1956.
106. Franklin, W., and Lowell, F. C. Failure of ragweed pollen extract to destroy white cells from ragweed-sensitive patients. *J. Allerg.* 20:375, 1949.
107. Chambers, V. V., Hudson, B. H., and Glaser, J. A study of the reactions of human polymorphonuclear leukocytes to various allergens. *J. Allerg.* 29:93, 1958.
108. Shelley, W. B. New serological test for allergy in man. *Nature* (London) 195:1181, 1962.
109. Cruickshank, C. N. D., *et al.* Cited by Stanworth, D. R. Reagins. *Brit. Med. Bull.* 19: 235, 1963
110. Hoigné, R., and Storck, H. Ueber die Bedeutung der Thrombocyten bei allergischen Vorgängen. *Schweiz. Med. Wschr.* 83: 718, 1953.
111. Hoigné, R., Leoliger, A., Morandi, L., and Flückiger, P. Thrombocytopenische Purpura bei drei Fällen von medikamentöser Allergie. *Bull. Schweiz. Akad. Med. Wiss.* 10:438, 1954.
112. Hoigné, R., Grossmann, W., and Storck, H. New serological method for demonstrating sensitivity to allergens. *Int. Arch. Allerg.* 8:103, 1956.

113. Kleine, N., Matthes, M., and Müller, W. Untersuchungen über die Trübungsreaktion nach Hoigné zum Nachweis einer Allergensensibilisierung. *Klin. Wschr.* 35:132, 1957.
114. Cooke, R. A., Loveless, M. H., and Stull, A. Studies on immunity in a type of human allergy (hay fever): Serological responses of nonsensitive individuals to pollen injections. *J. Exp. Med.* 66:689, 1937.
115. Loveless, M. H. Immunological studies of pollinosis: I. The presence of two antibodies related to the same pollen antigen in the serum of treated hay fever patients. *J. Immun.* 38:25, 1940.
116. Sehon, A. H., Hollinger, H. Z., Harter, J. G., Schweitzer, A. E., and Rose, B. Localization of blocking antibody in sera of ragweed-sensitive individuals by starch electrophoresis. *J. Allerg.* 28:229, 1957.
117. (*a*) Sherman, W. B. Changes in serological reactions and tissue sensitivity in hay fever patients during the early months of treatment, *J. Immun.* 40:289, 1941. (*b*) Sherman, W. B. Reaginic and blocking antibodies, *J. Allerg.* 28:62, 1957.
118. Alexander, H. L., Johnson, A. B., and Bukantz, S. C. Studies on correlation between symptoms of ragweed hay fever and titer of thermostable antibody. *J. Allerg.* 19:1, 1948.
119. Loveless, M. H. Humoral antibody and tissue tolerance induced in pollen sensitive individuals by specific therapy. *Southern Med. J.* 33:869, 1940; Immunological studies of pollinosis: IV. The relationship between thermostable antibody in the circulation and clinical immunity, *J. Immun.* 47:165, 1943.
120. Delorme, P. J., Richter, M., Grant, S., Blumer, H., Leznoff, A., and Rose, B. Immunologic studies of ragweed-sensitive patients treated by a single repository antigen injection. *J. Allerg.* 32:409, 1961.
121. Arbesman, C. E., and Reisman, R. E. Repository Pollen Therapy: Clinical and Immunologic Studies. Ref. 77, p. 187.
122. Friedman, H., and Criep, L. H. Effect of repository therapy on immunologic responses to pollen extract. *J. Allerg.* 33:215, 1962.
123. Feinberg, S. M., and Feinberg, A. R. Desensitization Therapy with Emulsified Extracts: Its Present Status. Ref. 77, p. 161.
124. Connell, J. T., and Sherman, W. B. The effects of treatment with the emulsions of ragweed extract on antibody titers. *J. Immun.* 91:197, 1963.
125. Bernton, H. S., Chambers, D. C., and Querry, M. V. Therapy of ragweed pollenosis with blocking antibody. *J. Allerg.* 33:356, 1962.
126. Sherman, W. B. Skin-Sensitizing and Blocking Antibodies. Ref. 45, p. 155.
127. Perelmutter, L., Lea, D. J., Freedman, S. O., and Sehon, A. H. Determination of rabbit and human anti-ragweed antibodies by the precipitin method. *Int. Arch. Allerg.* 21:1, 1962.
128. Nisonoff, A., Wissler, F. C., Lipman, L. N., and Woernley, D. L. Separation of univalent fragments from the bivalent rabbit antibody molecule by reduction of disulfide bonds. *Arch. Biochem.* 89:230, 1960.
129. Porter, R. R. Separation and isolation of fractions of rabbit gamma-globulin containing the antibody and antigen combining sites. *Nature* (London) 182:670, 1958.
130. Loveless, M. H., and Cann, J. R. Distribution of "blocking" antibody in human serum proteins fractionated by electrophoresis-convection, *J. Immun.* 74:329, 1955.
131. Webb, T., and Lapresle, C. Study of the adsorption on and desorption from polystyrene-human serum albumin conjugates of rabbit anti-human serum albumin antibodies having different specificities. *J. Exp. Med.* 114:43, 1961.
132. Perelmutter, L., Lea, D. J., Freedman, S. O., and Sehon, A. H. Demonstration of precipitating antibodies in sera of ragweed-allergic individuals by the agar gel technique, *Int. Arch. Allerg.* 20:355, 1962.
133. Lea, D. J., and Sehon, A. H. The chemical characterization of nondialyzable constituents of ragweed pollen. *Ibid.,* p. 203.
134. Spitzer, R. H., and Kaplan, M. A. Precipitating antibodies of human antisera elicited by a purified dwarf ragweed fraction. *J. Allerg.* 34:295, 1963.
135. Fisher, J. P., and Connell, J. T. Passive cutaneous anaphylaxis in the guinea pig with serum of allergic patients treated with ragweed extract emulsions. *J. Allerg.* 33:59, 1962.

SECTION II. DIAGNOSTIC PROCEDURES AND FACTORS WHICH COMPLICATE DIAGNOSIS

42. Skin Tests

RAY F. BEERS, JR.

SKIN TESTS FOR IMMEDIATE REACTIVITY

Skin tests that induce an immediate wheal can be performed by a variety of techniques, i.e., scratch and its variants (scarification, prick, multiple puncture), intradermal, and iontophoresis, all of which by-pass the keratin layer so that the antigen can combine with antibody in the deeper skin layers and produce a controlled, visible, allergic reaction in miniature without danger to the patient. Since scratch tests are safer and not so readily influenced by primary irritation, they are commonly performed first, intradermal testing being reserved for materials that fail to cause a reaction to the scratch test. With certain materials that cause a particularly violent reaction, the scratch test is often the only method employed.

SKIN TESTING FOR ATOPY

This procedure is frequently helpful in the diagnosis of seasonal and perennial rhinitis and asthma, often useful in the diagnosis of infantile eczema and acute urticaria, and rarely of much value in the elucidation of adult eczema and chronic urticaria. The wide variety of materials available for testing purposes makes two approaches possible: (1) the mass or barrage approach, which involves the use of batteries of tests with numerous substances, the clinical significance of the materials causing positive reactions being established later, and (2) the selected approach, based on the clinical leads supplied by the primary clinical tool, a painstaking history. In agreement with Alexander [5], we prefer the latter approach, since skin reactivity, even if undoubtedly immunological, does not, without ancillary information, allow the conclusion that the substance giving rise to the reaction has any bearing on the patient's complaints. The demonstration of immediate skin reactivity to an allergen identifies the patient as atopic, an important initial step in diagnosis. Most, but not all, atopic individuals will show one or more skin reactions to the following materials: the locally prevalent tree, grass, and weed pollens; molds of the genera *Alternaria, Hormodendrum, Aspergillus,* and *Penicillium* (species is unimportant); house dust, and cat, dog, and horse danders. These materials therefore comprise a perfectly adequate list of "routine materials," to which additions can be made as indicated by the history; i.e., cereal grains, milk, and eggs should be added for bakers, since these materials are often inhaled; granary workers, farmers, and flour-mill workers require the addition of cereal grains and smuts; tomato handlers should be tested with *Cladosporium* (a mold which grows exclusively on tomatoes), and so on.

TEST MATERIALS

The ideal material for skin tests would be a solution of a chemically identified allergen dissolved in sufficient water or saline to be completely devoid of irritant properties when introduced into normal tissue. Unfortunately, this ideal state does not exist; most of the testing extracts in common use represent approximate concentrations of unknown substances, including, in addition to allergens, substances which might be irritating to normal tissue. Since not a single allergen has been isolated and completely identified, real standardization of test materials is, at the moment, impossible. On the other hand, some rough measure of potential activity is necessary. Several methods of standardization have been devised: weight by volume, total nitrogen concentration, and protein nitrogen concentration. Units based on these methods, i.e., pollen units, Noon units, total nitrogen units, and protein nitrogen units, are roughly interchangeable. Since there is no clear advantage to any one method over another, the use of the most familiar method is advisable.

Pollen Extracts. These are potent and usually free from irritants, so positive skin reactions to the usual testing strengths are almost always specific and usually of clinical significance. Negative reactions usually signify lack of clinical sensitivity, although exceptions may be noted, especially in young children, who may show a lag of several years between clinical sensitivity and the development of positive skin reactions.

Mold Spore Extracts. These are not as free from irritants as extracts of pollens, but they are potent, and the irritants can be rendered innocuous by dilution. Positive skin reactions to the usual testing strengths are usually immunological and often clinically significant. This is not true of skin reactions which are demonstrable intradermally only with high concentrations (1 : 400).

House Dust Extracts. These vary widely in potency and freedom from irritation; it is therefore always difficult to evaluate critically the implications of a positive reaction to a given material. In general, positive reactions elicited by scratch may be significant; by the intradermal route, positive reactions are, more often than is generally realized, of doubtful significance.

Dander Extracts. Such extracts are generally potent and reasonably free from irritation. Positive skin reactions are usually of immunological and often of clinical significance. Goat, cattle, and hog danders are the exceptions, providing relatively weak extracts with a high irritation potential. Positive skin reactions to these materials are therefore not nearly so reliable as those to other danders.

Extracts of Miscellaneous Inhalants (Feathers, Wool, Kapok, Silk, Insects). All are, on the whole, weak (excepting insects) and irritating. The significance of positive skin reactions is therefore usually dubious.

Egg White, Nuts, Seeds, Fish, Shellfish Extracts. These are the most potent testing extracts known. They are potentially dangerous, since deaths have occurred after their use, and severe systemic reactions have appeared with scratch tests. Irritation is no problem, because most physicians, for safety, confine the test to the scratch method. Positive reactions are almost universally immunological and usually of clinical significance.

Extracts of All Other Foods. These are highly variable, often weak, quite irritating in high concentrations, and therefore useless for intradermal testing. Positive reactions obtained by scratch test, which tends to obviate the irritation potential, may be immunological but often have no clinical significance except in the child of 3 or under.

INDIRECT TESTING

In 1919, Ramirez [2] transfused the blood of a patient with horse dander asthma into a nonallergic recipient, who promptly had an asthmatic attack on the way home from the hospital in a horse-drawn carriage. In 1921, this transfer factor was successfully passed to the skin of nonatopic recipients by Prausnitz and Küstner [3], using Küstner's serum, which was fish-sensitive. When antigen was injected into the recipient at the serum-transfer site, a typical wheal and erythema reaction appeared. The transfer factor was named reagin by Coca [4]. Transferability and skin fixation were rapidly confirmed by DeBesche [2], Coca and Grove [4], and others. As a clinical method, it was brought to its greatest refinement by Walzer [6], who also demonstrated the ability of the antibody to fix in a wide variety of tissues, e.g., nasal, ophthalmic [7], and rectal mucosa, and gallbladder [8]. The passive transfer (or P-K) test has had a profound effect on the development of theoretical allergy. Its diagnostic usefulness is limited because the technique requires potent sera free from syphilis, hepatitis virus, and bacterial contamination and a nonallergic recipient (preferably not related to the patient) whose skin will accept reagin [4]. Furthermore, after all these rather difficult requirements are met, a positive response to the P-K test proves only that the reaction is immunological but not, any more than with a direct test, that the tested allergen has any bearing on the patient's symptoms.

Reagins have also been demonstrated to nonatopic antigens, e.g., worm polysaccharides [9], animal sera [10], liver extracts [11], pancreatic extracts [12, 13], and penicillin [14].

ANAPHYLACTIC AND ARTHUS REACTIVITY

These may be associated with two types of antibodies, reagins and anaphylactic antibody. Direct and indirect tests, including passive cutaneous anaphylaxis (PCA), may be useful, at times, to predict the development of serum sickness. Methods for detecting skin-sensitizing antibodies have already been described. To induce PCA, the sensitizing dose is given intradermally in the skin of the recipient animal and the eliciting dose intravenously with 2.5 mg. of Evans blue in the solution of antigen. Maximal localization of the dye at the sensitization site occurs within fifteen minutes. The reaction is not species-specific and can be induced by use of the serum of one species and the skin of several others, but in the case of human serum, only the guinea pig and monkey will accept sensitization [15]. The method has been used to demonstrate human antibody to horse serum and diphtheria toxin [16]. Layton and Yamaraka's demonstration [17] of PCA-like reactions in monkeys to a variety of allergens confirms the potential usefulness of the method which, so far, is still experimental.

Skin-sensitizing antibody is demonstrable regularly in serum reactions, usually in stinging-insect reactions, in a significant number of pencillin reactions, occasionally with other biologicals, and in association with some living disease agents.

NONPRIMARY SERUM REACTIONS

About 70 percent of human beings given heterologous serum (horse, rabbit) develop demonstrable skin-sensitizing antibody [18]. Skin tests with dilutions of the respective sera are therefore of considerable value in predicting the nonprimary reactions. A history of previous exposure to serum or the presence of the atopic trait makes such testing mandatory before serum is given. Deaths occur more frequently in the atopic individual spontaneously sensitive to horse dander after a first injection of horse serum than in normal individuals after secondary injections because of immunological cross-reactivity between horse serum and dander [19].

STINGING-INSECT REACTIONS

Stinging-insect reactions usually, but not always, occur in the presence of skin-sensitizing antibody. Direct skin tests with the venom or whole body extract, which contains venom antigen, are usually performed with the common stinging insects, i.e., bee, wasp, hornet, and yellow jacket, since a patient's description of the offending insect is often unreliable and there is cross-reactivity between the various antigens. Such extracts are fairly irritating but so potent that this is a minor problem. Systemic reactions have been recorded on scratch to dilutions of whole body extract as high as 1 : 100,000 [20]. Although this is unusual, the test materials must be treated with respect. The skin reactions usually correlate roughly with the clinical history, but negative skin reactions in the presence of full-blown anaphylaxis do occur.

PENICILLIN REACTIONS

Since penicillin is by far the most frequent cause of serum sickness-type reactions, it is unfortunate that the presence of skin-sensitizing antibody is so variable. The reasons for this variability and a possible approach to effective skin tests for the screening of penicillin-sensitive patients are discussed in detail in Chapter 59.

SKIN TESTS BASED ON ALLERGY OF INFECTION

Allergy of infection accounts for a large variety of skin test procedures. Those performed with tuberculin, histoplasmin, blastomycin, and coccidioidin are the most widely used and will be discussed first.

Tuberculin Tests. These are usually performed with Koch's old tuberculin [21] or Seibert's trichloroacetic acid-precipitated purified protein derivative [22] prepared from human strains of *Mycobacterium tuberculosis.* They are elaborated on in Chapter 30.

Histoplasmin Test. The intradermal route is used exclusively for this test. The skin test material commonly employed is an extract of the growth of the mycelial phase of *Histoplasma capsulatum* at room temperature for four to five months. For a full discussion, see Chapter 32.

Blastomycin Test. Blastomycin is prepared from the broth filtrate of the mycelial phase of *Blastomyces dermatitidis.* It is performed and read in the same way as the tuberculin test; i.e., induration greater than

10 mm. is considered specific. The reaction is not specific for infection with *B. dermatitidis,* since cross-reactions occur with other molds, e.g., *H. capsulatum, Haplosporangium parvum* [23], and *Blastomyces brasiliensis* [24]. A yeast phase antigen which is a polysaccharide rather than protein has been prepared which causes typical delayed reactions of the tuberculin type. Although of great theoretical interest, the polysaccharide antigen does not seem more specific than crude blastomycin.

Coccidioidin Test. Coccidioidin is prepared from the broth filtrate of the mycelial phase of ten strains of *Coccidioides immitis* grown on an asparagin medium and standardized in normal and hypersensitive individuals [25]. For a description of skin tests with coccidioidin, see Chapter 31.

SKIN TESTS IN BACTERIAL DISEASES

Brucellin Test. This test is performed intradermally with brucellin, the active principle obtained from a broth filtrate of *Brucella melitensis.* Broad variations in results that have been reported are due to differences in antigen and techniques. Positive reactions bear no relation to the activity of infection and may stimulate the formation of agglutinins, interfering with subsequent serological diagnosis. Consequently its diagnostic use has been discouraged [26]. The same considerations hold for brucellergen, the antigen obtained from the ground whole body extracts and heat-killed vaccines (see Chapter 33).

Chancroid. Since the time of Ito and Reenstierna [27], attempts have been made with various antigens to produce a worthwhile skin test for the diagnosis of chancroid. None has been successful.

Mallein Test. Mallein is prepared for and primarily used in ungulates affected by glanders. The test is performed with an active principle obtained from a peptone-broth culture of *Actinobacillus (Malleomyces, Pfeifferella) mallei.* Although little used in man, it has wide usage in veterinary medicine, where it is considered relatively specific. The few recorded cases in man indicate its potential usefulness [28].

Schick Test. Skin tests are of no value in the diagnosis of diphtheria, but the intradermal injection of active diphtheria toxin, the Schick test, discloses immunity or susceptibility to the disease. Culture filtrate, 0.10 ml., containing 1/50 MLD of toxin is injected, and reactions are read at 24 and 48 hours and seven days. Heat-inactivated culture filtrate serves as a control, since several reactions other than that due to toxin are commonly observed.

1. The *positive reaction* begins in 24 to 36 hours, is maximal at 96 hours, and persists for one week. It may be followed by brown pigmentation that persists for several weeks. There is no reaction at the control site. It is a manifestation of the pure destructive effect of diphtheria toxin on tissue and indicates susceptibility to the disease.

2. The *negative reaction* is characterized by absence of any response at either the test or the control site. It indicates the presence of sufficient antitoxin antibody to prevent disease, i.e., nonsusceptibility.

3. In the *pseudoreaction* there is immediate or delayed allergic reactivity at both test sites. The reactions subside in 72 hours or even sooner, and no further reaction occurs at either site. It indicates antitoxic immunity plus allergic reactivity to other constituents of the culture filtrate.

4. The *combined reaction* is characterized by the appearance of immediate or delayed allergic responses at both control and test sites. The reaction at the control site subsides in 72 hours or less, but at the test site it continues for 7 days, producing a typical toxic reaction. It probably indicates susceptibility to antitoxin plus allergic reactivity to nontoxic components of *Corynebacterium diphtheriae.* It is most often seen in adults and is thought to be due to previous exposure. Individuals who have a combined reaction are probably less susceptible to infection than individuals with positive reactions. Attempts to establish further immunity in these hypersensitive individuals can give rise to systemic reactions, including urticaria and asthma.

Test for Gonorrhea. The various skin test antigens developed for the diagnosis of gonorrhea have proved to be of little value and have been abandoned.

Test for Granuloma Inguinale. Skin test materials have been prepared from human tissue and from chick embryos infected with *Donovania granulomatis* have not proved to have any real value, so are not obtainable today.

Lepromin Test. Mitsuda's lepromin test, introduced in 1924, utilized boiled ground-up lepromatous nodules as the test material [29]. Since then, lepromins have been separated from the skin by Fernandez and Castro [30] and Dharmendra [31], the latter using chloroform and ether extract. Skin reactions are of two types: (1) a typical tuberculin-type delayed reaction coming on in 24 to 28 hours (Fernandez reaction), and (2) a long-delayed, granuloma-type reaction coming on in 3 to 4 weeks (Mitsuda reaction). Mitsuda's (integral) lepromin gives rise to more Mitsuda reactions than Fernandez reactions. With Fernandez and Dharmendra lepromins, the situation is reversed. Neither reaction is especially useful in the diagnosis of leprosy, but it is helpful in typing and prognosis. Both types of positive reactions are obtained in patients with tuberculoid leprosy, and, in general, the stronger the reaction the better the prognosis. Patients with lepromatous leprosy do not give either type of skin reaction.

Test for Pertussis. Various antigens have been utilized in an effort to diagnose and predict immunity or susceptibility to *Bordetella pertussis.* They include whole body vaccine (Sauer) [32], sonically disrupted vaccine (agglutinogen-Flosdorf) [33], and thermostable and the thermolabile toxins [34]. None has proved to be entirely satisfactory. In addition, a single test dose of agglutinogen causes a rise in the agglutinin titer of the "immune" individual and promptly converts a negative skin reactor to a positive one.

Tests for Pneumococcal Infection. Of the numerous antigens prepared from pneumococci for skin test purposes, none has any diagnostic importance, but the polysaccharide antigen is of interest because it was the first nonprotein shown to be antigenic [35]. The skin reaction is of the immediate wheal and erythema type. For a while it was thought that immediate reactivity was characteristic of polysaccharide antigens, but this has been shown to be false. As noted earlier, the delayed reactions to some of the molds are caused by polysaccharide antigen. Skin reactions to pneumococcal polysaccharide appear at about the time of crisis in pneumonia. Failure of development of the response, which is type-specific, suggests a poor prognosis [36]. Unfortunately, skin tests themselves with pneumococcal polysaccharides will induce formation of antibodies in noninfected individuals [37]. This severely limits the utility of the Francis test.

Dick Test. The introduction of 0.10 ml. of a 1 : 1,000 dilution of culture filtrate of beta-hemolytic streptococci produces, in susceptible individuals, an erythema greater than 10 mm. in diameter in about 24 hours [38]. The reaction fades rapidly and may be gone in 3 days. Unfortunately, the Dick test response has meaning only for the particular toxin being used, and a wide variety of erythrogenic toxins is produced by different strains of beta-hemolytic streptococci [39]. The test cannot predict susceptibility to infection and is unreliable in determining liability to toxin action. Its use, therefore, has largely been abandoned.

The injection of 0.50 ml. of scarlet fever convalescent serum or 0.10 ml. of erythrogenic antitoxin blanches the erythema of scarlet fever within six to eight hours. This reaction (Schultz-Carlton) [40] has limited usefulness, but occasionally has served to differentiate scarlet fever erythema from that due to German measles or drug eruptions.

Tests for Syphilis. Various skin test materials have been prepared for the diagnosis of syphilis. The best known is probably Noguchi's luetin [41], prepared from culture-grown *Treponema pallidum.* None of the materials proved to be of value. On the other hand, Pearson *et al.* [42] reported recently that a treponemin extracted from virulent Nicholas strain *T. pallidum* rabbit testicular syphilomas converted negative serological reactions (TPI and TPCF) to positive in syphilis-suspect patients. They feel that this is an anamnestic reaction that does not occur in nonsyphilitic individuals. The serological conversion is associated with a positive skin reaction of the delayed type which they believe has definite specificity. The reaction may be of value in differentiating the biological false positive reactor from the individual who has latent syphilis. Its usefulness remains to be established, but the method does not seem to have been taken up with any great degree of enthusiasm.

Test for Tularemia. Three types of skin tests have been described by Foshay. All are specific and diagnostically important because a reaction to them antedates considerably the development of a positive result of the agglutination test. The tests use a polysaccharide antigen [43], a protein antigen [44], and goat anti-*Pasteurella tularensis* antibody [45], respectively. The soluble polysaccharide antigen gives rise to typical wheal and erythema reactivity that appears in the second week of infection.

Antibody against *P. tularensis* is developed in goats until high titers of agglutinating antibodies are demonstrable. This serum is injected intradermally in 0.04 ml. amounts, with normal goat serum as a control. Since, in the diseased patient, antigen is already circulating, this amounts to a form of PCA. An immediate whealing reaction develops in the antibody-containing serum site but not in the control site. Since antigen is probably circulating in significant amounts shortly after invasion of the patient by *P. tularensis,* positive reactions develop very quickly, often within 5 days. Since the test requires circulating antigen, the reaction disappears shortly after remission of the disease. The protein antigen causes a tuberculin-type delayed reactivity, is highly specific, and induces a positive response within 7 to 10 days after infection. Once developed, the reaction persists for long periods, probably for life, so this preparation cannot be used to differentiate active from past disease. This is not much of a problem because repeated episodes of tularemia are quite uncommon.

The usual hospital laboratory makes no attempt to isolate *P. tularensis,* since the procedure is difficult and dangerous for laboratory personnel. The agglutination test is highly specific, but diagnostically positive titers are slow to develop, rarely appearing before the third to fifth week of the illness. It is therefore surprising that these excellent skin tests are rather uncommonly used.

Tests for Typhoid Fever. Many antigens have, in the past, been prepared for skin test purposes, but none has proved to be of any practical value, and their use has been abandoned.

SKIN TESTS FOR VIRAL AND RICKETTSIAL DISEASES

The skin tests applicable to the diagnosis of viral disease have been covered in Chapter 36.

Skin tests have not been of value in the study of rickettsial diseases.

SKIN TESTS IN FUNGUS DISEASES

The skin test methods for the three major fungus diseases have already been considered, but a few more need to be covered here.

Actinomycosis. Skin tests are of no value in the study of this disease. Much of the early work was done with aerobes or questionable anaerobes of no etiological importance, and more recent work has shown that normal individuals reacted more than patients with the disease [46].

Aspergillosis; Candidiasis. Skin tests used in these diseases are described in Chapter 34.

Cryptococcosis. Until recently, skin tests have been useless in the study of this disease, but the picture may change. Salvin and Smith [47] reported the isolation from living fungus cells, subjected to high pressure and subsequently extracted with glycine, of an antigen which, in infected guinea pigs, gives rise to typical delayed skin reactions. Epidemiological studies with this material are planned.

Chromoblastomycosis. A delayed skin reactive principle is extractable from the mycelial phase of *Hormodendrum pedrosoi.* The positive reaction indicates hypersensitivity, but it has been so little investigated as to be meaningless at the present time.

Nocardiosis. One instance of skin hypersensitivity among many tests has been recorded [48]. This single observation, although important, does not provide clinically useful information.

Sporotrichosis. Suspensions of killed *Sporotrichum schenckii* and culture filtrates provide skin test material which produces typical delayed reactions in man. The reactions are believed to be more specific than the serological tests that have been used in the study of this disease and are therefore potentially useful [49]. Like most delayed reactions, this one persists for at least two years and probably longer. It cannot be used, therefore, to differentiate past from active infection.

Dermatomycoses. The superficial cutaneous mycoses may be caused by organisms of at least three genera, i.e., *Trichophyton, Microsporum,* and *Epidermophyton.* The broth filtrates of all provide skin test-active materials (trichophytins) that seem to have a strong common denominator; therefore trichophytin derived from any one of the species will induce positive skin reactions in patients infected with any of the genera [50]. The organisms are so ubiquitous, infection probably being universal, that positive reactions are of little diagnostic use. Negative responses, on the other hand, may be useful in demonstrating the delayed reaction anergy of Hodgkin's disease. Wheal and erythema reactivity occasionally develops to trichophytin and may sometimes cause clinical symptoms, i.e., urticaria [51].

SKIN TESTS IN PARASITIC DISEASES

Amebiasis. Although positive delayed skin reactions have been demonstrated with saline extracts of *Entamoeba histolytica* in patients with extraintestinal disease, tests have never been used in a serious way clinically.

Trypanosomiasis. Skin tests are not available for the study of African sleeping sickness, but skin tests have been used in the study of Chagas' disease. Washed cultures of *Trypanosoma cruzi* apparently give rise to typical delayed skin reactions in infected human beings and rabbits [52], but little real information is available.

Leishmaniasis. Saline-merthiolate suspensions of the whole organisms of *Leishmania brasiliensis* or *L. tropica* and a polysaccharide antigen isolated from cultured *L. brasiliensis* provide highly specific skin test material of the delayed type that is very useful in the diagnosis of cutaneous and mucocutaneous leishmaniasis [53]. The Montenegro test [54] (with killed whole organisms) has been widely utilized in Brazil. Skin test materials are not available for the study of visceral leishmaniasis (kala-azar).

Trichomoniasis. Intradermal tests have been used in veterinary medicine in the study of *Trichomonas foetus* infections, but such tests have seen little or no use in man.

Toxoplasmosis. Frenkel [55] described skin reactions to toxoplasmins in 1948 and noted that the reaction may not become positive until months after infection has taken place. The specificity of the test is still being investigated, but all indications seem to point to reasonable accuracy. A commercial preparation is available for investigational purposes.

Trichinosis. Since its introduction by Bachman [56] in 1928, the *Trichinella* skin test has been widely used in man and hogs. Test material is made of extracts of dried ground trichinae. Typical immediate wheal reactions are considered to indicate a positive response. Delayed reactions also occur occasionally, but their significance is unknown. Due to widespread exposure to *Trichinella* and immunological cross-reactions with *Ascaris* and *Trichuris trichiuria* as well as, probably, unknown helminths, the test is of little value in either hogs or man. With first infections, conversion from negative to positive reactions can at times be demonstrated, but it is slow in developing. In a recently reported case, it is of interest that trichinosis was diagnosed, treated, and reported cured before a positive skin reaction appeared [57].

Filariasis. There are common antigens shared by all six species of filarial worms known to infect man as well as by a variety of heterologous filarids and other nematodes, particularly hookworms and ascarids. It is difficult to obtain human filarids, therefore the dog heartworm *Dirofilaria immitis* is used to prepare skin test material [58]. The normal saline extract has proved useful in assessing exposure to infection but is of no value in judging the activity of the disease. In highly sensitized patients, 0.01 ml. of the 1 : 10,000 dilution may induce an episode of filarial fever.

Ascariasis. A polysaccharide is extractable from adult ascarids or their intestinal tissues that gives rise to immediate wheal and erythema reactivity in the skin of sensitized animals and human beings. Unfortunately there is very little correlation between positive skin reactions and the presence of active infection.

Skin tests with ascarid antigens can be of some help in the differential diagnosis of visceral larva migrans. This disease of children is caused by migration of the dog ascarid *Toxocara canis.* Infected children will show positive skin reactions not only to extracts of *T. canis* but to *Ascaris lumbricoides* and *A. suum* [59]. Positive reactions to any of the test materials therefore reveal sensitization to ascarids, but the species cannot be determined by skin tests.

Hydatid Disease (Echinococcosis). The intradermal injection of 0.05 to 0.10 ml. of sterile undiluted cyst fluid obtained from human beings or lower animals (sheep, cow, rabbit), the Casoni test [60], gives rise to both immediate and delayed allergic reactivity in infected human patients. Both the immediate wheal and the delayed papule are considered strong evidence of active disease, even though the reactions can be demonstrated for some time after surgical removal of the cyst.

Schistosomiasis. Skin test materials extracted from adult schistosomes, cercariae, and eggs have found some use in epidemiological studies, but no significant differences between the various antigen sources have been noted [61]. The test is of no value in diagnosis.

SKIN TESTS IN GRANULOMATOUS DISEASES

Boeck's Sarcoid. In the differential diagnosis of granulomatous disease, a positive Kveim reaction supports the diagnosis of sarcoidosis [62]. The test material consists of a particulate suspension from the lymph nodes or spleen of a patient with sarcoidosis after passage through a bacterial filter. For technical details and interpretation of the Kveim test, see Chapter 28.

Zirconium and Beryllium. The lesions caused by these chemicals are granulomatous, and the introduction of minute amounts of very dilute solutions will, in susceptible individuals, provoke the appearance of a slowly developing epithelioid granuloma. Although not widely studied, the reactions seem specific.

ALLERGIC CONTACT DERMATITIS

The diagnostic problems of contact dermatitis and the use of the patch test are discussed in Chapter 57.

REFERENCES

1. Alexander, H. L. Overemphasis on skin tests in allergy. *Tristate Med. J.* 1:85, 1929.
2. Ramirez, M. A. Horse asthma following blood transfusion. *J.A.M.A.* 73:984, 1919.
3. Prausnitz, C., and Küstner, H. Studien über die Ueberempfindlichkeit. *Zbl. Bakt.* [Orig.] 86:160, 1921.
4. Coca, A. F., and Grove, E. F. Studies in hypersensitiveness: Study of atopic reagins. *J. Immun.* 10:445, 1925.
5. DeBesche, A. Studies on the reactions of asthmatics and on passive transfer of hypersusceptibility. *Amer. J. Med. Sci.* 166:265, 1923.
6. Walzer, M. Indirect method for testing for conditions of atopic hypersensitiveness: Second preliminary report. *J. Allerg.* 1:231, 1930.
7. Walzer, M., Sherman, H., and Feldman, L. A. Studies in mucous membrane hypersensitiveness: I. Passive local sensitization of the ophthalmic mucous membrane. *J. Allerg.* 6:215, 1935.
8. Walzer, M., Gray, I., Henry, W., and Livingston, S. Studies in experimental hypersensitiveness in the rhesus monkey: IV. The allergic reaction in passively locally sensitized abdominal organs (preliminary report). *J. Immun.* 34:91, 1938.
9. Brunner, M. Immunological studies in human parasitic infection: I. Intradermal testing with parasitic extracts as an aid in the diagnosis of parasitic infestations. *J. Immun.* 15: 83, 1928.
10. Tuft, L., and Ramsdell, S. G. Antibody studies in serum sickness: I. With special reference to the Prausnitz-Küstner reaction. *J. Immun.* 16:411, 1929.
11. Feinberg, S. M., Alt, H. L., and Young, R. H. Allergy to injectable liver extracts: Clinical and immunological considerations. *Ann. Intern. Med.* 18:311, 1943.
12. Cohen, A. E., and Simon, F. Insulin hypersensitivity. *J. Allerg.* 9:503, 1938.
13. Lowell, F. C. Skin sensitizing antibody and allergy resistance to insulin. In Pappenheimer, A. M., Jr. (Ed.), *The Nature and Significance of the Antibody Response.* New York: Columbia University Press, 1953.
14. Siegel, B. B., and Coleman, M. Studies in penicillin hypersensitivity. *J. Allerg.* 28:264, 1957.
15. Ovary, Z. Immediate reactions in the skin of experimental animals provoked by antibody-antigen interaction. *Progr. Allerg.* 5:459, 1958.
16. Kuhns, W. J., and Pappenheimer, A. M., Jr. Immunochemic studies of antitoxin produced in normal and allergic individuals hyperimmunized with diphtheria toxoid: I. Relationship of skin sensitivity to purified diphtheria toxoid to the presence of circulating, non-precipitating antitoxin. *J. Exp. Med.* 95:363, 1952.
17. Layton, L. L., and Yamanaka, E. Demonstration of human reagins to foods, cat dander, an insect, and ragweed and grass pollens. *J. Allerg.* 33:271, 1962.
18. Longcope, W. T., O'Brien, D. R., and Perlzweig, W. A. The antigenic properties of ex-

tracts of horse dander: II. The isolation of two antigenic proteins from extracts of horse dander. *J. Immun.* 11:253, 1926.
19. Tuft, L. Further studies in serum allergy: VI. Antigenic relationship between horse dander and horse serum sensitivity. *J. Allerg.* 6:25, 1934.
20. Mueller, H. L. Serial intracutaneous testing for bee and wasp sensitivity. *J. Allerg.* 30:123, 1959.
21. Seibert, F. B., and Dufour, E. H. Comparison between the international standard tuberculins, PPD-S, and old tuberculin. *Amer. Rev. Tuberc.* 69:585, 1954.
22. Seibert, F. B., Aronson, J. D., Reichal, J., Clark, L. J., and Long, E. R. The isolation and properties of the purified protein derivative of tuberculin. *Amer. Rev. Tuberc.* 30 (supp.): 713, 1934.
23. Friedman, L., and Conant, N. F. Immunologic studies on the etiologic agents of North and South American blastomycosis: I. Comparison of hypersensitivity reactions. *Mycopathologia* 6:317, 1953.
24. Edwards, P. Q., Knight, R. A., and Marcus, S. Skin sensitivity of human beings to *Histoplasma capsulatum* and *Blastomyces dermatitidis* polysaccharide antigens. *Amer. Rev. Resp. Dis.* 83:528, 1961.
25. Smith, C. E., Whiting, E. G., Baker, E. E., Rosenberger, H. G., Beard, R. R., and Saito, M. T. The use of coccidioidin. *Amer. Rev. Tuberc.* 57:330, 1948.
26. Spink, W. W. The diagnosis of brucellosis. *Conn. Med. J.* 12:406, 1958.
27. Reenstierna, J. Ein Serum gegen weichen Schanker, insbesondere dessen Bubonen. *München. Med. Wschr.* 56:895, 1920.
28. Rowe, C., and Miller, W. R. Human glanders: report of six cases. *Ann. Intern. Med.* 26:93, 1947.
29. Mitsuda, K. In *Troisième Conférence Internationale de la Lèpre: Communications et Debits.* Paris: J. B. Baillière et fils, 1924.
30. Fernandez, J. M., and Castro, N. O. Standardization of lepromin. *Rev. Argent. Derm.* 25:435, 1941.
31. Dharmendra, L. J. The lepromin test: A review. *Leprosy Rev.* 19:92, 1947.
32. Sauer, L. W. Whooping cough: A study in immunization. *J.A.M.A.* 100:239, 1933.
33. Felton, H. M., and Flosdorf, E. W. The detection of susceptibility to whooping cough: I. Institutional experience with the pertussis agglutinogen as a skin test reagent. *J. Pediat.* 29:677, 1946.
34. Flosdorf, E. W., and Kimball, A. C. Separation of the phase I agglutinogen of *Hemophilus pertussis* from toxic components. *J. Immun.* 39:475, 1940.
35. Tillett, W. S., and Francis, T., Jr. Cutaneous reactions to the polysaccharide of pneumococci in lobar pneumonia. *J. Exp. Med.* 50:687, 1929.
36. Finland, M., and Sutliff, W. D. Specific cutaneous reactions and circulating antibodies in the course of lobar pneumonia. I. Cases receiving no serum therapy. *J. Exp. Med.* 54:637, 1931; II. Cases treated with antipneumococcic sera. *Ibid.*, p. 653.
37. Finland, M., and Dowling, H. F. Cutaneous reactions and antibody response to intracutaneous injections of pneumococcus polysaccharide. *J. Immun.* 29:285, 1935.
38. Dick, G. F., and Dick, G. H. Results with the skin test for susceptibility to scarlet fever, *J.A.M.A.* 84:1477, 1925.
39. Stock, A. H., and Vernly, E. Properties of the scarlet fever toxin of the N.Y. 5 strain. *J. Immun.* 69:373, 1952.
40. Schultz, W., and Carlton, W. Serologische Beobachtungen am Scharlachexanthem, *Z. Kinderheilk.* 17:328, 1918.
41. Noguchi, H. A cutaneous reaction in syphilis. *J. Exp. Med.* 14:557, 1911.
42. Pearson, R. W., Portnoy, J., Magnuson, H. J., and Wheeler, A. H. The combined use of treponemin skin testing and specific serological tests in the diagnosis of syphilis. *J. Invest. Derm.* 31:75, 1958.
43. Foshay, L. The nature of the bacterial specific intradermal reaction. *J. Infect. Dis.* 59:330, 1936.
44. Foshay, L. Tularemia: Accurate and early diagnosis by means of the intradermal reaction. *J. Infect. Dis.* 51:286, 1932.
45. Foshay, L. Intradermal antiserum tests: A bacterial specific response not dependent upon serum sensitization but confused with it. *J. Allerg.* 6:360, 1935.
46. Mathieson, D. R., Harrison, R., Hammond, C., and Henrici, A. T. Allergic reactions of the actinomycetes. *Amer. J. Hyg.* 21:405, 1935.
47. Salvin, S. B., and Smith, R. F. An antigen for the detection of hypersensitivity to *Cryptococcus neoformans. Proc. Soc. Exp. Biol. Med.* 108:498, 1961.
48. Glover, R. P., Herrell, W. E., Heilman, F. R., and Pfuetze, K. H. Nocardiosis: *Nocardia asteroides* infection simulating pulmonary tuberculosis. *J.A.M.A.* 136:172, 1948.
49. Norden, A. Sporotrichosis: Clinical and laboratory features and a serological study in animals and humans. *Acta Path. Microbiol. Scand.*, supp. 89, 1951.
50. Sulzberger, M. B., and Baer, R. L. *Office Immunology—Including Allergy.* Chicago: Year Book Publishers, Inc., 1947. P. 339.
51. Sulzberger, M. B., and Kerr, P. S. Trichophytin hypersensitiveness of urticarial type with

circulating antibodies and passive transference. *J. Allerg.* 2:11, 1930.

52. Mayer, M., and Pifano, F. O diagnostico da molestia de Chagas por intra-dermo-reaccao com cultura de *Schizotrypanum cruzi. Trop. Dis. Bull.* 38:640, 1941.
53. Pellegrino, J. Nota preliminar sobre a reacao intradermica feita com fracao polissacaridea isolada de formas de cultura de *Leishmania brasiliensis. Trop. Dis. Bull.* 50:696, 1953.
54. Montenegro, J. Cutaneous reaction in leishmaniasis. *Arch. Derm. Syph.* 13:187, 1926.
55. Frenkel, J. K. Dermal hypersensitivity to toxoplasma antigens. *Proc. Soc. Exp. Biol. Med.* 68:634, 1948.
56. Bachman, G. W. A precipitin test in experimental trichinosis. *J. Prev. Med.* 2:35, 1928.
57. Stone, O. J., Stone, C. T., Jr., and Mullins, J. F. Thiabendazole—probable cure for trichinosis. *J.A.M.A.* 187:536, 1964.
58. Bozicevich, J., and Hutter, A. Intradermal and serological tests with *Dirofilaria immitis* antigen in cases of human filariasis. *Amer. J. Trop. Med.* 24:203, 1944.
59. Soulsby, E. J. L. Diagnosis of Helminth Infections. In Gell, P. G. H., and Coombs, R. R. A. (Eds.), *Clinical Aspects of Immunology*. Philadelphia: F. A. Davis Company, 1963. P. 123.
60. Casoni, T. La diagnosi biologica dell echinococcosi umana mediante l'intradermoreazione. *Folia clin. chim. microscop.* 4:5, 1911.
61. Kagan, I. G., Pellegrino, J., and Memoria, J. M. P. Studies on the standardization of the intradermal test for the diagnosis of bilharziasis. *Amer. J. Trop. Med.* 10:200, 1961.
62. Kveim, A. En ny og spesifik-kutan reakjon ved Boechs sarcoid. *Nord. Med.* 9:169, 1941.

43. *Other Diagnostic Procedures*

KENNETH P. MATHEWS

MANY OR MOST ATOPIC PATIENTS are clinically sensitive to more than one agent, their degree of sensitization may fluctuate from time to time, the extent of exposure to individual allergens or combinations of clinically significant allergens varies markedly, cumulative effects may be important, and the influence of nonspecific agents may fluctuate widely. This formidable array of variables indicates why the determination of the specific cause(s) of clinical atopic diseases can present a taxing challenge to even the most expert in the field, although in many instances it is possible to ascertain the clinically important allergens with relative ease.

The available specific diagnostic tests for the causes of atopic diseases unfortunately are subject to error in performance or interpretation, and many are cumbersome for routine clinical use. Hence clinical evaluation, largely by an expertly taken history, remains the cornerstone of the study of the patient. In addition to its own diagnostic value, it is essential for the intelligent selection of appropriate diagnostic tests and provides a warning to take special precautions in testing patients with extreme degrees of sensitivity.

HISTORY TAKING

Procedures for history taking are described in standard texts on allergy. Although different techniques have been suggested, it seems likely that the skill of the interviewer is more important than the particular technical approach which he has adopted. The history has two objectives: (1) to determine whether the patient has, in fact, an atopic disease, and (2) to ascertain the factors which contribute to the development of symptoms in any individual patient.

Regardless of procedure, the following comments apply to allergy histories in general. (1) Adequate information cannot be obtained without the investment of a substantial amount of time. (2) It is as important to establish that a patient does not have an atopic disease as to determine that he does. (3) The history can mislead unless the information which has been obtained is precise; this refers particularly to the exact dates of seasonal symptoms. (4) Patients must be persuaded to report their own observations. Otherwise their statements tend to be biased by what they have been told by former physicians or by their knowledge of previous skin tests. (5) On the other hand, since atopic diseases commonly are chronic, useful additional information about previous diagnostic procedures and therapy often can be obtained. (6) Forms may be helpful (e.g., a checklist of the patient's environment and habits) but should be used as a supplement to and not as a substitute for the narrative description of the disease.

At the most, the history can provide almost diagnostic information, particularly if the patients are observant and the symptoms seasonal. At the least, the history can limit the range of etiological possibilities which require further studies. Strategically timed *follow-up visits* may be of major assistance, especially if the patient is encouraged to keep a record of time, place, and circumstances of his subsequent symptoms. Occasionally, when there has been little variation in the patient's environment, it is useful to *create history*. For instance, vacations from work or home or both may be instructive. Hospitalization of patients with severe illness of obscure cause in an air-filtered, "allergen-free" room with minimal medication might clarify the role of environmental factors. *Home visits* or inspection of the patient's work environment may be helpful if the history suggests an important but unidentified exposure at home or at work. Temporary removal or avoidance of suspected items might establish their clinical significance as allergens.

IN VIVO TESTS

PROVOCATIVE TESTS FOR INHALANT ALLERGY

Bronchial Tests. Although attempts are made occasionally to reproduce asthmatic attacks by observing patients as they are exposed to suspected inhalant allergens under natural conditions or in test rooms, ordinary bronchial tests attempt to induce controlled, subclinical asthma by the inhalation of aerosolized allergenic extracts. Although widely used for investigational purposes, bronchial tests have been applied clinically most extensively in Europe.

Several techniques have been employed in these tests. In most, the patient simply inhales aerosolized allergenic extracts delivered from a suitable nebulizer by compressed air or oxygen flowing at a rate of about 6 liters per minute. To conserve extract, a Y-tube generally is introduced into the circuit between the pressure source and the nebulizer. It is important that the nebulizer deliver aerosolized particles in the size range of 0.5 to 3 or 5 μ, since larger droplets do not penetrate down into the lower respiratory tract. When a high degree of sensitivity is suspected, testing is started with only a few inhalations of moderately concentrated extract or 1 ml. of suitably diluted extract. If there is no response, a larger number of inhalations or a more concentrated extract is tried. If, on the other hand, responses to intracutaneous tests with the extract are negative, it is generally safe to start by nebulizing the skin test strength of extract. If this evokes no response, tenfold more concentrated extract is used. Several investigators have found it necessary to nebulize 1 ml. of concentrated extracts to induce responses with or without positive skin test reactions; e.g., Colldahl [1] found that 56 percent of the provocative reactions observed by him required the use of a 1 : 10 dilution of allergenic extracts. If a strong response is elicited, the test is terminated (e.g., by aerosolized isoproterenol), and further testing is deferred until the following day. Control tests are performed with the extract diluent.

Open techniques allow for only a very rough estimate of the amount of allergen delivered to the patient. Better measurement is obtained with closed circuit systems [2], and Itkin *et al.* [3] have suggested the addition of phenol red to the allergen solution as a tracer which permits quantitation of the inspired aerosol. Pronounced responses can be recognized clinically, but subclinical changes, particularly with small amounts of allergen, can be discerned with ventilatory function tests. Lowell and Schiller [4] used the recorded timed vital capacity for this purpose, and this simple method is still popular. Other techniques have also been used [5–8]. Positive responses often occur within about 10 minutes after the allergen has been inhaled, and frequently spontaneous recovery is observed within 1 hour if excessive amounts of allergen are not given. However, delayed reactions can occur after 4 to 20 hours [2, 3, 9], particularly, in Herxheimer's experience, after aerosolization of house dust extracts. Juhlin-Dannfelt [10] reported that positive reactions to provocative tests could be induced a second time in 25 of 27 cases and three or more times in 12 of 13 instances. In some patients, repeated aerosol challenges produce changes in the threshold of reactivity.

With some exceptions, the usual outcome of provocative tests shows a close correlation with the clinical history (Table 43-1).

Reactions to these tests are more likely to be positive when the skin test reactions are pronounced than when they are weak, but it has been uniform experience that many allergens which elicit skin reactions fail to induce asthma or significant changes in pulmonary function in patients who have no clinical sensitivity to the test material. Usually bronchial reactions require extract concentrations about two orders of magnitude higher than those re-

TABLE 43-1. Correlation of Provocative Tests and History

Clinical History	Skin Tests	Provocative Inhalation Tests
+	+	+
−	+	−
−	−	−
+	−	− or +

quired for positive reactions to intracutaneous skin tests, but in occasional cases the reverse pattern has been observed [11]. Some investigators have failed to obtain positive responses to bronchial tests when the skin reactions were negative [4, 10], but others have reported that even in the absence of positive skin responses, bronchial reactions can occur if the clinical history is suggestive of allergy [1, 9, 12, 13]. However, positive responses in these circumstances may require rather prolonged nebulization of very concentrated extracts. Support for the specificity of some of these reactions is provided by Nilsson and Kaude's [13] observation that constitutional reactions could be evoked in four of six such patients by injecting relatively concentrated extracts intracutaneously even though the skin reactions remained negative.

The use of provocative bronchial tests is helpful because they actually reproduce the patient's symptoms and do not rely on a test response in a distant organ. Sufficient experience has accrued that these tests can be done with reasonable safety, and if minimal changes, which are not discernible by the patient, are measured, much of the subjective element is eliminated. Objectivity can also be enhanced by matching the color (if any) of the test solutions by adding inert material to the control solutions and masking the taste with peppermint water. Thus provocative bronchial tests are useful for investigational purposes, particularly in the evaluation of uncommon allergens or drugs for treating asthma. On the other hand, they are time-consuming, especially if several different allergens must be evaluated. Since most allergic individuals are evaluated as outpatients, this is particularly disadvantageous. In addition, the possibility of delayed reactions has discouraged the more extensive use of these tests in ambulatory patients in this country. Although most observers have advised that provocative bronchial tests be deferred until patients are free from asthma, Colldahl [9] reported satisfactory results in patients with some "rough breathing" at the time of the tests. Some other problems are obvious: the simpler tests require patient cooperation; cough interferes; accurate regulation of the allergen dosage is difficult; and, in our experience, results may be influenced by the time interval since the patients last had symptoms. It should be noted that reactions to prolonged inhalation of concentrated extracts in patients who do not react to the inhalation of diluent might not be specific but represent a bronchial response to an irritant. Finally, it must be recognized that there are differences between provocative inhalation tests and natural exposure to allergens. In nature, exposure is usually prolonged, and the allergens are particulate substances in the air rather than aqueous extracts. Indeed, there are major uncertainties regarding how substances as large as pollen grains induce asthma, since they would not be expected to reach the bronchioles. Consequently, it should not be surprising that there are occasional discrepancies between the clinical history and the results of provocative bronchial tests.

Nasal Tests. As in bronchial testing, the nasal response of allergic individuals can be observed by exposing them to suspected allergens under natural conditions or in test rooms [12], but generally the allergens are introduced directly into the nose by a variety of techniques. When tests are conducted with dry pollen grains or powdered allergens, the material may be applied directly to the nasal mucosa; others have used powder blowers, have blown the test substance off a cone of paper into the nose, or have had the patient insufflate the allergen from the blunt end of a toothpick (the sniff test) [14]. When extracts are employed, they are sprayed into the nose by atomizers or by syringe and needle or placed on cotton pledgets which are inserted in the nose. Although intramucosal testing by injecting the allergenic extract into the inferior turbinates has been reported, it is rarely done. When dry pollen is used for testing, some innocuous pollen is used as a control in the other nostril; diluent serves as a control for tests with allergenic extracts. If the skin reactions are negative, the nasal tests should be done with dry pollen or, as in bronchial tests, with concentrated extracts.

Subjective responses (sneezing, etc.) and objective criteria (appearance of mucous membranes) are used to evaluate nasal tests. It is hoped that the development of improved techniques, such as the methods for measuring resistance to nasal air flow reported by Seebohm and Hamilton [15], will enhance the value of these tests. Although the test reactions, when properly controlled, appear to be immunologically specific, Wolff *et al.* [16] pointed out that similar changes can be produced in the nasal mucous membranes by irritants and by emotional stress. In spite of these and other variables, however, Feinberg *et al.* [6] obtained quite reproducible results, under suitable conditions, in nasal titration tests carried out in ragweed-sensitive patients.

Properly performed, nasal testing is a reasonably safe procedure. Its greatest value at present is in deciding which skin tests are clinically significant [12], especially when the history is vague. However, the crude techniques for controlling and evaluating these tests show little progress from the pollen-sniffing described by Kirkman and Blackley a century ago.

Conjunctival Tests. The eye has been widely used for diagnostic testing not only in atopic disease but also in relation to serum hypersensitivity. A drop of allergenic extract may be placed in the conjunctival sac, or dry pollen or powdered allergens may be tapped in off a toothpick or other applicator. The patient keeps his eye closed for a few moments, and then it is observed for the development of redness, which often is especially evident at the caruncle. Chemosis occurs with pronounced reactions, and there frequently are accompanying tearing and itching. Homolateral rhinorrhea is not infrequently associated with positive responses as the allergen is washed down the nasolacrimal duct. The eye is observed for ten minutes. Pollen or powdered allergens are removed by taking out the mucus in which they become entrapped with a cotton-tipped applicator. If the reaction is positive, the conjunctival sac is washed out with saline solution and a drop or two of 1 : 1,000 epinephrine is applied. Further testing must then be postponed to a subsequent day. Delayed reactions are rare. Pine pollen is often used as a control in the opposite eye when dry pollen is the test agent; the diluent serves as the control for allergenic extracts. It is difficult or impossible to evaluate eye tests in the presence of pre-existing conjunctival inflammation. As with nasal tests, very concentrated extracts or preferably dry pollen [17] is used in testing patients with negative or equivocal intracutaneous test reactions, while most clinicians use diluted allergenic extracts, if eye testing is done at all, when allergens cause positive reactions to intracutaneous tests. Eye tests are more time-consuming than skin tests, and only one allergen can be evaluated at a time.

In comparing the results of conjunctival and skin tests, many investigators have agreed that intracutaneous tests require less concentrated extracts, and scratch tests more concentrated extracts, than ophthalmic tests [17, 18]. It is unusual to obtain a positive ophthalmic response when the reaction to the intracutaneous test with the same allergen is negative, but this has been recorded [17, 19]. Ophthalmic reactions more frequently are correlated with the clinical history than are positive reactions to intracutaneous tests, but the former are less often associated with clinical difficulty than are positive nasal (and probably bronchial) reactions. Because of the small size of the conjunctival sac, tests expose it to more allergen per unit of surface area than when allergens are applied to nasal or bronchial surfaces, and this may in part explain why eye tests are more likely to reflect "latent allergy" [6]. It might be expected that they would be of particular value in patients who have prominent eye symptoms but negative skin test reactions. Surprisingly, however, there is no good correlation between results of eye tests and the occurrence or severity of ocular symptoms [17, 18].

EVALUATION OF FOOD ALLERGY

Possible food allergy might be suspected from the patient's observations, suggestive symptoms, prominent skin reactions to food allergens, or simply the presence of an atopic disease of uncertain etiology. Foods tend to cause sporadic or continuous perennial symptoms, but seasonal foods may produce confusing seasonal patterns. When foods (e.g., fish, shellfish, nuts, and berries) produce immediate reactions, the relationship is often so conspicuous that patients themselves make the proper diagnosis. Recognition of more delayed reactions may be difficult not only because of the delayed onset of symptoms but because of other factors: multiple sensitization, fluctuating reactivity, cumulative effects, sometimes almost continuous exposure, and nonspecific factors. It also should be remembered that cooking can change the allergenicity of a food.

Patients often have preconceived ideas about food sensitivities, and it may be difficult to convince them that they are *not* allergic to numerous foods. However, if food allergy exists, it is so readily treated by elimination that the evaluation of food allergy is justified whenever there is reason to suspect its possible occurrence.

Procedures for evaluating food allergy are

described in many standard texts and treatises [20, 21]. Experience with these has yielded the following observations: (1) Patients' food suspects may be correct but can be influenced by suggestion, especially if previous skin tests to foods have been carried out. Numerous suspects are particularly open to question. (2) Patients' food likes and dislikes do not correlate well with clinical sensitivity. (3) Except with foods that cause immediate reactions, skin tests are not a good indicator of clinical sensitivity to food. (4) A diet diary occasionally clarifies the cause of intermittent urticaria but rarely is of value in establishing food as an etiological factor in respiratory atopic disease. (5) Success with elimination diets depends not only on the proper manipulation of foods but also on timing of the procedure to mimimize other variables (e. g., pollen or mold seasons, infection). Explicit instructions are essential. (6) The longer the time required to achieve apparent benefit on an elimination diet, the greater the possibility that improvement may be due to other factors or the natural course of the disease. Diagnostic elimination diets must have specified time limits: they should not be carried out indefinitely. (7) The longer the interval between reintroduction of a food and the precipitation of symptoms, the greater the chance that the symptoms are not actually due to the food. A single observation that reintroduction of a food apparently precipitates symptoms does not establish a cause-and-effect relationship: reaction might have happened by coincidence. A firm diagnosis requires reproducibility of the pattern on three separate occasions (unless the reaction is alarming).

With adequate instruction, patients ordinarily can carry out elimination diets at home, but occasionally *ingestion tests* under the physician's direct observation may be helpful, particularly in patients who are unobservant or who claim to have bizarre reactions which need to be verified.

It is obvious that relatively rigid elimination diets offer more likelihood of improvement than a half-hearted regimen. The ultimate would be to take the patient off food altogether. This is approached by the occasional use of "synthetic diets," especially in hospitalized patients. Casein hydrolysates have often been used for this purpose. Although fairly nutritious, their unpleasant taste makes them unacceptable for more than three or four days. Subsequently, every food may be added to the patient's diet, one at a time.

Patients who have strong convictions that they are afflicted with numerous food sensitivities on the basis of insubstantial evidence present a difficult problem. Most of them have been told to eliminate foods merely because of positive skin responses. When symptoms persist, they restrict their diet even further. It may be necessary to test them with foods in a disguised form (e.g., mixed in mashed potatoes, special puddings [22], or highly seasoned food). In rare instances, particularly for academic reasons, the food could be given by gastric gavage. If the tests are negative, psychiatric considerations should influence what the patient is told.

Of additional techniques used in the diagnosis of food allergy, the *leukopenic index* has been discussed extensively in the literature. Although there is no doubt that the peripheral white blood cell count sometimes falls after food is eaten, the consensus is that this response is not a reliable index of an immunological food hypersensitivity. The same statement applies to changes in the *pulse rate* after food ingestion.

IN VITRO TESTS

SPECIFIC SEROLOGICAL TESTS FOR SKIN-SENSITIZING ANTIBODY

Quite naturally, the development of increasingly sensitive techniques by experimental immunologists has encouraged the attempt to demonstrate and quantitate skin-sensitizing antibodies *in vitro*. Important as this quest is from both the experimental and the practical points of view, there has been no unequivocal demonstration of skin-sensitizing antibodies in serum by an *in vitro* test system, and there are some doubts that these antibodies combine firmly with allergens unless they are attached to cells. A variety of serological techniques has yielded positive reactions between sera of atopic persons and various allergens, but it remains to be established that the skin-sensitizing antibodies are responsible for these reactions. From the large amount of information currently accruing in this area, brief mention is made of some approaches being utilized in this work, since herein lies a major hope for improving clinical laboratory procedures for atopic diseases. The heterogeneity of most allergen preparations is a limiting factor in interpreting many of these data.

Numbers of investigators have observed

that sera of atopic persons may specifically produce *hemagglutination* of red cells sensitized with pollen or food allergens by the tannic acid or bis-diazotized benzidine techniques or by special antiglobulin methods. It now seems quite clear, however, that the hemagglutination is not produced primarily by the skin-sensitizing antibodies [23]. Similarly, *precipitation* of allergens, especially milk proteins, has frequently been demonstrable with human sera, but this seems to have no relationship to skin-sensitizing antibodies or the presence of atopic disease [24]. Older work with *complement fixation* tests showed irregular reactions with atopic sera. Relatively specific reactions between *isotopically tagged* pollen, dust, and horse allergens and the serum globulins of sensitive patients have been demonstrated by increased radioactivity in precipitates obtained with either ammonium sulfate or antiglobulin serum [25]. Diffusion in gel of isotopically tagged pollen extracts against serum of pollen-sensitive patients has sometimes shown bands on radioautographs even in the absence of visible bands of precipitate [26]. Also, in *radio-immunoelectrophoresis* of atopic serum against antihuman serum, isotopically tagged allergens mixed with the antiserum may specifically localize to some arcs of precipitate, as shown by autoradiography [27]. The serum factor responsible for some of these recently studied reactions has not been clearly identified, but the possibility that it might be skin-sensitizing antibody, at least in some instances, has not been excluded.

IN VITRO HISTAMINE RELEASE

The addition of allergens *in vitro* to the whole blood of atopic individuals produces a release of histamine from the leukocytes into the plasma [28]. This phenomenon depends not on serum antibodies but on antibodies associated with the leukocytes. The quantity of histamine released is not closely related to skin reactions, but there is a significant, inverse relationship between the latter and the amount of allergen required to produce maximal histamine release [29].

Basophil degranulation tests provide microscopic visualization of this phenomenon, which occurs with several types of specific hypersensitivity reactions involving peripheral blood leukocytes. Wider experience will be needed to assess the value and limitations of this technique [30].

REFERENCES

1. Colldahl, H. A study of provocative tests on patients with bronchial asthma: II. The outcome of provocation tests with different antigens. *Acta Allerg.* 5:143, 1952.
2. Herxheimer, H. Bronchial obstruction induced by allergens, histamine and acetyl-beta-methylcholinechloride. *Int. Arch. Allerg.* 3:189, 1952.
3. Itkin, I. H., Anand, S., Yau, M., and Middlebrook, G. Quantitative inhalation challenge in allergic asthma. *J. Allerg.* 34:97, 1963.
4. Lowell, F. C., and Schiller, I. W. Measurement of changes in vital capacity as a means of detecting pulmonary reactions to inhaled, aerosolized allergenic extracts in asthmatic subjects. *J. Allerg.* 19:100, 1948.
5. Engstrom, I., Karlberg, P., Koch, G., and Kraepelien, S. Use of analysis in mechanics of breathing in provocation test in bronchial asthma. *Acta Paediat.* (Stockholm) 47:441, 1958.
6. Feinberg, S. M., Stier, R. A., and Grater, W. C. A suggested quantitative evaluation of the degree of sensitivity of patients with ragweed pollinosis. *J. Allerg.* 23:387, 1952.
7. Colldahl, H., and Lundin, G. Ventilatory studies of the lungs in asthma. *Acta Allerg.* 5:37, 1952.
8. Schleinzer, R. Pathophysiologische Studien der Pollenallergie. *Acta Allerg.* 4:7, 1951.
9. Kaude, J. Inhalation and skin tests in asthmatic children. *Helv. Paediat. Acta* 15:580, 1960.
10. Juhlin-Dannfelt, C. On the significance of exposure and provocation tests in allergic diagnostics. *Acta Med. Scand.* 239 (supp.): 320, 1950.
11. Colldahl, H. A study of provocation tests on patients with bronchial asthma: I. The reliability of provocation tests performed under different conditions. *Acta Allerg.* 5:133, 1952.
12. Harris, L. H. Experimental reproduction of respiratory mold allergy. *J. Allerg.* 12:279, 1941.
13. Nilsson, H., and Kaude, J. Inhalation and skin test in the diagnosis of asthma bronchiale. *Dis. Chest* 37:535, 1960.
14. Tuft, L., and Blumstein, G. I. Pollen tolerance nasal tests in hay fever. *J. Allerg.* 21:326, 1950.

15. Seebohm, P. M., and Hamilton, W. K. A method for measuring nasal resistance without intranasal instrumentation. *J. Allerg.* 29:56, 1958.
16. Wolff, H. G., Holmes, T. H., Goodell, H., and Wolf, S. Life situations, emotions and nasal disease. *Trans. Ass. Amer. Physicians* 59:88, 1946.
17. Peshkin, M. M. XI. A dry pollen ophthalmic test in pollen asthma and hay fever patients negative to intracutaneous tests. *J. Allerg.* 3:20, 1931.
18. Fineman, A. H. Studies on hypersensitiveness: XXIII. A comparative study of the intradermal, scratch and conjunctival tests in determining the degree of pollen sensitivity. *J. Immun.* 11:465, 1926.
19. Abram, L. E. An evaluation of conjunctival testing in extrinsic respiratory allergy. *J. Allerg.* 20:66, 1949.
20. Rowe, A. H. *Elimination Diets and the Patient's Allergies* (2nd ed.). Philadelphia: Lea & Febiger, 1944.
21. Rinkel, H. J., Randolph, T. G., and Zeller, M. *Food Allergy*. Springfield, Ill.: Charles C Thomas, Publisher, 1951.
22. Loveless, M. H. Allergy for corn and its derivatives: Experiments with a masked ingestion test for its diagnosis. *J. Allerg.* 21:500, 1950.
23. Perelmutter, L., Freedman, S. O., and Sehon, A. H. Demonstration of multiple hemagglutinating factors in sera of ragweed-allergic individuals with the help of immunosorbents. *J. Immun.* 89:623, 1962.
24. Peterson, R. D. A., and Good, R. A. Antibodies to cow's milk proteins—their presence and significance. *Pediatrics* 31:209, 1963.
25. Lidd, D., and Farr, R. S. Primary interaction between I^{131}-labeled ragweed pollen and antibodies in the sera of humans and rabbits. *J. Allerg.* 33:45, 1962.
26. Patterson, R., Pruzansky, J. J., and Feinberg, S. M. Studies on reactions of human allergic serum with protein antigens: I. Methods of passive immune elimination and gel diffusion autoradiography. *Ibid.*, p. 236.
27. Yagi, Y., Maier, P., Pressman, D., Arbesman, C. E., and Reisman, R. E. The presence of the ragweed-binding antibodies in the β_2A-, β_2M- and γ-globulins of sensitive individuals. *J. Immun.* 91:83, 1963.
28. Noah, J. W., and Brand, A. Correlation of blood histamine release and skin test response to multiple antigens. *J. Allerg.* 26:385, 1955.
29. Van Arsdel, P. P., Jr., Middleton, E., Jr., Sherman, W. B., and Buchwald, H. A quantitative study on the *in vitro* release of histamine from leukocytes of atopic persons. *J. Allerg.* 29:429, 1958.
30. Shelley, W. B. Indirect basophil degranulation test for allergy to penicillin and other drugs. *J.A.M.A.* 184:171, 1963.

44. Nonspecific Factors in Allergic Disease

MAX SAMTER AND A. S. MARKOWITZ

SOME PREVIOUS CHAPTERS HAVE DEscribed, in considerable detail, the components of the immunological sequence as well as the components of the tissue injury which the antigen-antibody complex sets in motion. We propose here to examine the nonspecific factors which modify the clinical manifestations of immunological events.

Immunological mechanisms are not, per se, immunological diseases. Some of our difficulties in coping with atopic diseases are clearly the result of our tendency to apply limited immunological findings to the interpretation of the disease in man.

Nonspecific factors may affect antigen, antibody, or the localization of the antigen-antibody complex. Nonspecific factors may influence the nature, rate, and extent of injury of the tissue involved in antigen-antibody interactions. In other words, a discussion of nonspecific factors is concerned with the handling of immunological problems by the host. It is likely that our clinical awareness of these factors has preceded our efforts to understand them: the selective bibliography of this chapter combines early observations with recent efforts to define this twilight area.

The anaphylactic shock of the guinea pig is a reproducible experiment because (1) we use genetically similar animals of equal age and sex, kept in an identical environment and maintained on identical diets; (2) we select dose and type of the antigen; (3) we establish the maximal titer of antibody; and (4) we challenge at the optimal date by the optimal route. Under these experimental conditions, we accomplish explosive release of a known chemical mediator which overwhelms the physiological balance of mucous glands, capillaries, and smooth muscles and produces bronchoconstriction, broncho-obstruction, and death.

The capriciousness of human allergic disease, on the other hand, reflects our experience (1) that the antigen is rarely known; (2) that its uptake at the site of exposure and its subsequent removal to the site of antibody formation is haphazard; (3) that the immunological competence of lymphocytes may vary; (4) that the fate of the antigen-antibody complex is not uniformly predictable; (5) that the reaction of the cell to contact with antigen or antibody might be either protective or harmful; (6) that the chemical mediators which are set free by the antigen-antibody complex are variable from individual to individual and also within the individual from tissue to tissue; and (7) that smooth muscles, mucous glands, and vascular bed of man are subject to complex autonomic controls which may diminish or exaggerate their response.

THE ANTIGEN

Occasionally, man develops anaphylactic reactions which are comparable to anaphylactic reactions in experimental animals: if this occurs, the antigen, as a rule, can be identified. In some forms of spontaneous human allergy, we are still aware of the nature of the antigen, e.g., in sensitivities to milk or egg protein, but we do not know the reason why ingested protein of this type is an antigen in some people but not in others. So far, on the other hand, no one has succeeded in identifying the antigenic component of even a single airborne allergen.

In immune reactions caused by bacteria and, in some instances, by viruses, we might be able to evaluate the relative significance of specific and nonspecific factors more adequately than in atopic diseases. Antigens of bacterial wall and somatic antigens have been reasonably well analyzed, and the differences in response are probably not so much that of the antigen as of the host.

The host assumes increasing importance in the largely uncharted area of autoimmune diseases. Classically, the antigen of autoimmune disease has been thought to be a tissue component removed from its normal location by (traumatic, microbial, enzymatic) injury and, perhaps, sufficiently altered (by degradation or by coupling with chemicals) to be treated as a heterologous substance.

The chemical configuration which permits simple chemicals to combine with protein and to become "antigenic determinants" has been more clearly postulated than the structural characteristics of the host-molecule which accepts them [1, 2]. In spite of ample opportunity, drug reactions are comparatively infrequent: the host does not appear to be eager to cooperate in the formation of antigenic conjugates.

Autoimmune reactions induced in experimental animals, e.g., by the injection of homologous protein in Freund's adjuvant, differ significantly from autosensitization in man. Rheumatoid lesions are not rheumatic fever. The unpredictable course of human autoimmune disease has encouraged the search for alternate explanations.

It has been suggested, for instance, that human autoimmune disease might require a breakdown of homologous cells. Released cellular material might induce the formation of a family of antibodies with several specificities, including specificity against red blood cells [3]. Or, the antigen might be exogenous but immunologically related to one or several tissue components. Consequently, the resulting antibody will cross-react with these tissues which, by definition, are not antigens but "endogenous receptors." An experimental counterpart to the concept of cross-reactivity in man is the injection of a heterophil antiserum (against sheep red cells, dog lung, pneumococci) into the carotid artery of guinea pigs (Forssman). With this technique, it is possible to produce cerebral vascular damage which resembles human allergic encephalitis at least as much as, if not more than, allergic encephalitis produced by the injection of brain in Freund's adjuvant [4].

The genetic propensity for autoimmune diseases, the tendency to form multiple autoimmune antibodies [5], adds another dimension to the study of nonspecific factors which influence specific events. It is not certain, however, whether genetic predisposition refers to the handling of the antigen, the vulnerability of cells, the antibody-forming system, or the "endogenous receptors" for autoimmune antibodies.

Transport. Antigen will be taken up at the site of initial contact by macrophages. Increasing evidence suggests that the type of cells which remove the antigen influences the development of sensitivity. Soluble antigens, for instance, are taken up by different cells when injected in solution than when injected in an emulsion with Freund's adjuvant: the role of the mycobacteria in these changes is not yet clear. Macrophages might do more than deliver antigen to the lymphatic system. They might modify it on the way or even add a factor necessary for the stimulation of antibody synthesis, e.g., some form of ribonucleic acid (RNA) [6–8]. Airborne inhalants which happen to be absorbed by a mucous membrane rich in macrophages might prove to be "strong" antigens, while antigen injected into an environment poor in macrophages might fail to induce antibody formation. Rebuck *et al.* [9] called attention to the "trophocytic" function of leukocytes in the acceleration of tumor growth. A similar function might apply to the rate of antibody formation which relies on active participation of migratory cells.

THE ANTIBODY

The behavior of the lymphatic system which, exposed to antigen, reacts with the synthesis of antibodies is a specific phenomenon and not within the scope of this review. Whatever the specific state, antibody synthesis is protein synthesis, and factors which affect protein synthesis will equally affect the synthesis of antibodies [10]. Uremic rabbits show a marked delay in antibody response [11], possibly because of the depletion of the amino acid pool by urinary excretion of amino acid conjugates [12].

Of the nonspecific factors which influence protein synthesis, hormones have received considerable attention. Hypothysectomized animals show a decrease in protein synthesis by microsomes which can be partly restored by the addition of growth hormone and completely restored by the addition of growth hormone and insulin [13, 14]. In thyroidectomized animals, thyroid hormone (which controls release and activity of growth hormone) does not restore protein synthesis, but triiodothyronine does. Sex hormones are known to affect protein synthesis of their target tissues, i.e., of primary or secondary sex organs, but there is increasing evidence that they also influence the synthesis of enzymes and proteins in nonsex-connected organs [15]. Whether or not this has any bearing on the sex distribution of immunological diseases is at present a matter of speculation. Adrenal corticosteroids in substantial doses depress antibody formation, but the capacity of the hormone to act on a wide variety of cells makes it difficult to interpret the biological meaning of this depression.

Hormones might influence protein synthesis at various sites. They might act on the transfer of amino acids from the pool to the synthesizing cells. They might modify either the secondary or tertiary structure of protein. They might alter RNA synthesis in general, the synthesis of mRNA, the activity of mRNA, or even the coding site of the desoxyribonucleic acid molecule.

ANTIGEN-ANTIBODY COMPLEX AND COMPLEMENT

Acceptable evidence suggests that nonspecific factors, for instance, inflammatory lesions produced during the period of sensitization, influence the localization of the antigen-antibody complex: the eye in particular has been studied extensively for these relationships [16, 17]. Tissues are not necessarily passive recipients of antigen-antibody interactions: in some instances, at least, they must be permissive, if not selective. Atopy might be based on a genetic ability to form univalent antibodies to substances which are innocent for the non-atopic population, but the "atopic trait" per se does not predict in which tissue the atopic disease will become manifest. It is certain that, within the atopic group, we find eczema families, hay fever families, bronchial asthma families, but the biochemical basis for this predilection is not known [18].

Complement (C′) is another nonspecific factor which modifies the effect of the antigen-antibody complex. It is rather surprising that our *in vitro* acquaintance with complement has not given us more insight into its *in vivo* significance for the natural history of immunological disease. In atopy, the role of complement is uncertain, but it has been suggested that C'_3 (or an esterase similar to it) might be necessary for the release of histamine [19]. Exhaustion of complement might prevent the response of tissue to antigen-antibody interactions, but by and large, only the *Komplementschwund* of acute glomerulonephritis has been used as a possible measure for a prediction of the clinical course of the disease [20–22].

THE CHEMICAL MEDIATORS

The nature of chemical mediators which are released in human atopic disease is only partially known (Chap. 15): almost with a sense of shock, the clinical community realized some years ago that antihistamines failed to provide the therapeutic answer to the management of diseases which had been assumed to be caused by histamine. Histamine appears to be the established mediator in certain acute forms of atopy, but its role in subacute and chronic atopic disease remains uncertain.

Elegant studies have clarified the intricate process which leads to a release of free histamine when mast cells disintegrate. It can be expected that this amount is variable since it is based on a number of variables, e.g., the intake of histidine, decarboxylation, and, finally, the distribution of mast cells. Mast cells are perivascular cells, but their numbers are not uniform or predictable: "the existence of many patterns, even among the various organs and tissues within the same species, gives evidence that the mast cell population of any tissue is controlled largely by local factors, either physiological or pathological" [23]. The mystery of the mast cell is complicated by our growing suspicion that the release of histamine and the resulting changes in surrounding tissues are probably not their primary physiological function: Riley [24] believes that mast cells produce mucopolysaccharides and that histamine is only a pacemaker which encourages the cells of the connective tissue to accept and engulf their heparin-containing granules.

Other chemical mediators which appear to participate in the pathogenesis of spontaneous and induced immunological diseases have been identified. It has not yet been possible to define their place in allergic diseases with precision. Whatever their role, they resemble histamine in the unevenness of their distribution. It seems possible that more than one mediator is involved in allergic disease, and that it will become necessary to establish a ratio between various mediators, e.g. slow-reacting substance, histamine, and bradykinin, before treatment of allergic conditions can become rational.

THE MILIEU INTERNE OF ALLERGIC REACTIONS

The site of release of chemical mediators is not necessarily the site where they act. It is likely that they must penetrate protective barriers—components of connective tissue (ground substance and basement membrane)—before they reach target cells. Ground substance appears to be a primary instrument for the maintenance of homeostasis. Careful studies suggest that it represents a two-phase system, a water-rich (less dense) and a colloid-rich (denser) phase which are in effective equilibrium and control water and ion exchange. The ground substance is indeed versatile; it can form colloid complexes with ions and with amines.

Ground substance contains acid mucopolysaccharides, neutral heteropolysaccharides, protein, and soluble collagen (probably of local origin) which serves as a reservoir for nutrients, metabolites, ions, and water (which originate from plasma). Gersh and Catchpole [25] emphasize that "the significant functional feature of basement membrane is that all exchanges between blood plasma, ground substance, and epithelium must take place through two basement membranes."

It seems reasonable to assume that ground substance and basement membranes represent a protective barrier which, if intact, should be able to inactivate chemical mediators before they reach the cell. By the same token, severe and progressive allergic diseases might be based upon or have caused an impairment of the integrity of the ground substance which abolishes its protective potential.

The ground substance is subject to hormonal control. Specifically, adrenal corticosteroids appear to be able to reverse edema and inflammation of immunological diseases. "Normal ground substance and basement membrane of the respiratory tract appear to be unaffected by adrenal corticosteroids." Respiratory allergies are characterized by a loss of definition of perivascular basement membranes. Adrenal corticosteroids will restore normal structure, i.e., return of PAS staining, and presumably normal function [26]. Cyclic nasal symptoms and cyclic urticaria which recur with the menstrual cycle are interesting examples of hormone-induced changes in reactivity.

SYMPATHETIC AND PARASYMPATHETIC CONTROLS

Factors which, by their effect on alpha or beta receptors, decrease or increase autonomic responses have been clarified in extensive studies (Chap. 16). As a rule, the "responsiveness" of autonomic structures varies significantly during each twenty-four hour period. The physiological behavior of the autonomic structures which participate in human "immediate" allergic disease reflects physiological demands. The extent of the changes induced by the chemical mediators of allergy must depend on the autonomic equilibrium at the moment of impact. Emotional factors, weather, infection, and, probably, various ill-defined factors of everyday living are likely to alter the autonomic balance.

The effect of weather has been carefully studied [27]. It is surprising that we still have not established which of the components of weather increase the incidence of bronchial asthma. Agreement appears to exist that high humidity (within the narrow range) in the absence of pronounced temperature changes increases the incidence of bronchial asthma. Several explanations have been offered; none has been confirmed [28, 29]. It is certain that temperature and humidity are not the only factors. During sirocco weather in Israel, one half of the patients who have bronchial asthma did not note any change, 30 percent responded with marked aggravation of symptoms, and the rest showed an equally striking improvement [30].

The shift in autonomic controls, for instance, under "stress" [31] or during wakefulness and sleep, has been substantiated: its significance for allergic manifestations, however, is not clear. An interesting example of a phenomenon which has been attributed to autonomic imbalance is the diurnal fluctuation of peripheral eosinophil levels. Rud [32] showed that there is an average midmorning fall of about 20 percent below the 8:00 A.M. level, and a night-time peak about 30 percent above it. It is likely that many of these observations will acquire a new meaning if they are translated into our more sophisticated terms and insights.

By and large, the literature on nonspecific factors favors the immediate type of allergic response, but it might apply equally to the Arthus phenomenon and to "delayed" inflammation. Rich used to say that the development of rheumatoid lesions in rabbits can be predicted within a few days after intravenous injection of horse serum by a cursory examination of the rabbits' ears. Rabbits with ears which "flicker" when held against the light were prone to develop typical changes, in contrast to rabbits with "stable" peripheral circulation which yielded a significantly higher rate of "failures." Kallós and Pagel [33] studied the role of the vascular bed in the pathogenesis of rheumatoid changes. Using rabbits they injected hog serum and, simultaneously, caffeine every four hours during the period of sensitization. The cardiovascular changes produced with this technique are impressive, and the authors concluded that the "functional stress" had "localized" the allergic reaction. It might be well to remember that Smadel and Farr [34] showed that the fate of Masugi-nephritic rats given injections of antikidney serum depends on their diet at the moment of injection. One can only guess whether these observations apply to man, but it is tempting to assume that some of our habits might make the difference between asymptomatic handling and the development of symptoms after exposure to antigens to which most of us must be exposed, at one time or another.

Our approach to the assessment of the role of nonspecific factors in the pathogenesis of allergic disease has been slow and hesitant. Clinicians have been inclined to prefer "specific" tests. This preference is hardly justified, for if one considers the incredible sequence of nonspecific events which is necessary to make even a skin test possible, it is a miracle that skin tests are of any clinical value at all. It is possible to measure many, if not most, of the nonspecific factors which are part of the allergic syndrome. Some of the necessary techniques are simple and should become part of the examination of the allergic patient. Others, e.g., the assessment of the functional state of ground substance, are the subject of intensive investigation in the laboratory but cannot yet be adapted to routine clinical use. It can be expected, however, that the technical problems will be solved, that the nonspecific factors which influence allergic disease will gain the attention which they deserve, and that our increasing awareness of the protective potential of the tissue in which the allergic reaction occurs might eventually provide us with the means for a more comprehensive therapeutic approach.

REFERENCES

1. Metzger, H., Wofsy, L., and Singer, S. J. A specific antibody-hapten reaction with novel spectral properties. *Arch. Biochem.* 103:206, 1963.
2. Samter, M., and Berryman, G. H. Immune Mechanisms in Drug Hypersensitivity. In Brown, E. A. (Ed.), *Allergology* (Proceedings of 4th International Congress). New York: Pergamon Press, 1962. P. 99.
3. Brand, K. Persistence and stability of species-specific hemagglutinogens in cultivated mammalian cells. *Nature* (London) 194:752, 1962.
4. Leibowitz, S., Morgan, R. S., Berkinshaw-Smith, E. M. I., and Wright, G. P. Cerebral vascular damage in guinea pigs induced by various heterophile antisera injected by the Forssman intracarotid technique. *Brit. J. Exp. Path.* 42:455, 1961.
5. Holmes, M. C., and Burnet, F. M. The natural history of autoimmune disease in NZB mice: A comparison with the pattern of human autoimmune manifestations. *Ann. Intern. Med.* 59:265, 1963.
6. Fishman, M., and Adler, F. L. Antibody formation initiated *in vitro:* II. Antibody synthesis in x-irradiated recipients of diffusion chambers containing nucleic acid derived from macrophages incubated with antigen. *J. Exp. Med.* 117:595, 1963.
7. Fishman, M., Hammerstrom, R. A., and Bond, V. P. *In vitro* transfer of macrophage RNA to lymph node cells. *Nature* (London) 198: 549, 1963.
8. Uhr, J. W. Actinomycin D: Its effect on antibody formation *in vitro. Science* 142:1476, 1963.
9. Rebuck, J. W., Brennan, M. J., and Hall, J. A. Some aspects of leukocyte behavior as studied by the human skin window technique with reference to their trophocytic functions in the responses of inflammation and to autochthonous and homologous cancer cells in man. *Ann. N.Y. Acad. Sci.* (in press).
10. Dubos, R. J., and Schaedler, R. W. Effect of dietary proteins and amino acids on the susceptibility of mice to bacterial infections. *J. Exp. Med.* 108:69, 1958.
11. Gowland, G., and Smiddy, F. G. The effect of acute experimental uremia on the immunological responses of the rabbit to bovine serum albumin. *Brit. J. Urol.* 34:274, 1962.
12. Frimpter, G. W., Thompson, D. D., and Luckey, E. H. Conjugated amino acids in plasma of patients with uremia. *J. Clin. Invest.* 40:1208, 1961.
13. Korner, A. The effect of hypophysectomy of the rat and of the treatment with growth hormone on the incorporation *in vivo* of radio-

active amino acids into the proteins of subcellular fractions of rat liver. *Biochem. J.* 74: 462, 1960.
14. Wagle, S. R. The influence of growth hormone, cortisol and insulin on the incorporation of amino acids into protein. *Arch. Biochem.* 102:373, 1963.
15. Bond, H. E. A sex-associated protein in liver tissue of the rat and its response to endocrine manipulation. *Nature* (London) 196:242, 1962.
16. Riehm, W. *Erkrankungen des Auges und Allergie.* In Hansen, K. (Ed.), *Allergie* (3rd ed.). Stuttgart: Georg Thieme Verlag, 1957.
17. Woods, A. C. Immune reactions following injuries to the uveal tract. *J.A.M.A.* 77:1317, 1921.
18. Samter, M. The state of allergy, International Forum, *Therapeutic Notes,* p. 134, 1955.
19. Austen, K. F., and Brocklehurst, W. E. Anaphylaxis in chopped guinea-pig lung: III. Effect of carbon monoxide, cyanide, salicylaldoxime and ionic strength. *J. Exp. Med.* 114: 29, 1961.
20. Kellett, C. E., and Thomson, J. G. Complementary activity of blood serum in nephritis. *J. Path. Bact.* 48:519, 1939.
21. Freedman, P., and Markowitz, A. S. Isolation of antibody-like gamma globulin from lupus glomeruli. *Brit. Med. J.* 1:1175, 1962.
22. Lange, K., Wasserman, E., and Slobody, L. B. The significance of serum complement levels for the diagnosis and prognosis of acute and subacute glomerulonephritis and lupus erythematosus disseminatus. *Ann. Intern. Med.* 53: 636, 1960.
23. Simpson, W. L. Distribution of mast cells as a function of age and exposure to carcinogenic agents. *Ann. N.Y. Acad. Sci.* 103:16, 1963.
24. Riley, J. F. Functional significance of histamine and heparin in tissue mast cells. *Ibid.,* p. 159.
25. Gersh, I., and Catchpole, H. R. The nature of ground substance of connective tissue. *Perspect. Biol. Med.* 3:282, 1960.
26. Rappaport, B. Z., Samter, M., Catchpole, H. R., and Schiller, F. The mucoproteins of the nasal mucosa of allergic patients before and after treatment with corticotropin. *J. Allerg.* 24:35, 1953.
27. Petersen, W. F. *The Patient and the Weather.* Ann Arbor, Mich.: Edwards Brothers, Inc., 1934–37 (various volumes).
28. Rappaport, B. Z., Nelson, T., and Welker, W. H. The effect of low relative humidity at constant temperature on pollen asthma. *J. Allerg.* 6:111, 1935.
29. Ordman, D. The "climate" group of respiratory allergy patients. *Int. Arch. Allerg.* 12:162, 1958.
30. Gutmann, M. J. The influence of sirocco weather on bronchial asthma in Jerusalem (based on meterological records during a period of 19 years). *Acta Med. Orient.* 16:255, 1957.
31. Wolff, H. G., Holmes, T. H., Goodell, H., and Wolf, S. Life situations, emotions, and nasal disease changes in nasal functions associated with varying emotional states and life situations. *Trans. Ass. Amer. Physicians* 59:88, 1946.
32. Rud, F. The eosinophil count in health and in mental disease: Biometrical Study, *Acta Psychiat. Neurol.,* supp. 40, 1947.
33. Kallós, P., and Pagel, W. *Acta Med. Scand.* 91:292, 1937; quoted by Pagel, W. In Kallós, P. (Ed.), *Fortschritte der Allergielehre.* Basel: S. Karger, 1939. P. 116.
34. Smadel, J. Z., and Farr, L. E. Experimental nephritis in rats induced by injection of antikidney serum: II. Clinical and functional studies. *J. Exp. Med.* 65:527, 1937.

45. Physiology of the Nose and Pathophysiology of Allergic Rhinitis*

BEN Z. RAPPAPORT

PHYSIOLOGY

The nose is an olfactory and air-processing organ. The olfactory sense is limited to small portions of the nasal mucosa in the upper part of the vault that is covered by nonciliated neuroepithelial cells. These specialized cells are capable of detecting and transmitting odor information to the brain. Heating, moistening, and cleansing of inspired air for which the structure of the nose is suited are essential for oxygen and carbon dioxide gas exchange and for protection of the delicate pulmonary alveoli. The mouth is a poor substitute as an airway, and its use as such is not established within the first two weeks of life [1].

HEATING OF AIR

Inspired air is heated as it passes over the highly vascular turbinates and septum. The latticed, parallel arrangement of the closely spaced vessels in the turbinates provides a radiator-like structure which is highly effective for heat and moisture exchange [2]. In addition to heat derived from the blood vessels, there is heat transfer from the warmer expired and residual air to the inspired air [2]. So effective is the thermostatic process that with an outdoor temperature of 0° C., the air delivered to the pharynx is warmed to a temperature between 36° and 37° C. [3, 4], a remarkable degree of heating efficiency in view of the large air volume delivered in a brief period of time.

CLEANSING OF AIR

Cleansing of the air begins with the removal of coarse foreign particles by the stiff hairs lining the preturbinal part of the nares; fine particles are entrapped by the mucous blanket and action of the cilia. Except for the small olfactory area in the vault, the nasal mucosa, including that of the septum, is lined by ciliated cells that extend into the paranasal sinuses. The cilia form a closely packed covering like the pile of a carpet. Although hardy, these cell processes are expendable: they are shed during infection but can regenerate in hours [5].

The cilia move with a quick, lashlike stroke followed by a slow recovery, beating at the rate of 8 to 12 cycles per second. The wavelike, synchronous movement of groups of adjacent cilia produces a continuous flow of the mucous blanket and its entrapped foreign matter toward the pharynx, from which it is expectorated or swallowed [5]. In the sinuses, the mucous blanket covering the walls moves in a spiral toward the ostia and then to the nasopharynx. The rate of the continuous flow of mucus varies in different regions of the nasal mucosa; from the farthest sinus, it reaches the pharynx in about 20 minutes [5, 6]. The mucous blanket is renewed about every 10 minutes by a new cover derived from the glands and the goblet cells [5]. Its tenacious, adhesive properties and continuous flow lead to entrapment and removal for disposal of foreign particles, including bacteria. Dry cultures sprayed into the nasal cavity are swept quickly and completely into the nasopharynx for disposal in a few minutes [7]. The chemical and immunological properties of mucus give additional protection against bacterial invasion of the respiratory tract.

The chemical barriers against infection

* The work reported here was supported by U.S. Public Health Service grant No. A1-04422-03.

consist of the pH of the mucus [8, 9] and its lysozyme content [10]. The importance and significance of the acidity of nasal secretions were established by measurement of its pH in situ [8, 9]. Recently designed instruments demonstrated that the mucus is much more acid than previous studies had indicated. In early studies, the pH had been estimated by relatively inaccurate methods at varying periods after removal of mucus from the nose. The results reported varied with the loss of carbon dioxide content during the varying intervals between removal of the mucus and measurement of the pH. Far more alkaline readings were recorded than those obtained by determinations in situ. These later studies indicated that the pH of nasal secretions in normal adults varies from 5.5 to 6.5 and in infants from 5 to 6.7, an unfavorable medium for bacterial growth [11, 12]. The secretions become alkaline during either acute rhinitis or allergic episodes [13].

In addition to its acidity, normal nasal mucus contains lysozyme, a lytic enzyme against bacterial proteins [10]. Lysozyme is present in higher concentration in the upper and posterior parts of the nose, and its higher activity there may explain the lower concentration of bacteria in these areas than in the rest of the nose [11].

HUMIDIFICATION OF AIR AND PHYSIOLOGICAL NASAL ENGORGEMENT

The relative humidity of inspired air after its passage through the nose is raised to 79 percent. An additional 15 percent rise occurs in passage through the bronchi [14]. A high water vapor content in the inspired air is essential for oxygen and carbon dioxide gas exchange in the alveoli and for maintenance of the liquidity of the mucous blanket covering the epithelium. As much as 2 qts. of fluid per day are required for adequate air moistening [15]. The moisture is derived largely from the blood vessels of the turbinates and to a lesser degree from the seromucinous glands. Wright [16] stated that under favorable conditions the turbinates on one side of the nose are swelling while those on the opposite side are shrinking and delivering the squeezed-out fluid into the nasal fossae in a slow cycle, requiring fifty minutes to four hours for completion.

The physiological turbinal swelling and shrinking are due to vasodilatation and constriction. Because of the parallel arrangement of the numerous closely spaced arteries and veins in the turbinates, the veins are compressed as the arteries dilate. The effect is to dam the venous flow, thereby elevating the intracapillary pressure which leads to transudation of fluid [17]. The smooth muscle and elastic tissue in the turbinates permits these structures to swell during the transudation process. When the artery constricts, vascular engorgement is reduced and the contractile tissue squeezes the transudated fluid, as from a wet sponge, into the nasal fossae [17].

During the early process of engorgement and swelling, while the vessels are still near the surface, the turbinates become red and hyperemic. Increased and sustained swelling leads to widening of the spaces between blood vessels and to their shift to a deeper position below the surface, resulting in pallor of the nasal mucosa unless infection is present. As the fluid is squeezed out of the edematous turbinates and the blood vessels come closer together nearer the surface, the normal pink color of the mucosa returns [17].

In addition to the cyclic physiological engorgement, a variety of local and reflex causes can produce swelling of the nasal mucosa. Turgescence of the turbinates can be due either to reflex stimulation of the vascular dilator center or, less frequently, to inhibition of the tonic activity of the vasoconstrictor nerves. The following causes, either alone or in conjunction with allergy or infection, can increase nasal edema: (1) irritants, as dusts, fumes or liquids; (2) strong odors and bright lights [18]; (3) chilling of the surface of the body [19, 20]; (4) endocrine factors associated with menstruation, pregnancy, and sexual excitement [18]; and (5) emotional disturbances related to experiences of conflict, resentment, and frustration [18].

PATHOPHYSIOLOGY OF EDEMA IN ALLERGIC RHINITIS

Although swelling of the turbinates may be due to diffusion of fluid from the capillaries, the edema of allergy and infection is associated with changes in ground substance of the nasal mucosa.

The matrix surrounding organized structures, such as vessels, cells, and fibers, is called ground substance. Since routinely used stains do not combine with the mucoproteins composing ground substance, its characteristics were not demonstrable until 1946–48 when special staining methods, such as periodic acid-fuchsin (PAS) stain and more recently cationic stains, permitted visualization and histological study of these mucoproteins.

When stained by the McManus-Hotchkiss (PAS) method [21, 22], the ground substance of the allergic nasal mucosa which has not been exposed to antigen does not differ from that of normal (nonallergic) nasal mucosa (Fig. 45-1). It stains pink except for more intense zones at the junction of the surface epithelium with the tunica propria and around blood vessels and glands [23]. These deeper staining zones form sheaths called basement membranes, which are composed of denser, more highly polymerized mucopolysaccharides similar in composition to the adjacent ground substance [24].

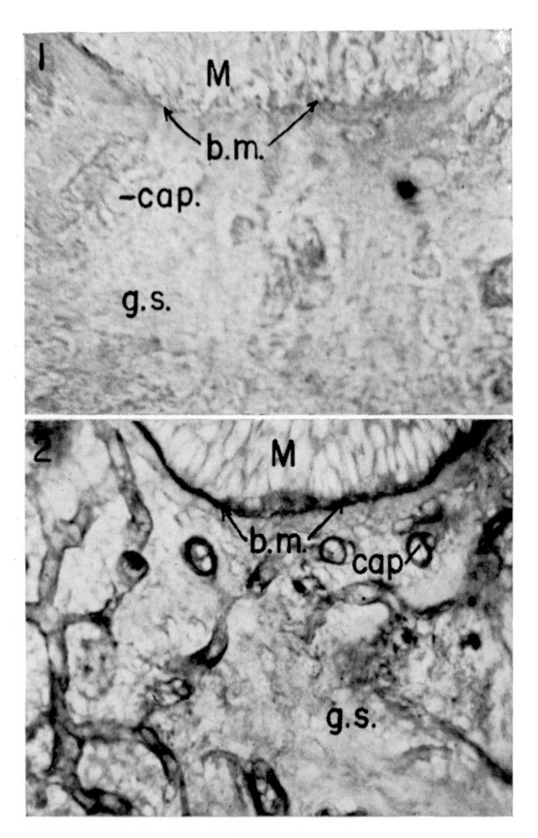

Fig. 45-1. Stain for mucoproteins by PAS method. (*1*) Nasal mucosa from ragweed-sensitive patient removed at height of the allergic reaction (August 31). (*2*) Nasal mucosa from nonallergic individual. Note difference in staining intensity of ground substance (*g.s.*), basement membrane (*b.m.*), and pericapillary basement membrane (*cap*). Sections were from frozen-dried tissues; 4 μ. (× 400 before 20% reduction.)

During the reaction induced by specific allergen and during inflammatory processes, changes in ground substance occur in proportion to the severity and duration of the allergic or inflammatory reaction [23]. The mucopolysaccharides composing the ground substance lose stainability until, in severe allergic reactions, the periodic acid–Schiff stain is barely visible. The sheaths forming the subepithelial, periglandular, and perivascular basement membranes correspondingly lose stainability and width.

When corticosteroids are used to relieve nasal congestion in allergy, the staining intensity of ground substance and basement membranes is restored to normal.

The interpretation that we have made of these changes is based on other studies [24–26] which suggest that the ground substance is in constant and sometimes rapid change from a semisolid to a relatively fluid state.

The changes in the hydrophilic properties of the mucopolysaccharides lead to variations in fluidity of ground substance. The mucopolysaccharides that compose the solids of ground substance are probably formed in fibroblasts and mesenchymal cells [25, 26, 36]. These cells can produce a variety of molecular groupings of mucopolysaccharides to form colloids of various sizes; the smaller the colloidal aggregates, the greater their hydrophilic properties. It has also been suggested that after ground substance is formed, it can undergo either disaggregation or, reversibly, aggregation [25, 26].

The mucoproteins and mucopolysaccharides of ground substance are in equilibrium with tissue fluids; this state has been described as a two-phase system which is, in turn, in equilibrium with the blood [27]. In nonedematous mucosa, the larger colloidal aggregates of mucopolysaccharides predominate and form a colloid-rich, water-poor phase which is in equilibrium with tissue fluids in a water-rich, colloid-poor phase. This theory, based on electrochemical observations [27], is in accord with electronmicroscopic observations which describe the ground substance as a system of submicroscopic vacuoles of 600 to 1,200 A diameter (the water-rich, colloid-poor phase) enclosed in a denser substance (the colloid-rich, water-poor phase) [28, 29].

Abnormal states characterized by edema lead either to colloidal disaggregation or to production of smaller molecular aggregates by the cells, or, simultaneously, to both processes. With the formation of smaller, more hydrophilic colloidal aggregates, the composition of the ground substance changes to a water-rich, colloid-poor phase that requires for equilibrium an increased hydration with tissue fluids. To restore phase equilibrium, water is absorbed from the blood [30].

As edema subsides, the colloidal state is restored to the normal colloid-rich, water-poor phase with reduced hydrophilic properties; water is resorbed into the blood stream, and the edema subsides.

Changes in ground substance are not limited to allergy. They have been described in such unrelated conditions as scurvy [31], inflammation, growing tumors [32], exfoliative gingivitis [33], and ulcerative colitis [34].

This summary of the ground substance changes in nasal allergy is based on our work with biopsy specimens prepared by freeze-drying immediately after removal. The histological sections prepared from these tissues were denatured in 95 percent ethanol to render the highly soluble mucopolysaccharides insoluble, thus preventing their loss in the aqueous PAS reagent during staining [23]. Freeze-drying is essential because the highly soluble proteins of ground substance do not lend themselves to fixation with aqueous solutions like formaldehyde [38], the fixative used in some of the studies of nasal mucosa ground substance [35, 37]. The mucopolysaccharides are largely dissolved in the 96 percent water of 4 percent formaldehyde (10 percent formalin) before the chemical can make them insoluble [38].

PATHOGENESIS OF POLYPS

In an attempt to explain the pathogenesis of polyps, Eggston and Wolff [39] stated that they are formed because of venous and lymphatic obstruction in sites with unobstructed arterial flow. The venous and lymphatic stasis leads to edema and formation of polyps. This explanation disregards the rich anastomosis in the nasal mucosa. Localized venous stasis in such tissue is improbable except in unusual cases of massive venous thrombosis.

An effort to relate nasal edema of allergy or infection with polyps must account for the greater severity of polypoid edema, its localized character, its irreversibility, and its recurrence after surgical removal. Only during the administration of corticosteroids does the edema of nonfibrotic polyps subside as does that of nasal allergy.

Polyps occur most frequently in severe, persistent, perennial nasal allergy and, more notably, when the allergy is complicated by purulent sinusitis. The prolonged nature of the edema of perennial allergy, especially when it is complicated by infection, requires continuous formation of hydrophilic types of colloids by fibroblasts and mesenchymal cells.

In speculating about the similarity of the changes in ground substance of nasal polyps and in that of severe nasal allergy, one must keep in mind, of course, the fact that histological similarity does not constitute proof of common pathogenesis.

It is possible that after prolonged stimulation, some of the fibroblasts become preferentially predisposed to form smaller hydrophilic colloids rather than the larger colloidal aggregates. Continuous formation of the more hydrophilic colloids may result from stimulation of embryonic types of cells or from acquired characteristics by adult cells. It has been noted that in the skin of pigs, the ground substance of mucopolysaccharides differs greatly in the embryo from that in the adult [40]. If cells with the preferential capacity to form a hydrophilic type of colloid are dispersed in a mosaic pattern with cells capable of forming normal, less hydrophilic colloid, edema will be diffuse and no polyposis will result. If, however, such cells are grouped at some sites to form cell loci which produce abnormal, hydrophilic mucopolysaccharides, prolonged stimulation will result in severe, localized edema and polyposis. Surgical removal of polyps will not eliminate the foci of abnormal cells, and the polyps will recur.

PROTECTIVE MECHANISMS OF THE NASAL MUCOSA

The defense of the respiratory tract begins with the cleansing of air by ciliary movement and by the activity of the flowing mucous blanket, which have been described. Below the mucous blanket is the second line of defense, the epithelial cells of the surface-covering layer, of the seromucinous glands, and the goblet cells.

The protective function of the epithelium is exercised in two major ways. First is its ability to proliferate and form an anatomical barrier against invasion [5]. The "normal," nonirritated nasal lining, present probably only in infants, is a single layer of columnar cells. With normal, physiological function, irritation results in various degrees of stratification and multiplication of cell layers up to the stratified squamous form characteristic of skin epithelium. The effect is greater with inflammation [41]. Exfoliation of severely injured epithelium and of cilia is followed rapidly by regeneration [5].

In addition to its function as an anatomical barrier to invasion by noxious elements, the nasal epithelium, like that of the allergic skin [42], contains antibodies. Recent immunofluorescent studies have demonstrated that the epithelial cells composing the glands and surface cells of the nasal mucosa contain reaginic antibodies that participate in the allergic reaction [43]. These findings in allergic mucosa parallel the observations in the epithelial cells of allergic skin, including those of sweat glands, sebaceous glands, and hair follicles [42].

When an allergic reaction is produced by contact with a specific antigen, the antigen, presumably bound to antibody, is demon-

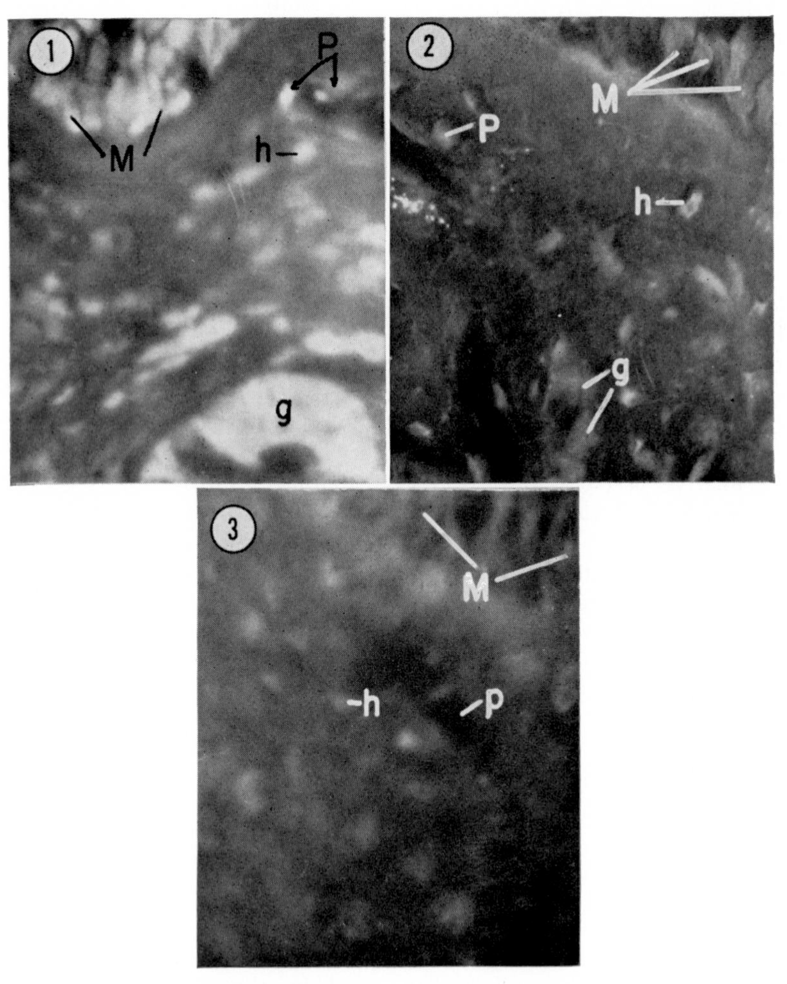

Fig. 45-2. Immunofluorescent staining of nasal mucosa with fluorescein-isothiocyanate conjugated reagins. (*1*) Mucosa from ragweed-sensitive patient after topical challenge with ragweed antigen. Specific staining of mucosa cells (*M*), histiocytes (*h*), gland cells (*g*), and pericapillary cells (*p*). (2) Mucosa from same patient as in *1* after topical application of 1:100,000 histamine solution. Note much lesser fluorescence (nonspecific) of the structures indicated in *1*. (*3*) Mucosa from nonallergic individual after topical application of ragweed pollen. Stain with conjugated reagins is negative, as in *2*. All sections cut at 4 μ and photographed under dark-field illumination. ($\times$ 400 before 20% reduction.)

strable in the surface epithelial cells, in the epithelial cells forming the glands, in histiocytes, fibrocytes, and endothelial cells, and antigen is demonstrable in ground substance and in association with fibrous tissue bundles (Fig. 45–2). The presence of antibody in the surface epithelial cells and in gland cells of the allergic nasal mucosa is not due to overflow of antibody into these cells following exposure to specific antigen. In biopsy specimens from allergic nasal mucosa removed without exposure to antigen, the binding of antigen by antibody within surface epithelial and gland cells can be demonstrated. When sections from such unchallenged mucosa are coated with specific antigen, fluorescence can be shown in surface epithelial and gland cells.

Since reaginic antibody is present in the epithelial cells which form the seromucinous glands, it is not surprising that it has been found in nasal secretions [44]. Similarly, after experimental induction of an infectious common cold, γ-globulins are found in nasal secretions, which ordinarily contain only albumin [45].

REFERENCES

1. Durward, A., Lord, O. C., and Polson, C. J. Congenital choanal atresia. *J. Laryng.* 60:461, 1945.
2. Swindle, P. F. Architecture of blood vascular networks in erectile and secretory lining of nasal passages. *Ann. Otol.* 44:913, 1935.
3. Proetz, A. W. *Applied Physiology of the Nose.* St. Louis: Annals Publishing Co., 1953.
4. Fabricant, N. D. The topical temperature of clinically normal nasal and pharyngeal mucous membranes. *Arch. Otolaryng.* 66:275, 1957.
5. Hilding, A. Four physiologic defenses of the upper part of the respiratory tract: Ciliary action, exchange of mucin, regeneration and adaptability. *Ann. Intern. Med.* 6:227, 1932.
6. Hilding, A. Physiology of drainage of nasal mucus: Flow of mucus currents through drainage system of nasal mucosa and its relation to ciliary activity. *Arch. Otolaryng.* 15:92, 1932.
7. Fabricant, N. D. Physiology of Nasal Mucosa. In Coates, G. M., Schenck, H. P., and Miller, M. V. (Eds.), *Otolaryngology.* Hagerstown, Md.: W. F. Prior Company, Inc., Vol. 3. 1955.
8. Fabricant, N. D. Significance of the pH of nasal secretions in situ. *Arch. Otolaryng.* 34: 150, 1941.
9. Fabricant, N. D. Significance of the pH of nasal secretions in situ: Further studies. *Ibid.,* p. 297.
10. Hilding, A. Changes in the lysozyme content of the nasal mucus during colds. *Arch. Otolaryng.* 21:38, 1934.
11. Tweedie, A. R. Nasal flora and reaction of nasal mucus. *J. Laryng.* 49:586, 1934.
12. Grannoni, E., and Bernicchi, L. Ricerea della catalassi nella mucosa nasale del coniglio. *Minerva Otorinolaring.* 5:302, 1955.
13. Buhrmester, C. C. A study of the hydrogen ion concentration, nitrogen content and viscosity of nasal secretions. *Ann. Otol.* 42:1041, 1933.
14. Perkowitzschky, R. Quoted in Ref. 3.
15. Foster, E. E. The influence of imperfect nasal respiration on the oral cavity. *Ann. Otol.* 16:661, 1907.
16. Wright, J. The contractile elements in the connective tissue: II. The elastic fibre in the nasal mucosa in health and disease. *New York Med. J.* 91:729, 1910.
17. Heetderks, D. R. Observations on reaction of normal nasal mucous membrane. *Amer. J. Med. Sci.* 175:231, 1927.
18. Holmes, T. H., Goodell, H., Wolf, S., and Wolff, H. G. *The Nose,* Springfield, Ill.: Charles C Thomas, Publisher, 1950.
19. Mudd, S., Goldman, A., and Grant, S. B. Reaction of the nasal cavity and postnasal space to chilling of the body surface, vasomotor reactions. *J. Exp. Med.* 34:11, 1921.
20. Spiesman, I. G. Vasomotor reactions. *Arch. Otolaryng.* 17:829, 1933.
21. McManus, J. F. A. The histological demonstration of mucin after periodic acid. *Nature* (London) 158:202, 1946.
22. Hotchkiss, R. D. A microchemical reaction resulting in the staining of polysaccharide structures in fixed tissue preparations. *Arch. Biochem.* 16:131, 1948.
23. Rappaport, B. Z., Samter, M., Catchpole, H. R., and Schiller, F. The mucoproteins of the nasal mucosa of allergic patients before and after treatment with corticotropin. *J. Allerg.* 24:35, 1953.
24. Gersh, I., and Catchpole, H. R. The organization of ground substance and basement membrane and its significance in tissue injury. *Amer. J. Anat.* 85:457, 1949.
25. Gersh, I. Some Functional Considerations of Ground Substance in the Connective Tissues. In Ragan, C. (Ed.), *Second Conference on Connective Tissues.* New York: Josiah Macy, Jr., Foundation, 1951.
26. Gersh, I. Ground substance and the plasticity

of connective tissues. *Harvey Lect.* 45:211, 1950.
27. Joseph, N. R., Engel, M. B., and Catchpole, H. R. Interaction of ions and connective tissue. *Biochim. Biophys. Acta* 8:575, 1952.
28. Bondareft, W. Submicroscopic morphology of connective tissue ground substance with particular regard to fibrillogenesis and aging. *Gerontologia* 1:222, 1957.
29. Chase, W. H. Extracellular distribution of ferrocyanide in muscle. *Arch. Path.* 67:525, 1959.
30. Catchpole, H. R. Present Concept of the Vascular Environment in Blood Vessels and Lymphatics. In Abramson, D. I. (Ed.), *Blood and Lymphatics.* New York: Academic Press, Inc., 1962.
31. Pirani, C. L., and Catchpole, H. R. Serum glycoproteins in experimental scurvy. *Arch. Path.* 51:597, 1951.
32. Catchpole, H. R. Serum and tissue glycoproteins in mice bearing transplantable tumors. *Proc. Soc. Exp. Biol. Med.* 75:221, 1950.
33. Engel, M. B., Ray, H. G., and Orban, B. The pathogenesis of desquamative gingivitis: A disturbance of the connective tissue ground substance. *J. Dent. Res.* 29:410, 1950.
34. Levine, M. D., Kirsner, J. B., and Klotz, P. A new concept of the pathogenesis of ulcerative colitis. *Science* 114:552, 1951.
35. Weisskopf, A., and Burns, F. H. The ground substance of the nasal turbinates. *Ann. Otol.* 67:292, 1958.
36. Weisskopf, A., and Burns, F. H. Histochemical studies of the pathogenesis of nasal polyps. *Ann. Otol.* 68:509, 1959.
37. Hlavácek, Vl. and Lojda, Zd. Histologisches Bild der allergischen Nasenschleimhaut vor und nach ACTH und Cortison Behandlung. In Eigler, G., and Findeisen, D. G. R. (Eds.), *Der Schupfen.* Leipzig: Johann Ambrosius Barth, Verlag, 1959.
38. Szirmai, J. A. Quantitative approaches in the histochemistry of mucopolysaccharides. *J. Histochem. Cytochem.* 11:24, 1963.
39. Eggston, A. A., and Wolff, D. *Histopathology of the Ear, Nose and Throat.* Baltimore: Williams & Wilkins Company, 1947.
40. Loewi, G., and Meyer, K. The acid mucopolysaccharides of embryonic skin. *Biochim. Biophys. Acta* 27:453, 1958.
41. Hilding, A. Experimental surgery of the nose and sinuses; Changes in the morphology of the epithelium following variations in ventilation. *Arch. Otolaryng.* 16:9, 1932.
42. Rappaport, B. Z. Antigen-antibody reactions in allergic human tissues: II. Study by fluorescence technique of the localization of reagins in human skin and their relation to globulins. *J. Exp. Med.* 112:725, 1960.
43. Rappaport, B. Z. Antigen-antibody reactions in allergic human tissues. III. Immunofluorescent study of allergic nasal mucosa. *J. Immun.* 93:792–797, 1964.
44. Samter, M., and Becker, E. L. Ragweed reagins in nasal secretions. *Proc. Soc. Exp. Biol. Med.* 65:140, 1947.
45. Anderson, T. O., Reff, L. J. M., and Jackson, G. G. Immunoelectrophoresis of nasal secretions collected during a common cold: Observations which suggest a mechanism of seroimmunity in viral respiratory infections. *J. Immun.* 89:691, 1962.

46. Allergic Rhinitis—Diagnosis

SAMUEL M. FEINBERG

THE SYNDROME OF PERENNIAL SNEEZing, nonpurulent rhinorrhea, and nasal blocking has been called by many names, such as vasomotor rhinitis, hyperesthetic rhinitis, atopic rhinitis, allergic rhinitis, and perennial rhinitis. Because an allergic etiology is detected in only 50 or 60 percent of individuals having these symptoms, with uncertainty as to what the causative factor may be in many of the remaining, we [1] prefer to include the entire group in the general term "hyperesthetic rhinitis" and limit the use of the term "allergic" to those in whom an allergic etiology is established. Nevertheless we shall discuss here all aspects of this syndrome, whether allergic or not.

SYMPTOMS AND COMPLICATIONS

The major symptoms of hyperesthetic rhinitis are those of hay fever, i.e., any combination of the following manifestations: itching of the nose, sneezing, rhinorrhea, and nasal stuffiness. In some instances, itching of the palate, pharynx, ears, or eyes also occurs. There is an impression that itching implies an allergic etiology. In the early phases of an attack, sneezing and rhinorrhea may be more pronounced than in the later stages, when nasal obstruction may be most conspicuous. The poor response of the chronic obstructive stage to antihistamines gives one the feeling that mediators other than histamines are involved in the mechanism, particularly in this phase.

Periodicity of the manifestations is the rule. Most individuals are worse on arising, gradually improving some time in the morning. In a large number, only morning symptoms are present. Most individuals feel worse in the recumbent than in the upright position, the side of the nose that is lowermost being the most affected. Others, for reasons difficult to understand, note clearing when lying down. In the more severe cases, of course, the condition, with slight variation, may be present at all times. Many women note an aggravation of symptoms in the premenstrual period, and an occasional one has symptoms only at that time. Periodicities may occur as a result of diminished physical activity (evenings or weekends), increased exposure to an allergen, or conditions of the atmosphere. But frequent variations in intensity of symptoms occur which cannot be explained.

In the acute phase of the syndrome, the secretions are watery, clear, and may be profuse. Later they become mucoid but remain clear. In a prolonged episode or in chronic cases with stagnation and poor drainage, the secretions may become flecked with solid material or become actually discolored.

Other symptoms or complications may accompany, or result from, hyperesthetic rhinitis. Headache is not uncommon. It is usually due to a closure of the sinus openings or a diminution of the air space in the sinus cavities from extension of the edematous reaction into the sinus mucosa. The headache is often located over the bridge of the nose or in the frontal or occipital region. There may be pain also over the maxillary areas. Acute or chronic infection of the sinuses is not a rare complication. Involvement of the Eustachian tubes is likely when there is itching or a feeling of "fulness" in the ears, pain, or impaired hearing or a sensation of abnormal noises. Chronic eustachitis, with serious loss of hearing, is not uncommon and may indeed constitute the major complaint, while the nasal symptoms responsible for it may be so slight as to be of no concern to the patient. In some instances, particularly in children, the eustachitis may lead to recurring episodes of purulent otitis media.

In persistent cases, postnasal discharge is quite common. Although most individuals with a postnasal syndrome without the conventional symptoms of hyperesthetic rhinitis are not allergic, occasionally postnasal discharge is the sole manifestation of an allergic nose. The postnasal secretions may cause a cough. On the other hand, since asthma develops in about one third of subjects with hyperesthetic rhinitis, the possibility that a cough is on a bronchial basis must always be kept in mind.

In chronic cases of perennial rhinitis, nasal polyps occur frequently; estimates vary between 10 and 25 percent. They may appear as outpouchings (polypoid) or as mature pedunculated structures. They are comparatively rare in young children and occur ordinarily when the allergy is complicated by infection. In some instances polyps are diagnosed without previous evidence of hyperesthetic rhinitis. There are conflicting opinions as to the significance of polyps in relation to allergy of the nose [2]. Our experience does not indicate that the presence of polyps speaks more strongly for extrinsic allergy than their absence. There appears to be an individual predilection to polyp formation. Many patients with severe chronic nasal symptoms do not have polyps, whereas many others with rather inconsequential rhinitis develop them readily. There is a special type of subject who is particularly prone to recurring polyp formation. Characteristically, he has severe asthma, pronounced nasal symptoms, the syndrome usually of recent development, and a history of allergy to aspirin [1]. In addition, usually no cause for the persistent allergic symptoms can be found.

Anosmia is one of the most disturbing complications of this syndrome. It may occur with persistent chronic rhinitis or even be the first symptom; it is more apt to appear after polyp formation or after surgery for removal of polyps.

CAUSATIVE FACTORS

Extrinsic allergic causes can be identified in 50 to 60 percent of cases of nonseasonal hyperesthetic rhinitis. For the most part, they are inhalants, most commonly house dust and frequently animal danders. In tropical and subtropical areas, molds, insect dusts, and pollen may induce a nonseasonal pattern. Foods are not common causes in adults but are relatively more important in early childhood. Occasionally, an allergy may be traced to such causes as *Ascaris* or pinworm infestation. There is also reason to believe that chronic infection of the paranasal structures may cause symptoms. Whether or not this is on the basis of a bacterial allergy is not certain. Nevertheless in 30 to 40 percent of individuals with symptoms of hyperesthetic rhinitis no allergic or any other primary cause can be determined.

A number of secondary factors aggravate the condition. Cold air and particularly drafts are disturbing. At times, temperature changes seem to be a sole primary cause. High humidity or very dry air usually makes the condition worse. The process of eating will sometimes clear the nose, whereas a full stomach is apt to increase the discomfort. Exercise is likely to improve it, but quiet and repose may aggravate it. Acute emotional upsets, fright, or excitement may temporarily improve the symptoms, whereas persistent emotional distress may worsen them. Some have claimed that hypothyroidism is a cause [3]; we are not particularly impressed by this association. Marked septal deviations increase the symptoms, and it may even be that nasal spurs of themselves can be responsible for setting off reflexly this syndrome.

PHYSICAL AND LABORATORY FINDINGS

The inferior turbinates usually appear to be swollen and may actually meet the septum. They are of a bluish or pearly gray color and look water-logged. The rest of the mucosa may assume a similar color, although in some instances the mucous membrane is red. Polyps may be seen on simple inspection, or their visualization may require complete nasal examination. The upper lip and the skin on the tip of the nose may show inflammation and excoriation from the discharge and from nose-wiping. Transillumination may disclose clouding or a fluid level, particularly if the sinuses are infected. Roentgen examination gives frequent information regarding infection, the presence of a thickened membrane, and even polyps not readily seen on nasal examination. Sinus lavage to determine infection is indicated in some instances. In patients who have had the nasal condition since early childhood, structural changes in the upper jaw frequently are evident as a result of mouth-breathing. The palate is high and narrow and the upper jaw is elongated, resulting in an overbite that almost certainly eventually requires orthodontic correction.

Nasal smears are often helpful. Characteristically, there are numerous eosinophils in the secretions. A smear showing almost all neutrophilic polymorphonuclear cells implies acute infection or other marked irritation or stasis. In the case of an infection complicating an allergic condition, both types of cells may be present in large numbers or neutrophils may predominate. If there is a small number of eosinophils and they occur in groups, this suggests allergy. Sometimes one must search for a clump of eosinophils. Many times the secretions are watery and contain almost no cells. It is important to look for the solid flecks in the secretion where the cells are apt to be found. One sees many patients with typical symptoms of allergic rhinitis, with eosinophils in nasal secretions, yet totally without evidence of extrinsic allergic factors, as determined by skin tests, elimination diets, and environmental changes. No one knows whether these symptoms are caused by unknown extrinsic allergens, intrinsic allergic mechanisms, or by other factors which, through release of histamine or of other mediators, produce the nasal manifestations and eosinophil chemotaxis.

One of the most common problems in connection with allergic rhinitis is to distinguish an acute exacerbation from the advent of a common cold. In the latter, the symptoms and watery rhinorrhea in the first two days may be indistinguishable from allergy. It is here in particular that a nasal smear may be helpful. Staining can be done with either Wright or Giemsa stain. A stained blood smear showing an increased eosinophil count may also be helpful, but it is to be remembered that blood eosinophilia does not indicate where the allergic inflammation occurs, and, furthermore, a normal count is quite common in nasal allergy.

SPECIFIC TESTS

This general subject is covered extensively elsewhere in this volume. Here we need only to make several points that apply to hyperesthetic rhinitis. Positive reactions to skin tests, scratch or intradermal, are noted in 50 to 60 percent of cases, as against 98 or 99 percent of seasonal cases. The percentage may be higher in a select group, e.g., children.* Inhalants are the most common reactors although foods cause reactions in some. Eye or nose tests with inhalants have been recommended by some either to show mucous membrane sensitivity when skin reactivity is not present [5] or to indicate the clinical significance of a skin reactor [6]. We feel that in most instances the clinical evaluation of a skin reactor by this means can be misleading. Usually an inhalant antigen which causes a strong reaction on the skin will also cause a conjunctival or nasal reaction if the concentration is adequate, and yet, under clinical conditions, the substance may not be a source of symptoms. Our experience also indicates that a positive mucous membrane reaction in the presence of a negative skin reaction is exceptional.

Only history (past), observation (present), and planned changes (future) can disclose the clinical significance of suspected allergenic substances. In many instances, the positive skin (or eye or nose) reactions are not clinically significant or at least do not signify the sole cause of the disease, since elimination of the reactors does not give complete relief. Significance of the seasonal reactors is seldom difficult to assess.

Hyperesthetic rhinitis is easily diagnosed. Only rare conditions may be confused with it. Although many patients fail to give positive reactions to skin tests or respond to clinical trials, most of them have the stigmata of allergy, such as a family history, other atopic symptoms, and nasal eosinophilia. It is suspected, though not proved, that most of this group are allergic, that the unknown factor might be an atmospheric but unrecognized antigen, or, perhaps, that hyperesthetic rhinitis might, at times, be an "intrinsic" allergic disease.

It appears that other than cases of atopy in which the offending allergen is detected and which thereby present a recognizable pattern,

* Recent investigations [4] have shown that subjects with delayed skin hypersensitivity reactions induced by an injection of emulsified pollen extract develop rhinorrhea and nasal obstruction associated primarily with mononuclear infiltration of the nasal tissue six hours or later after the pollen extract is placed in the nose. These findings tend to cast doubt on the necessity for the presence of a classic antigen-antibody interaction to explain atopic-like symptoms.

hyperesthetic rhinitis involves a bewildering array of contradictions. Numerous physical and other environmental circumstances, for reasons unknown, benefit some patients and make others worse. Periodicities are only partially explained. Polyps appear inexplicably in some individuals, in others, not; and cases that point to allergy may not be proved to be allergic. There are those who would identify hypothyroidism as an etiological factor; others disagree.

With this partial list of uncertainties, it becomes important to recognize that mucosal edema is the constant lesion in all cases. Edema, of course, is the common denominator of many atopic lesions. Hyperesthetic rhinitis, then, may be an example of an "atopic state" in which atopy cannot be clinically identified. The recognition of this situation by clinicians will obviate disappointments when specific treatment is applied to all cases.

REFERENCES

1. Feinberg, S. M., Durham, O. C., and Dragstedt, C. A. *Allergy in Practice* (2nd ed.). Chicago: Year Book Publishers, Inc., 1946.
2. Kern, R. A., and Schenck, H. P. Allergy, a constant factor in the etiology of so-called mucous nasal polyps. *J. Allerg.* 4:485, 1933.
3. Huber, H. L., and Harsh, G. F. The so-called "nonallergic" vasomotor rhinitis. *J. Allerg.* 5:432, 1934.
4. Slavin, R. G., Fink, J. N., Becker, R. J., Tennenbaum, J. I., and Feinberg, S. M. Delayed response to antigen challenge in induced delayed reactivity. *J. Allerg.* 35:499, 1964.
5. Rudolph, J. A., and Cohen, M. B. Vasomotor rhinitis with negative skin tests: Local nasal allergy. *J. Allerg.* 5:476, 1934.
6. Fineman, A. H. Studies in hypersensitiveness: XXIII. A comparative study of the intradermal, scratch, and conjunctival tests in determining the degree of pollen sensitivity. *J. Immun.* 11:465, 1926.

47. *Allergic Rhinitis—Relation to Sinusitis and Polyps*

RUSSELL CLARK GROVE

THE RELATION OF ALLERGIC RHINITIS to sinusitis and polyps has been for many years one of the most controversial of the manifestations of allergy. Many allergists and otolaryngologists disregard the importance of sinusitis; others, among whom the late Robert Cooke was the leading exponent, emphasize its importance.

Several points must be clarified. The following discussion applies to allergic rhinitis of the perennial type, often called vasomotor rhinitis, not to pollen or seasonal rhinitis. The term simply means that the nasal membranes have the capacity of vasodilatation and vasoconstriction when subjected to certain extrinsic or intrinsic factors. Whether or not sinusitis and polyps are the result of the allergic rhinitis has been a point of debate. The investigation reported later favors the view that sinusitis and polyps are often the cause of rhinitis, possibly through the mechanism of bacterial allergy.*

Sinusitis may be the primary or secondary cause of allergic rhinitis. In the secondary type, sinusitis is associated with allergens which also contribute to the rhinitis under certain conditions. The diagnosis and management of these allergic patients can be achieved only by thorough combined allergic and rhinological examinations.

To obtain an understanding of the relation between allergic rhinitis and sinusitis, 225 patients were studied in terms of history, allergy skin tests, laboratory tests, and rhinological and x-ray examinations. In 95 (42.2 percent) the rhinitis was associated with allergens, as demonstrated by positive skin reactions, or with foods, as determined by elimination diets. The other 130 had negative skin reactions or the allergic factors were mildly contributory. In these 130 patients, sinusitis and, in many, polyps were present and were either a primary or a secondary factor.

Hansen-Pruss [1] made two separate studies, one, in patients with what he called allergic rhinitis, which included pollinosis, and a second in patients with perennial rhinitis. In the first group of 287 patients, 214 (74.8 percent) had sinusitis and polyps. In the second group of 93 patients, 61 (64.5 percent) also had sinusitis and polyps. Kern [2] stated that 89 percent of his patients with allergic rhinitis had sinus involvement.

To show that the relation of allergic rhinitis to sinusitis and polyps is comparable to other allergic situations, a comprehensive study was made of the 130 patients mentioned earlier in whom the infection of sinusitis was considered the primary or secondary cause of the allergic rhinitis. There were 73 men and 57 women. (Rackemann [3] found that 73 percent of his patients were women, and Winkenwerder and Gay [4] 64.6 percent.) Average age of the 130 patients when first seen was 40 years. Only 27 (20 percent) were in the first three decades. In contrast to this incidence, the age of these patients at the time of onset of the disease is interesting; in fact, 56 percent had their onset of symptoms in the first three decades and 70 percent in the first four decades. In Rackemann's group of 257 patients, only 11 percent had their onset after age 40, and in Winkenwerder and Gay's 158 patients, approximately 83 percent had their onset in the first four decades.

There was a family history of allergy in 42

* *Editor's comment:* The chapter summarizes the clinical evidence which links allergic rhinitis to sinusitis and to nasal polyps. It does not attempt to discuss the pathogenesis of these diseases, but includes opinions—based on the author's extensive experience—about possible cause and effect relationships. It acknowledges the controversy about the etiologic significance of co-existing atopic disease and suggests that much work remains to be done before a confident decision about the most feasible approach to therapy can be made.—M. S.

percent of 99 patients who were definite about their antecedent history. Rackemann [3] found the family history positive in 25 percent of his group, and Winkenwerder and Gay [4] stated that less than one half of their patients had a family history of allergy.

The duration of the symptoms varied from 3 months to 50 years or a complete lifetime. Only seven patients had had symptoms less than 6 months; 76, from 1 to 10 years, and 28 had a duration of over 20 years.

A history of associated allergies was obtained in 60 percent of 113 patients from whom a definite past history was obtained. Asthma was the most common, occurring in 47 percent and in 15 percent having developed in early life. However, in a good many cases, the asthma and allergic rhinitis developed at the same time, with the onset of an upper respiratory tract infection. Seasonal hay fever was second in incidence, with 16.5 percent; urticaria was present in 13.5 percent and eczema in 1.5 percent. Clarke and Rogers [5] reported that among 162 patients with allergic rhinitis, men were more likely to have asthma and hay fever than women. Winkenwerder and Gay [4] found asthma to be a complication of allergic rhinitis in 51 percent, hay fever in 32 percent, eczema in 10 percent, and urticaria in 6 percent. It is interesting that Weille [6] expressed the opinion that sooner or later asthma would develop in 15 percent of the patients with allergic rhinitis, a rather conservative estimate.

Examinations of the nasal secretions for eosinophils showed that 56 percent of 70 patients had values of 1 to 4 plus. Winkenwerder and Gay [4] found eosinophils in only 12 percent. Hansel [7] has emphasized the importance of this method of diagnosis if examinations are made during or immediately after an acute attack. Of 80 patients, 65 percent had a blood eosinophil count over 5 percent, usually below 15 percent. Others also have commented on the association of high eosinophil values with infection [8–10].

All 130 patients had skin tests: 68 (51.5 percent) had no appreciable positive reactions; the others gave single or multiple positive reactions of varying intensity. Thirteen were sensitive to house dust alone, and 42 to house dust and other allergens; 34 were sensitive to pollens, 20 to chicken feathers, the remainder to miscellaneous allergens. Positive reactions to food were few; Cooke [11] stated that not more than 2 to 3 percent of cases of nasal allergy are caused by foods. Rowe [12] and Tuft [13], however, emphasized the importance of foods in this condition.

Drug reactions are frequent in these patients with infection. Histories disclosed hypersensitivity to: alcohol, procaine, bromides, pentobarbital sodium, codeine, oxytetracycline, demethylchlortetracycline, 1 each; sulfonamides, 2; cocaine and iodides, 3; penicillin, 12; and aspirin, 19. Apparently, the infective group is more often sensitive to aspirin than the noninfective group. Cooke [14] in 1919 had observed only 1 positive skin reaction to aspirin in a patient clinically sensitive to it. Duke [15] in 1933 had never seen one. Tissue reactions to iodides, penicillin, sulfonamides, alcohol, and cocaine applied locally were significant.

On rhinological examination of the 130 patients, one or both maxillary sinuses were cloudy on transillumination in 104 (80 percent). In the rest, however, the sinuses were clear, indicating that this method of examination does not give conclusive diagnostic evidence. This observation was made in 1940 by Grove and Cooke [16], who injected a radiopaque solution into the sinuses (Fig. 47-1).

Nasal polyps were present in 77 (59 percent) of the patients, being bilateral in 62 and unilateral in 15; pus was found in 33 and mulberry hypertrophy of the posterior tip of the inferior turbinate in 6 patients. Woodward and Swineford [17] in 128 patients found only 12.5 percent with nasal polyps, a seemingly small number. Hansen-Pruss [1] reported a greater incidence.

These 130 patients with infection selected from the 225 individuals with allergic rhinitis all had x-ray evidence of sinusitis of varying degrees (Fig. 47-2). Maxillary and ethmoidal sinusitis, unilateral or bilateral, was present in 55 patients. Six had cysts in the maxillary sinuses. Since 80 percent of the total group were in the age group 30 to 60 years, it is not surprising that sinusitis was so extensive.

After the skin tests and the clinical and x-ray examinations of the nose and sinuses, the question of etiology was considered in terms of the points of view of both the rhinologist and the allergist who saw these patients. It was decided that demonstrable allergy was a factor in less than one fourth of the patients.

From the foregoing observations, it seems apparent that polyps and sinusitis are not al-

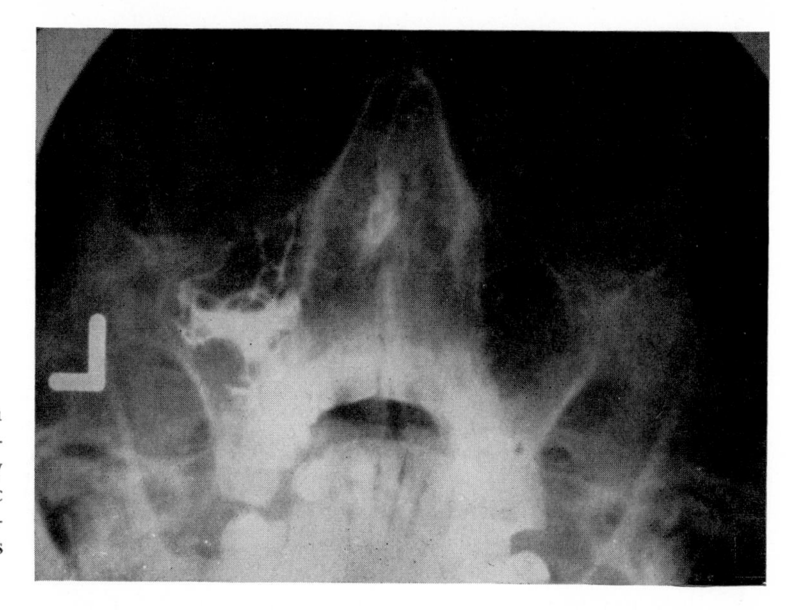

Fig. 47-1. Roentgenogram made after injection of Lipiodol into the left maxillary sinus, showing characteristic polypoid changes in the mucous membrane. This sinus transilluminated clearly.

ways secondary to allergic rhinitis but may be considered primary diseases of the nasal and paranasal mucous membranes. With an overwhelming exposure of the nose to skin-sensitizing types of allergens, such as pollens or house dust, polyps may appear in the ethmoid regions, but these do not often become permanent unless associated with infection. Eagle [18] emphasized the importance of infection in these patients and has been a strong exponent of bacterial allergy as an etiological factor, and Grove and Cooke [19] reported bacteriological findings in chronic sinusitis.

Polyps are rarely observed in the maxillary sinuses as the result of nonbacterial allergens. For instance, during or immediately after constitutional reactions to an injection, x-ray films of sinuses known previously to be normal did not reveal so-called "allergic sinusitis." Moreover, injection into the maxillary sinuses of a radiopaque substance during severe nasal reactions to pollen revealed no abnormality.

It has been observed that polyps in the maxillary sinuses only occasionally disappear with antihistamine and steroid therapy. When they diminish (rarely disappear), it is probable that early edema is present; or if in cases of long duration antibiotics are used in conjunction with steroids, the infection is

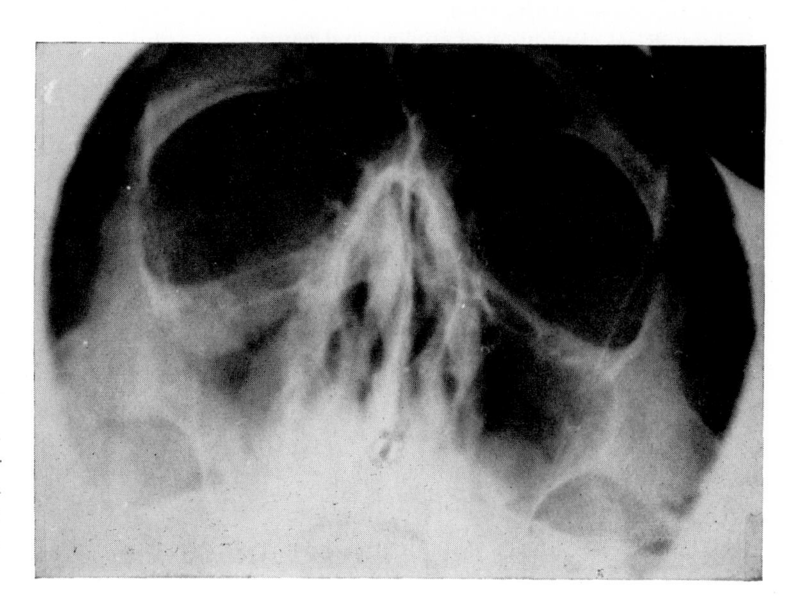

Fig. 47-2. Roentgenogram showing extensive hyperplastic polypoid pathology seen often in patients with allergic rhinitis and sinusitis with polyps.

controlled and not the allergy. The ethmoid polyps are more responsive to steroid therapy than are maxillary polyps.

In the past few years, not many articles have been written about nasal polyps, and those few concern their relation to systemic diseases rather than to allergic rhinitis [20]. The pathogenesis of allergic rhinitis and polyps is discussed in Chapter 45.

Samter [21] has stressed the fact that atopic patients may have perennial rhinitis and bronchial asthma from early childhood whereas nonatopic patients may not develop nasal polyps and asthma until later life. The importance of infection in the later group as well as in the atopic group should be emphasized. Samter pointed out that acetylsalicylic acid sensitivity is found frequently in the nonatopic patients.

In a comprehensive presentation dealing with nasal polyps, Lederer [22] gave a short discussion of vasomotor (allergic) rhinitis and stated: "Many clinicians deem vasomotor rhinitis to be of functional or psychosomatic origin. These same observers are of the opinion that continued vasomotor rhinitis may lead to polyps and they consider psychotherapy prominent in the management of recurrent polyps." Whereas psychosomatic problems are very important in the symptoms of allergic rhinitis, it is unlikely that they influence the development of nasal polyps.

Hollender [23] quoted Yago, who believes that nasal polyps have a closer relation to sinusitis than to allergic rhinitis or bronchial asthma. A study of 102 pathological specimens, however, showed edema and eosinophilic infiltration, which suggested a close relation to allergy. Marked eosinophilia of the sinus membranes is frequently present in patients with bacterial infection.

Textbooks on allergy make little mention of the relation of allergic rhinitis to polyps and sinusitis. Chait [24] gives a good, though brief, discussion of nasal polyps. He stated that only one third of the total number of patients with polyps had atopic nasal symptoms alone (hay fever and allergic rhinitis), but he did not emphasize the relation to perennial rhinitis. He did contend that nasal polyps would appear concurrently with an upper respiratory infection and disappear spontaneously when the infection had subsided, an observation that has been made by others. Chait found that polyps may subside permanently after conventional specific and nonspecific management. There is controversy about this prognosis, since apparently a large number of these patients eventually will need surgery.

REFERENCES

1. Hansen-Pruss, O. C. Bacterial allergy and the importance of otolaryngological procedures. *Laryngoscope* 59:540, 1949.
2. Kern, R. A. Discussion of etiology and nature of chronic hyperplastic sinusitis. *J. Allerg.* 4:545, 1933.
3. Rackemann, F. M. *Clinical Allergy, Particularly Asthma and Hay Fever: Mechanism and Treatment.* New York: Macmillan Company, 1931.
4. Winkenwerder, W. L., and Gay, L. N. Perennial allergic rhinitis: An analysis of 198 cases. *Bull. Hopkins Hosp.* 2:90, 1937.
5. Clarke, J. A., Jr., and Rogers, H. C. Statistical study of allergic (vasomotor) rhinitis. *Arch. Otolaryng.* 25:124, 1937.
6. Weille, F. L. Studies in asthma: Surgical treatment of chronic sinusitis in asthma. *J.A.M.A.* 100:241, 1933.
7. Hansel, F. K. Further observations on the cytology of the nasal secretions in allergy. *J. Allerg.* 10:251, 1959.
8. Spain, W. C. Allergic Rhinitis: Perennial. In Cooke, R. A. (Ed.), *Allergy in Theory and Practice.* Philadelphia: W. B. Saunders Company, 1947.
9. Feinberg, S. M., and Durham, O. C. *Allergy in Practice.* Chicago: Year Book Publishers, Inc., 1944.
10. Coca, D. F., Walzer, M., and Thommen, A. A. *Asthma and Hay Fever in Theory and Practice.* Springfield, Ill.: Charles C Thomas, Publisher, 1931.
11. Cooke, R. A. Allergy in rhinology. *Laryngoscope* 40:210, 1930.
12. Rowe, A. H. Nasal allergy. *Arch. Otolaryng.* 28:98, 1938.
13. Tuft, L. *Clinical Allergy.* Philadelphia: W. B. Saunders Company, 1937.
14. Cooke, R. A. Allergy and drug idiosyncrasies. *J.A.M.A.* 73:759, 1919.
15. Duke, W. W. Aspirin allergy: A method of testing for aspirin sensitivity and a method of avoiding aspirin catastrophes. *J. Allerg.* 4:426, 1933.
16. Grove, R. C., and Cooke, R. A. The use of thorium dioxide in roentgenography of the sinuses. *Amer. J. Roentgen.* 44:680, 1940.

17. Woodward, F. D., and Swineford, O. Allergic rhinitis: Analysis of 128 cases in which rhinologist and allergist collaborated. *Arch. Otolaryng.* 34:1103, 1941.
18. Eagle, W. W. Bacterial allergy: Otolaryngological aspects. *Southern Med. J.* 10:908, 1942.
19. Grove, R. C., and Cooke, R. A. Etiology and nature of chronic hyperplastic sinusitis. *Arch. Otolaryng.* 18:622, 1933.
20. Samter, M. Nasal polyps: An inquiry into the mechanism of their formation. *Arch. Otolaryng.* 73:334, 1961.
21. Samter, M. Nasal polyps: Their relationship to allergy, particularly to bronchial asthma. *Med. Clin. N. Amer.*, p. 175, 1958.
22. Lederer, F. L. The problem of nasal polyps. *J. Allerg.* 30:420, 1959.
23. Hollender, M. D. Nasal polyps. *Eye, Ear, Nose, Throat Month.* 41:922, 1962.
24. Chait, R. A. Allergic Rhinitis and Nasal Polyps. In Prigal, S. J. (Ed.), *Fundamentals of Allergy*. New York: McGraw-Hill Book Company, Inc., 1960.

48. Physiology and Pathology of Bronchial Asthma

ELLIOTT MIDDLETON, JR.

BRONCHIAL ASTHMA IS CHARACTERized by episodic bronchial obstruction and ventilatory insufficiency and production of mucoid sputum. The essential pathological changes in the bronchi and bronchioles are mucosal edema, hypersecretion of a viscid, tenacious mucus, and smooth muscle contraction. Two types of bronchial asthma are recognized clinically: extrinsic asthma, for which the underlying immunological, biochemical, and pharmacological mechanisms are reasonably well defined, and intrinsic asthma, about which the causal mechanisms are poorly understood. However, both types share essentially the same physiological and pathological features; these will be considered in detail after a review of the normal anatomy and physiology of the bronchial tree.

NORMAL ANATOMY AND PHYSIOLOGY OF THE BRONCHIAL TREE

The lung is a vast capillary bed separated from the alveolar spaces by a vital delicate membrane across which gas exchange occurs. Transport of air to and from the air–blood junction is provided by the branched tracheobronchial system, the main successive divisions of which are: primary bronchi, secondary bronchi, bronchioles, terminal bronchioles, and respiratory bronchioles, followed by alveolar ducts, alveolar sacs, and alveoli [1, 2]. The bronchi and bronchioles are nonrespiratory, air-conducting, semirigid tubes irregularly girdled by cartilage. They have their own blood supply and innervation, both sensory and motor. A sheath of connective tissue enveloping the larger bronchi and their early subdivisions permits them to change in length and in diameter without directly affecting adjacent lung parenchyma. This connective tissue sheath becomes sparse at the periphery of the bronchial subdivisions and, at about the point where cartilage disappears, freely interlaces with the connective tissue of the surrounding lung parenchyma. Since the smallest airways and terminal air spaces have no cartilaginous support, their patency depends on constant tractional forces afforded by the intricate latticework of elastic, collagenous, and reticular fibers. The mechanical stability of the lung is also determined in part by the unique surfactant properties of a lecithin-containing film lining the alveoli [3, 4]. Figure 48-1 shows a cross-section of a normal bronchus.

INNERVATION OF THE AIRWAYS

Branches of the autonomic nervous system provide the innervation of the airways [5]. *Efferent* parasympathetic (vagal) and sympathetic nerves coming through the cardiac and pulmonary plexuses enter the lung and spread throughout its ramifications to innervate the smooth muscle, glands, blood vessels, and mucous membrane. The plexus around the large pulmonary vessels gives origin to parasympathetic postganglionic nerve fibers. Two main types of *afferent* end-organ found in the bronchial wall are known to have physiological importance. Subepithelial receptors, considered responsible for the cough reflex, are found concentrated at points of branching from the trachea to the proximal end of the respiratory bronchioles. Smooth muscle endings, which are responsible for the Hering-Breuer inflation reflex, occur throughout the smooth muscle of the respiratory tract and are

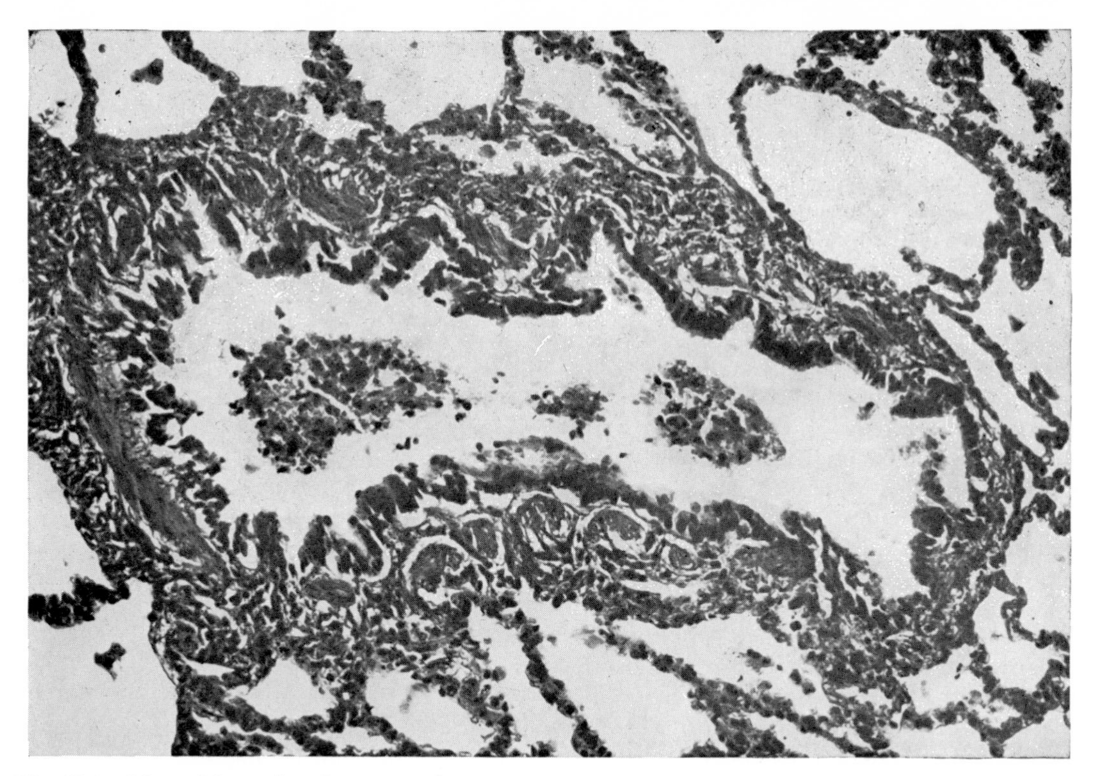

Fig. 48-1. Normal bronchus for comparison with Figure 48-2. (× 144.)

smaller and less numerous in the narrower passages.

TRACHEOBRONCHIAL AND BRONCHIOLAR EPITHELIUM

Throughout the respiratory tree there is an epithelial lining. In the larger tracheobronchial passages, a pseudostratified columnar epithelium is found which rests upon the lamina propria. The following types of cells and structures make up the epithelium and mucosa [1, 2, 6]. *Ciliated columnar cells* are tall cells with about 270 cilia per cell. Extending into the lumen, the cilia are bathed in a watery fluid beneath the overlying mucous blanket. The ciliary processes do not actually extend into the mucous film, but their moving tips impinge upon its under surface. *Goblet cells,* found singly or in groups among the ciliated cells, are the tall nonciliated vacuolated cells. The mucus secreted by them joins that produced by the submucosal mucous glands to form the sheet of mucus which overlies the cilia. *Brush cells* are best seen with the aid of the electron microscope. The nonciliated brush cells are found between goblet cells with which they are in close contact by cytoplasminic projections that suggest a nutritive function. Possibly they provide some of the low-viscosity fluid which bathes the cilia. *Basal cells* are short cells stationed on the basement membrane between the tapered ends of the tall columnar cells. Basal cells may, on demand, be capable of differentiating into ciliated or nonciliated tall cells.

All of these specialized cells rest on a *basement membrane,* composed of reticulin and collagen fibers, that is 4 to 7 μ in thickness. The *lamina propria* lies beneath the basement membrane and consists of a small amount of reticular and collagenous connective tissue and many elastic fibers, especially in its deeper portions, resting on the smooth muscle layer. A network of capillaries, lymphatics, and the fine ramifications of nerves is found in the lamina propria. Scattered lymphocytes are normally seen also. Human lung connective tissue also has an abundant complement of mast cells [7, 8], a rich source of histamine. Beneath the smooth muscle lie the deep bronchial mucous glands and beyond this the cartilaginous layer.

As the peripheral bronchioles are approached, the epithelium becomes simple columnar and finally cuboidal in type. Cilia are not present in these fine ramifications. Mucus-producing glands and goblet cells decrease in number in the smaller bronchi and disappear, as does cartilage, in the narrow-lumen bronchioles of about 1 mm. diameter.

MUCUS FORMATION AND CILIARY ACTION

The mucous film normally covering the epithelium of the lower respiratory tract originates from goblet cells and mucus-producing glands. It consists in part of mucopolysaccharides and mucoprotein [9] and serves as a protective barrier for the epithelium. Two types of glandular acini may be distinguished, mucous and serous [6]. Serous glands predominate, mucous acini usually being few and scattered. Serous acini characteristically show minute granules which fill the cytoplasm, are basophilic, and give a positive reaction with the periodic acid–Schiff stain (PAS), but occasionally are eosinophilic. Cytoplasm of the mucous cells contains large, weakly basophilic granules which stain strongly with PAS and mucicarmine. Adhering to the periphery of both types of glands are flat, elongated myoepithelial cells which may facilitate mucus secretion in a contractile manner. The gland ducts, lined by goblet cells, penetrate to the surface through the smooth muscle layer, lamina propria, and epithelium.

All of the factors which control secretion of mucus are not known, but glandular activity is influenced by cholinergic nerves [10], and hypersecretion is evoked by histamine, bradykinin, and acetylcholine.

The warmed and humidified air which passes from the nose to the lower respiratory tract is not entirely devoid of particulate matter, the removal of which is one of the functions of the mucous blanket which overlies the epithelium of the lower tract. This blanket is constantly moving upward toward the larynx and pharynx by the propelling action of the cilia, which beat in coordinated wavelike movements about 1,000 times each minute [11]. The cilia are not under nervous control, and the mechanism controlling their activity is unknown. There is a suggestion that ciliary action is governed by the acetylcholine-cholinesterase system [12], and others have implicated 5-hydroxytryptamine [13]. The movement of the mucous blanket (ciliary action) is very susceptible to drying and is affected by irritants such as smoke. Beginning with a sheet of mucus that must be meters in area extent at the periphery, there is a progressive increase in rate of flow and in thickness as the mucous blanket travels orad.

The deposition of particulate matter, which includes common allergens, in the respiratory tract depends on the combined forces of gravity, inertia, velocity, diffusion, the viscosity of the medium, and the density and nature of the particles. Those in the size range 0.25 to 0.50 μ have the lowest probability of being deposited in the respiratory tract. Elimination of deposited particulate matter is accomplished in part by phagocytosis [11]. Pulmonary phagocytes arrive in the air spaces after migrating from alveoli, capillaries, or tissue spaces and then either are swept out on the mucous blanket or return to the tissue. Digestible particulates may be broken down, but insoluble ones may remain in the lung for long periods.

SMOOTH MUSCLE OF THE LOWER RESPIRATORY TRACT

Beneath the mucosa lies a layer of smooth muscle which laces in all directions around the bronchi and bronchioles, never forming a closed ring, however [1]. Numerous elastic fibers are intimately associated with the smooth muscle cells throughout their extent in the bronchial tree. The mesh of smooth muscle is distinct to the end of the respiratory bronchioles, which begin with a diameter of about 0.5 mm., and even continues in the walls of the alveolar ducts. In these smaller tubes, the smooth muscle is thicker relative to the diameter of the lumen [14], suggesting that changes in bronchomotor tone might influence the diameter of these airways more because of the greater bulk of smooth muscle.

Control of Airway Smooth Muscle Tone. In quiet normal breathing, the airway muscle is in tonic contraction. This state of tonicity can be decreased by injection of atropine [15–18], by aerosol administration of isoproterenol [16, 17, 19, 20], and by vagotomy [21], as shown by increase in anatomical dead space, decrease in airway resistance, and increase in bronchial caliber. Airway muscle tone thus appears to be mediated by cholinergic vagal pathways. The normal tone provides a baseline for variations in tracheobronchial caliber in either direction, as, for example, bronchoconstriction in asthma.

Nervous regulation of airway smooth

muscle includes local and axon reflexes, central nervous control, the action of parasympathetic and sympathetic nerves, and reflex regulation (see Ref. 5 for detailed review). The anatomy of innervation of the lungs suggests the existence of *axon or local synaptic* reflexes which may play a part in the pulmonary vascular changes following inhalation of nebulized histamine. The *central* nervous origin of constrictor or dilator fibers remains unknown, but it seems reasonable to assume that constrictor fibers, like other vagal efferent nerves, may arise in the medulla. The activity of these nerves may in turn be influenced by nervous activity originating in higher (psychic) centers and thus account in part for the variability in bronchomotor tone as related to emotional states. *Parasympathetic* nerve overactivity leads to bronchoconstriction. Vagal stimulation causes displacement of air from the lungs, decreases airway caliber, and increases airway resistance—effects which are blocked by atropine, potentiated by eserine. On the other hand, stimulation of the *sympathetic* pathways produces a bronchodilator response. When the sympathetic nerves to the lungs are stimulated, catecholamines are released into the venous effluent: an isoproterenol-like substance has been identified. The possible importance of this finding to the identification of the sympathetic mediator in the airways is obvious. *Reflex* regulation is responsive to such influences as asphyxia, hypercapnia, hypoxemia, lung inflation, irritation of the respiratory epithelium and pulmonary vascular bed, the action of drugs on chemoreceptors, and the effects of intravascular pressure changes on baroreceptors. The most important among these are probably hypercapnia, hypoxemia, and reflexes due to irritation of respiratory epithelium. Hypercapnia apparently produces parasympathetic airway constriction. General hypoxemia acts to increase tracheobronchial tone, an effect which may be mainly mediated by stimulation of carotid body chemoreceptors. Irritation of the respiratory epithelium from the nose to the bronchi almost uniformly produces a bronchoconstrictor response, confirming the presence of nasobronchial, laryngobronchial, and bronchobronchial reflex arcs. Since atropine or vagotomy, or both, generally block the bronchoconstrictor response, it is evident that the response is vagal and cholinergic in nature. A great variety of stimuli evoke the bronchoconstrictor response, e.g., mechanical, chemical, electrical, cold, and inhalation of inert dusts. Possibly some of these mechanisms are operative in asthma induced by inhaled irritants. It is well recognized that nonallergenic dusts and fumes, and cold air may induce bronchoconstriction in subjects with asthma [22].

PHYSIOLOGICAL AND PATHOLOGICAL CHANGES IN BRONCHIAL ASTHMA

Bronchial obstruction with impaired air flow and ventilatory insufficiency are the basic physiological alterations of respiration in asthma. The severity of obstruction to air flow varies with the degree of bronchial pathology: mucosal edema, mucus hypersecretion, and smooth muscle spasm. In severe forms of the disease, the ventilatory insufficiency may be great enough to cause hypoxemia, hypercapnia, cor pulmonale, and death from widespread obstruction of the bronchial passages by inspissated mucus. The normal tendency of the bronchial tree to narrow and shorten during expiration accounts for the acute overinflation of the lungs which tends to develop during bouts of severe asthma and also explains why the respiratory distress is primarily expiratory. During symptom-free intervals, lung function may be normal.

SPUTUM

Tenacious, stringy mucoid sputum causes coughing and contributes to the wheezing and dyspnea. Grossly, this mucus may form small grayish pearls which appear as tiny Curschmann spirals when spread on a glass slide. Superimposed bronchial infection causes the typical asthmatic sputum to become purulent. Methodological problems have hampered progress in investigations of the physical and chemical properties of sputum in asthma. This sputum consists not only of mucus secreted by tracheobronchial glands but also of contributions from epithelial cells lining the respiratory tract, eosinophils which accumulate as a result of allergic reactions, and, with infection, of bacteria and leukocytes and the products of their metabolism. Perhaps some of the pharmacologically active end products of the allergic stimulus also accumulate in sputum. The most important element in this composite material is the mucus.

Intrabronchial accumulation and stagnation of mucus is a cardinal cause of respiratory embarrassment. Normally, disposition of the mucus depends on ciliary activity for mechanical removal and perhaps some resorptive and digestive capacities of lung tissue for chemical removal. Excessive accumulation of intrabronchial mucus depresses ciliary activity, and the reverse is also true [23]. Whether there is some impairment of the chemical mechanisms of disposition of mucus in asthma is unknown.

Chemical studies of asthmatic sputum by Bukantz and Bern [24] have shown it to contain hexosamine, N-acetylhexosamine, and fucose, but neither uronic acids nor nucleoprotein. A large portion of sputum appeared to be a mucopolysaccharide, fractions of which had blood substance activity as determined by hemagglutination inhibition experiments. In some studies, no chemical differences between asthmatic and normal bronchial mucus have been demonstrated [24, 25]. Mendes *et al.* [26] have reported that asthmatic sputum may contain serum proteins and other proteins not immunologically related to them. Although the state of hydration affects the viscosity of mucus, this factor alone may not account entirely for its highly viscid nature in asthma. Possibly a higher state of polymerization of normal mucus constituents contributes to the high viscosity. Improvement of analytical techniques may provide answers to many of these questions.

GROSS AND MICROSCOPIC PATHOLOGY

The histopathology of asthma has been carefully examined by a number of workers since the basic description of Huber and Koessler in 1922 [27]. Recently, the subject has been reviewed by Cardell and Pearson [28], who correlated the clinical and pathological findings. Certain characteristic pulmonary lesions are found in subjects dying of asthma. The lungs are distended with air and do not collapse when the chest is opened. The extremely viscid, tenacious mucus is found in abundance in bronchi of all sizes and completely occludes the lumen of some. Often there are some congestion of the lung and small areas of collapse.

The histological lesions are most readily observed in bronchi measuring 2 to 5 mm. in diameter. Within the mucus are many eosinophils, variable numbers of shed bronchial epithelial cells, and, occasionally, Charcot-Leyden crystals. Shedding of clusters of epithelial cells, many of them bearing cilia, has been shown to occur with greater frequency in asthma than in other respiratory diseases and increases considerably during asthmatic attacks [29]. It appears to hinder recovery from attacks, for in severe asthma, ciliated cells that desquamate may not be replaced, and this might facilitate bronchial infection. It probably is caused by subepithelial edema.

Thickening, congestion and edema of the bronchial wall are also seen, and, with smooth muscle contraction, the inner aspect of the bronchioles appears folded. The smooth muscle appears to be thickened. In the epithelial layer, areas of shedding and squamous metaplasia may be seen. Mucous glands are prominent and distended, and mucus-engorged goblet cells are common. Thickening and hyalinization of the basement membrane is also a common feature but not specific [30]. Chronicity of asthma is probably important in determining the degree of thickening of the basement membrane, since it was not apparent in an infant dying of asthma. The whole thickness of the bronchial wall reveals cellular infiltration which consists mainly of eosinophilic leukocytes and quite frequently of numerous plasma cells. The bronchiolar pathology is similar but may not show as much contraction or folding of the mucous membrane. Often the bronchioles are completely filled with mucus, which may extend into the alveoli. Figure 48-2 shows the microscopic changes in a bronchus from an asthmatic.

The changes just described are the principal findings in uncomplicated fatal asthma. True pulmonary emphysema with breakdown of alveolar walls and coalescence of alveoli is not found in uncomplicated asthma. Nor is bronchiectasis a common accompaniment. Additional pulmonary lesions occur from chronic bronchitis, with which some degree of peribronchial and pulmonary fibrosis is encountered. The cardinal features of the pathology are: bronchial plugging by mucus, infiltration of the mucous membrane by eosinophils, and thickening of the basement membrane.

Biopsy studies obtained during life from asthmatic patients have revealed that the extent of these changes correlates well with the

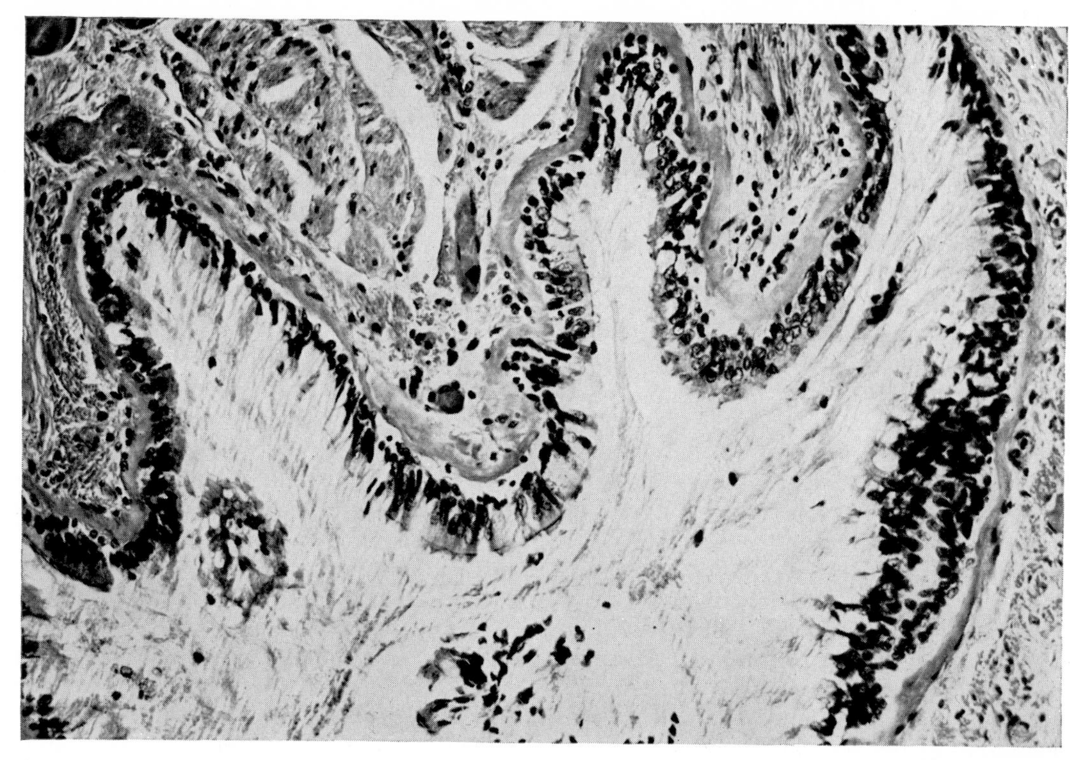

Fig. 48-2. Bronchial asthma. The lumen of the bronchus is filled with mucus which is streaming from the bronchial epithelium. Note very thick hyalinized basement membrane beneath the epithelial layer and slight chronic inflammation of the peribronchial connective tissue. The muscle appears thicker than in the normal bronchus. (× 144.)

activity of the asthma [6]. Indeed, in symptom-free subjects, biopsy material may show little or none of the "typical" pathology. Goblet cell hyperplasia was found on biopsy in asthma and bronchitis, but asthmatics had a preponderance of morphologically normal deep serous glands. In chronic bronchitis, the mucous acini were increased in size and number. It is interesting that in biopsies, thickening of the basement membrane was not a constant finding. In fact, thinning, and reduplication, as well as thickening of the basement membrane in asthmatics were reported by Glynn and Michaels. A characteristic feature in asthmatic tissue was eosinophilic infiltration of the lamina propria.

CHEMICAL PATHOLOGY

Most of the biochemical changes which produce allergic (and, conceivably, nonallergic) bronchial asthma have been identified [31–34]. It is certain that asthma is distinguished not only by the release of active substances but also by the exaggerated response of the bronchial tree to the chemical mediators of anaphylaxis (see Chap. 15). A number of published reports testify to the fact that the asthmatic bronchial tree is overly sensitive to the actions of inhaled histamine [35, 36], acetylcholine [36], slow-reacting substance [37], and bradykinin [38, 39]. Whether this heightened reactivity is due to some special property of capillaries, mucous glands, smooth muscle, or some other structure in asthmatic lung is unknown.

It is evident, however, that histamine, and any other mediators of bronchoconstriction, once released or formed as a result of the antigen-antibody interaction, must traverse a finite intercellular space before reaching an effector cell (capillary, mucous gland, smooth muscle, sensory nerve ending). Perhaps the chemical characteristics of the intercellular space and the ground substance filling it are of critical importance in determining the activity of these chemicals on the effector cells. There is some reason to believe that the chemical pathology of asthma may involve ground substance rather than unique cell responsiveness. It is in this region of microanatomy that extracellular acid-base balance and the ionic environment of cells (which affects their response to stimuli) is maintained. To a significant degree the ionic environment will be determined by the state of aggregation of the intercellular colloidal ground substance. The fundamental changes that occur in this colloid as a result of allergic reactions in the mucous membrane of the nose is reviewed in Chapter 45. Briefly, the ground substance mucopolysaccharides lose normal stainability (PAS) as a result of allergic reactions [40], indicating disaggregation of the colloid [41]. It seems entirely plausible to assume that similar changes may occur in the ground substance of the bronchial tree. With disaggregation of the colloid, its capacity to bind organic and inorganic ions and its effect on local water balance may be altered. Thus it seems conceivable that the effector cell activity of histamine, other mediators, and inorganic ions such as potassium and calcium may be influenced by the degree of colloid aggregation.

Finally, mention should be made of the importance of the acetylcholine-cholinesterase system and the autonomic nervous system in asthma. Acetylcholine has long been an enigma with regard to its possible participation in the pathogenesis of asthma. Some early workers considered asthma to be a disease of dysautonomia [42], suggesting that it represented a state of parasympathetic preponderance. (Recent speculation [43] regarding the importance of the autonomic nervous system has centered on the hypothesis that asthma may in part result from a functional imbalance between two types of *adrenergic* effector systems, the alpha and beta [44]. A more detailed description of this subject appears in Chapter 16.) Cholinergic nerves are known to be important in the control of normal bronchial smooth muscle tone and to influence the secretory activity of bronchial mucous glands. As with histamine, many subjects with asthma are overly sensitive to inhaled acetylcholine or Mecholyl, developing acute bronchoconstriction on exposure to these agents [36]. Tiffeneau [45] has carefully examined the threshold of excitability of the bronchomotor system and found it to be decreased to variable degrees in asthmatic patients. Thus the threshold dose of acetylcholine (administered by aerosol) required to bring about bronchoconstriction was moderately or markedly reduced in asthmatics, in some cases to one one-thousandth of the amount required to cause ventilatory changes in normal subjects. The threshold of excitability was reduced by allergic reactions, bronchopulmonary infection, psychic trauma, and by inhaled irritants which stimulate bronchoconstrictor reflexes.

Although Scudamore *et al.* [46] reported increased levels of acetylcholine in venous blood of asthmatic subjects, Michelson and Lowell [47] were unable to confirm these results. Of course, the rapidity with which acetylcholine is destroyed by its specific enzymatic inactivator, cholinesterase, might account for failure to detect increased liberation at the cellular level. Brocklehurst [48], however, failed to show release of acetylcholine during *in vitro* anaphylaxis in guinea pig lung. Nakamura [49], on the other hand, marshaled impressive evidence that acetylcholine is an important mediator of anaphylaxis in experimental animals. Absolute chemical identification was not achieved, however, and many interesting effects observed by Nakamura—augmentation of the Schultz-Dale reaction or *in vivo* anaphylaxis by eserine—might be explained by reflex activity involving cholinergic nerves. Along these lines is the suggestion of Samter [50] that depressed cholinesterase activity, either by natural variation or by drugs which inhibit cholinesterase (e.g., prostigmine), may enhance bronchoconstriction or urticarial reactions in patients sensitive to acetylsalicylic acid, and morphine, a notoriously dangerous drug for asthmatics and a known inhibitor of cholinesterase, might cause severe bronchoconstriction. Indeed, the experiments of Karczewski [51] showed that anaphylactic shock in guinea pigs was accompanied by marked increase in the electrophysiological pattern of activity of the vagus nerve, involving both afferent and efferent pathways. It was concluded that the increase in afferent activity was directly related to the anaphylactic reaction taking place in the lung, i.e., to bronchoconstriction and stimulation of pulmonary stretch receptors. Increased activity in the efferent motor fibers was attributed to reflex stimulation which produced further bronchoconstriction. Further study of these effects and other aspects of the chemical pathology of asthma will enhance understanding of the complexities of this disease.

REFERENCES

1. Maximow, A. A., and Bloom, W. *A Textbook of Histology*. Philadelphia: W. B. Saunders Company, 1944.
2. Krahl, V. E. Microstructure of the lung. *Arch. Environ. Health* 6:37, 1963.
3. Clements, J. A. Surface tension in the lungs. *Sci. American,* December, 1962.
4. Radford, E. P. Mechanical stability of the lung. *Arch. Environ. Health* 6:128, 1963.
5. Widdicombe, J. G. Regulation of tracheobronchial smooth muscle. *Physiol. Rev.* 43:1, 1963.
6. Glynn, A. A., and Michaels, L. Bronchial biopsy in chronic bronchitis and asthma. *Thorax* 15:142, 1960.
7. Riley, J. F. *The Mast Cells*. Edinburgh: E. & S. Livingstone, Ltd., 1959.
8. Salvato, G. Mast cells in bronchial connective tissue of man. *Experientia* 15:308, 1959.
9. Brogan, T. D. The carbohydrate complexes of bronchial secretion. *Biochem. J.* 71:125, 1959.
10. Goodman, L. S., and Gilman, A. *The Pharmacological Basis of Therapeutics* (2nd ed.). New York: Macmillan Company, 1955.
11. Hilding, A. C. Phagocytosis, mucous flow, and ciliary action. *Arch. Environ. Health* 6:61, 1963.
12. Kordik, P., Burn, J. H., and Bulbring, E. Ciliary movement and acetylcholine. *Brit. J. Pharmacol.* 7:67, 1952.
13. Gosselin, R. E. The cilioexcitatory activity of serotonin. *J. Cell. Comp. Physiol.* 58:17, 1961.
14. Miller, W. S. *The Lung* (2nd ed.). Springfield, Ill.: Charles C Thomas, Publisher, 1947.
15. Severinghaus, J. W., and Stupfel, M. Respiratory dead space increase following atropine in man, and atropine, vagal or ganglionic blockade and hypothermia in dogs. *J. Appl. Physiol.* 8:81, 1955.
16. Butler, J., Caro, C. G., Alcala, R., and DuBois, A. B. Physiological factors affecting airway resistance in normal subjects and in patients with obstructive respiratory disease. *J. Clin. Invest.* 39:584, 1960.
17. Tulou, P. Influence du calibre de la trachée et des grosses bronches sur la ventilation pulmonaire: Apport des méthodes d'évaluation fonctionnelle et en particulier de la mesure de l'éspace mort anatomique. *Bronches* 11:55, 1961.
18. Widdicombe, J. G., Kent, D. C., and Nadel, J. A. The mechanism of bronchoconstriction during inhalation of dust. *J. Appl. Physiol.* 17:613, 1962.
19. DuBois, A. B., and Dautrebande, L. Acute effects of breathing inert dust particles and of carbachol aerosol on the mechanical characteristics of the lungs in man: Changes in response after inhaling sympathomimetic aerosols. *J. Clin. Invest.* 37:1746, 1958.
20. Nadel, J. A., and Comroe, J. H., Jr. Acute effects of inhalation of cigarette smoke on airway conductance. *J. Appl. Physiol.* 16:713, 1961.
21. Klassen, K. P., Morton, D. R., and Curtis, G. M. The clinical physiology of the human bronchi: III. The effect of vagus section on the cough reflex, bronchial caliber and clearance of bronchial secretions. *Surgery* 29:483, 1951.
22. Wells, R. E., Walker, J. E. C., and Hickler, R. B. Effects of cold air on respiratory air flow resistance in patients with respiratory-tract disease. *New Eng. J. Med.* 263:268, 1960.
23. Gordonoff, T. Physiologie und Pharmakologie des Expektorationsvorganges. *Ergebn. Physiol.* 40:53, 1938 (cited in Ref. 24).
24. Bukantz, S. C., and Bern, A. W. Studies with sputum: I. Initial observations on the chemical nature and blood group substance content of asthmatic sputum. *J. Allerg.* 29:29, 1958.
25. Tappan, V., and Zalar, V. The pathophysiology of bronchial mucus, in mucous secretions. *Ann. N.Y. Acad. Sci.* 106:722, 1963.
26. Mendes, E., Strauss, A., Ferri, R. G., and Ulhoa Cintra, A. B. Immunochemical studies of the asthmatic sputum. *Acta Allerg.* 18:17, 1963.
27. Huber, H. L., and Koessler, K. K. The pathology of bronchial asthma. *Arch. Intern. Med.* 30:689, 1922.
28. Cardell, B. S., and Pearson, R. S. B. Death in asthmatics. *Thorax* 14:341, 1959.
29. Naylor, B. The shedding of the mucosa of the bronchial tree in asthma. *Thorax* 17:69, 1962.
30. Crepea, S. B., and Harman, J. W. The pathology of bronchial asthma: I. The significance of membrane changes in asthmatics and nonallergic pulmonary disease. *J. Allerg.* 26: 453, 1955.
31. Mongar, J. L., and Schild, H. O. Cellular mechanisms in anaphylaxis. *Physiol. Rev.* 42: 226, 1962.
32. Ungar, G., and Hayashi, H. Enzymatic mechanisms in allergy. *Ann. Allerg.* 16:542, 1958.
33. Salvato, G. Asthma and mast cells of bronchial connective tissue. *Experientia* 18:330, 1962.
34. Brocklehurst, W. E. Slow reacting substance and related compounds. *Progr. Allerg.* 6:539, 1962.
35. Weiss, S., Robb, G. P., and Blumgart, H. L. The velocity of blood flow in health and dis-

ease as measured by the effect of histamine on the minute vessels. *Amer. Heart J.* 4:664, 1929.
36. Curry, J. J., and Lowell, F. C. Measurement of vital capacity in asthmatic subjects receiving histamine and acetyl-beta-methyl choline. *J. Allerg.* 19:9, 1948.
37. Herxheimer, H., and Streseman, E. The effect of slow reacting substance (SRS-A) in guinea pigs and in asthmatic patients. *J. Physiol.* 165: 78P, 1963.
38. Mélon, J., and Lecomte, J. Étude comparée des effets de la bradykinine et des réactions anaphylactiques locales chez l'homme. *Int. Arch. Allerg.* 21:89, 1962.
39. Lecomte, J., Petit, J. M., Mélon, J., Troquet, J., and Marcelle, R. Propriétés broncho-constrictrices de la bradykinine chez l'homme asthmatique. *Arch. Int. Pharmacodyn.* 137: 232, 1962.
40. Rappaport, B. Z., Samter, M., Catchpole, H. R., and Schiller, F. The mucoproteins of the nasal mucosa of allergic patients before and after treatment with corticotropin. *J. Allerg.* 24:35, 1953.
41. Pearse, A. G. E. *Histochemistry: Theoretical and Applied.* Boston: Little, Brown, 1953.
42. Eppinger, H., and Hess, L. Zur Pathologie des vegitativen Nervensystems. *Z. Klin. Med.* 67: 345, 1909. (Cf. also Ref. 45.)
43. Cookson, D. U., and Reed, C. E. A comparison of the effects of isoproterenol in the normal and asthmatic subject. *Amer. Rev. Resp. Dis.* 88:636, 1963.
44. Ahlquist, R. P. A study of the adrenotropic receptors. *Amer. J. Physiol.* 153:586, 1948.
45. Tiffeneau, R. Hiperexcitabilidad del Aparato Broncomotor del Asmatico. Excitaciones Broncoconstrictivas Asmogenas. *Rev. Argent. Alerg.* 8:33, 1961.
46. Scudamore, H. H., Vorhaus, H. J., and Kark, R. M. Acetylcholine and cholinesterase in the blood of patients suffering with bronchial asthma. *J. Lab. Clin. Med.* 37:860, 1951.
47. Michelson, A. L., and Lowell, F. C. Blood acetylcholine in bronchial asthma. *J. Lab. Clin. Med.* 47:119, 1956.
48. Brocklehurst, W. E. Histamine and Other Mediators in Hypersensitivity Reactions. In Halpern, B. N., and Holtzer, A. (Eds.), *Allergology* (Proceedings of the 3rd International Congress). Paris: Éditions Médicales Flammarion, 1958. P. 361.
49. Nakamura, K. *Allergy and Anaphylaxis.* Tokyo: Department of Bacteriology, Nippon Medical School, 1954.
50. Samter, M. Pathophysiology of Bronchial Asthma. In Jamar, J. M. (Ed.), *International Textbook of Allergy.* Copenhagen: Munksgaard, 1959. Pp. 224–239.
51. Karczewski, W. The electrical activity of the vagus nerve in anaphylactic shock. *Acta Allerg.* 17:334, 1962.

49. *Respiratory Changes in Bronchial Asthma*

PAUL M. SEEBOHM

BRONCHIAL ASTHMA PROVIDES ONE of the most common and dynamic examples of abnormal pulmonary physiology seen in clinical medicine. In its simpler form it is almost entirely a problem of disturbed function, with only minimal changes in tissue morphology strategically located to elicit maximal derangement of respiration. That structural change is minimal is borne out by the rapidity of onset as well as sudden cessation of some attacks. Long before pulmonary function tests were available, clinicians had known that the primary functional disturbance in bronchial asthma was small-airway obstruction because of the prolonged expiration, sibilant expiratory rales, and hyperresonance. The absence of these findings between attacks further supported the impression of the reversible nature of the obstruction. Patients with isolated seasonal attacks of asthma and all other asthmatics may well begin with this simpler form of the disease. With the help of physiological tests, the clinician can measure subtle changes in lung function not detected by a physical examination [1–3]. It is now evident that some attacks subside neither quickly nor completely and leave a residual obstruction of the airway that may persist in the absence of symptoms or physical signs.

If the bronchiolar airways become narrowed from fibrotic changes or collapse on expiration because of the loss of supporting elastic tissue and alveolar septa, the interference to air flow will mimic that seen with bronchial asthma. The similarity in physiological impairment of respiration in these conditions is so nearly complete that function tests alone often cannot separate them. Since the obstructive lesion in asthma is usually reversible with either bronchodilating or anti-inflammatory drugs and the fibrotic and inelastic states are not, serial measurements of airway patency showing relief of obstruction suggest the presence of bronchial asthma.

Since disturbed function of respiration dominates the clinical problems arising from bronchial asthma, this discussion will summarize some of the physiological principles and tests that may be useful in the understanding of this disease.

AIRWAY RESISTANCE

The physiological lesion of bronchial asthma is in the bronchioles. On inspiration, air flows into the lung because of a hypoatmospheric pressure created in the alveoli by thoracic expansion. On expiration, the air flows in the opposite direction because of the hyperatmospheric pressure in the alveoli resulting from elastic recoil of the lung. The resistance in this tubular system can be calculated if the volume flow and the alveolar-atmospheric pressure difference are determined, for resistance (R) is equal to pressure difference (ΔP) divided by volume flow ($\dot{V}$).

$$R = \frac{\Delta P}{\dot{V}}$$

The body plethysmograph provides a means of measuring flow and alveolar pressure without influence from pressures relating to elastic recoil or tissue friction [4]. The normal airway resistance measured with this device during breathing at the resting expiratory level is 1 to 1.5 cm. H_2O per liter per second [3–5].

In addition to pressure difference and volume flow, resistance to the flow of a gas is greatly influenced by the size of the tube through which the gas passes. It varies directly with length and inversely with the fourth power of the radius in smooth, straight tubular systems with laminar flow patterns. The bronchial airways are neither straight nor smooth, and air flow is usually both laminar and turbulent. Nevertheless the radius of the bronchioles has a dominant effect on airway resistance. On inspiration, there is roentgenographic evidence of both elongation and dilatation of the bronchial tree [6]. These changes could produce opposite and equalizing effects on resistance, but direct measurements have shown dilatation to reduce resistance in excess of any increase from elongation [7].

The degree of bronchiolar dilatation varies directly with the volume of air in the lungs. When the chest is fully inflated, the airway resistance is decreased fourfold over that found after complete expiration [7]. This relationship is very important technically when serial determinations of airway resistance are made by the direct method, for a shift in the residual lung volume may give a false impression of a change that has not occurred [3, 7].

Patients with asthma frequently state that they are breathing "on the top of the lungs." Spirograms of induced attacks show that the subjects attain this position by inflating the chest with 1 to 2 liters of additional air within a few minutes after exposure to the bronchospastic stimulus [8]. This is ordinarily considered to be the result of "air trapping" behind partially obstructed bronchioles which open on inspiration and close before air escapes on expiration. It is not always certain whether the resting expiratory level is pulled up to the inflated position to ease the effort of breathing or whether it climbs because of progressive trapping of air. In either case, breathing with a nearly full chest of air is preferred because maximal dilatation of the bronchial system affords a much-needed reduction of airway resistance and thereby partially compensates for the constrictive effect of the asthmatic process.

Physical examination of the patient during an asthmatic attack reveals that he is breathing with his thorax in an elevated position and that his residual lung volume has increased. He is assisted by the accessory muscles of respiration and elevation of the shoulders. The breath sounds are characterized by marked prolongation of the expiratory phase accompanied by the sibilant rales of bronchiolar obstruction. The respiratory rate may be only slightly increased, if at all, because of the increase in time required to exhale each breath of air. If the obstruction worsens, inspiration too becomes prolonged and sibilant rales occur, but always to a lesser degree than heard on expiration. Although tissue resistance may be increased in some asthmatic patients studied, the obstructed airway is the major defect and constitutes the chief interference with free exchange of air [9].

After asthmatic attacks subside and patients are free from physical signs or symptoms, measurements of airway resistance may still show elevated values. Some of these will return to normal after administration of bronchodilators [3]. In view of the susceptibility of asthmatic patients to nonspecific bronchospasm-producing stimuli, a possible explanation may lie in this latent obstructive state.

VENTILATION

The disturbance in airway resistance during an asthmatic attack promptly changes the relationship of the lung volumes. The functional residual capacity (FRC) is increased and the vital capacity is reduced. The spirogram of the induced attacks shows an early reduction in tidal volume, although later the tidal volume may return toward normal before the increased FRC declines [8]. The respiratory rate may increase very little, if at all. The fall in tidal volume causes a decline in the alveolar ventilation (minute volume minus anatomical dead space [100 to 150 ml.] times respiratory rate) by as much as 50 to 60 percent. If the tidal volume returns to normal, the alveolar ventilation will be restored to pre-attack levels. Inspired air may be, however, inefficiently distributed, in which case the physiological dead space may be much greater than the anatomical and the effective alveolar ventilation will remain reduced.

Measurements of the distribution of inspired air in patients with asthma show abnormalities in both the symptomatic and the nonsymptomatic group [1, 10]. If good perfusion of the alveoli is assumed and poor distribution of inspired air does not supply sufficient O_2 to poorly ventilated areas of the lungs, O_2 tension in the blood will fall [5, 8, 11]. This cannot be compensated for by increasing the exchange in the well-ventilated areas because excess O_2 beyond the normal amount dissolving and combining with hemoglobin cannot be stored in the blood for redistribution to the less oxygenated blood leaving the poorly ventilated areas. The O_2 saturation of arterial blood may be below normal by 5 to 10 percent in patients with moderately severe attacks of bronchial asthma but of course may fall further in status asthmaticus [1, 11, 12].

The increased ventilation of unobstructed alveoli can remove excess CO_2 to offset the reduced elimination in the poorly ventilated areas, and as a result most patients who have hypoxemia from asthma do not have hypercapnia [1, 5]. If, however, the obstruction of airways becomes more nearly complete and generalized hypoventilation of all or most of the alveoli occurs, elimination of CO_2 also becomes inadequate [12, 13].

CARBON DIOXIDE RETENTION

If the CO_2 tension in the alveoli increases, the amount of CO_2 dissolved in the plasma also increases. Normally, the CO_2 is dissolved as carbonic acid in the blood under a tension of 38 to 40 mm. Hg pressure and provides with bicarbonate (HCO_3^-) a buffering system which determines the pH of the blood. The relation between the bicarbonate ion and the dissolved CO_2 is usually about 20 : 1 when pH is a normal 7.40. The first effect of CO_2 retention is to lower pH and produce what is called respiratory acidosis. If the lungs were normal, any increase in CO_2 would provide a stimulus to the medullary respiratory center and be compensated for by hyperventilation; however, in the case of an obstructive airway disease, such as asthma, the ventilatory effort is already at a maximum. Since the dissolved CO_2 cannot be eliminated, the increased acidity is compensated for by increasing the bicarbonate ions, which occurs as follows: (1) The ionized plasma carbonic acid provides more bicarbonate ions ($CO_2 + H_2O \rightleftarrows H_2CO_3 \rightleftarrows H^+ + HCO_3^-$), and (2) the kidneys excrete the H^+ and Cl^- ions and retain the HCO_3^-. The HCO_3^-/CO_2 ratio of 20 : 1 is thus maintained, and the pH returns toward normal; however, the total plasma (venous or arterial) CO_2 content is increased [5].

Respiratory acidosis, compensated or uncompensated, coupled with hypoxemia results in a less responsive medullary respiratory center to the pCO_2 stimulus. On the other hand, the hypoxemia that is always associated with hypercapnia is a stimulus to the carotid body which may then serve as the major drive to respiration.

If the asthmatic lesion is corrected, respiration quickly restores oxygenation and CO_2 elimination, but if it is not and further obstruction develops in the face of growing muscular fatigue or respiratory depressant drugs, or both, death may follow from severe CO_2 narcosis and anoxia.

The pulmonary circulation is affected by asthma in that pulmonary hypertension may be present during attacks. This is thought to result from increased intra-alveolar pressure secondary to airway obstruction [12]. If asthma progressively impairs ventilation over a period of months or years, death may result from heart failure secondary to cor pulmonale; but in the uncomplicated patient, this is unusual.

PULMONARY FUNCTION TESTS

During an acute attack of asthma, clinical observations will detect many of the physiological changes taking place, so that special lung function measurements are often not necessary for proper assessment of the clinical problem and treatment of the patient. The exception is the presence of severe hypoxia and hypercapnia, for then analyses of the arterial blood for the pCO_2, pH, and O_2 saturation may become essential to proper treatment and prognosis [13].

Pulmonary function tests are most valuable in determining the amount of residual airway obstruction present in asthmatic patients during convalescent or symptom-free periods. Serial measurements may be useful guides to therapy, especially when adrenal corticosteroids have been given to induce complete suppression of the asthmatic lesion after other measures have failed. Testing before and after therapy may assist in distinguishing the reversible obstruction of bronchial asthma from fixed fibrotic or inelastic changes or in assessing the degree of respiratory deficiency attributable to each when both occur in the same patient.

LUNG VOLUMES

One of the simpler measurements of lung function is the determination of the lung volumes. At the end of a normal expiration, the lungs are at the *resting expiratory level,* and the air remaining in the lungs is the *functional residual capacity* (FRC). If expiration is forced beyond the resting level, the *expiratory reserve volume* (ERV) is expelled. The remaining air is the *residual volume* (RV), which cannot be removed with any expiratory effort. The ERV plus the RV constitutes the FRC. On inspiration from the resting expiratory level, the first 300 to 500 ml. is the *tidal volume* (TV), and additional air to the maximal capacity of the chest is the *inspiratory reserve volume* (IRV). The IRV, TV, and ERV constitute the *vital capacity* (VC). The VC can be measured with gas flowmeters and bellows or cylindrical spirometers. In general, a spirometer-kymograph unit is preferable, for it measures all volumes, except RV, and inscribes a pattern of the respiratory cycle. This spirogram will disclose the presence of air trapping with forced respirations and provide a record for calculating flow rates or forced expiratory volumes.

Residual Volume (RV). This cannot be measured directly but can be calculated from gas "wash-out" or body plethysmographic methods. The nitrogen remaining in the chest at the end of expiration can be determined by having the subject breathe 100 percent oxygen for 7 to 20 minutes, collecting all of the expired gas, and assaying the nitrogen content. Considering 80 percent of the FRC to be nitrogen permits a calculation of its volume. FRC − ERV = RV [5].

The VC is reduced during an asthmatic attack and RV increased. After symptoms disappear, there is a gradual return to normal. During this period of change, VC may be a useful measure of response to therapy.

AIR DISTRIBUTION

The distribution of inspired air is normally almost uniform throughout the lungs. It can be measured by determining the concentration of nitrogen in a forced expiration after breathing of 100 percent O_2 for seven minutes. More than 2.5 percent of nitrogen is considered abnormal. Another method consists of having the subject take a single breath of 100 percent O_2 and measuring the nitrogen concentration in the expired air. A rise in nitrogen concentration of over 1.5 percent in the expired gas between the 750 ml. and the 1,250 ml. portion of the expired volume indicates uneven distribution. A nitrogen meter which records nitrogen concentration immediately is used to make a continuous analysis and record of the nitrogen concentration in different portions of the expired air and thus provide a graphic picture of the nitrogen concentration in the alveolar air. If distribution is even, this curve will be flat; if uneven, it will become steeper as the poorly ventilated alveoli with undiluted nitrogen empty into the expired sample. The uneven distribution detectable in bronchial asthma is evidence of a variable degree of bronchiolar obstruction and may persist during an asymptomatic period [1].

MECHANICS OF VENTILATION

Although the serial measurement of lung volumes may reflect changes in airway patency, the time required to move given volumes of air becomes a more sensitive index of airway resistance, especially when the vital capacity is normal. There are many tests designed to assess airway resistance both directly and indirectly.

Forced Expiratory Volume (FEV). Forced expiratory volume, or timed vital capacity, is a maximal effort test that measures the volume of air exhaled in one, two, and three seconds, which should normally represent 83, 94, and 97 percent of the vital capacity, respectively. Bronchiolar obstruction will reduce these values considerably.

Maximal Expiratory Flow Rate (MEFR). This is a sensitive indirect measure of airway resistance. The vital capacity is expelled with a maximal effort into a spirometer-kymograph with an accelerated recording speed. The rate of flow between 200 and 1,200 ml. of expired air is calculated from the tracing. In adults, this value is normally about 400 liters per minute but may fall to as low as 20 liters in obstructive bronchial disease. It is reduced when bronchial asthma is symptomatic, and if it remains abnormal during asymptomatic periods, it indicates residual bronchiolar obstruction.

Maximal Midexpiratory Flow (MMF). This rate also can be calculated from the spirogram by determining the flow rate for the middle half of the forced vital capacity.

Maximal Breathing Capacity (MBC). Maximal breathing capacity is the amount of air breathed per minute with a maximal effort. This is usually done with a tidal volume equal to one-half the vital capacity and an average frequency rate of 50 to 60 per minute. Naturally, motivation, muscular tone, and general physical stamina may influence the results. Normal standards must be calculated for each patient because of the wide range of variations related to sex, age, and body surface area [5]. The actual test of MBC is now called maximal voluntary ventilation (MVV), and the designation should include a suffix indicating the breathing frequency used in performing the test.

In comparative studies with direct body plethysmographic methods for measuring airway resistance in normal subjects who had had bronchiolar obstruction artificially induced with dust aerosols, MBC and MMF showed a better correlation than the forced timed vital capacity [14]. Although these indirect methods are not as sensitive as the direct measurement of airway resistance, they are useful for clinical evaluation. Maximal midexpiratory flow can be estimated repeatedly with less patient effort and inconvenience than tests for MBC. Since increased airway resistance is the primary defect in bronchial asthma, this test provides a practical quantitative measure of the clinical status of the asthmatic patient.

DIFFUSING CAPACITY

Neither the alveolar-capillary membrane nor the size of the alveolar-capillary surface area should be altered in uncomplicated bronchial asthma, and the diffusing capacity as measured by the CO method is usually normal [10, 12]. Significant change in airway resistance does not alter diffusing capacity. A normal diffusing capacity in patients with bronchial asthma indicates integrity of the alveoli of the lungs, in spite of the degree of ventilatory impairment. Reduction of diffusing capacity in asthma suggests complicating conditions, such as emphysema or interstitial fibrosis.

ARTERIAL BLOOD OXYGEN, CARBON DIOXIDE, AND pH

The normal O_2 saturation is approximately 96 percent, but during an asthmatic attack this value is frequently reduced in accordance with severity. The fall follows an alteration in the ventilation and perfusion relationships in the lung. Well-perfused areas of the lung carry blood through poorly ventilated alveoli with low O_2 tensions. The O_2 saturation can be accurately measured manometrically by the Van Slyke and Neill method on arterial blood. If less accurate absolute values can be tolerated and it is desirable to measure rapid changes in saturation, such as may occur with induced asthmatic attacks in experimental or diagnostic tests, an ear oximeter can be used to detect changes in the relative amounts of oxygenated and nonoxygenated hemoglobin flowing through the subcutaneous capillaries [11].

The O_2 tension in arterial blood (pO_2) can now be measured directly with an O_2 electrode, a technique that is likely to bring the scientific estimation of oxygenation of the blood closer to the bedside than has been possible with the manometric method of Van Slyke.

The hypoventilation of bronchial asthma must be generalized and uniform to produce CO_2 retention. This is a constant threat to patients with chronic persistent asthma and may follow the administration of sedatives in patients with asthma of any severity. The tension of the dissolved CO_2 in the blood reflects the adequacy of ventilation of the lungs, and detection of its elevation should alert the clinician to the probability that medullary respiratory control may no longer be responsive to it. The normal tension of CO_2 is 38 to 40 mm. Hg in arterial plasma. This represents about 1.25 mEq. per liter of CO_2. The $[HCO_3^-]$ is about 25 mEq. per liter. Since there is a constant relationship between these two values and the plasma pH, one can calculate one value if the other two are known. The relationship is stated in the classic equation of Henderson-Hasselbalch.

$$pH = 6.10 + \log \frac{HCO_3^-.}{CO_2}$$

The pH and total CO_2 content of arterial plasma can be determined in the laboratory more easily than the pCO_2, or HCO_3^-. Since the $HCO_3^- = \text{total } CO_2 - pCO_2$, the substitution of the values for pH and total CO_2 in the formula provides all the factors needed for solving the equation for pCO_2.

The Astrup method [15] of measuring pH of blood without and with two known tensions of CO_2 provides data for immediate reading of pCO_2 and bicarbonate values from nomograms. Using capillary blood, one group has found this a useful method in monitoring the progress of response to treatment of severe status asthmaticus [13].

The CO_2 electrode designed by Severinghaus [16] provides a direct method for measuring blood pCO_2 and will undoubtedly come into general use in the evaluation of clinical problems relating to respiratory acidosis.

It would be desirable to have the data from all pulmonary function tests on all patients with bronchial asthma, but usually for many reasons this is not possible. It therefore becomes necessary to select those measurements that can be expected to be most useful to clinical management at certain times in the course of the disease. During prolonged status asthmaticus, arterial blood O_2 saturation, pH, and pCO_2 might be very helpful in directing therapy. In symptom-free convalescent periods, lung volumes, flow rates, and distribution studies may be needed to determine the presence or absence of residual airway obstruction after clinical signs and symptoms have disappeared. In some patients, the vital capacity alone is sufficiently sensitive to reflect gross changes in airway obstruction during recovery periods. Aside from specific clinical indications, pulmonary function tests convert qualitative clinical impressions into quantitative physiological concepts for an improved understanding of this dynamic respiratory disease.

REFERENCES

1. Beale, H. D., Fowler, W. S., and Comroe, J. H., Jr. Pulmonary function studies in 20 asthmatic patients in the symptom-free interval. *J. Allerg.* 23:1, 1952.
2. Bernstein, I. L., and Kreindler, A. Lung compliance and pulmonary flow resistance: I. Clinical studies in symptomatic and asymptomatic asthmatic children. *J. Allerg.* 34:127, 1963.
3. Ruth, W. E., and Andrews, C. E. Airway resistance studies in bronchial asthma. *J. Lab. Clin. Med.* 54:889, 1959.
4. DuBois, A. B., Botelho, S. Y., and Comroe, J. H., Jr. A new method for measuring airway resistance in man using a body plethysmograph: Values in normal subjects and in patients with respiratory disease. *J. Clin. Invest.* 35:327, 1956.
5. Comroe, J. H., Jr., Forster, R. E., DuBois, A. B., Briscoe, W. A., and Carlsen, E. *The Lung: Clinical Physiology and Pulmonary Function Tests* (2nd ed.). Chicago: Year Book Medical Publishers, Inc., 1962.
6. Heinbecker, P. A method for the demonstration of calibre changes in the bronchi in normal respiration. *J. Clin. Invest.* 4:459, 1927.
7. Briscoe, W. A., and DuBois, A. B. The relationship between airway resistance, airway conductance and lung volume in subjects of different age and body size. *J. Clin. Invest.* 37:1279, 1958.
8. Lowell, F. C., Schiller, I. W., and Lowell, A. The use of a closed system in the study of asthma and emphysema. *J. Allerg.* 23:335, 1952.
9. Marshall, R., and DuBois, A. B. The viscous resistance of lung tissue in patients with pulmonary disease. *Clin. Sci.* 15:473, 1956.
10. Bates, D. V. Impairment of respiratory function in bronchial asthma. *Clin. Sci.* 11:203, 1952.
11. Lowell, F. C., Schiller, I. W., Lynch, M. T., and Lowell, A. Change in the rate of oxygen saturation of the arterial blood associated with induced asthmatic attacks. *J. Allerg.* 24:499, 1953.
12. Williams, H. M., Jr., and Zohman, L. R. Cardiopulmonary function in bronchial asthma. *Amer. Rev. Resp. Dis.* 81:173, 1960.
13. Bukanz, S. C. Residential center for children with intractable asthma. *J.A.M.A.* 185:75, 1963.
14. Lloyd, T. C., Jr., and Wright, G. W. Evaluation of methods used in detecting changes of airway resistance in man. *Amer. Rev. Resp. Dis.* 87:529, 1963.
15. Astrup, P. A simple electrometric technique for the determination of carbon dioxide tension in blood and plasma, total content of carbon dioxide in plasma, and bicarbonate content in "separated" plasma at a fixed carbon dioxide tension (40 mm. Hg). *Scandinav. J. Clin. Lab. Invest.* 8:33, 1956.
16. Severinghaus, J. W. Respiratory System: Methods; Gas Analysis. In Glasser, O. (Ed.), *Medical Physics*. Chicago: Year Book Medical Publishers, Inc., 1960. Vol. 3, p. 550.

50. Infection in Bronchial Asthma

STANLEY F. HAMPTON

ASTHMA MAY BE CLASSIFIED INTO two distinct types, based on differences in underlying factors. One, due to atopic influences, often is called "atopic asthma" [1] but is also labeled extrinsic [2], immunological [1], sensitive [3], noninfective [4], allergic [5], and exogenic [6]. It is caused primarily by hypersensitivity to noninfective antigens, such as pollens, to other inhalants, and occasionally to foods. The second type might be designated "infective asthma" [7], but it is also referred to as nonatopic [1], intrinsic [2], nonimmunological [1], nonsensitive [3], nonallergic [5], and endogenic [6]. Infection per se, or possibly nonpathogenic bacteria that are ubiquitous to the respiratory tract, may cause it, but there also may be unknown intrinsic factors. Here, the terms "atopic asthma" and "infective asthma" will be used to denote the two types under consideration.

Historically, Salter first used the word "intrinsic" [8, 9] as early as 1864 and "extrinsic" [9] in 1868, but their meanings differed from the present connotations. For his intrinsic asthma Salter referred to exciting causes as "those which apply directly to the bronchial tubes, or affect them primarily," including such specific factors as animal emanations as well as nonspecific factors, such as chemical and mechanical irritants. His extrinsic asthma referred to "sources of remote nervous irritation" and "physical stimuli—excitement, fear, or other violent emotions."

The differentiation between atopic and infective asthma is important in terms of treatment and prognosis. The characteristics of each type are outlined in Table 50-1.

ATOPIC ASTHMA

Atopic asthma is characterized by a prominent genetic influence; usually there is a family history of asthma or of other atopic disease. The onset is at an early age, most cases beginning in the first two decades. Onset after age 35 is unusual. Seasonal hay fever and perennial allergic rhinitis, not necessarily due to the same etiological factors as the asthma, frequently coexist.

Atopic asthma is characterized by positive immediate wheal and erythema reactions to skin tests and presence in the serum of skin-sensitizing antibodies [10] to the offending antigenic factors. It usually responds to treatment, both symptomatically with drugs and specifically by elimination of the antigen or antigens or hyposensitization with extracts thereof [11]. There may be a tendency, although slight, to outgrow it or have permanent spontaneous remissions, especially when it first occurs in infancy [12].

Sputum examinations reveal a prominence of eosinophils and, as a rule, show no evidence of infection. Infection, in fact, is absent or, if present, is secondary. Intractable asthma and death are uncommon [13–15].

INFECTIVE ASTHMA

Infective asthma is characterized by a less prominent genetic influence than in the atopic type, but occasionally there is a family history of atopic disease. The onset usually is either under age 5, with sporadic attacks associated with acute febrile respiratory infection and with complete remissions between episodes; or over 35, when the asthmatic state tends to become persistent and chronic and complicated by chronic bronchitis, subsequent pulmonary emphysema, and cor pulmonale.

Reactions to skin tests with identifiable common antigens, involved in atopic asthma, are not positive. Although skin-sensitizing antibodies to antigenic fractions of respiratory bacteria have been demonstrated in some cases, as discussed later, no definite immunological mechanism has been established in this type of asthma.

TABLE 50-1. Characteristics of Atopic and Infective Asthma

Characteristics	Atopic	Infective
Genetic influence	Present	Variable
Age of onset	Usually under 35	Under 5, over 35
Associated hay fever	Frequent	Uncommon
Skin tests	Usually pos.	Neg.[a]
Skin-sensitizing antibody	Usually present	None[a]
Response to antiatopic therapy	Good	None
Sputum	Eosinophils	Eosin., bacteria, PMN. leukocytes
Associated infection	Secondary, when present	Apparently primary
Intractable asthma	Uncommon	Common
Death	Rare	More frequent

[a] Excluding those to bacterial antigens.

Infective asthma usually is not as amenable to treatment and certainly not to specific antiatopic therapy. There is little tendency to spontaneous remissions.

Sputum examinations, as a rule, reveal a prominence of pus cells and bacteria as well as eosinophils.

Infections of the respiratory tract are common and are associated not only with the onset of the first attack of asthma but frequently with repeated bronchial infections, and most cases of intractable asthma as well as of deaths are of this type [13–19]. It has been reported that about one third of the patients who die do so within two years of onset [15].

COMBINED ATOPIC AND INFECTIVE FACTORS

Although the separation of asthma into "atopic" and "infective" groups [20, 21] is useful, the two often occur in combination. Cooke [21] found that the asthma in 50 percent of his patients was due to inhalant, food, or drug allergens, in about 35 percent to infection and in 15 to 20 percent to both infective and noninfective causes. Williams *et al.* [22], in England, reported multiple type causes, including psychogenic, in 38 percent of his cases. Swineford *et al.* [23], in an analysis of Swineford's "asthmagram," considered 88 percent of asthmatic patients to have combined allergy.

Rackemann [20] pointed out an important relation between extrinsic and intrinsic asthma in the same patient. First, intrinsic asthma is likely to develop in the patient who has had unabated extrinsic asthma for many years. Second, infective asthma commonly develops many years after complete remission of earlier asthma due to specific antigens.

Moreover, a number of nonspecific factors, unrelated to the fundamental underlying causes, may precipitate attacks of asthma. Sherman [24] describes this relationship: "Once the asthmatic pattern has developed through allergy to extrinsic agents or infection, paroxysms of asthma may be precipitated by many factors unrelated to the original causes." Such secondary factors include emotional stress, irritating smoke, fumes and odors, physical exertion, and weather conditions, particularly changes in temperature and humidity.

ROLE OF INFECTION

The association of respiratory infection in infective asthma is the rule, but the role of infection in terms of etiology is controversial. One question is whether the infectious agents per se induce hypersensitivity or whether the infection is a nonspecific factor. Some investigators [25–29] have felt that there is no primary relationship between asthma and infection but rather that the infection is a secondary factor that may increase the severity of the asthmatic state by increasing obstruction in the bronchi and bronchioles by virtue of bronchial edema and cellular infiltrates and particularly by increasing the volume and tenacity of the sputum. Others [12, 31–36] believe the relationship to be primary and specifically one of bacterial allergy. Still others [37–40] recognize a primary relationship but question the specificity. Feinberg [37] hypothesized that ". . . it is possible that the antigen is not the bacterial body itself but the product of its action on tissues" or "the infection may merely prepare the tissues for development of a specific extrinsic allergy." Glaser [39] stated: "It is further possible that the infection lowers, in some way, the allergic resistance of the mucous membranes so that allergens which would not normally cause asthma may do so." It has been suggested that several alternatives must be considered, e.g., autosensitization, induction of sensitization not previously present, conversion of latent or subclinical to active or clinical sensitization, and perhaps the induction of bronchospasm by pharmacodynamic substances produced by infectious agents [40] (see also Chap. 16). Lowell [41] suggests that, in intrinsic asthma, there merely is an increased reactivity of the bronchial tree to nonspecific factors and "absence of allergy."

Cooke [21] stressed the mechanism of bacterial hypersensitivity in asthma associated with infection. He based his opinion on the high incidence of allergy in the histories of children and young adults (not of older adults) with infective asthma, the occurrence of asthma as a result of infection only, the frequent occurrence of blood eosinophilia and the induction of asthma in patients following injections of respiratory bacterial vaccine.

BACTERIOLOGY OF THE RESPIRATORY TRACT

Numerous pathogenic bacteria, particularly *Hemophilus influenzae, Diplococcus pneumoniae,* beta hemolytic streptococci, and coagulase-positive yellow staphylococci [42–50], have been isolated from the sputum and bronchoscopic aspirates and swabs of patients with asthma, presumably due to infection with the particular organisms.

There is disagreement regarding the normal flora of the bronchial tree and whether sputum cultures reveal the true bacteriological picture of the lower respiratory tract or contaminants from the mouth and oropharynx. There are reports that the bronchial tree is sterile [43–51]. May [52] reported that in bronchitis, *Neisseria catarrhalis,* and nonhemolytic streptococci, *Streptococcus viridans,* were found almost universally in both purulent and mucoid sputum as a result of their extension from the upper respiratory tract into a damaged bronchial tree, where they colonized.

The reader is referred to reviews of Kortekangas [44] in Europe and Rosebury [53] in the United States for detailed discussions of the bacteriology of the upper and lower respiratory tract in health and disease.

A study of bacterial hypersensitivity in asthma [54] recorded cultures of sputum of 29 patients taken during 82 episodes of asthma, which were apparently precipitated by acute respiratory infection. *Neisseria* were present in all 82 specimens and growth was moderate to heavy in 79. Other organisms, both pathogens and nonpathogens, were also encountered. Differential fermentation of the *Neisseria* isolated from 41 sputum specimens revealed the following species in 74 subcultures: *N. catarrhalis,* 10; *N. flava,* 11; *N. flavescens,* 4; *N. perflava,* 20; *N. pharyngis,* 10; *N. sicca,* 10; *N. subflava,* 9.

The high incidence of *Neisseria* and other normally present bacteria and low incidence of pathogens in the sputum of some asthmatic patients [45, 54] is suggestive, but not conclusive, evidence that there may be a significant change, qualitatively and quantitatively, in the nonpathogenic bacteria of the bronchial tree during asthmatic attacks.

FIRST ATTACK OF ASTHMA AND ACUTE INFECTION

The first attack of asthma in many patients has been reported to be associated with acute respiratory infection [20, 55], including pneumonia [56], influenza [57], measles and whooping cough [58]. During World War II in military personnel the first attack was observed to occur with primary atypical pneumonia, the symptoms and signs of asthma developing as the pneumonia was clearing. Fagerberg [55] studied 748 patients with asthma, 615 of whom were considered to have endogenous and 133 exogenous asthma, and found that respiratory infection precipitated the first attack in 61.9 percent of the former group. On the other hand, asthma has been observed to subside at the time of acute specific infectious diseases, such as measles [59].

Although asthma is commonly associated with obvious infectious disease at the onset, occasionally neither infective nor atopic factors are apparent. Consequently, other factors, largely unknown, might be responsible for some cases of nonatopic asthma. Aspirin intolerance [60], often manifested by severe, and even fatal, asthma [61–65], is a case in point. It occurs apparently in nonatopic patients, and has been thought to be part of the "infective" group [66–69].

POSSIBLE ROLE OF BACTERIAL ALLERGY

Whether or not bacterial hypersensitivity can induce asthma is still uncertain. The roles of the many antigenic fractions of the bacterial cell, the selective antibodies induced, the sites of the antigen-antibody interaction, and the relevant mediators that may induce asthma are among the unsolved problems.

Since the tuberculin-type skin reaction to specific antigen is associated with several infectious diseases, the question arises whether this delayed, cellular type of allergy [70] may be involved in the etiology of asthma. While theoretically attractive, the concept of "delayed-type" asthma is not supported by acceptable evidence. Since the symptoms of both atopic and infective asthma are essentially the same, both types, theoretically, should be identified with similar immunological mechanisms and chemical mediators. Thus, since extrinsic asthma clearly is a manifestation of the immediate type of hypersensitivity with circulating antibody, so should intrinsic asthma be.

The immediate or anaphylactic type of reaction to a variety of bacteria, including colon, hay, typhoid, anthrax and tubercle bacilli, was first demonstrated in 1907 by Rosenau and Anderson [71] and two years later was shown to be transferable by serum [72]. Baldwin [73] induced anaphylaxis, but not the tuberculin reaction, in the guinea pig with aqueous extract of the tubercle bacillus. Some fractions of bacteria, such as the pneumococcus [74–76], will cause positive skin reactions and elicit shock and contraction of the isolated uterine muscle of the guinea pig but, like haptens, are not antigenic.

Kuhns and Pappenheimer [77–79] demonstrated that a skin-sensitizing antibody could be induced with diphtheria toxoid. It seems reasonable to assume that common respiratory bacteria might be capable of inducing an immediate type of hypersensitivity. The demonstration by Swineford and Holman [80] of immediate wheal skin reaction and skin-sensitizing antibodies to soluble fractions of respiratory bacteria, the induction of anaphylactic shock and desensitization in sensitized guinea pigs with bacterial antigens [81–83], and the accidental or intentional induction of asthma in man by inhalation of various bacterial substances [84–88] lend support to the concept. There is one report of the induction of asthma by aerosolization of influenza virus vaccine [57].

The concept that some bacterial antigens may be comparable to noninfectious agents in their capacity to induce asthma was strengthened by a study of bacterial hypersensitivity carried out in our laboratories in which asthma was induced by aerosolization of specially prepared antigenic fractions of *N. catarrhalis* in patients who had asthma associated with acute respiratory infections [89]. Positive immediate local wheal and erythema skin reactions were present in 12 of 14 patients (55 positive reactions in 81 tests performed with all fractions). The size of the wheal, however, was small and, as a rule, did not have pseudopodia, characteristic of the typical skin reaction to pollen. On the other hand, only 3 of 21 nonasthmatic controls had such positive skin reactions. Skin-sensitizing antibodies were demonstrable in the sera of 5 of the 16 patients to one or more fractions. After the patients were exposed to the antigens by aerosol as well as by periodic injections every one to four weeks for several years, however, there was no serological evidence of blocking antibody [90] or inhibition of complement fixation [91], as has been shown with ragweed pollen antigen.

Inasmuch as the clinical symptoms and signs of the two types of asthma are indistinguishable, presumably there is a common chemical mediator. In atopic asthma, such a mediator appears to be released from the tissues as a result of an antigen-antibody interaction which involves skin-sensitizing antibody. The demonstration of direct counterparts with some bacteria, particularly with those recorded in asthmatic individuals, is a tempting argument for the role of bacterial allergy.

REFERENCES

1. Walzer, M. Asthma. In Coca, A. F., Walzer, M., and Thommen, A. A. (Eds.), *Asthma and Hay Fever in Theory and Practice*. Springfield, Ill.: Charles C Thomas, Publisher, 1931.
2. Rackemann, F. M. A clinical study of one hundred and fifty cases of bronchial asthma. *Arch. Intern. Med.* 22:517, 1918.
3. Walker, I. C. A clinical study of 400 patients with bronchial asthma. *Boston Med. Surg. J.* 179:288, 1918.
4. Spain, W. C. Non-Infective Asthma. In Cooke, R. A. (Ed.), *Allergy in Theory and Practice*. Philadelphia: W. B. Saunders Company, 1947.
5. Tuft, L. *Clinical Allergy* (2nd ed.). Philadelphia: Lea & Febiger, 1949.
6. Fagerberg, E. Studies in bronchial asthma: I. Occurrence of asthma without and with specific allergy as the cause of the disease. *Acta Allerg.* 11:293, 1957.
7. Cooke, R. A. Infective asthma: Indications of its allergic nature. *Amer. J. Med. Sci.* 183:309, 1932.
8. Salter, H. H. *On Asthma: Its Pathology and Treatment*. Philadelphia: Blanchard & Lea, 1864.
9. (*a*) Salter, H. H. *On Asthma. Its Pathology and Treatment* (2nd ed.). London: John Churchill & Sons, 1868. (*b*) *Ibid.* (1st American from the last English edition.) New York: William Wood, 1882.
10. Prausnitz, C., and Küstner, H. Studien über die Ueberempfindlichkeit. *Zbl. Bakt.* [Orig.] 86:160, 1921.
11. Rackemann, F. M., and Edwards, M. C. Asthma in children: A follow-up study of 688 patients after an interval of twenty years. *New Eng. J. Med.* 26:815 and 856, 1952.
12. Sherman, W. B., and Kessler, W. R. *Allergy in Pediatric Practice*. St. Louis: C. V. Mosby Company, 1957.
13. Rackemann, F. M. Death from bronchial asthma. *J. Allerg.* 15:249, 1944.
14. Bullen, S. S. Correlation of clinical and autopsy findings in 176 cases of asthma. *J. Allerg.* 23:193, 1952.
15. Alexander, H. L. A historical account of death from asthma. *J. Allerg.* 34:305, 1963.
16. Earle, B. V. Fatal bronchial asthma: A series of fifteen cases with a review of the literature. *Thorax* 8:195, 1953.
17. Houston, J. C., de Navasquez, S., and Trounce, J. R. A clinical and pathological study of fatal cases of status asthmaticus. *Ibid.*, p. 207.
18. Alexander, H. L. Death from Bronchial Asthma. In Halpern, B. N., and Holtzer, A. (Eds.), *Allergology* (Proceedings of 3rd International Congress). Paris: Éditions Médicales Flammarion, 1958. P. 109.
19. Williams, D. A., and Leopold, J. G. Discussion of Ref. 18, p. 119.
20. Rackemann, F. M. Intrinsic asthma. *J. Allerg.* 11:147, 1940.
21. Cooke, R. A. Ref. 4.
22. Williams, D. A., Lewis-Fanning, E., Rees, L., Jacobs, J., and Thomas, A. Assessment of the relative importance of allergic, infective, and psychological factors in asthma. *Acta Allerg.* 12:376, 1958.
23. Swineford, O., Johnson, E. R., Jr., Cook, H. M., Jr., and Ochota, L. Infectious asthma: An analysis of the asthmagrams of 100 cases and a critical review. *Ann. Allerg.* 20:155, 1962.
24. Sherman, W. B. Asthma. In Beeson, P. B., and McDermott, W. (Eds.), *Cecil-Loeb Textbook of Medicine* (11th ed.). Philadelphia: W. B. Saunders Company, 1963.
25. Alexander, H. L. Bronchial Asthma. In Harrison, T. R. (Ed.), *Principles of Internal Medicine* (2nd ed.). New York: McGraw-Hill Book Company, Inc., 1954.
26. Alexander, H. L. *Bronchial Asthma: Its Diagnosis and Treatment*. Philadelphia: Lea & Febiger, 1928.
27. Hansel, F. K. *Clinical Allergy*. St. Louis: C. V. Mosby Company, 1953.
28. Vaughan, W. T., and Black, J. H. *Practice of Allergy* (3rd ed.). St. Louis: C. V. Mosby Company, 1954.
29. Feingold, B. F. Infection in the Allergic Child. In Ratner, B. (Ed.), *Allergy in Relation to Pediatric Practice*. St. Paul, Minn.: Bruce, 1951.
30. Thomas, W. S. *Asthma: Its Diagnosis and Treatment*. New York: Paul B. Hoeber, Inc., 1928.
31. Rackemann, F. M. *Clinical Allergy*. New York: Macmillan Company, 1931.
32. Sodeman, W. A. Differential Diagnosis. In Derbes, V. J., and Engelhardt, H. T. (Eds.), *Treatment of Bronchial Asthma*. Philadelphia: J. B. Lippincott Company, 1946.
33. Unger, L. *Bronchial Asthma*. Springfield, Ill.: Charles C Thomas, Publisher, 1945.
34. Benson, R. L. The role of bacteria in allergy, with special reference to asthma. *Ann. Intern. Med.* 6:1136, 1933.
35. Baldwin, H. S. Infectious Factors in Asthma. In Prigal, S. J. (Ed.), *Fundamentals of Modern Allergy*. New York: McGraw-Hill Book Company, Inc., 1960.
36. Urbach, E., and Gottlieb, P. M. *Allergy*. New York: Grune & Stratton, Inc., 1946.
37. Feinberg, S. M., Durham, O. C., and Drag-

stedt, C. A. *Allergy in Practice* (2nd ed.). Chicago: Year Book Publishers, Inc., 1946.
38. Segal, M. S. *The Management of the Patient with Severe Bronchial Asthma.* Springfield, Ill.: Charles C Thomas, Publisher, 1950.
39. Glaser, J. *Allergy in Childhood.* Springfield, Ill.: Charles C Thomas, Publisher, 1956.
40. Grossman, R., and Prigal, S. J. Bronchitis, Emphysema and Other Diseases in Relation to Asthma. Ref. 35.
41. Lowell, F. C. Bronchial asthma. *Amer. J. Med.* 20:778, 1956.
42. Prigal, S. J. The Interrelationship of Allergy, Infection and the Psyche: A "United Field Theory" for the Allergist. Ref. 35.
43. Pecora, D. V., and Yegian, D. Bacteriology of the lower respiratory tract in health and chronic disease. *New Eng. J. Med.* 258:71, 1958.
44. Kortekangas, A. E. Investigations of the bacterial flora of the respiratory tract. *Acta Otolaryng.* (Stockholm), supp. 150, 1959.
45. Brown, C. C., Jr., Coleman, M. D., Alley, R. D., Stranahan, A., and Stuart-Harris, C. H. Chronic bronchitis and emphysema: Significance of bacterial flora in sputum. *Amer. J. Med.* 17:478, 1954.
46. Wilmer, H. B., and Cobe, H. M. Vaccine therapy: The uses and misuses. *J. Allerg.* 4:414, 1933.
47. Stevens, F. A. The treatment of infectional asthma in children with filtrates of cultures of upper respiratory pathogenic bacteria. *J. Pediat.* 4:307, 1939.
48. Bergquist, G. Vaccine therapy in bronchial asthma. *Acta Allerg.* 9:97, 1955.
49. Bergman, S., Colldahl, H., and Nilsson, E. Bronchial infection and B. S. R., in asthma with a description of a method for sterile removal of bronchial secretion. *Acta Allerg.* 8:163, 1955.
50. Shinefield, M. A. The use of autogenous acellular bacterial antigen complex in the treatment of recurrent respiratory infections and asthma in infants and children. *New York J. Med.* 56:1468, 1956.
51. Laurenzi, G. A., Potter, R. T., and Kass, E. H. Bacteriologic flora of the lower respiratory tract. *New Eng. J. Med.* 265:1273, 1961.
52. May, J. R. The bacteriology of chronic bronchitis. *Lancet* 2:534, 1953.
53. Rosebury, T. *Microorganisms Indigenous to Man.* New York: McGraw-Hill Book Company, Inc., 1962.
54. Hampton, S. F., Galakatos, E., and Johnson, M. C. Unpublished results.
55. Fagerberg, E., Studies in bronchial asthma: IV. A comparative examination between patients with endogenous and exogenous bronchial asthma respectively with regard to the part played by infection for the first onset of the complaint. *Acta Allerg.* 12:17, 1958.
56. Harkavy, J. Role of unresolved pneumonia in bronchial asthma. *J.A.M.A.* 79:1970, 1922.
57. Hajos, M. K. Influenza virus sensitization in bronchial asthma. *Acta Allerg.* 16:347, 1961.
58. Peshkin, M. M. Asthma in children: III. The incidence and significance of various diseases and infections and of tonsillectomy and adenoidectomy. *Amer. J. Dis. Child.* 33:880, 1927.
59. Adler, F. L. Competition of Antigens. In Shaffer, J. H., LoGrippo, G. A., and Chase, M. W. (Eds.), *Mechanisms of Hypersensitivity.* Boston: Little, Brown, 1959.
60. Cooke, R. A. Allergy in drug idiosyncrasy. *J.A.M.A.* 73:759, 1919.
61. Sheldon, J. M., Lovell, R. G., and Mathews, K. P. *A Manual of Clinical Allergy.* Philadelphia: W. B. Saunders Company, 1953.
62. Lamson, R. W., and Thomas, R. Some untoward effects of acetysalicylic acid. *J.A.M.A.* 99:107, 1932.
63. Dysart, B. R. Death following ingestion of five grains of acetylsalicylic acid. *J.A.M.A.* 101:446, 1933.
64. Francis, N., Ghent, C. T., and Bullen, S. S. Death from ten grains of aspirin. *J. Allerg.* 6:504, 1935.
65. Greenberg, L. A. An evaluation of reported poisonings by acetylsalicylic acid. *New Eng. J. Med.* 243:124, 1950.
66. Friedlaender, S., and Feinberg, S. M. Aspirin allergy: Its relationship to chronic intractable asthma. *Ann. Intern. Med.* 26:734, 1947.
67. Van Leeuwen, W. S. Pathognomonische Bedeutung der Ueberemfindlichkeit gegen Aspirin bei Asthmatikern. *Munchen. Med. Wschr.* 75:1588, 1928.
68. Sherman, W. B. Drug allergy. *Amer. J. Med.* 3:586, 1947.
69. Salen, E. B., and Arner, B. Some views on the aspirin-hypersensitive allergy group. *Acta Allerg.* 1:47, 1948.
70. Lawrence, S. H. The delayed type of allergic inflammatory response. *Amer. J. Med.* 20:428, 1956.
71. Rosenau, M. J., and Anderson, J. F. Studies in hypersusceptibility and immunity. *U.S. Marine Hosp. Service Hyg. Bull.* No. 36, 1907.
72. Kraus, R., and Holobut, T. Ueber die Wirkung des intraokular injizierten rabiziden Serums. *Z. Immunitaetsforsch.* 3:130, 1909.
73. Baldwin, E. R. Studies in immunity to tuberculosis: I. Hypersusceptibility or anaphylaxis. *J. Med. Res.* 22:189, 1910.
74. Heidelberger, M., and Avery, O. T. The soluble specific substance of pneumococcus. *J. Exp. Med.* 38:73, 1923.
75. Avery, O. T., and Tillett, W. S. Anaphylaxis with the type specific carbohydrate of pneumococcus. *J. Exp. Med.* 49:251, 1929.
76. Tillett, W. S., and Francis, T. Cutaneous reactions to the polysaccharides and proteins of

pneumococcus in lobar pneumonia. *J. Exp. Med.* 50:687, 1929.
77. Kuhns, W. J., and Pappenheimer, A. M., Jr. Immunochemical studies of antitoxin produced in normal and allergic individuals hyperimmunized with diphtheria toxoid: I. Relationship of skin sensitivity to purified diphtheria toxoid to the presence of circulating, non-precipitating antitoxin. *J. Exp. Med.* 95:363, 1952.
78. Kuhns, W. J., and Pappenheimer, A. M., Jr. Immunochemical studies of antitoxin produced in normal and allergic individuals hyperimmunized with diphtheria toxoid: II. A comparison between the immunological properties of precipitating and non-precipitating (skin sensitizing) antitoxins. *Ibid.,* p. 375.
79. Kuhns, W. J. Immunological properties of a form of non-precipitating diphtheria antitoxin which does not sensitize human skin. *J. Immun.* 75:105, 1955.
80. Swineford, O., Jr., and Holman, J. Studies in bacterial allergy: III. Results of 3,860 cutaneous tests with 34 crude polysaccharide and nucleoprotein fractions of 14 different bacteria. *J. Allerg.* 20:420, 1949.
81. Swineford, O., Jr., and Reynolds, R. J. Studies in bacterial allergy: V. Persistence of desensitization, with bacterial haptens, of guinea pigs sensitized passively with heterologous serum. *J. Allerg.* 22:350, 1951.
82. Swineford, O., Jr., Tull, L., and Westervelt, F. B. Studies in bacterial allergy: VII. Bronchial desensitization and resensitization in passively sensitized guinea pigs. *J. Allerg.* 26:157, 1953.
83. Friebel, H., and Lund, B. Bakterien als Ursache allergeischer Asthmaanfalle. *Naunyn-Schmiedeberg Arch. Exp. Path.* 228:189, 1956.
84. Bousfield, G., and King-Brown, W. W. Diphtheria immunization with finely atomized toxoid. *Lancet* 1:491, 1938.
85. Baker, A. G. Treatment of chronic bronchial asthma: Aerosol of *Staphylococcus* bacteriophage lysate as an adjunct to systemic hyposensitization. *Amer. Pract.* 9:591, 1958.
86. Aas, K. Nasal eosinophilia in so-called bacterial hypersensitivity in asthmatic children: Preliminary Report. *Acta Paediat.* 50:1, 1961.
87. Pernis, B., Viglianai, E. C., Cavagna, C., and Finulli, M. The role of bacterial endotoxins in occupational diseases caused by inhaling vegetable dust. *Brit. J. Industr. Med.* 18:120, 1961.
88. Hajos, M. K. A comparative study of skin tests and bronchial tests with bacterial solutions in infective bronchial asthma. Preliminary communications. *Acta Allerg.* 55:517, 1960.
89. Hampton, S. F., Johnson, M. C., and Galakatos, E. Studies of bacterial hypersensitivity in asthma: I. The preparation of antigens of *Neisseria catarrhalis,* the induction of asthma by aerosols, the performance of skin and passive transfer tests. *J. Allerg.* 34:63, 1963.
90. Cooke, R. A., Barnard, J. H., Hebald, S., and Stull, A. Serological evidence of immunity with co-existing sensitization in a type of human allergy: Hay fever. *J. Exp. Med.* 62: 733, 1935.
91. Portnoy, J., and Sherman, W. B. Complement fixation studies in ragweed allergy: II. Determination of antibody in human sera to ragweed antigen by means of a complement fixation inhibition test. *J. Allerg.* 25:229, 1954.

51. Rationale of Treatment with Injected Aqueous Extracts of Air-Borne Allergens

FRANCIS C. LOWELL

CONVENTIONAL TREATMENT WITH aqueous allergenic extracts entails repeated injections given over periods of months or years. The injections are given in the expectation that they will enhance tolerance of the mucous membranes of the eyes and respiratory tract to air-borne allergens. The experience with injected extracts of grass and ragweed pollens far exceeds that with extracts of other inhalant allergens, and the discussion here is concerned with this experience. Treatment of pollinosis by repeated injections of aqueous extracts of pollens is referred to as injection therapy. The extracts represent a complex mixture of water-soluble substances contained in pollen which is expected to call forth an immune response to one or more of them, and this indeed occurs. A relation between these immunological responses and the clinical efficacy of such injections is widely considered to be the rationale for this form of treatment. The immunological responses have been detected and measured with some success. Before we can state that injection therapy produces clinical improvement, we must be able to recognize and measure such improvement under appropriate experimental conditions.

Any discussion of injection therapy for pollinosis is beset by difficulties arising from the clinical context in which such treatment is given. The patient demands relief from symptoms; and if, in his opinion, this is achieved, he is satisfied, and treatment is considered to have been effective irrespective of such objective measurements as one may choose to make. Since conventional treatment requires months and and may extend over years, the patient's course may be influenced by spontaneous changes in the disease, variations in the environment, and the giving of medication. The patient's opinion is also influenced by medication given and the distortion and blurring which accompany the passage of time. To these may be added bias in both patient and physician. Finally, uncertainty in etiological diagnosis is inherent in the clinical situation. One cannot know with certainty that symptoms occurring in the course of seasonal exposure to a pollen in a patient fulfilling the usual criteria for clinical sensitivity to it are indeed caused by this exposure and not by some coincident, unrelated, or unrecognized allergen.

In the first reports of injection therapy [1, 2] pollen was described as containing a toxin, and the injections were given to induce an antitoxic immunity. These first extracts were prepared from grass pollen by boiling, a step which today would be expected to inactivate the allergenic activity or alter the specificity of the pollen antigens. These reports, and many to follow over the half-century of experience with injection therapy, describe a protective or therapeutic effect of injections, and injection therapy has been widely accepted as effective. Since the evidence of effectiveness has not been based on controlled clinical trials, there have been many doubts as to its value [3]. This will be discussed further.

Among the hypotheses advanced to explain how injections of pollen extracts might benefit the patient, desensitization and immunization have received most attention. A nonspecific effect has also been postulated, but there is little evidence of such a mechanism [4].

By desensitization is meant the lowering of

the state of allergic reactivity by the injection of antigen in amounts which diminish or eliminate antibody. This has been assumed to occur in patients in a manner analogous to the induction of a refractory state in animals with anaphylactic sensitivity to an antigen. One or more injections of antigen can induce a transitory state of tolerance to the antigen, and during this period the level of circulating antibody is reduced or antibody may disappear completely. Although a reduction of the amount of circulating antibody may follow the repeated injection of an allergen in man [5], there is no evidence that this occurs in significant degree in patients receiving therapeutic injections of allergenic extracts. Indeed, there appears to be little consistent change in the specific reactivity of the skin, and the level of skin-sensitizing antibody may rise [6, 7]. Deliberate intravenous injection of amounts of allergenic extract sufficient to induce a systemic allergic reaction in six untreated subjects failed to alter the level of skin-sensitizing antibody measured by either dilution or the neutralization technique [8]. It is also noteworthy that in the report just cited, the amount of extract that induced a constitutional reaction was equivalent, based on titration by the neutralization technique, to the amount of antibody contained in less than 1 ml. of serum. This would represent one two-thousandth or less of the total circulating antibody.

In addition to antibodies present in the plasma, significant quantities are presumably fixed in tissue, so that the fraction of total antibody represented by 1 ml. of serum is certainly very small. It therefore seems very unlikely that extracts can be safely administered in amounts that would measurably and significantly influence the titer of antibody in the recipient. It is not surprising that the frontal attack on the allergic state in pollinosis as carried out in the so-called rush treatment [9a] was abandoned. Nevertheless rapid desensitization by progressive increases in the dose of heterologous therapeutic sera, as given for the treatment of diphtheria or for the prevention of tetanus, has been regarded as a rational and useful procedure [9b]. This procedure is also regarded as desensitization in the sense that administration of progressively larger amounts of antigen neutralizes or eliminates circulating antibody responsible for allergic reactions. However, such attempts at desensitization are usually unsuccessful in those "spontaneously" serum-sensitive patients who also show clinical manifestations on exposure to the dander of the species from which the serum is obtained; in other words, among those who present clinical and immunological features most closely simulating pollinosis. On the other hand, success is most often achieved in those who have become allergic as a result of previous injections of serum from the animal serving as the source of therapeutic antiserum. Thus experience with therapeutic antisera may not bear on the question at hand. But even here, critical appraisal of reportedly successful desensitization by this means should include the possibility that, rather than achieving desensitization, the administration of progressively larger doses of antiserum merely uncovered a misconception as to the level of allergy and that, after all, allergy of a degree to preclude administration of clinically significant amounts of antiserum was not present.

What has been said regarding changes in skin reactivity applies in patients treated over short or relatively short periods of time. There is evidence, however, that injections continued over several years will bring about a gradual reduction of skin reactivity [10]. Patients reactive on skin tests to several pollen extracts who received injections of only one or two of the extracts showed a progressive decline in skin reactivity to the extracts with which they were treated over a period of years while retaining a relatively constant level of reactivity to the other extracts. This, indeed, suggests that desensitization in a quite literal sense may take place, but it seems unlikely that it is related to the refractory state that can be temporarily induced in sensitive animals by the injection of large doses of antigen. There is no evidence that the benefits claimed for injection therapy are linked to this slow loss of skin reactivity.

Induced tolerance to *injected* allergenic extracts appears to be the rule among patients with pollinosis receiving weekly serial injections of pollen extracts, and treatment schedules are based on the assumption that this occurs. Injections given repeatedly in a single site induce a lowering of tissue reactivity which appears to be nonspecific [11–14]. Increased tolerance, as judged by susceptibility to constitutional allergic manifestations, also develops in most patients so treated, although no systematic study of this has been made. Similar changes, however, were observed in a patient with both sensitivity and resistance to insulin [5]. When insulin was withheld for several months, the pronounced sensitivity to small doses of insulin gave way, on treatment with insulin, to a high degree of tolerance along with the appearance of both resistance to insulin and insulin-inactivating activity in the serum. Inactivation appeared to be due to the formation of antibody to insulin analogous to "blocking" antibody to pollen extracts [15], and it was later shown that the serum contained an insulin-binding γ-globulin [16]. An incidental observation during a study of skin-sensitizing antibody to allergenic fractions of castor bean may also bear on this point [17]. It was noted that, in the course of repeated testing, the subjects changed in their response to the testing procedure in that a remote subcutaneous injection of the allergen would no longer induce a reaction at a passively sensitized site. This change was attributed to an interfering ("blocking") antibody developing as an immune response to repeated subcutaneous injections of antigen.

It may be concluded, therefore, that injections of allergenic substances can induce heightened tolerance to injected allergen and that this tolerance is mediated by a change in the blood which is in all probability a binding [18], neutralizing, or blocking [15] antibody.

Therapeutic injections of pollen extracts lead to the appearance of antibody to components of pollen extract. Since pollen extracts contain a multiplicity of antigens, some of which may be inactive in the causation of allergic symptoms, the mere demonstration that antibody has appeared in the serum is not in itself evidence that the patient's clinical level of allergic reactivity has been modified. However, as already stated, one of the serological changes induced by injections of pollen extract is the appearance of neutralizing or blocking antibody which, as the name suggests, seems particularly well suited to mediate the desired clinical effect of injections. Nevertheless it remains to be proved that the appearance of this antibody does establish a reduced level of susceptibility to *inhaled* pollens. We are confronted here with the difficulty in assessing the reduction of the level of susceptibility referred to at the outset. Controlled studies (see later) carried out in recent years have shown that one cannot rely on an opinion regarding the clinical response. Therefore the individual patient is unsatisfactory as an indicator of a therapeutic effect of injection therapy. Since conclusions regarding a relation between the appearance of blocking activity in the serum and the efficacy of the therapeutic procedure have been based on observations of small numbers of patients—considered, for the most part, individually—a reliable answer is not to be anticipated from the studies which have been reported to date, and the evidence is conflicting [7].

The foregoing discussion has been presented without a clear indication as to whether or not injections of aqueous pollen extracts are indeed effective in decreasing seasonal allergic symptoms. It clearly reflects the difficulties presented by clinical trials in this field that this question has remained unsettled in the more than fifty years since this form of treatment was first described and advocated [1, 2]. Many of the variables to be considered in the assessment of results were acknowledged and enumerated at that time. Since there was no experimental control and since 8 of the patients described received coseasonal and 20 received preseasonal treatment, this report is far from conclusive. However, like the great majority of similar clinical trials which have followed these early reports, the results were regarded as indicative of a therapeutic effect of the injections. This conclusion has been supported by recent studies carried out with varying degrees of experimental control [19–23].

Based on an analysis of the problems of experimental control, the selection of patients and the means of assessing the frequency and intensity of symptoms [23], a study of ragweed pollinosis was conducted in 1963 [24]. A highly significant difference was observed between treated and untreated groups in favor of a therapeutic effect of injections. The arrangement of the experiment was such as to show that this effect was a specific one and that protection was lost wholly or in part within five months after injections were stopped. The cumulative experience indicates, however, that at the present level of clinical understanding, a correlation between the efficacy of injection therapy and any of the several observed serological changes occurring in patients so treated will not be possible by considering patients individually. Rather, a statistical approach will be required in which groups of patients are compared under conditions of strict experimental control. At the present time the rationale for injection therapy remains unsettled.

REFERENCES

1. Noon, L. Prophylactic inoculations against hay fever. *Lancet* 1:1572, 1911.
2. Freeman, J. Further observations on the treatment of hay fever by hypodermic inoculations of pollen vaccine. *Lancet* 2:814, 1911.
3. Lowell, F. C. American Academy of Allergy Presidential Address, *J. Allerg.* 31:185, 1960.
4. Samter, M., and Kofoed, M. A. On the rationale of treating allergic diseases with bacterial pyrogens. *J. Allerg.* 23:327, 1952.
5. Lowell, F. C. Immunologic studies in insulin resistance: I. Report of a case exhibiting variations in resistance and allergy to insulin. *J. Clin. Invest.* 23:225, 1944.
6. Tuft, L., and Heck, V. M. Studies in sensitization as applied to skin test reactions: I. Do skin test reactions change? *J. Allerg.* 25:340, 1954.
7. Sherman, W. B. Reaginic and blocking antibodies. *J. Allerg.* 28:62, 1957.
8. Lowell, F. C., Franklin, W., Schiller, I. W., and Follensby, E. M. Acute allergic reactions induced in subjects with hay fever and asthma by the intravenous administration of allergens with observations on blood clot lysis. *J. Allerg.* 27:369, 1956.

9a. Freeman, J. "Rush" inoculation, with special reference to hay-fever treatment. *Lancet* 1:744, 1930.

9b. Rackemann, F. M. *Clinical Allergy, Particularly Asthma and Hay Fever: Mechanism and Treatment.* New York: Macmillan Company, 1931.

10. Sherman, W. B., Sprecace, G., Pomper, S. G., Lemlich, A., and Ziffer, H. The effect of antigen injections on skin reactivity to antigens. Presented at the Annual Meeting of the American Academy of Allergy, February, 1964.
11. Cooke, R. A. Studies in specific hypersensitiveness: IV. On the phenomenon of hyposensitization (the clinically lessened sensitiveness of allergy). *J. Immun.* 7:219, 1922.
12. Bowman, K. L., and Walzer, M.: The response of specific and histamine wheal sites in atopic skins to restimulation with specific and nonspecific excitants. *J. Immun.* 29:81, 1935 (abst.).
13. Bowman, K. L., and Walzer, M. Studies in reaginic and histaminic wheals: I. The effects of reaginic and histaminic wheals upon the subsequent responsiveness of passively sensitized cutaneous sites. *J. Allerg.* 24:126, 1953.
14. Lowell, F. C., and Williams, M. The effect of subcutaneous injections of allergenic extract on the local reactivity to intracutaneously injected extract. *J. Allerg.* 34:35, 1963.
15. Loveless, M. H. Immunological studies of pollinosis: I. The presence of two antibodies related to the same pollen-antigen in the serum of treated hay-fever patients. *J. Immun.* 38:25, 1940.
16. Burrows, B. A., Peters, T., Lowell, F. C., Trakas, A. N., and Reilly, P. Physical binding of insulin by gamma globulins of insulin-resistant subjects. *J. Clin. Invest.* 36:393, 1957.
17. Spies, J. R., and Bernton, H. S. Response of nonallergic persons to injected castor bean allergen, CB-1A. *J. Allerg.* 33:73, 1962.
18. Follensby, E. M., and Lowell, F. C. Removal of a skin-reactive component in ragweed pollen extract by human serum protein present as an immunologic precipitate. *J. Allerg.* 28:307, 1957.
19. Bruun, E. Control examination of the specificity of specific desensitization in asthma. *Acta Allerg.* 2:122, 1949.
20. Frankland, A. W., and Augustin, R. Prophylaxis of summer hay fever and asthma: A controlled trial comparing crude grass pollen extracts with the isolated main protein component. *Lancet* 1:1055, 1954.
21. Johnstone, D. E. Study of the role of antigen dosage in the treatment of pollenosis and pollen asthma. *Amer. J. Dis. Child.* 94:1, 1957.
22. Johnstone, D. E. Value of hyposensitization therapy for perennial bronchial asthma in children. *Pediatrics* 27:39, 1961.
23. Lowell, F. C., Franklin, W., and Williams, M. A "double blind" study of treatment with aqueous allergenic extracts in cases of allergic rhinitis. *J. Allerg.* 34:165, 1963.
24. Lowell, F. C., Franklin, W., and Williams, M.: A double blind study on the specificity of injection therapy with aqueous extracts in ragweed pollenosis. Ref. 10.

52. Rationale of Desensitization by Injections of Emulsions of Antigens

ALAN R. FEINBERG AND SAMUEL M. FEINBERG

THE RATIONALE FOR THE USE OF antigens in emulsion for desensitization is based on the principles (1) that it provides slow absorption of the antigen, thus reducing the number of injections required, and (2) that antigen in the emulsified state enhances antibody formation.

Although the major discussion here concerns the use of antigens emulsified in mineral oil, it is pertinent to point out that the concept of slow absorption has been considered and tried for many years. For example, in 1944, Feinberg [1] stated: ". . . if a slowly absorbed antigen were deposited in the tissues . . . diminution in constitutional reactions would definitely be expected; reduction in the number of injections would undoubtedly be possible; and by more continuous stimulation of antibodies a more complete immunity might be attained." Further: "These considerations prompted us in 1931 to begin the search for a medium which would effectively reduce the rate of absorption of an antigen such as pollen. . . . In the course of fourteen years we have made and experimented with various preparations in order to achieve the aforementioned objective. Preparations included precipitated pollen suspended in oil, whole ground pollen suspended in oil or normal saline, and oil-in-water and water-in-oil emulsions. One of the most successful preparations was an oil-continuous emulsion with gum dammar as the emulsifying agent." It was concluded, however, that none of these preparations was sufficiently effective, safe, or acceptable.

During the same period pollen emulsified in lanolin and olive oil was suggested by Naterman [2]. Later he substituted pollen tannate [3]. Pollen extracts dissolved in gelatin for slow absorption were proposed by Spain *et al.* [4].

Freund *et al.* [5] are generally credited with introduction of the concept of use of antigens emulsified in hydrocarbon oils to increase antibody formation. Beginning in 1937, Freund showed that antibody formation could be enhanced in animals by incorporating antigens in a mineral oil emulsion with or without tubercle bacilli. He found also that although the incomplete adjuvant (without tubercle bacilli) would raise antibody titer which determines the immediate type of sensitivity, the complete adjuvant was required to induce the delayed type of sensitivity.

The use of emulsified influenza vaccine was begun by Salk *et al.* [6, 7] in 1950. They used Arlacel-A (mannide mono-oleate) and a lighter mineral oil than Freund. By 1953, more than 12,000 injections of emulsified influenza vaccine had been given, with good results and without serious local reactions [8]. In 1958, Berlin and McKinney [9] described an apparatus consisting of two syringes connected by a double-hub needle so that the mixture would pass from one syringe to the other through this needle and emulsify in the process. Davenport *et al.* [10, 11] continued with such influenza vaccination for several years and showed that the emulsion produced a higher and longer lasting antibody titer and more lasting clinical immunity than aqueous preparations. They did call attention to the fact that despite systematic testing of the vaccine components in animals, abscesses occasionally occurred in man, mainly in Negroes and children.

Our clinical experience for the last three or four years with emulsified influenza vaccine resembles the foregoing accounts. With 0.25 ml. of the emulsified preparation, containing equal parts of aqueous vaccine and emulsifying agent, given in a single injection, the protection provided in the 1962–63 season exceeded that obtained with two injections of 1 ml. of aqueous vaccine in control patients. However, such an achievement depends simply on the production of a good titer of antibody. We shall discuss later the differences between this simple mechanism and desensitization.

Using Freund's animal work as a basis, Loveless [12] in 1947 described her results of treating thirty-three ragweed hay fever patients with an emulsion of Falba, mineral oil, and ragweed extract. Of fifty-four injections, nine caused constitutional reactions. Her later efforts resulted in fewer reactions. Although Loveless stated that this method produced effective results, she made no claim that they were better than with the multiple aqueous injections. In 1957, Brown [13] reported on his first use of emulsified pollen extract. Since then a number of publications concerning emulsions by Brown and by others [14–32] have appeared, dealing with results of treatment, modifications of technic and preparations, evaluation of tolerance, examination of the emulsions, and the use of various antigens.

PREPARATION AND TESTING OF MATERIALS

PRESENT METHOD

Extracts. Pollen is defatted with ethyl ether, dried, then extracted with a sorbitol extracting fluid (sorbitol 18.2 gm.; K_2HPO_4, 1.7 gm.; KH_2PO_4, 0.27 gm.; phenol, 0.4 gm.; diluted to 100 ml. in distilled H_20) for 24 to 48 hours. The mixture is then filtered by pressure through a Seitz or Polypore bacteriological filter and tested for sterility. Subsequent dilutions are made with sorbitol diluting fluid (sorbitol 18.2 gm., phenol 0.4 gm. to 100 ml. distilled H_20) which has been run through a Seitz filter for sterilizing. Extracts are labeled according to pollen units (1 pollen unit = 0.001 mg. of pollen or 1 ml. of a 1 : 1,000,000 extract w/v [weight : volume]). Extracts and emulsions are kept refrigerated.

Emulsions. The emulsion base is prepared by thorough mixing of 1 part Arlacel A,* specially treated of recent date, with 6 parts of Drakeol 6 VR.† This oil-Arlacel mixture is Seitz-filtered, then 2.33 ml. is dispensed with an automatic pipette under sterile precautions into 5 ml. sterile, previously unused vials and capped with a Neoprene closure. At this point, all apparatus should be perfectly dry or the oil will appear cloudy from a small amount of emulsion, although this is actually not harmful. To this vial is added 1.67 ml. of the pollen extract in a concentration 2.4 times that desired for the final emulsion. For example, if the final emulsion should have 10,000 pollen units per milliliter, 1.67 ml. of a 24,000 unit per ml. of extract is added. This mixture is then shaken a few seconds by hand to obtain a crude emulsion so that the contents are distributed evenly. The mixture is then withdrawn as completely as possible into a 5 ml. plastic syringe and the barrel of the syringe drawn to the 5 ml. mark. The needle is removed and the end of the syringe closed with a Neoprene closure which is then taped on tightly. The syringe is placed in a Spex apparatus‡ and emulsified for 10 minutes in the case of pollen, or in 3 minute intervals in the case of heat-labile material, with a period for cooling between runs. For convenience, the emulsion is then transferred through a double-hubbed needle to 10 ml. glass syringes. From these syringes, emulsion is dispensed for use into 1 ml. disposable tuberculin syringes. A 23 × 1 in. disposable needle is used for injection, which is given intramuscularly in the deltoid.

The Spex mixer mill apparatus emulsifies the material by shaking it in three planes so that the ends of the container move about 100 times a second. Before use, the emulsion may be shaken again in the Spex apparatus or passed by hand several times back and forth through the No. 18 double-hubbed needle.

OTHER METHODS

There are actually dozens of apparatus available or invented for preparing emulsions. Basically they all act by achieving a rapid mixing of the oil and water components by breaking them into small particles. This may be achieved by forcing the material through a small opening such as a needle or through multiple small openings such as a sieve. Or it may be mixed rapidly in a blender or squeezed between rapidly moving plates. It may be subjected to ultrasonic force. The limitations of the apparatus to be used are that the material must be kept sterile, the heating

* Hill Top Laboratories, Cincinnati.

† Pennsylvania Refining Co., Butler, Pa.

‡ Hollister-Stier Laboratories, Spokane, Wash.

in the process of emulsification must be kept minimal, and the procedure must be reproducible.

We have used both defatted and undefatted pollen to prepare extracts and can detect no difference in therapeutic effect or stability of emulsion. Ragweed extract filters more easily if it is defatted, and we have returned to that procedure. Many variables have been tried in the extracting fluid. The best emulsions are prepared when the salts are kept at a minimum.

TESTING OF EMULSIONS

We have tried various methods of testing emulsions and have reduced our procedure to the following routine: (1) Prepared emulsions are placed in the refrigerator and not used for 24 hours. If there is breakdown in 24 hours, the emulsion is discarded. If there is no breakdown, the emulsion appears to be stable for many months and possibly years. (2) On handling the emulsion in the glass syringe, a feeling for the viscosity is developed. If the viscosity feels different from normal, the emulsion is discarded. (3) On microscopic examination the emulsion has a "ground-glass" appearance under high power, is homogenous, and the particles are extremely small. There is no Brownian movement of the particles. Such a motion may be observed in an inverted emulsion.

To test new types of emulsions or those prepared by variations in technic, several other physical methods are used. High-speed centrifugation of the emulsion should reveal no aqueous portion at the bottom of the tube. Water-soluble and oil-soluble dyes and radioactive tracer have been used to advantage. Testing of an emulsion by incorporating a pharmacological agent such as a toxin or an immunizing agent such as bovine serum albumin will give evidence as to its effectiveness. However, results obtained in such ways cannot be directly translated to a substance such as ragweed pollen, which differs physically and chemically from the other substances used.

To the procedures for testing an emulsion noted above should be added its test for treatment and for local and systemic tolerance by the patient. When investigating an experimental procedure in preparing emulsions, we have found that by testing several sensitive subjects with the emulsion by scratch test and comparing the reaction or lack of it with threefold serial dilutions of the aqueous antigen we can estimate the amount of antigen that is immediately released and active.

ASSESSMENT OF TOLERANCE

Since antigen emulsions now in use release the first significant dose of the antigen within several hours, it is necessary to know whether the amount thus released exceeds the particular patient's tolerance. There is no certain method of measuring such tolerance. Loveless suggested quantitative conjunctival tests. However, the ratio of quantitative response of conjunctival, nasal, and bronchial tissues differ in given individuals, depending mainly on the clinical sensitivity of the particular tissue. Some rely on the size of an individual skin reaction, but quantitative skin tests have been used more frequently.

We have the impression that measurement of tolerance depends on a number of factors: the severity of the patient's symptoms, his reaction to previous desensitization therapy, modification of his tolerance by previous treatment, and the titer of the quantitative skin test. Scratch tests are made with pollen extract dilutions composed of a series of 10 vials of threefold dilutions beginning with 1 : 20 (50,000 pollen units per ml. or approximately 25,000 protein N units per ml.). The average patient will react to about 500 or 160 pollen units per ml.; the most sensitive will react to 5 or 2 pollen units or even less. Patients with average skin sensitivity can begin repository therapy with 1,000 pollen units or higher. Those with higher sensitivity are best begun with 500 units, whereas those with extreme skin sensitivity may need to begin with only 100 units. As a rule, tolerance is increased by the first repository treatment, so that the second dose one month later can be about five times the first. The skin test titration is an approximate measure of tolerance, but only if the patient is not under desensitization treatment.

TREATMENT

Our experience, and that of many others, indicates that the incidence of good results is greater with the conventional treatment with aqueous extract than with the repository method, although there are exceptions. Patients selected for repository treatment are chiefly those who for any number of reasons find it difficult to carry out multiple-dose therapy. We prefer to avoid treating younger children by this method, especially Negro children. If the patient has had poor results with the emulsion in spite of an adequate dose of the allergen to which he is clinically sensitive, we then try aqueous treatment. We also recommend this when a large number of allergens are involved or when frequent visits are important for the continuous treatment and observation of the chronic asthmatic.

Our usual procedure is to give 1,000 units or more, followed by a second injection about four weeks later which, as has been stated, is five times the first dose, unless there was undue local or any systemic reaction to the first injection. In some instances, we give a third dose of about 10,000 units. If but 500 units are given in the first dose, a second dose, three to five times the first, is given three weeks later, followed in another three weeks by about 5,000 or more units, again depending on the reaction to each dose. Some patients tolerate only the smaller doses.

When should the initial dose of an allergen be given? In a cooperative study, comparison of the timing of a single dose of emulsion with therapeutic results suggested that emulsions given eight to twelve weeks before onset of the ragweed season were most effective. In practice, we prefer to give the first injection of ragweed extract in May and the second in June. We give no injections after July. The volume of emulsion injected has varied from 0.2 to 1.0 ml.

Certain allergens, including house dust and molds, have been the cause of most of the local delayed reactions and failed to give beneficial results. Although we use these in emulsion form on occasion, we generally avoid their use. We feel also that emulsified insect extracts should not be used. We insist on a clear clinical correlation of symptoms with the allergen to be employed, as well as unequivocally positive responses to scratch tests.

Administration of 20,000 to 30,000 pollen units divided in multiple doses of emulsion to a small group of very allergic patients gave poorer than average results.

REACTIONS

The possible hazards from administration of emulsified antigens are: (1) "immediate" local or constitutional reactions; (2) local reactions of delayed onset or long duration; (3) induced immediate or delayed type of sensitivity, and (4) possible other remote effects.

Slight soreness or stiffness at the site of injection is fairly common and is generally due to introduction of foreign body (emulsified oil) in the tissue spaces causing distention and some irritation. A pronounced local swelling, frequently associated with hot skin and sometimes with erythema, may occur in one-half to several hours, if the immediately released portion of the antigen is excessive. Systemic reactions include erythema, urticaria, or angioedema, less frequently asthma, and sometimes chills and fever. Whereas aqueous extracts usually cause systemic reactions in minutes, "immediate" reactions to emulsions usually appear not earlier than two hours after injection and sometimes not for several more hours. The preponderance of angioedema is characteristic. We do not know of any method (or any preparation) by means of which constitutional reactions can be avoided in all cases. Attention to the principles outlined for the assessment of tolerance and the use of three or four primary doses of aqueous extract or of one priming dose of emulsion several weeks prior to the large dose will minimize such reactions to 5 percent or less, and they are rarely severe. Comparing the frequency of reactions with those to conventional aqueous extract therapy, one can say that reaction occurs more often per number of injections but in a lower percentage of patients. Most reactions can be managed with antihistamines; an occasional one requires epinephrine, and, rarely, a persisting effect requires corticosteroids.

Prolonged local reactions appear to be of two types. One, due to foreign body tissue response, may be noted soon after injection or may not be observed until weeks or even months later. The reaction may consist of a diffuse hard swelling, frequently as one or more nodular areas, or a small nodular area may be the first observation. These swellings do not, as a rule, lead to discomfort or breakdown. They diminish with time, although some evidence of swelling may be present even after a year or two. Although swellings may occur if the injection has been intramuscular, they are more apt to appear when the subcutaneous technic is used. Some individuals are more prone to these swellings than others; it is usually wise, therefore, to refrain from further emulsion therapy in those who have had them previously. In the early stages, systemic corticosteroid therapy may be helpful.

The second type of prolonged local reaction begins 10 days or more after the injection, progressively enlarges, causes some increased warmth of the skin, and finally tends to break down to form a sterile abscess although the process may resolve without abscess formation. From clinical observation, skin tests on patients with a history of emulsion-produced abscess, and experimental studies in induced sensitivity, we believe that many of these cases represent an induced (or already present) delayed sensitivity to an antigen to which there were no skin-sensitizing antibodies originally. Undoubtedly other factors are involved, and it is widely accepted that children and Negroes are particularly prone to this complication. Corticosteroids may be helpful in the early stages. When the area becomes fluctuant, aspiration or incision is indicated.

In an extensive study of induced hypersensitivity with emulsified antigens (pollens and molds) [31, 34–37], we found that the immediate type of skin reactivity could be induced in 32 of 34 atopic individuals and 8 of 22 nonatopic subjects, and a delayed type of hypersensitivity in 14 of 34 atopic and 12 of 22 nonatopic subjects. None of the atopic individuals who were given an emulsion of the antigen to which they had spontaneous immediate type sensitivity developed a delayed skin reaction, although the peripheral leukocytes of 40 percent of them were able to transfer the delayed hypersensitivity state. By quantitative passive transfer studies, Sherman and Connell [38] have shown that an injection of emulsified ragweed extract increases titers of sensitizing antibody in ragweed hay fever sufferers. In some of our cases of experimentally induced delayed reactivity, the original emulsion injection site became swollen and in a few instances resulted in sterile abscesses.

The clinical importance of these observations is not clear. None of our subjects has had hay fever in the season. Fisher and Connell [26] produced a systemic reaction with a second emulsion of pollen extract, and it is not unlikely that clinical immediate type of sensitivity may be induced when it had not been present previously. The clinical aspects of induced delayed sensitivity are also not clearly defined. It is possible that delayed sensitivity might produce symptoms when the antigen (pollen or mold spores) is inhaled. A recent report [38a] shows that in subjects with induced delayed skin reactivity to pollen, delayed symptoms of rhinorrhea and nasal stuffiness could be produced by a tampon of pollen extract. At any rate, it would be well to take care that emulsion therapy should not be given with any antigen to which the individual has not been proved to be allergic.

A discussion of other possible remote effects of emulsions is, at present, purely speculative. The materials have not been proved to be carcinogenic. Some experiments in animals [39] which seem to indicate distant inflammatory effects lack sufficient control or confirmation. Nevertheless one must give thought to the possible fate of the foreign material, particularly if a number of injections are repeated for some years.

EVALUATION OF RESULTS

Immunization with an antigen (such as influenza virus) in emulsified form augments and prolongs antibody formation and is comparable to increased antibody formation from the use of antigen with adjuvants in animals. The problem in allergy is somewhat different, however. Antibodies (sensitizing) are already present, and it has been shown that the emulsified antigen actually increases them, a fact we would expect to be harmful. In the absence of antibodies, an emulsified antigen in man can produce new sensitizing antibodies or delayed sensitivity. It would seem, therefore, that if any benefit is derived from emulsion injections it must be because of the production of blocking antibodies or because of some other, unknown, compensating protective mechanism.

Evaluating the benefits of treatment is the most difficult and controversial part of both repository emulsion and aqueous type treatment [40, 41]. The difficulty lies in lack of adequate quantitative objective methods for measuring response. Antibody studies by hemagglutination methods and other techniques do not seem to correlate with results. Skin-testing by titration does not give indication of the amount of relief to be expected. We have observed a reduction in skin reactivity after treatment in most cases, but this cannot be used to predict clinical response. Titration of the nasal mucosa or the bronchi is a more promising method of evaluating such response. Another possible indication of increased resistance to allergen is the determination of tolerance of aqueous injections after a repository emulsion injection is given. It might be assumed that much larger doses of aqueous antigen would be tolerated than would be the case before treatment, but we have found in limited testing that only moderate increases in tolerance are to be expected. These methods are promising but, at present, reports of the patient are our chief means of evaluating results. This, for many obvious reasons, is far from simple, if the evaluation is to be truly impartial.

In correlating the results of treatment reported by different investigators, many variables make it difficult to decide what the comparative immunological responses are from year to year, since the natural history of the disease is not clear. Such variables include pollen counts, weather conditions, and variations in sensitivity. Furthermore, treatment with conventional aqueous injections in previous seasons may produce benefit the following season with pollen emulsion or with no treatment at all. Other allergies modify results, as in the patient allergic to ragweed and molds who is treated for ragweed only. To evaluate adequately this type of treatment a large group of previously untreated patients must be observed by impartial investigators using the double blind technique. The patients must be proved to be clinically sensitive to the allergen investigated and must not be significantly allergic to other allergens prevalent at the same time. They must be adequately observed during the season of study, whether or not they say they have symptoms.

RESULTS OF TREATMENT

In view of the aforementioned difficulties, only a general impression can be given of results of treatment. A nationwide collaborative study was conducted in 1960 on the treatment of ragweed patients with pollen emulsion. There were 1,777 subjects, of whom 200 were given placebo emulsions [25]. Of those receiving pollen emulsions, 74 percent had moderate to complete relief of hay fever and 77 percent of asthma; with placebo injections, 44 percent of patients with hay fever and 40 percent of those with asthma had comparable results. A comparison of the results of emulsion treatment in those who had had previous conventional treatment indicated that 52 percent of patients fared better with the latter method, 35 percent were the same, and 13 percent were worse.

The reports of others on results from repository therapy vary. Many experienced observers believe that emulsion therapy has usefulness in selected cases, particularly because of convenience for the patient, yet they feel that over-all reliability is greater with the multiple-dose aqueous therapy. Others have made excessive claims for superior results from repository treatment. In some, but not all instances, such differences in apparent results are attributable to variable pollen counts, since obviously reports of experiences in areas of widely differing exposure can hardly be compared.

REFERENCES

1. Feinberg, S. M. *Allergy in Practice.* Chicago: Year Book Publishers, Inc., 1944. P. 595.
2. Naterman, H. L. The treatment of hay fever by injection of pollen extract emulsified in lanolin and olive oil: A preliminary report. *New Eng. J. Med.* 218:797, 1938.
3. Naterman, H. L. Pollen tannate suspended in peanut oil with aluminum monostearate in the treatment of hay fever. *J. Allerg.* 22:175, 1951.
4. Spain, W. C., Fuchs, A. M., and Strauss, M. B. A slowly absorbed gelatin-pollen extract for the treatment of hay fever. *J. Allerg.* 12:365, 1941.
5. Freund, J., Casals, J., and Hosmer, E. P. Sensitization and antibody formation after injection of tubercle bacilli and paraffin oil. *Proc. Soc. Exp. Biol. Med.* 37:509, 1937.
6. Salk, J. E., Lewis, L. J., Bennett, B. L., Younger, J. S., and Bubash, G. R. The use of an adjuvant to facilitate studies on the immunologic classification of poliomyelitis viruses. *Bact. Proc.,* p. 80, 1950 (abst.).
7. Salk, J. E., Laurent, A. M., and Bailey, M. L. Direction of research in vaccination against influenza: New studies with immunologic adjuvants. *Amer. J. Public Health* 41:669, 1951.
8. Salk, J. E. Use of adjuvants in studies on influenza immunization: 3. Degree of persistence

of antibody in human subjects two years after vaccination. *J.A.M.A.* 151:1169, 1953.

9. Berlin, B. S., and McKinney, R. W. A simple device for making emulsified vaccines. *J. Lab. Clin. Med.* 52:657, 1958.
10. Davenport, F. M., Hennessy, A. V., and Bell, J. A. Immunologic advantages of emulsified virus vaccines. *Milit. Med.* 127:95, 1962.
11. Davenport, F. M. Applied immunology of mineral oil adjuvants. *J. Allerg.* 32:177, 1961.
12. Loveless, M. H. Application of immunological principles to the management of hay fever, including a preliminary report of the use of Freund's adjuvant. *Amer. J. Med. Sci.* 214:559, 1947.
13. Brown, E. A. Prevention of reactions to repository injection treatment. *Ann. Allerg.* 15: 499, 1957.
14. Brown, E. A. The treatment of pollinosis by means of a single annual injection of emulsified extract: V. Preparation, standardization and administration. *Ann. Allerg.* 17:34, 1959.
15. Brown, E. A. The treatment of allergy to ragweed pollen by means of a single annual injection of emulsified pollen extract: Discussion of results, relationship and some miscellaneous factors. *Ibid.,* p. 358.
16. Sobel, G. Repository treatment of ragweed pollinosis. *J. Allerg.* 32:288, 1961.
17. Mitchell, W. F., Mitchell, J. H., Sivon, I., and Wilson, W. M. Clinical response to emulsified pollen extract in the Midwest: A five year study. *J. Allerg.* 34:107, 1963.
18. Arbesman, C. E., and Reisman, R. E. Repository therapy: Further clinical and immunological studies. *Ibid.,* p. 39.
19. Sherman, W. B., Brown, E. B., Karol, R. S., Myers, P. A., Kessler, W. R., Chapin, H. B., Goodman, A. A., Barnard, J. H., and Popovitz, C. J. Repository emulsion treatment of ragweed pollinosis. *J. Allerg.* 33:473, 1962.
20. Furstenberg, F. F. Repository method for the treatment of ragweed pollinosis. *Ann. Allerg.* 18:866, 1960.
21. Prigal, S. J. Studies with medicated water-in-oil emulsions: I. Use of a high speed shaker for the production of emulsions under sterile conditions. *J. Allerg.* 33:295, 1962.
22. Friedlaender, S., and Friedlaender, A. S. Clinical effects of ragweed antigen emulsion: A double blind study. *Ibid.,* p. 412.
23. Eisenberg, B. C., and MacLaren, W. R. Adverse reactions to injected emulsified pollen extract in allergic patients on the west coast: Relationship to the total dosage of antigen. *J. Allerg.* 32:373, 1961.
24. Loveless, M. H. Recent advances in repository therapy in allergy. *J. Amer. Med. Wom. Ass.* 15:955, 1960.
25. Feinberg, S. M. Repository antigen therapy: Its present status. *J. Allerg.* 32:271, 1961 (editorial).
26. Fisher, J. P., and Connell, J. T. A study of immunological responses of a normal individual to injections of ragweed pollen emulsified in mineral oil adjuvant. *J. Allerg.* 34:250, 1963.
27. Barlow, P. P., and Bortz, A. I. Studies on repository antigen preparation: I. Retention of antigen at the injection site in rats. *Med. Bull. Univ. Michigan* 26:138, 1960.
28. Arbesman, C. E., and Reisman, R. E. Immunologic studies of repository ragweed pollen therapy. *J. Allerg.* 32:435, 1961.
29. Feinberg, S. M., and Feinberg, A. R. Desensitization Therapy with Emulsified Extracts: Its Present Status. In Brown, E. A. (Ed.), *Allergology* (Proceedings of 4th International Congress). New York: Pergamon Press, 1962. P. 161.
30. Feinberg, S. M., Rabinowitz, H. I., Pruzansky, J. J., Feinberg, A. R., and Kaminker, A. Repository antigen injections: Absorption studies by immunological and radioactive methods. *J. Allerg.* 31:421, 1960.
31. Feinberg, A. R., Feinberg, S. M., and Fisherman, E. W. Repository antigen injections: Preparation and therapy. *Ibid.,* p. 433.
32. Grolnick, M., Pelz, H. H., and Chao, I. Absorption pattern of ragweed antigens and active sensitization in man following repository pollen injections. *J. Allerg.* 32:327, 1961.
33. Berlin, B. S. Gross physical properties of emulsified influenza virus vaccine and the adjuvant response. *J. Immun.* 85:81, 1960.
34. Sparks, D. B., Feinberg, S. M., and Becker, R. J. Immediate skin reactivity induced in atopic and non-atopic persons following injection of emulsified pollen extracts. *J. Allerg.* 33:245, 1962.
35. Becker, R. J., Sparks, D. B., Feinberg, S. M., Patterson, R., Pruzansky, J. J., and Feinberg, A. R. Delayed and immediate skin reactivity in man after injection of antigen in emulsion: Cell transfer and delayed sensitivity. *J. Allerg.* 32:229, 1961.
36. Feinberg, S. M., Becker, R. J., Slavin, R. G., Feinberg, A. R., and Sparks, D. B. The sensitizing effects of emulsified pollen antigens in atopic subjects naturally sensitive to an unrelated antigen. *J. Allerg.* 33:285, 1962.
37. Slavin, R. G., Tennenbaum, J. I., Becker, R. J., Feinberg, A. R., and Feinberg, S. M. Cell transfer of delayed hypersensitivity to ragweed from atopic subjects treated with emulsified ragweed extracts. *J. Allerg.* 34:368, 1963.
38. Sherman, W. B., and Connell, J. T. Presented at Conference on Evaluation of Repository Therapy, New York, 1962.

38a. Slavin, R. G., Fink, J. N., Becker, R. J., Tennenbaum, J. I., and Feinberg, S. M. Delayed response to antigen challenge in induced delayed reactivity. A clinical and cytologic study in man. *J. Allerg.* 35:499, 1964.

39. Steiner, J. W., Langer, B., and Schatz, D. L. The local and systemic effects of Freund's adjuvant and its fractions. *Arch. Path.* 70:424, 1960.

40. Lowell, F. C., and Franklin, W. A "double blind" study of treatment with aqueous allergenic extracts in cases of allergic rhinitis. *J. Allerg.* 34:165, 1963.

41. Fontana, V. J. The scientific approach to allergy. *New York J. Med.* 63:933, 1963.

53. Pharmacological Approach to Treatment of Atopic Disorders*

DOMINGO M. AVIADO

SYMPTOMATIC CONTROL OF IMMUNOLOGICAL diseases interrupts the allergic reaction by means of drugs. The sequence by which normal tissue undergoes an allergic reaction has been identified, the functional characteristics of allergic tissue are understood, and we know some of the drugs that convert the latter to the former.

The use of drugs in specific allergic reactions is discussed in other chapters; this chapter summarizes the effects of various drugs on the allergic reaction in general and on lung tissue in particular [1, 2].

The allergic response consists of (1) the primary events following the introduction of antigen and resulting in the appearance of antibodies, (2) intermediate events in which there is a release of humoral agents, and (3) the functional impairment of the tissue. In Figure 53-1, drugs are grouped in accordance with this sequence. It will be noted that the primary events can be interrupted by drugs introduced before the antigen-antibody response (radiomimetic drugs), during the inductive phase (antimetabolites), and during both phases as well as immediately following the antigen-antibody interaction (cortisone). Some secondary events can be controlled by depletion of the humoral agents (histamine-releasers) and by blocking of the action of the humoral agent (antihistaminics). Neither approach controls the allergic response in the lung, so that discussion here will be on the reversal of the functional abnormalities, e.g., by sympathomimetics, musculotropics, opiates, and antitussives.

INTERFERENCE WITH THE PRIMARY EVENTS

Several drugs have been used to bring about a state of "immunological tolerance," in this chapter considered to be an "atypical state of unresponsiveness to an antigenic stimulus." Although this term was originally intended to refer to the state of the recipient of a homograft which was retained, Hitchings and Elion [3] have used it in a broader sense to characterize the individual who fails to respond to an antigenic stimulus which gives rise to good responses in the majority of individuals. Drugs which induce tolerance can be grouped according to the time of their administration in relation to administration of the antigen.

DRUGS WITH MAXIMAL EFFECTS WHEN GIVEN BEFORE THE ANTIGENIC STIMULUS

The radiomimetic drugs are the best examples of drugs which interfere with the immunological response if administered prior to administration of the antigen. Like x-rays, the radiomimetic agents have been especially useful in controlling the rejection of homografts and heterografts by the recipient. Such agents depress the bone marrow and are too potent for use in the prevention of minor allergic responses.

Cortisone seems to exert its maximal protective effect when its administration is begun before the initial exposure to the antigen. However, Fischel *et al.* [4] observed the hor-

* Supported in part by the U.S. Army Medical Branch and Development Command, Department of the Army, under Contract No. DA-49-193-MD-2093.

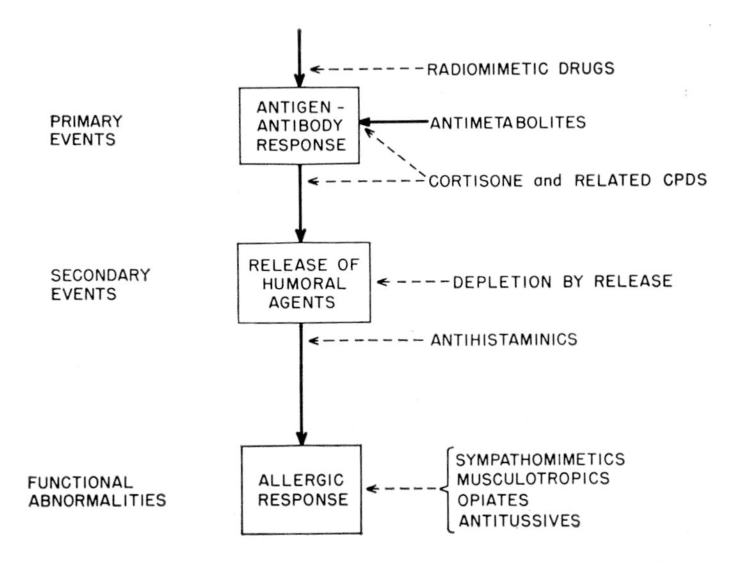

Fig. 53–1. Action of drugs on the allergic response.

mone to influence established immunity. In rabbits, the production of antibodies against egg albumin associated with the specific anamnestic or secondary response was inhibited by cortisone. There are at least three steps in the formation of antibody at which cortisone probably exerts an inhibitory effect: the assimilation of antigen by the tissues, the inflammatory reaction that is associated with injection of antigen, and the synthesis of antibody globulin. Fischel and his collaborators have raised the possibility that all of these steps have a common biochemical denominator.

ANTI-IMMUNE EFFECTS OF ANTIMETABOLITES

Antimetabolites induce immunological tolerance primarily during the inductive period, i.e., the interval between the introduction of antigen and the appearance of the antibody. At present, antimetabolites are used to suppress homograft reaction. In the dog, lung homotransplants have exhibited prolonged survival after suppression of immunological response by methotrexate, an antagonist of folic acid and useful in bringing about a remission of acute leukemia [5]. Another antimetabolite, azathioprine, has been shown to prolong the survival of lung homotransplants [6]. The review article by Hitchings and Elion [3] contains other examples of chemical suppression of the immune response, but none of them has yet been applicable to clinical allergy.

CORTISONE AND RELATED COMPOUNDS

The efficacy of corticosteriods in the treatment of bronchial asthma has been documented by numerous reports. The exact mechanism of action, however is not clear, and observations in animals suggest three types. The first is a primary inhibition of the response of sensitized tissue to antigen, as previously mentioned and demonstrated in the sensitized guinea pig lung by Stormorken [7], who observed that cortisone blocked the bronchoconstriction when administered before the constricting stimulus. On the other hand, Lefcoe [8] described a second action which relaxes the tracheal ring of the guinea pig directly, following the addition of a water-soluble hydrocortisone preparation to the isolated organ bath. The same preparation administered to patients by inhalation in aerosol form had beneficial effects, presumably from a direct relaxation of the smooth muscle.

The third action of corticosteroids is suppression of inflammation in the walls of the bronchioles and a consequent increase in their caliber. The most direct evidence pertaining to the diseased lung tissue was obtained by Franklin *et al.* [9] in 58 patients with obstructive pulmonary emphysema. The improvement in lung function brought about by inhalation of a powerful bronchodilator (isoproterenol) was compared before and after the administration of corticosteriods (cortisone, cortisol, prednisone, and prednisolone). The improvement in ventilatory function of the lung was greater when isoproterenol was administered following corticosteroids than where isoproterenol was given alone.

INTERFERENCE WITH RELEASE OF HUMORAL AGENTS

The role of histamine and other humoral agents in mediating the allergic response is discussed in Chapter 15. From the pharmacological standpoint, one possible means of blocking the allergic response is to deplete the tissue depots. Paton [10] reviewed the compounds that release histamine in tissues, but none of them is useful clinically for a number of reasons. Some of them, like morphine and tubocurarine, have primary actions other than the release of histamine. One compound (48/80) is the closest approach to a chemical compound that will release only histamine in the tissues, but the initial release brought about by such a drug causes histamine shock. So far, it has not been possible to deplete the stores of histamine in patients by means of chemical compounds.

Recent experiments have suggested a more practical way of controlling the release of histamine in the lung [11]. It has been possible to collect blood from vessels which supply the tracheobronchial tree in the dog lung in situ and to assay it chemically for histamine. Histamine is constantly released into the blood, and in eight anesthetized dogs, the release amounted to a mean value of 6 μg/liter of bronchial blood. If the vagal branches supplying the lung were stimulated electrically while bronchial blood flow was maintained at the same rate, there was a reduction in release of histamine in the lung—3 μg/liter of bronchial blood; thus the release of histamine can be reduced by excitation of the vagus nerve. It appears, then, that the release of histamine in the lung can be influenced by autonomic nerves. Hitherto, the release of histamine has been studied by perfusion of the isolated and excised lung, so that the influence of nerves could not be studied.

The role of the vagus nerve in regulating the tracheobronchial passages will have to be investigated in patients with bronchial asthma. If demonstrated, the autonomic drugs can be applied to the treatment of asthma. However, drugs that increase vagal tone (methacholine, eserine) cannot be used safely because they initiate a primary bronchoconstrictor response. It is, of course, conceivable that a drug will be developed that can mimic the vagal action of inhibiting the release of histamine, yet is without bronchoconstrictor action.

Blockade of the vagal fibers by atropine would mean a disruption of vagal control on the release of histamine. This action of atropine has just become apparent and can be added to other reasons for not using atropine in the treatment of bronchial asthma: inspissating action on tracheobronchial secretion, dryness of mouth and nasal cavity, abnormalities in vision, and so on.

BLOCKADE OF HISTAMINE BY ANTIHISTAMINICS

The efficacy of antihistaminic drugs in relieving the allergic responses in the nasal mucosa and skin is well documented. The accepted explanation of their action is that antihistaminics compete with the histamine released during an allergic response for the special "receptors" in the tissue. The phenomenon has been referred to as "competitive inhibition" of the histaminic receptor sites, in the same manner that atropine blocks the receptor site for acetylcholine.

The antihistaminics fail in the treatment of bronchial asthma for several reasons. Failure is not due to the resistance of bronchial muscle to the antihistaminic action, in the way that gastric glands are not blocked by antihistaminic drugs. In man and animals, the bronchoconstrictor action of administered histamine is effectively inhibited by prior administration of an antihistaminic drug. Human bronchial asthma is more complex than bronchial reactions caused by administered histamine. Possibly, the histamine released in the allergic response acts on receptors that are not accessible to blocking drugs, or humoral agents other than histamine may have more conspicuous effects in bringing about bronchoconstriction in bronchial asthma. Other features of antihistaminics also account for their limited use in bronchial asthma, e.g., the relative lack of a "pure" antihistaminic drug. Most of them have an atropine-like action so that there is a loss of the important vagal control of histamine release mentioned earlier. Hawkins [12] described a direct bronchoconstrictor action of most antihistaminic drugs which is in part due to a histamine-releasing action limited only to the bronchial muscle.

ANTIALLERGIC ACTION OF SYMPATHOMIMETICS

The sympathomimetic drugs reverse the functional manifestations of the allergic response. As commonly known, epinephrine is of primary importance in the treatment of a number of acute allergic disorders, including urticaria, serum reactions, serum sickness, and angioneurotic edema. The exact mechanism of its antiallergic reaction is not clear; only the bronchodilator action of epinephrine has been extensively studied. Symptomatic relief and improvement in lung ventilation caused by epinephrine have been shown in patients with bronchial asthma. The mechanism for relaxation is the activation of sympathetic receptors of the bronchial muscle. Such receptors exist in all organs supplied by the sympathetic nervous system, so that the action of epinephrine includes stimulation of the heart, constriction of vessels of skin, kidney, and lung, as well as dilatation of others.

INHALATION OF EPINEPHRINE

The inhalation of epinephrine in aerosol form has been relied on to relax bronchioles with minimal absorption of the drug. This procedure is effective in most asthmatic patients, but a few become tolerant to epinephrine. *Status asthmaticus* cannot be explained in simple terms of tolerance or tachyphylaxis because, in laboratory preparations, epinephrine can be relied on repeatedly to relax the bronchioles. Blumenthal *et al.* [13] drew the analogy between epinephrine-fastness in asthma and the poor pressor response to epinephrine in acidosis. They succeeded in overcoming *status asthmaticus* by injecting a molar solution of sodium lactate, which increased blood pH.

Another possible explanation of the lack of bronchodilator action of epinephrine may be found in recent observations on the effects of epinephrine on the bronchial circulation. Epinephrine injected directly into the bronchial artery of the dog causes relaxation of the bronchial muscle but congestion of the bronchial mucosa by constriction of the bronchial veins [14]. It is possible that, in *status asthmaticus,* the vascular effects become more conspicuous than the effects on bronchial muscle so that the end result might be an increase of airway resistance (Fig. 53-2).

INHALATION OF ISOPROTERENOL

A simple substitution of the amine of epinephrine has produced isoproterenol, which is a more potent bronchodilator than epinephrine. The increase in activity applies also to cardiac stimulation, but the vascular effects are different; isoproterenol is a pure vasodilator, whereas epinephrine is a dilator for most vessels but a constrictor for the vessels of kidney, skin, and lung. In other words, renal shutdown [15] and pulmonary edema may be encountered with excessive dosage of epinephrine but not of isoproterenol.

Inhalation of isoproterenol has been widely used in recent years (Fig. 53-3). Several convenient methods of producing aerosol are available [16]. When isoproterenol is administered by aerosol, the bronchomotor effects are accompanied by dilatation of the pulmonary vessels, which is desirable [17]. The pulmonary arterial pressure falls, and the load on the right ventricle is therefore reduced.

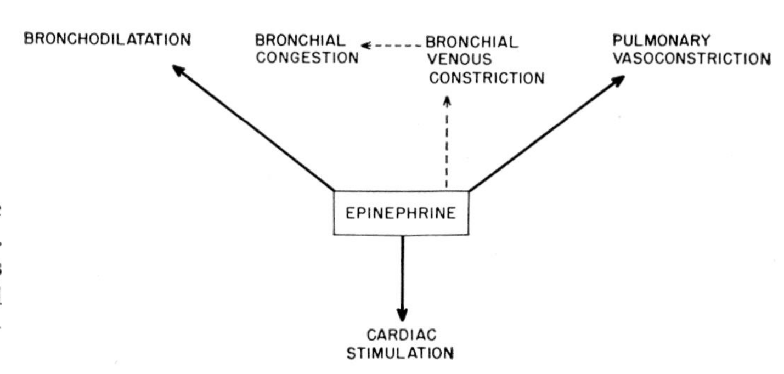

Fig. 53-2. Action of epinephrine on the cardiopulmonary system. Constriction of the bronchial veins can lead to congestion of bronchial mucosa and increase in airway resistance.

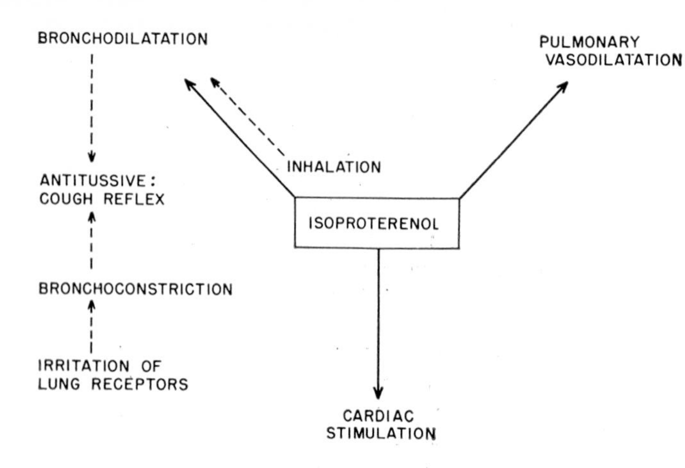

Fig. 53-3. Action of isoproterenol on the cardiopulmonary system. *Broken lines* pertain to effects of inhalation in aerosol form leading to bronchodilatation and antitussive action. The new theory discussed in the text pertains to the importance of bronchoconstriction in initiation of the cough reflex.

ORAL ADMINISTRATION OF EPHEDRINE AND PSEUDOEPHEDRINE

Until about thirty years ago, epinephrine was the only available bronchodilator. The major limitation in its clinical use was its ineffectiveness by the oral route. The discovery of the sympathomimetic action of ephedrine and its optical isomer, pseudoephedrine, by Chen and Schmidt [18] led to the introduction of drugs which are effective orally and have a duration of action longer than that of epinephrine. Both ephedrine and pseudoephedrine have bronchodilator action, which is accompanied, however, by some stimulation of the central nervous and cardiovascular systems. Pseudoephedrine has a weaker vasoconstrictor action than ephedrine, but their cardiac effects are about equal [19].

METHOXYPHENAMINE AND PROTOKYLOL

These two synthetic amines were introduced after the discovery of ephedrine. Given orally, both reduce airway resistance in patients with bronchial asthma. Both are free from any stimulation of the central nervous system, in contrast to ephedrine, but neither is more selective than ephedrine; protokylol is capable of stimulating the heart, whereas methoxyphenamine is a depressant.

Both drugs have one common feature: they relax the bronchial smooth muscle by an action on the beta receptors. This term has been introduced to include actions of epinephrine which are not blocked by ordinary adrenergic blocking agents (such as dihydrogenated ergot alkaloid), which block alpha receptors exclusively. More specifically, the beta receptors are located in organs in which the smooth muscles are relaxed by epinephrine (bronchi, heart, blood vessels, iris, and gut), whereas the alpha receptors are located in organs in which the smooth muscles are constricted by epinephrine (blood vessels, gastrointestinal sphincters).

Compared with epinephrine, these drugs are distinguished by increased potency, prolonged duration of action, and efficacy by the oral route. Unfortunately, it has not been possible to dissociate the bronchodilator action from the action on the cardiovascular system. The vasoconstriction and pressor effects (alpha receptor action) have been abolished, but vasodilatation and cardiac stimulation (beta receptor action) remain features of sympathomimetic bronchodilatation.

AMINOPHYLLINE AND OTHER MUSCULOTROPIC DRUGS

Although aminophylline has been used for several decades as a bronchodilator, its vasodilator action has only recently become apparent. In the presence of bronchial asthma, a reduction of pulmonary arterial pressure has been observed by several investigators [20–24]. Aminophylline increases pulmonary blood flow by cardiac stimulation (Fig. 53-4), but the blood pressure falls despite the rise in flow because of local pulmonary vasodilatation, which has been documented in several perfusion experiments [25–27].

The major shortcomings of aminophylline are its poor absorption when taken orally and its actions on the heart and peripheral blood vessels, which accompany the bronchodilatation. An alcoholic solution of theophylline

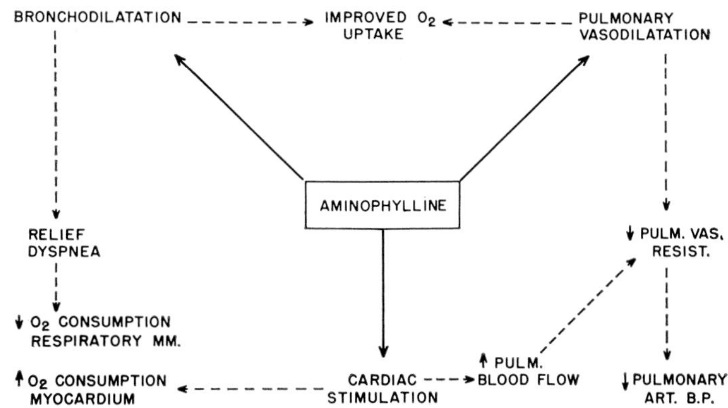

Fig. 53-4. Action of aminophylline on the cardiopulmonary system. *Broken lines* specify the functional consequences of the primary actions of the drug. The fall in pulmonary arterial blood pressure is largely the consequence of pulmonary vasodilatation.

(aminophylline minus ethylenediamine) has been reported to be rapidly absorbed in the gastrointestinal tract [28]. When aminophylline is given intravenously, a fall of systemic blood pressure by peripheral vasodilatation is likely to occur. Other related xanthines have been tested for more selective action, but the compounds so far tested dilate both lung and peripheral vessels. It has not been possible to dissociate the reactivity of the two vascular beds.

Other musculotropic drugs have been shown to be effective in relaxing bronchospasm. Nitroglycerin [29], erythrol tetranitrate [29], and khellin [30] have bronchomotor actions and vascular effects. Actually, their relaxing effects on the pulmonary vessels are not undesirable, because they would reduce the load on the right ventricle. However, the combined relaxing action of musculotropic drugs on bronchial and pulmonary vascular smooth muscles has raised the question of which of the two effects is more important in the control of an acute asthmatic attack of cardiac origin.

SEDATION BY OPIATES

The use of opiates in bronchial asthma has been repeatedly criticized because of the danger of respiratory depression. The sensitivity of the respiratory center to carbon dioxide is depressed by ordinary therapeutic doses of morphine and meperidine. Many clinicians believe that as long as the danger is recognized, the opiates can be depended on in acute asthma or in status asthmaticus when the usual methods of treatment have failed.

It is possible to present a reasonable comparison between morphine and meperidine [31]. The former has a potential bronchoconstrictor action because of its histamine-releasing properties, but the latter has a bronchodilator action by atropine-like and antihistaminic actions. Equivalent analgesic doses, however, will induce about the same degree of respiratory depression, sedation, euphoria, and central antitussive action.

ANTITUSSIVES

Coughing may be triggered by the allergic response of the tracheobronchial passages. The accepted concept of the initiation of the cough reflex is that the cough receptors in the airways are stimulated by toxic inhalants, mechanical irritation, local inflammation, and secretions. A new theory proposes that the common triggering mechanism for the cough reflex is bronchoconstriction and that the receptors are intimately related with the bronchial muscles [32]. The basis for this theory is that (1) almost all stimuli of the cough reflex initiate bronchoconstriction, and (2) the bronchodilators administered by inhalation (e.g., isoproterenol and propylhexedrine) and orally (ephedrine, phenylpropanolamine) have antitussive actions but no central depressant action on the cough center (Fig. 53-3, *broken lines*).

The theory that bronchospasm triggers the cough reflex has important therapeutic implications. The sympathomimetic and musculotropic bronchodilators discussed earlier should be expected to relieve cough reflex not by a simple blockade of cough receptors in the bronchial passages but by relieving bronchospasm and inactivating the corresponding receptors. One of the opiates (meperidine) has a bronchodilator action which may contribute to its antitussive action. If this theory is supported in additional studies, there is no need to use any of the numerous other remedies in the management of cough associated with the allergic response.

REFERENCES

1. Aviado, D. M. Pharmacology of the pulmonary circulation. *Pharmacol. Rev.* 12:159, 1960.
2. Aviado, D. M. General Principles in the Therapy of Diseases on the Pulmonary Circulation: Medical and Surgical Procedures. In *The Lung Circulation.* Oxford: Pergamon Press, 1965.
3. Hitchings, G. H., and Elion, G. B. Chemical suppression of the immune response. *Pharmacol. Rev.* 15:365, 1963.
4. Fischel, E. E., Vaughan, J. H., and Photopoulos, C. Inhibition of rapid production of antibody by cortisone: Study of secondary response. *Proc. Soc. Exp. Biol. Med.* 81:344, 1952.
5. Blumenstock, D. A., Collins, J. A., Thomas, E. D., and Ferrebee, J. W. Homotransplants of the lung in dogs. *Surgery* 51:541, 1962.
6. Hardy, J. D., Eraslan, S., Dalton, M. L., Alican, F., and Turner, M. D. Reimplantation and homotransplantation of the lung: Laboratory studies and clinical potential. *Ann. Surg.* 157: 707, 1963.
7. Stormorken, H. On the pharmacology of the isolated sensitized guinea pig lung. *Arch. Int. Pharmacodyn.* 119:238, 1959.
8. Lefcoe, N. M. The effect of hydrocortisone hemisuccinate on tracheal smooth muscle of the guinea pig and cat. *J. Allerg.* 27:352, 1956.
9. Franklin, W., Michelson, A. L., Lowell, F. C., and Schiller, I. W. Bronchodilators and corticosteroids in the treatment of obstructive pulmonary emphysema. *New Eng. J. Med.* 258: 774, 1958.
10. Paton, W. D. M. Histamine release by compounds of simple chemical structure. *Pharmacol. Rev.,* 9:269, 1957.
11. Aviado, D. M. Pharmacology of the Bronchial Circulation. With Special Reference to a New Homeostatic Mechanism for Bronchomotor Tone. In *Proceedings of the First International Pharmacological Meeting.* Oxford: Pergamon Press, 1963. P. 125.
12. Hawkins, D. F. Bronchoconstrictor and bronchodilator actions of antihistamine drugs. *Brit. J. Pharmacol.* 10:230, 1955.
13. Blumenthal, J. S., Blumenthal, M. N., Brown, E. B., Campbell, G. S., and Prasad, A. Effect of changes in arterial pH on the action of adrenalin in acute adrenalin-fast asthmatics. *Dis. Chest* 39:516, 1961.
14. Martinez, L., de Letona, J., Castro de la Mata, C., and Aviado, D. M. Local and reflex effects of bronchial arterial injection of drugs. *J. Pharmacol. Exp. Ther.* 133:295, 1961.
15. Aviado, D. M., Wnuck, A. L., and De Beer, E. J. The effects of sympathomimetic drugs on renal vessels. *J. Pharmacol. Exp. Ther.* 124: 238, 1958.
16. Freedman, T. Medihaler therapy for bronchial asthma: A new type of aerosol therapy. *Postgrad. Med.* 20:668, 1956.
17. Buhr, G. Ueber den Einfluss der Aludrin-Aerosol-Inhalation auf die Druckverhältnisse in der Arteria pulmonalis beim Menschen. *Z. Kreislaufforsch.* 42:669, 1953.
18. Chen, K. K., and Schmidt, C. F. The action of ephedrine, the active principle of the Chinese drug, ma huang. *J. Pharmacol. Exp. Ther.* 24:339, 1924.
19. Aviado, D. M., Wnuck, A. L., and De Beer, E. J. Cardiovascular effects of sympathomimetic bronchodilators: Epinephrine, ephedrine, pseudoephedrine, isoproterenol, methoxyphenamine and isoprophenamine. *J. Pharmacol. Exp. Ther.* 122:406, 1958.
20. Foscarini, M., and Galassi, L. Comportamento della pressione del piccolo circolo all'azione della aminofillina. *Clinicia* (Bologna) 14:167, 1953.
21. Schuman, C., and Simmons, H. G. Cardiac asthma: Its pathogenesis and response to aminophylline. *Ann. Intern. Med.* 36:864, 1952.
22. Storstein, O., Helle, I., and Rokseth, R. The effect of theophylline ethylenediamine on the pulmonary circulation. *Amer. Heart J.* 55:781, 1958.
23. Zimmerman, H. A. Preliminary report on the pulmonary circulation in bronchial asthma. *Amer. J. Med.* 46:667, 1949.
24. Zimmerman, H. A. A study of the pulmonary circulation in man. *Dis. Chest* 20:46, 1951.
25. Borst, H. G., Berglund, E., and McGregor, M. The effects of pharmacologic agents on the pulmonary circulation in the dog: Studies on epinephrine, nor-epinephrine, 5-hydroxytryptamine, acetylcholine, histamine and aminophylline. *J. Clin. Invest.* 36:669, 1957.
26. Quimby, C. W., Jr., Aviado, D. M., and

Schmidt, C. F. The effects of aminophylline and other xanthines on the pulmonary circulation. *J. Pharmacol.* 122:396, 1958.

27. Sai, Y. The action of certain bronchial asthma remedies on the pulmonary circulation. *Acta Med.* (Fukuoka) 24:165, 1954.
28. Spielman, A. D. Therapeutic effectiveness of elixophyllin for the oral treatment of acute and chronic bronchial asthma. *Ann. Allerg.* 15:270, 1957.
29. Hirshleifer, I., and Arora, Y. Nitrites in the treatment of bronchial asthma. *Dis. Chest* 39: 275, 1961.
30. Brown, E. B. Intramuscular crystalline khellin for management of chronic bronchial asthma. *Amer. Pract.* 7:609, 1956.
31. Herschfus, J. A., Salomon, A., and Segal, M. S. The use of Demerol in patients with bronchial asthma. *Ann. Intern. Med.* 40:506, 1954.
32. Salem, H., Greene, L. C., and Aviado, D. M. Antitussive drugs: A new theory for the initiation of the cough reflex and the influence of bronchodilators. *Am. J. Med. Sci.* 247:585, 1964.

54. Symptomatic Treatment of Atopic Disorders

SAMUEL O. FREEDMAN

THE PHARMACOLOGIST WHO EVALUATES the effect of a drug over a measured period of time on a single organ or disease process is in a more fortunate position than the practicing physician, who may have to consider the effect of several drugs administered for a protracted period on a whole sequence of biological events. In the case of the allergic diseases, the accepted sequence of abnormal response is: (1) the antigen-antibody interaction, (2) the release of chemical mediators, and (3) the characteristic functional changes of the allergic inflammatory response in shock organs such as the lungs, nasal mucosa, and skin. The clinician may choose to interrupt the abnormal pathway at one or more of these three stages, or he may choose to employ therapy such as sedation or oxygen which has no specific antiallergic activity.

The selection of drugs in an individual case is usually determined both by the nature of the clinical problem and by the treating physician's past successes and failures with commonly used antiallergic drugs. For example, antihistamine drugs which block chemical mediators are often effective in the treatment of hay fever but are of little benefit in bronchial asthma, where the nature of the chemical mediator is unknown. However, once the decision has been made to employ an antihistaminic, the choice of a specific preparation is largely a matter of individual preference. The complexity of the clinical situation is further increased by the common observation that different patients with the same disease process may react differently to the same medication. For instance, epinephrine, which reverses the functional abnormality in bronchial asthma, provides prompt and effective symptomatic relief in most cases, but the acutely ill, dehydrated, "dry" asthmatic, whose problem is primarily that of retained secretions rather than bronchospasm, may actually be made worse by the drying action of epinephrine on the bronchial mucosa.

No drugs are available, at present, for clinical use which primarily inhibit antigen-antibody interactions. Therefore drugs which block chemical mediators, drugs which reverse the functional consequences of allergic reactions in shock organs, and drugs which have a nonspecific effect on allergic diseases will be considered in that order.

ANTIHISTAMINE AND ANTISEROTONIN DRUGS

This class of drugs finds its greatest application when administered by mouth for the treatment of allergic rhinitis, urticaria, and atopic eczema. A wide variety of antihistamine drugs is manufactured, and despite many claims to the contrary, increased potency is almost always associated with increased toxicity. Consequently there is no one preparation which is outstanding in its ratio of clinical effectiveness to side-effects of nausea or drowsiness [1]. However, different patients vary in their susceptibility to these side-effects, and the choice of the most suitable drug for the individual patient is often a matter of trial and error. Of considerable interest is the recent observation that orally administered chlorpheniramine acts as a peripheral vasoconstrictor in man. It is conceivable that its decongestant effect on the human nasal mucosa is at least partially attributable to its vasoconstrictor activity [2]. Topically applied antihistaminics exert their action primarily because of their local anesthetic properties rather than because of their antiallergic action. Furthermore, antihistaminics applied topically are potent sensitizers which occasionally induce a severe secondary contact dermatitis.

Hydroxyzine is an ataractic drug with antihistamine properties. It has been shown that experimental human histamine skin wheals are better inhibited by hydroxyzine than by chlorpheniramine or by phenothiazine derivatives [3]. In clinical practice, hydroxyzine not infrequently provides effective control of chronic urticaria and angioedema [4].

Recently two drugs, cyproheptadine and homochlorcyclizine, which possess antiserotonin as well as antihistamine activity, have been subjected to extensive clinical trials. In laboratory animals, cyproheptadine has antihistamine, antiserotonin and adrenergic blocking activities [5], and homochlorcyclizine has been found to be an antagonist of histamine, serotonin, acetylcholine, and slow-reacting substance [6]. However, these agents have proved to be generally disappointing in the treatment of human allergic diseases. Cyproheptadine and homochlorcyclizine are sometimes useful in the management of chronic urticaria [7, 8], and homochlorcyclizine is held to be of mild benefit in bronchial asthma in children [9]. Clinical studies have shown that the antiallergic effect of homochlorcyclizine is not directly attributable to its known antagonism to serotonin, histamine, or acetylcholine or to its bronchodilator action [8]. It is possible that its clinical activity is due primarily to its antagonism to slow-reacting substance. Another unexpected observation was the finding that cyproheptadine produced a marked increase in appetite, weight gain, and linear growth in asthmatic children [10].

CORTICOSTEROIDS

The mode of action of corticosteroids in allergic diseases is not well understood, but it is generally agreed that their immediate effect is due to a blocking or suppression of the allergic inflammatory response in susceptible tissues. When administered over a longer period, corticosteroids may also interfere with antibody production.

The systemic side-effects of corticosteroids are well known and for clinical purposes may be divided into three categories: (1) those which are potentially fatal, e.g., adrenal collapse, and peptic ulceration with hemorrhage; (2) those which may lead to serious functional disability, e.g., osteoporosis, increased bruising, induction of diabetes mellitus in predisposed individuals, fluid retention, mental changes, increased intraocular pressure [11], increased susceptibility to infection, and poor wound healing, and (3) those which alter the patient's appearance, e.g., acne, moon facies, excessive weight gain, and hirsutism. Side-effects may even occur with locally applied corticosteroids. For example, elevated intraocular pressure has been reported following the use of corticosteroid eye drops [12], local tissue atrophy following subcutaneous injection of triamcinolone [13], and systemic anaphylaxis following intra-articular injection of hydrocortisone [14].

Nevertheless these drugs have a definite place in the treatment of allergic diseases because they frequently produce dramatic relief of otherwise uncontrollable and incapacitating symptoms.It often requires fine clinical judgment to decide whether the anticipated hazards of giving corticosteroids are likely to be greater than the hazards of withholding them. For instance, it can be predicted that certain side-effects are more likely to occur in some patients than in others, e.g., peptic ulceration in patients with a previous history of peptic ulcer disease, steroid diabetes in patients with a family history of diabetes mellitus, reactivation of pulmonary tuberculosis in patients with old tuberculous disease, fluid retention in patients with cardiac failure, cirrhosis of the liver or renal disease, and osteoporosis in postmenopausal females. However, when the indication for corticosteroids is strong enough, these anticipated side-effects may be effectively controlled in most instances by the administration of other forms of medical treatment concomitantly with corticosteroids. For example, an ulcer regimen may be prescribed for the peptic ulcer patient, isonicotinic acid hydrazide for the patient with old tuberculosis, diuretics for the cardiac, cirrhotic, or renal patient, and oral hypoglycemic agents for the patient predisposed to diabetes.

It has recently been suggested that the death rate from bronchial asthma has been significantly reduced since the introduction of corticosteroid therapy [15], but others have pointed out that this apparent decline in mortality may be due to a revision of the International Code of listing of deaths [16]. Long-term follow-up studies of cases of intractable asthma have shown a considerable morbidity but a surprisingly low mortality rate associated with protracted corticosteroid therapy. In a retrospective study of 87 patients with severe asthma on continuous or intermittent corticosteroid therapy over a period of ten years, it was found that 6 had died but in only 1 was there a connection between corticosteroids and death [17].

A particular problem related to systemic corticosteroid therapy is the inhibition of linear growth which occurs in children given this form of medication. The inhibition of growth occurs to a much lesser extent with cortisone than with other corticosteroids [18]. However, when considering the growth-suppressing effects of corticosteroids, one should note that inhibition of growth in children with severe asthma occurred in the presteroid era and that it is often difficult to separate this phenomenon by statistical methods from steroid-induced growth inhibition [19]. One possible solution to the problem of growth retardation when corticosteroids must be given to children is to give them in conjunction with anabolic hormones. Methandienone, administered to a group of such children, produced a marked increase in linear growth without significant virilization, salt retention, or hepatotoxicity [20].

The use of aerosolized corticosteroids in chronic asthma has been suggested as a means of reducing the side-effects caused by their systemic administration. After extensive clinical trials, it has been found that aerosolized dexamethasone phosphate controls asthma and reduces requirements for systemic steroids in some patients whose symptoms are not excessively severe. However, significant systemic absorption of medication and adrenal suppression do occur. Therefore the usual precautions associated with systemic steroid therapy must be observed [21]. Candidiasis of the oropharynx and larynx may also be a hazard with this form of medication [22]. Another possible method of reducing the harmful side-effects of corticosteroids is the use of an intermittent dosage regimen. In this form of treatment, the total corticosteroid requirement for a forty-eight hour period is administered in a single dose every other day. The clinical effectiveness is reported to be identical with conventional dosage schedules, and adrenal suppression is appreciably lessened [23].

Adrenal suppression may persist for many months after corticosteroid therapy is discontinued. On the other hand, pituitary function (ACTH secretion) usually recovers more rapidly than adrenocortical function [24]. Therefore the administration of ACTH following cessation of corticosteroid therapy may provide a useful stimulus to endogenous adrenocortical hormone production, but it provides no assurance of permanent restoration of adrenal function [25].

BRONCHODILATOR DRUGS

Numerous drugs exist which are capable of reversing, to a greater or lesser extent, the functional consequences of allergic inflammation in human bronchi. The bronchodilator drugs commonly prescribed for this purpose are of two principal types: (1) adrenergic drugs such as epinephrine and related compounds, and (2) aminophylline.

The action of these drugs on bronchospasm alone will not provide a full explanation of their clinical effectiveness or clinical failure. Their therapeutic action in reversing airway resistance in bronchial asthma also depends on their decongestant effect on the bronchial mucosa and on the moistening effect of aerosol bronchodilators on the mucus in the bronchial lumina. In addition, the route of administration exerts a profound influence on the therapeutic properties of adrenergic drugs.

When administered systemically, the principal action of epinephrine and related substances on human bronchi appears to be that of muscular relaxation with very little change in mucosal edema or secretion [26]. On the other hand, adrenergic drugs produce an intense vasoconstriction when applied locally (i.e., by aerosol) to the bronchial mucosa. In the evaluation of the relative merits of aerosol or systemic administration of bronchodilator drugs, it should be remembered that inhaled medication does not affect bronchioles that are completely occluded by mucus, whereas systemically administered drugs reach every bronchiole. When aerosol and oral administration of isoproterenol are compared in human subjects, it is found that aerosol medication has an optimal effect earlier, but its activity is of shorter duration than oral medication [27]. Side-effects and bronchodilator activity are the same for both routes of administration.

When the bronchodilator actions of aerosolized epinephrine and aerosolized isoproterenol are compared, it is found that there is no significant difference in their effect on airway resistance, despite their different pharmacological activities [28]. In experimental animals, isoproterenol is ten times more effective than epinephrine as a bronchial antispasmodic [29], but isoproterenol acts as a vasodilator of the bronchial mucosa in contrast to the vasoconstrictor action of epinephrine [30]. Thus, in the clinical situation, the superior muscle relaxant properties of isoproterenol compared to epinephrine are counterbalanced by increased mucosal congestion.

Some patients with severe bronchial asthma may become completely refractory to the actions of adrenergic drugs. This may occur as the result of extensive mucous plugging of bronchioles or as the result of changes in blood pH. It has been demonstrated that lowered blood pH due to CO_2 retention may lead to resistance to the bronchodilator effects of epinephrine [31]. It has also been suggested that intravenously administered sodium lactate may restore the patient's sensitivity to epinephrine. However, the clinical effectiveness of sodium lactate in this regard has not been proved by adequately controlled studies.

One of the major disadvantages of the use of adrenergic drugs in treatment of bronchial asthma is their tendency to produce tachycardias, arrhythmias, and hypertension in certain patients. However, it is possible that clinicians have been overly cautious in withholding adrenergic drugs in the presence of ectopic cardiac rhythms. In animals, epinephrine given intravenously in the presence of experimentally induced ventricular tachycardia produces transitory ectopic arrhythmias but never fibrillation or prefibrillatory arrhythmias [32]. It is conceivable that the deleterious effects of adrenergic drugs on a damaged myocardium may be less harmful than the increased muscular work, transitory asphyxia, and pulmonary hypertension which occur with severe asthma resistant to other forms of drug therapy.

In experimental animals, aminophylline has a moderate antispasmodic action on the bronchial musculature. In addition, increased respiration results from the central nervous system-stimulating activity of aminophylline, and the cardiac output is increased. In clinical practice, aminophylline given intravenously produces a greater improvement in pulmonary function than isoproterenol inhaled or taken orally [33]. The mode of action of aminophylline in man is not well understood inasmuch as the degree of clinical improvement obtained is out of proportion to its muscle-relaxing activity. It is possible that the increased respiratory rate produced by the drug promotes the more effective removal of mucous plugs. Aminophylline given intravenously or rectally is usually highly effective. The principal disadvantage of aminophylline in the management of bronchial asthma is that it is much less effective when taken by mouth because of uncertain absorption and gastrointestinal irritation. Aminophylline suppositories may, rarely, cause granular proctitis after prolonged usage. A more serious side-effect is the toxicity which occasionally occurs in children as the result of aminophylline overdosage. Central nervous stimulation may produce convulsions, drowsiness, and coma; increase in gastric secretion due to the drug may cause recurrent vomiting; and increased urine output may result in albuminuria and dehydration [34].

MUCOLYTIC AGENTS

One of the major functional abnormalities in the asthmatic lung is the accumulation of thick, tenacious secretions in the bronchioles. There are several recognized methods of liquefying or loosening mucous plugs, none of them entirely effective.

Although many experienced physicians will attest to their clinical effect, there is little experimental evidence that traditional expectorant drugs such as potassium iodide and ammonium chloride actually liquefy or "thin" the sputum of asthmatic patients [35].

Proteolytic enzymes such as trypsin and chymotrypsin have been administered in aerosol, aqueous, and parenteral form in an attempt to make sputum less viscous and hence less difficult to raise and expectorate. However, detailed clinical investigation has failed to show that these enzymes effectively reduce the viscosity of sputum [36]. Furthermore, it has been reported that aerosolized trypsin may cause rash, fever, or hemoptysis in a small percentage of individuals and injected chymotrypsin may cause acute anaphylactoid reactions [37].

The use of intermittent positive-pressure breathing with aerosolized bronchodilator drugs represents one of the more rational techniques for relieving bronchial obstruction due to mucous plugs. The method has the advantage of simultaneously moistening inspissated secretions, distributing bronchodilator medication evenly throughout the bronchial tree, and reinflating atelectatic lobules. The net effect is a more liquid mucus in dilated bronchioles, thereby producing conditions which favor the eventual expulsion of mucous plugs by coughing. Intermittent positive-pressure breathing is usually most effective when combined with other therapeutic measures such as postural drainage, systemically administered antibiotics, and adequate hydration. The addition of detergent compounds to aerosol solutions does not seem to improve the efficacy of this form of treatment [38], nor does oxygen have any advantage over compressed air. Furthermore, the prolonged administration of oxygen may result in CO_2 narcosis in patients whose asthma is associated with pulmonary emphysema. Patients with bullous emphysema are not usually considered to be candidates for intermittent positive-pressure breathing because of the danger of rupturing bullae under conditions of positive pressure.

TOPICAL NASAL DECONGESTANTS

Topically applied adrenergic drugs are often highly effective in providing temporary relief from nasal congestion in allergic rhinitis, but their continuous use is not infrequently associated with a worsening of the condition for which they were originally prescribed.

A particular offender in this respect is naphazoline hydrochloride, which almost invariably results in "rebound" nasal congestion if used for longer than four or five days [39]. It is of interest that the chemical formula of naphazoline is structurally quite different from that of other adrenergic drugs. It is a representative of the imidazoline class of compounds and as such is related both to phenylethylamine, the chemical prototype of epinephrine, and to histamine. It is known that epinephrine possesses both vasoconstrictor and vasodilator elements and thus exerts a biphasic action on small blood vessels. The vasodilator effect of epinephrine is weaker but more prolonged than the vasoconstrictor component. It is because of this vasodilatation secondary to intense vasoconstriction that epinephrine is unsuitable for routine intranasal application. On the other hand, drugs such as ephedrine and amphetamine do not possess the vasodilator factor and therefore are much more useful as nasal decongestants. It is possible that the "rebound" congestion resulting from the frequent use of naphazoline is the result of secondary vasodilatation similar to that which occurs with epinephrine [40]. It is also conceivable that the delayed aggravation of allergic rhinitis provoked by this compound is in some way related to its chemical similarity to histamine.

Other nasal vasoconstrictors occasionally have similar effects but to a less striking degree. The increased nasal congestion in these cases is probably due to secondary irritation in sensitive mucous membranes or to interference with the normal ciliary activity of the nasal mucosa.

SEDATION AND PSYCHOTHERAPY

Emotions such as frustration, anger, insecurity, embarrassment, panic, and dejection may cause nonspecific vasomotor changes in allergic shock organs through the action of the autonomic nervous system [41]. Therefore any therapeutic measure which allays or suppresses these emotional reactions may favorably influence the course of allergic diseases. The use of mild sedation such as that provided by the barbiturates or chloral hydrate is often a valuable adjunct to therapy. In the evaluation of the therapeutic significance of tranquilizing drugs in the management of allergic diseases, it should be remembered that many of these drugs (e.g., the phenothiazine derivatives) possess antihistamine, anticholinergic, or adrenergic blocking activities. Therefore not all of the clinical improvement produced by them can be attributed to their sedative or tranquilizing properties. The usefulness of meperidine and related drugs as sedatives in bronchial asthma is severely limited by their activity as respiratory depressants. Ether given rectally exerts its action in acute status asthmaticus by providing profound sedation and hypnosis as well as by promoting expectoration through its irritant effect on the bronchial mucosa.

The role of psychotherapy in the treatment of allergic disorders is much more controversial. Some authorities feel that psychological disturbances frequently are primary causes of the allergic state [42], whereas others contend that these changes are for the most part secondary to the physical, social, and economic disability brought about by protracted illness. In a recent study of intrapersonal relationships between asthmatic children and their families, no correlation was found between emotional disturbance in the family and the development or severity of asthma in children, but there was a definite correlation between emotional disturbance in the family and psychiatric illness in asthmatic children [43]. On this basis, it would seem that psychotherapy may be helpful in the management of psychiatric illness occurring in allergic patients either as a result of their primary allergic disease or coincidentally. However, psychotherapy alone is unlikely to reverse the complex series of immunological and biochemical events which lead to the allergic state.

REFERENCES

1. Dragstedt, C. A. Histamine and Antihistaminics. In Drill, V. A. (Ed.), *Pharmacology in Medicine* (2nd ed.). New York: McGraw-Hill Book Company, Inc., 1958.
2. Abramson, D. I., Tuck, S. Jr., Chu, L. S. W., and Donatello, T. M. Vascular effects of chlorpheniramine maleate (Chlor-trimeton). *J. Allerg.* 34:258, 1963.
3. Dundas, E., Toogood, J. H., and Wanklin, B. A. Inhibition of experimental skin wheals by some ataractic and antihistaminic drugs. *J. Allerg.* 32:1, 1961.
4. Feinberg, A. R., Pruzansky, J. J., Feinberg, S. M., and Fisherman, E. W. Hydroxizine (Atarax) in chronic urticaria and in allergic manifestations. *J. Allerg.* 29:358, 1958.
5. Stone, C. A., Wenger, H. C., Ludden, C. T., Stavorski, J. M., and Ross, C. A. Antiserotonin-Antihistamine Properties of Cyproheptadine. *J. Pharmacol. Exp. Ther.* 131:73, 1961.
6. Kimura, E. T., Young, P. R., and Richards, R. K. Pharmacologic properties of homochlorcyclizine: A serotonin antagonist. *J. Allerg.* 31:237, 1960.
7. Baily, I. S. Cyproheptadine in the treatment of urticaria. *Brit. Med. J.* 2:430, 1961.
8. Fisherman, E. W., Feinberg, S. M., Feinberg, A. R., and Pruzansky, J. J. Homochlorcyclizine, an antiallergic drug with multiple clinical properties. *J. Allerg.* 31:232, 1960.
9. Beaudry, P. H., and Becklake, M. R. A trial of SA-97 in the treatment of asthma in children. *J. Allerg.* 33:210, 1962.
10. Lavenstein, A. F., Dacaney, E. P., Lasagna, L., and Van Metre, T. E. Effect of cyproheptadine on asthmatic children. *J.A.M.A.* 180:912, 1962.
11. Bernstein, H. N., and Schwartz, B. Long-term steroid therapy and ocular pressure. *Arch. Ophthal.* 68:742, 1962.
12. Becker, B., and Mills, D. W. Elevated intraocular pressure following corticosteroid eye drops. *J.A.M.A.* 185:170, 1963.
13. Fisherman, E. W., Feinberg, A. R., and Feinberg, S. M. Local subcutaneous atrophy. *J.A.M.A.* 179:971, 1962.
14. O'Garra, J. A. Anaphylactic reactions to hydrocortisone injections. *Brit. Med. J.* 1:615, 1962.
15. Alexander, H. L. A historical account of death from asthma. *J. Allerg.* 34:305, 1963.
16. Richards, W. Deaths from asthma. *J. Allerg.* 35:86, 1964.
17. Baldwin, H. S., Dworetzky, M., and Isaacs, N. J. Evaluation of steroid treatment of asthma since 1950. *J. Allerg.* 32:109, 1961.
18. Van Metre, T. E., Jr., Niermann, W. A., and Rosen, L. J. A comparison of the growth suppressive effect of cortisone, prednisone, and other adrenal cortical hormones. *J. Allerg.* 31:531, 1960.
19. Falliers, C. J., Tan, L. S., Sventivanyi, J., Jorgenson, J. R., and Bukantz, S. C. Influence of asthma and steroid therapy on growth. *Amer. J. Dis. Child.* 105:127, 1963.
20. Evans, R. G. Methandienone in long term corticosteroid therapy. *Acta Allerg.* 17:220, 1963.
21. Crepea, S. B. Inhalation corticosteroid (Dexamethasone PO_4) management of chronically asthmatic children. *J. Allerg.* 34:119, 1963.
22. Dennis, M., and Itkin, I. H. Effectiveness and complications of aerosol Dexamethasone phosphate in severe asthma. *J. Allerg.* 35:70, 1964.
23. Harter, J. G., Reddy, W. J., and Thorn, G. W. Studies on an intermittent corticosteroid dosage regimen. *New Eng. J. Med.* 269:591, 1963.
24. Meakin, J. W., Tantongco, M. S., Crabbe, J., Bayles, T. B., and Nelson, D. H. Pituitary-adrenal function following long-term steroid therapy. *Amer. J. Med.* 24:459, 1960.
25. Carreron, G. G., Canary, J. J., Meyer, R. J., and Kyle, L. H. Adrenocortical function after long-term corticoid therapy. *J. Lab. Clin. Med.* 56:235, 1960.
26. Farber, S. M., and Wilson, R. H. L. The rational approach in the use of bronchodila-

tors in chronic respiratory disease. *Ann. Intern. Med.* 50:1241, 1959.

27. Morton, J. W., and Ostenoe, L. G. A comparative study of aerosol, oral and intravenous administration of bronchodilators in asthma with the use of isoproterenol (Isuprel), Th 152, and aminophylline. *J. Allerg.* 34:16, 1963.
28. Simonsson, B. A comparison between the ventilatory effect of two types of adrenalin, administered through different nebulizers. *J. Allerg.* 33:166, 1962.
29. Hebb, C. O., and Konzett, H. Vaso- and bronchodilator effects of N-isopropyl-norepinephrine in isolated perfused dog lungs. *J. Pharmacol. Exp. Ther.* 96:229, 1949.
30. Dautrebande, L. *Preparing Solutions for Pneumodilating Aerosols,* Research and Development Report, UR 530. Rochester, N.Y.: University of Rochester, 1958. P. 235.
31. Blumenthal, M. N., Braun, E. B., Campbell, G. S., and Prasad, A. Effect of changes in arterial pH on the action of adrenalin in acute adrenalin-fast asthmatics. *Dis. Chest.* 39:516, 1961.
32. Sherf, D., Taner, D., and Yildiz, M. Effect of epinephrine on experimental ectopic ventricular tachycardias. *Proc. Soc. Exp. Biol. Med.* 105:30, 1960.
33. Cander, L., and Comroe, J. H., Jr. A method for the objective evaluation of bronchodilator drugs: Effects of Dapanone, Isuprel, and aminophylline. *J. Allerg.* 26:21, 1955.
34. Bacal, H. L., Linegar, K., Denton, R. L., and Gourdeau, R. Aminophylline poisoning in children. *Canad. Med. Ass. J.* 80:6, 1959.
35. Simon, S. W., and Harmon, G. A. A comparison of various expectorant drugs employing a new method for determining sputum viscosity. *J. Allerg.* 32:493, 1961.
36. Editorial. The reduction of sputum viscosity. *Brit. Med. J.* 1:929, 1962.
37. Ferrara, A., Finke, S. R., Grieco, M. H., Connell, J. T., and Sherman, W. B. Anaphylactic reactions to aqueous chymotrypsin. *J. Allerg.* 34:460, 1963.
38. Palmer, K. N. V. A new mucolytic agent for inhalation in chronic bronchitis. *Lancet* 2:802, 1961.
39. Schiller, I. W. Deleterious effects of privine hydrochloride. *New Eng. J. Med.* 232:333, 1945.
40. Feinberg, S. M., and Friedlaender, S. Nasal congestion from frequent use of privine hydrochloride. *J.A.M.A.* 128:1095, 1945.
41. Holmes, T., Goodell, H., Wolf, S., and Wolff, H. *The Nose.* Springfield, Ill.: Charles C Thomas, Publisher, 1950.
42. Abramson, H. A. Psychotherapy in Allergy. In Brown, E. A. (Ed.), *Allergology* (Proceedings of Fourth International Congress). New York: Pergamon Press, 1962. P. 422.
43. Dubo, S., McLean, J. A., Ching, A. Y. T., Wright, H. L., Kauffman, P. E., and Sheldon, J. M. A study of relationships between family situation, bronchial asthma, and personal adjustment in children. *J. Pediat.* 59:402, 1961.

SECTION VII. ALLERGIC DISEASES OF THE SKIN; REACTIONS TO SERUM, DRUGS, AND INSECTS

55. Urticaria and Angioedema

JAMES A. MCLEAN AND JOHN M. SHELDON

URTICARIA IS A LOCALIZED SWELLING of the skin associated with erythema, itching, and, at times, wheal formation. The main area of involvement is the upper corium and superficial skin layer. Angioedema, on the other hand, is characterized by similar edematous swelling in the deep skin structures, namely, the dermis and subcutaneous tissues. The lesion is consequently more extensive than urticaria. Since the two conditions are essentially the same, they will be described together, and the term angioedema (proposed first by Cooke [1] and later by Bruun [2]) will be used here instead of the more conventional "angioneurotic edema."

Hippocrates described urticaria from mosquito bites. Sydenham, in 1685, described some lesions resembling those occasioned by stinging nettles—probably urticaria. Junker described urticaria in 1718, and Bateman, in 1814, noted its frequent occurrence with the eating of certain foods, especially shellfish. Although Quincke's edema is the term commonly found in the European literature to denote angioedema since Quincke's publication in 1882 [3], three earlier descriptions were published between 1848 and 1876.

It has been stated that the word urticaria is derived from the Latin word *urere,* meaning to burn; others believe it comes from the name of the common nettle plant, *Urtica urens,* the hairs of which cause a nettle rash after brushing the skin. (Interestingly, these plant hairs contain histamine, acetylcholine, and serotonin.)

The true incidence of urticaria is difficult to determine, since many acute cases recognized by patients as being due to food sensitivity are never seen by physicians. A survey of 1,424 college students revealed that 15.1 percent had had at least one episode of hives [4]. Schwartz [5] found that bronchial asthma, urticaria, and Quincke's edema coexist frequently. Swinny [6] reported an incidence of 22.3 percent in 958 nonallergic patients, whereas 52.9 percent of 633 patients with either hay fever or asthma had urticaria. In absolute terms, urticaria was almost ten times more common in the nonallergic population, although its relative frequency was higher in atopic individuals. Acute urticaria is more common in the younger age groups (children and young adults) than is chronic urticaria, which is encountered frequently in the middle-aged, especially women [7].*

MECHANISM OF WHEAL FORMATION

The initial investigations into the mechanism of urticarial wheal formation date back to the classic experiments of Sir Thomas Lewis [8] in which he demonstrated that urticarial wheals can be explained on the basis of a triple response: dilatation of the capillaries and venules, increased capillary permeability, and arteriolar dilatation due to an axon reflex which produces the "flare." The active dilatation of the minute vessels of the skin (terminal arterioles, capillaries, and venules) is independent of the central nervous system and local nervous reflexes and is followed by a relaxation of the arterioles, resulting in a flare extending beyond the local response. The final wheal and edema result from exudation of fluid into the tissues due to increased capil-

* Since the completion of this chapter, an extensive review of laboratory findings and clinical observations in urticaria has been published (Beall, G. N. *Medicine* 43:131, 1964).

lary permeability of the vessel walls. Mechanical, electrical, chemical, and thermal stimuli all produce the response, presumably by liberating "H-substance," now identified as histamine, which initiates the reflex vascular reaction. Injections of allergens into sensitized individuals induce urticarial wheals, and histological examination reveals that histamine injections in allergic individuals have an "effect almost indistinguishable from that produced by the injection of an allergen" [9]. Katz [10] studied the histamine and protein contents of cantharidin blisters on allergic patients before and after local reactions were induced by the injection of allergens. Both histamine and protein contents rose sharply in a few minutes. Conflicting evidence concerning the histamine content in human skin biopsies from urticarial wheals has been reported. Nilzen [11] concluded that the decreased skin histamine content noted 10 to 25 minutes after mechanical stimulation of the skin of healthy subjects and patients with dermographism, as well as in spontaneously occurring wheals in patients with urticaria, is due to the histamine's being carried away. He also found a decrease of blood histamine level in patients with chronic urticaria, the blood level becoming higher as the urticaria diminished. However, Beall [12], Rose [13], and Rorsman [14] have found no significant change from normal of the plasma histamine concentration in patients with urticaria. In a reported case of urticaria and angioedema following D-tubocurarine administration, plasma and blood histamine levels were elevated to twice "normal" approximately 45 minutes after the acute reaction. Although D-tubocurarine itself will cause histamine release which results in a slight rise in the plasma level, it was inferred that the urticarial reaction had caused a rise in plasma histamine beyond "normal levels" in other patients receiving the same preanesthetic medication [15].

Antihistamines furnish further indirect proof that histamine participates in the pathogenesis of urticarial wheal formation. All of the foregoing observations support the concept of an allergic etiology for urticaria due to histamine liberation following an antigen-antibody interaction. Histamine liberators have also been shown to produce a triple response in the skin, and this reaction, too, is reduced by antihistaminic drugs. The many histamine-releasing agents have been classified into the following types [16]: material that damages tissue (venoms, toxins, traumatic agents), proteolytic enzymes (trypsin), surface-acting agents (Tween 20, bile), substances with large molecules (egg white, dextran, horse serum), morphine and other drugs, and monobasic compounds (alkylamines). It has been suggested that any of these histamine-releasing agents may play a role in chronic urticaria without an antigen-antibody mechanism [17].

Studies of wheal formation by measurements of fluorescence curves after ultraviolet light exposure revealed increased capillary permeability in histamine wheal formation; the response in normal subjects and allergic patients was identical [18]. It was postulated that precapillary sphincter relaxation causes capillary dilatation and that the enlarging pores allow capillary permeability to increase. Cooper [19] studied patients with spinal cord lesions and found that the production of the spreading flare phase of the triple response induced by histamine injections is not present following complete transection of the cord, thus confirming the axon reflex theory of arteriolar dilatation following histamine initiation of local vasodilatation. However, Cooper does not believe that the axon reflex alone will explain the flare phenomenon, basing this assertion on his findings in other neurological situations.

Histamine liberation has also been demonstrated in some cases of physical allergy. Rose [21] and Beall [12] have noted elevated plasma histamine levels in cold urticaria, but passive transfer was positive in only some cases. Studies with C^{14}-labeled histamine have revealed that histamine metabolism and excretion are the same in healthy individuals and in patients with cold urticaria [22]; however, the lack of histaminuria despite the pronounced elevation of plasma histamine level is unexplained. Punch biopsies and peripheral blood basophil smears were obtained from two patients with cold urticaria; the tissue mast cells and basophils showed degranulation after cooling of the skin [23]. It was postulated that in these cases of acquired, essential, cold urticaria, the local and systemic signs were due to histamine release from the mast cells in the skin and basophilic granules in the blood. However, Rorsman *et al.* [24] have shown that circulating basophils decrease, as does the blood histamine level, in cases of urticaria due to "nonphysical" causes, whereas the basophils do not decrease in urticaria due to "physical agents," e.g., cold urticaria. These studies confirm the earlier conclusion of Horton that the reaction in cold urticaria is due to the liberation of histamine in the exposed tissues. However, an immunological mechanism cannot be postulated for all cases. The same also applies in solar urticaria, in which a positive passive transfer is often obtained only in patients who are sensitive to wavelengths of light less than 3,700 A (and presumably an immunological mechanism is involved), whereas sensitivity to light wavelengths greater than 3,700 A is not associated with a positive passive transfer reaction. One finds little experimental proof of an immunological basis for the reactions in "physical allergy," although it cannot be completely excluded.

In "cholinergic urticaria," another chemical mediator is involved: patients having this condition respond in an abnormal manner to acetylcholine released from efferent nerves in apparently normal amounts after exposure to heat and after exertion, emotional stress, and parasympathetic activity. Grant *et al.* [25] showed that the cholinergic nerve fibers of the autonomic nervous system, when stimulated by heated blood, will release acetylcholine, which in turn liberates histamine, causing urticaria. Cholinesterase levels of the skin are significantly reduced in cholinogenic urticaria [26] (as contrasted with dermographism and chronic urticaria) even though serum cholinesterase levels remain normal. However, other work disputes the idea that the histamine flare is due to acetylcholine release at vascular endings [27]. Herxheimer [28], after studying patients with cervical sympathetic blocks, suggested the possible release of an intermediate agent which, while not yet identified, is neither acetylcholine nor histamine.

Experimental studies of psychological influences on wheal formation were carried out by Graham and Wolf [29], who measured skin temperatures, reactive hyperemia thresholds, and the sensitivity of the skin to histamine and pilocarpine iontophoresis in thirty subjects with chronic urticaria. They found that urticaria was due to extreme dilation of arterioles and minute vessels and was part of the individuals' reaction to stress situations, just as with actual skin trauma. They believed that a dilated capillary per se is more permeable and that only capillary dilation is necessary for wheal formation. Kepecs *et al.* [30] studied the rate of exudation into sites of cantharidin blisters on the skin of patients with eczema and urticaria and found an increase with certain emotional states. These exudation rates could be depressed with antihistamines. Further investigation in the laboratory under controlled conditions is needed to elicit and quantitate the psychological factors in wheal formation.

Angioedema can be produced in unsensitized rats by injections of egg white, dextran, globulin, and other substances. This may be augmented as well as inhibited by various drugs. The significance of these experiments in human angioedema remains to be determined.

PATHOLOGY

Histologically, the wheal is an edema in the superficial layer of the corium. The collagen fibers, which are swollen and pale, are widely separated by edema fluid, the dermal papillae are widened, and the rete pegs are inflated. It has been stated that the marked dermal edema in the absence of any other appreciable pathological changes is diagnostic [31]. Blood and lymphatic vessels are dilated. Several biopsies taken at an allergen (ragweed) injection site in allergic patients revealed the following sequential morphological picture: slight edema and vessel enlargement occurs at 5 minutes, and about 10 percent of the perivascular infiltration is eosinophilic at 10 minutes; early inflammatory changes are noted at 15 minutes, as well as moderate congestion and edema. At the same time, about 25 percent of the wandering cells are eosinophilic, and this figure increases to 90 percent in 30 minutes, when severe inflammatory changes are noted. Monocytic infiltration is noted at 6 hours, and at 22 hours plasma cells, some lymphocytes, tissue fragments, and cellular debris are conspicuous [9].

DIAGNOSIS

The recognition of urticaria and angioedema is not difficult. Urticarial lesions have an erythematous base, and there may be flat-topped papules with sharp borders. The lesions vary in size from a small dot to an area which may encompass the whole side of the thorax or abdomen, or an extremity, particularly when several individual lesions have coalesced. Angioedema may be associated with urticaria or may occur alone; it consists of swelling and erythema, again varying in size and being more firm and nonpitting on pressure. Since cutaneous nerve endings are most prominent in the superficial layers of the skin, itching is more evident with hives than with angioedema. However, some patients experience a burning or stinging sensation, whereas itching is less common in angioedema. Individual lesions usually occur in crops and are more transitory (a few hours to a day) in urticaria than in angioedema, and one crop usually fades before the next appears. The swelling of angioedema persists for a day or two or more, and when it disappears there are usually no residual markings. The lesions have an asymmetrical distribution, and when at times urticaria and angioedema fuse, a true differentiation is not possible. Swelling may occur on the eyelids, lips, tongue, genitalia, or the hands and feet as well as on the trunk. Pharyngeal involvement may produce asphyxia; gastrointestinal involvement has also been noted.

In the *differential diagnosis* of angioedema, several conditions should be considered. Urticaria and angioedema may occur as an integral component of *serum sickness.* The edema occurring in congestive heart failure, renal disease, and myxedema is usually readily identified. *Elephantiasis nostras* resembles angioedema of the lips; it is, however, a lymphedema resulting from a low-grade skin and lymphatic infection usually caused by a streptococcus. The swelling persists for days and usually responds to antibiotic therapy. *Erythema multiforme* has a definite urticarial component and may be associated with systemic disease. *Atopic dermatitis* and *contact dermatitis* may also exhibit areas of erythema and slight edema on rare occasions, but the clinical course is quite different. *Insect bites* may resemble wheals and are believed to be a cause of urticaria in childhood.

Another condition that should be kept in mind is *urticaria pigmentosa.* The lesion consists of pigmented macules and papules which are persistent and thus different from ordinary hives, even though transitory wheals may also occur. The wheals may be produced by vigorous rubbing of the skin near the area of the pigmented lesions; they are due to liberation of histamine from mast cells.

ETIOLOGICAL FACTORS

PHYSICAL AGENTS

Dermographism (urticaria factitia) is produced by light stroking of the skin and usually appears within a few minutes after the trauma [32]. Thus it is differentiated readily from ordinary urticaria. The wheal produced by stroking is similar to the reaction to an injection of histamine. It could, therefore, be considered a true "physical allergy," although vasomotor instability has been suggested as an underlying mechanism. The lesions may also occur on pressure areas, under shoulder straps, buckles, girdles, wristbands, and on other areas of friction, and initially they may be linear. Lesions usually appear within a few minutes after trauma. In some instances, they may persist for 24 hours [33]. No allergic factors are etiologically significant, but it should be noted that dermographism has a high incidence in patients who have had penicillin reactions and may remain after other signs of the reactions have disappeared.

In addition to friction, other physical agents such as *heat, sunlight,* and *cold* may induce whealing and angioedema. (For underlying mechanisms, see Chapter 57.) Occasionally, cryoglobulinemia is associated with cold urticaria as well as with cold hemolysins and cold agglutinins. Urticaria and erythema have been reported in a patient sensitive to both heat and cold [34]. Systemic disease may be accompanied by urticaria from physical agents, e.g., multiple myeloma, Raynaud's syndrome, malignant tumors, syphilis, and lupus erythematosus. Light sensitivity may be tested by exposure to sun and ultraviolet light, since the sensitizing wavelengths are at the ultraviolet end of the spectrum. Ice applied to the skin or immersion of an extremity may bring out the lesions.

EMOTIONAL STRESS

Although well documented as a cause of urticaria in isolated cases, the importance of emotional stress in individual cases must be carefully assessed. Graham and Wolf [29] were able to reproduce psychogenic urticaria under experimental conditions. Attempts are still being made to find a specific personality type and affective determinants which characterize patients with chronic urticaria [35]. The remarks of Dubo *et al.* [36] concerning the need for disciplined evaluation in investigations of the relationships between childhood asthma and family and personal adjustments might well be applied to chronic urticaria.

Some observers [37] have reservations about the role of emotions except in *cholinergic urticaria,* which occurs mostly in young females following exertion or in emotional situations. It is a form of diffuse heat urticaria. The lesions are small, multiple, and may be surrounded by large axon reflexes.

Rees [38] analyzed 100 cases and concluded that personality—general stability and capacity for adjustment—had an indirect role in urticaria to the extent that it is related to emotional tension, which in turn influences the autonomic reactions and vasomotor stability.

It has been observed that the urticarial lesions produced by stress tend to appear in the late afternoon and disappear overnight.

HEREDITY

Hereditary angioedema is characterized by recurring episodes of acute edema of the skin, subcutaneous tissues, and underlying muscle and mucous membranes, especially of the gastrointestinal tract, where it may cause symptoms of intestinal obstruction. Acute laryngeal edema is a frequent cause of death in this condition.* The prognosis is poor. The disease is familial, rare, and transmitted as a Mendelian dominant trait. Allergy plays no role, but recent studies [39] reveal that the inborn biochemical defect is probably a deficiency of a serum inhibitor to plasma kallikrein or a serum globulin permeability factor, or both. In addition, an absence of the serum inhibitor of C′1-esterase has been noted [40] in several members of three families (in members clinically exhibiting hereditary angioedema and in asymptomatic members). It is postulated that it is the function of C′1-esterase to increase vascular permeability, and there may be some relation between the action of the serum inhibitor of C′1-esterase and kallikrein.

ALLERGY

Allergy is generally recognized as the most important etiological factor in acute urticaria, but it contributes also to the chronic form.

Acute urticaria is usually self-limited, and the cause is often discovered by the patient himself. Most individuals are aware of the fact that berries, fish, or penicillin may cause an acute outbreak of hives. The chronic cases pose the more difficult diagnostic problems. There is no simple means of determining the cause; diligent inquiry and an intensive study are required, and even then, an allergic basis or the exact cause is not always detected.

A careful history is the most useful diagnostic tool. It cannot be overemphasized that all other diagnostic procedures are of secondary importance and that many laboratory tests are unnecessary if the physician takes the time to obtain a complete history. In general, the usual causes of chronic urticaria are drugs, foods, infections, and emotional stress. Each should be carefully sought during the initial history taking.

Allergy to Drugs. Although many patients are aware of the drugs they are taking, those in proprietary products purchased over the counter may be overlooked. Often it is wise to use common names and trade names while talking to the patient about medications, for he may take these preparations as part of his daily routine and not look upon them as medicines. It should also be noted that sensitization can occur after a drug has been taken for years.

In general, antibiotics, sedatives, tranquilizers, hormones, and vaccines are the commonest offenders. Penicillin sensitivity may present itself in varied forms, and persistent urticaria associated with other symptoms of serum sickness that occurs with penicillin allergy is a frequent occurrence. Besides preparations prescribed by the physician, penicillin may be encountered in food, since cattle with cystic mastitis are given penicillin that can be detected in the milk in significant amounts for about three days. Penicillin and other antibiotics also are included in poultry and cattle feed and are used in fowl preservatives.

* E.g., fatalities have been described by R. Richards, and H. M. Crombie (*Brit. Med. J.* 2:1787, 1960) after dental extraction in two patients who suffered from familial angioedema.

A reported case of chronic penicillin urticaria with exacerbation following ingestion of dairy products and clearing of the lesions by penicillinase [41] illustrates this type of drug sensitivity. Simple chemicals, such as aspirin, Decholin, and bromsulphalein, may also induce urticaria by acting as haptens. If a drug is suspected, skin-testing is usually unreliable [42] except with high molecular weight drugs, e.g., insulin, ACTH, and liver extract. Some drugs cause urticaria through their action as histamine liberators and induce positive skin reactions even though the patient had not encountered them clinically.

On the basis of clinical impression, it has been suggested that giant lesions occurring on the trunk with violaceous hue and serpiginous borders are seen in drug allergy, as are lesions grouped in an umbrella or pyramid pattern. Large wheals which progressively enlarge at the periphery with clearing in the central areas may be seen with penicillin reactions.

Food Allergy. This is a frequent cause of acute urticaria and at times may play a role in chronic urticaria. This usually occurs when the ingested food has not been recognized as an allergen. For example, hives after the ingestion of grapes may come from a meat sauce or a chewing gum which contains grape extract. Food allergy is further complicated by the fact that some foods tend to cause a delayed reaction, several hours to a day after the food is ingested. On rare occasions, the patient may know that he is sensitive to a certain food such as peanuts but does not realize that he also is sensitive to other members of the same food family (legumes). Seafood, nuts, berries, egg, chocolate, milk, and pork are common offenders. Others are pink-colored beverages and foods that contain phenolphthalein.

Diet manipulation can substantiate the diagnosis of food allergy, since skin tests with food are rarely helpful. At times, skin tests may be useful by suggesting the trial elimination of vegetable gums, orris root, or foods that may contain molds. Positive reactions must be corroborated by diet manipulation, and a negative skin response does not rule out food allergy.

Alcoholic beverages cause urticaria in some patients. Whether this is a specific allergy to grains or yeast or the result of nonspecific vasodilatation must be assessed in individual patients.

How foods induce urticaria is not established. In some instances, systemic absorption through the oral mucosa apparently occurs in exquisitely sensitive individuals. Whether products of enzymatic digestion produce urticaria after passage from the portal vein through the liver into the systemic circulation or whether they reach the blood stream via the thoracic duct are questions which are not clearly answered.

Contact Allergy. Contact allergens may induce urticaria, e.g., wool, animal hair and saliva, and metal. These instances are unusual, and patch tests are helpful when the response is checked for both immediate and delayed reactions.

Allergy to Inhalants. Urticaria caused by air-borne allergens such as pollen has been described [43] but is rare. Inhalation of flour, dander, and cosmetics may induce whealing. The term "osmylogenic urticaria" refers to urticaria induced by odors, e.g., of fish [44]. Formaldehyde, aldehydes in cigarette smoke, and ammonia fumes have also been implicated in the etiology of osmylogenic urticaria.

Allergy to Infection. An acute infection may cause the onset of urticaria; a minor infection may trigger an exacerbation in a patient who previously suffered from it. A comprehensive history and physical examination should be directed particularly to the sinuses, gums, chest, gallbladder, urinary tract, and the female genital tract as well as the skin (pyoderma) in search of an active or smoldering infection or of infestation with parasites. Urticarial lesions due to infection may have a stinging or burning sensation rather than pruritus, usually involve the deeper subcutaneous tissues, and may be slightly painful to light pressure after the erythematous appearance has subsided.

TREATMENT

Specific therapy is the same as for all other atopic conditions, i.e., removal of the offending agent. However, it should be stressed that frequently there are multiple triggers in an individual patient, e.g., both heat and cold sensitivity, or cold urticaria with emotional upsets, or chronic urticaria due to penicillin with recurrent flares on inhalant, ingestant, and contactant exposures to mold [45]. All too often (frequently more than 50 percent of the time), the exact cause of chronic urticaria cannot be discovered despite careful evaluation.

Complete elimination of the offending substance from the system usually takes several days and perhaps, as in penicillin sensitivity, several months. If use of suspected or implicated drug is essential, e.g., of insulin, recrystallized products may be tried, or "rapid desensitization" may be attempted. Hyposensitization should not be tried unless urticaria is a part of systemic symptoms caused by inhalant allergens or by stinging insects. Obviously, infections and parasitic infestations should be treated adequately. Avoidance of exposure to sunlight, use of light-filtering ointments, and increasing daily exposures to light have been advocated for solar urticaria, and daily baths in progressively cooler water for patients who have urticaria due to cold.

Other symptomatic measures are similar to those for atopic disorders in general (Chap. 54).

The treatment of dermographism consists of reassurance and the symptomatic use of hydroxyzine or antihistamines.

COMPLICATIONS

Although urticaria and angioedema are reversible and are thus considered benign, serious complications may arise that are related to acute compression by the edematous swelling in critical areas. The danger of acute laryngeal edema is well known. Gastrointestinal distress, with pain, vomiting, and diarrhea, may occur. Cerebral edema, peripheral neuropathy, cardiac involvement, and exophthalmos have been reported with the urticaria and angioedema associated with serum sickness. Angioedema has been stated to involve bile ducts, salivary glands, lungs, joints, and the genitourinary tract [46]. Persistent progressive renal disease has been associated with angioedema following severe penicillin reactions [47].

REFERENCES

1. Cooke, R. A. *Allergy in Theory and Practice.* Philadelphia: W. B. Saunders Company, 1947.
2. Bruun, E. The so-called angioneurotic edema. *J. Allerg.* 24:97, 1953.
3. Quincke, H. Ueber akutes umschriebenes Hautödem. *Mschr. Prakt. Derm.* 1:129, 1882.
4. Mathews, K. P., Hemphill, F. M., Lovell, R. G., Forsythe, W. E., and Sheldon, J. M. A controlled study on the use of parenteral and oral antihistamines in preventing pencillin reactions. *J. Allerg.* 27:1, 1956.
5. Schwartz, M. Heredity in bronchial asthma. *Acta Allerg.* 2 (supp.):1, 1952.
6. Swinny, B. The atopic factor in urticaria. *Southern Med. J.* 34:855, 1941.
7. (*a*) Dratler, S. Critical review of fifty cases of urticaria. *Virginia Med. Monthly* 73:510, 1946. (*b*) Fink, A. I., and Gay, L. N. A critical review of 170 cases of urticaria and angioneurotic edema followed for a period of from two to ten years. *Bull. Hopkins Hosp.* 55:280, 1934.
8. Lewis, T. *The Blood Vessels of the Human Skin and Their Responses.* London: Shaw & Sons, Ltd., 1927.
9. Kline, B. S., Cohen, M. B., and Rudolph, J. A. Histologic changes in allergic and nonallergic wheals. *J. Allerg.* 3:531, 1932.
10. Katz, G. Histamine release in the allergic skin reaction. *Proc. Soc. Exp. Biol. Med.* 49:272, 1942.
11. Nilzen, A. Studies in histamine (H-substance) with special reference to the conditions obtaining in urticaria and related skin-changes. *Acta Dermatovener.* 17 (supp.):1, 1947.
12. Beall, G. N. Plasma histamine concentrations in allergic diseases. *J. Allerg.* 34:8, 1963.
13. Rose, B. Studies on blood histamine in patients with allergy: II. Alterations in the blood histamine in patients with allergic disease. *J. Clin. Invest.* 20:419, 1941.
14. Rorsman, H. Basopenia in urticaria. *Acta Allerg.* 16:185, 1961.
15. Westgate, H. D., Schultz, E. A., and Van Bergen, F. H. Urticaria and angioneurotic edema following D-tubocurarine administration: Report of a case, with observations on blood and plasma histamine levels. *Anesthesiology* 22:286, 1961.
16. Paton, W. D. M. The Mechanism of Histamine Release. In Wolstenholme, G. E. W., and O'Connor, C. M. (Eds.), *Ciba Foundation Symposium on Histamine.* Boston: Little, Brown, 1956. P. 59.
17. Winkelmann, R. K. Chronic urticaria. *Proc. Mayo Clin.* 32:329, 1957.
18. Criep, L. H., and Levine, M. I. Studies of capillary permeability in allergy with the dermofluorometer. *J. Allerg.* 20:185, 1949.
19. Cooper, I. S. A neurologic evaluation of the cutaneous histamine reaction. *J. Clin. Invest.* 29:465, 1950.

20. Gözsy, B., and Kátó, L. Factors other than histamine affecting capillary permeability. *Int. Arch. Allerg.* 19:168, 1961.
21. Rose, B. Histamine, hormones, and hypersensitivity. *J. Allerg.* 25:168, 1954.
22. Lindell, S. E., Nilsson, K., and Rorsman, H. Metabolism of histamine in cold-urticaria. *J. Invest. Derm.* 36:17, 1961.
23. Juhlin, L., and Shelley, W. B. Role of mast cell and basophil in cold urticaria with associated systemic reaction. *J.A.M.A.* 177:371, 1961.
24. Rorsman, H., Slatkin, M. W., Harber, L. C., and Baer, R. L. The basophile leukocyte in urticarial hypersensitivity to physical agents. *J. Invest. Derm.* 39:493, 1962.
25. Grant, R. T., Pearson, R. S. B., and Comeau, W. J. Observations on urticaria provoked by emotion, by exercise and by warming the body. *Clin. Sci.* 2:253, 1936.
26. Magnus, I. A., and Thompson, R. H. S. Cholinesterase levels in the skin in cholinogenic urticaria and pruritus. *Brit. J. Derm.* 68:283, 1956.
27. Lorincz, A. L., and Pearson, R. W. Studies on axon reflex vasodilatation and cholinergic urticaria. *J. Invest. Derm.* 32:429, 1959.
28. Herxheimer, A. The nervous pathway mediating cholinogenic urticaria. *Clin. Sci.* 15:195, 1956.
29. Graham, D. T., and Wolf, S. Pathogenesis of urticaria: Experimental study of life situations, emotions and cutaneous vascular reactions. *J.A.M.A.* 143:1396, 1950.
30. Kepecs, J. G., Robin, M., and Brunner, M. J. Relationship between certain emotional states and exudation into the skin. *Psychosom. Med.* 13:10, 1951.
31. Robbins, S. L. *Textbook of Pathology* (2nd ed.) Philadelphia: W. B. Saunders Company, 1962.
32. Johnston, T. G., and Cazort, A. G. Dermographia—clinical observations. *J.A.M.A.* 169: 91, 1959.
33. Baughman, R. D., and Jillson, O. F. Seven specific types of urticaria with special reference to delayed persistent dermographism. *Ann. Allerg.* 21:248, 1963.
34. Rajka, G., and Vincze, E. Occurrence of urticaria (erythema) due to both cold and heat. *Acta Allerg.* 12:30, 1958.
35. (*a*) Shoemaker, R. J., Levine, M. I., Shipman, W. G., and Mally, M. A. A search for the affective determinants of chronic urticaria. *Amer. J. Psychiat.* 119:358, 1962. (*b*) Kraft, B., and Blumenthal, D. L. Psychological components in chronic urticaria. *Acta Allerg.* 13: 469, 1959.
36. Dubo, S., McLean, J. A., Ching, A. Y. T., Wright, H. L., Kauffman, P. E., and Sheldon, J. M. A study of relationships between family situation, bronchial asthma, and personal adjustment in children. *J. Pediat.* 59:402, 1961.
37. (*a*) Sulzberger, M. B., and Baer, R. L. (Eds.). *1950 Year Book of Dermatology and Syphilogy*. Chicago: Year Book Publishers, Inc. 1951. P. 164. (*b*) Rothman, S., and Walker, S. A. The problem of emotional factors in the allergies. *Int. Arch. Allerg.* 1:306, 1951.
38. Rees, L. An aetiological study of chronic urticaria and angioneurotic edema. *J. Psychosom. Res.* 2:172, 1957.
39. Landerman, N. S., Webster, M. E., Becker, E. L., and Ratcliffe, H. E. Hereditary angioneurotic edema: II. Deficiency of inhibitor for serum globulin permeability factor and/or plasma kallikrein. *J. Allerg.* 33:330, 1962.
40. Donaldson, V. H., and Evans, R. R. A biochemical abnormality in hereditary angioneurotic edema: Absence of serum inhibitor of C'1-esterase. *Amer. J. Med.* 35:37, 1963.
41. Zimmerman, M. C. Chronic penicillin urticaria from dairy products: Proved by pencillinase cures. *Arch. Derm.* 79:1, 1959.
42. Sherman, W. B. Drug allergy. *Amer. J. Med.* 3:586, 1947.
43. Waldbott, G. L., and Merkle, K. Urticaria due to pollen. *Ann. Allerg.* 10:30, 1952.
44. Derbes, V. J., and Krafchuk, J. D. Osmylogenic urticaria. *Arch. Derm.* 76:103, 1957.
45. Shelley, W. B., and Florence, R. Chronic urticaria due to mold hypersensitivity: A study in cross-sensitization and autoerythrocyte sensitization. *Arch. Derm.* 83:549, 1961.
46. Bruun, E., and Dragsted, P. J. Edema circumscriptum. Quincke. I. A historical and clinical survey. *Acta Allerg.* 3:257, 1950.
47. Sheldon, J. M., Mathews, K. P., and Lovell, R. G. The vexing urticaria problem: Present concepts of etiology and management. *J. Allerg.* 25:525, 1954.

56. *Atopic Dermatitis and Infantile Eczema*

ADOLPH ROSTENBERG, JR., AND DIANA R. BOGDONOFF

THE CONDITION COMMONLY KNOWN as atopic dermatitis was first set off from other eczemas and prurigos about 1885 by the French dermatologists, Besnier and Brocq. It has been variously labeled prurigo diathésique, prurigo Besnier, neurodermatitis, allergic eczema, eczema pruriginosum allergicum, flexural eczema, diathetic eczema, and endogenous eczema. Over the years it was noted that the skin changes were often associated with certain allergic manifestations, especially hay fever and asthma. About 1930, it was hypothesized that these skin lesions were the cutaneous analogues of asthma and hay fever, and the label "atopic dermatitis" was coined. It is questionable that this is the most suitable designation, but it is so well entrenched in the United States that it is not likely to be changed. In England, France, and Scandinavia, the most popular label seems to be "prurigo Besnier."

It is usually stated that the condition begins in infancy as a more or less acute exudative eczema which, with the passage of years, ultimately becomes a dry lichenified dermatitis. Although the sequence from exudative eczema to lichenified dermatitis is often observed, we are not certain that it is the same condition that undergoes this metamorphosis. There is good reason to believe that there may be two separate conditions, namely, infantile eczema and atopic dermatitis, which are related in the sense that they often coexist or develop sequentially in the same person. An individual apparently often inherits the genetic capacity for developing both. About 25 percent* of the children who manifest infantile eczema later have a dry, lichenified dermatitis, which we label by the general term atopic dermatitis or prurigo Besnier. Conversely, a high percentage of older children or adults with the dry lichenified flexural eczema of which we speak had infantile eczema, but this was neither a necessary nor a sufficient condition for the development of these lesions.

The phrase, "infantile eczema," strictly speaking, merely means an infant with an eczematous process. Insofar as one can name a single pathognomonic feature, it is spongiosis (epidermal intercellular edema), which can develop by a variety of means. The most usual is external irritation. Dermatitis venenata is a classic example of this. There has been much debate, still unresolved, as to whether an eczema can develop because of an endogenous irritant. We believe that this clearly is the case. By an endogenous irritant is meant any material coming from within that can ultimately alter the metabolic processes of the epidermis so as to lead to intercellular edema. An example of an eczema that seemingly develops via such a mechanism is that seen in phenylketonuria, in which the eczematous lesions presumably develop because of abnormal, or abnormal concentrations of, metabolites.

Traditionally, the eczemas of infants are divided into three main categories: (1) atopic, (2) seborrheic, and (3) contact. The term infantile eczema is usually reserved for the atopic variety. We consider the distinction between infantile atopic eczema and infantile seborrheic eczema usually (possibly always) to be spurious. In the vast majority of cases designated as seborrheic eczema in an infant, the condition is the same as atopic infantile eczema. Many do not share this view, but the alleged morphological differences between the two do not stand up in practice. Over the years, the senior author has seen many infants in whom he and other dermatologists made a diagnosis of seborrheic dermatitis only subsequently to change the label to atopic dermatitis. In this connection we should like to quote

* This figure is based on children with infantile eczema who are seen at a hospital or clinic. Presumably, there are many others with milder cases who are not seen. The incidence of further skin trouble in these children is unknown.

from Meara [1]: "In watching the progress of infants with eczema one becomes very conscious of the fact that children who present in infancy with a nondescript pattern of eczema, or eczema in sites and of such nature that the diagnosis of seborrheic eczema has been entertained, are often found to develop other atopic manifestations, or the characteristic picture of juvenile atopic eczema may appear as the child grows older."* A true contact eczema can develop in an infant, but then there is, as a rule, no great problem in distinguishing it on the basis of location and history from other varieties of eczema.

CLINICAL ASPECTS

INCIDENCE

The exact incidence of atopic dermatitis is not known, but it surely is a relatively common disease. Hellerström and Hjördis [2] stated that Besnier's prurigo comprises one sixth to one fifth of all cases of skin disease seen at Karolinska Institute, Stockholm. Walker and Warin [3] estimated that 3.1 percent of children in Bristol, England, had eczema, and believed that this figure was on the low side. Brereton *et al.* [4] estimated that 1.1 percent of the children in the area of Cambridge, England, had eczema. Regardless of the exact incidence, infantile eczema and adult atopic dermatitis are not uncommon diseases. Their frequency plus their long-term morbidity adds to their importance.

COURSE

Our discussion of infantile eczema will be confined here to the atopic variety,† including what some may call seborrheic eczema. The eruption commonly begins about the third month of life, having as sites of predilection the cheeks and scalp. The first sign is often a rosy flush which may be mistaken by doting parents for the glow of health, but this glow soon becomes unmistakably a disease process. The flush becomes less and less rosy and develops more of a brownish color. Simultaneously, the patch furnishes mute testimony of the underlying eczematous process by developing superficial fissures with overlying crust formation. A similar involvement may be manifest on the scalp, where it is known as "milk crust." We believe that infantile eczema primarily localized to the scalp is no more indicative of seborrheic eczema than one not so localized. The eczematous process may then extend to any area of the body, but sites of predilection are the wrists, antecubital areas, and popliteal spaces. The infant is evidently quite uncomfortable, as shown by his attempts to rub or otherwise handle the affected parts. There usually is fretfulness, which may interfere with sleeping.

When a child with infantile eczema is seen, we know of no way of foretelling whether he will later have the adult form of prurigo Besnier or whether the condition will regress early in life. We have the impression, though no documentary evidence, that the longer the eruption lasts in childhood, the more likely it is to persist into adult life. This is a more reliable prognostic sign than is the severity of the infantile eczema or its distribution.

With passage of time, the process, as a rule, spreads to involve more of the body. This is not inevitable, but the eczematous process does not remain constant. It improves and exacerbates, without concrete assignable reason. There may be almost complete remissions but small telltale patches of eczema or lichenification over the wrists or the antecubital areas remain. This is the usual course until the child is 2½ or 3 years old, when a fair percentage of patients improve. At this age, the disease in many seemingly disappears. Even in those in whom it does not completely disappear, there is a period of relative quiescence which lasts until the child is 8 or even 12 years old, when often the disease breaks out with new vigor.

At age 2 to 3 years, the process becomes drier and the lesions increasingly lichenified (although occasionally lichenified patches are present almost from the beginning). Thus, as the years pass, exudative lesions are not present except possibly very early at times of bursts of activity; hence the phrase "adult type atopic dermatitis" is used, although it does not necessarily mean that the condition is occurring in an adult. The first symptom

* We shall not consider the difficult problem of whether there is a true independent entity of seborrheic eczema in infants. If such exists, and we are not certain that it does, it is: (1) rare, (2) a superficial infection, and (3) morphologically indistinguishable from atopic infantile eczema.

† We are using the word "atopic" in this connection merely as a convenient designation. No pathogenic or immunological mechanism is implied.

that presages the flaring up of old patches or the development of new patches is intolerable itching. This is unquestionably the most important feature of this disease. Jacquet stated many years ago: "It is not the eruption that is itchy, but the itchiness that is eruptive." This is the key to the understanding of this condition, and we shall revert to it several times. The process continues during the teens and into the early twenties when again there may seem to be a remission, although the incidence of remissions at this age is considerably lower than was believed some years ago. Furthermore, with remission at about age 20, the skin does not return completely to normal. The dry, sallow appearance of the skin remains, often associated with fair-sized patches of lichenification in the antecubital and popliteal areas. In a significant number of patients, the disease persists indefinitely; in these, the lichenification may become quite extreme and generalized.

STIGMATA

Individuals with adult atopic dermatitis tend to have a rather easily recognized physical appearance. They commonly are thin, giving the impression of being hyperkinetic and nervous. The facial expression appears to be set or rigid, the "atopic facies." The eyes are deeply set and in an inordinately high percentage are brown [5]. The skin is usually xerotic, frequently ichthyotic, and shows hyperkeratotic follicular papules. The complexion is sallow and nearly always of a dull-gray hue. There may be spotty hyperpigmentation, and vitiligo is not uncommon. Mongolian folds (Morgan), a fold of the lower lid radiating laterally and slightly down from the inner canthus, are a feature of chronic cases. There often is loss of the lateral half of the eyebrows (Hertoghe's sign). The nails may be polished, eburnated, and worn but are not otherwise dystrophic. There is evidence of scratching and excoriation out of proportion to noticeable dermatitis.

In general, individuals with adult atopic dermatitis have certain constitutional alterations apart from the skin disease. These seem to be mainly mildly abnormal responses of the vascular system. White dermographism is a common feature but by no means unique. A more specific alteration is the delayed blanch phenomenon, which consists of the development of a blanching three to five minutes after the intradermal injection of acetylcholine or pharmacologically related materials. This occurs in about 70 percent of the subjects with atopic dermatitis [6].

Patients with atopic dermatitis do not respond normally to mild alterations of ambient temperature. They show a greater degree of cooling and a smaller rate of warming of fingers and toes than do control subjects [7, 8]. However, the skin in the antecubital and popliteal fossae does not behave the same way. In these areas the skin of those with atopic dermatitis shows less cooling and faster warming than in normal individuals.

LABORATORY INVESTIGATION

Fewer laboratory studies have been done in infantile atopic eczema than in the adult form. Fontana *et al.* [9] studied complement titers, serum protein patterns, presence of C-reactive protein, and latex fixation tests in 42 children with infantile eczema. On the whole they did not find any alterations. When changes were found, they were considered to be nonspecific, i.e., unrelated to the eczema.

A variety of biological and immunological studies have been made in individuals with atopic dermatitis. Occasional claims have been made of one or another abnormality, but, in general, either they have not been confirmed or the abnormality is not unique for atopic dermatitis.

Immunologically, 70 to 80 percent of individuals with atopic dermatitis are atopic; i.e., they tend to develop the atopic antibody (reagin) in response to the inhalation or ingestion of common protein allergens. It is our firm impression that these antibodies are never directly or causally responsible for the production of skin lesions. Such antibodies may, of course, be causally related to concomitant atopic manifestations, as asthma and hay fever.

DIFFERENTIAL DIAGNOSIS

The differential diagnosis of infantile eczema seldom presents a problem, assuming that one does not try to make the dubious distinction between atopic and seborrheic infantile eczema. As already mentioned, contact dermatitis in an infant rarely presents a diagnostic problem. A rather common dermatitis of infancy is diaper rash, but its location and appearance (erythema which may go on to erosions) plus the correlation between the wearing of the diaper and the eruption, make the diagnosis easy. Rather rarely, mycotic eruptions develop in infants. When they occur, a scraping from the lesions will show mycelial elements.

There are several quasi-eczematous processes in infants which, though rare, are serious and must be differentiated from an ordinary banal infantile eczema. These are (1) Ritter's disease, (2) Leiner's disease, (3) the Letterer-Siwe syndrome, and (4) the Aldrich syndrome.

Ritter's disease, or dermatitis exfoliativa neonatorum, is considered to be a bacterial infection developing in the newborn at a time when the stratum corneum is imperfectly developed. Potter [10] believes that the condition is essentially the same as that described by Lyell under the name toxic epidermal necrolysis. Organisms are found as a more or less continuous layer in the uppermost portions of the epidermis. The epidermis tends to peel off in sheets, yielding a scalded appearance. As the noneponymous label implies, the condition is essentially an exfoliative dermatitis. It develops at birth or within the first two weeks of life. The prognosis before the days of antibiotics was extremely grave, and even today there is a high mortality.

Leiner's disease, or erythroderma desquamativum, is a generalized scaling dermatitis (eczema) involving scalp, eyebrows, face, and trunk plus gastrointestinal disturbances. It comes on after the first few weeks of life or even somewhat later. It is often classified as seborrheic dermatitis with gastrointestinal complications. We regard it as an extremely severe form of infantile eczema. The gastrointestinal upsets may be on the basis of allergic reactions to foods or intolerance arising because of an imperfectly matured intestinal tract. Various investigators have suggested that the condition arises because of a biotin deficiency, but we know of no adequate documentation for this view. Hill [11] attempted to segregate a condition he termed atopic erythroderma as intermediate between Leiner's disease and infantile atopic eczema. Although the cases Hill described are intermediate in severity between the two, we regard all three as a continuous spectrum of the same underlying disease, the differences being determined by the genetic constitution of the individual in whom they are displayed.

The *Letterer-Siwe syndrome* (histiocytosis X, a nonlipid reticuloendotheliosis) begins as a rule at a slightly later age than do other infantile eczemas. The child is usually 5 months to 1 year old before the obvious manifestations appear. The cutaneous lesions are of variable morphology. There is a tendency to a rather banal-appearing eczema, but careful observation will detect petechial spots in the eczematous patches. In addition, there may be pyogenic and noduloulcerative lesions. Signs of systemic involvement such as hepatosplenomegaly, generalized enlargement of the lymph nodes, and localized tumors of the bone may be present. There is usually secondary anemia. The pathognomonic feature is, however, the finding in the skin of abnormal reticulum cells which contain large nuclei with one or two nucleoli and an eosinophilic cytoplasm. The course is, as a rule, slowly downhill, nearly always to fatal termination.

The *Aldrich syndrome* consists of the triad of thrombocytopenia, eczema, and recurrent infections. It usually begins later than the other conditions discussed. Indeed, some cases have appeared after the first year of life. Again, the eczema is banal in appearance, but scattered among the eczematous lesions are petechiae or other evidence of bleeding into the lesions which should put one on guard that this is not an ordinary infantile eczema. In addition to the eczema, evidence of systemic involvement is present. The child's general development is below par, and there is a history of repeated infections, such as purulent otitis media and pneumonia. In addition, there may be bleeding from the bowel. There is said to be a familial tendency. All cases of the syndrome have been in male infants. The condition has a gloomy prognosis in that practically all patients with this diagnosis have died within the first few years of life.

The differential diagnosis of atopic dermatitis in the adult usually is quite easy. The characteristic appearance of individuals with this condition has already been mentioned. On occasion, however, chronic contact or seborrheic dermatitis may present diagnostic difficulties. It is important to realize that all three of these conditions converge toward a common morphological mean. Table 56-1 presents the salient differential features. The history of the development of the condition may be of value in suggesting which label is the most appropriate. It is not always possible to distinguish among them.

TABLE 56-1. Comparison of Features of Atopic Dermatitis, Allergic Dermatitis Venenata, and Seborrheic Dermatitis

Characteristics	Atopic Dermatitis	Allergic Dermatitis Venenata	Seborrheic Dermatitis
Age of onset	Infancy and/or early childhood	Any age, but more in adulthood	Adolescence and adulthood
Family history	High incidence of respiratory allergy and/or atopic dermatitis	None	Very questionable
Personal history	High incidence of respiratory allergy and/or atopic dermatitis	None	Possibly a slight increase of acne and/or oily skin
Skin appearance apart from lesions	Dry, mottled pigmentation; lichenification	Normal	Some tendency to oiliness, greasiness, and possibly swarthiness
Site of predilection	Flexures	Exposed areas	Scalp, nasolabial folds, ears, intertriginous areas, sternum
Usual features of eruption	Individual papules coalesce to form large lichenified areas with indefinite margins	Erythema, papules, vesicles, often sharply marginated	Irregular patches covered with greasy brownish scale or crust not sharply marginated; on scalp, flakes of dandruff and crusts
Pruritus	Marked; precedes new lesions	Variable; follows lesions	Not prominent
Eye complications	Cataracts	None	Blepharitis, styes (?)
Skin tests	Multiple positive immediate wheal reactions; not of clinical utility	Positive patch test to specific agent; of clinical utility	None

PATHOLOGY

There is nothing pathognomonic about either infantile or adult atopic eczema. The members of the eczema family present a common histological denominator. On microscopic section, an area of chronic atopic dermatitis cannot be distinguished with accuracy from an area of chronic contact dermatitis. A slide from a patient with infantile eczema shows the same microscopic features whether from a case of "infantile" atopic dermatitis or ones of seborrheic dermatitis, or even dermatitis venenata. Without clinical information, all the pathologist can safely report is that the section shows an eczema or dermatitis which is acute, subacute, or chronic, as the case may be.

Acute eczema, microscopically, is characterized by intraepidermal vesicles (spongiosis) along with inter- and intracellular edema. The dermis contains dilated blood vessels, edema, and perivascular infiltration by acute inflammatory cells. There is nothing specific about the infiltrate.

With chronicity, the epidermis shows pronounced hyperkeratosis, areas of parakeratosis (retention of nuclei in the cells of the horny layer), and regular acanthosis, or hyperplasia of the Malpighian layer (the neurodermatitic reaction), with elongation and thickening of the rete ridges. There is no vesicle formation and minimal, if any, edema. The perivascular infiltrate consists of chronic inflammatory cells, usually lymphocytes, but mast cells, tissue eosinophils, and fibroblasts may be numerous.

COMPLICATIONS

The principal complications of atopic dermatitis are infections and ocular disturbances. It has often been stated that patients with atopic dermatitis are not particularly susceptible to pyogenic infections, but this statement must be taken relatively. Possibly they do not have pyogenic infections as frequently as might be expected of individuals who constantly scratch the skin, but they certainly have pyogenic infections more frequently than does the normal population.

Sedlis and Prose [12] studied 169 children with infantile eczema and stated: "Skin infection was a frequent complication in our series. We have had twenty-eight patients with impetiginous eczema. An additional five patients developed multiple abscesses. Four of these had lesions requiring incision and drainage. Among infections other than that of the skin, the single largest group was otitis media. We have had fourteen patients with otitis, and in some of them recurrences were observed."

Patients with atopic dermatitis are also singularly vulnerable to certain viruses, specifically the vaccinia and herpetic. Infection with these causes either eczema vaccinatum or eczema herpeticum. Groups of tense purulent vesicles with umbilicated centers develop anywhere, but the face is a favorite site. The lesions cannot be differentiated on morphological grounds. Immunological or inoculation studies are required to distinguish them. Accompanying the rash is a high fever, and the patient is quite toxic. This complication is more frequent in childhood but can occur at any age. An unfortunate sequel is scarring, although each lesion does not necessarily produce a scar. Both infections have a serious outlook, although with antibiotic therapy, the prognosis is not nearly as ominous as it once was.

In the older literature there was frequent reference to "eczema death." Children with infantile eczema would die suddenly, often 24 to 48 hours after becoming ill. There has been much speculation as to the cause of these deaths, but the best-informed opinion attributed them to overwhelming infections, usually bronchial pneumonia. Today, with improved care of eczematous children and with the availability of antibiotics, this dreaded complication is no longer seen.

Children with infantile eczema often have pronounced enlargement of the peripheral lymph nodes, which is known as dermatopathic lymphadenitis or lipomelanotic reticulosis of Pautrier and Woringer. This is a benign lymphoid hyperplasia developing in the nodes draining affected areas. Its importance is that it may seriously mislead and alarm the inexperienced observer. Consider a child who is somewhat emaciated and who has enlarged nodes. A node may be removed for pathological study and an inexperienced pathologist interprets the reticulum activity as evidence of true reticulosis. An ominous diagnosis such as Hodgkin's disease may be made.

Ocular complications occur much more frequently with prurigo Besnier than they do with other common skin disease, but still only a small percent (5 or less) of patients with atopic dermatitis have them. Of the ocular complications, by far the most frequent is the formation of cataracts.

Brunsting *et al.* [13] examined 1,158 patients with atopic dermatitis and found that 136 had typical cataracts. In 79, the cataracts were visible grossly or the patients were aware of visual impairment, but 57 in whom opacities were seen by slit lamp had no visual impairment. Of the 136 patients, 40 were between age 10 and 19 and 65 were between age 20 and 29 when the cataract was discovered. It is thus obvious that this complication occurs in relatively young people, with peak incidence in the twenties. This cataract has distinctive morphological features, which were described in detail by Cowan and Klauder [14]. Various theories have been advanced as to why the development of cataracts is a relatively frequent complication of atopic dermatitis, but none is very convincing. Our own view is that this predisposition is part of the genetic make-up of these individuals.

Keratoconus is a much rarer complication than cataracts, but it develops more frequently in atopic dermatitis than in other skin diseases.

PROGNOSIS

Two important questions for which exact answers cannot be given are: (1) what is the duration of an eczema starting in infancy, and (2) are such children likely to develop certain conditions as adults? A number of studies have dealt with the prognosis of infantile eczema, but all were retrospective; i. e., some years after the children were seen with eczema, an attempt was made to evaluate their present condition. This is unsatisfactory in that information is obtained at the time of the follow-up on only a relatively small percentage (usually less than 50) of the total number of children treated for infantile eczema during that period. Furthermore, all such studies were of children whose eczema was severe enough to have brought them to a skin clinic or hospital for treatment. No follow-up figures exist for all eczemas.

Within the limitations set forth, 25 percent of children with eczema severe enough to be brought to a clinic for treatment will have eczema well into adulthood or possibly for the rest of their lives. In somewhat more than 25 percent of them, asthma will develop. A small but significant percentage (possibly 5) will be susceptible to recurrent respiratory infections.

PATHOGENESIS

Surely the most controversial aspect of atopic dermatitis is its pathogenesis. We shall divide the pathogenic theories into three main categories: (1) atopic, (2) psychosomatic, (3) diathetic. Our discussions of these views will be condensed and simplified, but the salient features of each will be taken up.

ATOPIC HYPOTHESIS

As mentioned earlier, ever since Besnier and Brocq's early description, it had been noted that individuals with this skin condition often had asthma or hay fever, or both. Around 1930 it was hypothesized that the skin lesions of prurigo Besnier were the cutaneous analogues of asthma and hay fever, the lesions developing presumably because of the union in the skin of the antigen with the atopic antibody (reagin). Feinberg [15] described the atopic hypothesis as follows: "Generally, there is a constitutional background, usually a distinct hereditary history of allergy. From previous contact with a specific allergen, such as a food, a specific reagin develops which attaches itself to tissue cells. Reintroduction of the specific antigen into the body causes an antigen-antibody reaction. When this reaction takes place in the cells of the capillary loop of the corium, subsequent inflammatory and exudative changes result in the entity recognized as atopic dermatitis. Wheal formation takes place beneath the epidermis with resulting irritation and thickening." This seemed a clear and useful concept of the pathogenesis, for here was an explanation that not only offered a reasonable interpretation but furnished a rationale for direct attack on the condition that should improve or prevent the cutaneous alterations. Unfortunately, time has not borne out this optimistic hope. Elsewhere, one of us has set forth reasons why the atopic hypothesis seems incorrect [16]. A few of the arguments will be discussed briefly.

Before considering them, we might point out that atopy is neither a necessary nor a sufficient condition for the production of the cutaneous lesions of prurigo Besnier. It is not necessary in that between 20 and 30 percent of adults with atopic dermatitis do not have a personal or family history of atopy. It is not sufficient for if it were, every patient with atopic asthma and hay fever would present the cutaneous lesions of prurigo Besnier. Furthermore, individuals with hypo- or agammaglobulinemia may have the skin lesions of atopic dermatitis even though they do not have antibodies or have them in markedly reduced concentration.

The major objection to the atopic hypothesis, apart from the pragmatic fact that neither removal of the alleged offending allergens nor "desensitization" to them has yielded worthwhile results, is the fact that the only known cutaneous reaction between the atopic antibody and its antigen is an urticarial wheal. There is no doubt that when patients with atopic dermatitis are tested with a variety of protein allergens, many immediate wheals are produced; but none of the myriad of wheals so produced has converted into the lichenified lesions of atopic dermatitis. This is the great paradox. For if the lesions develop as a consequence of the antigens reacting with the atopic antibody in the shock tissue—the skin—why, then, are the lesions of the disease not produced when the antigen is deliberately introduced into the skin?

Furthermore, in those in whom a given substance allegedly causes an exacerbation, the exacerbation is limited to areas of pre-existing dermatitis. New lesions do not develop. This is difficult to explain with the atopic theory. If the exacerbation occurs directly because of union of the atopic antibody with its antigen, it would be expected that new lesions should develop. The atopic antibody can be found over the entire cutaneous surface; and the antigen is presumably distributed to the entire integument. Therefore, wherever it comes in contact with the antibody, new lesions should be produced. A partial explanation for this is afforded by the experiment of Engman *et al.* [17]. They studied a child with atopic dermatitis and a history of a violent exacerbation every time the child ate wheat. They were able to corroborate this on several occasions. Once, while relatively free from eczema, the child was hospitalized and fed wheat. Before the feeding, one half of the body was wrapped in a heavy occlusive dressing so that the child could not scratch that half. After the wheat was eaten, there was a pronounced exacerbation on portions of the body accessible to the child. In other words, the wheat caused pruritus but did not cause the development of lesions, which were exacerbated only where the child was able to scratch. Such an experiment clearly shows that, as a practical measure, such a child should avoid wheat, but it also demonstrates that the union of the atopic antibody with its antigen does not suffice to produce the skin lesions.

PSYCHOSOMATIC THEORY

We shall consider briefly the psychodynamics of atopic dermatitis since it has been claimed that the disease is basically "psychosomatic." Individuals with this condition are said to have a special temperament or personality profile which makes them prone to develop the skin lesions or somehow conduces to their genesis. The proponents of these views have not spelled out the mechanism by which the psychosomatic influences could produce the lesions, nor is there any consistency regarding the precise nature of the psychogenic alterations which yield these lesions. The major point advanced is that correlations can be made between exacerbations of the skin lesions and tensional situations. In a review elsewhere [18], it was pointed out that these theories do not provide an adequate explanation of the pathogenesis of the disease. Many of the psychosomatic views are perversions of the original ideas advanced by Besnier and Brocq that the lesions develop primarily because of an altered capacity of the cutaneous sensory receptors to respond to a variety of pruritic stimuli. To this was given the label "neurodermatitis," but in modern parlance this has been interpreted as being equivalent to psychosomatic influences.

DIATHETIC HYPOTHESIS*

When Besnier first segregated this condition from other eczemas and prurigos, he thought it developed because of some inborn constitutional difference, hence the label prurigo diathésique. Subsequently, he called the condition pruritus with lichenification (note the word sequence; Brocq was aware that pruritus came first). Ultimately, Brocq changed this to neurodermatitis, meaning by this that the cutaneous receptors for itching sensations were particularly susceptible. We believe that the enhanced liability to develop pruritus is based on a genetic alteration; this and the tendency to lichenification constitute the heritable basis for the condition. The gene that determines this is believed to be physically close to the gene that determines that the individual will be atopic; consequently, a child often inherits both, but not necessarily.

Although there is no satisfactory explanation for the enhanced susceptibility to itching, it seems to be a well-established clinical fact that the threshold for itch sensations is conspicuously lowered in individuals with atopic dermatitis. Arthur and Shelley [19] furnished experimental evidence of this. Using a chemical pruritic stimulus, they observed that the amount of the agent required to induce itching was far less and the persistence of the sensation far longer in an atopic subject than in subjects with hand eczema and in normal controls. The disparity between individuals with atopic dermatitis and those with hand eczema (mostly dermatitis venenata) seems extremely significant in that it suggests a special cutaneous pruritic susceptibility in atopic dermatitis and that not any cutaneous inflammation, even though pathologically close to atopic dermatitis, is an appropriate substrate for the genesis of pruritic sensations.

Further evidence of the importance of itching in determining activity of the disease is furnished by a clinical observation. On sev-

* Since this chapter was written there has been increasing evidence that one of the basic genetically determined biochemical deviations in this disease is an abnormality in the handling of norepinephrine. This material apparently exists in a higher concentration in the skin and in a lesser concentration in the blood of persons with atopic dermatitis than in others.

eral occasions we have seen patients with paraplegia who had severe atopic dermatitis before development of the paraplegia. It is fascinating to note that in areas not involved by the paraplegic process the atopic dermatitis is active and unchanged, but over the popliteal areas and on sites below the level where the paraplegia begins, the atopic dermatitis has vanished except for occasional slight lichenification. Gans [20] observed similar consequences after nerve injury.

THERAPY

Because the basic mechanism in atopic dermatitis is not known, all therapy is symptomatic. The paramount symptom is itching, and all therapeutic efforts must be directed against it. It is here that the physician's concept of the disease becomes of more than academic importance, for if he focuses on a single aspect, be it allergenic or psychogenic, he will fail because he overlooks other equally important factors. He must realize that the basic alteration increases vulnerability to itching; consequently, all the factors that promote itching must be simultaneously controlled to effect a favorable result. For simplicity of discussion, therapy will be divided into various forms, but for the reasons just given, an integrated approach is necessary.

TOPICAL THERAPY

The most important of all drugs for topical therapy are the corticosteroids. Hydrocortisone in a concentration of 0.5 to 1 percent or the synthetic steroids in appropriately lower concentrations are extremely efficient in controlling itching and reducing inflammation. At comparable dose levels, it is questionable that any corticosteroid can be singled out as having unique effects. Although valuable, these drugs do not affect the basic abnormality nor, for the matter, do any others.

Next to the steroids, tars are most useful. Crude coal tar, 1 percent in a hydrophilic ointment or a cold cream, is as good as any. In general, the more refined and elegant the tar, the less its therapeutic effect. Occasionally, an antibacterial agent is needed, obviously when there is some secondary impetiginization. Neomycin and bacitracin are efficient for this purpose.

The skin of the patient with prurigo Besnier often reacts capriciously. At times, it is difficult to predict just what will be tolerated. The vehicle is frequently the stumbling block. An appropriate vehicle is as important as the active ingredient, although this is not as true with the corticosteroids as with other drugs. In general, creams are better tolerated than ointments. The more acute the inflammation, the more this is true; but for an indolent, heavily lichenified patch, an ointment may be desirable, and indeed an occlusive dressing may add to the efficacy. Nevertheless patients with atopic dermatitis in general do not tolerate occlusion.

Topically applied antihistaminics are used by some, but we mention them only to condemn them. They have no place in the treatment of atopic dermatitis.

SYSTEMIC THERAPY

The chief aim of systemic therapy is to provide the patient with sufficient equanimity to refrain from excoriating his skin. Any of the many tranquilizing agents are of some value; no one has unique virtues. Modest doses of barbiturates (e.g., phenobarbital 0.015 to 0.032 gm.) can also be used. Antihistaminics are often given orally, seemingly with some slight effect, probably due to a side action that promotes somnolence.

Steroids given systemically have a rapid therapeutic effect. But we deprecate their use because of their inherent dangers, for a patient with atopic dermatitis will require treatment over a long period. Furthermore, once systemic steroid therapy is initiated, the patient may become difficult to manage, because it is much simpler and pleasanter to swallow a few pills than to anoint oneself with a relatively greasy preparation. It becomes difficult to persuade the patient that he should sacrifice speed for safety and comfort for caution. The many other drugs that were used in the past, such as calcium gluconate, sodium thiosulfate, and arsenic, have no place in today's therapy.

The foregoing remarks apply primarily to the adult form of atopic dermatitis. In infantile eczema, the same basic principles apply. The primary difference is that the condition is more exudative, so ointments are rarely well tolerated. The use of creams, or even lotions, may be desirable. Steroids should not be given systemically to children.

A difficult task in the management of children is the prevention of scratching. Occasionally some form of mild restraint may be necessary. Rather than full arm splints we prefer to put heavy dressings over the skin or sedate the child sufficiently to reduce the scratching. An essential feature is the handling of the parents, who must be made to realize that the condition may persist for a long time. The child, as he grows older, must not be treated as if he were a pariah; yet he must be made aware of the fact that his skin is vulnerable, and to some degree it has to be protected.

ENVIRONMENTAL CONTROL

It is necessary, insofar as possible, to control the multitudinous ambient pruritic stimuli.

Hot, muggy weather is badly borne by patients with this condition. There seems to be some impairment of the ability to deliver sweat to the skin surfaces. As a consequence, conditions which promote much sweating often cause intolerable itching. Cold weather is a burden because of dry, ichthyotic skin that is vulnerable to cold. Painful chapping and fissuring may develop. In general, the ideal climate for those with prurigo Besnier is a warm dry one.

Fabrics that come in contact with the skin may cause itching. By far the most important is wool, which is tolerated very poorly. Some believe that wool acts as an allergen which causes an antigen-antibody interaction when woolen particles are inhaled, but this view seems unjustified. Nylon is a runner-up to wool in terms of its pruriginous property. The best tolerated of all fabrics in this respect is cotton.

Detergents and other mildly irritating chemicals can cause difficulty. The skin should not be washed too frequently, for in many it is inherently dry. Washing tends to defat the skin and thereby conduces to itching and inflammation.

ANTIALLERGIC THERAPY

As already pointed out, we do not believe that allergic factors play a significant role in the development or perpetuation of atopic dermatitis. Occasionally, but very rarely, itching sufficient to induce a paroxysm of scratching may develop as a consequence of an antigen-antibody interaction. In such an instance, it is, of course, desirable to eliminate the responsible allergen, but skin-testing is not the way to identify it. Numerous immediate reactions will be obtained, but there is no reliable method to determine what is responsible for the itching. By the same token, it follows that desensitization therapy is not warranted. On rare occasions, a food may cause itching, but food sensitivity per se does not produce the cutaneous lesion. In our management of the adult form of atopic dermatitis, we do not interfere with the diet, and we have seen younger children who have become nutritionally impoverished by vain efforts to improve the skin condition by elimination of foods.

RADIOTHERAPY

Superficial x-ray therapy will give some temporary relief. Its use is not recommended, because atopic dermatitis is a protracted condition, and sooner or later irreversible skin changes will develop with x-radiation. Ultraviolet radiation has little or no value.

CONTROL OF EMOTIONIAL FACTORS

Tensional, conflictual situations may induce itching, but we do not believe that psychotherapy is indicated. We agree that tranquility is a desideratum, but the preferable approach to this is via pharmacology rather than psychiatry.

REFERENCES

For a general reference, see Baer, R. L., *Atopic Dermatitis* (New York: New York University Press, 1955). This small monograph covers many aspects of atopic dermatitis.

1. Meara, R. H. Eczema in infancy and childhood. *Proc. Roy. Soc. Med.* 55:558, 1962.
2. Hellerström, S., and Hjördis, L. Studies of Besnier's prurigo (atopic dermatitis). *Acta Dermatovener.* 36:11, 1956.
3. Walker, R. B., and Warin, R. P. The incidence of eczema in early childhood. *Brit. J. Derm.* 68:182, 1956.
4. Brereton, E. M., Carpenter, R. G., Rook, A. J., and Tyser, P. A. The prevalence and prognosis of eczema and asthma in Cambridgeshire school children. *Med. Officer,* p. 317, Dec. 18, 1959.
5. Carney, R. G. Eye color in atopic dermatitis. *Arch. Derm.* 85:17, 1962.

6. Lobitz, W. C., and Campbell, C. J. Physiologic studies in atopic dermatitis (disseminated neurodermatitis). *Arch. Derm.* 67:575, 1953.
7. Eyster, W. H., Jr., Roth, G. M., and Kierland, R. R. Studies on the peripheral vascular physiology of patients with atopic dermatitis. *J. Invest. Derm.* 18:17, 1952.
8. Weber, R. G., Roth, G. M., and Kierland, R. R. Further contributions to the vascular physiology of atopic dermatitis. *J. Invest. Derm.* 24:19, 1955.
9. Fontana, V. J., Sedlis, E., Prose, P., Messina, V. P., and Holt, L. E., Jr. Complement titer, C-reactive protein, and electrophoretic serum protein patterns in eczematous children. *New York J. Med.* 62:2801, 1962.
10. Potter, B. Ritter's disease (toxic epidermal necrolysis). *Lancet* 2:458, 1962.
11. Hill, L. W. Nomenclature, classification, and pathogenesis of "eczema" in infancy. *Arch. Derm.* 66:212, 1952.
12. Sedlis, E., and Prose, P. Infantile eczema with special reference to the pathologic lesion. *Pediatrics* 23:802, 1959.
13. Brunsting, L. A., Reed, W. B., and Bair, H. L. Occurrence of cataracts and keratoconus with atopic dermatitis. *Arch. Derm.* 72:237, 1955.
14. Cowan, A., and Klauder, J. V. Frequency of occurrence of cataract in atopic dermatitis. *Arch. Ophthal.* 43:759, 1950.
15. Feinberg, S. M., Durham, O. C., and Dragstedt, C. A. *Allergy in Practice* (2nd Ed.). Chicago: Year Book Publishers, Inc., 1946.
16. Rostenberg, A., Jr. Atopic Dermatitis: A Discussion of Certain Theories Concerning Its Pathogenesis. In Baer, R. L. (Ed.), *Atopic Dermatitis*. Philadelphia: J. B. Lippincott Company, 1955.
17. Engman, M. F., Weiss, R. S., and Engman, M. F. L. Eczema and environment. *Med. Clin. N. Amer.* 20:651, 1936.
18. Rostenberg, A. Psychosomatic concepts in atopic dermatitis—a critique. *Arch. Derm.* 79: 692, 1959.
19. Arthur, R. P., and Shelley, W. B. The nature of itching in dermatitic skin. *Ann. Intern. Med.* 49:900, 1958.
20. Gans, O. Pathogenesis of Besnier's prurigo. *Trans. St. John Hosp. Derm. Soc.*, winter issue, 1956.

57. Allergic Eczematous Contact Dermatitis*

RUDOLF L. BAER AND LEONARD C. HARBER

ALLERGIC ECZEMATOUS CONTACT dermatitis (aecd), the clinical expression of allergic eczematous contact sensitization, is a form of delayed hypersensitivity. It was first established as a clinical entity in 1896, the year Josef Jadassohn [1] introduced the patch test as a clinical diagnostic and investigative tool.

Clinical changes depend on the acuteness or chronicity of the eruption. In the acute phase, papules and vesicles predominate along with erythema and edema and at times also bullae. In the subacute phase, vesicular changes are less pronounced and intermingle with crusting, scaling, and early thickening of the skin. The chronic phase is characterized by thickening, lichenification, and scaling, with minor or no papulovesicular features.

The clinical course is characterized by exacerbations following exposures to the allergen and remissions following cessations of exposures. The localizations of the eruption depend almost entirely on the sites of major exposure to an allergen (Table 57-1), secondary lesions developing in less exposed sites. Lesions may also be seen in sites without conspicuous opportunities for exposure [2]. In appropriate conditions, flare-ups and recurrences follow systemic administration of allergens.

Similar eczematous changes may be seen in other eczematous dermatoses of different pathogeneses (primary irritant contact dermatitis, nummular eczema, atopic dermatitis in infants, solar eczema, eczematous fungous infections, etc.) as well as in noneczematous dermatoses with superimposed eczematous changes. These eczematous changes, however, together with the characteristic clinical course, localizations, and immunological features, make it possible to distinguish aecd from other eczematous dermatoses.

Causal agents generally are small molecular compounds ("simple" chemicals), such as dyes, cosmetics, plant oleoresins, topical medicaments, industrial substances, and plastics, but in exceptional cases may be as large as proteins. Sensitization to more than one contact allergen is not uncommon, as some individuals appear to have an unusual susceptibility to this form of allergic change. The three principal categories of multiple sensitizations are shown in Table 57-2 [3]. As a rule, the entire integument is sensitive, although localized sensitivity, e.g., of the hands or face, or localized lack of sensitivity may occur. On a nonspecific basis, however, the scalp, palms, and soles are notoriously less reactive than the rest of the integument, while the eyelids, sides of the neck, and genitals are notoriously reactive.

Familial tendency to allergic eczematous contact sensitization has never been demonstrated in man. The existence of such genetic strains, however, cannot be ruled out, since relative insensitivity to tuberculin has been reported as an inherited trait in some families sensitized with BCG [4]. Further, selective inbreeding in guinea pigs has produced a strain highly sensitizable to dinitrochlorobenzene (DNCB) and other substances [5].

The *reaction time,* i.e., the interval between exposure to an allergen and occurrence of clinical manifestations, is usually 12 to 48 hours but may vary from 4 to 72 hours. The *incubation period* of sensitization clinically is at least 5 days. A *spontaneous flare-up* phenomenon may occur (1) at the site of the sensitizing exposure if sufficient allergen remains in situ to react with the now sensitized skin after the incubation period has elapsed, and (2) as an anamnestic response in previously (weeks to many years) involved sites after exposure at distant sites to the homologous allergen.

It is not known whether the reaction in sen-

* Supported in part by Grant No. DA-49-193-MD-2275 from the U.S. Army Medical Research and Development Command.

TABLE 57-1. Characteristic Localizations of Allergic Eczematous Contact Dermatitis and Common Causal Allergens Suggested by Each Site

Localization	Suggested Causes
Scalp	Lotions, scalp tonics, pomades, hair dyes, wave-sets, etc.[a]
Lobes of ears	Earrings of nickel, white gold, other metals, Bakelite, other plastics; perfumes, etc.
Trunk, various sites	Clothing, brassieres, girdles, underwear, night clothes, sweaters, bathing materials, bath salts, soaps, perfumes, massage creams, etc.
Thighs, legs, ankles	Dyed materials and materials of trousers, underdrawers, socks, etc; match boxes, cigaret lighters, coins, and other metallic objects carried in trouser pockets, etc.; volatile and airborne substances, dusts inside trousers, etc.; garters (rubber, elastic, dyes, metal clasps)
Feet (particularly dorsa of great toes), sides and dorsa of feet, sometimes soles (often with little interdigital involvement)	Shoes, leather dyes, tanning agents, shoe polishes, chemicals in shoe materials, rubbers, sock and stocking dyes and finishes, etc.

[a] The scalp is often remarkably resistant to external irritants and allergens. Thus dermatitis caused by substances used on the scalp often appears not primarily on the scalp but predominantly or exclusively on other, more sensitive, skin areas, such as eyelids, ears, and retroauricular areas, nape and other parts of the neck, the face in general, and even the hands.

SOURCE: Extracted from Sulzberger, M. B., Wolf, J., and Witten, V. H., *Dermatology, Diagnosis and Treatment* (2nd Ed.). Chicago: Year Book Medical Publishers, Inc., 1961. Table 10, p. 170.

TABLE 57-2. Characteristics of Multiple Eczematous Sensitivities

Characteristics	Multiple Nonspecific	Multiple Primary Specific	Multiple Secondary Specific
Mechanism	Low threshold for effects of primary irritants; not an immunological phenomenon	Abnormal capacity to undergo primary allergic sensitizations	Capacity to develop allergic secondary or cross-sensitizations or primary sensitization to allergen which obligatorily produces cross-sensitization
Role of nonspecific factors	Usually highly important	Sometimes contributory	Usually not contributory
Immunochemical relation of materials producing multiple sensitivities	Usually none	Usually none	Always present
Duration	Evanescent—weeks to months	Relatively persistent	Relatively persistent

Source: Baer [3].

sitized skin has its inception in the epidermis or in the dermis. Histologically, perivascular accumulation of small round cells and histiocytes in the uppermost dermis within six hours is the first visible change [6–8]. These cells then migrate via a disturbed basal cell layer into the epidermis. Subsequently, there develops intra- and intercellular edema in the epidermis leading to spongiosis—the hallmark of "eczema." Large intraepidermal areas of edema are seen clinically as vesicles and bullae.

A reaction similar to or identical with that which occurs clinically can be reproduced deliberately for diagnostic or investigative purposes by the patch test technic. This involves application of the allergenic material under a semiocclusive dressing to unaffected skin (usually on the arm or back) in a concentration which is *nonirritating to normal skin* (for listings of proper concentrations and vehicles, see Ref. 3).

A great deal of knowledge of the pathogenic mechanism in aecd has been culled from experiments in guinea pigs. Many, but not all, of the results from these investigations appear to be applicable to man. For example, it is important to remember that unaltered guinea pig skin is incapable of consistently reacting with the spongiosis which is so characteristic of aecd in man [7].

The concept that allergic contact sensitivity is dependent on alterations in organ systems other than the skin was demonstrated in transplantation studies between identical twins [9]. These showed that sensitized skin, when transplanted to a nonsensitive host, loses its sensitivity and that, conversely, nonsensitized skin transplanted to a sensitized host within a short time acquires his contact sensitivity. Sensitization develops as long as the regional lymph nodes and the lymphatic pathways between these and the cutaneous site of allergen application remain intact, even after the nerve supply has been deliberately cut [10]. If the lymphatic pathways are cut or the regional lymph nodes removed within forty-eight hours after the sensitizing exposure, sensitization does not develop. Thus the regional lymph nodes are necessary for the development, but not for the maintenance, of sensitization. Lymph node cells are capable of concentrating the hapten up to 300 times [11], and this provides an opportunity for adequate exposure of those cells of the lymphocytic series which are actively involved in the sensitization process.*

The changes which occur in the regional lymph nodes of guinea pigs during conversion to the contact allergic state [12–14] correspond to those seen in other forms of delayed "cellular" hypersensitivity: a pronounced weight increase of the regional lymph nodes regularly precedes sensitization to DNCB. This hyperplasia is due to an increase of lymphatic reticulum cells (stem cells) followed by an increase of large lymphocytes. Apparently, lymphatic reticulum cells are responsible for initiation of antibody formation and then transmit this capacity to large lymphocytes. Cells from the regional lymph nodes which enter the blood stream "seed" other parts of the lymphatic system, thus giving rise to distant foci of antibody production [10].

Allergic eczematous contact-type sensitivity is not dependent on humoral antibodies, and passive transfer cannot be achieved with serum. However, in guinea pigs, successful passive transfer is possible with suspensions of mononuclear blood cells or lymph node cells [15–18]. It is noteworthy that in contradistinction to the ease with which tuberculin sensitivity and other types of bacterial hypersensitivity can be transferred in man [19], attempts to transfer passively allergic eczematous contact sensitivity to "simple" chemicals in man have produced conflicting results. Negative findings by some [20–24] are opposed by positive findings of others [5, 6]. It has been suggested that in order for passive transfer to occur, a self-replicating unit which is available with bacterial antigens but not with "simple" chemicals might be required [27]. It appears possible, however, that the white blood cells of sensitive donors may contain a factor which facilitates active sensitization to the homologous allergen in human recipients of these cells [22, 23]. One might speculate that this facilitated *active* sensitization is made possible by the passively transferred cells which provide such self-replicating units.

Recently it was postulated that "delayed" responses, like "immediate" responses, are

* The findings in guinea pigs by Fishman (*Nature* [London] 198:549, 1963) tend to support a hypothesis of Rostenberg (*Arch. Derm. Syph.* 56:222, 1947) that the high incidence of sensitization after application of the antigen to the skin may be due to richness of the cutis in macrophages.

mediated through humoral antibodies, since if the serum concentration of antibody is as low as 10^{-10} M and the cellular avidity for fixing antibody is as high as 10^{-10} M, all of the immunological findings of delayed sensitivity would be plausible, despite the failure of present-day methods of antibody detection to demonstrate humoral antibodies [28]. Perhaps of relevance in this connection is the recent finding that the "transfer factor" of delayed allergy in man is a dialyzable material of low molecular weight (< 40,000), that it is not a protein or a globulin fragment by chemical or immunological tests, and that it is, therefore, not an antibody in the conventional sense [29]. While this evidence could be taken to speak against the Karush-Eisen hypothesis, the possibility remains that the "transfer factor" could induce in the recipient the synthesis of another material which in turn mediates the delayed response.

Hapten conjugation with proteins is a prerequisite to evoking contact sensitization to "simple" chemicals [30–32]. In the past, it was thought that the specificity in allergic eczematous contact sensitization depends on the hapten, with the protein being relegated to the role of a carrier (*Schlepper*), but now the protein is thought to have a more important role in determining antigenic specificity [32].

Depending on the particular proteins in the epidermis and cutis involved in the union of the reactive hapten, hapten-epidermal protein conjugates and hapten-dermal protein conjugates might be formed. Differences in these conjugates also could result in epidermal or dermal delayed hypersensitivity. Why does contact with "simple" chemicals engender a delayed rather than an immediate form of sensitization? It has been proposed that the type of protein with which the hapten links determines whether an immediate or delayed type of hypersensitivity is induced [33]. Thus the union of contact allergens with the insoluble fibrous protein of the skin (keratin, collagen) would engender a delayed eczematous sensitivity, whereas conjugation of hematogenously distributed drug allergens with globular proteins of the serum (e.g., globulin and albumin) would be more likely to result in an immediate hypersensitivity associated with humoral antibodies. Relatively minor variations in antigenic structure determine whether a delayed or an immediate type of hypersensitivity or both will ensue [34, 27]. For example, by using a moderately sized hapten (picryl chloride), a transitory immediate type of hypersensitivity directed against the "simple" chemical was produced, whereas long-lasting delayed hypersensitivity directed against the carrier was evoked. The nature of the complete antigen in terms of the number and chemical structure of the hapten combining sites influences the induction of an immunological response directed against the hapten (in the form of humoral antibodies) or against the carrier protein (in the form of a delayed reaction). A large "area of recognition" on the antigen seems a requirement for the delayed response, but only a small area is needed for antibody formation leading to immediate sensitivity.

Wide variations exist in the ability of different substances to cause allergic contact sensitization. Chemically quite similar substances may vary greatly in this respect. A striking example of this is the high *sensitizing index** of 1-2-4 trinitrobenzene as compared with that of the 1-3-5 analogue [35, 36]. The physicochemical properties which determine the ability of a compound to sensitize have been a matter of interest for many years [35, 36]. *In vivo* conjugation of the hapten with protein is a prime requisite to inducing contact sensitization [11]. With DNCB, chemical union of the hapten or its oxidation products with protein occurs in the Malpighian layer of the epidermis, the amino acid sites of lysine and cysteine being most reactive [37]. Conjugation with the keratin of the horny layer, however, does not result in sensitization. Twenty-four hours following exposure, little or no DNCB or derivatives are demonstrated in the cutis, whereas significant amounts remain in the epidermis. The hapten probably must conjugate with protein not only to sensitize but also to elicit a reaction in already sensitized skin [11]. It has been clinically observed and experimentally confirmed [38] that disease processes which provide partially or wholly denatured skin proteins increase susceptibility to allergic contact sensitization (burned, eczematous, "varicose" skin). Adjuvant procedures, usually involving simultane-

* The sensitizing index, i.e., the capacity of a substance to engender allergic contact sensitization, should not be confused with the *index of sensitivity*, which reflects the existing incidence of sensitivity to a substance in a given population at a given time and which is influenced by a host of nonimmunological factors.

ous exposure to killed mycobacteria [30, 39], also cause remarkable increases in sensitizing capacity.

The concept that the protein component of the conjugate is not merely an inert carrier but plays an important role in determining antigenicity [32] logically leads to the conclusion that allergic eczematous contact sensitivity is a form of autosensitization.* Probably many different antigenic complexes are formed, since the hapten presumably denatures different cutaneous proteins [32]. These then become "foreign" and can be thought of as "autologous homografts" [40–42].

The relationship between eczematous sensitivity and tuberculin-type sensitivity still requires further exploration. These two forms of delayed sensitivity share many points of identity or resemblance and they frequently coexist [43–45]. However, there is not yet enough justification to consider them identical.

Dermal (tuberculin-type) sensitivity may be sensitization mainly to hapten complexes with dermal proteins, whereas eczematous (contact) sensitivity may be sensitization principally to hapten complexes with epidermal proteins. The relationship of contact sensitivity and tuberculin-type sensitivity to "simple" chemicals also has been expressed in terms of two cross-reacting systems with different carrier specificity [27]. These differences in carrier specificity in contact and tuberculin sensitivity alone, however, do not explain why two such morphologically different forms of delayed reactivity are produced in the same individual exposed to the same "simple" chemical allergen. Nor do they explain the fact that contact sensitivity cannot be engendered in certain species of laboratory animals in which tuberculin-type sensitivity can be induced (e.g., rabbits).

Several procedures have been reported which appear to be capable of specifically reducing the capacity of guinea pigs to undergo active sensitization to contact allergens. This has been achieved in adult guinea pigs by intravenous injection [46] and feeding [47, 48] of the allergen prior to the sensitizing exposure. Feeding or intraperitoneal injection of the contact sensitizer into pregnant guinea pigs also has been shown to reduce specifically the sensitizability of the offspring [49, 50]. The effects of prenatal exposure, however, are very moderate in degree as far as can be judged from tests in 4- to 6-week-old guinea pigs.

The administration of ACTH and glucocorticoids does not inhibit the induction of contact sensitization but has at times decreased allergic eczematous contact reactivity in already sensitized human beings and guinea pigs. In man, however, the patch test reaction is completely suppressed only very rarely.

The ability of agammaglobulinemic individuals to undergo contact allergic sensitization appears to be unimpaired in contrast to their inability to develop sensitizations mediated by humoral antibodies [26]. On the other hand, patients with certain lymphomas [51] and with sarcoidosis [52, 53] appear to have a marked diminution in their sensitizability to "simple" chemical contact allergens although γ-globulins are present in normal or, in sarcoidosis, even in increased concentration. This paradox has been paraphrased as follows: "The hypogammaglobulinemic patient without plasma cells can develop delayed reactivity, while patients with sarcoid and Hodgkin's disease possess plasma cells but cannot develop this reactive state" [54]. Sensitizability to contact allergens also is conspicuously reduced in aged cachectic individuals.

* The concept of "partial" autosensitization to skin is relatively new, but autosensitization to skin was described by Whitfield in 1921. It should be noted that his term "autosensitization" makes much more sense for disease processes where the patient has become *sensitized* to autologous materials than the now-fashionable term "autoimmunity." Although Whitfield referred to several clinical phenomena, the one that has gained most attention among clinicians is an acute, patchy, eczematous eruption which occurs secondarily to a pre-existing chronic localized dermatitis. The latter is commonly a varicose symptom complex on the lower extremity. Exacerbation or irritation of the localized eczematous process on the leg is accompanied or followed by a vesiculopapular eczematous eruption often on the extensor aspects of the upper extremities.

The mechanism producing the disorder is not known, but it has been variously attributed to autosensitization to skin, to sensitization to microbial antigens commonly found in the skin, to sensitization to medications used in therapy, and to skin "denatured" by microorganisms or topical medicaments. Experimental work in this field is difficult because, except for fetal skin and skin from "germ-free" animals, it is impossible to obtain skin not containing microbial antigens. Among the pertinent references are: Voisin and Maurer (*Sem. Hop. Paris* 33:1909, 1955), Rosenthal, Baer, and Hagel (*Proc. Soc. Exp. Biol. Med.* 97:279, 1958), Parish (*Clinical Aspects of Immunology* [Philadelphia: F. A. Davis Company, 1963], p. 695), and Wilhelmj, Owens, and Kierland (*Arch. Derm.* 86:161, 1962).

Under clinical conditions, allergic eczematous contact sensitivity, once established, often persists for many years. However, loss of sensitivity after a few years is not uncommon [55] and seems to vary somewhat with different allergens. Continued exposure or lack of exposure to the allergen does not appear to be decisive. Under experimental conditions, early spontaneous loss of contact sensitivity has been observed [56].

The keystone of effective management of aecd is the discovery and elimination or avoidance of the causal agent. This is possible through clinical observation, including clues from localizations and periodicity of the eruption and a detailed and well-focused history. If necessary, this can be combined with the use of patch tests [57]. As with other laboratory procedures, however, the results of such tests must be closely correlated with the history and clinical course before they are accepted as being significant, since positive results of patch tests may be totally unrelated to the presenting eruption.

Nonspecific topical and systemic therapy should be instituted as quickly as possible, whether or not the etiological factor has been discovered. For toxicological reasons, attempts to abolish specifically an existing sensitivity by oral or parenteral hyposensitization procedures generally are impractical. However, even in dermatitis due to plant oleoresins, for which such procedures have been in use for many years, they have doubtful value [58, 59] unless they are carried out for a long and often impractical period of time [60].

REFERENCES

1. Jadassohn, J. Zur Kenntnis der medicamentösen Dermatosen. *Verh. Deutsch. Derm. Ges.* 5:103, 1895.
2. Marcussen, P. V. The rise in incidence of nickel sensitivity. *Brit. J. Derm.* 71:97, 1959.
3. Baer, R. L. Multiple eczematous sensitizations. *J.A.M.A.* 170:1041, 1959.
4. Palmer, C. E., and Meyer, S. N. Research Contributions of B.C.G. Vaccination Programs: I. Tuberculin Allergy as a Family Trait. *Public Health Rep.* 66:259, 1951.
5. Chase, M. W. Models for Hypersensitivity Studies. In Lawrence, H. S. (Ed.), *Cellular and Humoral Aspects of the Hypersensitive States.* New York: Paul B. Hoeber, Inc., 1959. P. 253.
6. Miescher, G. In Charpy, J. (Ed.), *Le Mécanisme Physiopathologique de l'Eczema.* Paris: Masson et Cie, 1954.
7. Baer, R. L., Rosenthal, S. A., and Sims, C. F. The allergic eczema-like reaction and the primary irritant reaction: A histologic comparison of their evolution in the acanthotic skin of guinea pigs. *Arch. Derm.* 76:549, 1957.
8. Waksman, B. H. A Comparative Histopathological Study of Delayed Hypersensitivity Reactions. In Wolstenholme, G. E. W. (Ed.), *Cellular Aspects of Immunity.* Boston: Little, Brown, 1960.
9. Haxthausen, H. Allergic dermatitis: Studies in identical twins. *Acta Dermatovener.* 23:438, 1943.
10. Frey, J. R., and Wenk, P. Experimental studies on the pathogenesis of contact eczema in the guinea pig. *Int. Arch. Allerg.* 11:81, 1957.
11. Eisen, H. N., Orris, L., and Belman, S. Elicitation of delayed allergic skin reactions with haptens. *J. Exp. Med.* 95:473, 1952.
12. Macher, E. Die Reaktion der regionaeren Lymphknoten beim tierexperimentellen allergischen Kontaktekzem. *Hautarzt* 13:18, 1962.
13. Macher, E. *Ibid.,* p. 136.
14. Macher, E. *Ibid.,* p. 174.
15. Landsteiner, K., and Chase, M. W. Studies on sensitization of animals with simple chemical compounds: Skin sensitization induced by injection of conjugates. *J. Exp. Med.* 73:431, 1941.
16. Landsteiner, K., and Chase, M. W. Experiments on transfer of cutaneous sensitivity to simple compounds. *Proc. Soc. Exp. Biol. Med.* 49:688, 1942.
17. Chase, M. W. The cellular transfer of cutaneous hypersensitivity to tuberculin. *Proc. Soc. Exp. Biol. Med.* 59:134, 1945.
18. Haxthausen, H. Studies on the lymphocytes as "transmitter" of the hypersensitiveness in allergic eczema. *Acta Dermatovener.* 27:275, 1947.
19. Lawrence, H. S. The Transfer of Hypersensitivity of the Delayed Type in Man. Ref. 5, p. 279.
20. Haxthausen, H. Experiments on passive transfer of eczematous allergy. *J. Invest. Derm.* 19:293, 1952.
21. Haxthausen, H. Attempts on passive local sensitization by intracutaneous injection of cells from freshly excised lymph nodes of eczema allergics. *J. Invest. Derm.* 21:237, 1953.

22. Baer, R. L., and Sulzberger, M. B. Attempts at passive transfer of allergic eczematous sensitivity in man. *J. Invest. Derm.* 18:53, 1952.
23. Baer, R. L., Serri, F., and Kirman, D. Attempts at passive transfer of eczematous sensitivity in man by means of white cell suspensions. *J. Invest. Derm.* 19:217, 1952.
24. Harber, L. C., and Baer, R. L. Attempts to transfer eczematous contact-type allergy with whole blood transfusions. *J. Invest. Derm.* 36:55, 1961.
25. Epstein, W. L., and Kligman, A. M. Transfer of allergic contact-type delayed sensitivity in man. *J. Invest. Derm.* 28:291, 1957.
26. Good, R. A., Zak, S. J., Jensen, D. R., and Pappenheimer, A. M., Jr. Delayed allergy and agammaglobulinemia. *J. Clin. Invest.* 36:894, 1957.
27. Gell, P. G. H., and Benacerraf, B. Studies on hypersensitivity: IV. The relationship between contact and delayed sensitivity. *J. Exp. Med.* 113:571, 1961.
28. Karush, R., and Eisen, H. A theory of delayed hypersensitivity. *Science* 136:1032, 1962.
29. Lawrence, H. S., Askari, S., David, J., Franklin, E. C., and Zweiman, B. Transfer of immunological information in humans with dialysates of leucocyte extracts. *Trans. Ass. Amer. Physicians* 76:84, 1963.
30. Landsteiner, K., and Chase, M. W. Studies on the sensitization of animals with simple chemical compounds: VII. Skin sensitization by intraperitoneal injections. *J. Exp. Med.* 71:237, 1940.
31. Landsteiner, K., and Jacobs, J. Studies on the sensitization of animals with simple chemical compounds: II. *J. Exp. Med.* 64:625, 1936.
32. Epstein, S. The antigen-antibody reaction in contact dermatitis. *Ann. Allerg.* 10:633, 1952.
33. Mayer, R. L. Significance of cross-links in the formation of hapten-carrier complex. *Int. Arch. Allerg.* 8:115, 1956.
34. Gell, P. G. H., and Benacerraf, B. Delayed hypersensitivity to simple protein antigens. *Advances Immun.* 1:332, 1961.
35. Landsteiner, K., and Jacobs, J. Studies on sensitization of animals with simple chemical compounds. *J. Exp. Med.* 61:643, 1935.
36. Sulzberger, M. B., and Baer, R. L. Sensitization to simple chemicals: III. Relationship between chemical structure and properties and sensitizing capacities in the production of eczematous sensitivity in man. *J. Invest. Derm.* 1:45, 1938.
37. Eisen, H. N., and Belman, S. Studies of hypersensitivity to low molecular weight substances: Reactions of some allergenic substituted dinitrobenzenes with cysteine or cystine of skin proteins. *J. Exp. Med.* 98:533, 1953.
38. Landsteiner, K., and DiSomma, A. A. Studies on the sensitization of animals with simple chemical compounds: VIII. Sensitization to picric acid; subsidiary agents and mode of sensitization. *J. Exp. Med.* 72:361, 1940.
39. Frey, J. R., and Wenk, P. The influence of Calmette-Guérin bacillus infection on dinitrochlorobenzene contact eczema of guinea pigs. *Dermatologica* 117:154, 1958.
40. Mitchison, N. A. Passive transfer of transplantation immunity. *Proc. Roy. Soc.* [Biol.] 142:72, 1954.
41. Lawrence, H. S. Some Biological and Immunological Properties of Transfer Factor. Ref. 8, p. 243.
42. Baer, R. L. The Mechanism of Cutaneous Reactions to Contact Allergens. *Proc. 12th Int. Congress Dermatology Excerpta Medica Foundation.* 1:44.
43. Epstein, S. Contact dermatitis from neomycin due to dermal delayed (tuberculin-type) sensitivity: Report of 10 cases. *Dermatologica* 113:191, 1956.
44. Epstein, S. Dermal contact dermatitis: Sensitivity to rivanol and gentian violet. *Dermatologica* 117:287, 1958.
45. Marcussen, P. Eczematous allergy to metals. *Acta Allerg.* 17:311, 1962.
46. Sulzberger, M. B. Hypersensitiveness to neoarsphenamine in guinea pigs: Experiments in prevention and desensitization. *Arch. Derm. Syph.* 20:669, 1929.
47. Chase, M. W. Inhibition of experimental drug allergy by prior feeding of the sensitizing agent. *Proc. Soc. Exp. Med. Biol.* 61:257, 1946.
48. Sulzberger, M. B. Arsphenamine hypersensitiveness in guinea pigs: II. Experiments demonstrating the role of the skin, both as originator and as site of the hypersensitiveness. *Arch. Derm. Syph.* 22:839, 1930.
49. Baer, R. L., Rosenthal, S. A., and Hagel, B. The effect of feeding simple chemical allergens to pregnant guinea pigs upon sensitizability of their offspring. *J. Immun.* 80:429, 1958.
50. Harber, L. C., Rosenthal, S. A., and Baer, R. L. Actively acquired tolerance to dinitrochlorobenzene. *J. Immun.* 88:66, 1962.
51. Schier, W. W., Roth, A. A., Ostroff, G., and Schrift, M. H. Hodgkin's disease and immunity. *Amer. J. Med.* 20:94, 1956.
52. Rostenberg, A., Jr. Etiologic and immunologic concepts regarding sarcoidosis. *Arch. Derm.* 64:385, 1951.
53. Leider, M., and Sulzberger, M. B. Studies in allergy of infection: Responses of skin to BCG vaccination in various categories of tuberculin sensitivity. *J. Invest. Derm.* 13:249, 1949.
54. Raffel, S. *Immunity* (2nd ed.). New York: Appleton-Century-Crofts, Inc., 1961. Chap. 14.
55. Baer, R. L., and Witten, V. H. Allergic Eczematous Contact Dermatitis. *1956–57 Year Book of Dermatology and Syphilology.* Chicago: Year Book Publishers, Inc., 1957.

56. White, W. A., Jr., and Baer, R. L. Failure to prevent experimental eczematous sensitization: Observations on the "spontaneous" flare-up phenomenon. *J. Allerg.* 21:344, 1950.
57. Fisher, A. A. Some immunologic phenomena in treatment of and patch testing for ragweed oil dermatitis. *J. Invest. Derm.* 19:271, 1952.
58. Kligman, A. M. Hyposensitization against *Rhus* dermatitis. *Arch. Derm.* 78:47, 1958.
59. Kanof, N., and Baer, R. L. Hyposensitization to poison ivy. *Ann. Allerg.* 22:161, 1964.
60. Morgan, J. K. Observations on persistence of skin sensitivity with reference to nickel eczema. *Brit. J. Derm.* 65:84, 1953.

58. *Clinical Anaphylaxis and Serum Sickness* *

CARL E. ARBESMAN

ANAPHYLACTIC REACTIONS IN MAN

Anaphylaxis in animals is discussed in Chapter 10. Anaphylaxis is induced by a primary sensitizing dose of antigen and, after an incubation period when precipitating antibodies are produced, followed by a secondary or challenging injection of the same antigen.

Anaphylaxis-like reactions in man have been known for many years. The offending substances may be drugs, chemicals, pollens, venom from stinging insects, foreign sera, viral vaccines, and even foods. Usually the antigen must be injected parenterally but there are many reports [1–3] of anaphylactoid reactions after ingestion of chemicals and antibiotics.

Man may develop (1) the guinea pig type of anaphylaxis which involves the bronchial tree and might cause severe dyspnea, asthma, and even death; (2) pulmonary reactions similar to those of rabbit anaphylaxis, with respiratory decompensation and collapse; and (3) the shocklike picture of sharp drop in blood pressure, vasomotor collapse, nausea, and diarrhea, as seen in the dog. Therefore man can respond with untoward reactions that involve one or many shock organs as well as one or several chemical mediators (see Chap. 15).

I prefer the term "anaphylactoid" reactions in man, rather than anaphylactic reactions, because of the absence of demonstrable precipitating antibodies. The serum from man will not passively sensitize animals, nor can he be readily desensitized by sublethal dosages of the offending antigen. There often is no history of a primary or sensitizing dose or exposure to the antigen which presumably induces this systemic reaction. Frequently, as in anaphylaxis-like penicillin reactions, skin-sensitizing antibodies (reagins) are found in the serum. Whether or not one calls the systemic reaction anaphylactic, anaphylactoid, allergic, or constitutional, the clinical syndrome resembles that in the experimental animal.

Anaphylactoid reactions occur most frequently in atopic individuals with skin-sensitizing antibodies in their sera. Examples are the constitutional reactions of the anaphylaxis-type following an overdose of an allergen such as pollen, fungus, or dander extracts, or the inadvertent venous seepage from a small dose of allergen in an individual clinically sensitive to it. It is most difficult to sensitize a nonatopic individual to any of these allergens. However, skin-sensitizing antibodies can be induced experimentally in human subjects by injections of *Ascaris* extract [4], tetanus and diphtheria toxoids [5], oil emulsions of pollens [6], and horse serum. I do not know of any reports of such individuals being deliberately challenged with a large amount of the antigen intravenously.

Another common anaphylactoid reaction is that produced by stinging insects in hypersensitive individuals. Their sera contain reagins (skin-sensitizing antibodies). However, we [7] have recently noted hemagglutinating antibodies in the sera of previously untreated patients who were allergic to insect stings. It is known that the hemagglutination test is 1,000 to 10,000 times as sensitive as the precipitin test. Perhaps, then, the only difference between anaphylaxis in animals and the shocklike picture in man may be quantitative. Another evidence of the presence of precipitating antibody in small amounts is the positive hemagglutination titer against a "purified" ragweed pollen fraction in approximately 80 percent of previously untreated ragweed-sensitive patients [8]. Sera from these patients also have precipitation bands on radio-immunoelectrophoresis [9].

* Supported in part by Grant AI-1303 from the National Institute of Allergy and Infectious Diseases, National Institutes of Health, Bethesda, Md.

They will not, however, passively sensitize a guinea pig. Perhaps here, too, quantitative factors are involved.

Undoubtedly, the systemic reactions produced by penicillin are the most common and disturbing. Unfortunately, intradermal tests for skin-sensitizing antibody are not completely satisfactory. Parker [10] and Levine [11] and their co-workers have described the use of a metabolite of penicillin, penicilloyl, conjugated to a nonantigenic substance, polylysine, for skin testing to detect allergy to penicillin. We and others are unable to verify the high degree of reliability claimed for this test. Similarly, hemagglutination tests for penicillin antibodies [12–14] are not a reliable measure of clinical sensitivity to the drug.

Severe and even fatal anaphylactoid reactions have been reported to injections of milk extract [15], Decholin [16], Furadantin [17], and ACTH [18]. The various types of reactions and the drugs and chemicals involved have been excellently classified by Alexander [19].

TREATMENT

Obviously, avoidance of known offenders is the best prophylactic treatment. As mentioned previously, results of skin tests for drug sensitivity are not of great significance. At times, despite a history of a previous reaction to a drug such as penicillin, its use may be required as a life-saving measure, as in subacute bacterial endocarditis. In such an instance, it may be possible to desensitize a patient by starting with small amounts and gradually increasing increments of the agent until therapeutic amounts can be tolerated [12]. This procedure is not without its hazards, however, and remedies and equipment for emergency use, such as epinephrine, antihistaminics, oxygen, and a tracheotomy set, should be kept at the bedside.

Treatment of an anaphylactoid reaction in man is the same as that of severe asthma. However, corticosteroids cannot be relied on to control the immediate life-threatening symptoms.

SERUM SICKNESS

Almost sixty years ago, von Pirquet and Schick [20] published a classic description of reactions that follow injections of horse serum in man. Since then, many investigators have reported on the incidence, types of reactions, immunological findings, and complications associated with the disease. Although the clinical use of commercially prepared immune horse serum has greatly diminished since the introduction of antibiotics, chemotherapeutic agents, and toxoids, a great amount of foreign sera, primarily in the form of tetanus antitoxin, is administered each year. Toogood [21] reported that about 146,000 doses of tetanus antitoxin were given in Canada during 1957. Smaller amounts of botulinus antiserum, gas gangrene antiserum, rabies antiserum, and snake venom antiserum are used clinically. It is therefore important that we have an understanding of serum sickness.

As already stated, true anaphylaxis (immunological definition) in man comparable to that in animals is rarely seen. Probably the closest analogy to anaphylaxis in man, from an immunological point of view, is serum sickness.

TYPES OF REACTIONS

There are three types of clinical reactions that can follow an injection of foreign serum.

Primary Serum Sickness. This occurs 7 to 12 days after an injection of serum. It is characterized by fever, arthralgias, urticaria, and maculopapular eruptions. Usually the site of the injection or the initial skin test site, or both, become erythematous and edematous 1 to 3 days before onset of systemic manifestations. The symptoms may be mild and transitory, lasting only 2 to 4 days, or may be very severe and continue for several weeks, during which a variety of complications can develop. The most frequent are brachial plexus neuritis, carditis, optic neuritis, nephritis, Guillain-Barré syndrome [22, 23], and periarteritis nodosa. Laboratory studies may disclose albumin and hyaline casts in the urine, eosinophilia, and several types of antibodies, which are discussed later. Barnett *et al.* [24] recently reported plasmacytosis in a case of serum sickness.

The occurrence of primary serum sickness depends on the amount of serum administered, its purity, and the route of administration. If 100 ml. of "native" horse serum were given, over 90 percent of the recipients would have serum disease, whereas if 10 ml. or less were injected, approximately 10 percent would be so afflicted [25]. When foreign serum is injected intravenously or intrathecally, the incidence increases. In recent years, tetanus antitoxin has been "purified" and concentrated by enzymatic and chemical treatment, so that this so-called despeciated horse serum globulin can contain 1,500 units of tetanus antitoxin in 0.5 ml. of serum. Despite this small amount given for prophylaxis against tetanus infections, the incidence of primary serum sickness is still between 1.6 [26] and 20 percent [27, 28] following administration of 1,500 units (0.5 ml.) of tetanus antitoxin to subjects with negative skin reactions to horse serum.

Accelerated Serum Sickness. This occurs in individuals who had previously received an injection of horse serum. The symptoms are essentially those described for primary serum sickness but occur 1 to 3 days after the injection instead of after the classic 7 to 12 day period. Occasionally the patient may have dyspnea and wheezing. This type of reaction is rarely fatal. As in animal anaphylaxis, there usually was a previous sensitizing dose, then a second or challenging injection. The laboratory findings are approximately the same as in primary serum sickness, but a positive skin reaction develops earlier (with onset of symptoms).

Atopic Type Serum Reaction. This usually occurs in individuals who have had or have some allergic disorder and are known to be sensitive to animal danders or sera. They give a positive skin reaction to horse serum before its injection. Were such a patient given horse serum, within minutes he might have severe wheezing, dyspnea, generalized urticaria and erythema, and vasomotor collapse, and even death might occur.

IMMUNOLOGICAL MECHANISMS

It was demonstrated many years ago that individuals who develop serum sickness after an injection of horse serum produce heterophil, skin-sensitizing, precipitin [29, 30], and anaphylactic antibodies.

Heterophil Antibodies. Years ago, when large amounts of native horse serum were given therapeutically, these antibodies were frequently seen in relatively high titers. This was due to the fact that the foreign serum contained a relatively large amount of heterophil (Forssman) antigen. (These antibodies can be differentiated from the "heterophil antibodies" found in the serum of patients with infectious mononucleosis because the former, but not the latter, are absorbed out with guinea pig tissue.) With the more purified, concentrated tetanus antitoxin in present use, one rarely encounters an increase in heterophil titer in serum sickness [31].

Skin-sensitizing Antibodies. These appear in the serum with the onset of symptoms and are present a relatively short time, although a positive reaction to an intradermal test may persist for many years.

Precipitins. Precipitins have been detected in the serum of individuals who have received relatively large amounts of horse serum. Nevertheless, even with this type of therapy, several investigators were unable to demonstrate precipitins consistently in serum of patients with serum sickness. These precipitins, when demonstrable, are evident only *after the onset* of symptoms but remain detectable for years. Many workers in this area of study have mentioned the inadequacy of the precipitin test [32, 33].

Anaphylactic Antibodies. These may be demonstrated soon after symptoms of serum sickness appear. As little as 1 ml. of the patient's serum injected parenterally into a normal guinea pig can passively sensitize the animal. Challenge with horse serum twenty-four hours later causes typical fatal anaphylaxis. These antibodies may or may not be related to the precipitin titer of the serum, but they tend to disappear much quicker than do the precipitins [31].

Serum from patients with serum sickness can also passively sensitize the skin of normal guinea pigs, demonstrable by positive passive cutaneous anaphylaxis (PCA).

Hemagglutinating Antibodies. These antibodies were studied by tanned cell hemagglutination technique [28, 31, 34, 35]. It was found that all patients whose titer of hemagglutinating antibody was greater than 200 (despite a negative reaction to an intradermal test) before an injection of 0.5 ml. of tetanus antitoxin (horse serum) would develop primary serum sickness 7 to 10 days after the inoculation (Fig. 58-1). Patients whose titer was below 200 did not manifest this condition. Furthermore, all patients who did develop serum sickness had hemagglutinins in their serum *after* the onset of the disease in titers greater than 10,000 and often as high as 5,000,000. Elevated titers were demonstrated in sera of patients who had had serum sickness as long as 16 years previously. A small

TABLE 58-1. Hemagglutination of Serum from Patients with Serum Sickness and Various Mammalian Sera as Antigens

Serum	Titer
Mouse	800
Guinea pig	800
Cat	500
Rabbit	1,600
Hog	2,000
Lamb	200
Rat	0
Horse	512,000

percentage who had initial pretreatment titers below 200 had a relatively small increase in hemagglutination titers (less than 10,000) after the injection of serum but did not develop serum sickness. Yet in most individuals, antibodies were not demonstrable by this technique even after antitoxin administration.

In these studies, it was demonstrated that patients in whom serum sickness developed also had hemagglutinating antibodies to many other mammalian sera (Table 58-1). This verified an earlier observation of a common antigenicity among all mammalian sera [36].

It has been recommended that antitetanus bovine serum be used for patients who need protection against tetanus and are sensitive to horse serum [37]. This procedure, however, must be approached with caution because of the known cross-antigenicity of mammalian sera. For example, a patient clinically sensitive to horse serum was, after proper intradermal testing, given antitetanus bovine serum [38]. The immunological findings (hemagglutination and skin-sensitizing antibody titers against both horse serum and bovine serum) are illustrated in Figure 58-2. Particularly notable are the anamnestic response with the horse serum titer and the presence of the skin-sensitizing antibody before production of hemagglutinating antibodies against bovine and horse serum.

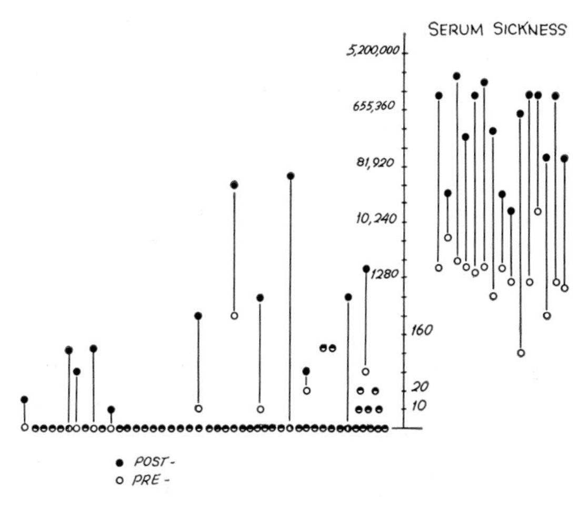

Fig. 58-1. Hemagglutination titers of patients' sera before and after administration of TAT. O sera before injection; ● sera 8 to 14 days after injection. Patients with serum sickness had higher titers before the initial injection as well as after the appearance of symptoms.

SIGNIFICANCE OF HEMAGGLUTINATING ANTIBODIES

As mentioned earlier, patients who have a pretreatment horse serum titer greater than 200 develop serum sickness within 7 to 10 days. If this information were available to the physician, perhaps certain prophylactic procedures would be employed to prevent the reaction. Germuth [39] and Dixon *et al.* [40] have shown that the pathological lesions produced in rabbits by large injections of foreign serum can be prevented by administration of corticosteroids before the injection of antigen.

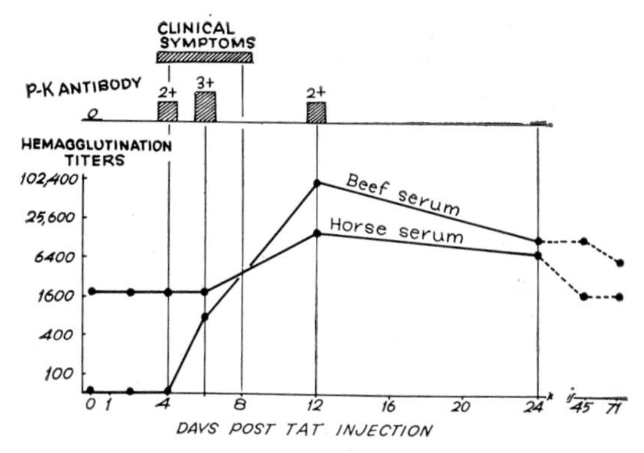

Fig. 58-2. Time relationship of clinical symptoms, hemagglutination titers, and presence of skin-sensitizing antibody in a horse serum sensitive patient who was given bovine antitetanus serum.

It seems logical to believe, therefore, that adequate doses of a corticosteroid given to individuals who have an initial hemagglutination titer over 200 may prevent serum sickness. Another important consideration is that the physician, with knowledge of the pretreatment hemagglutination titer, can at least warn the patient of the possible development of symptoms of serum sickness in 7 to 10 days.

Frequently, a patient who has been in an accident receives both tetanus antitoxin and penicillin. Either substance can produce identical symptoms of serum sickness. If, in such circumstances, the hemagglutination test of the patient's serum were utilized, and a titer greater than 10,000 against horse serum were demonstrated, one could assume that the patient's reaction was caused by horse serum. If the titer against horse serum were below 10,000, the reaction more probably was due to the penicillin.

The fact that the hemagglutination titer of the patient's serum rises *after* the onset of symptoms lends support to Dixon's findings in experimental serum sickness in animals (see Chap. 12). It is believed that soluble antigen-antibody complexes (in antigen excess) in the circulation cause mast cell degranulation with liberation of pharmacologically active substances such as histamine, which in turn can cause the various symptoms of serum sickness. Whether this theory is applicable to man is not proved.

Another important characteristic of human serum sickness is the development of a skin-sensitizing antibody when the symptoms appear. It is thermolabile and probably is not a γ_2-globulin (IgG). It is transitory, tending to disappear soon after the convalescent period, whereas the hemagglutinating antibody may persist for years. The relative duration of these two antibodies is illustrated in Figure 58-3. The possibility exists that the skin-sensitizing antibody that develops can, in turn, fix to certain tissues and that the small amount of circulating antigen (horse serum) still present could react with this type of antibody and cause serum sickness.

In our studies [28] there was no correlation between the titers of skin-sensitizing and hemagglutinating antibodies produced in serum sickness and the severity of the disease. However, it appears that patients with complications of serum sickness (such as Guillain-Barré syndrome) have extremely high hemagglutination titers over a long period. Whether these are the cause or result of the clinical syndrome remains to be elucidated.

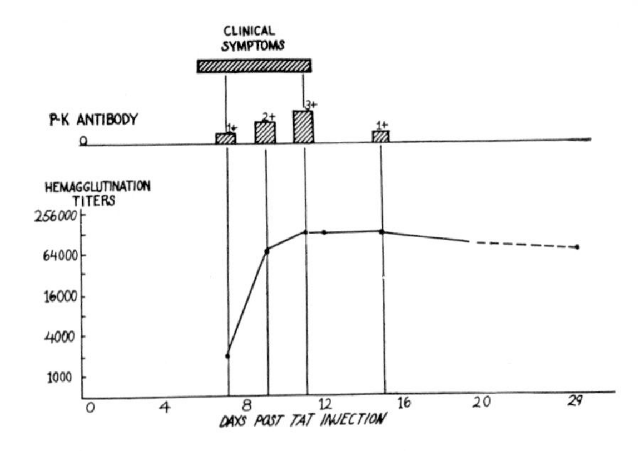

Fig. 58-3. Relationship of appearance of clinical symptoms of serum sickness, skin-sensitizing antibody and tanned cell hemagglutination titer.

Skin-sensitizing antibody may play a significant role in the pathogenesis of primary serum sickness, since the incidence of this disease is greatest in patients who had a positive skin reaction before horse serum administration [41].

Although the technique of tanned cell hemagglutination is of value for the prediction and diagnosis of serum sickness, it has certain limitations in that it requires a good serology laboratory and the result of the test is not known for several hours. Attempts to develop a more rapid, simple, and equally sensitive technique for determination of these antibodies have not been successful. Bentonite particles and formalinized cells, as well as slide techniques of agglutination, have been used, but although positive results are obtained, these procedures are not delicate enough to define titers less than 2,000 and so, for the purpose of predicting serum sickness, are of little value.

CHARACTERISTICS OF ANTIBODY AND ANTIGEN

By means of immunoelectrophoresis and studies of inhibition of hemagglutination it was demonstrated that either the α- or the γ-globulin fraction of horse serum, or both, are the antigenic constituents. Diagrams of representative human sera reacting with horse serum on immunoelectrophoresis are shown in Figure 58-4. To demonstrate the various precipitating bands by gel diffusion experiments, the hemagglutination titer of the pa-

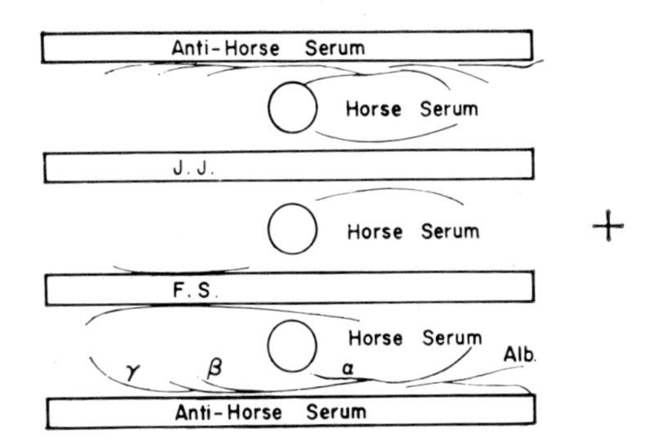

Fig. 58-4. Location of precipitating antigen in horse serum determined by immunoelectrophoresis. Serum from each of two patients was obtained in the recovery stage of primary serum sickness. Anti-horse serum rabbit serum was used as control.

tient's serum must be greater than 100,000 (Table 58-2). There was no correlation between the hemagglutination titer or clinical symptoms and the antigenic fraction of the horse serum demonstrated on immunoelectrophoresis. Of 17 sera so studied, 7 reacted only against the γ-globulin fraction of the horse serum, 3 against the α-globulin only, and 4 against both. When the PCA technique was used, a hemagglutination titer of 80,000 or greater was necessary to induce positive reactions, and there was a good correlation between the size of the PCA skin reaction and the hemagglutination titer.

The antibody of the patient's serum involved in these reactions is located (as would be expected) in the γ-globulin fraction (Fig. 58-5).

Several reports [42, 43] indicate that patients who receive tetanus antitoxin (TAT) and develop serum sickness are not adequately protected against tetanus due to rapid disappearance of the antitoxin from the circulation. We have not been able to demonstrate antibodies against the antitoxin portion of horse serum with regularity. This was attempted by the following experiment. Tetanus antitoxin was subjected to electrophoresis.

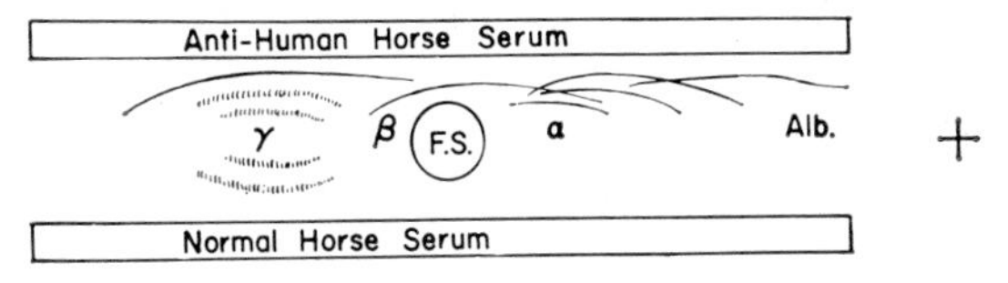

Fig. 58-5. Immunoelectrophoretic studies. After electrophoresis of patient's serum, normal horse serum was placed in one of the adjacent troughs, anti-human serum horse serum in the other. An arc of precipitate formed between horse serum and γ-globulin of human antiserum.

Serum from a patient known to react to the γ-globulin fraction of this antigen was added in one longitudinal trough and tetanus toxoid was placed in the other trough and in the terminal well (Fig. 58-6). The lines of pre-

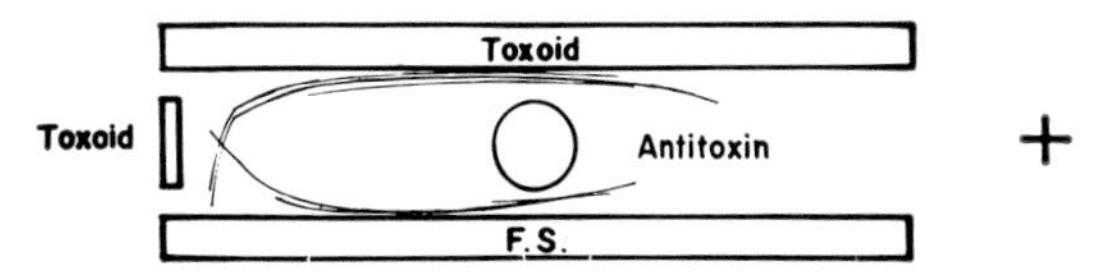

Fig. 58-6. Relationship of toxoid-TAT reaction and a serum sickness antiserum-TAT reaction. Crossed lines of precipitation indicate a reaction of nonidentity.

cipitate crossed, indicating a reaction of nonidentity. Thus, in this instance, the patient's serum seemed to have precipitated a horse serum component other than the flocculating antigen (antitoxin). However, in Ouchterlony studies with the sera from five patients recovering from serum sickness, it was noted that one serum appeared to have an antibody against TAT but the other sera did not [34].

IMMUNOLOGICAL MECHANISMS OF ACCELERATED SERUM SICKNESS

Inasmuch as accelerated serum sickness occurs in patients who have had a previous injection of horse serum, they may still contain minute amounts of precipitating (or hemagglutinating) antibody prior to the sec-

TABLE 58-2. Comparison of Hemagglutination Titer with Antigenic Fractions of Serum

No. of Patients	Hemagglutination Titer Range	Immunoelectrophoresis
7	130,000–1,300,000	Gamma
3	100,000–2,000,000	Alpha
4	130,000–1,300,000	Alpha and Gamma
3	32,000–100,000	No Ppt.

ond injection of horse serum. Because of the anamnestic response, these antibodies increase more rapidly than in primary serum sickness. This may explain why soluble antigen-antibody complexes appear in the circulation within 1 to 5 days rather than 7 to 10 days.

IMMUNOLOGICAL MECHANISMS OF ATOPIC REACTION

A positive skin reaction of the immediate type to horse serum prior to an injection of this substance usually indicates skin-sensitizing antibodies in the serum of such a patient.

We [44] made immunological studies of a patient who had an almost fatal reaction to a skin test to horse serum. Within five minutes after the test, he went into shock, with vasomotor collapse, marked erythema, and dyspnea. Serum samples were obtained daily during the course of the disease, and the skin-sensitizing and hemagglutinating antibody titers were determined. There was a pronounced increase in both titers as the disease progressed, and both titers continued to rise after the symptoms subsided. However, the skin-sensitizing antibody titer diminished much more rapidly than did the hemagglutination titer (Fig. 58-7). Therefore this type of reaction is different from both the primary

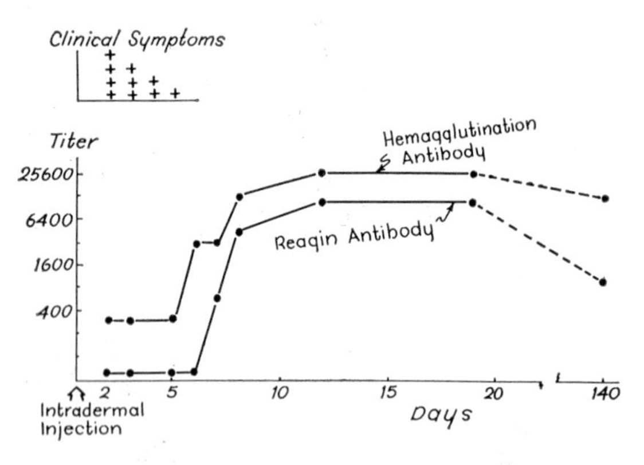

Fig. 58-7. Clinical course and immunological response following intradermal administration of test dose of TAT. Clinical symptoms had subsided by the sixth day. Antibody titers are expressed as the reciprocal of the highest serum dilution which gave a positive reaction.

serum sickness reaction described earlier and anaphylaxis in animals, as there was no sensitizing dose and no precipitating antibodies were present. Buff [45] reported a similar, but fatal, case without serological studies.

MANAGEMENT OF SERUM REACTIONS

Prophylaxis. Inasmuch as the chief therapeutic use of horse serum today is for protection against tetanus by means of antitoxin, serum reactions could readily be eliminated by routine prior active immunization with tetanus toxoid. Protection with tetanus toxoid should be as much a part of the immunization program for the general population as the prophylactic program against smallpox, diphtheria, pertussis, and poliomyelitis. It has been reported that a booster dose of toxoid as long as 15 years following the initial immunization will protect a patient adequately against tetanus [46, 47].

A careful history should be obtained prior to any injection of or test with horse serum. Skin tests should be performed before injection of serum. A positive response indicates the presence of skin-sensitizing antibodies and the possibility of an immediate, perhaps even fatal, reaction. Human tetanus antitoxin should be used [48, 49] for individuals who have never had active immunization with tetanus toxoid and give a positive reaction to horse serum on a skin test. This will eliminate the possibility of an acute reaction, yet protect the patient adequately.

If hemagglutination titers could be estimated in the sera of patients prior to an injection of horse serum, they could predict the possible development of primary serum sickness. Administration of corticosteroids during the incubation period conceivably could prevent this reaction.

Symptomatic Treatment. Most patients with primary serum sickness are adequately managed by the use of epinephrine, antihistamines, and acetylsalicylic acid and local application of antipruritic lotions. However, if arthralgias, fever, or other complications develop, it may be necessary to give corticosteroids. The amount and frequency will depend on the severity of the disease.

REFERENCES

1. Schoenfeld, M. R. Acute allergic reactions to morphine, codeine, meperidine hydrochloride, and opium alkaloids. *New York J. Med.* 60: 2591, 1960.
2. Lowell, F. C., and Krapin, D. Anaphylaxis to penicillin. *New Eng. J. Med.* 268:218, 1963.
3. Kern, R. A. Anaphylactic drug reactions: Their diagnosis, prevention and treatment. *J.A.M.A.* 179:19, 1962.
4. Brunner, M. Active sensitization in human beings. *J. Allerg.* 5:257, 1934.
5. Kuhns, W. J., Lawrence, H. S., and Pappenheimer, A. M., Jr. Immunochemical properties of antitoxin in normal and allergic individuals hyperimmunized with diphtheria toxoid. *Fed. Proc.* 10:413, 1951.
6. Becker, R. J., Sparks, D. B., Feinberg, S. M., Patterson, R., Pruzansky, J. J. and Feinberg, A. R. Delayed and immediate skin reactivity in man after the injection of antigen in emulsion. *J. Allerg.* 32:229, 1961.
7. Langlois, C., Arbesman, C. E., and Shulman, S. Stinging insects: Immunologic studies. *Fed. Proc.* 22:560, 1963.
8. Arbesman, C. E., Reisman, R. E., Bonstein, H. S., and Rose, N. R. Allergic and immunologic studies of a "purified" fraction of ragweed pollen. *J. Immun.* 90:612, 1963.
9. Yagi, Y., Maier, P., Pressman, D., Arbesman, C. E., Reisman, R. E. The presence of the ragweed-binding antibodies in the β_{2A}-, β_{2M}- and γ-globulins of sensitive individuals. *J. Immun.* 91:83, 1963.
10. Parker, C. W., Shapiro, J., Kern, M., and Eisen, H. N. Hypersensitivity to penicillenic acid derivatives in human beings with penicillin allergy. *J. Exp. Med.* 115:21, 1962.
11. Levine, B. B., and Ovary, Z. Studies on the mechanism of formation of the penicillin antigen: III. The N-(D-α-benzylpenicilloyl) group as an antigenic determinant responsible for hypersensitivity to penicillin G. *J. Exp. Med.* 114:875, 1961.
12. Reisman, R. E., Rose, N. R., Witebsky, E., and Arbesman, C. E. Penicillin allergy and desensitization. *J. Allerg.* 33:178, 1962.
13. Harris, J., and Vaughan, J. H. Immunologic reactions to penicillin. *J. Allerg.* 32:119, 1961.
14. VanArsdel, P. P., Jr., O'Rourke, T., Horan, D., and Kumasaka, Y. Serum hemagglutinating antibody in penicillin allergy. *J.A.M.A.* 185: 118, 1963.
15. Sachs, O. Anaphylaktischer Anfall nach Milchinjektion. *Deutsch. Med. Wschr.* 44:547, 1918.
16. Elliot, J. P., Jr., Vidrine, R., and Goldman, A. M. An anaphylactic reaction to sodium dehydrocholate. *Ann. Intern. Med.* 56:1228, 1960.
17. Khorsandian, R., Bremer, E. M., and Nodine, J. H. Anaphylactic reaction caused by treatment with nitrofurantoin. *J.A.M.A.* 184:500, 1963.
18. Zucker, A., and Bendo, D. Anaphylactic reaction to ACTH. *New York J. Med.* 61:623, 1961.
19. Alexander, H. L. *Reactions with Drug Therapy*. Philadelphia: W. B. Saunders Company, 1955.
20. Von Pirquet, C. F., and Schick, B. *Die Serumkrankheit*. Leipzig: Wier, 1905. (Translation by Schick, B. *Serum Sickness*. Baltimore: Williams & Wilkins Company, 1951.)
21. Toogood, J. H. Allergic reactions to antitetanus serum. *Canad. Med. Ass. J.* 82:907, 1960.
22. Arbesman, C. E., Hyman, I., Dauzier, G., and Kantor, S. Z. Immunologic studies of a Guillain-Barré syndrome following tetanus antitoxin. *New York J. Med.* 58:2647, 1958.
23. Miglets, A. W., Bartlett, W. G., Arbesman, C. E., and Loeser, W. D. Guillain-Barré syndrome resulting from tetanus antitoxin injection. *Neurology* 10:658, 1960.
24. Barnett, E. V., Stone, G., Swisher, S. N., and Vaughan, J. H. Serum sickness and plasmacytosis. *Amer. J. Med.* 35:113, 1963.
25. Mackenzie, G. M., and Hanger, F. M. Serum disease and serum accidents. *J.A.M.A.* 94:260, 1930.
26. Sansöe-Jensen, T., and Zachau-Christiansen, B. *Ugesk. Laeg.* Sept. 11, 1958 (cited in *J.A.M.A.* 168:1923, 1958).
27. Moynihan, N. H. Serum sickness and local reactions in tetanus prophylaxis: A study of 400 cases. *Lancet* 2:264, 1955.
28. Arbesman, C. E., Kantor, S. Z., Rose, N. R., and Witebsky, E. Serum sickness: Serologic studies following prophylactic tetanus antitoxin. *J. Allerg.* 31:257, 1960.
29. Hamburger, F., and Moro, E. Ueber die biologisch nachweisbaren Veränderungen des menschlichen Blutes nach Seruminjektion. *Wien. Klin. Wschr.* 16:445, 1903.
30. Wells, C. W. On the specific precipitin in the blood of persons injected with anti-diphtheria horse serum. *J. Infect. Dis.* 16:63, 1915.
31. Reisman, R. E., Rose, N. R., Witebsky, E., and Arbesman, C. E. Serum sickness: II. Demonstration and characteristics of antibodies. *J. Allerg.* 32:531, 1961.
32. Cannon, P. R., and Marshall, C. E. Studies on

the mechanism of the Arthus phenomenon. *J. Immun.* 40:127, 1941.

33. Tuft, L., and Ramsdell, S. G. Antibody studies in serum sickness. *J. Immun.* 17:539, 1929.
34. Rose, N. R., Reisman, R. E., Witebsky, E., and Arbesman, C. E. Serum sickness: III. Characterization of antigens. *J. Allerg.* 33:250, 1962.
35. Arbesman, C. E., Rose, N. R., and Reisman, R. E. Immunologic Studies of Serum Sickness. In Brown, E. A. (Ed.), *Proceedings of 4th International Congress.* New York: Pergamon Press, 1962.
36. Beede, R. B., Rose, N. R., and Arbesman, C. E. Sensitivity to animals: A case report with immunologic studies. *J. Allerg.* 29:139, 1958.
37. Glaser, J. Use of bovine antitoxin for prophylaxis of tetanus. *J. Pediat.* 19:403, 1941.
38. Reisman, R. E., Rose, N. R., and Arbesman, C. E. Immunologic studies of serum sickness from bovine antitetanus toxin. *J.A.M.A.* 176: 104, 1961.
39. Germuth, F. G., Jr. A comparative histologic and immunologic study in rabbits of induced hypersensitivity of the serum sickness type. *J. Exp. Med.* 97:257, 1953.
40. Dixon, F. J., Vazquez, J. J., Weigle, W. O., and Cochrane, C. G. Immunology and Pathogenesis of Experimental Serum Sickness. In Lawrence, H. S. (Ed.), *Cellular and Humoral Aspects of the Hypersensitive States.* New York: Paul B. Hoeber, Inc., 1959. P. 354.
41. Kojis, F. G. Serum sickness and anaphylaxis. *Amer. J. Dis. Child.* 64:93, 313, 1942.
42. Mahoney, L. J., and Moloney, P. J. On the prophylaxis of tetanus. *Canad. J. Surg.* 1:127, 1958.
43. Godfrey, M. P., Parsons, V., and Rawstron, J. R. Rapid destruction of antitetanus serum in a patient previously sensitized to horse serum. *Lancet* 2:1229, 1960.
44. Reisman, R. E., Arbesman, C. E., and Rose, N. R. Anaphylactoid reaction following an intradermal test of tetanus antitoxin. *Ann. Intern. Med.* 59:883, 1963.
45. Buff, H. B. Fatal anaphylactic shock following intradermal skin test with dilute horse serum antitoxin. *J.A.M.A.* 174:122, 1960.
46. Goldsmith, S., Rosenberg, E., and Pollaczek, E. H. A study of the antibody response to a booster of tetanus toxoid. *New Eng. J. Med.* 267:485, 1962.
47. Kaiser, G. C., King, R. D., Lempke, R. E., and Roster, M. H. Delayed recall of active tetanus immunization. *J.A.M.A.* 178:914, 1961.
48. McComb, J. A., and Dwyer, R. C. Passive immunization with tetanus immune globulin (human). *New Eng. J. Med.* 268:857, 1963.
49. Rubbo, S. D. Human globulin for tetanus immunization. *Brit. Med. J.* 5297(Vol. 2):79, 1962.

59. Drug Reactions*

CHARLES W. PARKER

EXPERIMENTAL ASPECTS

Studies with Simple Chemical Determinants

The use of simple chemical structures or haptens as antigenic determinants in the experimental animal has provided a powerful method of investigation of the structural basis of immunological specificity. Although the antigenic determinants examined most extensively are not used therapeutically in man, the information obtained appears to be relevant to the study of human drug allergy. Certain features of this work which are pertinent to the present discussion will be reviewed briefly. Chapter 9 gives a detailed description of immunological reactions involving simple chemical determinants.

The discussion of hypersensitivity reactions involving simple chemical determinants is divided into two parts. The first portion is concerned primarily with how a simple chemical induces antibody formation. In the second, the mechanism of elicitation of manifestations of allergy in an animal which has already formed antibody is considered.

INDUCTION OF THE PRIMARY IMMUNOLOGICAL RESPONSE

Antibody formation to a simple chemical or hapten may be induced by injection of the hapten in combination with a protein or, less reliably, by administration of the uncombined simple chemical. Hapten-protein conjugates are prepared *in vitro* by reacting a purified protein with a simple chemical capable of combining covalently† with functional amino acid residues of the protein.

Although proteins substituted with simple chemicals have been very useful as immunizing antigens, drug allergy in man begins with administration of the simple chemical itself. Simple chemicals vary greatly in their ability to induce hypersensitivity. Some rarely, if ever, produce allergy; others can cause an immunological response in virtually every test subject. Because hapten-protein conjugates are such effective antigens, it was long suspected that conjugation of simple chemicals to proteins *in vivo* might account for their antigenicity. The strong evidence to support this has been provided by the studies of Landsteiner and Jacobs, Eisen, Gell, and others [1–3]. A brief summary follows. (1) The most consistent property among diverse simple chemicals which are potent sensitizers is a high order of protein reactivity.‡ Simple chemicals which are unable to react with protein *in vitro* to form a covalent bond have a low incidence of sensitization. Although the ability of a simple chemical to combine covalently with protein can be correlated with its immunogenicity, the

---

* Supported by grants from the National Institute of Allergy and Infectious Diseases, U.S. Public Health Service.

† In this discussion, an important distinction is made between covalent binding of simple chemicals to proteins and reversible binding. In the formation of a covalent bond, a portion of the simple chemical molecule must be activated. Examples of the many simple chemicals with the required reactivity are acid chlorides, anhydrides, diazonium salts, and certain halonitrobenzenes. The reaction takes place with functional amino acid residues of the protein. In conjugating with a functional group of a protein, a reactive simple chemical undergoes structural modification, which may be extensive or, more often, is limited to a deletion of a small portion of its molecule. The bond that is formed is nonionic and is stable because electrons are shared between the simple chemical and the amino acid residue to which it is attached. In many instances, the stability of the attachment to protein exceeds that of a peptide bond. In contrast, in the reversible combination of a simple chemical with a protein, the simple chemical need not be activated; it does not undergo structural modification; the number of groups which can be combined is not correlated with the number of functional amino acids present on the protein; and the chemical can be separated from the protein by various means, including prolonged dialysis.

‡ The assumption that a simple chemical which

extent to which a simple chemical is bound reversibly by serum proteins has no apparent influence on the ability to immunize [2]. (2) A comparison may also be made among members of a single family of simple chemicals which differ in protein reactivity but form identical substituents on protein; there is a distinct correlation between rate of conjugation with protein, as measured *in vitro,* and frequency of induction of contact and anaphylactic sensitization by the simple chemical [2]. Moreover, the maximal incidence of sensitization is obtained with a hapten-protein conjugate prepared *in vitro.* (3) In a few instances, antibodies formed after administration of a simple chemical have been characterized in regard to whether specificity is for the simple chemical itself, for derivatives of the chemical not covalently bound by protein, or for derivatives which would become linked covalently with the protein of the host animal, and it has been found that antibody specificity is for the covalently bound derivatives [2, 4–6]. (4) In special circumstances it has been possible to show that protein of the host animal contributes to the specificity of a hypersensitivity response involving a haptenic determinant (e.g., in contact skin sensitivity; see later, under Elicitation of Contact Skin Hypersensitivity [7]).

Based on evidence of the type just described, the statement that the reaction of a simple chemical with protein is obligatory for the induction of an immunological response seems very reasonable. Admittedly, there are apparent exceptions in which simple chemicals that do not possess protein reactivity *in vitro* induce antibody formation. However, these may be plausibly ascribed to contaminants or to metabolic degradation of administered material to reactive intermediates.

ELICITATION OF HYPERSENSITIVITY

The ability of simple chemicals to induce antibody formation does not necessarily correlate with their efficacy in elicitation of manifestations of hypersensitivity. Moreover, the factors required for elicitation of immediate type reactions appear to differ significantly from those involved in the delayed response.

Elicitation of immediate type hypersensitivity

Elicitation by Multivalent Antigens. Hapten-specific immediate type hypersensitivity responses are elicited in immune animals on challenge with the appropriate hapten in stable combination with protein (or some other carrier) and, in occasional instances, by the simple chemical itself. The basis of the unreliability of unconjugated simple chemicals as elicitors of immediate type hypersensitivity has become evident from study of the influence of antigen and antibody valence on the production of manifestations of hypersensitivity. It has been found that the requirements for elicitation of immediate type reactions are similar to those for the *in vitro* precipitin reactions between antigen and antibody. The precipitating or challenging antigen must contain two or more haptenic groups per molecule (e.g., it must be multivalent) [8–10]. Uncombined or univalent hapten in a form which is not protein-reactive specifically inhibits the hypersensitivity reaction, just as it blocks precipitation in the test tube.

Inhibition by Univalent Hapten. Inhibition of a hypersensitivity reaction by univalent hapten affords direct evidence that the reaction is mediated by that group or one closely related in structure. If wheal and erythema are used for tests, antigen and hapten may be injected locally as a mixture. For complete inhibition, a large excess of univalent hapten (a 50- to as much as 1,000-fold molar excess over haptenic groups present on the multivalent antigen) must be used [4, 10]. The relatively high concentration of univalent hapten needed for inhibition may relate to the rapid diffusion of hapten away from the site of local injection and nonspecific binding of hapten to proteins other than antibody.

Elicitation by a Simple Chemical. An unconjugated or univalent simple chemical in nearly all instances specifically inhibits immediate type hypersensitivity responses. In two special circumstances it elicits an allergic response. The more important of these is when the simple chemical possesses a relatively high degree of protein reactivity. Here it may be assumed that the reactive chemical couples covalently with body protein at the

---

reacts to form a covalent bond with protein *in vitro* under mild conditions would also do so *in vivo* has been documented on a number of occasions (e.g., Ref. 2). The possibility that a reaction of relatively little consequence *in vitro* would be favored *in vivo* because of selective reactivity on the part of certain tissue proteins, as influenced by their local environment, is largely unexplored.

site of injection to create a multivalent hapten-protein conjugate [4].* A relatively high degree of protein reactivity is required to produce an immediate response, since significant amounts of the conjugate must be formed within a relatively short time. Moreover, even when this requirement is met, ordinarily the unconjugated chemical will still be present in large excess; it will inhibit the local reaction to a variable extent, depending on its structural similarity to the protein-bound derivative responsible for immunization.† It is not surprising, therefore, that a hapten with a relatively high order of protein reactivity, although capable of eliciting an immediate type allergic response, often fails to do so.

In addition to the condition in which hapten combines chemically with protein *in vivo,* there is a second circumstance in which a simple chemical produces allergic symptoms: it was recently reported that stable univalent dinitrophenyl derivatives of a special type could elicit passive cutaneous anaphylaxis (PCA), although most univalent dinitrophenyl derivatives inhibit the reaction [11]. The univalent elicitors differed from univalent inhibitors in that they contained an unrelated, large organic substituent, well separated from the dinitrophenyl group. As a possible explanation of this phenomenon, it seems reasonable to assume that the ability of the unrelated group to adsorb nonspecifically to protein is involved. Following the intravenous injection of the hapten and its localization in the cutaneous site by the specific interaction of the dinitrophenyl group with antibody, the unrelated substituent could then interact nonspecifically with antibody or other proteins present locally. In this manner, an aggregate composed in part of specific and in part of nonspecific bonds could be produced.

Desirable Properties of Conjugates. It is evident that in the study of hapten-specific allergic responses of the immediate type, multivalent conjugates prepared and characterized *in vitro* should be used. Certain factors must be considered in the choice of a conjugate.

1. Degree of substitution. Although a multivalent antigen is prerequisite for the provocation of an allergic reaction, it should not be inferred that all multivalent derivatives have the same potency as elicitors. A relatively small bivalent derivative with the two haptenic groups in close juxtaposition elicits poorly in some instances, especially when antibody of relatively low affinity is involved [9, 12–13]. This effect in part can be related to steric interference to the attachment of two antibody molecules simultaneously to the same bifunctional hapten.‡ When steric interference between haptenic groups is not a factor, however, an increase in the valence of the eliciting antigen in some instances increases its effectiveness as an elicitor [14, 15]. Presumably this relates to the requirement that a given antigen molecule must be combined with at least two antibody molecules in order to provoke manifestations of hypersensitivity; an increase in the number of haptenic groups per antigen molecule increases the likelihood that at least two of these will be combined with antibody.

2. The macromolecular carrier. Traditionally, a purified protein has been used as the macromolecular carrier for haptenic groups in the *in vitro* synthesis of an antigen for eliciting allergic responses. When antibodies have been formed to a hapten-protein conjugate, an immunologically unrelated protein is used for synthesis of the eliciting antigen. Hapten-protein conjugates are effective elicitors if adequately substituted, and usually they do not give rise to nonspecific reactions. There are two disadvantages to their use in human subjects, however. First, and more important, they are quite capable of inducing antibody formation both to the haptenic substituent and to the protein carrier. Therefore, with relatively large-scale testing, they would be expected to induce drug allergy in a significant number of normal subjects. Second, in view of the many different types of functional

* The simple chemical could induce an allergic response without coupling to protein if it were capable of polymerizing with itself to form multivalent antigen.

† The protein-bound derivative may differ substantially in structure from its precursor and, as a consequence, will induce an antibody which interacts weakly with the precursor. This situation obtains in penicillin allergy and may account in part for the fact that the injection of penicillin itself at times elicits an allergic response.

‡ The possibility cannot be excluded that the bifunctional hapten is bound specifically at one haptenic site and nonspecifically at the other, as suggested earlier for certain univalent derivatives. Nonetheless, in *in vitro* studies it is clear that both haptenic sites in a given bivalent molecule can be combined simultaneously with antibody.

groups on a protein, there is the possibility of substitution by a number of different haptenic molecules, some of which may not be characterized. Both of these disadvantages can be obviated in considerable measure by the use of a polymer of a functional amino acid as the carrier [4, 9, 16]. Polymers of L-amino acids (the isomeric configuration of natural amino acids) containing haptenic substituents vary in their immunogenicity, depending on the conjugate and the animal strain; in many instances, they appear to have less immunizing capacity than the corresponding hapten-protein conjugates [4, 9, 17–19]. Moreover, hapten-polyamino acid conjugates synthesized by use of D-amino acids (the unnatural configuration) appear to be nonimmunogenic and may provide a means by which any haptenic derivative of a drug could be tested in man without danger of induction of drug allergy [17, 20]. The use of polymers of L- and D-lysine as carriers for the penicilloyl group (penicilloyl-polylysines) in studies of penicillin allergy is described later.

Elicitation of contact skin sensitivity and delayed cutaneous reactions to hapten-protein conjugates

Apart from the Arthus reaction, which clearly is mediated by serum antibody, delayed cutaneous reactions in which simple chemical specificity is involved fall into two categories: delayed hypersensitivity to hapten-protein conjugates and delayed hypersensitivity to the simple chemicals themselves (termed contact skin sensitivity since the simple chemical is usually applied topically). By analogy with what has been found in regard to elicitation of immediate type reactions, it might have been anticipated that following sensitization with a hapten-protein conjugate, delayed skin reactions would be elicited by injection of hapten conjugated with heterologous protein as well as by the immunizing conjugate itself. That this has generally not been the case is explicable in terms of a contribution by the protein portion of the immunizing conjugate to the specificity of the delayed cutaneous response [7]. Also consistent with the concept of a contribution by the protein carrier in delayed cutaneous reactions are the results obtained in guinea pigs with contact skin sensitivity: challenge with the simple chemical is much more effective in eliciting a response than challenge with the hapten in combination with proteins not found in the host animal. In contact reactions in the guinea pig, it may be assumed that the immunizing conjugates are composed of hapten in combination with various proteins present in guinea pig skin. Reapplication of the simple chemical permits the resynthesis of the hapten-protein conjugates involved in the original immunological response, thereby permitting a maximal reaction. If hapten conjugated *in vitro* with guinea pig serum albumin (one of the more prominent proteins in guinea pig skin) is used for challenge, a sizable response is obtained; as expected, the response is less than that obtained with the simple chemical itself, since other prominent skin proteins which were involved in immunization are not conjugated to hapten.

Apart from mode of evolution, morphology, and transferability by cells rather than serum, delayed cutaneous hypersensitivity to simple chemicals differs from reactions of the immediate type in the nature of the antigenic determinant involved (hapten + protein versus hapten alone) in the following respects: (1) The requirement of the hapten-protein conjugate used for immunization in order to elicit delayed reactions is not evident in immediate type reactions in which conjugates of the hapten with a variety of proteins elicit perfectly well. (2) The importance of multivalent conjugates in elicitation of immediate type responses is in striking contrast to their ineffectiveness in elicitation of reactions in contact skin sensitivity. In the latter, the unconjugated chemical must be used; it is quite effective as an elicitor, presumably because there is ample time for formation of the required amount of conjugate in the skin. (3) Temporary inhibition of the reaction by means of a stable, univalent hapten is readily accomplished with immediate type reactions but not with delayed reactions.

Studies with Therapeutic Agents

SPECIAL PROBLEMS

It is an apparent paradox that studies with simple chemical determinants have contributed considerably to our knowledge of immune mechanisms but that simple diagnostic measures for detection of drug allergy generally are not available. This discrepancy is due primarily to the problem of identification of the antigenic determinants responsible for drug reactions. In model studies, the immunologist is able to choose from a variety of simple chemicals which react with proteins *in vitro,* and presumably *in vivo,* in well-defined ways. In studies of human drug allergy, it is seldom possible to demonstrate a reaction between the drug and the protein *in vitro.* It is therefore necessary to assume that the derivative responsible for the required reaction with protein arises *in vivo* or is present as a contaminant in the product as it is administered.

The problem of identifying the antigenic precursor if the unmodified drug does not possess protein reactivity is compounded by the fact that microgram quantities of antigen often suffice to induce an immunological response. With the therapeutic administration of many drugs in gram amounts, it is apparent that the allergen responsible for a drug reaction may be derived from a minor impurity in the product, or from a metabolic pathway which is of little significance in terms of the over-all degradation of the drug.

Although some data are available on *in vivo* degradation products of drugs that are prominently involved in human drug allergy, it is clear that this information is far from complete. In many instances, the steps involved in the formation of antigen may be multiple, and the reactivity of the immediate precursor to antigen may preclude its isolation in the free state. Moreover, the possibility of genetically determined differences among individuals in regard to pathways of drug degradation must always be considered. The complexity of the problem may be illustrated by the fact that 4-dimethylaminoazobenzene

$$C_6H_5{-}N{=}N{-}C_6H_4{-}N\begin{matrix} CH_3 \\ CH_3 \end{matrix}$$

has been demonstrated to give rise in the experimental animal to at least thirteen different products [21]. These arise primarily by hydroxylation, reductive cleavage of the $N = N$ group, and demethylation. The products have either one or two benzene rings and contain OH, NH_2, $N(CH_3)_2$, $NHCH_3$, and $NHCOCH_3$ groups in various combinations. It is apparent that a single drug could give rise to a number of antigenic determinants, and that these might differ considerably in configuration from one another and from the original molecule. One could further infer that drugs with relatively little structural similarity (at least in an immunological sense) could give rise to identical antigenic determinants, thereby causing unexpected allergic cross-reactions [22].

The likely requirement for one or more enzymatic steps in the degradation of many drugs in order to produce antigen explains why incubation of the drug with protein *in vitro* in the absence of enzyme fails to provide an active conjugate. It may also explain the fact that certain drug reactions in man which appear to be allergic in origin are sharply limited to a single organ system or even to a single cellular type. This could occur when the enzymatic or degradative step leading to the immediate precursor of antigen was largely limited to a single organ.*

Short of the preliminary identification of possible antigenic determinants, and the preparation of appropriate conjugates and univalent haptens, diagnostic procedures in drug allergy are usually unsuccessful. In lieu of characterized conjugates, attempts have been made to obtain hapten-protein conjugates without identifying the nature of the chemical reaction involved in their formation. (1) Leftwich [23] utilized serum proteins from patients receiving substantial doses of sulfonamides for testing; the presumption was that hapten might have combined with serum protein *in vivo* to the extent that the protein would elicit hapten-specific responses in subjects allergic to sulfonamides. Although he reported the induction of wheal and erythema responses by certain sera in subjects with sulfonamide allergy, others were unable to confirm this observation [24]. (2) The incubation of protein with a drug *in vitro,* followed by dialysis to remove unconjugated material, occasionally has been reported to result in a product which elicits hypersensitivity responses. Such procedures may be useful as a preliminary step in the identification of an antigenic determinant. (3) One may conjugate drugs to protein by "artificial" means, e.g., using a type of covalent bond which would not be expected to form *in vivo.* For example, Wedum [25] conjugated sulfonamides to pro-

* One explanation of the localization of symptoms in this event would be that the bulk of the antigen is formed and remains in a single area. Allergic symptoms would occur in other organs in relation to the extent to which antigen is disseminated. Alternatively, the combination of hapten with organ-specific protein could give rise to an immunological response with specificity for the protein as well as the haptenic group.

teins via the azo linkage. The conjugates formed apparently were not of value in the study of sulfonamide allergy in man. Nevertheless this approach is potentially of value provided there is definite structural similarity between substituents on the "artificial" conjugate and the actual antigenic determinant.

Other difficulties attend the investigation of drug reactions. Attempts at induction of drug allergy in lower animals often have been unsuccessful. In part, this may relate to species differences in mechanisms of drug degradation. The very infrequency of many drug reactions in man creates a serious problem in the induction of the experimental counterpart in animals. Moreover, without the appropriate hapten-protein conjugates for testing, hypersensitivity may well remain undetected. Despite these problems, it is clear that animal experimentation can provide important clues to the mechanism of human drug reactions. Indeed, the results of animal investigation in penicillin allergy are entirely consistent with those obtained by human testing.

STUDIES IN PENICILLIN ALLERGY

Penicillin allergy is an ideal model system for the investigation of allergy to therapeutic agents in man because of its frequency and medical importance and because there is usually no real difficulty in discerning when allergy is involved in an untoward reaction to this drug. Since principles established by animal experimentation should be applicable to human drug allergy, the following experimental approach has been used [4–6, 16, 26–28]: (1) The scrutiny of known penicillin derivatives for possible precursors of protein-bound antigen. (2) The synthesis and characterization of suspected precursors, the conjugates formed by their reactions with protein, and appropriate univalent haptens. (3) Immunization of animals with protein conjugates and suspected intermediates in order to establish immunogenicity and evaluate the extent to which various derivatives cross-react immunologically with one another. (4) (*a*) Establishment of the efficacy and specificity of protein and polyamino acid conjugates as elicitors of cutaneous reactions with animal sera of known specificity; (*b*) evaluation by means of these conjugates of immediate skin reactions in human beings allergic to penicillin and in guinea pigs sensitized with rabbit antisera to penicillin; (*c*) validation of the specificity of positive reactions by hapten inhibition. (5) The evaluation of globulin fractions from human subjects allergic to penicillin and animals immunized with penicillin in regard to hapten inhibition of hemagglutination and precipitation, and comparison of the inhibition curves obtained with those obtained with globulin fractions specific for protein conjugates.

The results substantiate the premise that principles discussed earlier are applicable to penicillin allergy. For example, one of the penicillin derivatives examined, the penicilloyl group (Fig. 59-1, IVa and IVb),* clearly is an important antigenic determinant in penicillin allergy. In addition, there is suggestive evidence that as many as five other penicillin derivatives are less commonly involved (derivatives V, VII, X, XI, and XII); the probable mechanisms of their formation are shown in Fig. 59-1) [6]. All of them are capable of existing in covalent linkage to protein. Penicillin itself and other derivatives of penicillin bound reversibly by serum albumin (e.g., VIII) apparently do not induce antibody formation.

Apart from the theoretical implications of recent studies in penicillin allergy, a number of practical or potentially practical considerations can be raised:

1. The intradermal injection of a multivalent penicilloyl conjugate (penicilloyl-polylysine) provides a convenient and valuable screening procedure for penicillin allergy in man [4, 29]. The cutaneous reaction is of the wheal and erythema type and can be evaluated within 15 to 20 minutes.

2. The penicilloyl group can arise either from penicillenic acid or directly from penicillin (Fig. 59-1, pathways 1b and 2). Penicillenic acid is much more reactive than penicillin, and when it is present in the injection solution, penicilloyl-protein conjugates can form very soon after injection. The precipitate development of serious systemic reactions to penicillin may be explicable on this basis. Since penicillenic acid can be demonstrated to form in the injection solution on prolonged storage [26], greater use of single-injection disposable units may be desirable. Moreover,

* Depending on the mechanism of formation (pathway 1 vs. pathway 2), the penicilloyl derivative may retain the D-α configuration of the parent penicillin (IVa) or form as a random mixture of diastereoisomers (IVb).

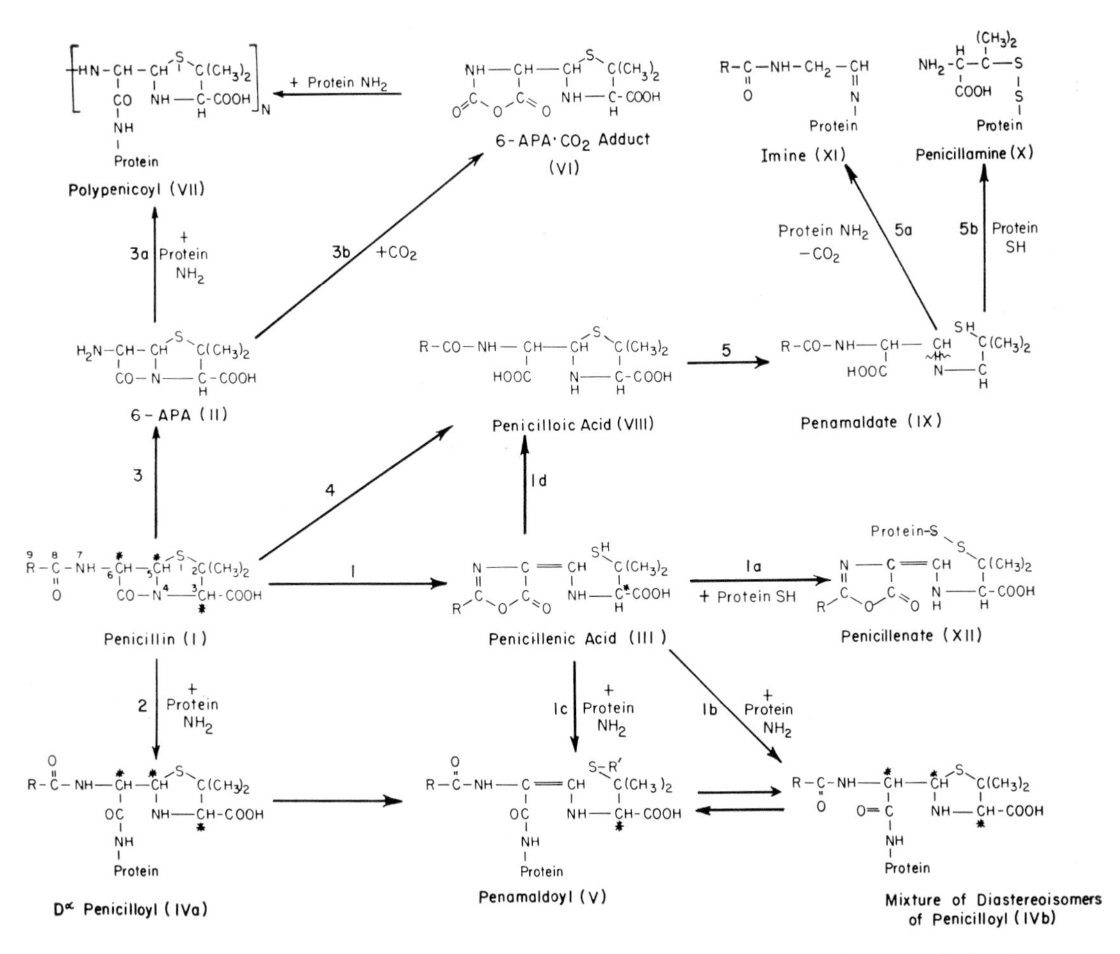

Fig. 59-1. Mechanisms of formation of antigen in penicillin allergy. In VII, the group in brackets may be polymerized. Asterisk refers to asymmetrical carbons. 6-APA is 6-aminopenicillenic acid.

previous reports that certain penicillin preparations are associated with an inordinate number of allergic reactions [30] are subject to re-evaluation. It may be that in some instances a relatively high degree of contamination with penicillin derivatives such as penicillenic acid was responsible rather than any special properties of the penicillin salt per se.

3. Stable univalent penicilloyl haptens are of potential value in the prophylaxis and treatment of penicillin reactions. Their nontoxicity in man is not, however, established; moreover, their efficacy in a given individual would not be assured unless it were firmly established that penicillyol was the only penicillin derivative to which antibodies had been formed.

4. The reported salutary effect of penicillinase in some subjects with penicillin allergy is readily explicable when the penicilloyl group is the antigenic determinant involved. Penicillinase hydrolyzes penicillin to free penicilloic acid (VIII, pathway 4, Fig. 59-1), removing a source of protein-bound penicilloyl and creating a univalent derivative capable of competing with the protein-bound antigen. If an important antigenic determinant in a given subject were X or XI, however, the rapid formation of penicilloic acid in the presence of penicillinase might accelerate formation of antigen and cause aggravation of allergic symptoms.

5. The mechanism of "desensitization" in penicillin allergy presumably is more complex than that of allergy to a foreign protein. During the administration of graded doses of penicillin to a subject with penicillin allergy, the absence of allergic symptoms up to a given point may be due to the fact that sufficient amounts of protein-bound penicilloyl have not yet formed or that penicillin and penicilloic acid are competitively blocking the

reaction. Clearly, interruption of therapy even for only a few hours is undesirable because the univalent inhibitors would be largely excreted during this time.

DETECTION OF PENICILLIN ALLERGY IN MAN

Skin Tests. The initial documentation of hypersensitivity to the penicilloyl group in man was through the elicitation of wheal and erythema responses on intradermal injection of penicilloyl-protein conjugates. In subsequent studies, penicilloyl-polylysine has been employed for cutaneous testing in order to minimize the possibility that the skin test reagent might induce antibody formation, thereby producing penicillin allergy.* The incidence of cutaneous reactions to penicilloyl-polylysine in subjects with a history of penicillin allergy has ranged between 35 and 75 percent in various series [4, 29, 31]. Positive responses are obtained in many instances when testing with penicillin produces negative results, as discussed later. An important factor in the extent to which reactivity to penicilloyl-polylysine is correlated with history of an allergic response is the nature of the patient population examined. Important variables probably include age, the amounts and type of penicillin received, the time interval since the penicillin reaction, and the degree of certainty that previous symptoms were actually due to penicillin allergy [29].

Positive cutaneous reactions to penicilloyl-polylysine occur in about 4 percent of individuals with no history of penicillin allergy [7]. Among individuals with no history of penicillin allergy, the one with a positive cutaneous reaction to penicilloyl-polylysine has a 10- to 300-fold greater chance of having a reaction on subsequent penicillin administrations (8 to 40 percent incidence of reactions) than the subject with a negative skin reaction [4, 29, 31, 32a].† Allergic reactions to penicillin in individuals with negative skin reactions characteristically develop hours to days after the penicillin injection; anaphylaxis has not been observed in this group of subjects. There has, however, been at least one immediate urticarial reaction without hypotension [32b].

Hemagglutination Reactions. Although precipitating antibody specific for penicilloyl very seldom is demonstrable in the serum of subjects with penicillin allergy, hemagglutinating activity can be demonstrated in many instances [33]. Depending on the exact technique of preparing cells, hemagglutination at a serum dilution of 1 : 16 or higher can be obtained with sera from as many as 65 percent of subjects with a history of penicillin allergy and from about 10 percent of subjects without historical evidence of allergy to the drug [6, 35].‡

REMAINING PROBLEMS IN DIAGNOSIS

Despite the identification of several antigenic determinants in penicillin allergy and the elaboration of useful diagnostic techniques both *in vivo* and *in vitro,* it is evident that problems in diagnosis still exist. Some of these now will be discussed.

1. From studies in penicillin allergy, it is evident that the drug may cause an immunological response without the development of allergic symptoms. The occurrence of penicillin antibodies in asymptomatic subjects is not surprising when one considers that many vaccines induce a protective titer of antibodies in a high percentage of subjects whereas allergic reactions are unusual. It hardly need be emphasized that in the subject with a clinical syndrome possibly due to penicillin, a positive cutaneous or serological response is

---

* In 200 human subjects there has been no evidence of induction of penicillin allergy by penicilloyl-poly-L-lysine, even on repeated injection [29, 31]. In the experimental animal, lightly substituted penicilloyl-poly-L-lysine in adjuvant can give rise to antibody formation in at least one animal strain [17, 19]. In similar conditions of animal experimentation, penicilloyl-poly-D-lysine appears to be nonimmunogenic [17].

† The most impressive statistics on the potential value of routine screening with penicilloyl-polylysine in prevention of penicillin reactions have been obtained at the St. Louis City Health Clinic by Shapiro [32a] and Summar [32b]. They have noted a more than 25-fold decrease in incidence of observed penicillin reactions when patients were excluded from therapy on the basis of both skin test and history as opposed to history alone [32b].

‡ In addition to hemagglutination, two other techniques have been employed for the detection of antibody in the serum of human subjects allergic to penicillin. One involves the coprecipitation of an I^{131}-labeled penicilloyl antigen when rabbit antihuman γ-globulin is added to a mixture of the antigen and human γ-globulin containing antibodies specific for penicilloyl [6]. Shelley [34] has recently described an assay involving degranulation of rabbit basophils by sera from subjects with penicillin allergy in the presence of penicillin.

suggestive, but not conclusive, evidence that penicillin allergy is responsible for symptoms.

2. In many instances, the subject with penicillin allergy will have both a high hemagglutination titer and cutaneous responsiveness to penicilloyl-polylysine. However, the result of one test may be strongly positive in the face of a completely negative result by the other technique [6, 36]. This can be related to the fact that the immune globulins responsible for direct hemagglutination in penicillin allergy appear to be predominantly 19S macroglobulins [6], whereas antibodies responsible for cutaneous reactions seem to be mainly in the B_{2A} fraction [37]. The evidence suggests that systemic anaphylaxis is related to the same type of antibodies which mediate immediate cutaneous reactions. Since there is considerable evidence that 19S macroglobulins have little or no activity in PCA [38], their presence in relatively large amounts in serum need not be necessarily associated with cutaneous responsiveness or with an unusually high risk of systemic anaphylaxis. On the other hand, a role of 19S antibody in the development of symptoms of serum sickness is not excluded. Nor is it clear that potential anaphylaxis would always be detected by cutaneous testing provided the appropriate antigen and proper technique were employed.

3. A further problem in diagnosis of penicillin allergy is related to the fact that multiple antigenic determinants are sometimes involved. When antibody specificities other than penicilloyl are present, the subject frequently is sensitive to penicilloyl as well, but this is not always true. Short of identification of all possible antigenic determinants and routine cutaneous testing with each of them, the possibility must be considered that despite a negative skin response to penicilloyl-polylysine, skin-sensitizing antibodies specific for other penicillin derivatives are present.

Although positive cutaneous reactions to penicilloyl-polylysine are much more common in penicillin allergy than are local responses to penicillin itself, some instances have been reported in which the latter produced a wheal and erythema response but penicilloyl-polylysine and other conjugates were inactive [36, 39].* Accordingly, penicillin itself may still have a definite place as a skin test reagent in the diagnosis of penicillin allergy. However, if penicillin is to be used for this purpose, two points must be kept in mind: (*a*) penicillin induces nonspecific reactions in some subjects, particularly at concentrations above 10,000 units per ml., and (*b*) skin testing with penicillin probably entails a substantially greater risk than testing with penicilloyl-polylysine, because of the former's greater diffusibility. The rapid entry of a portion of the injected penicillin into the circulation is a hazard, because the rapidity of formation of penicilloyl-protein conjugates from penicillin is not predictable and the amounts of penicillin used often are relatively large.†

4. The loss of cutaneous reactivity to penicilloyl-polylysine following penicillin therapy may be attributed to the combination of antibody with antigen and hapten. Positive cutaneous reactions to penicilloyl-polylysine may convert quickly to negative (within a few hours) after penicillin therapy, but in other instances, reactions may continue to be elicited for some days after the initial penicillin injection. This "desensitization" phenomenon must be considered in evaluating the subject during or after symptoms of penicillin allergy. A negative cutaneous reaction to penicilloyl-polylysine at this time is not proof that cutaneous reactivity would not have occurred

* One explanation of this occurrence might be that penicillin derivatives other than penicilloyl are responsible for penicillin hypersensitivity in these subjects. A second possibility is that in some instances a form of carrier specificity is involved, e.g., that the full antigenic determinant is penicilloyl (or some other penicillin derivative) combined with human protein. In this circumstance, pencilloyl-polylysine would elicit poorly because the carrier portion of the molecule differs from that of the immunizing conjugate. We have observed two subjects in whom penicilloyl-human serum albumin elicited somewhat larger reactions than comparably substituted penicilloyl conjugates with albumins of other species; both did have substantial reactivity to penicilloyl-polylysine, however [14].

In view of the size of the penicillin molecule, the possibility cannot be excluded that penicillin and penicillin derivatives might function on occasion as univalent elicitors. For example, in subjects with antibodies to X (Fig. 59-1), IX might function in this manner, assuming the R group (benzyl) in IX might act as an unrelated substituent. In subjects with penicilloyl-specific antibodies, the univalent penicilloyl derivatives tested have been inhibitory [4], although complete inhibition is not necessarily observed.

† To obtain a positive cutaneous response with penicilloyl-polylysine, the injection of 3 mμM penicilloyl or less is usually sufficient. To elicit a cutaneous reaction with penicillin, 400 mμM penicillin or more is often used.

had the test been performed before penicillin therapy or during early symptoms of allergy. In the absence of cutaneous reactivity to penicilloyl derivatives, the serum may contain hemagglutinating activity specific for penicilloyl in high titer, indicating that penicilloyl-specific antibody may well be involved in the production of allergic symptoms. Cutaneous reactivity to penicilloyl-polylysine may return or be demonstrated for the first time days to months after acute allergic symptoms have subsided. Because of the variation in results of *in vivo* or *in vitro* assays with time, several practical considerations arise: (*a*) The desirability of utilizing several different assays for antibody activity in the diagnosis of drug allergy is evident. (*b*) When a subject is suspected of having an allergic reaction to penicillin but clear substantiation is not obtained, re-evaluation at a later time will be indicated if a necessity for further therapy arises. (*c*) The evaluation of the efficacy of penicilloyl-polylysine and other test reagents in predicting penicillin reactions must be done prospectively, i.e., testing before penicillin therapy rather than after allergic symptoms have developed.

CLINICAL ASPECTS OF DRUG ALLERGY

Problems in Classification of Drug Reactions

In the classifying of drug reactions in man, a clear distinction must be made whenever possible between manifestations due to allergy and those due to other forms of drug toxicity. Allergic manifestations (1) have no linear relationship to drug dosage, often being produced by small amounts of the drug; (2) require an induction period on primary exposure but not on readministration; (3) occur in a minority of persons receiving the drug (with a few exceptions) [24]; (4) have no correlation with the known pharmacological properties of the drug; (5) often include anaphylaxis, the serum sickness syndrome, urticaria, contact dermatitis, and asthma as prominent clinical features, and (6) usually reappear on readministration of the drug in small amounts. On the other hand, toxic symptoms on a nonallergic basis often are (and often are not) an exaggeration of the desired pharmacological action of the drug, are correlated reasonably well with drug dosage, for the most part do not require an induction period, can be induced in the great majority of individuals if a substantial overdose is given, and usually reappear only with drug levels that caused symptoms first to appear.

Although the distinction between an allergic and a toxic action of a drug ordinarily is not difficult, at times the points of differentiation outlined above partially break down. (1) Manifestations apparently due to drug allergy may be largely limited to a single organ or organ system, taking the form of hepatitis, a blood dyscrasia, nephritis, vasculitis, dermatitis, or fever. Classic symptoms of allergy may be totally lacking in such instances. Symptoms suggestive of allergy, e.g., urticaria and asthma, occasionally are elicited nonspecifically by drugs. This is especially true in the patient with recurrent urticaria or asthma due to etiological factors other than drugs. For example, aspirin apparently can cause attacks of urticaria on a nonspecific basis in the patient with chronic urticaria, as well as induce urticaria as a manifestation of aspirin allergy. (2) A latent period of one to several weeks before symptoms appear may be required for development of cumulative drug toxicity as well as for induction of antibody formation. Reactions which begin within several days after the first known exposure to a drug may be due to allergy when there has been unwitting previous exposure or when there is unexpected cross-reactivity with another drug received previously. (3) A number of instances have been documented of isolated enzymatic defects which cause heightened susceptibility to a drug in a genetically determined segment of the population.* (4) Prompt exacerbation of symptoms on readministration of a drug in small amounts, when much larger quantities were tolerated originally, could in some instances indicate persistent subclinical damage at the cellular or subcellular level rather than allergy. (5) Careful studies of the histology of the lesions and the response to "antiallergic" therapy are always of interest but only rarely provide diagnostic informa-

* Perhaps the best-known example is that of glucose-6-phosphate dehydrogenase deficiency of red cells, in which a variety of drugs produce hemolytic anemia after a short latent period.

tion. The presence of eosinophilia is suggestive of allergy, but its absence does not militate at all against the diagnosis.

As a whole, the mechanism of many drug reactions remains obscure. This is especially true of many of the reactions involving visceral organs and the hemopoietic system. Immunological studies with the drug in question provide a potential answer but, without knowledge of the antigenic determinants involved, frequently will be unsuccessful. Many of the drug reactions which at present are unclassified may ultimately be shown to be due to allergy. There is little doubt that some will emerge as manifestations of idiosyncrasies in which an inborn enzymatic deficiency affects drug metabolism.

Clinical Manifestations

The clinical manifestations of drug allergy are legion and can only be discussed briefly here. For a detailed discussion of allergic manifestations due to individual drugs, the reader is referred to the very useful monograph by Alexander [40].

ANAPHYLAXIS

Anaphylactic reactions to foreign serum and to extracts of tissue and environmental antigens are well known and are discussed in appropriate chapters. We are concerned here with life-threatening reactions of rapid onset characterized chiefly by shock which occurs in response to a variety of therapeutic and diagnostic agents of nonprotein nature. The most notable causes are penicillin, the radiopaque organic iodides, local anesthetic agents, and, to a lesser degree, mercurials, streptomycin, vitamin K_1 oxide, bromsulphalein, and sodium dehydrocholate (Decholin) [40].

Anaphylaxis due to penicillin has been estimated to cause from 100 to 300 deaths per year in this country [41]. Fortunately, most anaphylactic reactions to penicillin are not fatal, and it seems probable that many such reactions are so mild that they are not detected.*

* It is important, but not always easy, to distinguish a vasovagal reaction due to injection trauma from a mild anaphylactic reaction. If hypotension responds promptly to recumbency and there are no associated allergic symptoms, a neurogenic mechanism is probably responsible for symptoms.

From observations of allergy to penicillin and foreign serum, it is evident that hypotension and its attendant signs, symptoms, and pathological changes may be the sole manifestations of anaphylaxis in man. It is not surprising, therefore, that the etiology of hypotensive episodes due to agents other than penicillin is not clear in most instances. The evidence that streptomycin, organic mercurials, sodium dehydrocholate, and bromsulphalein can cause anaphylaxis is rather convincing [40–42]; in a few instances, patients who have had systemic reactions to these drugs had an immediate reaction on cutaneous testing. The role of allergy in hypotensive states produced by local anesthetic agents and organic iodides is less clear. Some of the points for and against an allergic basis for these reactions will be listed briefly. (1) Clinical or pathological changes consistent with acute allergy occasionally are present in instances of fatal reactions to these agents but more often are absent. (2) Fatal or severe reactions appear to be most common in individuals with a history of severe allergy. On the other hand, the elicitation of urticaria and asthma in allergic individuals by nonspecific stress or cholinergic stimuli must be kept in mind. (3) Local anesthetic agents, and probably organic iodides as well, can cause allergic reactions other than anaphylaxis. (4) Organic iodides and local anesthetic agents cause hypotension and cerebral symptoms in animals by a nonallergic mechanism. (5) Serious reactions often occur in individuals with no known previous exposure to these agents or to closely related structures. (6) Cutaneous tests or preliminary intravenous injection of small doses of the agent have not been helpful in predicting and preventing reactions caused by the administration of the full amount.

SERUM SICKNESS SYNDROME

A syndrome indistinguishable clinically from serum sickness is produced by a variety of nonprotein drugs, among which the most common offenders are penicillin, streptomycin, sulfonamides, and the thiouracils.

CUTANEOUS MANIFESTATIONS

Skin manifestations occur in most patients with drug allergy and include urticaria, exanthemas, purpura, lesions of the contact type, exfoliative dermatitis, fixed eruptions, erythema nodosum and multiforme, and photosensitivity eruptions. The appearance of an eruption generally is not sufficiently characteristic to implicate one particular drug or to distinguish a drug-induced eruption from dermatitis due to other causes. Many drugs, e.g., penicillin and the sulfonamides, are capable of producing many types of cutaneous lesions. Cutaneous manifestations due to a given drug may change in character from day to day, sometimes beginning as an insignificant maculopapular eruption and progressing to a hemorrhagic or exfoliative lesion if exposure to the drug is continued or it is readministered. Cutaneous changes due to some drugs are primarily of only one or two types and may be sufficiently distinctive to suggest the diagnosis. Examples include the acneiform and bullous eruptions produced by iodides and bromides, and fixed drug eruptions due to phenolphthalein [43].

HEMATOLOGICAL CHANGES

Thrombocytopenia. At present, the commonest causes of drug-induced thrombocytopenia, apparently on an allergic basis, are quinidine or its diastereoisomer quinine, the sulfonamides, and sulfonamide derivatives without antibacterial activity such as chlorothiazide, chlorpropamide, tolbutamide, and acetazolamide [44]. Less commonly, chloramphenicol, meprobamate, and phenylbutazone have been found to cause thrombocytopenia, and in England, allyl-isopropyl-acetylcarbamide (Sedormid) has been a relatively frequent cause [45].

The clinical manifestations are primarily those of thrombocytopenia, e.g., hemorrhage and petechial skin lesions, but associated symptoms attributable to allergy, such as fever and arthralgia, may also be present. After withdrawal of the responsible drug, bleeding manifestations usually subside within a week. Rarely, death has resulted despite discontinuation of the drug on appearance of symptoms of thrombocytopenia. In an individual who has recovered from thrombocytopenia, readministration of the drug in small amounts usually causes prompt recrudescence of thrombocytopenia, sometimes within an hour. Manifestations of bleeding may be preceded by fever and chills. Less commonly, thrombocytopenia does not recur until therapeutic quantities of the drug have been given for at least several days [45]. The rapidity of the fall of the platelet count in many subjects following drug readministration is consistent with accelerated destruction of platelets in the peripheral circulation as opposed to decreased synthesis and release of platelets from the bone marrow; the latter may also occur to a limited extent.

The most impressive evidence that an immunological mechanism can be responsible for drug-induced thrombocytopenia has been obtained by Ackroyd [45] and Shulman [46], with confirmation by others, in patients with thrombocytopenia due to Sedormid, quinidine, and quinine. During or after recovery from symptoms of thrombocytopenia there is present, in the serum, a globulin capable of causing agglutination and lysis of normal platelets in the presence of the drug. In the absence of the drug, agglutination is not observed. It is assumed that a similar combination between antibody and the hapten-platelet complex takes place *in vivo,* rendering platelets unusually susceptible to destruction during transit through the circulatory system. In addition to assays involving platelet agglutination and lysis, sera from subjects with quinidine- and Sedormid-induced thrombocytopenias can mediate complement fixation in the presence of normal platelets and the appropriate drug.* A useful rapid screening test for a drug-induced thrombocytopenia on an allergic basis involves the incubation of the patient's serum with whole blood from a normal subject in the presence and absence of the suspected causative agent. Pronounced inhibition of clot retraction in the presence of the drug strongly suggests that there is a relation between bleeding manifestations and administration of the drug.

Although there is no doubt that purpura is primarily due to thrombocytopenia in these

* It is of interest that the phenomenon of hapten inhibition is not readily demonstrated in these reactions except at very high drug concentrations [45, 46]. Several explanations might be advanced to account for this: (*a*) The drug itself may differ substantially in structure from the actual protein-bound derivative of the drug responsible for immunization. (*b*) The drug may react with platelet protein (or with plasma protein which in turn is adsorbed to the platelet), producing an antigenic determinant requiring both protein and hapten moieties for strong interaction with antibody [45]. (*c*) The natural adhesiveness and adsorptive capacity of platelets may provide a mechanism by which antibody, once reacted with hapten or with a hapten-protein complex, might become more or less fixed.

subjects, it has been observed that patch tests with the drug may produce local purpura in the absence of systemic thrombocytopenia. It has been suggested that the drug in combination with capillary endothelium represents an antigenic complex similar to the hapten-platelet complex and is thereby capable of reacting with antibody, producing local tissue damage [45]. There is no direct substantiation of this concept, however.

Agranulocytosis. Formerly, aminopyrine was the commonest cause of drug-induced agranulocytosis. With decreased usage of this derivative, the phenothiazines have become the major causes of this condition. Other drugs implicated in a significant number of cases include phenylbutazone, dipyrone (the sulfonated derivative of aminopyrine), chloramphenicol, the sulfonamides, the thiouracils, methimazole, phenindione, and tolbutamide [44]. Following cessation of drug therapy, improvement may be expected within one to two weeks, provided death due to infection is forestalled during the interim. As in drug-induced thrombocytopenia, readministration of the drug, in low dosage with recrudescence of agranulocytosis, has been used to substantiate the role of the drug in leukocyte depression. With the development of acute changes in leukocyte levels, peripheral destruction of leukocytes is indicated, although it is also evident that during the initial bout of agranulocytosis, leukocyte precursors in the bone marrow are abnormal in number and morphology. Moeschlin [47] has attributed these changes in marrow morphology to excessive stimulation and perhaps exhaustion of the marrow in the face of rapid leukocyte destruction peripherally; however, a maturation arrest produced by the interaction of drug, antibody, and granulocyte precursors in the marrow is not excluded.

Direct substantiation of the presence of serum antibody and its role in destruction of granulocytes has been accomplished by passive transfer in a few instances. In the first study of this kind, Moeschlin and Wagner [48] found that serum from a patient who had had aminopyrine agranulocytosis and had received a further dose of the drug three hours previously, produced acute agranulocytosis in two normal recipients. With the sera of a number of patients with aminopyrine and sulfonamide agranulocytosis as well as in scattered instances in which other drugs were involved, agglutination of normal leukocytes has been demonstrated. Usually, the patient's serum is not effective unless the drug was readministered to the patient within several hours before the sample was taken. This is in contrast to results with platelet agglutinins in quinidine and Sedormid allergy, in which serum, normal platelets, and drug may be mixed *in vitro* to induce a positive response.

Hypoplastic Anemia. The commonest cause of drug-induced aplastic anemia is chloramphenicol. Other drugs not infrequently associated with this complication are various sulfonamides, both with antibacterial and with nonbacterial activities, phenylbutazone, the anticonvulsants Mesantoin and trimethadione, and a variety of organic solvents including benzene and materials used as insecticides and pesticides [44]. A few such reactions have also been associated with gold and quinacrine therapy [40].

The etiology of the aplastic anemia associated with therapy with the aforementioned drugs is unclear. Chloramphenicol, the principal causative agent, may produce bone marrow hypoplasia when given in large doses, but there is some doubt that this effect is relevant to blood changes seen in some patients receiving much smaller doses.

Hemolytic Anemia. Hemolytic anemias due to drug allergy must be distinguished from drug-induced hemolytic anemia on a genetic basis. The latter is associated with therapy with certain drugs, notably primaquine and other antimalarials, sulfonamides, antipyretic drugs (including acetophenetidin and aspirin), sulfones, and nitrofurans [44, 49]. In most such instances, it can be demonstrated that red blood cells are deficient in glucose-6-phosphate dehydrogenase activity and, as a result, are most susceptible to the action of drugs which have an oxidative capacity. Much less commonly, it appears that drug therapy causes hemolytic anemia on an immunological basis. This has been reasonably well documented with Mesantoin, Fuadin, quinidine, and quinine, acetophenetidin, para-aminosalicylic acid, Antazoline, and penicillin therapy, but only single cases are described in most instances. Substantiation of a relationship between drug therapy and red cell destruction has been obtained by demonstration of recurrence of the anemia and other signs of blood destruction on readministration of the drug. In most instances, the patient's serum has agglutinated compatible normal red cells in the presence of the drug and antihuman globulin. One case has been described in which drug-dependent thrombocytopenia and hemolytic anemia apparently related to quinidine therapy were present simultaneously [44].

VASCULITIS AND INFLAMMATION OF CONNECTIVE TISSUE

Acute Vasculitis. In subjects with serum sickness, drug fever, and drug-induced syndromes in which damage is primarily in a single organ, vascular changes often are readily demonstrated. The damage is predominantly in the smaller vessels and ranges in degree from mild cellular infiltration to acute necrosis [50]. Mild vasculitis does not necessarily give rise to local symptoms or gross pathological changes. When severe inflammatory changes and necrosis are present, vessels in many organs are usually involved, including those in the skin and kidneys. Apart from petechial skin lesions, proteinuria, hematuria, and manifestations of renal failure, symptoms often include fever, dermatitis, arthralgia, edema, and less frequently myositis, coronary arteritis, pneumonitis, and gastrointestinal bleeding [50–52]. Death is due primarily to renal failure. The drugs most frequently implicated in severe vasculitis are penicillin, the sulfonamides, and the thiouracils [40, 52]. A history compatible with drug allergy was obtained in seven of thirty patients with pathological changes of "allergic vasculitis" studied by McCombs *et al.* [51].

Chronic Vasculitis. In any patient with polyarteritis or some other variant of chronic inflammatory vascular disease, the possibility that a drug might be involved must be carefully considered. At least some of the drugs which cause acute vasculitis appear to be capable of causing a more chronic form of vascular inflammation, provided drug administration is continued for many weeks or more (examples include hydralazine and the thiouracils) [53, 54]. In one patient with arteritis during propylthiouracil therapy, an exacerbation of symptoms followed readministration of the drug on three separate occasions [54]. Despite the indication that drugs can cause subacute or chronic vasculitis, the available evidence (which admittedly is inadequate in many of the published case reports) suggests that drug allergy usually does not play a role in the pathogenesis of polyarteritis [53]. It is true that in some instances the patient was receiving medications at the time symptoms first appeared. Nevertheless there is no experimental evidence that a short course of therapy with a drug would produce a chronic vascular disease in which fresh lesions appear months or even years after the drug has been withdrawn.

Syndromes Resembling Systemic Lupus Erythematosus. A clinical syndrome resembling systemic lupus erythematosus (SLE), with or without the LE cell phenomenon, has been described in connection with prolonged hydralazine therapy [55] and much less frequently with therapy with other drugs (Mesantoin, isoniazid, procaine-amide, the tetracyclines). It is not established that hydralazine disease is due to drug allergy. Moreover, the nature of the association between the hydralazine-induced syndrome and SLE is obscure. Systemic manifestations in the main subside promptly after the drug is withdrawn provided irreversible tissue damage has not occurred, but minor abnormalities may persist for some years in a few patients. When this occurs, the question may be raised as to whether subclinical SLE preceded drug therapy [56].

Polymyositis. Although Symmers [52] stated that there is no evidence that polymyositis is caused by drug allergy, in two patients observed personally there was a very suggestive relationship between penicillin therapy and onset of this disease [14]. No attempt was made, however, to produce an exacerbation of symptoms by readministration of penicillin.

Thrombotic Thrombocytopenic Purpura. Symmers [52] has described several patients in whom it was felt that thrombotic thrombocytopenic purpura was probably caused by drug allergy, but in no instance was a causal relationship established.

HEPATIC DAMAGE

Among the more prominent causes of drug-induced liver damage in man are chlorpromazine (and other phenothiazines), the sulfonylureas, para-aminosalicylic acid, iproniazid, alkylated anabolic agents, novobiocin, gold, the thiouracils, streptomycin, isoniazid, Phenurone, and quinacrine [40, 57, 58].* Clinical syndromes fall primarily into three main categories, with damage which is primarily hepatocellular, hepatocanalicular, or a combination of the two.

The role of allergy in the development of liver changes cannot be stated with certainty in many instances. There is, however, highly suggestive evidence in a few instances that hypersensitivity is involved. For example, para-aminosalicylic acid has been reported to cause hepatic parenchymal damage, usually beginning after several weeks of treatment. Allergy is strongly suggested by concurrent fever, rash, lymphadenopathy, and eosinophilia; in many instances by provocation of symptoms on reinstitution of the drug in low dosage, and by the fact that a number of patients have been successfully restored to tolerance of full therapeutic levels of the drug by a desensitization program [58].

FEVER

Fever is a common manifestation of drug allergy. Although usually associated with other symptoms of allergy, occasionally it is the only prominent manifestation. Despite the absence of local symptoms, at autopsy prominent small vessel inflammation and focal necrosis in visceral organs may be noted. These changes indicate the possibility of serious complications should drug therapy be continued [43]. Among the more prominent causes of "drug fever" are quinidine, the sulfonamides, hydralazine, the thiouracils, and the arsenicals. A drug known as Nirvanol, used at one time in treatment of Sydenham's chorea, caused fever in virtually every subject to whom it was given in adequate dosage [43].

PULMONARY MANIFESTATIONS

Bronchial asthma, pulmonary infiltration by eosinophilia, hilar adenopathy, and so-called antigenic pneumonitis (with pulmonary edema most pronounced in perihilar areas) can all be manifestations of drug allergy.

NEPHROPATHY

Glomerulonephritis is often associated with the serum sickness syndrome or acute vasculitis due to drugs. A less common form of renal damage, probably due to allergy, is acute interstitial nephritis [59]. Acute tubular necrosis may occur secondary to prolonged hypotension in acute anaphylactic reactions, but it is a secondary rather than a primary complication of drug allergy. The role of drug allergy in chronic interstitial nephritis due to Phenacetin is unclear.

LYMPHADENOPATHY

Lymphadenopathy is common in the serum sickness syndrome. Rarely, patients receiving long-term diphenylhydantoin therapy have clinical and pathological changes highly suggestive of lymphoma [60]. Lymph node enlargement fades rapidly after cessation of therapy.

CARDIOPATHY

Myocarditis, coronary arteritis, and pericarditis are occasionally associated with allergic symptoms in other than cardiac areas. When documentation is based solely on serial electrocardiographic changes, however, there is the possibility that the observed abnormalities were due to hypotension or fever in a patient with pre-existing heart disease.

Diagnosis of Drug Allergy

The prompt diagnosis of an allergic reaction to a drug will decrease mortality, eliminate needless diagnostic procedures, and forestall serious, potentially fatal, complications.

CORRELATION OF SYMPTOMS WITH DRUG ADMINISTRATION

In many instances, a reasonable suspicion that drug allergy is present will justify discontinuation of the drug unless the disease being treated is serious and a satisfactory substitute is not available. Allergic manifestations due to a drug usually subside or improve within 24 to 48 hours after its discontinuation, providing tentative substantiation of the clinical impression of drug allergy. There are exceptions, however, in which manifestations continue unabated or even intensify temporarily in the week following cessation of drug therapy. When the allergic reaction has produced tissue necrosis, recovery may be slow and incomplete. When an unusually persistent antigen is involved (as following an injection of a long-acting penicillin preparation), al-

* It seems probable in retrospect that in some of the earlier reports in which hepatic damage was attributed to drug allergy, viral hepatitis was responsible for symptoms [40].

lergic symptoms may persist for several months or more.

SKIN TESTS

Attempts to elicit immediate cutaneous reactions in subjects with drug allergy by using the drug itself are seldom successful and involve a very significant risk to the patient (see p. 671).* If testing is done, the initial procedure should be the scratch test at very low concentrations of the drug: control tests on normal subjects should be done. Tests by passive transfer involve relatively little risk, but positive results are rarely obtained and hepatitis remains a significant hazard to the recipient.

In contact dermatitis due to drugs, positive skin reactions to patch tests are common. Nonspecific irritation must be excluded. Contact skin reactions or positive reactions to patch tests occasionally are obtained in systemic allergic syndromes of the immediate type, e.g., serum sickness and drug fever.

SEROLOGICAL REACTIONS

Apart from a few special instances (e.g., in penicillin allergy and certain drug-induced purpuras, thrombocytopenias, and hemolytic anemias), serological tests for antibodies to drugs generally are not available. However, a promising hemagglutination assay for detection of antibodies to salicylate recently has been reported [61].

PROSPECTS IN DIAGNOSIS

From studies of penicillin allergy, it seems evident that the primary problem in diagnosis of drug reactions is that of identifying antigenic determinants and preparing appropriate conjugates for testing, rather than any special properties of the antibodies involved. Although the characterization of major antigenic determinants in drug reactions is a rather formidable task, this problem will become less difficult as information concerning mechanisms of drug metabolism continues to accumulate.

Ultimately it should be possible to accurately diagnose the more important allergic drug reactions by use of *in vivo* and *in vitro* assays to supplement clinical impressions. Even with such assays, however, there will continue to be individuals in whom a definitive judgment cannot be made.

* Immediate cutaneous reactions in subjects with suspected drug allergy, using the drug in question, have been obtained most frequently with penicillin. Other drugs are streptomycin, quinidine, quinine, organic mercurials. In some reports, the possibility that reactions were elicited nonspecifically cannot be excluded.

Other Factors Involved in Development of Drug Reactions

DOSAGE, DURATION, AND NUMBER OF COURSES OF THERAPY

There is a general impression that the incidence of sensitization increases as the daily dose of a drug is increased. It is worthy of emphasis, however, that small doses may sensitize, and, in the patient who is already allergic, an extremely small amount of the drug may produce serious symptoms of hypersensitivity [62].

It is clear that the incidence of sensitization rises as therapy is prolonged or courses of therapy are repeated. The fact that a subject has tolerated a drug on numerous previous occasions is no assurance that allergic symptoms will not occur after the next injection. It is true, however, that the patient who receives chronic treatment with a drug is more prone to a reaction during the first six weeks of therapy than at a later time.

ROUTE OF ADMINISTRATION

Generally speaking, the route of injection does not influence the type of allergic syndrome produced by a drug; exceptions include contact dermatitis and local reactions in muscle, subcutaneous tissue, and the gastrointestinal tract. There is some evidence that with certain drugs, the incidence of allergic reactions is relatively low when the oral route is used [63]. The explanation for this phenomenon is not entirely clear, however, and it may be unwise to assume that this would hold true for all drugs. For example, one might visualize the following as possible factors in the reported low incidence of reactions to oral penicillin: (1) A course of orally administered penicillin often has been associated with lower blood levels than those obtained by the parenteral route (poor absorption and omission of dose in some subjects). This is less true with the newer oral preparations, however. (2) The acid pH of the stomach could destroy labile precursors of antigen present as contaminants in the penicillin solution.* The relatively low incidence of anaphylaxis to penicillin given orally may relate to destruction of labile intermediates in the stomach or to a relatively low rate of absorption of penicillin (as compared to the parenteral route).†

Administration of a drug by the topical route appears to be associated with an unusually high incidence of sensitization.

ADJUVANTS

Adjuvants predispose to an increased incidence of sensitization by delaying absorption and excretion of the drug and by causing local inflammation.

HOST FACTORS

Age and Sex. Allergic reactions to drugs in general are less frequent in children than in adults [43]. It is not known whether this is due to a less vigorous antibody response in the child (owing, in part, to less previous exposure to drugs) or whether some additional step in the chain of events leading to manifestations of hypersensitivity is involved. It must be kept in mind that sensitization incurred in childhood without overt symptoms may cause serious difficulties in later life.

With a few exceptions, drug reactions appear with about equal frequency in the two sexes.

Underlying Diseases. Certain underlying diseases influence the incidence of drug allergy because the drug is metabolized or excreted more slowly (chronic hepatic and renal disease). In certain diseases, the risk of an allergic drug reaction is lessened because immune responsiveness is impaired (e.g., hypogammaglobulinemia, tumors of the hemopoietic system); nevertheless drug reactions do occur in some instances [65].

It has been suggested that subjects with systemic LE have a higher incidence of allergic drug reactions than other chronically ill patients requiring similar medications because of heightened immunological responsiveness [66]. In a recent report, however, there was no indication that the response of patients with LE to several standard antigens differed quantitatively from that of normal subjects [67].

In the patient with severe dermatitis, topical medications are more likely to sensitize [62].

The apparent increase in incidence of allergic reactions to drugs in subjects with bronchial asthma and urticaria may be due in part to the frequency with which drugs are administered to these individuals. There is little doubt, however, that certain types of serious drug reactions (e.g., anaphylaxis and angioneurotic edema) have a high incidence in patients with asthma or urticaria [40, 43]. Although special caution is desirable in the subject with an allergic history, it should be stressed that most patients with life-endangering drug reactions have no indication of an allergic background.

Genetic Factors. Apart from genetic predisposition to the development of certain diseases such as asthma and hypogammaglobulinemia, there is no clearly defined genetic influence in man on the development of drug allergy. There is little doubt, however, that such influences ultimately will be identified, because it is clear that there can be genetically determined differences in rates of metabolism of a drug among human subjects, as demonstrated in persons receiving isoniazid [68], and because genetic influences on immunological responsiveness to certain antigens have been demonstrated in animals [19, 69].

REFERENCES

1. Landsteiner, K. *The Specificity of Serological Reactions* (rev. ed.). Cambridge, Mass.: Harvard University Press, 1945.
2. Eisen, H. N. Hypersensitivity to Simple Chemicals. In Lawrence, H. S. (Ed.), *Cellular and Humoral Aspects of the Hypersensitive States.* New York: Paul B. Hoeber, Inc., 1959.
3. Gell, P. G. H., Harington, C. R., and Rivers,

* The principal acid degradation product of penicillin, penillic acid, apparently is not involved in penicillin allergy; if it were, penicillin given orally quite conceivably could lead to a greater incidence of sensitization than parenteral preparations.

† An additional factor to be considered in the immunogenicity of oral preparations are reports that adult animals fed dinitrochlorobenzene become specifically unresponsive to sensitization to dinitrochlorobenzene by the contact route or to conjugates prepared by reacting the chemical with homologous proteins [64]. The explanation for this phenomenon and its relevance to human drug allergy are not clear.

R. P. The antigenic function of simple chemical compounds: Production of precipitins in rabbits. *Brit. J. Exp. Path.* 27:267, 1946.
4. Parker, C. W., Shapiro, J., Kern, M., and Eisen, H. N. Hypersensitivity to penicillenic acid derivatives in human beings with penicillin allergy. *J. Exp. Med.* 115:821, 1962.
5. Levine, B. B., and Ovary, Z. Studies on the mechanism of formation of the penicillin antigen. III. The N-(D-α-benzylpenicilloyl) group as an antigenic determinant responsible for hypersensitivity to penicillin G. *J. Exp. Med.* 114:875, 1961.
6. Thiel, J. A., Mitchell, S., and Parker, C. W. Unpublished data, 1964.
7. Gell, P. G. H., and Benacerraf, B. Delayed hypersensitivity to simple protein antigens. *Advances Immun.* 1:319, 1961.
8. Campbell, D. H., and McCasland, G. E. *In vitro* anaphylactic response to polyhaptenic and monohaptenic simple antigens. *J. Immun.* 49:315, 1944.
9. Parker, C. W., Kern, M., and Eisen, H. N. Polyfunctional dinitrophenyl haptens as reagents for elicitation of immediate type allergic skin responses. *J. Exp. Med.* 115:789, 1962.
10. Farah, F. S., Kern, M., and Eisen, H. N. Specific inhibition of wheal-and-erythema responses with univalent haptens and univalent antibody fragments. *J. Exp. Med.* 112:1211, 1960.
11. Amkraut, A. A., Rosenberg, L. T., and Raffel, S. Elicitation of PCA by univalent and divalent haptens. *J. Immun.* 91:644, 1963.
12. Parker, C. W. Antibody-hapten Reactions as Measured by a Spectrofluorometric Method. In *Conceptual Advances in Immunology and Oncology*. New York: Hoeber Med. Div., Harper & Row, 1963.
13. Ovary, Z. *In Vitro* and *in Vivo* Interactions of Anti-hapten Antibodies with Monovalent and Bivalent Haptens (Antibodies Against the 2,4 Dinitrophenyl Group with N-2,4 Dinitrophenyl-ε-L-lysine and N-di-2,4 Dinitrophenyl-L-lysine). *Ibid.*
14. Parker, C. W. Unpublished data, 1963.
15. Benacerraf, B., and Levine, B. B. Immunological specificity of delayed and immediate hypersensitivity reactions. *J. Exp. Med.* 115: 1023, 1962.
16. Parker, C. W., DeWeck, A. L., Kern, M., and Eisen, H. N. The preparation and some properties of pencillenic acid derivatives relevant to penicillin hypersensitivity. *Ibid.*, p. 803.
17. Parker, C. W., and Thiel, J. A. Immunogenicity of penicilloyl-polylysines. *J. Lab. Clin. Med.* 62:998, 1963 (abst.).
18. Kantor, F. S., Ojeda, A., and Benacerraf, B. Studies on artificial antigens: I. Antigenicity of DNP-polylysine and DNP copolymer of lysine and glutamic acid in guinea pigs. *J. Exp. Med.* 117:55, 1963.
19. Levine, B. B., Ojeda, A., and Benacerraf, B. Basis for the antigenicity of hapten-poly-L-lysine conjugates in random-bred guinea pigs. *Nature* (London), 200:544, 1963.
20. Benacerraf, B., Ojeda, A., and Maurer, P. H. Studies on artificial antigens: II. The antigenicity in guinea pigs of arsanilic acid conjugates of copolymers of D or L-α-amino acids. *J. Exp. Med.* 118:945, 1963.
21. Clayson, D. B. *Chemical Carcinogenesis.* Boston: Little, Brown, 1962.
22. Mayer, R. L. Compounds of quinone structure as allergens and cancerogenic agents. *Experientia* 6:241, 1950.
23. Leftwich, W. B. An intradermal test for the recognition of hypersensitivity to the sulfonamide drugs. *Bull. Hopkins Hosp.* 74:26, 1944.
24. Sherman, W. B. Drug allergy. *Amer. J. Med.* 3:586, 1947.
25. Wedum, A. G. Immunological specificity of sulfonamide azoproteins. *J. Infect. Dis.* 70:173, 1942.
26. DeWeck, A. L., and Eisen, H. N. Some immunochemical properties of penicillenic acid: An antigenic determinant derived from penicillin. *J. Exp. Med.* 112:1227, 1960.
27. Levine, B. B. Studies on the mechanism of the formation of the penicillin antigen: I. Delayed allergic cross-reactions among penicillin G and its degradation products. *Ibid.*, p. 1131.
28. DeWeck, A. L. Studies on penicillin hypersensitivity: I. The specificity of rabbit "anti-penicillin" antibodies. *Int. Arch. Allerg.* 21:20, 1962.
29. Parker, C. W. Penicillin allergy. *Amer. J. Med.* 34:747, 1963 (editorial).
30. Carr, E. A. Drug allergy. *Pharmacol. Rev.* 6:365, 1954.
31. Rytel, M. W., Klion, F. M., Arlander, T. R., and Miller, L. F. Penicillin hypersensitivity with penicilloyl-polylysine. *J.A.M.A.* 186:894, 1963.
32a. Shapiro, J. Unpublished data, 1963.
32b. Summar, A. Unpublished data, 1963.
33. Ley, A. B., Harris, J. P., Brinkley, M., Liles, B., Jack, J. A., and Cahan, A. Circulating antibody directed against penicillin. *Science* 127:1118, 1958.
34. Shelley, W. B. Indirect basophil degranulation test for allergy to penicillin and other drugs. *J.A.M.A.* 184:171, 1963.
35. Thiel, J. A., and Parker, C. W. Hemagglutination studies in human penicillin allergy. Proc. Amer. Acad. Allergy 19th Annual Meeting, Montreal, Canada, 1963. Abst. 37.
36. Van Arsdel, P. P., Jr., Tobe, A. D., and Pasnick, L. J. Association of hemagglutinat-

ing antibodies with skin sensitivity in penicillin allergy. *J. Allerg.* 34:526, 1963.

37. Fireman, P., Vannier, W. E., and Goodman, H. C. The association of skin-sensitizing antibody with the B_2A globulins in sera from ragweed-sensitive patients. *J. Exp. Med.* 117:603, 1963.
38. Josephson, A. S., Franklin, E. C., and Ovary, Z. The characterization of antibodies to penicillin. *J. Clin. Invest.* 41:588, 1962.
39. Siegel, B. B., and Levine, B. B. Antigenic specificities involved in immediate systemic reactions to penicillin. Ref. 35.
40. Alexander, H. L. *Reactions with Drug Therapy*. Philadelphia: W. B. Saunders Company, 1955.
41. Feinberg, S. M. Allergy from therapeutic products. *J.A.M.A.* 178:815, 1961.
42. Brown, W. J., Simpson, W. G., and Price, E. V. Re-evaluation of reactions to penicillin in venereal disease clinic patients. *Public Health Rep.* 76:189, 1961.
43. Sherman, W. B., and Kessler, W. R. *Allergy in Pediatric Practice*. St. Louis: C. V. Mosby Company, 1957.
44. Huguley, C. M., Jr. Drug-induced Blood Dyscrasias. *Disease-A-Month.* Chicago: Year Book Medical Publishers, Inc., October, 1963.
45. Ackroyd, J. F. The immunological basis of purpura due to drug hypersensitivity. *Proc. Roy. Soc. Med.* 55:30, 1962.
46. Shulman, N. R. Immunoreactions involving platelets: I. A steric and kinetic model for formation of a complex from a human antibody quinidine, as a haptene, and platelets; and for fixation of complement by the complex. *J. Exp. Med.* 107:665, 1958.
47. Moeschlin, S. Agranulocytosis Due to Sensitivity to Drugs. In Rosenheim, M. L., and Moulton, R. (Eds.), *Sensitivity Reactions to Drugs.* Oxford: Blackwell Scientific Publications, 1958.
48. Moeschlin, S., and Wagner, K. Agranulocytosis due to the occurrence of leukocyte-agglutinins. *Acta Haemat.* 8:29, 1952.
49. Dacie, J. V. Haemolytic reaction to drugs. *Proc. Roy. Soc. Med.* 55:28, 1962.
50. Zeek, P. M. Periarteritis nodosa and other forms of necrotizing angiitis. *New Eng. J. Med.* 248:764, 1953.
51. McCombs, R. P., Patterson, J. F., and MacMahon, H. E. Syndromes associated with allergic vasculitis. *New Eng. J. Med.* 255:251, 1956.
52. Symmers, W. St. C. The occurrence of angiitis and of other generalized diseases of connective tissues as a consequence of the administration of drugs (with a note on drug allergy as a cause of thrombotic purpura). *Proc. Roy. Soc. Med.* 55:20, 1962.
53. Rose, G. A., and Spencer, H. Polyarteritis nodosa. *Quart. J. Med.* 26:43, 1957.
54. McCormick, R. V. Periarteritis occurring during propylthiouracil therapy. *J.A.M.A.* 144:1453, 1950.
55. Morrow, J. D., Schroeder, H. A., and Perry, H. M., Jr. Studies on control of hypertension by Hyphex: Toxic reactions and side effects. *Circulation* 8:829, 1953.
56. Holley, H. L. Drugs and the lupus diathesis. *J. Chron. Dis.* 17:1, 1964 (editorial).
57. Zimmerman, H. J. Drugs and the Liver. *Disease-A-Month* Chicago: Year Book Medical Publishers, Inc., May, 1963.
58. Simpson, D. G., and Walker, J. H. Hypersensitivity to para-aminosalicylic acid. *Amer. J. Med.* 29:297, 1960.
59. Baker, S. B. de C., and Williams, R. T. Acute interstitial nephritis due to drug sensitivity. *Brit. Med. J.* 1:1655, 1963.
60. Saltzstein, S. L., and Ackerman, L. V. Lymphadenopathy induced by anticonvulsant drugs and mimicking clinically and pathologically malignant lymphomas. *Cancer* 12:164, 1959.
61. Weiner, L. M., Rosenblatt, M., and Howes, H. A. The detection of humoral antibodies against salicylates in hypersensitive states. *J. Immun.* 90:788, 1963.
62. Wood, W. S., and Lepper, M. H. Drug Reactions. *Disease-A-Month.* Chicago: Year Book Medical Publishers, Inc., August, 1958.
63. Chancey, R. L., Morris, A. J., Conner, R. H., Catanzaro, F. J., Chamovitz, R., and Rammelkamp, C. H. Studies of streptococcal prophylaxis: Comparison of oral and benzathine penicillin. *Amer. J. Med. Sci.* 229:165, 1955.
64. Chase, M. W. Inhibition of experimental drug allergy by prior feeding of the sensitizing agent. *Proc. Soc. Exp. Biol. Med.* 61:257, 1946.
65. Gitlin, D., Janeway, C. A., Apt, L., and Craig, J. M. Agammaglobulinemia. Ref. 2.
66. Harvey, A. M., Shulman, L. E., Conley, C. L., and Schoenrich, E. H. Systemic lupus erythematosis: Review of the literature and clinical analysis of 138 cases. *Medicine* 33:291, 1954.
67. Muschel, L. H. Systemic lupus erythematosis and normal antibodies. *Proc. Soc. Exp. Biol. Med.* 106:622, 1961.
68. Hughes, H. B. On the metabolic fate of isoniazid. *J. Pharmacol. and Exp. Therap.* 109:444, 1953.
69. Chase, M. W. Models for Hypersensitivity Studies. Ref. 2.

60. Insect Allergy

HARRY LOUIS MUELLER

IT HAS BEEN SAID THAT BY SHEER numbers and adaptation, insects shall inherit the earth. With recent reports that the cockroach is almost impervious to irradiation, along with man's ability and threat to destroy himself by this means, such a statement may be more than idle comment. Certainly, insects have attacked man from nearly every angle, and one of their most subtle approaches, which went almost unnoticed until a relatively few years ago, is in the field of hypersensitivity. Insect allergy occurs in two major forms: the inhalant and contact type, in which bits or particles of the insect act as atopic antigens, and the stinging or biting type, in which venom or saliva is the antigen, injected through the intact skin into an individual who may or may not be atopic.

INHALANT AND CONTACT INSECT ALLERGY

The numbers of insects are so tremendous that the figures, if obtainable, would be impossible to comprehend. Their distribution ranges from the poles to the equator in both terrestrial and aquatic forms, constantly multiplying and dying to provide an antigenic litter, by their disintegration, which exposes everyone to the possibility of sensitization. Although such sensitivity frequently occurs [1], it is surprising that it does not constitute one of the commonest forms of clinical allergy when one considers the vast numbers of the class Hexapoda, with more than a million varieties and their fantastic rate of reproduction. Some insects may produce up to 40,000 eggs daily, and others with multiple progeny from 1 egg may have as many as several thousand from a dozen eggs [2].

Individually and in swarms, whole [3] or disintegrated [4], insects may produce allergic symptoms by inhalation and contact. Patients with seasonal symptoms that do not fit pollen or mold seasons should be suspected of having insect allergy. Insect activity is not limited to warm weather and to the out-of-doors. Patients with perennial symptoms may be sensitized to such indoor insects as carpet beetles, roaches, silverfish, spiders, flies, and moths. When diagnosis and treatment fail with the usual environmental allergens, one should consider and pursue the possibility that insects may be involved.

Certain orders of the Hexapoda, because of their breeding places, habits, and numbers, are probably more important than most of the others. The caddis fly of the order Trichoptera [3] and the May fly of the order Ephemeroptera [5] cause a great deal of respiratory allergy in regions where they appear in swarms, as in the Great Lakes area. However, insects of the order Orthoptera, which includes the locusts and grasshoppers, have not been shown to be frequent allergic troublemakers, although they too may appear in huge numbers.

The number and identity of the substances that cause the allergic reaction in insect-sensitive individuals have not been established, but they probably are contained in the integument. Of three substances studied, orthopodin, chitin, and sclerotin, orthopodin is the protein which most probably represents the excitant of the allergic reaction [6]. Lack of precise knowledge and the many species of insects make the selection and preparation of extracts for testing and treatment a major problem. Most allergists have used either a limited number of the commoner species or mixtures of various orders. As indicated later, in the discussion of stinging insect allergy, there probably are common antigens and cross-sensitivities at the classification level of order and possibly even a common antigen in the class Hexapoda.

Skin testing should be done first by the scratch method. If responses to scratch tests are negative, intracutaneous testing may be indicated, although false positive reactions are common by this method unless high dilutions of testing material are used [1]. In one study with use of only intracutaneous testing for ten insects, with extracts of 1 : 1,000 dilution, there were 30 positive skin reactors among 60 patients with allergic symptoms [6]. These positive results may include a large number of false positive reactions, since passive transfer was possible in only 3 subjects, whereas Feinberg *et al.* [4] obtained positive passive transfers from all of their patients who gave positive reactions to the scratch method. It has also been suggested that false positive reactions and cross-reactivity with insect extracts might be due to microbial contamination on the appendages or in the gut of the extracted insects [4, 7]. Prompt processing and careful extraction are necessary to prepare suitable material for testing and treatment [8].

If specific sensitivity to an individual insect can be demonstrated by clinical correlation, treatment by conventional hyposensitization with extracts of the insect is justified and has been shown to be successful in appreciable numbers of cases [1, 3, 5, 8]. When more than one insect of the same order are involved, mixed extracts are probably preferable, but the mixing of extracts of insects from different orders is less desirable, at least during the period of building up to maximal tolerated dosage. Skin reactions serve as a guide for the selection of starting doses, and dilutions tend to be higher than average beginning doses for pollens and molds. Constitutional reactions do not seem to occur with any greater frequency than during hyposensitization with other inhalant allergens. Perennial treatment with maintenance of maximal tolerated doses every three or four weeks during seasons of clinical symptoms and every five to six weeks out of season is recommended, but dosage and interval schedules may have to be adjusted to the results in individual patients. Success, as in all hyposensitization treatment, depends primarily on the accuracy of the diagnosis and secondarily on methods of administration.

BITING INSECT ALLERGY

The injection or deposition of foreign material by biting insects in the act of feeding is probably a universal experience. Skin reactions may be immediate or delayed. Toxicity has been thought to play a part, but allergy is accepted as playing the more important role [9]. Allergic reactions to the bites of insects are usually induced by the injected saliva, which prevents clotting and facilitates feeding. The mechanisms vary according to the mouth parts, which range from the needle form of the mosquito to the blade type of the black fly and the louse [10].

Climate governs the presence of species that are troublesome in various areas. Sand flies and black flies are very prevalent on the east coast of the United States and in the Caribbean area [11]. Fleas are a frequent problem on the west coast, as is also the conenose or kissing bug, which may cause severe systemic reactions [12]. Other insects, notably mosquitos [13, 14], various flies, and spiders [12], are the source of systemic sensitivity, and we have had four patients with unpleasant and incapacitating reactions to Diptera, none of which have been life-threatening.

The reactions to biting insects are usually urticarial and may be followed by papular, vesicular, or eczematous lesions accompanied by edema and erythema resembing cellulitis. Papular urticaria in children is almost always due to insect bites, chiefly involving bed bugs or fleas. Sensitivity may develop rapidly on initial exposure, but some individuals lose much of their sensitivity through prolonged contact with the offending insect. Attempts at hyposensitization by use of insect extracts have met with some success and are justified when reactions are very troublesome and exposure to the insect cannot be avoided. Whole body insect extracts are employed in the same manner as that described for the treatment of inhalant insect allergy, with dose and time intervals adjusted to the clinical response. Local applications and internally administered antiallergic drugs are not consistently helpful in preventing reactions or relieving symptoms in biting insect allergy except for the use of sympathomimetic drugs for systemic anaphylactic reactions.

Thiamine hydrochloride taken internally has been reported to be a repellant for mosquitoes [15] and fleas [16]. In our experience, over 70 percent of 100 insect-sensitive patients given doses of 75 to 150 mg. of thiamine hydrochloride daily reported that insects bothered them little or not at all while taking it, but the effect wore off rapidly if the thiamine was omitted.

STINGING INSECT ALLERGY

The recording of instances of allergy to stinging insects began in 2641 B.C. with hieroglyphics in the tomb of an Egyptian king depicting the occupant's fatal wasp sting [17]. Scattered reports of sudden death from insect stings appeared in the medical literature during the Nineteenth Century, and Gould and Pyle [18] listed one dating back to 1811. Poisonous effects of venom were the suspected cause and the subject of various investigations until 1914, when the anaphylactic nature of these reactions was recognized by Waterhouse [19].

Although Braun [20] in 1925 described the progressive severity of reactions and successful desensitization of a patient, it was the classic paper of Benson and Seminov [21] in 1930 that stimulated the many therapeutic and immunological studies of insect allergy in the past 30 years. Questions arose over the relative protective values of venom and whole body extract and the use of single species or mixed extracts. Our experience with more than three hundred patients over a fifteen-year period and the published reports of others have provided information on which can be based a reasonable understanding of these problems, but there remain many unanswered questions.

Hypersensitivity to stinging insects with serious and fatal anaphylactic reactions is confined almost entirely to the order Hymenoptera, with honey bee, paper wasp, hornet, and yellow jacket providing most of the trouble since they all attack readily when disturbed. The easily identifiable bumble bees, as their name implies, are rather sluggish and inoffensive, stinging rarely, and we have collected only five instances of bumble-bee stings among the many stings sustained by over three hundred insect-sensitive patients. Ants, particularly the fire ant in the southern states, have occasionally been reported to cause anaphylactic reactions [12, 22–24].

Since stinging insects inject venom into their victims, it is obvious that the venom contains the sensitizing antigens, but venom also contains many other substances, possibly including microorganisms. It has been suggested that pollen adhering to the shaft of the stinger could be the cause of reactions in pollen-sensitive patients, but pollen has not been found on the stingers of these insects. Venom is formed by an acid gland and an alkaline gland, with the injected fluid being a mixture of products of the two glands that may vary in composition, concentration, and proportion. This variation may possibly explain the occasional history of patients who had a systemic reaction to a sting, then little or no reaction to a subsequent sting by what was probably the same species, whereas a third similar sting resulted in a more severe reaction than the original one.

Studies of the biochemistry of venom and of its pharmacological effects have demonstrated the presence of histamine, serotonin, acetylcholine, and kinin, which is similar to bradykinin [25–29]. Other constituents are a hemolysin, a neurotoxin, a convulsant factor, hyaluronidase, and other enzymes. The presence of formic acid presumably accounts for most of the pain that accompanies Hymenoptera stings. For a detailed review of the chemistry and pharmacology of venom, the reader is referred to reviews by Brock [2] and to Perlman [30]. Present research, with its quantitative emphasis, may reveal compounds yet unsuspected in the venoms of Hymenoptera [29].

IMMUNOLOGY

Hypersensitivity to insects results in two types of reactions. The immediate allergic reaction, ranging from simple urticaria to anaphylactic shock, constitutes the majority and in our experience accounts for 98 percent of such reactions. Its occurrence presupposes a previous sensitizing sting. The delayed reaction, appearing in from 24 hours up to 10 days, is similar to serum sickness, with fever, joint symptoms, and urticaria, and may occur with an initial sting. A subsequent sting may then induce an immediate reaction, and indeed did in one of our six patients with delayed reactions.

Benson and Seminov [21] and Benson [31], comparing venom with extracts of whole bee bodies and bodies from which stingers and poison sacs had been removed, presented evidence that in the stinging act the venom carries with it a minute amount of antigen peculiar to the bee's body and capable of sensitizing the victim. This antigen was present throughout the bee's body and was independent of venom or pollens. Passive transfer, although difficult, was possible in some patients and was related to the immediate reaction but not to the delayed reaction. The antigen could be species- or order-specific. Rockwell and Johnson [32], working with mosquitoes, reached similar conclusions concerning the source and specificity of the antigens.

Our experience with venom and whole body extracts is similar. By comparing intracutaneous skin reactions to venom with those to whole body extract, we found that 0.5 ml. of a 1 : 100 extract of whole insect body has an antigenic content approximately equivalent to an average sting of 0.005 ml. of venom. Although almost all of the patients will have immediate skin reactions with wheal and flare on intracutaneous testing with serial dilutions of whole insect extracts [33], we have found that only 20 percent have delayed 24- to 48-hour reactions. Benson reported that all of his patients gave delayed reactions, and he considered this a more important diagnostic test than the immediate reaction. We have cautiously used much more dilute testing extracts than Benson, which might explain this difference. Positive passive transfers can be shown in some, but not all patients and are not necessarily demonstrable in the patients with positive skin tests at high dilutions. It seems to us that the amount of circulating antibody varies among patients, and at various times in the same patient.

The Hymenoptera contain some antigens in common, some antigens common to two or three species, and some antigens that are species-specific. This can be demonstrated by intracutaneous testing and subsequent sting challenge. It has been confirmed experimentally by Foubert and Stier [34], who used the Ouchterlony gel diffusion method with the serum of rabbits sensitized with antigen mixed with Freund's adjuvant and diffused against antigen from whole body extracts of each of five different Hymenoptera species. This study indicated that bee, wasp, yellow hornet, black hornet, and yellow jacket extracts each contain from four to six antigenic fractions. Probably two of these are immunologically identical in all of these insects. However, the remaining two to four antigenic fractions are either common with one or two other species or are specifically characteristic of one insect and are not shared with other species.

The same investigators [34], using guinea pigs sensitized with bee, wasp, hornet, and yellow jacket whole body antigens, shocked the animals with homologous and heterologous antigens. Homologous antigens almost uniformly produced fatal shock, whereas heterologous antigens produced anaphylaxis with a greater incidence of survival, except in yellow jacket–sensitized animals, in which shock was invariably fatal. Bee-sensitized animals had the highest survival rate when shocked with heterologous antigen. This correlates with our clinical experience that patients "probably" stung by yellow jackets have the greatest number and severity of systemic reactions to subsequent stings by any of the Hymenoptera, whereas bee-sensitized patients, easily identified among bee keepers, have the largest percentage of reports of no reaction when stung by the other Hymenoptera.

Attempts by Terr and McLean [35] to identify the antibodies in the serum of hypersensitive patients by gel diffusion studies were unsuccessful, and we, too, have been unable to demonstrate precipitins in human sera by this method. They reported, in the same paper, on passive cutaneous anaphylaxis (PCA) studies in guinea pigs, using serum from rabbits given injections of bee extract emulsified in Freund's adjuvant and challenged with bee, yellow jacket, wasp, and hornet extracts, producing pronounced reactions. However, when sera from 27 untreated patients with anaphylactic reactions to Hymenoptera stings were tested by PCA, only 16 gave positive reactions, and no correlation was found between the PCA specificity and the insect which presumably caused the clinical reaction. Patients with positive reactions to intracutaneous tests at high dilutions are almost invariably exquisitely sensitive clinically, but a few with severe clinical sensitivity show little or no skin sensitivity on direct testing. It therefore seems probable that we have not established which type of antibody is responsible for the clinical reaction. There may also be other explanations for the systemic reactions in patients who show no evidence of the presence of antibodies by direct testing or immunochemical methods.

Even less is known about the immunological mechanism developed by treatment of these patients with graduated doses of insect extracts. Since it has not been possible to measure the sensitizing antibodies *in vitro,* we have been unable to measure any changes that might be produced by treatment. Retesting of treated patients by the intracutaneous method has failed to show any consistent changes in the skin reaction even though the patients have been proved to be protected by challenging stings.

IDENTIFICATION

Most patients are sure that they know what insect caused the sting and become quite indignant when this is questioned. Actually, it is a rare individual, layman or physician, who is familiar with the intricate differentiation of the Hymenoptera. Our experience in taking careful, detailed histories from hundreds of patients indicates that most have no knowledge whatever of the identity of the stinging insect, although all have definitely preconceived ideas about it.

This is not intended to mean that careful, detailed histories are meaningless, for one can turn up useful information at times. Circumstances at the time of the sting, including evidence of a nest, numbers of insects, and presence of a stinger, are helpful in presumptive identification. Polistes wasps build open comb or mud nests in protected places, such as eaves of buildings, yellow jackets nest under the ground, and hornets build hanging papier-mâché-type nests in bushes or trees. Honey bees are the only species that leave their stinger in the victim, but these are usually brushed off by rubbing before there is careful examination of the wound.

Identification cannot be certain unless the stinging insect is captured and brought for identification. Capture of a similar insect in the area where the sting occurred is not reliable, since all of these insects may mingle in some places, particularly where food is available. Since most patients have multiple or cross-sensitivities and there is no reliable way of determining the exact situation in a given patient, it seems wise to use an extract with a mixture of the four insects in treatment of all cases.

DIAGNOSIS

The diagnosis of systemic reactions to insect stings is seldom difficult on the basis of history and physical findings, but it is likely that rapidly fatal reactions are frequently misdiagnosed, with deaths perhaps attributed to heart disease. Most fatalities from insect stings occur within 15 to 30 minutes, and the victims do not have time to summon medical aid. Parrish [36] found that 92 percent of the fatalities he gathered from studies of vital statistics occurred within 5 hours following the sting. Many of our patients with systemic reactions, particularly of the severe and shock grades, reported onset of symptoms almost immediately, and one death reported to us occurred in less than 1 minute, before the victim could take his prescribed emergency medication. This suggests that in such cases the stinger may enter a capillary or venule, and we have suspected this because some of our patients with rapid onset of symptoms have reported the appearance of a tiny drop of blood at the site of the sting.

Patients move to or take vacations in warm climates, but stings are not confined to warm seasons. For example, the polistes wasp is an indoor attic dweller at times and becomes active quickly when the heat is turned on.

Systemic reactions are occasionally preceded by increasingly large local reactions to previous stings, but many people have large local reactions to successive stings for years without ever developing systemic sensitivity. In doubtful cases, serial testing is recommended, but there are no reliable criteria for determining which local reactions are the prelude to, or a beginning of, systemic sensitivity. Most local reactions are an inflammatory response to the toxic chemical substances in the venom. Some local reactions that increase in severity over a 24- to 48-hour period with erythema, swelling, tenderness, and regional adenitis are the result of infection. Patients having had many simultaneous stings may have systemic symptoms of a toxic reaction. Their appearance is usually delayed several hours or more after the stings and may include edema (without urticaria), headache, fever, drowsiness, weakness, involuntary muscle spasm, and convulsions. Although this differentiation from allergic systemic reactions may be useful, if the question of anaphylaxis is involved, measures to combat it should be undertaken without delay, regardless of suspected toxicity. Brock [2] stated that the toxicity of venom is not great enough to account for systemic symptoms, since bee keepers may have multiple daily stings with no ill effects; but that is different from the patient who suddenly receives large numbers of stings without previous conditioning [37].

Patients with systemic allergic reactions

TABLE 60-1. Classification of 303 Patients with Systemic Reaction to Insect Stings

Grade	Percent	Signs and Symptoms
1. Slight general reaction	31	Generalized urticaria, itching, malaise, anxiety
2. General reaction	38	Any of above plus 2 or more of: generalized edema; constriction in chest; wheezing; abdominal pain, nausea, vomiting; dizziness
3. Severe general reaction	20	Any of above plus 2 or more of: dyspnea; dysphagia; hoarseness or thickened speech; confusion; feeling of impending disaster
4. Shock reaction	11	Any of above plus 2 or more of: cyanosis; fall in blood pressure; collapse; incontinence; unconsciousness

have been classified into four groups according to the severity of symptoms, as listed in Table 60-1, which shows a larger percentage of grade 1 and 2 reactions than previously reported [38]. This probably reflects increased awareness of the problem on the part of referring physicians over the past five years.

Serial intracutaneous testing [33] with graduated dilutions of whole insect extracts seems to be the best available method of determining the approximate degree of sensitivity present in a given patient at a given time. Once developed, systemic sensitivity seems to increase in severity as time passes, but it is impossible to predict the speed of this increase.

Since severe reactions have been reported in patients given intracutaneous tests with whole insect extracts in 1 : 1,000,000 dilution [33], it is wise to start with dilutions of 1 : 100,000,000 for serial testing. If one is interested in learning the various degrees of skin sensitivity to the individual insects, separate extracts of bee, polistes wasp, hornet, and yellow jacket should be used. We have required a minimal erythema of 2.0 cm. diameter at the site of testing and a negative control for interpretation as a positive test. Test sites should be examined after 24 and 48 hours for a delayed, tuberculin-type reaction.

Testing within two weeks of the acute systemic reaction is not recommended because patients may be in a refractory period with little or no available antibody to react, and give false negative reactions [33].

In general, the more severe the sting reaction, the greater the skin sensitivity, but there are exceptions. In rare cases, no skin sensitivity could be demonstrated in dilutions as concentrated as 1 : 100, yet clinical sensitivity was present, as shown by another allergic systemic reaction to a subsequent sting. Only 6 percent of patients react to one insect alone, and these are either bee or polistes wasp. Less than 3 percent of patients show no skin sensitivity, immediate or delayed. Over 75 percent with systemic reactions to insect stings have a family or personal history of allergy, and they have a higher incidence of severe sting reactions. Stinging insect hypersensitivity can occur in any individual, but atopic subjects are more likely to develop it than nonatopic individuals.

TREATMENT

In view of the life-threatening nature of these reactions, desensitization should be attempted. The principles are the same as those of desensitization to inhalants described elsewhere in this volume, but are complicated by the fact that the natural history of insect sensitivity is not clear. Therefore the apparent possibility of a sudden increase in sensitivity must be considered and may require constant re-evaluation of dosage. Moreover, the patient must at all times be prepared to handle emergencies. We know of no published studies on blocking antibody in these patients, but Barnard [39] reported a personal communication from Loveless that blocking antibody had been demonstrated after treatment with venom. Treatment seems to afford lasting protection in most patients, and for these reasons we believe it to be a form of desensitization. Dosages are suggested in Table 60-2.

Emergency kits have been recommended for self-treatment of the acute attack [2, 39, 40]. Our experience with such equipment, relying on epinephrine and a syringe, has been unsatisfactory. In many instances, when the emergency arises the individual instructed in its use for a child is not available or the reaction is so severe that the patient is too ill to accomplish self-administration. Sublingual tablets of isoproterenol, 10 or 15 mg. as indicated according to age, have provided protection until medical attention could be obtained. Epinephrine, 1 : 200 solution in a dispenser to use by inhalation, should also be kept on hand to use for obstructive respiratory symptoms and for shock. These measures are recommended not as a substitute for specific injection treatment but only for protection in the event such specific treatment is not effective. Patients who have reached a maintenance dose of injection therapy should be instructed not to take any medication if stung, unless systemic symptoms appear.

Protective measures against stinging have been advised [41]. These include the wearing of light-colored clothing, avoidance of sweaty or other objectionable odors, hair oils, and perfumes, and avoidance of rapid evasive tactics. However, treated patients should not be encouraged to avoid stings, since it is valuable for both the patient and the physician to know that the patient is protected and will not have a reaction.

TABLE 60-2. Weekly Dosage Increments for Treatment with Each Dilution of Whole Insect Body Extract

Above 1 : 100,000 (ml.)	1 : 100,000 to 1 : 100 (ml.)	1 : 10 (ml.)
0.05	0.05	0.05
0.1	0.1	0.075
0.2	0.2	0.1
0.4	0.35	0.15
	0.5	0.2
		0.25

REFERENCES

1. Feinberg, S. M., Feinberg, A. R., and Pruzansky, J. J. Insect Allergy. In Halpern, B. N., and Holtzer, A. (Eds.), *Allergology* (Proceedings of the 3rd International Congress). Paris: Éditions Médicales Flammarion, 1958. P. 293.
2. Brock, T. Résumé of insect allergy. *Ann. Allerg.* 19:288, 1961.
3. Osgood, H. Allergy to caddis fly. *J. Allerg.* 28:292, 1957.
4. Feinberg, A. R., Feinberg, S. M., and Benaim-Pinto, C. Asthma and rhinitis from insect allergens. *J. Allerg.* 27:437, 1956.
5. Figley, K. D. Asthma due to the May fly. *Amer. J. Med. Sci.* 178:338, 1929.
6. Hellreich, E. Evaluation of skin tests with insect extracts in various allergic diseases. *Ann. Allerg.* 20:805, 1962.
7. Mueller, H. L. Insect allergy. *Pediat. Clin. N. Amer.* 6:917, 1959.
8. Perlman, F. Insects as inhalant allergens. *J. Allerg.* 29:302, 1958.
9. McKiel, J. A., and West, A. S. Nature and causation of insect bite reactions. *Pediat. Clin. N. Amer.* 8:795, 1961.
10. Goldman, L., Johnson, P., and Ramsey, J. The insect bite reaction. *J. Invest. Derm.* 18: 403, 1952.
11. Arean, V. M., and Fox, I. Dermal alterations in severe reaction to the bite of the sand fly. *Amer. J. Clin. Path.* 25:1359, 1955.
12. Micks, D. Insects and other Arthopods of medical importance in Texas. *Texas Rep. Biol. Med.* 18:624, 1960.
13. Benson, R. L. Diagnosis and treatment of sensitization to mosquitos. *J. Allerg.* 8:47, 1936.
14. Rockwell, E. M. Some investigational studies concerning reactions to insect bites. *Ann. Allerg.* 10:404, 1952.
15. Shannon, W. R. Thiamine chloride as an aid in the solution of the mosquito problem. *Minnesota Med.* 26:799, 1943.

16. Eder, H. L. Flea bites: Prevention and treatment with thiamine chloride. *Arch. Pediat.* 62:300, 1945.
17. Woddell, L. S. *Egyptian Civilisation: Its Summerian Origin and Real Chronology and Summerian Origin of Egyptian Hieroglyphics.* London: Luzak & Co., 1930.
18. Gould, G. M., and Pyle, W. L. *Anomalies and Curiosities of Medicine.* Philadelphia: Saunders Company, 1900.
19. Waterhouse, A. T. Bee stings and anaphylaxis. *Lancet* 2:946, 1914.
20. Braun, L. I. B. Notes on desensitization of a patient hypersensitive to bee stings. *S. Afr. Med. Rec.* 23:408, 1925.
21. Benson, R. L., and Seminov, H. Allergy in its relation to bee sting. *J. Allerg.* 1:105, 1930.
22. Caro, M. R., Derbes, V. J., and Jung, R. Skin responses to the sting of the imported fire ant. *Arch. Derm.* 75:475, 1957.
23. Favorite, F. G. The imported fire ant. *Public Health Rep.* 73:445, 1958.
24. Allington, H. V. Ant bite. *J.A.M.A.* 176:477, 1961.
25. Flury, R. Ueber die chemische Natur des Bienengiftes. *Arch. Exp. Path.* 85:319, 1920.
26. Lyssey, R. Experimental studies on the poison of the bee. *Arch. Intern. Physiol.* 16:272, 1921.
27. Phisalix, M. *Animaux Venimeux et Venins.* Paris: Masson et Cie, 1922. Vol. I.
28. Jacques, R., and Schacter, M. The presence of histamine, 5 hydroxytryptamine and a potent, slow contracting substance in wasp venom. *Brit. J. Pharmacol.* 9:352, 1954.
29. O'Connor, R., and Rosenbrook, W. The venom of the mud dauber wasps. *Canad. J. Biochem. Physiol.* 41:1943, 1963.
30. Perlman, E. Near fatal reactions to bee and wasp stings: A review and report of seven cases. *J. Mount Sinai Hosp., N.Y.* 22:336, 1955.
31. Benson, R. L. Diagnosis of hypersensitiveness to the bee and to the mosquito. *Arch. Intern. Med.* 64:1306, 1936.
32. Rockwell, E. M., and Johnson, P. The insect bite reaction. *J. Invest. Derm.* 19:137, 1952.
33. Mueller, H. L. Serial intracutaneous testing for bee and wasp sensitivity. *J. Allerg.* 30:123, 1959.
34. Foubert, E. L., and Stier, R. A. Antigenic relationships between honeybees, wasps, yellow hornets, black hornets, and yellow jackets. *J. Allerg.* 29:13, 1958.
35. Terr, A. I., and McLean, J. A. Studies on insect sting hypersensitivity. *J. Allerg.* 35:127, 1964.
36. Parrish, H. M. Analysis of 460 fatalities from venomous animals in the United States. *Amer. J. Med. Sci.* 245:35, Feb. 1963.
37. James, E. S., and Walker, W. G. ACTH in the treatment of multiple wasp stings. *Canad. Med. Ass. J.* 67:50, 1952.
38. Mueller, H. L. Further experiences with severe allergic reactions to insect stings. *New Eng. J. Med.* 261:374, 1959.
39. Barnard, J. H. Allergic reaction to insect stings and bites. *New York J. Med.* 57:1789, 1957.
40. Shaffer, J. H. Stinging insects—A threat to life. *J.A.M.A.* 177:477, 1961.
41. Morse, R. A., and Ghent, R. L. Protective measures against stinging insects. *New York J. Med.* 59:1546, 1959.

SECTION VIII. OTHER DISEASES CAUSED BY ATOPY

61. Cerebral Allergies, Including Migraine

ARNOLD P. FRIEDMAN

DURING THE PAST FORTY YEARS, A number of investigators have implied that allergy plays an important role in headache. Studies by many competent investigators indicate that allergy is an uncommon cause of chronic, recurring headaches [1]. The exact relation of allergy to headache is difficult to define because, in an allergic individual, not all coexisting disease syndromes need be of allergic origin. Furthermore, if in a single patient some allergenic material can be shown to produce a headache, it must be understood that under different conditions the same headache can be elicited by other factors.

Accurate diagnosis of the allergic state is a delicate task. It should be emphasized again that, even in an allergic individual, the presence of headache does not necessarily indicate that it is allergic in origin. The diagnosis is established on carefully conducted exposures to the allergens, including inhalants and ingested foods.

Much of the early work regarding the role of allergy in the causation of headache was done by Pagniez *et al.* [2], who, in 1919, implicated an allergic mechanism in migraine. This was followed by the report of Vaughan [3] in the United States, who developed a concept that allergy was an important factor in the causation of most cases of migraine. He, Balyeat and Brittain [4], and Rowe [5] reported that methods based on desensitization or removal of the allergic agent were the principal factors in successful management of patients with migraine. Eyermann [6] stated that allergy played an important part in the causation of headache and that allergic headache could result from edema of the mucosa of the nose and paranasal sinuses as a result of ingestion of allergenic foods. Wolf and Unger [7] not only induced headache by feeding allergens which caused positive skin reactions but failed to induce headache by administration of harmless extracts presented to the patient as a known offending allergen. The investigation was not carried out by a double-blind control, so that their evidence is not conclusive. On the other hand, Loveless [8], in a series of well-controlled studies, gave a variety of foods in disguised forms and placebos to patients alleged to have headaches precipitated by ingestion of some of the foods administered to them. Her study did not confirm the result of previous investigators that ingestion of food was a factor in the production of headache. However, Kallós and Kallós-Deffner [9] reported that a small, highly selected group of patients had true migraine headaches induced by exposure to specific allergens (injection, inhalation, or ingestion). In these patients, headache was always associated with asthma, hay fever, and/or angioneurotic edema. Hay fever and asthma were prevented by antihistamine agents given just before injection of an allergen. The headache was not prevented. Administration of ergotamine tartrate, on the other hand, did not prevent the allergic manifestations but prevented the occurrence of migraine when the allergen was given. Walker [10] was not able to demonstrate a significant therapeutic effect of elimination diets. She stated that the occurrence of allergic phenomena in some patients was so distressing and exhausting as to constitute a sufficient basis for the precipitation of migraine by other mechanisms.

Three types of chronic, recurring headache are said to be commonly related to allergic factors: classic migraine, cluster headaches, and headaches associated with vasomotor rhinitis.

MIGRAINE

Classic Migraine. The headache is periodic and recurrent, and familial and personality factors are important in its pathogenesis. The prodromata are sharply defined and neurological in nature and are contralateral and usually visual, but may be motor or sensory. Classic migraine occurs in about 10 percent of migraine patients.

Common Migraine. The prodromata of common migraine are vague and may precede the attack by several hours or days; they may include disturbances of the psyche, the gastrointestinal tract, and fluid balance. The actual headache lasts for hours to days, with a steady unilateral aching or throbbing pain. Other symptoms—nausea, vomiting, fatigue, chills, localized or general edema, diuresis—occur, often with nasal signs that may lead the physician to believe that the nasal involvement is the cause of the headache. This type of migraine is the more common.

Both types of migraine involve the cranial vascular system. For some not fully understood reason, tensions, stresses, and emotional conflicts affect the blood vessels, but there is no clear-cut definition of the essential nature of migraine. Generally, the prodromata of most migraine headaches are assumed to be caused by vasoconstriction of cerebral blood vessels. There then follow arterial and arteriolar dilatation of the cranial vessels, local tissue changes, an increase in the number of patent capillaries, edema, and tenderness, all of which act to produce the symptoms of migraine. Arterial dilatation during the headache can be observed (and recorded) by plethysmography in the scalp and forehead, and arteriolar dilatation and increase of capillary numbers can be observed during a frontotemporal headache in the bulbar conjunctivae by means of a slit lamp [11].

The mechanism of local tissue change is thought to be the release of a polypeptide, neurokinin, which has the capacity to induce arteriolar dilatation and edema and to cause reversible tissue damage [12]. The highly localized nature of these tissue changes during headache strongly suggests that they are of neurogenic origin.

With any prolonged vascular headache, sustained contraction of the neck and scalp muscles may occur and produce "muscle-contraction" pain. The pain of migraine is transmitted to consciousness by way of the trigeminal, glosspharyngeal, vagus, and three upper cervical nerves. It is postulated that the vasodilator fibers are carried by sympathetic vasodilator neurons that originate in the motor cortex or by other cholinergic vasodilator fibers in the facial nerve. Either or both could initiate the cranial vasodilatation and local biochemical changes that cause migraine headaches.

The criteria listed in Table 61-1 help to distinguish migraine from allergic headaches. It is true that many features of the migraine attack resemble localized allergic responses, e.g., the vascular nature of the headache, the vasodilatation of the conjunctiva, and edema of the nasal mucosa, but certain differences are apparent [13] (Table 61-2). Although theoretically the concept of allergy as an etiological agent in migraine offers many hopeful and suggestive possibilities, substantial proofs are too few and inconclusive to warrant acceptance of it.

MIGRAINE HEADACHE OF THE CLUSTER TYPE

The clinical syndrome characterized by paroxysmal attacks of cluster headache has been well documented in the literature of the past 90 years under a variety of eponyms, including ciliary or migrainous neuralgia, histaminic cephalalgia, and petrosal neuralgia. Headache in cluster migraine occurs in a series of closely spaced attacks, which may be separated by headache-free periods of months or even years. Prodromata are uncommon: the onset of pain is sudden and may awaken the patient after an hour or two of sleep. Congestion, tearing, nasal stuffiness, and occasionally ptosis and miosis follow, sometimes with unilateral or bilateral sweating. The pain stops as suddenly as it begins, after 20 to 90 minutes. Men are more often affected than women, and the attacks usually occur later in life in both.

Almost as many theories of etiology exist as

TABLE 61-1. Differential Features of Allergic Headache and Migraine

General Characteristics	Allergic Headache	Migraine
Family history	Uncommon	Common
Character of pain	Variable	Pulsatile
Prodromata	Uncommon	Common
Gastrointestinal symptoms	Occasional	Common
Response to allergens, inhalants, ingestants	Common	Uncommon
Relief by allergic management	Usual	Not usual

TABLE 61-2. Differences Between Migraine and Localized Allergic Responses

Physical Characteristics	Migraine	Localized Allergic Response
Periorbital discomfort	Severe	Moderate
Eye (bulbar, conjunctival vasodilatation)	Unilateral	Bilateral
Nose (edema, hyperemia, increased secretion)	Unilateral	Bilateral
Sneezing	Rare	Common
Associated symptoms (G.I., etc.)	Prominent	Infrequent
Pharmacology		
Antihistamine	No relief	Frequent relief
Steroids	No relief	Frequent relief
Vasoconstrictors	Relief	Relief
Pathology (cellular infiltration)	Present	Present

SOURCE: Friedman [13].

authors who have described the syndrome. Most seem to agree that we are dealing with periodic attacks of local dilatation of extracranial vessels in areas mainly supplied by branches of the external carotid arteries. However, this alone does not explain the secretory phenomena and other manifestations of a disturbance in the autonomic nervous system. Again, in this type of headache, the always-appealing theory of some kind of allergy to foods or inhaled allergens as a cause has been advocated. Nevertheless the percentage of these patients who show evidence of allergy in their history or on tests is always small. Skin tests alone do not provide satisfactory evidence of food allergy in cluster headaches. Allergy and headaches may coexist. The incidence of allergy is not greater in this group than in the general population. In addition, treatment with antihistaminic drugs and dietary or other antiallergic measures has always given poor results; when successful, improvement was temporary.

The most successful treatment of an attack of cluster headache is the use of dihydroergotamine or of ergotamine tartrate by injection, inhalation, or rectal suppositories. In some patients, the inhalation of 100 percent oxygen during the headache may prove effective. As with other types of migraine headaches, interim treatment has been successful with methysergide [14].

The importance of psychological factors in patients with cluster headache presents a problem in therapy, and in a number of instances formal psychological treatment has eliminated their recurrence. However, it must be remembered that such headaches may disappear for years without any therapy.

HEADACHES DUE TO ALLERGIC RHINITIS

Engorgement of the nasal mucosa in allergic rhinitis [15] may be associated with headache. Rhinitis in adults is usually due to inhaled allergens or infection, rarely to food. The actual causative allergens may in some instances be disclosed by skin tests. Pain may result from a variety of factors, including pressure of edematous membranes, nasal polyps, or closure of the openings of the paranasal sinuses.

Severe pain in face or frontal region may occur in chronic, allergic rhinitis in which acute infections of the sinuses develop. The headache is usually bilateral and may be located in the frontal, vertex, and/or temporal region.

The presence of allergic rhinitis may be manifested by obstruction of the nares, paroxysmal sneezing, the development of a clear mucoid nasal discharge, and predominance of eosinophils in smears of the stained discharge.

On rhinoscopic examination, the mucosa is swollen and moist and of a dull, red, pearly gray color. Attention is called to the fact that both headache and allergic rhinitis are common conditions and their coexistence may suggest, but does not always have, a cause-and-effect relationship.

Headache due to rhinitis usually can be relieved temporarily by shrinkage with neosynephrine or other vasoconstrictors. Such temporary relief may be useful in judging the importance of allergy as a cause of the headache. Although allergy is not a frequent cause of chronic, recurring headache, allergic factors should be given due consideration, especially in instances of headache associated with allergic rhinitis.

EPILEPSY

Idiopathic epilepsy in some cases has been suspected of being of allergic etiology (food was the suspected allergen). In general, neither allergists nor neurologists have been enthusiastic about this possibility. Several children have been observed and reported on whose electroencephalographic abnormalities waxed and waned in the absence of or with the success of treatment of the child's allergy. Others have found no significant electroencephalographic abnormalities in children with allergic symptoms.

Prigal [16] observed that some cases of epilepsy are due to allergy and cited the following cases. As early as 1919, a case of epilepsy of six years' duration was described [17] and was finally traced to chocolate. A well-known and well-established case of chocolate allergy resulting in convulsions was described by Pardee [18], and others were collected and reported by Clarke [19]. The most extensive and critical review of the subject is that of Davison [20].

Penfield and Jasper [21] reported that an occasional, rare patient, usually a child, has convulsions associated with widespread urticaria or other symptoms of allergy. They concluded that "where there is evidence of an allergic response, particularly to certain foods, it is worthwhile trying to eliminate the offending allergens, though this is not often effective in controlling seizures."

MENIERE'S DISEASE

In a small number of patients, Meniere's disease has been attributed to foods, inhalants, and other types of allergens. It was found in only 6 percent of 350 cases studied by Wright [22]. Furthermore, Meniere's disease is not often encountered with other allergic conditions. Duke [23] was among the first to observe this combination, and Atkinson [24] and Hansel [25] commented on the significance of allergy in vertigo and Meniere's disease. In these patients, deafness, tinnitus, and paroxysmal, episodic vertigo were part of the clinical picture. Vomiting, severe nausea, sweating, bradycardia, hypotension, visual disturbances, and, occasionally, loss of consciousness may be associated with the vertigo. The deafness of Meniere's disease is of the perceptive type and affects the lower tones in the first phase between 250 and 2,000 cps. Headache may be present during the attack. It should be noted that the order of the symptoms has little significance in the diagnosis of this disease.

REFERENCES

1. Friedman, A. P., and Von Storch, T. J. C. A review of headache. *New York J. Med.* 56: 3883, 1956.
2. Pagniez, T., Valléry-Radot, P., and Nast, A. Thérapeutique préventive de certaines migraines. *Presse Med.* 27:152, 1919.
3. Vaughan, W. T. Allergic migraine. *J.A.M.A.* 88:1383, 1927.
4. Balyeat, R. M., and Brittain, F. L. Allergic migraine, based on study of 55 cases. *Amer. J. M. Sci.* 180:212, 1930.
5. Rowe, A. H. Food allergy, its manifestations, diagnosis, and treatment. *J.A.M.A.* 91:1623, 1928.
6. Eyermann, C. H. Allergic headache. *J. Allerg.* 2:106, 1931.

7. Wolf, A. A., and Unger, L. Migraine due to milk: Feeding tests. *Ann. Intern. Med.* 20:828, 1944.
8. Loveless, M. H. Milk allergy: Survey of its incidence; experiments with masked ingestion test. *J. Allerg.* 21:489, 1950.
9. Kallós, P., and Kallós-Deffner, L., Allergy and migraine. *Int. Arch. Allerg.* 7:367, 1955.
10. Walker, V. B. *Report to the Ciba Foundation Conference on Migraine,* Nov. 1960.
11. Ostfeld, A. M., and Wolff, H. G. Behavior of conjunctival vessels in vascular headache. *Trans. Amer. Neurol. Ass.* 80:216, 1955.
12. Chapman, L. F., Ramos, A. O., Goodell, H., Silverman, G., and Wolff, H. G. A humoral agent implicated in vascular headaches of migraine type. *Arch. Neurol.* 3:223, 1960.
13. Friedman, A. P. Differentiation between allergic and nonallergic headache. *New York J. Med.* 62:3105, 1962.
14. Elkind, A. H., and Friedman, A. P. A review of headache, 1955 to 1961. *New York J. Med.* 62:1649, 1962.
15. Sherman, W. B. in Friedman, A. P., and Merritt, H. H. (Eds.), *Headache: Diagnosis and Treatment,* Philadelphia: F. A. Davis Company, 1959.
16. Prigal, S. J. (Ed.) *Fundamentals of Modern Allergy.* New York: McGraw-Hill Book Company, 1960.
17. Pagniez, T., and Lieutand, P. Phénomènes de type anaphylactique dans la pathogénie de certaines crises comitiales. *Presse Med.* 27:693, 1919.
18. Pardee, I. Allergic reactions in the central nervous system: report of two cases. *Arch. Neurol. Psychiat.* 36:1360, 1938.
19. Clarke, T. W. Allergic manifestations in central nervous system. *New York J. Med.* 39: 1498, 1939.
20. Davison, H. M. Allergy of nervous system. *Quart. Rev. Allerg.* 6:157, 1952.
21. Penfield, W., and Jasper, H. *Epilepsy and the Functional Anatomy of the Human Brain.* Boston: Little, Brown, 1954.
22. Wright, A. J. Ménière's disease—critical review. *Proc. Roy. Soc. Med.* 39:809, 1946.
23. Duke, W. W. Ménière's syndrome caused by allergy. *J.A.M.A.* 81:2179, 1933.
24. Atkinson, M. Observations on the etiology and treatment of Ménière's syndrome. *J.A.M.A.* 116:1753, 1941.
25. Hansel, F. K. *Allergy of the Nose and Paranasal Sinuses.* St. Louis: C. V. Mosby Company, 1936.

62. *Atopic Diseases of the Eye*

FREDERICK H. THEODORE

IN OPHTHALMOLOGY, AS IN OTHER specialties, allergy has come to be accepted as a major etiological mechanism. An increasing number of apparently unrelated ocular disturbances can be explained on the basis of hypersensitivity. This is not surprising in view of the fact that the eye and its adnexa offer a unique opportunity to observe and study, both clinically and experimentally, all of the fundamental allergic reactions to an extent not possible elsewhere in the body. However, because ocular allergies often resemble inflammations of nonallergic origin, on many occasions allergy is not recognized when it is present or is erroneously diagnosed when it does not exist.

Most of the difficulties that arise in the recognition and classification of allergies, especially of the external eye, stem from the fact that allergy itself is not a single entity, but may assume a number of forms. If, however, the clinical manifestations of these allergies are correlated and classified in accordance with the various allergic mechanisms involved, many otherwise troublesome diagnostic problems may be clarified.

Except for the avascular vitreous body, it is now accepted that allergic reactions may occur in every ocular structure. Such reactions may be of four types: (1) atopic and anaphylactic; (2) microbiallergic, secondary to infection and infestation; (3) contact reactions, and (4) autogenous. This chapter is concerned with the first category, namely, atopic allergic reactions of the eye and its adnexa. For the purposes of differentiating such reactions from other types, tables classifying all forms of allergy that affect a particular portion of the eye are included (all tables are from Ref. 1). However, discussion is limited primarily to atopic manifestations.

ALLERGIC REACTIONS OF THE CONJUNCTIVA

The conjunctiva affords a unique site for the study of allergic reactions. The juxtaposition of readily accessible mucous membrane and the adjacent thin and delicate skin of the eyelids provides the opportunity for all types of allergic reactions to occur to an extent, and with a frequency, that do not exist elsewhere. Although the nasal mucosa is often the site of explosive air-borne allergies, contact allergy is relatively rare. The reverse is true of the skin. Only in the conjunctiva are both of these forms of allergy, as well as reactions to microbial allergens, commonly encountered (Table 62-1). Such allergic responses may result either from local exposure to excitants or as part of a generalized hypersensitivity.

ATOPIC CONJUNCTIVITIS

This conjunctival reaction, occurring in atopy and in anaphylaxis, represents an antigen-antibody response and should not be confused with the conjunctivitis associated with so-called atopic dermatitis. As indicated in Table 62-1, atopic conjunctivitis may be acute or chronic.

ACUTE ATOPIC CONJUNCTIVITIS

This is characterized by sudden or immediate hyperemia and edema. Pronounced chemosis of a "glassy" appearance occurs, associated usually with a watery, but sometimes mucopurulent, discharge. It is the conjunctival prototype of the immediate type of allergic response and usually is caused by the air-borne group of allergens, pollens, animal danders and feathers, mold spores, dusts, insects, and scents. The conjunctival reaction is similar to the general inflammatory edema that involves the upper respiratory tract.

A similar picture may occur in food allergies, such as allergies to egg and milk, but in that event the ocular reaction has only a minor role in a dramatic systemic reaction. A family history of allergy (atopy) is usual.

As in the nasal symptoms of hay fever, the reaction may be so intense that a profuse mucopurulent discharge occurs. Itching and burning may be intolerable. Eosinophils are

TABLE 62-1. Conjunctival Allergy

1. Atopic conjunctivitis
   Atopic (familial history of allergy); rarely anaphylactic
   Immediate allergic response (in a few minutes) after contact
   Positive intradermal wheal reaction in 15–30 min.
   Due to inhalants (pollens, dusts, fungi, animal epidermals)
   a) Acute atopic conjunctivitis
      Major characteristics: chemosis, eosinophilia, itching, burning
   b) Chronic atopic conjunctivitis
      Major characteristics: itching, slight edema, eosinophilia
2. Microbiallergic conjunctivitis
   Atopy not essential
   Delayed allergic response
   Delayed positive intradermal reaction (24–48 hr.); immediate urticarial reaction may occur
   Due to products of microorganisms: bacteria, fungi, parasites, possibly viruses
      Major characteristics: irritation, burning, some follicles
3. Allergic dermatoconjunctivitis
   Atopy not essential
   Delayed allergic responses (24–48 hr.)
   Positive patch test in 1–5 days
   Contact allergy to locally applied drugs or chemicals
      Major characteristics: eczema, eosinophilia
4. Vernal conjunctivitis

often abundant in the secretions. The reaction usually subsides rapidly once the excitant is removed.

Skin tests of the intradermal type cause an immediate wheal response in most patients in this group. Ophthalmic tests, i.e., direct instillation of the suspected allergen in weak dilution, are generally not safe in these cases, because severe, and possibly permanent, ocular damage may result. Because of chemosis, early epidemic keratoconjunctivitis (adenovirus type 8) may be confused with acute allergic conjunctivitis. The virus infection, however, is differentiated by the presence of preauricular lymphadenopathy. Moreover, on scrapings, mononuclear cells are found instead of eosinophils.

CHRONIC ATOPIC CONJUNCTIVITIS

In contrast to the often dramatic and generally severe reactions of acute atopic conjunctivitis, the chronic form frequently shows little or no objective evidence of inflammation in comparison to the irritating subjective symptoms of itching, burning, photophobia, and dryness that are usually present [2]. As a result, the patients often are considered to be psychoneurotic or are thought to have chronic catarrhal conjunctivitis. Actually, since in many cases of chronic conjunctivitis no bacteria can be demonstrated, it may be that a significant number of such so-called cases actually are overlooked forms of chronic atopic conjunctivitis. In fact, even when the ophthalmologist is alerted to the frequency of chronic atopic conjunctivitis and performs routine epithelial scrapings, he is often surprised to find numerous eosinophils in cases that clinically did not appear to be allergic [3].

The conjunctiva often looks rather pale. A minor degree of edema may be suggested by the somewhat juicy appearance of the conjunctiva, especially in the lower fornix in its temporal portion. Although the response is essentially papillary, follicles may appear in long-standing cases, especially when there is relatively little inflammatory reaction. In other patients, with a more subacute process, there may be significant injection, as well as slight chemosis. Corresponding to the grade of the reaction in general, there may be a slight watery discharge or a mucopurulent one. In either event, eosinophils are found in epithelial scrapings, always in diagnostic numbers, although less numerous than in the acute atopic form. Chronic atopic conjunctivitis is often known as simple allergic conjunctivitis.

The diagnosis is often difficult because the

condition may resemble other forms of chronic conjunctivitis, in particular microbiallergic conjunctivitis due to staphylococci. The conjunctival inflammation often is not readily distinguished in the two types, although there generally are slight differences. However, more important than the appearance of the conjunctiva itself are the history, the finding of eosinophils, and the response to certain forms of therapy and, if possible, to elimination of the causative factor. These clues afford the framework for differentiating chronic atopic conjunctivitis from other forms of chronic inflammation of the conjunctiva.

VERNAL CONJUNCTIVITIS

This is a recurrent, bilateral, interstitial inflammation of the conjunctiva that occurs in warm weather. Although the exact cause is unknown, it is included among allergies of the eye because the condition has so many allergic facets. The most likely hypothesis is that vernal conjunctivitis is a form of physical allergy, that it is the ocular reaction to the warm season in especially predisposed atopic individuals. The disease is often confused with chronic atopic conjunctivitis.

Clinical Aspects. Vernal conjunctivitis is a disease of warm climates. In the Mediterranean area, an incidence of up to 2 percent in all patients examined in eye clinics has been reported; in New York City, the probable figure is less than one tenth of 1 percent [4]. The condition almost always affects boys more than girls, in a proportion of over 3 to 1. After puberty, the incidence is about equal in the sexes. It is a disease of childhood, with the usual age of occurrence between 6 and 20 years. Colored races are particularly prone to the limbic form of the disease. In most patients, a familial incidence is usual, with an allergic background being present more than half the time. In addition, over 50 percent of all patients with vernal conjunctivitis have other types of allergic diseases of atopic nature, such as hay fever, asthma, atopic dermatitis, and allergies to foods, dust, and molds.

The outstanding symptom of the disease is extreme itching. Photophobia is also a common complaint.

Objective Findings. Vernal conjunctivitis is a bilateral disease which occurs in two main forms: palpebral and limbal. In a significant percentage of patients a mixed type occurs in which both conjunctiva and corneal limbus show changes. The palpebral form is nearly always limited to the tarsal conjunctiva of the upper lid, where large cobblestone vegetations appear in long-standing cases. Involvement of the conjunctiva of the lower lid indicates the extreme severity of the condition in that individual.

The disease is essentially proliferative, characterized by a conspicuous and continuously increasing formation of hyalinized connective tissue. This opaque tissue imparts a milky, bluish appearance to the conjunctiva by obscuring the capillaries, which normally give it a pink color. No matter how many years' duration of other forms of allergic conjunctivitis, the capillary markings are never obliterated. Sometimes patients with subjectively very severe vernal conjunctivitis have only slight conjunctival thickening and microscopic papillae containing central blood vessels (blood points). Usually, however, the proliferation progresses to formation of the classic excrescences, which are hard, flat, large, polygonal papillae of varying size, with a predilection for the tarsus of the upper lid. In some countries, vernal conjunctivitis, because of the predominant upper lid involvement, may be confused with trachoma. When in doubt, epithelial scrapings are helpful; however, the two conditions may coexist. Follicular conjunctivitis, despite its predilection for the lower lid, true follicular character, and preauricular adenopathy, is sometimes confused with vernal conjunctivitis.

The discharge that occurs in vernal conjunctivitis has great diagnostic value. The tenacious, thick, "chewing-gum" pseudomembrane, which may be peeled off the conjunctiva without bleeding, is characteristic. Even if a membrane is not present, exposure of the everted lid, massage, or the heat of a camera light or slit lamp will result in its formation. The extremely alkaline secretion is notable for the masses of eosinophils or eosinophilic granules that it contains [5].

The limbic proliferations of the bulbar type of vernal conjunctivitis may occur without palpebral lesions. They appear as yellowish gray gelatinous elevations in the palpebral fissure zone. Tranta's dots are white points which sometimes cap the excrescences and are pathognomonic of vernal conjunctivitis. As differentiated from phlyctenules, vernal lesions do not stain with fluorescein. Furthermore, there is, in general, less inflammatory reaction than in phlyctenular keratoconjunctivitis. Conjunctival eosinophilia is a valuable differential point in diagnosis.

Corneal Lesions. The most frequent and characteristic corneal lesion of vernal catarrh is superficial epithelial keratitis, requiring biomicroscopy for its recognition, located usually in the upper half of the cornea. The cornea looks white, as if flour had been blown over it, and stains in a punctate fashion. These lesions clear rapidly as the condition improves and thus offer an excellent index of the efficacy of treatment. Other types of corneal involvement are much less common, some occurring by direct extension of the limbal process, others being deeper and central, leaving serious opacities. Still others resemble dystrophies, such as pseudogerontoxon.

Etiology. On the basis of all the clinical characteristics of the disease and its clinical course, with exacerbations during warm weather and clearing in all but the most severe cases during the winter or on migration to a cold climate, it appears that vernal conjunctivitis is a form of physical allergy to the warm season which occurs only in atopic individuals [1]. The special factors that predispose these individuals may be endocrine, metabolic, allergic, and, possibly, infectious. In some way they all combine to condition atopic individuals so that the warm season acts as a trigger mechanism setting off a kind of chain reaction that precipitates the disease.

ALLERGIC REACTIONS OF THE EYELIDS

The eyelid proper is often the site of allergic reactions. In fact, such allergies, usually of the contact variety, are so common that they would appear to constitute, at least statistically, the most important form of ocular allergy encountered in clinical practice. Atopic reactions are less common. Because the eyelids represent a transitional structure consisting of conjunctiva and skin, with the lid margin between, allergies of both the conjunctiva and the eyelids often overlap and occur at the same time (Table 62-2).

ALLERGIC EDEMA OF THE EYELIDS

Anaphylactic and atopic allergic reactions of the eyelids manifest themselves as urticaria or angioedema. Such reactions may occur in serum sickness, from insect bites, from the ingestion of various types of foods and many drugs, and sometimes, although rarely, from inhalants and contactants. Even microbial allergens, particularly fungal products, may cause urticarial reactions around the eyelids. In addition, physical agents, such as cold and sunlight, may lead to such urticaria.

ALLERGIC REACTIONS OF THE CORNEA

A large part of corneal disease is allergic in nature [6]. The cornea manifests all recognized forms of allergic reactions, including the atopic, microbial, and contact types. Furthermore, other diseases which occur in allergic individuals, such as atopic dermatitis and, possibly, rosacea, demonstrate corneal lesions.

It is interesting that some of the fundamental experimental work in ocular allergy was performed with the cornea as a shock

TABLE 62-2. Allergy of the Eyelids

1. Anaphylactic and atopic allergy (immediate)
   Allergic edema (urticaria, angioedema, serum sickness, insect bites): drugs, animal sera, etc.
2. Contact allergy (delayed)
   a) Allergic dermatoconjunctivitis: drugs, chemicals
   b) Eczematous contact dermatitis: cosmetics, drugs, chemicals, apparel
3. Microbial allergy (delayed)
   a) Infectious eczematoid dermatitis
      (1) Bacterial: staphylococci, streptococci
      (2) Fungal: trichophytosis, candidiasis
   b) Infections of lid margin (usually staphylococcal)
      (1) Blepharitis
      (2) Meibomitis
      (3) Hordeolum
      (4) Chalazion

organ. As early as 1909, Weekers [7] produced phlyctenules in rabbits sensitized to bovine tuberculosis. During the following twenty years, this work was confirmed and expanded by many investigators. Wessely [8] in 1911 was a pioneer in demonstrating that the cornea is capable of reacting anaphylactically to produce parenchymatous keratitis. Thus, two of the most important corneal diseases of that era, interstitial keratitis and phlyctenular ophthalmia, were shown to have an allergic etiology.

CLASSIFICATION OF CORNEAL ALLERGY

As in allergies of the conjunctiva, eyelids, and other parts of the eye, the various manifestations of corneal allergy are best understood when they are considered on the basis of the allergic mechanism involved. In fact, this mechanistic approach has particular advantages in regard to the cornea, because different types of allergy may cause relatively similar clinical pictures, and because the type of reaction depends to a great extent on the degree of hypersensitivity, time of exposure, and other factors which alter the clinical picture. A classification of corneal allergy is presented in Table 62-3.

ATOPIC REACTIONS

Atopic reactions of the cornea are generally caused by pollen allergy or by certain ingestants. They are chiefly superficial, although occasionally deep keratitis does occur. The location of such atopic lesions (especially those due to ingestants) are often marginal, occurring at the corneal limbus. This is to be expected, because the limbus is the site where the avascular, yet reactive, cornea is most exposed to the vascular sclera. Superficial keratitis due to atopy is much more common than reports in the literature would seem to indicate. Because of the mildness of atopic corneal reactions, few cases are referred to the ophthalmologist. Others may be missed by physicians who have no experience in the use of the slit lamp. Also, many atopic reactions are self-limited or improve with treatment of the general atopy.

Corneal Reactions to Pollens and Dust. Although the conjunctiva is commonly affected in hay fever, corneal involvement is much less frequent and occurs in more severe cases. It is usually confined to superficial keratitis with a few isolated areas which stain with fluorescein. Mild keratitis may occur in conjunctival tests with pollen extract. Such keratitis is often self-limited and responds readily to the same treatment as the conjunctivitis. This mild lesion presents no problem either diagnostically or therapeutically and should give little cause for concern. More severe reactions may occur to corn and orris root. In severe generalized hypersensitivity to dusts, the cornea may become involved.

Corneal Reactions to Ingestants. Corneal allergies due to foods are generally more severe

TABLE 62-3. Allergy of the Cornea

1. Atopic allergy (immediate)
   a) Topical allergens: superficial keratitis (rarely ulceration)
   b) Generalized allergy: superficial and marginal keratitis (rarely deep)
2. Contact allergy (delayed)
   a) Drugs: superficial keratitis, deep ulceration
   b) Other contactants: superficial keratitis, deep keratitis
3. Microbial allergy
   a) Syphilis, tubercle bacilli (other bacteria): interstitial keratitis
   b) Tubercle bacilli, staphylococci, other bacteria, *Coccidioides immitis,* nematodes: phlyctenular ophthalmia
   c) Staphylococci, bacillary dysentery: marginal infiltrates and ring ulcers
   d) Virus of herpes simplex: disciform edema of corneal stroma
4. Keratitis of possible allergic origin
   a) Vernal catarrh
   b) Keratitis with atopic dermatitis
   c) Rosacea keratitis
   d) Periarteritis nodosa
5. Allergic reactions in corneal transplants
   Interstitial keratitis

than those due to inhalants. Although they may, at times, be superficial, they tend to involve the corneal stroma. In addition, corneal allergy has been reported from the internal use of a mixture containing Phenacetin and antipyrine.

KERATITIS OF POSSIBLE ALLERGIC ORIGIN

Vernal Catarrh. Except for the limbal proliferations, corneal lesions of vernal catarrh are an often overlooked feature of the disease. They may be divided into two groups: those occurring as direct extension of the limbic and conjunctival disease, and those in which there is no such direct extension. In the first group are included crescentic, raised, fleshy processes and pannus-like formations. Lesions that do not arise from direct extension of the conjunctival process may be toxic or possibly nutritional in origin. The most important of these is superficial epithelial keratitis. Corneal ulcers and dystrophies may occur [1].

Keratitis Associated with Atopic Dermatitis. Corneal involvement of varying intensity may complicate chronic atopic dermatitis. According to Hogan [9], the corneal reaction may occur simultaneously with, or follow, repeated exacerbations of conjunctivitis. The superficial third of the periphery of the cornea is affected first. The corneal stroma near Bowman's membrane becomes clouded. The lesion gradually spreads deeper into the stroma, and, after some time, blood vessels push in from the limbus. The corneal epithelium covering the area of keratitis becomes edematous and shows minute punctate staining with fluorescein. In some instances, the entire cornea becomes hazy and vascularized, with resultant diminished visual acuity.

Two other types of corneal lesion have been described in association with atopic dermatitis. Pillat [10] reported a case with superficial punctate keratitis. In rare instances, keratoconus is associated with atopic dermatitis. Patients with this condition have severe and extensive dermatitis with lichenification and pigmentation, severe bronchial asthma, and reactions to food and inhalant allergens. It is possible that by carefully studying such cases, ophthalmologists will gain better insight into the pathogenesis of keratoconus. The latter is also a complication of vernal catarrh. Corticosteroid administration, both local and systemic, is the indicated form of treatment.

Rosacea Keratitis. The etiology of rosacea is obscure. Although a few observers maintain that it is an allergic manifestation, there is little definite substantiation.

Keratitis in Periarteritis Nodosa. Keratitis has been described as a complication of periarteritis nodosa.

Allergic Reactions in Corneal Transplants. It is probable that allergy has a role in the clouding of corneal grafts, occurring from the tenth day to the sixth week. Castroviejo [11] believes that this corneal opacification is the result of uveitis, an allergic response to foci of infection in the nose or throat. Maumenee [12], on the other hand, showed experimentally that the recipient can become sensitized to donor material following corneal transplants, and he concluded that this allergic reaction is in large measure responsible for the clouding of grafts after the tenth day.

ALLERGIC REACTIONS OF THE SCLERA

The widespread use of anti-infective agents and the control of syphilis and tuberculosis have lessened the importance of infection in the causation of scleritis. Thus, although scleritis in itself is a relatively infrequent disease, the percentage of inflammations of the sclera of probable allergic origin is very high—perhaps higher than in any other ocular structure. However, since the sclera, unlike the conjunctiva, cornea, and uvea, does not lend itself readily to experimental study, it has been largely ignored by investigators. One is forced to depend chiefly on clinical observations, which suggest that allergy is indeed an important etiological mechanism but that many instances of scleritis are best explained on the basis of microbial allergy, which does not concern us here (Table 62-4).

ATOPIC REACTIONS

Most atopic allergic reactions causing scleritis arise from foods, generally fish and especially seafood. Inhalant allergies are rare but may occur from ragweed.

ALLERGIC REACTIONS OF THE UVEA

There is substantial evidence, based on anatomical, experimental, and clinical data, that allergy has an important role in endogenous uveitis [1, 13, 14]. Anatomically the extremely

TABLE 62-4. Allergy of the Sclera

1. Atopic allergy (immediate reaction)
   a) Inhalants: episcleritis
   b) Food allergy: episcleritis
2. Microbial allergy (delayed reaction)
   a) Streptococci, staphylococci: episcleritis, scleritis
   b) Tubercle bacillus: scleritis, sclerosing keratitis
   c) Other microorganisms: episcleritis, scleritis
3. Collagen diseases (mechanism?)
   Gout, rheumatic fever, rheumatoid arthritis, periarteritis nodosa: scleritis, episcleritis

vascular uvea offers a particularly favorable site for the concentration of proteins, antigens, and antibodies originating elsewhere in the body. Furthermore, it is known that local antibody formation can and does occur in the uvea itself. Since the uvea thus affords such an ideal shock organ for the study of allergic reactions, it is not surprising that investigators in the field of immunology have utilized it experimentally in the production of allergic reactions ever since the introduction of the concept of anaphylaxis. The subject is considered in depth in Chapter 72. The classification in Table 62-5 summarizes the clinical manifestations of uveal hypersensitivity.

Anaphylactic and atopic reactions of the uvea, although rare, offer the best clinical corroboration of the impression that the uvea may participate in generalized allergic reactions. A prime example of this is uveitis complicating serum sickness [15]. Other instances of atopic allergic uveitis may result from hypersensitivity to ragweed, house dust, cat dander, and other inhalants and to foods.

ANGIOEDEMA OF THE UVEA

Acute iridocyclitis of great severity, associated with edema of the cornea and elevation of intraocular tension (secondary glaucoma), has been observed in conjunction with angioedema, on rare occasions. Several reported instances responded dramatically to antihistamines [1].

CATARACT COMPLICATING ATOPIC DERMATITIS

In severe cases of atopic dermatitis, cataracts may occur, most commonly in the third decade of life. Such cataracts may either have a classic typical appearance or be of the complicated type that occurs in a variety of general disorders. They are almost always bilateral. Although many theories concerning their causation have been advanced, none has been proved. It is believed that, like atopic dermatitis, atopic cataract may be an allergic manifestation of a relatively complex and not yet elucidated nature occurring in specially predisposed and conditioned atopic individuals. The prognosis of surgery for atopic cataracts should be guarded, because an unusually high percentage of patients develop retinal detachments after the operation.

ALLERGIC REACTIONS OF THE RETINA AND OPTIC NERVE

The optic nerve and retina are frequently the site of reactions to various types of noxious

TABLE 62-5. Allergy of the Uvea

1. Anaphylactic and atopic reactions
   Uveitis from sera, pollens, animal proteins, foods, drugs, angioedema
2. Microbiallergic reactions
   a) Nongranulomatous uveitis (allergy apparently main factor): streptococci, tubercle bacilli, staphylococci, gonococci, pneumococci
   b) Granulomatous uveitis (allergy not primary factor but may alter nature of inflammatory response): tuberculosis, syphilis, toxoplasmosis, brucellosis
3. Autogenous allergic reactions
   a) Sympathetic ophthalmia (allergy to autogenous uveal pigment)
   b) Endophthalmitis phacoanaphylactica (allergy to autogenous lens protein)

agents. Although most of such phenomena are obviously toxic in nature, often definite allergic manifestations seem to occur. In general, allergic reactions of the retina and optic nerve appear to follow the usual pattern of allergy elsewhere. Except for contact allergy, which obviously is impossible, anaphylactic, atopic, and microbiallergic reactions have been noted.

In the evaluation of reactions in the retina and optic nerve, a distinction must be made between allergy and hyperreactivity, especially in regard to drugs. For example, most individuals given large doses of atropine manifest the classic pharmacological and toxic actions of the drug, such as vomiting, tachycardia, fever, and dilatation of the pupil. When, however, an individual reacts with the same symptoms when given a very small amount of atropine, or reacts similarly after its local instillation into the eye, this is a toxic effect following a minute dose, i.e., hyperreactivity. In other words, the reaction is quantitatively different. When, however, an individual is allergic to a drug, he responds with qualitatively different symptoms, e.g., asthma, rhinitis, urticaria, skin eruptions and other accepted allergic phenomena. Examples of hyperreactivity important to the ophthalmologist occur in quinine amblyopia, reactions to minute amounts of nicotine, and following the use of atropine and cocaine. Pronounced ciliary spasms from extremely small amounts of pilocarpine and other miotics should also be noted.

In toxic and hyperreactive reactions that involve the retina and optic nerve, there is little immediate objective evidence of tissue involvement, so that diagnosis depends on subjective findings, especially in the central vision and visual fields. In most instances of neuroretinal allergy, however, reactions are exudative and hemorrhagic, so that they are readily apparent on ophthalmoscopic examination. The only major exceptions seem to be the rare cases of retrobulbar neuritis which arise on an allergic basis. Table 62-6 classifies all known instances of neuroretinal allergy.

TABLE 62-6. Neuroretinal Allergy

1. Anaphylactic and atopic reactions
   a) Serum
   b) Food
   c) Pollen
   d) Drug
   e) Angioedema and urticaria
2. Microbiallergic reactions
   a) Tuberculin
   b) Other organisms
3. Other reactions of possible allergic origin
   a) Eye changes in periarteritis nodosa
   b) Central angiospastic retinopathy

Most instances of proved neuroretinal allergy have occurred in the course of serum sickness, but with the diminishing use of antisera, this is now seldom encountered. Food allergy as a cause of neuroretinitis has been reported from peanuts, fish, chocolate, milk, eggs, and Coca-Cola. Pollen, as of primrose and ragweed, has been incriminated. Sulfonamide drugs and procaine have been observed to give rise to allergic retinal reactions. Generalized angioedema due to a variety of agents has resulted in retinal exudative lesions. Instances of retrobulbar neuritis occurring on the basis of atopic reactions have also been reported, usually due to foods.

Periarteritis nodosa may cause neuroretinal lesions, and central angiospastic retinopathy must also be included in this category.

Retinal Detachment. Some rare instances of detachment of the retina have been interpreted as allergic reactions. Unfortunately, in almost every instance only presumptive evidence was available for the diagnosis.

REFERENCES

1. Theodore, F. H., and Schlossman, A. *Ocular Allergy*. Baltimore: Williams & Wilkins Company, 1958.
2. Theodore, F. H. The classification and treatment of allergies of the conjunctiva, *Amer. J. Ophthal.* 36:1689, 1953.
3. Theodore, F. H. Epithelial Scrapings in the Differential Diagnosis of the Conjunctivides. In Sorsby, A. (Ed.), *Modern Trends in Ophthalmology*. London: Butterworth & Co., Ltd., 1955. 3rd series, p. 98.
4. Beigelman, M. N. *Vernal Conjunctivitis*. Los Angeles: University of Southern California Press, 1950.
5. Theodore, F. H. The significance of conjunctival eosinophilia in the diagnosis of al-

lergic conjunctivitis. *Eye, Ear, Nose and Throat Month.* 30:653, 1951.

6. Schlossman, A., and Theodore, F. H. The Classification of Allergies of the Cornea. In *Acta XVIII International Congress of Ophthalmology, Brussels,* 1958. Vol. 2, p. 1136. Brussels: Imprimerie Médicale et Scientifique, S.A., 1959.
7. Weekers, L. Nouvelle pathogénie des phlyctènes. *Bull. Acad. Roy. Med.* (Belg.) 23:577, 1909.
8. Wessely, K.: Ueber anaphylaktische Erscheinungen an der Hornhaut (experimentelle Erzeugung einer parenchymatösen Keratitis durch artfremdes Serum). *München. Med. Wschr.* 58:1713, 1911.
9. Hogan, M. J. Atopic keratoconjunctivitis, *Amer. J. Ophthal.* 36:937, 1953.
10. Pillat, A. Zur Mitteilung der Hornhaut beim Ekzem. *Wien. Klin. Wschr.* 50:768, 1937.
11. Castroviejo, R. Ocular allergy, cornea and lens. *Trans. Amer. Acad. Ophthal. Otolaryng.* 54:242, 1952.
12. Maumenee, A. E.: The influence of donor-recipient sensitization on corneal grafts. *Amer. J. Ophthal.* 34:142, 1951.
13. Coles, R. S., and Theodore, F. H. Clinical aspects of uveal hypersensitivity, *A.M.A. Arch. Ophthal.* 62:223, 1959.
14. Silverstein, A. M., and Zimmerman, L. E. Immunogenic endophthalmitis produced in the guinea pig by different pathogenetic mechanisms. *Amer. J. Ophthal.* 48:435, 1959.
15. Theodore, F. H., and Lewson, A. C. Bilateral iritis complicating serum sickness. *Arch. Ophthal.* 21:82, 1939.

SECTION IX. HYPERSENSITIVITY TO PHYSICAL AGENTS

63. Reactions to Light, Heat, and Trauma*

RUDOLF L. BAER AND LEONARD C. HARBER

HYPERSENSITIVITY TO LIGHT

Hypersensitivity to light, i.e., to electromagnetic radiation in the ultraviolet and visible spectral ranges, is now recognized as one of the more common causes of cutaneous pathology. The mechanism in some diseases clearly is immunological (e.g., in some cases of light urticaria, in photocontact dermatitis, and photoallergic drug eruptions). Other photosensitive eruptions are based on a nonimmunological, phototoxic mechanism (e.g., porphyria, phototoxic contact dermatitis, phototoxic drug eruptions). In still other cases the pathogenic mechanism is unknown (e.g., the very large group of polymorphous light eruptions and some cases of light urticaria). Only the major forms of allergic light hypersensitivity are discussed here.

PHOTOALLERGIC ERUPTIONS DUE TO SIMPLE CHEMICALS

These eruptions can be engendered by systemic administration (e.g., ingested and injected drugs) or by topical application of the photosensitizing agent. Since photoallergic drug reactions and photocontact dermatitis are based on similar biophysical principles, they are considered together here.

The sites of predilection of photodermatitis due to simple chemicals include the face, "V" of the neck and chest, dorsa of the hands, and extensors of the forearms. Characteristically, there is sparing of less light-exposed areas, such as the region beneath the chin and an area on the upper lip shielded by the nose. However, the eruption may involve any skin area receiving light of sufficient intensity and an appropriate concentration of the photosensitizing chemical.

In photocontact dermatitis the clinical changes are principally erythema, edema, and eczematous (papulovesicular) and less frequently bullous and papulourticarial lesions. In photoallergic eruptions due to systemically administered drugs, lichen planus-like and other changes may be seen as well. The differential diagnosis of these photoallergic eruptions includes mainly phototoxic contact dermatitis, phototoxic drug eruptions, primary irritant contact dermatitis, allergic contact dermatitis, polymorphous light eruptions, lupus erythematosus, and seborrheic dermatitis.

It has been shown experimentally in man that the events in photoallergic sensitization due to simple chemicals fulfill the established postulates for allergic sensitization with respect to induction, incubation period, spontaneous flare-up phenomenon, and reaction time [1]. The role of light as an initiator of these reactions is crucial. It has been postulated that the simple chemical agent which sets off the photoallergic reaction is converted in the skin into a new compound after it absorbs photons of actinic radiation [2]. The specific wavelength of the light spectrum absorbed is a function of the physicochemical structure of the compound and the tissue constituent with which it may have become conjugated. The newly formed compound usually is an oxidation product of the parent compound [3]. It is this newly formed substance that acts as an antigen in a small percentage of those exposed.

Experimental verification of this hypothesis

* Supported in part by grant No. DA-49-193-MD-2275 from the U.S. Army Medical Research and Development Command.

would require that if the new compound formed by the oxidative effect of light were known and could be synthesized *in vitro,* exposure to this new compound should elicit an allergic response of the same morphological variety in the photoallergic individual *even in the absence of light.* Successful achievement of this requirement has been reported in patients with sulfanilamide in the absence of light [4]. These findings require confirmation, and further studies are needed to elucidate the biochemical pathways involved in the photoallergenic activity of other simple chemical substances. Examples of drugs which are known for their capacity to engender photoallergic reactions are certain sulfonamides and chlorothiazides. Examples of contactants which are known to engender photoallergic reactions are promethazine and certain sulfonamides. It is noteworthy that some of the substances known to be precursors of photoallergens also can induce allergic contact dermatitis, a fact which tends to support the hypothesis that they have become antigens or antigenic determinants.

The photoallergic sensitivity discussed here must not be confused with phototoxic (also called phototraumatic) reactions which are produced in the skin by certain compounds such as psoralens, tetracyclines, and coal-tar derivatives. These are nonimmunological reactions [5] which almost always consist of erythema and edema and, in their more severe form, of vesiculation and bulla formation. In appropriate conditions of light exposure and concentration of the phototoxic agent, such reactions can be engendered *upon first exposure* in a high percentage (and theoretically in all) of those exposed. Their pathogenic mechanism does not require any alterations in the chemical structure of the photosensitizer, except for those which occur during the extremely short period of molecular excitation following exposure to the specific wavelengths of light. The fact that a substance has phototoxic properties does not, of course, rule out the possibility that it may also engender photoallergic reactions. Thus it has been shown that a mild phototoxic reaction occurs in practically all who are exposed to sulfanilamide plus light [1], whereas a photoallergic reaction occurs only in a very small percentage of those similarly exposed.

The essence of treatment of all forms of photosensitivity to simple chemical agents is the discovery of the offending chemical and its elimination from the patient's environment. Other therapeutic measures follow principles similar to those discussed below for light urticaria.

LIGHT URTICARIA ("SOLAR" URTICARIA)

The first definitive clinical description of light urticaria apparently was published in 1904 [6], and a year later, the first tests with light were made in a patient with solar urticaria [7]. A recent review of the world literature [8] cites more than seventy cases of light urticaria documented since that time. The clinical histories reveal that light urticaria is usually acquired in the third and fourth decades of life but that the age of onset has varied from 3 to 52 years [9, 10]. Only in one instance has the disease been reported to have occurred in more than one sibling [11].

Clinical characteristics of the eruption are remarkably uniform regardless of the causal wavelength and pathogenic mechanism. The interval between exposure to light and the first manifestation—pruritus localized to the site of exposure—often is as short as 30 seconds and usually does not exceed a few minutes. This pruritus is followed within seconds by erythema confined sharply to the light-exposed area. In a few minutes, a solid area of urticarial edema without pseudopods replaces the erythema. This is also sharply confined to the light-exposed area and is surrounded by a large axon flare (erythema) with irregular borders. Cutaneous lesions do not occur distant from the site of exposure. The lesions usually persist for 1 to 4 hours. If a sufficiently large area of the body surface is involved in the reaction, systemic manifestations, including asthma, anaphylactoid reaction, and collapse, may ensue [12]. Areas frequently exposed to light (face, dorsa of hands) usually are clinically less sensitive than other areas, probably due to absorption of light by the relatively thick horny layer and increased melanin pigment. There is no evidence that a familial or personal background of atopy is particularly common in patients with solar urticaria.

The *action spectrum,* i.e., the specific part of the light spectrum which elicits the eruption, varies according to the type of light urticaria (Table 63-1). Studies with monochromatic light have shown that an individual may have several specific eliciting wave-

TABLE 63-1. Classification of Light Urticaria

Urticaria Type	Action Spectrum (A)	Passive Transfer	Reverse Passive Transfer	Mechanism
I	2,850–3,200	Pos.	Pos.	Allergic
II	3,200–4,000	Neg.	Neg.	Unknown: no serum factor demonstrable
III	4,000–5,000	Neg.	Neg.	Unknown: no serum factor demonstrable
IV	4,000–5,000	Pos.	Neg.	Unknown: probably allergic
V	2,800–5,000	Neg.	Neg.	Unknown: no serum factor demonstrable
VI	4,000	Not Reported	Not Reported	Protoporphyrin (IX) acts as photosensitizer; immunological studies not reported

lengths, depending on the particular substance or substances which are capable of capturing the quanta of radiant energy [13, 14].

Diagnostic tests for urticaria due to light consist of exposing a skin site to a given amount of electromagnetic radiation under standard conditions. When natural sunlight is not available, fluorescent tubes have proved superior to carbon arc or hot quartz mercury vapor lamps. They emit a continuous spectrum, are readily available, relatively inexpensive, and readily standardized. Special filters (Owens-Corning) can be interposed between the light source and the skin to define accurately the action spectrum. Ordinary window glass 3 mm. thick is a crude filter, since it has the property of absorbing most ultraviolet radiation below 3,200 A. Monochromators emit extremely narrow bands of electromagnetic radiation and, though very costly, are useful for investigative purposes.

The lumbar area (Fig. 63-1) usually is the most suitable site for testing since it is normally covered and thus protected against light. In type I light urticaria, one sixtieth of an erythema dose (3.10^5 ergs/cm.^{2}) is often sufficient to elicit pruritus. In many localities in temperate zones, this corresponds approximately to less than one minute of cloudless sunshine at noon of a summer day [15]. Five to ten times this amount of radiation often suffices to evoke a wheal.

MECHANISMS

Table 63-1 shows the six types of light urticaria which are readily differentiated and the inferences regarding their etiological mechanisms. In all cases of light urticaria, it must be assumed that the absorption of elec-

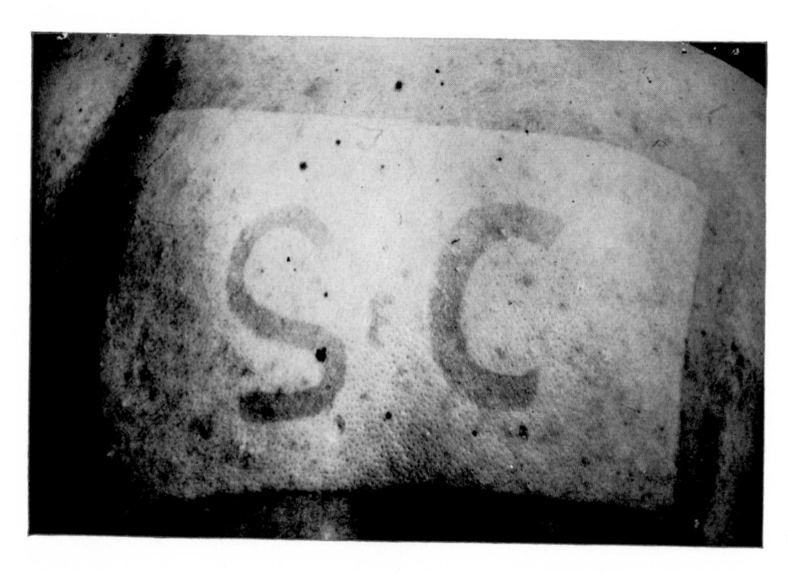

Fig. 63-1. Type I light urticaria elicited with 2,850–3,200 A radiation. There are sharply marginated edema limited to the light-exposed area and an axon flare (erythema) extending beyond the area of irradiation.

tromagnetic energy causes liberation or formation of a substance or substances in the skin capable of eliciting an urticarial response.

There is convincing evidence in some instances favoring an immunological process. It is not conceivable that quanta of radiant energy react directly with antibodies, and it has been proposed that radiation causes the release or formation of a substance in the skin which is the actual antigen involved in the immunological reaction [16, 17]. Furthermore, it seems likely in many instances that this substance is one which normally is released or formed in the skin of everyone who is exposed to the particular wavelengths of light [18]. The conclusion from this, therefore, is that the anomaly resides in an allergic sensitization to a normally occurring cutaneous metabolite to which other individuals do not form antibodies [17]. These cases represent striking examples of "autoimmune" disease. Type I would best fit in with such a concept.

In other instances, however, light urticaria might be based on release of a primary urticariogenic agent or on conversion of a precursor compound into a primary urticariogenic agent. This would not require involvement of an immunological mechanism. Type VI would best fit in with this possibility.

The following evidence supports the concept that light urticaria in some instances is based on an immediate type of allergic hypersensitivity: (1) *Passive transfer* of sensitivity by the patient's serum has been achieved in almost all cases of type I and some of type IV [19–22]. Type I passive transfer serum antibodies have characteristics apparently identical with Prausnitz-Küstner antibodies. They are found in the globulin fractions of serum proteins, are heat-labile, and are not destroyed by exposure to ultraviolet light. (2) *"Reverse" passive transfer* of sensitivity has been achieved in type I [19, 23]. Here the skin site is irradiated first and the serum is injected intradermally thirty minutes later.

The mechanism producing light urticaria types II, III, and V remains to be elucidated. No metabolic disturbances have been found, and although an allergic mechanism is possible, proof is still lacking [18, 20, 24]. Type VI light urticaria is due to disturbances in porphyrin metabolism which manifest themselves in the form of an increase in protoporphyrin [25–27]. The urinary porphyrin excretion levels remain normal, but the red blood cell and fecal protoporphyrin and the fecal coproporphyrin levels are elevated. Urticarial lesions occur on exposure to 4,000 to 4,100 A radiation, which closely corresponds to the 4,080 A absorption peak of the protoporphyrin molecule. Since studies on passive transfer, reverse passive transfer, heat lability, and so on, have not been reported, it is not possible to state whether immunological factors are involved in addition to the metabolic anomaly.

MANAGEMENT

Exposure to sunlight or other sources emitting reaction-producing wavelengths of light should be avoided as much as possible. Protective garments and other devices (e.g., veils) which cover the skin are helpful but not always practical. At times, one can augment the skin's capacity to block harmful radiation (via increase in the thickness of the horny layer and melanin pigmentation—not via specific desensitization!) by exposure first to minute amounts of radiation and then to gradually increasing doses.

Topically applied preparations which absorb or reflect light also afford partial protection in some cases. The most commonly used compounds for such protection in the 2,800 to 3,200 A ("sunburn spectrum") range are benzoic acid derivatives (e.g., para-aminobenzoic acid, glyceryl para-aminobenzoate, menthyl anthranilate, digalloyl trioleate, and phenylsalicylate). In our experience, the para-aminobenzoic acid molecule [28] is most effective [29]. The effectiveness of these compounds depends on their capacity to absorb or reflect the radiation and on various factors which influence the time during which effective concentrations remain on the skin surface (quantity, vehicle, substantivity, etc.). In light sensitivity in the spectral ranges above 3,200 A, ointments, creams, and lotions containing titanium dioxide are most effective. In some patients the reaction can be weakened by systemically administered adrenal corticosteroid, antimalarial, and antihistaminic compounds, but on the whole their therapeutic efficacy has been disappointing.

HYPERSENSITIVITY TO HEAT

Two distinct types of heat urticaria have been recognized since 1924 [30]. They are considered separately as the *localized* and the *generalized* forms.

LOCALIZED HEAT URTICARIA

In this form, the lesions are confined solely to areas exposed to heat and clinically are indistinguishable in appearance and symptomatology from urticaria due to light and cold. The incidence of this disorder appears to be exceedingly low; indeed, the number of reported cases [29, 31] is too small to permit any generalizations as to the age of onset, sex incidence, and duration. Table 63-2 gives the salient features in two of our patients. Localized urticarial lesions were induced in both patients by placing test tubes containing water at 118° F. on the flexor surface of the forearm for five minutes. In normal controls, this evoked only mild erythema. Neither patient had any evidence of cold, light, or trauma urticaria.

The etiological mechanism in localized heat urticaria is entirely unknown. In view of the resemblance in clinical appearance and symptomatology to light and cold urticaria, an allergic mechanism involving a normal metabolite, released in the skin on exposure to heat as the antigen, is an attractive hypothesis. Localized heat urticaria then would represent another instance of "autoimmune" disease. In neither of our patients nor in the few previously reported cases, however, was there any evidence of passively transferable serum antibodies.

GENERALIZED HEAT URTICARIA (CHOLINERGIC URTICARIA)

The generalized or diffuse form of heat urticaria, more aptly called cholinergic urticaria [31], is induced not only by heat but also by physical and emotional stress.

The whealing in cholinergic urticaria is very different in clinical appearance [31] from that seen in other forms of urticaria. There is a generalized eruption, most conspicuous on the trunk, which consists of discrete wheals 1 to 3 mm. in diameter surrounded by a flare of erythema up to ten times the size of the wheal. When viewed at a distance, the patient may give the appearance of having a generalized flush. Unlike cold, light, and localized heat urticaria, there is no tendency for the wheals to become confluent.

The term cholinergic urticaria has been used ever since it was shown [31, 32] that an abnormal response to acetylcholine is responsible for this type of urticarial reaction. Heating of an extremity to temperatures greater than the body temperature will not cause cholinergic urticaria if the circulation from that extremity is "occluded" by a cuff. When the cuff is released, however, a generalized reaction occurs within minutes. No lesions occur distal to the site of "occlusion," indicating that no urticariogenic agent is produced or released locally without a "central message." Whealing does occur, however, after the cuff has been released. Local and systemic reactions follow the injection of Doryl (carbamyl choline), Mecholyl (methacholine), and pilocarpine [32].

A similar mechanism can induce severe generalized itching, usually referred to as cholinergic itching [33], without urticarial lesions following exposure to heat, exercise, or emotional stimuli.

Several explanations have been offered for this abnormal response to acetylcholine and related compounds, but there is no evidence suggesting an underlying immunological reaction. Nor has it been shown that abnormally large quantities of acetylcholine are released. It is possible, however, that there is a lowered threshold of reactivity to this compound which alone is responsible for the whealing, or it may be that histamine or an H-like substance [34] is also necessary to obtain the vasodilation and whealing following antidromic impulse [35, 36]. It has been suggested also that a cholinesterase or histaminase deficiency might be the underlying defect [34]. Evidence of decreased cholinesterase levels has

TABLE 63-2. Localized Heat Urticaria in Two Patients

Sex	Age	Duration of Disease	Passive Transfer	Response to Acetylcholine and Mecholyl Injection	Response to Exercise and Emotion	History of Atopy	
						Family	Personal
F	62	24 mo.	Neg.	Normal	Normal	No	No
M	35	5 mo.	Neg.	Normal	Normal	Yes	Yes

been reported [37], although others have been unable to corroborate it.

The pathways resulting in acetylcholine release can be paraphrased as follows: Sufficient warming of a portion of the body will increase the temperature of the blood passing through that area; or increase of the general body temperature (e.g., by 0.4–1.2° F. rectally) will raise the blood temperature. When the warmed blood reaches the heat-regulating centers of the brain, excitation of the peripheral nervous system occurs with the release of acetylcholine at autonomic nerve endings. Acetylcholine or an H-like substance [34], or both, associated with its release, initiate the urticarial lesions and other symptoms of cholinergic urticaria. Since eccrine sweating is initiated via cholinergic fibers, it seems reasonable that physical and emotional stress associated with sweat-gland stimulation would be associated with urticaria in persons who have this abnormal response to acetylcholine. Furthermore, strenuous exercise could result in a sufficient increase of the body temperature to initiate the reaction at the regulatory brain center. The sequence of steps resulting from the onset of stimulation would thus include messages from the periphery via the blood stream to the brain, followed by messages from the brain via the peripheral nervous system leading to the release of acetylcholine in the skin and elsewhere. That acetylcholine release is associated with abnormal manifestations elsewhere is evident from the systemic reactions which clinically often occur with the skin lesions. These include diarrhea, abdominal cramps, syncope, general weakness, and hypersalivation [30, 31, 38].

The various methods for testing patients with cholinergic urticaria are listed in Table 63-3. The most consistent results appear to have been obtained with Mecholyl. Acetylcholine usually produces an equivocal response, probably because of its rapid hydrolysis, but may be used successfully together with physostigmine.

The ideal management of patients with localized heat urticaria is avoidance of contact with heat, and, with cholinergic urticaria, avoidance of physical and emotional stress in addition to heat. Application of cold and exposure to a cool environment appear to help in some cases. It should be noted, however, that cholinergic *and* cold urticaria in the same patient have been reported [39]. Pharmacological therapy has limited value, since the effects of antihistamines vary greatly in different patients. Trials with several compounds are suggested, however, before this therapy is abandoned.

HYPERSENSITIVITY TO TRAUMA

Cutaneous hypersensitivity reactions due to mechanical stimuli are seen in two forms. The most important, by far, is the occurrence of wheals following mechanical stimulation of the skin. This has been called variously

TABLE 63-3. Response in Localized and Cholinergic Heat Urticaria to Pharmacological and External Stimuli

			Response	
Agent	Mode of Administration	Dosage	Localized Heat Urticaria	Cholinergic Urticaria
Mecholyl	I.M.	12 mg.	Normal	Wheal
	I.D.	0.01 mg./0.05 ml.	Normal	Wheal
Pilocarpine	I.M.	5 mg.	Normal	Wheal
Histamine	I.M.	1 mg.	Normal	Normal
Acetylcholine	Iontophoresis	1/100,000	Normal	Wheal
	I.M.		Normal	Wheal
Heat	Topically	118° F, 5 min.	Wheal	Normal[a]
Exercise			Normal	Wheal
Emotion			Normal	Wheal

[a] Except when sufficiently extensive areas are exposed, resulting in elevation of blood temperature.

urticarial dermographism, urticaria factitia, and urticaria due to trauma. In parallel with our use of the terms light urticaria, cold urticaria, and so on, we will refer to this condition as trauma urticaria. The other form of hypersensitivity to mechanical stimuli is pressure urticaria, i.e., the appearance of wheals after prolonged pressure.

TRAUMA URTICARIA

The skin of all individuals responds with whealing to a sufficiently strong traumatic stimulus such as whipping or very forceful scratching. The skin of some persons, however, wheals after mild mechanical stimulation such as ordinary scratching [30]. The force required to elicit an urticarial response in such hypersensitive persons is about one-fifth that required in normal controls [40], as shown by the following procedure: a 2 mm. weighted, ball-like metal point is mechanically drawn over the skin. Normal individuals will tolerate up to 1,000 gm. of weight on the ball without whealing of the skin, whereas patients with trauma urticaria show threshold whealing with 200 gm. or less [40].

Clinically, trauma urticaria manifests itself as wheals corresponding in shape exactly to the pattern of the trauma. Because of this, the eruption is often linear. The reaction spreads at least slightly beyond the area of trauma but always retains the shape of the traumatic insult. Pseudopods are not seen. Systemic manifestations are a theoretical possibility, but we have never seen asthma or shocklike reactions, even in patients with extensive trauma urticaria. Most patients complain of more or less severe itching, but some have no itching whatever.

Trauma urticaria occurs in about 5 percent of the normal population [41, 42], with approximately the same incidence in persons with other forms of acute and chronic urticaria [40]. The condition is acquired and follows an unpredictable course of remissions and exacerbations. Contrary to earlier claims [29], there is no particular association with atopy and eosinophilia.

The pathogenic mechanism in trauma urticaria has been only partially elucidated. In close to 50 percent of the small number of subjects tested, passive transfer antibodies have been demonstrated [41, 42]. As in light urticaria, an autoimmune mechanism might be responsible. Trauma urticaria can also be demonstrated in urticaria pigmentosa (mastocytosis), e.g., in eight of eleven cases studied by us [43]. It seems possible, therefore, that some cases of trauma urticaria might be based on a cutaneous anomaly in which an excessive number of tissue mast cells are present in the skin without gross clinical evidence of urticaria pigmentosa or systemic mastocytosis.

The management of trauma urticaria, apart from avoidance of trauma, must rely mainly on antihistamine drugs. These often lessen the severity of the urticarial changes and the pruritus. Also, a temporary blocking of the whealing capacity can sometimes be engendered by deliberately producing the wheals every morning. This is done by "scrubbing" skin areas with a brush during bathing. The patient starts with one extremity, then daily treats larger skin areas until the entire trunk and the extremities are included. Whole body "scrubbing" then is continued on a daily basis.

PRESSURE URTICARIA

Pressure urticaria is inadequately studied, but it apparently is a distinct form of hypersensitive response to trauma. It is acquired, and no known genetic factors exist. It is characterized by the appearance of wheals or edematous plaques immediately following or as long as eight hours or more after persistent pressure. It may be associated with ordinary trauma urticaria [44]. The lesions may persist for periods up to 24 hours [45, 46]. The wheals and swellings have been evoked by a variety of stimuli that produce persistent pressure, including blood pressure cuffs, waist belts, sitting, and walking. The lesions occur at the sites of pressure, e.g., the arm, waist, soles, and gluteal area. Laboratory assays have shown no elevation of blood histamine levels either during or after an attack [44]. However, controlled studies have indicated that antihistamine drugs administered by mouth or by iontophoresis will diminish the intensity of the reaction [44].

REFERENCES

1. Epstein, S. Photoallergy and primary photosensitivity to sulfanilamide. *J. Invest. Derm.* 2:43, 1939.
2. Burckhardt, W. Untersuchungen über die Photoaktivität einiger Sulfanilamide. *Dermatologica* 83:63, 1941.
3. Thorpe, W. V., and Williams, R. T. Studies in detoxication: Synthesis of some possible biological oxidation products of sulphanilamide. *Biochemistry* 35:61, 1941.
4. Schwarz-Speck, M. Experimentelle Untersuchungen zur Frage der Photoallergie der Sulfonamide. *Dermatologica* 114:232, 1957.
5. Baer, R. L., and Harber, L. C. Photosensitivity to drugs: Studies in man and guinea pigs. *Arch. Derm.* 83:7, 1961.
6. Merklen, P. *Pratique dermatologique.* Paris: Masson et Cie, 1904.
7. Ward, S. B. Erythema and urticaria with a condition resembling angio-neurotic edema, caused only by exposure to the sun's rays. *New York Med. J.* 81:742, 1905.
8. Stevanovic, D. V. Urticaria solaris: A clinical and experimental study. *Acta Med. Jugosl.* 14: 144, 1960.
9. Rajka, E. *Physikalische Allergie.* Budapest: Akademiar Klads, 1950.
10. Sellei, J. Urticaria solare. *Arch. Derm. Syph.* (Berlin), 61:32, 1930.
11. Polano, K. Urticaria solare. *Dermatologica* 97:327, 1948.
12. Burckhardt, W. Ein Fall von Lichturticaria. *Dermatologica* 94:202, 1947.
13. Magnus, I. A. Action Spectra in Human Skin. In *Progress in Photobiology,* Børge Chr. Christensen and Bent Buchmann Editors (3rd International Congress). New York: Elsevier Publishing Co., P. 144, 1961.
14. Porter, A. D. Urticaria solaris. *Brit. J. Derm.* 66:417, 1954.
15. Daniels, F., Jr. Physical factors in sun exposure. *Arch. Derm.* 85:358, 1962.
16. Bernstein, F. Beitraege zu den physikalischen Idiosynkrasien der Haut: IV. Mitteilung. Spezifische Sensibilisierung als Ursache idiosynkrasischer Lichtdermatosen. *Arch. Derm. Syph.* (Berlin) 168:177, 1933.
17. Epstein, S. Allergische Lichtdermatosen. *Dermatologica* 80:291, 1939.
18. Blum, H. F., Baer, R. L., and Sulzberger, M. B. Studies in hypersensitivity to light: II. Urticaria solare ($\lambda < 3700$ A). *J. Invest. Dermat.* 7:99, 1946.
19. Epstein, S. Urticaria photogenica. *Ann. Allerg.* 7:443, 1949.
20. Rajka, E. Passive transfer in light urticaria: Pathomechanism of physical allergy. *J. Allerg.* 13:327, 1942.
21. Fidelsberger, G., and Lindemayr, W. Ueber Lichturticaria. *Int. Arch. Allerg.* 4:65, 1953.
22. Kesten, B. M. Urticaria solare (4200–4900A). *Arch. Derm. Syph.* (Chicago) 64:221, 1951.
23. Harber, L. C., Baer, R. L., Wheatley, V. R., and Holloway, R. M. Immunologic and biophysical studies in solar urticaria. *J. Invest. Derm.* 41:439, 1963.
24. Blum, H. F., and West, R.: Studies of an Urticarial Response to Blue and Violet Light in Man. *J. Clin. Invest.,* 16:261, 1937.
25. Magnus, I. A., Jarrett, A., Prankerd, R. A. J., and Rimington, C. Erythropoietic protoporphyria. *Lancet* 2:448, 1961.
26. Langhof, H., Muller, H., and Rietchel, L. Studies in familial protoporphyrinemic light urticaria. *Arch. Klin. Exp. Derm.* 212:506, 1961.
27. Redeker, A., Berke, M., and Levan, N. Erythropoietic protoporphyria with eczema solare. *Arch. Derm.* 86:569, 1962.
28. Rothman, S., and Rubin, J. Sunburn and paraaminobenzoic acid. *J. Invest. Derm.* 5:445, 1942.
29. Harber, L. C. Clinical evaluation of quantitative differences in ultraviolet absorption of compounds containing the substituted benzoic acid nucleus. *J. Invest. Derm.* 23:427, 1954.
30. Duke, W. W. Urticaria caused specifically by the action of physical agents. *J.A.M.A.* 83:3, 1924.
31. Hopkins, J. G., Kesten, B. M., and Hazel, O. G. Urticaria produced by heat or by psychic stimuli. *Arch. Derm. Syph.* (Chicago) 38:679, 1938.
32. Grant, R. T., Pearson, R. S. B., and Comeau, W. J. Observations on urticaria provoked by emotion, by exercise and by warming the body. *Clin. Sci.* 2:253, 1936.
33. Nomland, R. Cholinergic urticaria and cholinergic itching. *Arch. Derm. Syph.* (Chicago) 50:247, 1944.
34. Peters, G. A., and Silverman, J. J. The role of histamine and acetylcholine in the mechanism of heat allergy. *Arch. Intern. Med.* 77:526 1946.
35. Lewis, T., and Marvin, H. M. Observations relating to vasodilation arising from antidromic impulses to herpes zoster and trophic effects. *Heart* 14:27, 1927.
36. Lewis, T. *The Blood Vessels of the Human Skin and Their Responses.* London: Shaw & Sons, Ltd., 1927.

37. Morgan, J. K. Observations on cholinergic urticaria. *J. Invest. Derm.* 21:173, 1953.
38. Siegel, H. Urticaria caused by heat, exertion and excitement: Report on twenty-two cases among American soldiers in Japan. *Arch. Derm. Syph.* (Chicago) 57:204, 1948.
39. Rajka, E., and Vincze, E. Occurrence of urticaria (erythema) due to both cold and heat. *Acta. Allerg.* 12:30, 1958.
40. Lorincz, A. Hypersensitivity to Trauma. In Baer, R. L. (Ed.), *Allergic Dermatoses Due to Physical Agents.* New York: New York University Press, 1956, P. 11.
41. Rothman, S. Personal communication cited by Lorincz [40].
42. Walzer, A. Urticaria: III. Experimental urticaria factitia. *Arch. Derm. Syph.* (Chicago) 18:868, 1928.
43. Harber, L. C., Hyman, A. B., Morrill, S. D., and Baer, R. L. Urticaria pigmentosa, effects of reserpine. *Arch. Derm.* 83:199, 1961.
44. Kalz, F., Bower, C. M., and Prichard, H. Delayed and persistent dermographia. *Arch. Derm. Syph.* (Chicago) 61:772, 1950.
45. Rothman, S. Urticarielle Reaktionen auf Physikalische Reize. *Hautarzt* 10:4, 1959.

64. The Cryopathies

BRAM ROSE

AMONG THE PHYSICAL AGENTS CAPABLE of inducing allergy-like reactions in man, exposure to cold occupies an important position. Three conditions are recognized clinically: cold urticaria, paroxysmal hemoglobinuria, and cryoglobulinemia. Certain other cryopathies, such as the cryofibrinogenemias, cold intolerances, and occlusive arterial diseases, are not discussed in detail because this chapter deals primarily with cold urticaria: they must be kept in mind, however, and ruled out before one accepts a diagnosis of cold urticaria [1]. It has been suggested that the condition is one of true allergy [2] and more recently one of autoimmunity [3]. As will be seen, neither postulate can be substantiated fully.

COLD URTICARIA

The first record of urticaria related to cold exposure was published in 1866 by Bourdon [4], who described local and generalized manifestations in a woman. Since that time, many reports and reviews of this not uncommon condition have appeared [5, 6]. Several types are recognized, consisting of (1) localized urticaria occurring only at the point of contact, such as the hands, mouth, lips, or pharynx; (2) localized urticaria at the point of contact followed by generalized urticaria, and (3) localized urticaria followed by systemic manifestations, such as flushing, headache, nausea, vomiting, dyspnea, cough, chest pain, tachycardia, and syncope.

Generally, patients with cold urticaria are healthy, without manifestations of other diseases. However, sporadic cases associated with Raynaud's phenomenon have been described in patients with a variety of conditions such as purpura, cryoglobulinemia, and arthralgias, with multiple myeloma as the most frequently associated disease [6, 1]. Some unusual transitory cardiac abnormalities, such as altered T waves and premature beats, have been observed [7].

Cold urticaria occurs in two forms. The first is the familial, which tends to afflict several members of the family and usually begins in childhood [8, 9]. Joint pains may be present. Familial cold urticaria differs from acquired cold urticaria in two significant ways, namely, the cold test is negative, and the serum factor cannot be passively transferred (see later).

The second, and much more common, is the acquired form, which occurs equally in both sexes and has its onset at 10 to 60 years of age, the majority of patients being adults. Essentially, they complain of itchy swelling of the exposed parts of the body in cold or damp weather or when swimming in cold water. However, cases have been described in the tropics in individuals who have never traveled [10]. The inciting factor seems to be a drop in temperature only, and the actual temperature need not be low.

The onset of symptoms varies considerably, coming on during the cold in some, whereas in others the lesions appear only after the individual, having been exposed, enters a warm atmosphere. Generally, the lesions remain for an hour or two and then disappear as they came, in palindromic fashion. In the more sensitive, disturbing symptoms such as swelling of the lips, tongue, and pharynx may occur when cold foods are eaten. Drownings are presumed to have occurred, for many such individuals have been pulled out of the water covered with urticaria and in syncope [11]. As a rule, these patients are not reactive or sensitive to other physical agents, such as heat, trauma, and the sun's rays, nor do they manifest dermographism. About one-third have an atopic background, with rhinitis, asthma, and often a strong family history of allergy.

PHYSIOPATHOLOGY

The mechanism responsible for the sudden appearance of cold urticaria is obscure. Many factors have been suspected: these include viral and bacterial infection [12] and specific agents such as drugs and acetic acid [13, 19]. A well-documented case in which the condition appeared some two weeks after a bout of serum sickness subsequent to the injection of antitetanus serum has been recorded [14].

The reactions of the skin and its vasculature to cooling were studied in detail by Sir Thomas Lewis [15] and his co-workers. Their classic observations showed that in the normal subject, vasoconstriction is the prime event followed by pain and numbness of the exposed part. Fifteen to 20 minutes later, local vasodilatation supersedes vasoconstriction and produces relief from pain, redness, and rising skin temperature. The sequence requires an intact sensory innervation and is presumably dependent on an axon reflex. Temperatures must be as low as −5 to −10° C. This is in sharp contrast to the reaction observed in patients with cold hypersensitivity, in whom marked changes can occur on exposure to water at 30° C., although lower temperatures are usually required. It is also possible to

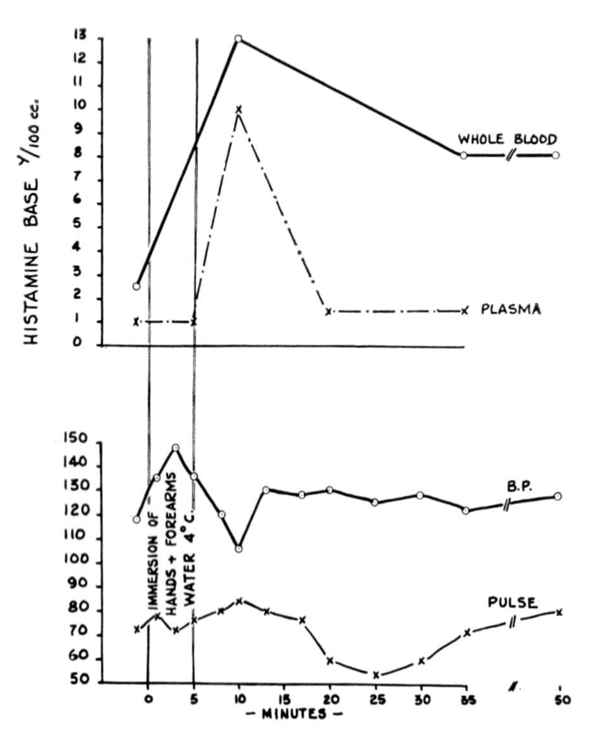

Fig. 64-1. Patient with cold urticaria. Release of histamine into the blood followed immersion of an extremity in water 4° C. for 6 minutes. Symptoms began to appear at 6–7 minutes and were at their maximum at the 20-minute period.

produce the lesion simply by placing an ice cube on the skin, usually the forearm, for 1 to 2 minutes, although from 15 to 20 seconds or less is sufficient in very sensitive subjects. In the normal subject, this gives rise only to a slight erythema which soon disappears. In sensitive individuals, a faintly erythematous swelling appears in 4 to 5 minutes, gradually increasing until an easily palpable and whitish wheal with sharply demarcated border is present only at the site of application, often extending over the area where the water has run down. In some subjects, the reaction occurs while the ice cube is in contact with the skin, but in the majority it is only after removal of the ice and rewarming that the characteristic wheal begins to form. There is generally no flare. Retesting of the site with another exposure to cold induces no response in some, but in others, a second wheal may form on top of the first, or, if the original wheal has disappeared, a fresh one forms.

Histamine release was suspected early and implicated indirectly by such means as the release of free hydrochloric acid into the gastric juice, flushing, tachycardia, and a drop of blood pressure following exposure of an extremity to water at 4° C. for 5 minutes [11]. In our own series, in which histamine contents of the whole blood and plasma were determined by the Code modification [16] of Barsoum and Gaddum's method [17] before and at intervals after the immersion of the hand and forearm in water at 4° C. for 5 minutes, a brisk release of histamine into the plasma could be observed in 5 of 10 subjects [18]. A typical example is shown in Figure 64-1. It can be seen that the histamine content of the plasma returns to normal well before the swelling is at its height. The swelling occurs universally over the exposed area and is usually maximal at 20 minutes. The dorsum of the hand may swell tremendously, so that the subject is unable to make a fist. The swelling is nonpitting and disappears within one half to three quarters of an hour. This procedure is not without hazard, for severe syncope can be produced associated with marked bradycardia (see Fig. 64-2).

An increase in the histamine content of the urine associated with histaminemia was reported by Sterky and Thoren [20], who used the method of Duner and Pernow [21] for their estimations. Similar observations have been reported by others [22], but it should be

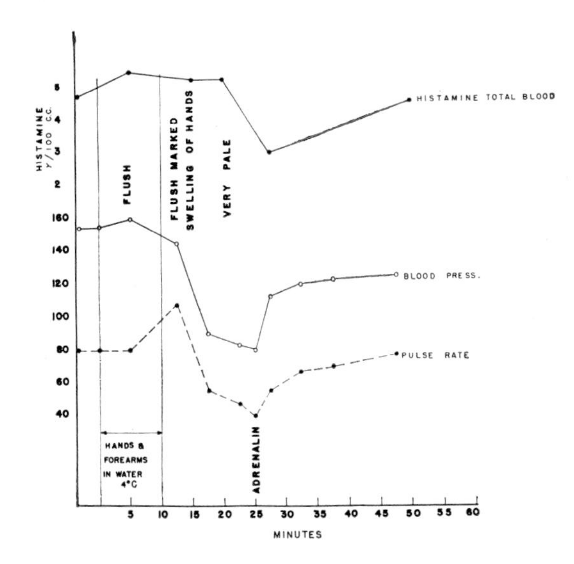

Fig. 64-2. Patient with cold urticaria. Immersion of hands and forearms for 10 minutes induced no change in blood histamine level. Marked swelling of the extremities occurred, followed by pallor, drop in BP, and pronounced bradycardia with syncope.

emphasized that the free or plasma histamine is the biologically active fraction [23].

A substantial proportion of patients do not respond to antihistaminics, and although the urticarial swellings occur in the usual fashion, there is no evidence of histamine release. Furthermore, the changes in the circulation may not be those of histamine. Such a case is illustrated in Figure 64-2. The total and blood histamine levels did not alter during exposure to cold, even though the lesions were striking. In addition, although the blood pressure fell, this was associated with profound bradycardia. It is of interest in this connection that the patient reported on by Herlitz [14] reacted to acetylcholine, which apparently reduplicated the lesions when injected intradermally. This patient was refractory to all forms of treatment save desensitization with this agent. It seems evident, therefore, that histamine release occurs in some 50 percent of patients, but other vasodilator agents such as acetylcholine and perhaps serotonin may be responsible in others.

It was shown earlier by Harris *et al.* [24] and confirmed by Sherman and Seebohm [2] as well as others [25] that one could transfer a factor in serum by the classic Prausnitz-Küstner method. Results are variable, and it has been stated that transfer is not possible in the familial form of cold urticaria. Heidelman *et al.* [22] believe that there is an allergic and a nonallergic form of cold urticaria. They were able to transfer the cold factor in the allergic type only: their patient had bronchial asthma as well as cold urticaria. The patient studied by Sherman and Seebohm was also sensitive to ragweed, which permitted a study of both ragweed reagin and the cold factor. Exhaustion of a passively transferred site with cold did not prevent the reaction to ragweed. When the serum was fractionated by free electrophoresis, ragweed reagin was localized in the γ-globulin, but none of the individual fractions were capable by themselves of passive transfer of the cold activity. Furthermore, when the serum was incubated with human skin, it was no longer capable of transferring the cold factor, although the transfer of reagin was not impaired. Samsøe-Jensen [25] was able to confirm that skin can bind the cold factor. These findings are difficult to interpret in the light of present concepts, since it is now believed that reagin is essentially a γ_{2A} fraction with high affinity for skin [26]. One would therefore have expected skin to bind both fractions. As compared to the stability of reagin, the cold factor could be demonstrated in serum for a few days only, and disappeared within a week or so when the serum was stored in the cold. Others have found it stable for longer periods [25], but the optimal time for testing was at 3 hours after transfer, although some activity could be observed as long as 24 hours with fresh serum. These findings are in considerable contrast with the properties of reagin. It is of interest that both fractions were inactivated when the serum was heated to 56° C. for 4 hours.

The fact that the reaction can be passively transferred cannot be taken as evidence that it is allergic unless one assumes that "cold" is an antigen or that the skin becomes antigenic when the temperature is lowered. It is possible that one is dealing here with a system somewhat analogous to the antibody system in paroxysmal hemoglobinuria. Such a concept would have to assume that the serum factor is an antibody with an affinity for skin to which it becomes bound when the temperature is lowered. On rewarming, the complex could then liberate the active agent in a manner similar to the Donath-Landsteiner antibody (see later).

Eosinophils implicated in allergic and histamine reactions [27, 28] have been reported to increase in the blood of a cold-sensitive patient following exposure, but our own studies carried out on five patients with cold urticaria failed to confirm these results, and opinion would seem to be divided [3]. An actual decrease of eosinophils, as well as platelets, has been reported during exposure to cold in such patients [22].

Juhlin and Shelley [3] observed degranulation and disruption of the tissue mast cells at the site of an induced lesion as well as lysis of basophils suspended in serum from patients with cold urticaria after exposure to lowered temperature.

In patients who are subject to cold urticaria, routine laboratory tests such as urinalysis, hemograms, serum electrophoresis, and blood chemical analysis of various types show values generally within normal limits. In some, cryoglobulinemia and more recently cryofibrinogenemia have been found [1]. It is of interest that histamine metabolism [29] appears to be normal.

Since other allergic manifestations coexist in a fair percentage of patients with cold urticaria, allergy has been considered a possible etiological factor. Food, pollen, as well as drugs have been implicated. It is conceivable, on the other hand, that there may be a localized hypersensitivity of the skin to histamine, similar, perhaps, to the sensitivity to histamine of the asthmatic lung as compared to the lung of normal subjects [30]. Since cold urticaria can be transferred by the Prausnitz-Küstner technique, we must assume that the serum contains a "sensitizing" factor. The nature of the factor is unknown, but other observations seem to confirm the existence of humoral substances which enhance or alter the response to histamine. Histamine injected into the skin of a normal recipient will not induce local eosinophilia. Nor does eosinophilia develop if histamine is injected into a site which has been pretreated by passive transfer of reaginic serum [31].

In the absence of demonstrable antigens, we do not have sufficient evidence to classify cold urticaria as a disease of autoimmunity.

APPROACHES TO TREATMENT

Administration of antihistaminics, if effective, is the treatment of choice. Desensitization to histamine or immersion of the extremities daily in water, gradually reducing the temperature each day until 4° C. for five minutes can be tolerated without the development of symptoms, is sometimes of use. More recently, treatment of the condition with intramuscular injections of penicillin has been reported [32]. Treatment of macrocryoglobulinemia by means of various agents such as penicillamine, penicillin intravenously, and vitamin B_6-SH is based on their ability to rupture SH bonds, thus dissociating macroglobulins into smaller components [33]. It is difficult to explain their effectiveness, since neither cryoglobulins nor macroglobulins can be demonstrated in most cases of cold urticaria.

We, as well as others [3], have been unable to alter the reaction to cold by the administration of ACTH (Duracton) in a dose of 40 units daily or of any of the orally active adrenocortical steroids in daily doses of the equivalent of 100 mg. of cortisone. This is in keeping with the observation that these compounds do not alter the conventional wheal and flare reaction due to the injection of histamine or of allergens in atopic subjects.

PAROXYSMAL COLD HEMOGLOBINURIA

Antibody systems which depend on lowering of the temperature for their activation have been recognized for many years in association with marked clinical sensitivity to cold. There are two essential forms.

COLD HEMOLYSIN SYNDROME

This syndrome, which has been termed by Witebsky [34] the disease of autoimmunity par excellence, is characterized by paroxysms of hemoglobinuria associated at times with chills, fever, malaise, and occasionally urticaria. It is quite variable and may appear in single or repeated attacks over the years whenever the weather turns cold. The attack is usually followed by the passing of dark, red or brown urine and has long been noted as a late manifestation of syphilis, acquired or congenital, with positive serologic reactions [35]. There is also a nonsyphilitic form in which severe anaphylactoid reactions and bronchial asthma have been described [36]. It is of interest that in the latter, a false positive Wassermann reaction may be present.

The underlying pathology is related to the

presence in the serum of an antibody system to red blood cells which is a hemolysin, activated by cooling to 16° C. or lower, during which time it apparently combines with the cells. Upon rewarming, hemolysis occurs. For this reason, it is referred to as a biphasic antibody. This is the so-called Donath-Landsteiner (D-L) reaction and is diagnostic for the condition [37].

The D-L antibody is much more active than the antibodies of the cold hemagglutinin syndrome at comparable titers (see below). Thus, brisk hemolysis can occur with titers in the range of 1:2 to 1:64. It is thought to be a 7S γ-globulin [38] and is not identical with Wassermann reagin (Chap. 37).

COLD HEMAGGLUTININ SYNDROME

The cold hemagglutinin syndrome represents a second type of "idiopathic" paroxysmal cold hemoglobinuria unrelated to syphilis [39]. Although cold hemagglutinins have been found in association with a number of diverse conditions, particularly virus infections, primary atypical pneumonia, malignant lymphoma, and systemic lupus erythematosus (SLE), the highest titers are found in cold hemagglutinin disease, in which values as high as 1 : 1,000,000 have been found [40]. This is in sharp contrast to those found in the cold hemolysin syndrome. Patients with the cold hemagglutinin syndrome may exhibit Raynaud's phenomenon—cyanosis as well as gangrene of an extremity or its digits. Local purpura and urticaria have been described. As with the cold hemolysin syndrome, hemolysis which may be quite profound, and hemoglobinuria may occur. Sometimes cryoglobulinemia is present.

The cold agglutinins are macroglobulins in the S19-S20 range and are nonspecific with reference to blood groups or species of erythrocytes [41]. Whereas the agglutinating effect is independent of serum complement, hemolytic activity depends on its presence. In contrast to DL antibody system, the reaction occurs simply on cooling of the serum, and rewarming is not required.

CRYOGLOBULINEMIA

The diagnosis of cryoglobulinemia is based on precipitation of protein when serum is cooled, provided the precipitate redissolves when the serum is rewarmed to body temperature. The condition may be primary, but this is uncommon. In most instances, cryoglobulinemia is associated with one of a variety of conditions, such as multiple myeloma, lymphogranuloma, Hodgkin's disease, subacute bacterial endocarditis, cirrhosis of the liver, SLE, chronic lymphatic leukemia, and kala-azar. Cold sensitivity is often a feature, and the symptoms, apart from those related to the associated disease, include purpura, epistaxis, superficial ulcers of the skin, Raynaud's phenomenon, chills, and urticarial eruptions.

Cryoglobulins may be single proteins of the 7S variety or of the 19S macroglobulin type. Some of the 19S varieties may consist of a soluble complex of 7S and 19S γ-globulins. Thus a cryoglobulin studied by LoSpalluto *et al.* [42] which was of the 22S variety could be split into two components, one of which was a 19S and the other a 7S. Neither component retained the property of precipitating in the cold, but on recombination, this was restored. Of further interest was the finding that the essential component was the 19S which, when combined with a 7S fraction from another serum, would also precipitate. However, the reverse did not occur, for when the 7S component of the original serum was combined with a 19S fraction from a second individual, no precipitation occurred on exposure to cold.

The lesions associated with cryoglobulinemia are thought to be due to local intravascular precipitation or gelification resulting in stasis and ischemia. It has also been suggested that the cryoglobulins are antigenic, leading to the formation of autoantibodies, or that histamine release consequent on the combination of the antigen with antibody may explain the chills and the urticarial reactions [41, 43]. However, the direct measurement of histamine seems for the most part to have been made in the cases of cold urticaria in which no cryoglobulins could be demonstrated. Further details on the cryoglobulins will be found elsewhere in this volume.

CRYOFIBRINOGENEMIA

Mention should be made briefly of cryofibrinogenemia, a condition first described by Korst and Kratochvil [44] in which a cryoprotein is found which, in this instance, consists of fibrinogen. Heparinized plasma is used, and on standing at 4° C., a precipitate with the properties of fibrinogen is formed. Like cryoglobulins, cryofibrinogens may be of the 7S or 19S (macro) types and redissolve if the plasma is rewarmed. These unusual proteinopathies are associated with bleeding tendencies, neoplasms in high percentage, and cold intolerance [45].

It is not known whether cryoglobulins or cryofibrinogens are related to mechanisms of hypersensitivity, but the fact that they are found in association with urticarial reactions related to cold exposure warrants their brief mention here.

REFERENCES

1. Ritzmann, S. E., and Levin, W. L. Cryopathies: A review. *Arch. Intern. Med.* 107:186, 1961.
2. Sherman, W. B., and Seebohm, P. M. Passive transfer of cold urticaria. *J. Allerg.* 21:414, 1950.
3. Juhlin, L., and Shelley, W. B. Role of mast cell and basophil in cold urticaria with associated systemic reactions. *J.A.M.A.* 177:371, 1961.
4. Bourdon, H. Note sur l'urticairea intermittent. *Bull. Mem. Soc. Med. Hop.* (Paris) 3:259, 1866.
5. Walzer, M. A critical review of the recent literature on physical allergy. *J. Allerg.* 9:64, 1937.
6. Kelly, F. J., and Wise, R. A. Observations on cold sensitivity. *Amer. J. Med.* 15:431, 1953.
7. Duke, W. W. Relationship of heat and effort sensitiveness and cold sensitiveness to functional cardiac disorders. *J. Allerg.* 4:43, 1932.
8. Kile, R. L., and Rusk, H. A. Case of cold urticaria and unusual family history. *J.A.M.A.* 114:1067, 1940.
9. Witherspoon, F. G., White, S. B., and Bazeniore, J. M. Familial urticaria due to cold. *Arch. Derm. Syph.* (Chicago) 58:52, 1948.
10. Muller, S. A. Urticarial sensitivity to cold in the tropics. *Arch. Derm.* 83:930, 1961.
11. Horton, B. T., Brown, G. E., and Roth, G. M. Hypersensitiveness to cold. *J.A.M.A.* 107:1265, 1936.
12. Kobacker, J. L., and Parkhurst, H. J. Cold urticaria following measles in three sisters. *J.A.M.A.* 105:662, 1935.
13. Herlitz, G. Cold urticaria on nutritional-allergic basis with contralateral urticarial reaction after exposure to cold. *Int. Arch. Allerg.* 4:10, 1953.
14. Herlitz, G. Cold allergy and acetyl-choline. *Ibid.*, p. 1.
15. Lewis, T. *The Blood Vessels of the Human Skin and Their Responses.* London: Shaw & Sons, Ltd., 1927.
16. Code, C. F. The quantitative estimation of histamine in the blood. *J. Physiol.* 89:257, 1937.
17. Barsoum, G. S., and Gaddum, J. H. The pharmacological estimation of adenosine and histamine in blood. *J. Physiol.* 85:1, 1935.
18. Rose, B. Unpublished results, 1948.
19. Blackman, N. S. Hypersensitivity to cold. *New York J. Med.* 59:2614, 1959.
20. Sterky, G., and Thoren, C. Cold urticaria. *Acta Paediat.* 49:185, 1960.
21. Duner, H., and Pernow, B. Determination of histamine in blood and urine by absorption on Amberlite. *Scand. J. Clin. Lab. Invest.* 10:233, 1958.
22. Heidelman, G., Preuss, E. G., and Kaiser, W. Zur Pathogenese und Klinik der Kalteurtikaria. *Deutsch. Med. Wschr.* 82:284, 1957.
23. Rose, B. Histamine, hormones and hypersensitivity. *J. Allerg.* 25:168, 1954.
24. Harris, K. E., Lewis, T., and Vaughan, J. Hemoglobinuria and urticaria from cold occurring singly or in combination. *Heart* 14:305, 1929.
25. Samsøe-Jensen, T. Cold urticaria: Report of a case: Passive transfer and *in vitro* experiments with skin cells. *Acta Dermatovener.* 35:107, 1955.
26. Stanworth, D. R. Reagins. *Brit. Med. Bull.* 19:235, 1963.
27. Kovacs, B. A. Antihistaminic effect of eosinophile leucocytes. *Experientia* 6:349, 1950.
28. Archer, R. K., Feldberg, W., and Kovacs, B. A. Antihistaminic activity in extracts of horse eosinophils. *Brit. J. Pharmacol.* 18:101, 1962.
29. Lindell, S. E., Nilsson, K., and Dorsman, H. Metabolism of histamine in cold urticaria. *J. Invest. Derm.* 36:17, 1961.
30. Rose, B., Rusted, I., and Fownes, J. A. Intravascular catheterization studies of bronchial asthma: I. Histamine levels in arterial and mixed venous blood of asthmatic patients before and during induced attacks. *J. Clin. Invest.* 29:1113, 1950.
31. Wilkinson, R., Milos, P., and Rose, B. To be published.
32. Obermayer, M. E. Treatment of cold urticaria with penicillin. *Arch. Derm.* 87:269, 1963.
33. Ritzmann, S. E., Colman, S. L., and Levin, S. C. The effect of some mercaptanes upon a macrocryogelglobulin: Modifications induced by cysteamine, penicillamine and penicillin. *J. Clin. Invest.* 39:1320, 1960.
34. Witebsky, E. Historical Roots of Present Concepts of Immunopathology. In Grabar, P., and Miescher, P. (Eds.), *Immunopathology* (2d In-

ternational Symposium). Basel: Benno Schwabe & Co., 1959.

35. Crosby, W. H. Paroxysmal nocturnal hemoglobinuria: Relation of clinical manifestations to underlying pathogenic mechanisms. *Blood* 8:769, 1953.
36. Becker, E. M. Paroxysmal cold hemoglobinurias. *Arch. Intern. Med.* 81:630, 1948.
37. Donath, J., and Landsteiner, K. Ueber paroxysmale Hämoglobinurie. *München. Med. Wschr.* 151:1590, 1904.
38. Dacie, J. V. *The Hemolytic Anemias: Congenital and Acquired.* London: J. & A. Churchill, Ltd., 1962.
39. Schubothe, H. Immunbiologische Probleme der gruppenunspezifischen Hämantikörper. *Schweiz. Med. Wschr.* 82:1102, 1952.
40. Christenson, W. N., Dacie, J. V., and Croucher, B. E. E. Electrophoretic studies on sera containing high-titre cold hemagglutinins. *Brit. J. Haemat.* 3:262, 1957.
41. Jolpe, R., Bruce-Robertson, A., Fletcher, A. A., and Charles, W. B. Essential cryoglobulinemia: Review of the literature and report of a case treated with ACTH and cortisone. *Amer. J. Med.* 20:533, 1956.
42. LoSpalluto, J., Dorward, B., Miller, W., and Ziff, M. Cryoglobulinemia based on interaction between a gamma macroglobulin and 7S gamma globulin. *Amer. J. Med.* 32:142, 1962.
43. Steinhardt, M. J., and Fisher, G. S. Cold urticaria and purpura as allergic aspects of cryoglobulinemia. *J. Allerg.* 24:335, 1953.
44. Korst, D. R., and Kratochvil, C. L. Cryofibrinogen in case of lung neoplasm associated with thrombophlebitis migrans. *Blood* 10:945, 1955.
45. McKee, P. A., Kalbfleisch, J. A., and Bird, R. M. Incidence and significance of cryofibrinogenemia. *J. Lab. Clin. Med.* 61:203, 1963.

PART FOUR: DISEASES WITH IMMUNOLOGICAL FEATURES

John H. Vaughan, Editor

Introduction

JOHN H. VAUGHAN

THIS PART DEALS WITH DISEASES OF unknown etiology, but marked by certain immunological manifestations. In some of these diseases, there is much evidence that the immunological factors contribute to pathogenesis; in others, there is little such evidence. In none of the diseases is it known that the primary etiology is immunological. Rather, evidence suggests that the immunological features often are secondary. Even so, secondary factors may contribute to pathogenesis, and it is of importance to know the extent to which this is so.

Serum sickness–like phenomena compose one form of immunological disease with which this section will deal. Serum sickness is due to exogenous antigens interacting with their antibodies in the tissues to form antigen-antibody complexes with consequent tissue damage [1]. The tissue damaged is, so to speak, an innocent bystander caught up in an immunological event not of its own making. Evidence suggests that polyarteritis may sometimes be a disease of this sort. Not only drugs or other iatrogens but conceivably also naturally invasive microbial agents may constitute the requisite exogenous antigen. Endogenous antigens, released from tissue sites recessed from the immunologically competent tissues, or "new" antigens formed from normal tissues by a denaturing process, might also react with antibodies resulting in a vasculitis similar to that in serum sickness. The nephritis of lupus erythematosus and the polyvasculitis of rheumatoid arthritis are possible examples.

The term *autoimmune* disease, by contrast, implies direct attack by immunological factors on the tissues toward which the immunological factors are directed. The concept of "autoimmunity" has gained a strong foothold in the laboratory. Experimental allergic encephalomyelitis and thyroiditis are the best-studied instances and are produced by injecting organ extracts in adjuvants into animals. Runting disease and homologous disease, which involve the implanting into tolerant animals of lymphoid tissues intolerant of the recipients, is a graft-versus-host reaction. Coombs-positive hemolytic anemia, polyarthritis, dermatitis, myocarditis, and other evidences of generalized disease develop in these animals. The fact of experimental "autoimmune" disease stands, therefore, on a firm foundation. Clinicians are now struggling with the difficulty of determining how far these examples in experimental pathology can be extrapolated into clinical pathology.

To a considerable extent, clinicians have been limited in their studies of immunological disease to the identification of antibodies that appear in the serum. We know from the experimental models, however, that serum antibodies themselves have an uncertain role in pathogenesis and that they may even in some instances protect against "autoimmune" diseases. Clinical devotees of autoimmunity have, therefore, often been inclined to regard serum autoantibodies as markers, or signals, of "autoimmunity," even though the antibodies not be themselves noxious. "Cellular hypersensitivity" then becomes the culprit; and this has been abetted by our knowledge that experimental allergic encephalomyelitis and thyroiditis can be transferred by cells but not by serum. But this orientation is a rather ill-advised convenience in that we now deal with a postulated mechanism of pathogenesis so shrouded in mystery that in man the postulate is generally untestable. As emphasized by Paterson (Chap. 71), two major uncertainties may be identified: (1) we do not know whether or not the effectiveness of the transfer of disease by cells is simply an expression of the cells' ability to make and more effectively deliver antibodies; and (2) we do not know enough about differences in cytopathogenicity of antibodies of one or another of the immunoglobulin classes or of specificity for one or another tissue antigen.

It must be noted that in some, if not all,

"autoimmune" hemolytic diseases of man (see Chap. 79), serum antibodies may indeed be autopathogenic. The Donath-Landsteiner antibody of paroxysmal cold hemoglobinuria is an example. The added prerequisite of exposure to cold need not detract from this example, but should alert us to what may be a common principle, i.e., that combinations of factors may be more important in pathogenesis than any one factor alone. It hardly need be said that this is equally true of diseases with well-established etiologies, such as tuberculosis and typhoid fever.

Thus Witebsky's postulates [2] for acceptance of a disease as an "autoimmune" disease may be difficult to fulfill in man, just as were Koch's postulates for infectious disease. Attention to Witebsky's postulates nevertheless is demanded of us, as they set a meaningful standard. The postulates are therefore given.

1. It should be possible to demonstrate either circulating antibodies, active at body temperature* in the serum of patients suffering from the disease, or cell-bound antibodies.
2. The antigen against which the antibody is directed should be characterized or even isolated.
3. Antibodies should be produced against the same antigen in experimental animals.
4. Pathological changes should appear in the corresponding tissue of an actively sensitized animal that are similar or identical to those seen in the human disease.

A word is needed in lament of the term "autoimmune." The word "immune," it will be recalled, comes from the Latin *immunis,* referring to exemption from public service. As applied in medicine, "immune" has been used to refer to exemption from infection. The term "autoimmune" does not fit this predecessor, in that the concept of protection inherent in the earlier word is reversed in the later word. The term "autoaggressive" would be better, if the presence of autoantibodies inevitably implied autopathogenicity; but autopathogenicity is not inevitable. "Autoreactive" would accommodate autoantibodies that are not autoaggressive, but this does not suit antibodies to intracellular antigens ordinarily protected from interacting with their antibodies by intact cell membranes.

For these reasons, we have recently preferred the term "autosensitivity" [3]. One definition of the word sensitivity is: "the capacity of an organism to respond to stimulation." The term "autosensitivity" suits the biological state, therefore, by implying a capacity for reaction, or a capacity for pathogenic sequelae, whether or not either of these capacities is realized. "Autoallergy" has the further implication of an *altered* capacity to respond, and some may prefer it to autosensitivity.

The diseases of "autosensitization," or "autoallergy," are an intriguing element in today's medicine. Despite the looseness of thinking and writing that has too often been evident in this field, and despite instances of regrettably careless experiment, one cannot ignore the fact that "autosensitization" exists. Its better understanding is therefore awaited with great interest.

REFERENCES

1. Dixon, F. J., Vazquez, J. J., Weigle, W. O., and Cochrane, C. G. Immunology and Pathogenesis of Experimental Serum Sickness. In Lawrence, H. S. (Ed.), *Cellular and Humoral Aspects of the Hypersensitive States.* New York: Paul B. Hoeber, Inc., 1959. P. 354.
2. Witebsky, E. Historical Roots of Present Concepts of Immunopathology. In Grabar, P., and Miescher, P. (Eds.), *Immunopathology* (1st International Symposium). Basel: Benno Schwabe & Co., 1959. P. 1.
3. Leddy, J. P., Hill, R. W., Swisher, S. N., and Vaughan, J. H. Observations on the Immunochemical Nature of Red Cell Autosensitization. In Grabar, P., and Miescher, P. (Eds.), *Immunopathology* (3rd International Symposium). Basel: Benno Schwabe & Co., 1963. P. 318.

* Which may include quite low temperatures in the superficial vessels of the skin!

65. Rheumatoid Arthritis

CHARLES L. CHRISTIAN

CLINICAL FEATURES

The term rheumatoid arthritis, introduced by Garrod a century ago, applies to a syndrome of polyarthritis which can, in most instances, be differentiated from acute rheumatic fever, gout, degenerative joint disease, pyogenic arthritis, and the other syndromes reviewed in Part IV. This chapter is limited to a review of "peripheral joint rheumatoid arthritis of adults." Juvenile rheumatoid arthritis is considered by most workers to be the childhood equivalent of this syndrome, but in several clinical respects it is unique. Rheumatoid spondylitis (Marie-Strümpell) and psoriatic arthritis are clinically distinct from peripheral joint rheumatoid arthritis and are not included in the discussion.

PROBLEM OF DEFINITION

Although precise definition of rheumatoid arthritis is lacking, a Committee of the American Rheumatism Association (ARA) proposed arbitrary criteria that have gained general acceptance. These criteria (see Reference 2) set definitions for classical, definite, probable, and possible rheumatoid arthritis. There is no problem in the recognition of classical disease, and there are relatively few uncertainties in the classification of definite rheumatoid arthritis. Diagnoses of probable and possible rheumatoid disease are arrived at largely by the process of exclusion, and it will be noted that a patient with involvement of one or more joints that persists for three weeks will arbitrarily be classified under "possible rheumatoid arthritis," if features listed under exclusions are absent. These standards, although of limited practical value, have led to somewhat improved characterization of patients included in clinical studies, and they are constant reminders of our ignorance concerning the etiology and pathogenesis of rheumatoid arthritis.

The ARA list of exclusions includes features usually associated with other connective tissue syndromes, i.e., systemic lupus erythematosus (SLE), polyarteritis, and scleroderma. Herein lies an insoluble problem. Two cases will illustrate, in part, the dilemma.

Case 1. A woman at age 35 developed symmetrical polyarthritis which involved, among other joints, those of the hands and wrists. Subsequent to sustained disease, deformities of the intercarpal, carpal-metacarpal, and interphalangeal joints developed. Subcutaneous nodules were noted, and the serological test for rheumatoid factor gave positive results. At age 47 (12 years after onset of polyarthritis), she had a febrile illness which was associated with an exacerbation of polyarthritis, pericarditis, leukopenia, and repeatedly positive results of LE tests.

There are three possible interpretations of this case: (1) the patient had two diseases, rheumatoid arthritis and SLE; (2) the patient had SLE, and the first manifestation was a polyarthritis which antedated by twelve years other features of the syndrome, and (3) the patient had rheumatoid arthritis which, in its severe systemic form, exhibited features that are commonly but not specifically associated with SLE.

Case 2. A 42-year-old man experienced fever, malaise, weight loss, and polyarthritis that fulfilled ARA criteria for definite rheumatoid arthritis. The manifestations were severe and were not controlled with a conservative medical regimen, so that adrenal corticosteroid therapy was initiated. Fifteen months after onset of the illness, he became febrile while receiving moderate doses of adrenocorticosteroids, and the following manifestations appeared: peripheral neuropathy, digital gangrene of fingers and toes, and mesenteric thrombosis which resulted in death. Postmortem examination disclosed necrotizing vascular lesions in the heart, pancreas, small intestine, and skeletal muscle which were indistinguishable from those seen in polyarteritis. The basic arguments cited regarding Case 1 are equally applicable here, and a definitive answer to the questions raised is not available.

Although each of the several connective tissue syndromes in "classical forms" can be distinguished from the others, it is apparent that their shared clinical and pathological features make syndrome-labeling of certain patients impossible. It seems likely that the arbitrary separation of such syndromes will lose significance as mechanisms of pathogenesis are elucidated.

CLINICAL MANIFESTATIONS

Constitutional symptoms (weakness, malaise, and anorexia) are frequent and may be severe, but in most patients polyarthritis is the sole objective clinical manifestation. Onset of the arthritis may be gradual or acute, the latter form resembling acute rheumatic fever. The usual features of inflammatory synovitis—pain, swelling, tenderness, warmth—are present. Fever is common in patients with acute onset. Moderate anemia (normocytic, slightly hypochromic), which is present in about one fourth of patients, usually does not respond to oral iron therapy. For reasons unknown, there is a predilection to symmetrical involvement of the small joints of the hands (particularly the proximal interphalangeal and metacarpal phalangeal joints) and the wrists, but any articular structure can be affected. Arthritis of the knees (unilateral or bilateral) occurs as the initial manifestation as commonly as hand and wrist involvement. Morning stiffness or stiffness after any period of inactivity is present in most patients. Weakness and atrophy of muscles adjacent to involved joints are usual. The muscle-wasting may result from disuse, but in some patients, striking muscle atrophy in the face of minor joint manifestations suggests that primary myopathy may be a manifestation of rheumatoid arthritis.* In 15 to 20 percent of cases, subcutaneous nodules are present. These occur predominantly over pressure points, such as the extensor aspects of the forearms. The histology of nodules (see later) is of some diagnostic importance.

Although most patients manifest only arthritis, other organ system involvement is sometimes evident. This is particularly true of subjects who exhibit features of what is commonly called "malignant rheumatoid arthritis" or "severe systemic rheumatoid disease." These are the patients who may have pleuritis, pericarditis, myocarditis, and ischemic vascular phenomena resulting in peripheral neuropathy, digital gangrene, and indolent cutaneous ulcers. The development of this type of disease seems to have increased since the advent of adrenal corticosteroid therapy, but there is no doubt that it was observed prior to the use of such drugs. The term "rheumatoid disease" has been suggested for patients with primarily nonarticular manifestations.

* In such individuals, the predominant clinical picture may be similar to that of polymyositis.

INCIDENCE, SEX, AGE, AND GENETIC CONSIDERATIONS

There are no reliable figures for the over-all incidence of rheumatoid arthritis in the United States. In the survey of a town of 9,500 individuals in Michigan, 1.24 percent of the population fulfilled ARA criteria for "definite" or "probable" rheumatoid arthritis. A collaborative study disclosed that 2 to 3 percent of each of seven European populations could be classified as having "definite" disease.

Rheumatoid arthritis is two to three times more common in females than in males. The disease occurs in individuals of all ages, but the peak incidence is in the decade from 30 to 40. In some series, a second and smaller peak has been noted in individuals 50 to 60 years of age. In a small percentage of cases of rheumatoid arthritis, multiple family members also have the disease, but in most instances, familial aggregation is not conspicuous. (See later for family studies of the rheumatoid factor.)

NATURAL HISTORY

The most extensive prospective study of rheumatoid arthritis was based on 293 cases followed at the Massachusetts General Hospital. From this and other studies, the following generalizations can be made: (1) The clinical course is highly variable: in some patients, manifestations are almost subclinical; in others, a rapid progression into severe disability occurs. (2) The prognosis for an individual patient at the outset of the disease is not predictable, but "classical" disease and seropositivity early in the course are significantly associated with sustained disease and hence a poorer prognosis. In a statistical sense, seronegative status at the outset favors an intermittent course, and therefore a better prognosis. (3) Spontaneous remissions and exacerbations occur in most patients. Remissions, which may be complete and persist for many years, can occur at any time, but they are infrequent in patients who have experienced sustained disease for years and are common in patients who have had the disease for less than one year. (4) The life span is not much shortened, and the causes of death, with a few exceptions, are not different from those in a random population. The exceptions are amyloidosis and the visceral manifestations of diffuse vasculitis ("severe systemic disease"). (5) In general, about 50 percent of patients with rheumatoid arthritis maintain fair to good functional capacity and can lead nearly normal lives; about 25 percent are partially incapacitated and, with sustained or intermittent disease, experience slowly progressing disability; and about 25 percent do poorly and lead greatly restricted lives. A small proportion (less than 10 percent) are totally disabled.

PATHOLOGY

Synovial Membranes. These membranes are inflamed, the intensity and character varying with duration and severity of the disease. Early lesions consist of nonspecific synovitis with polymorphonuclear cells and plasmacytes, and a villous or papillary thickening of the synovial structures. A vascular granulation tissue (pannus) deriving from the chronically inflamed synovium extends over the articular cartilage and erodes into the subchondral base. It is the destructive potential of the pannus which accounts for the deformities of chronic rheumatoid arthritis. Synovial membranes of tendon sheaths may demonstrate all of the foregoing features of the articular synovium.

Muscle. Nonspecific mononuclear infiltrates in a perivascular distribution have been observed with some frequency. Less commonly, necrotizing arteritis is seen.

Nodules. Subcutaneous nodules occur characteristically over pressure points and have unique histological features (central area of necrosis surrounded by palisading mesenchymal cells and an outer mantle of lymphocytes and granulation tissue). There is a significant association of nodules with the presence of rheumatoid factor and with severe and sustained disease. Granulomatous lesions comparable to subcutaneous nodules are observed, rarely, in the myocardium, valve leaflets, sclerae, and lungs. Histological studies of early subcutaneous nodules suggest that focal necrotizing vasculitis initiates the process. There are a few reports of subcutaneous nodules with the characteristic morphology in asymptomatic healthy individuals. Although the histology of chronic rheumatoid nodules is distinct from that of nodules appearing with acute rheumatic fever, the early acute rheumatoid nodules are frequently indistinguishable from rheumatic fever nodules.

Heart and Lungs. There is a controversy regarding the incidence of heart disease in rheumatoid arthritis. In one autopsy series, valvular changes indistinguishable from chronic rheumatic heart disease were demonstrated in over 50 percent of patients, but most other studies have not confirmed this observation. Old pericarditis is a common finding at autopsy (as high as 40 percent), but clinically apparent pericarditis is infrequently seen. Cardiovascular lesions that are probably a part of the rheumatoid process are (1) valvular nodules, (2) diffuse granulomatous myocarditis, and (3) aortitis pathologically resembling syphilitic aortitis. These are *unusual* manifestations, and the last is most frequently associated with Marie-Strümpell spondylitis.

Diffuse interstitial pulmonary fibrosis, a common manifestation of progressive systemic sclerosis (scleroderma), may be a significant feature of rheumatoid arthritis, but its frequency in the disease is low. The association of rheumatoid disease and multiple granulomatous nodules of lungs was noted first in Welsh coalminers (Caplan's syndrome) and is apparently a unique and exaggerated tissue response of rheumatoid subjects to the inhalation of silica dusts.

Miscellaneous. Uveitis has been observed in approximately 3 percent of patients with rheumatoid arthritis. Chronic scleritis is an infrequent complication. There is an intimate relationship between rheumatoid arthritis and Sjögren's syndrome (keratoconjunctivitis sicca), and chronic lymphadenoid thyroiditis

(Hashimoto's thyroiditis) seems to occur with a frequency that exceeds the expected incidence. Generalized lymphadenopathy and splenomegaly, to degrees which simulate the malignant lymphomas, are occasional manifestations. Amyloidosis has been observed in 10 to 20 percent of autopsy series. There is a controversy regarding the possible significant association between rheumatoid arthritis and chronic glomerulitis.

RADIOGRAPHIC FEATURES

X-ray films of involved joints and the adjacent osseus tissue reflect the histopathological changes in the synovial membrane. The earliest changes include soft tissue swelling and osteoporosis. Loss of radiolucent articular cartilage, secondary to pannus formation, causes joint space narrowing on x-ray films; and the pannus will result in juxta-articular erosions if it extends into subchondral bone. In the extreme, there may be extensive resorption of bone adjacent to involved joints. Subluxation deformities and bony ankylosis, if present, are visualized by x-rays.

GENERAL LABORATORY FEATURES

The "acute phase reactants" such as the erythrocyte sedimentation rate and the C-reactive protein test are nearly always abnormal and generally reflect the degree of disease activity. Leukocytosis and moderate anemia are less frequent features of active disease but, when present, usually correlate with the activity of disease. The majority of patients with active disease have significant elevations of serum γ-globulin on paper electrophoresis. Synovial fluid usually contains abnormal numbers of leukocytes (as high as 60,000 per $mm.^3$) and shows poor mucin clot formation when dilute acetic acid is added, but the main value of synovial fluid analysis is in ruling out infection when that is suspected.

MANAGEMENT

GENERAL

Lacking a cure for the disease, it is usual to refer to therapeutic efforts as management. A detailed knowledge of the patient and his environment and a sympathetic willingness to deal with the problems are hackneyed, yet valid, requisites to the management of any chronic disease. The patient must take an active role in the program of therapy and must be educated, if necessary, in avoiding a passive dependent attitude. The imparting of optimism is essential and not unrealistic in view of the natural history of rheumatoid disease. Therapy is, in good part, constructed around the thesis that a *spontaneous* remission may occur at *any* time. Of the numerous drugs administered, none is generally accepted as being capable of inducing remissions. The goals of present-day therapy are (1) to control pain as effectively as possible with agents which do as little harm as possible, and (2) to prevent, minimize, or reverse deformities of joints, while awaiting the hoped-for remission.

A listing of remedies which have been applied in the treatment of rheumatoid arthritis would include a sizable part of the pharmacopoeia. Even a compilation of those drugs alleged to have "curative" action would serve no purpose. Because of the spontaneous variations in disease activity, large numbers of patients are required for therapeutic trials, and such comments as "much improved," "improved," and "some improvement" often reflect nothing more than wishful thinking on the part of the patient or physician.

DRUGS

Anti-inflammatory agents

Salicylates. In doses of 3.0 gm. or more per day, the salicylates have the lowest incidence of serious toxicity. The effectiveness of adequate amounts of salicylates suggests that they have more than an analgesic action, but their anti-inflammatory effect observed with certain experimental models of inflammation has not been conclusively demonstrated in rheumatoid arthritis.

Adrenocorticosteroids. These are the most effective agents available for suppression of the inflammation and control of pain, but have a number of limitations. (1) Although pain may be dramatically suppressed by a given dose of steroid, the disease (including progression of deformities) is not controlled, and if the disease is sustained, the dose of drug may have to be progressively increased. (2) It is very difficult, if not impossible, to discontinue steroid therapy when the disease remains active, because of severe exacerbations which follow reduction in dosage. (3) Patients on long-term steroid therapy may develop serious life-threatening complications in frequencies and to degrees which make rheumatoid arthritis seem almost inconsequential. A recent proposal that steroids be administered in a single dose every 48 hours (in an effort to prevent complications of steroid therapy) has not been tested in more than a few rheumatoid patients.

Physicians who have had to cope with the limitations of long-term steroid therapy are generally reluctant to initiate it. If there were a reliable method for predicting, at the outset, the—intermittent or sustained—course of the disease there would be less fear of giving steroids to "intermittent" patients. Without such knowledge, one must assume that any patient with early disease may subsequently have sustained progressive rheumatoid arthritis. With these facts in mind, what are the indications for steroid therapy? There is no complete agreement, but if disease is very severe and the patient progresses rapidly toward invalidism, in spite of more conservative and less toxic therapy, most physicians will initiate steroid therapy, using the smallest dose* that will permit ambulation, together with physical rehabilitation.

Occasionally the disease may be less severe but affects the head of a family or a mother; consequently, a family unit is compromised. If there is no other solution and if low doses of steroid might keep the patient "on the job," steroid therapy may be indicated. The wish for immediate short-term improvement must always be tempered with the knowledge that long-term steroid therapy can lead to disaster.

Since the dissociation of mineralocorticoid from glucocorticoid effects, which resulted from the development of the delta-1 dehydrosteroids (prednisone and prednisolone), no major improvement has been accomplished in the reduction of undesired side effects. Of the several different steroids available, none stands out as superior. Triamcinolone, which is approximately equivalent to prednisone in potency, may have a greater propensity for inducing muscular wasting.

Intra-articular administration of steroid has a definite but limited role in therapy. When one or two involved joints are the main source of disability, 25 to 50 mg. of hydrocortisone, or its equivalent, may be injected into the joint space. Prednisolone t-butyl acetate, 20 to 30 mg., has been judged superior to hydrocortisone in duration of effect. A minority of patients so treated will experience less pain for periods in excess of a few days and can thus be maintained on injections every few weeks. In the author's experience, even patients who initially respond soon reach a point of diminishing returns.

Endogenous steroid therapy, stimulated by maintenance corticotropin (ACTH) therapy, is rarely used. There is still an unresolved issue regarding the usefulness of periodic ACTH injections in patients on long-term steroid therapy. Adrenal atrophy may be minimized by such treatments, but it is uncertain whether or not the normal response to stress is maintained.

Phenylbutazone and Its Analogues. These are potent anti-inflammatory agents but are not very effective in the average case of rheumatoid arthritis. Potential toxicity (myeloid depression and peptic ulceration) further limits their usefulness.

Other drugs

Antimalarial Drugs. Such antimalarials as chloroquine (125–500 mg. per day) have modest anti-inflammatory properties, but their alleged effectiveness in the treatment of rheumatoid arthritis may depend on some other action. Those who advocate the use of chloroquine maintain that improvement, if it occurs, is usually delayed for weeks to months after institution of therapy. Cooperative drug trials by a committee of the American Rheumatism Association suggested that antimalarial treatment was better than a placebo, but these conclusions were based on fine statistical differences. Reports of irreversible retinopathy in a small number of patients treated with antimalarials have discouraged but not stopped their use.

Gold Compounds. Gold thiol compounds (gold thioglucose and gold thiomalate) have been used in the treatment of rheumatoid arthritis for more than thirty years. It is still

* *Editor's comment:* This point should be emphasized. *Minimal* corticosteroid therapy is the only allowable course. No attempt should be made to relieve pain completely, for this can seldom be done for long, and the resultant maintenance dose often ends up much higher.—J. H. V.

not known how they act or, indeed, if they have any influence on the course. Therapeutic trials in Great Britain offered some support to the advocates of gold therapy, but controversy continues regarding its efficacy. The usual course of gold therapy is 50 mg. intramuscularly at weekly intervals. If a remission occurs, coincident to gold therapy, maintenance injections are continued (50 mg. every two to four weeks). If no remission ensues after a total dose of 1 to 2 gm., the treatment is called a failure and discontinued. Gold toxicity (myeloid depression, skin rash, and nephritis) is infrequent, but blood counts and urinalyses must be made at least once a month during therapy and treatment discontinued if evidence of toxicity appears. During the first few weeks of treatment, blood counts and urinalyses should be made weekly.

Experimental drugs

Preliminary reports on compounds which are chemically related to tryptophan or its metabolic products suggest that they may be useful agents in the treatment of rheumatoid arthritis. (The generic name of the drug, which has been most extensively evaluated, but not yet marketed, is indomethacin.) Certain of the alkylating drugs (nitrogen mustards) and antimetabolite compounds have been tried in patients with severe rheumatoid disease. The studies are incomplete, and whether an apparent improvement results from anti-inflammatory effect or a suppression of the immune response is not known.

PHYSICAL MEDICINE MEASURES

Emphasis should be placed on a simple exercise program that will minimize muscle weakness and loss of joint mobility. With proper indoctrination and periodic review by a physical therapist, these goals can usually be obtained by the patient's own efforts at home. Certain modalities of heat may be useful adjuncts to an exercise program; a hot soaking bath will usually suffice. When deformities and weakness are established, admission to a rehabilitation service for a more intensive program may be required.

ORTHOPEDIC SURGERY

Operative procedures such as arthrodeses, arthroplasty, prosthetic replacement, and osteotomies may, in *selected* situations, improve function. Synovectomies are advocated by some orthopedists, but their merit is unproved.

EXPERIMENTAL ARTHRITIS

Of the many types of experimental arthritis, the models which most closely mimic rheumatoid arthritis are mediated by either infectious agents or immunological responses. Pleuropneumonia-like organisms (PPLO) induce arthritis in several species which may superficially resemble rheumatoid arthritis. *Erysipelothrix rhusiopathiae* infection in hogs and rabbits and *Streptobacillus moniliformis* infection in rodents likewise may be expressed in part as chronic synovitis. Experimental models of arthritis which are probably immunological in character include adjuvant arthritis which results from intradermal injection into rats of complete Freund's adjuvant and a recently described chronic arthritis which follows the injection of heterologous fibrin clots into the joints of rabbits previously immunized with the fibrin plus complete Freund's adjuvant. A milder and less chronic arthritis was observed when autologous fibrin was used. Heterologous nephrotoxic antisera, when injected into rabbit joints, result in a synovitis which is probably mediated by the host's immune response to heterologous protein. In spite of certain similarities between these models and rheumatoid arthritis, none of them is the equivalent of the human syndrome.

SEROLOGICAL ABNORMALITIES

A significant number of patients with clinical rheumatoid arthritis exhibit antinuclear and biologically false positive Wassermann reactions (two apparent autoimmune phenomena which have much more striking associations with SLE). The incidence of antinuclear factors in rheumatoid subjects varies widely, depending on the techniques utilized and the arbitrary separation of the two syndromes—rheumatoid arthritis and SLE. From the literature, the incidence of positive LE cell reactions in rheumatoid subjects varies between 0 and 27 percent, and the reported incidence of antinuclear factors demonstrated by immunofluorescence techniques varies between 14 and 65 percent. (The study which yielded positive results in 65 percent of rheumatoid subjects noted positive results in 22 percent of patients with generalized osteoarthritis.) The antinuclear antibodies may be present in all three classes of immunoglobulins (γ_2-, γ_{1M}-, and γ_{1A}-globulins) in both rheumatoid and SLE subjects. Some studies have disclosed a significant incidence of splenomegaly, rheumatoid nodules, and severe disease in rheumatoid patients with positive LE cell reactions. Most rheumatoid subjects possess what is commonly called the "rheumatoid factor(s)" (RF). Because there is considerable heterogeneity of RF and because they are reactive with γ-globulins, they are often referred to as "anti-γ-globulin factors."

TECHNIQUES

Various particles which are "coated" with γ-globulin serve as indicator systems for RF. A partial list of agglutination systems includes: sensitized bacteria, sensitized sheep cells (amboceptor-coated), human Rh-positive cells coated with anti-Rh antibodies, and particles of polystyrene latex or bentonite which have reacted with γ-globulins. In all of these reactions, there is the requirement of some type of γ-globulin, usually of human or rabbit origin. Gamma-globulins denatured in such a way that aggregates form will visibly react with RF without the use of a carrier particle; i.e., precipitation of soluble aggregates occurs.

RHEUMATOID FACTOR

The factors which react with the foregoing systems are present in the macroglobulin fractions of γ-globulin (γ_{1M} or β_{2M} in two different nomenclatures). The sedimentation constant of this fraction is 19, but RF, in whole serum, exists as a complex (formed with low molecular weight 7S γ-globulin). Sedimentation studies of sera with very large amounts of RF demonstrate the complex (S constant of approximately 22) sedimenting ahead of the 19S component. There is recent evidence that 7S γ-globulins in some rheumatoid sera demonstrate anti-γ-globulin specificities (referred to as 7S rheumatoid factors). Complexes with intermediate sedimenting properties (7S to 19S) which are observed in these sera appear to result from the interaction of 7S RF with other 7S γ-globulin. Aside from this molecular inhomogeneity of anti-γ-globulin factors, there is abundant evidence of the heterogeneity of RF in its varied specificity for different animal γ-globulins and, in the system which utilizes sensitized Rh-positive human cells, varied specificity for different genetic types of human γ-globulin. (Present methods for study of the human Gm and Inv groups of γ-globulins exploit this varied anti-γ-globulin reactivity of rheumatoid arthritis and of certain other pathological and normal states.)

"REACTANT" GAMMA-GLOBULIN

The γ-globulin with which RF reacts has been called the reactant. In systems which utilize rabbit γ-globulin as the reactant, such as the sensitized sheep cell agglutination, the reactive part of the rabbit molecule is Porter's fraction III (papain digestion; see Chap. 3). The human equivalent of Porter's fraction III (piece B in Franklin's terminology) also exhibits reactivity with RF; the fragments which contain antibody combining sites are nonreactive.

In most serological systems, the reactant γ-globulin consists of antibody in specific combination with its respective antigen (e.g., rabbit amboceptor with sheep cells, antistreptococcal antibodies with streptococci, or anti-Rh antibodies with Rh-positive red cells), and it is usually impossible to demonstrate a reaction between the antibody alone and the RF. From such observations, it has been suggested that RF displays primary specificity for γ-globulin which has been denatured in the course of combining with antigen; i.e., RF is specific for immune complexes. There are controversies on this subject which cannot be reviewed here, but a tentative conclusion which is consistent with the facts is that there are several potentially antigenic configurations on a γ-globulin molecule against which different RF's may be directed. In the course of immune complex formation, certain of these potentially antigenic configurations on the γ-globulins are exposed. Their antigenic capabilities and their availabilities to react with RF's are then revealed. Optimal reactivity of "reactant" γ-globulin thus would result from either immune complex formation or other types of denaturation.

CLINICAL ASSOCIATIONS

In all of the many serological systems utilized, the majority of rheumatoid sera react positively. The incidence of positive reactions varies with different techniques. The most widely applied and the simplest procedure is the latex fixation test—latex particles coated with normal human γ-globulin (Cohn fraction II derived from large pools of human plasma).

Seventy percent or more of sera of patients with the clinical diagnosis of rheumatoid arthritis will agglutinate γ-globulin-coated particles at a dilution of 1:20 or higher. There is a high degree of correlation between the presence of RF and the following clinical features: (1) subcutaneous nodules, (2) symmetrical deforming arthritis of the hands and wrists, and (3) "severe systemic rheumatoid disease." Although, as noted earlier, seropositivity has a statistically significant association with sustained versus intermittent disease, this is not a striking relationship, and there are consistently seronegative patients who experience sustained disease with severe deforming changes.

Less than 5 percent of normal human sera give a positive reaction to the usual serological tests. An occasional healthy blood donor will have high titers of RF. It should be emphasized that RF is not specific for rheumatoid arthritis. A significant percentage of patients with other connective tissue syndromes are seropositive, and in a variety of illnesses (pulmonary tuberculosis, sarcoidosis, leprosy, syphilis, liver disease, leishmaniasis, and bacterial endocarditis), the seropositivity significantly exceeds the normal incidence. Patients with the syndromes sometimes classified as variants of rheumatoid arthritis (juvenile rheumatoid arthritis, Marie-Strümpell spondylitis, psoriatic arthritis, arthritis associated with ulcerative colitis, regional enteritis, agammaglobulinemia) are in general seronegative. An exception to this is the fact that the majority of patients with juvenile rheumatoid arthritis were judged seropositive on the basis of an inhibition test. This procedure is difficult to perform and interpret and remains, after several years of study, a research tool.

In general, patients who are seropositive remain so, and seronegative patients continue to be seronegative regardless of subsequent clinical events. There are a few exceptions; e.g., for a given serological system, subjects with borderline or low positive titers may fluctuate between negative and the low order of positivity, and patients experiencing complete remissions, in some studies, have changed from positive to negative.

FAMILY STUDIES

There is no general agreement regarding the relative incidences of rheumatoid arthritis and RF in family members of rheumatoid propositi and the family members of controls. Although there are reports of failure to demonstrate any significant aggregation of the disease or RF in blood relatives of rheumatoid patients, most family studies have suggested that the incidence of seropositivity in the relatives of seropositive patients exceeds the expected norm. In population and family studies in Great Britain, it appeared that RF and rheumatoid arthritis might be transmitted independently in that the incidence of seropositivity was comparable in the relatives of seropositive propositi regardless of whether or not arthritis was a feature of the propositi. Seropositivity increases with age, and in an English study was greater in an urban than in a rural population. A family study of agammaglobulinemia subjects revealed an unexpectedly high incidence of rheumatoid arthritis and RF. In the largest series of patients with agammaglobulinemia studied in the United States, approximately one third had seronegative arthritis indistinguishable from juvenile rheumatoid arthritis. The potential significance of these observations is considered later.

EXPERIMENTAL STUDIES

There are two general means of inducing, in experimental animals, anti-γ-globulin factors which mimic RF. In one, rabbits or guinea pigs are immunized with their own γ-globulin plus complete Freund's adjuvant, and in the other, long-term immunization of rabbits is accomplished with killed bacteria or with soluble proteins. With the former method, successful immunization has been accomplished by injecting autologous γ-globulin in the following forms: immune precipitates, denatured γ-globulin, and enzyme-treated γ-globulin. Animals given injections of denatured autologous γ-globulin develop anti-γ-globulin antibodies which are nonreactive with native autologous γ-globulin but demonstrate specificity for denatured autologous γ-globulin and certain heterologous γ-globulins. The present interpretation of these studies is that denaturation results in the acquisition of "new" antigenic determinates which are not present in native γ-globulin but which are similar to antigenic determinates of the heterologous γ-globulins.

Prolonged immunization of rabbits with

killed *Escherichia coli, Bacillus subtilis,* and *Salmonella typhimurium* and with egg albumin or horse spleen ferritin results in development of rheumatoid factor-like substances (RFLS) which more closely resemble the human RF than the factors that follow immunization with isolated autologous γ-globulin. The RFLS induced by immunization with bacteria are exclusively macroglobulin antibodies, and they demonstrate primary specificity against rabbit γ-globulin. Like human RF, their serological specificity for γ-globulin is detected only if the γ-globulin is in the form of an immune complex or is aggregated by other means, such as heat. When the immunizing stimulus is discontinued, RFLS greatly diminishes but returns in anamnestic fashion after reimmunization.* According to the current interpretation of these phenomena, prolonged immunization with an antigen results in a continuous formation *in vivo* of immune complexes and the "immunologic denaturation" of autologous γ-globulin is the stimulus for production of autoantibodies.

Although it is not possible to cite all the evidence here, one can conclude that the RF's are autoantibodies with specificity directed against multiple antigenic determinates of γ-globulin and that the closest experimental model of RF results from prolonged immunization with a variety of antigens.† How these observations may relate to the etiology and pathogenesis of rheumatoid arthritis will be considered.

* If this phenomenon is equivalent to the human RF, it suggests that an antigenic stimulus in rheumatoid arthritis must be sustained since serological titers in rheumatoid subjects usually remain constant. In a human model of hyperimmunization (bacterial endocarditis), titers of RF decreased subsequent to eradication of the infection.

† *Editor's comment:* Most workers in the field agree with this interpretation. Yet many continue to be bothered by the reported instances in which homo- or heteroreactivity of the rheumatoid factor is better exhibited than is autoreactivity (see Ref. 8). This feature may also mark the autoreactive antibodies in acquired hemolytic disease, in liver disease, and perhaps elsewhere. Since the RFLS elicited by hyperimmunization of rabbits exhibit this same strange behavior, however, many investigators are inclined to regard better homo- and heteroreactivity as artefact, possibly because of "internal consumption" of the most avidly autoreactive of the rheumatoid factor or because of the need for denaturation of the autologous "reactant" γ-globulin before the rheumatoid factor can properly react with it.—J. H. V.

ETIOLOGICAL CONSIDERATIONS

Every conceivable etiological concept has, at one time or another, been related to the pathogenesis of rheumatoid arthritis. An infectious etiology was favored for several decades; in older nomenclatures, rheumatoid arthritis was synonymous with "infectious arthritis," and it was studies of the possible relationship of streptococcal infection to rheumatoid arthritis in the 1930's which initiated investigations of RF.

For several years after the first experience with cortisone therapy of rheumatoid arthritis, investigations were predominantly in the endocrine sphere. In recent years, autoimmune bases have been postulated for most diseases of unknown etiology, including rheumatoid arthritis, and at present there is a revival of interest in the possible role of infectious agents in the pathogenesis of rheumatoid arthritis.

EVIDENCE OF AN IMMUNE BASIS

The evidence that the immune response in some way relates to rheumatoid arthritis may be summarized as follows: (1) There are certain clinical and pathological analogies between serum sickness (in which immunological bases are implicit) and the connective tissue syndromes, including rheumatoid arthritis. The host response to heterologous serum or certain drugs may closely mimic rheumatoid arthritis, rheumatic fever, or SLE. (2) Serological studies have demonstrated beyond doubt that autoimmune *phenomena* are operative in most patients with rheumatoid disease, although there is *no* evidence that RF mediates the pathogenesis of the disease. (3) If one considers the illnesses other than rheumatoid arthritis that are significantly associated with RF, a common feature of most of them is the presence of a chronic antigenic stimulus (leprosy, syphilis, tuberculosis, bacterial endocarditis, and leishmaniasis). These observations, together with studies of experimental RF induced by hyperimmunization, suggest that in rheumatoid disease there may be some unrecognized chronic antigenic stimulus. (4) In some patients, a respiratory infection or grippelike illness occurs as a prodrome to the development of arthritis, much as pharyngitis precedes the development of acute rheumatic fever. (5) Hypergammaglobulinemia, a common feature of rheumatoid arthritis, could be cited as evidence of an immunological process. (6) The involved synovial structures and subcutaneous nodules, in chronic cases, contain plasmacytes and lymphocytes in nodular aggregates that resemble lymphoid follicles.*

NATURE OF THE HYPOTHETICAL ANTIGENIC STIMULUS

If one accepts the premise that immunological events mediate the development of rheumatoid arthritis, it is admitted that the responsible antigen(s) has eluded detection. Two general possibilities exist: (1) the antigen is autologous and rheumatoid arthritis is an autoimmune disease, or (2) the antigen is exogenous (such as a microbial agent) and the disease might be analogous to chronic serum sickness.

Autoimmunity. The concept which involves some loss of tolerance for "self-antigens" remains theoretical, and except for autoantibodies with specificity for blood cell elements, there is no direct evidence linking human autoimmune phenomena to disease mechanisms. No evidence to date can attribute a pathogenic role to RF. Transfusion of high-titer rheumatoid sera was accomplished without event, and there are instances of normal healthy persons with large amounts of circulating RF. A report of cytopathogenic properties of rheumatoid sera for cells growing in tissue culture has not been corroborated. The chronic arthritis which frequently complicates agammaglobulinemia occurs in the absence of detectable RF.† It is true that the small number of patients with diffuse vasculitis almost invariably have high serological titers, but, in our experience, the great majority of patients with serum titers of 1:56,000 or higher (FII tanned sheep cell agglutination test) are not clinically separable from patients with lower titers. Individuals with very large amounts of RF—those whose sera contain the heavier than 19S complex in analytical ultracentrifuge studies—frequently have anemia, leukopenia, and hepatosplenomegaly (features of Felty's syndrome). It is possible that the relative insolubility of these complexes may contribute to secondary pathological manifestations. There is continued interest in the pathological potential of low molecular weight anti-γ-globulin factors. As previously noted, 7S RF's in whole sera appear to exist as intermediate complexes with sedimentation constants between 7 and 19, and correlations have been made between the presence of such intermediate complexes and disease activity, especially pulmonary lesions.

Exogenous Source of Immunological Stimulus. If the immune response to an environmental antigen were responsible for the pathogenesis of rheumatoid arthritis, the closest experimental models would be chronic serum sickness induced by continued injection into rabbits of heterologous serum proteins) and the changes resulting from hyperimmunization of rabbits with killed bacteria (Chap. 12). In neither of these models is arthritis a feature, but in both there are anti-γ-globulin factors which mimic RF. (The predominant pathological changes are in the kidney.) Dissimilarities between the lesions in man and in the rabbit could reflect nothing more than species variations in tissue responses to a common event. Furthermore, if certain antigens (microbial or otherwise) exhibited tropism for synovial structures, the inflammatory response would be concentrated in these tissues. Man must continually cope with a multitude of antigens which include dietary substances, the microbial flora of the gastrointestinal tract, pathogenic microorganisms, and a variety of materials which can gain access to the body via the skin and mucous membranes. Under normal conditions, the host's responses do not permit the induction

* *Editor's comment:* Two recent observations deserve attention. The hemolytic complement activity of joint fluid has been found to be depressed in rheumatoid arthritis, as compared with other arthritides (Pekin, J., Jr. Zvaifler, N.J., *J. Clin. Invest.,* 43:1372, 1964), and there are cytoplasmic inclusions of γ-globulins in the joint fluid polymorphonuclear leukocytes (Hollander, J. L., *et al., Arthritis Rheum.,* 7:314, 1964). The possibility that immune complexes are being actively phagocytosed and that this may lead to release of leukocytic lysosomal enzymes is under active study (Astorga, G. and Bollet, A. J., *Arthritis Rheum.,* 7:288, 1964). —J. H. V.

† *Editor's comment:* An infrequently appreciated fact about patients with severe hypogammaglobulinemia is that they may be exquisitely sensitive to aggregated γ-globulins (Barandum, *Vox Sang.* 7:157, 1962) and therefore perhaps also to antigen-antibody complexes. One is reminded that the susceptibility of animals to passive cutaneous anaphylaxis is inversely related to the amount of nonantibody γ-globulin present at the test site. Is it possible that patients with severe hypogammaglobulinemia are inordinately susceptible to hypersensitivity from whatever very small amounts of circulating γ-globulins they have?—J. H. V.

of disease. The questions are, in rheumatoid arthritis: Might some unique type of antigenic stimulus occur, or might certain individuals, because of a genetic or acquired defect in their host responses, react abnormally to an otherwise innocuous antigenic substance? In the sphere of clinical allergy, certain types of contact sensitivity would be examples of the former, and ragweed sensitivity an example of the latter. There are other possible examples involving microbial agents. Rheumatoid arthritis is not limited to, or even concentrated in, one or more environments, and attempts to relate a specific microbial agent to the pathogenesis of the disease have been unsuccessful. In the light of current difficulties in characterizing the almost limitless variety of viral agents, negative results should not discourage further efforts to isolate microorganisms from patients with rheumatoid arthritis.*

The possibility that a common microbe might, in a host with the proper genetic trait, be the stimulus for the development of rheumatoid arthritis deserves consideration. (Might there be an analogy to the observation that no more than 2 to 3 percent of patients with streptococcal pharyngitis develop acute rheumatic fever, or to the situation with salmonella infections in which about 2 percent of patients chronically harbor the microorganism in intracellular sites? A genetic basis is not proved for either of these phenomena, but something, presumably the character of the host, influences the course of the disease in a small minority of cases.) The potential significance of genetic factors in the pathogenesis of rheumatoid arthritis is suggested by the family studies of patients with rheumatoid arthritis and with agammaglobulinemia. In the latter state, in which incompetence of the immune response is marked, there is an unexpected frequency of rheumatoid arthritis, RF, and either high or low serum γ-globulin levels in blood relatives. Is it possible that the relatives have a more subtle qualitative deficiency in the immune response? With such a concept, the varied "dose" or expressivity of a genetic abnormality might account for a wide spectrum of immunologic disorders. (A high incidence of atopic dermatitis has been noted in agammaglobulinemia subjects.)

* In a recent study (Bartholemew, L., *Arthritis Rheum.* 7:291, 1964 [abst.]), *Mycoplasma* were isolated from synovial fluids of five of seven rheumatoid subjects after the primary inocula were carried through tissue culture phases for several weeks. The recognized latency of *Mycoplasma* in certain tissue culture lines and the ever-present risk of artefactual contamination are bases for reservation, but of note is the fact that this study included controls from which *Mycoplasma* were not isolated.

DELAYED HYPERSENSITIVITY

In the immunological sphere, most attention has been directed to changes in circulating immunoglobulins. The cell-mediated response (delayed hypersensitivity), because it is poorly characterized and difficult to ascertain, has been neglected. Since evidence implicates delayed responses in the development of experimental autoimmune disorders, the possible role of delayed hypersensitivity in the pathogenesis of rheumatoid arthritis requires further study.

OTHER ETIOLOGICAL CONSIDERATIONS

Although the prevailing theories regarding the etiology of rheumatoid arthritis center on interrelating aspects of genetics, infection, and in the immune response, other concepts remain of potential importance. In consideration of microbial agents as possible etiological factors, stress was placed on the host's immune response to the microbe's antigens as the mediator of tissue inflammation. A virus, or a pleuropneumonia-like organism, might induce chronic synovitis, and the immunological events could be secondary phenomena without pathogenetic significance. In the metabolic sphere, there are the observations that some rheumatoid subjects hyperexcrete certain products of tryptophan metabolism; and there are a few patients with rather chronic atypical gout that closely resembles rheumatoid arthritis. Psychological factors have been studied. Emotional problems are frequent, and an occasional subject experiences the initial onset or exacerbations of disease following emotional upset; but there is little to make the psyche suspect as a primary factor in the development of rheumatoid arthritis.

REFERENCES

GENERAL

1. Fourteenth rheumatism review. *Ann. Intern. Med.* 56:15, 1962.
2. American Rheumatism Association on Criteria for Rheumatic Arthritis: Primer on the Rheumatic Diseases. *J.A.M.A.* 171:1213, 1959.

CLINICAL ASPECTS

3. Short, C. L., Bauer, W., and Reynolds, W. E. *Rheumatoid Arthritis.* Cambridge, Mass.: Harvard University Press, 1957.

EFFECTS OF PROLONGED STEROID THERAPY

4. Howell, D. S., and Ragan, C. The course of rheumatoid arthritis during 4 years of induced hyperadrenalism (IHA). *Medicine* 35:83, 1956.
5. Berntsen, C. A., and Freyberg, R. H. Rheumatoid patients after five or more years of corticosteroid treatment: A comparative analysis of 193 cases. *Ann. Intern. Med.* 54:938, 1961.

EPIDEMIOLOGY AND FAMILY STUDIES

6. Symposium: *The Epidemiology of Chronic Rheumatism.* Philadelphia: F. A. Davis Company, 1963. Edited (under direction of J. H. Kellgren) by M. R. Jeffrey and J. Ball.

SEROLOGICAL PHENOMENA

7. Vaughan, J. H. Serum responses in rheumatoid arthritis. *Amer. J. Med.* 26:596, 1959.
8. Transactions of the Conference on the Immunologic Aspects of Rheumatoid Arthritis and Systemic Lupus Erythematosus. *Arthritis Rheum.* 6:402, 1963.
9. Fudenberg, H. The hereditary human gamma globulin (Gm) groups: Interpretations and extensions. *Progr. Allerg.* 7:1, 1963.

EXPERIMENTAL ARTHRITIS

10. Gardner, D. L. The experimental production of arthritis: A review. *Ann. Rheum. Dis.* 19:297, 1960.

66. *Systemic Lupus Erythematosus*

HALSTED R. HOLMAN

SYSTEMIC LUPUS ERYTHEMATOSUS (SLE) is a disease of unknown cause at present considered to be a member of the rheumatic disease family. Until about 1950 it was thought to be a rare and usually fatal disease. The development of new diagnostic tests and heightened awareness of physicians have now established that the disease is more common than formerly believed and that it exists in mild to rapidly fatal forms. The introduction of corticosteroids in management has radically changed the patterns of the disease and the outcome for the individual patient. More recently, numerous autoimmune phenomena have been demonstrated in SLE, and it has become fashionable to consider it an autoimmune disease.

Various thorough reviews of the clinical and experimental features of SLE have been published in the past decade [1–4]; most notable is that by Harvey and his colleagues [1]. We shall attempt here to present the various facets of our understanding of the illness.

CHARACTER AND NATURAL HISTORY

The disease usually affects women in the child-bearing age, although the very young and the very old, male and female, may develop it. The salient features of SLE are involvement of many different tissues and wide variation in clinical expression. The first form to be recognized was a rapidly advancing, usually fatal systemic illness characterized by high fever, skin rash, polyarthritis, effusion from pleural, pericardial, and peritoneal surfaces, and central nervous system abnormalities. At the other end of the spectrum lies an indolent, remitting disease characterized by arthralgia, myalgia, and malaise. Degrees of severity between these extremes are more common. Virtually every organ system in the body may be affected individually or in concert. The patient may combine, for instance, rash, arthritis, grand mal seizures, nephrosis, hemolytic anemia, and unexplained abdominal pain. Alternatively, a patient may have solely the clinical picture of acute nephritis or isolated pleural effusion. He may appear to have idiopathic thrombocytopenic purpura or may have only tender, painful muscles.

Not only is the disease characterized by enormous variability in its clinical forms, but the extent and severity of involvement of different organ systems may change during the illness. At one time in the experience of an individual patient, arthritis may predominate, whereas a year later, hemolytic anemia or nephritis or peripheral neuropathy may be the central feature.

The clinical course is characterized by spontaneous remissions and exacerbations. After a remission, the disease may reappear in another organ system. Thus, a first attack may resemble acquired hemolytic anemia, and the second may be predominantly polyserositis. Occasionally, the clinical characteristics change so dramatically as to lead to the suspicion of a different disease, such as polyarteritis nodosa or rheumatoid arthritis. This probably reflects not an actual change in the nature of the illness but rather the facts that there are many features common to all diseases in the rheumatic category and that precise clinical classification is often difficult. However, in certain instances there is an apparent decisive change in the type of illness, for the clinical picture of a lymphoma has been reported to evolve into SLE or vice versa over the period of a few years.

Despite the variability in clinical characteristics, a reasonable definition of the disease is possible. It is a remitting, febrile, and presumably noninfectious illness of unknown etiology which usually affects young women. It involves predominantly serous and synovial surfaces, skin and kidney, and has characteristic hematological and serological changes (see later). The natural evolution of the illness will often lead to subsequent expression of the illness in other systems.

PATHOLOGICAL CHANGES

The pathological features are surprisingly meager for a disease that involves so many organ systems. When the fulminant lupus "crisis" was common, it was not unusual for a patient to die with clinical evidence of disease in the brain, skin, muscles, joints, and serosal surfaces without any distinctive pathological findings.

Two characteristic tissue lesions do exist and, when found, are strongly suggestive of the diagnosis. The first is a lesion of the glomerulus of the kidney which consists of thickening of the basement membrane, with hyaline thrombi and hematoxylin bodies in the capillaries. The second is periarteriolar fibrosis in the spleen. The thickened glomerular basement membrane has fibrinoid staining characteristics and has been shown to contain γ-globulin on immunofluorescent microscopy [5, 6]. The hematoxylin bodies are swollen cell nuclei devoid of cytoplasm and coated with γ-globulin. Often the morphological picture of lupus nephropathy is indistinguishable from that of membranous glomerulonephritis.

A less distinctive lesion that is frequently seen is thickening and necrosis of the walls of medium-sized arterioles with periarteriolar inflammatory infiltrations. The vasculitis may be diffuse and devastating, affecting medium-sized arterioles in many organs, or it may be relatively restricted to a few arteries, resulting in such syndromes as mesenteric artery occlusion or aseptic necrosis of the femoral head. A patient may have a history of seizures and the appearance of hemiparesis or hemiplegia before death and be found at postmortem examination to have minimal, if any, cerebral vasculitis or brain damage detectable by light microscopy.

The pathological changes in the skin are not unique. They consist of patchy atrophy of the epidermis and nuclear change in the epidermal cells, with collagen degeneration and elastic tissue proliferation in the dermis. These alterations are difficult to distinguish from those seen in simple actinic dermatitis. Infrequently, the lungs may show interstitial pneumonitis with infiltration by many types of inflammatory cells or, at a later stage, interstitial fibrosis.

Lack of major morphological changes in SLE had been recognized prior to the introduction of corticosteroids, and therefore this is not the result of suppressive therapy.

The paucity of pathological findings on light microscopy and the identification of γ-globulin localized on the glomerular basement membrane and on the hematoxylin bodies have encouraged the view that an immunological mechanism is responsible for tissue damage. Although this is a reasonable supposition, it has not been established. Recovery of the γ-globulin from the glomerular basement membrane has shown the existence of a number of different antibodies, including antinuclear antibodies localized in an area where there are no known nuclear constituents [7]. This suggests a trapping of γ-globulin or of circulating antigen-antibody complexes (see later) rather than a specific attachment of antibody to antigens of the glomerular membrane. Many patients have large numbers of circulating autoantibodies capable of reacting *in vitro* with cytoplasmic and nuclear constituents. After death, however, such antibodies are not found localized on the vast majority of cells.

The mechanism of cell damage remains an enigma. The minimal visible change strongly suggests that influences are at work which alter cell function without altering cell morphology. Identification of these influences would assist in an understanding not only of the pathogenesis of SLE but, conceivably, of other harmful biological processes known to cause human disease.

IMMUNOLOGICAL ABNORMALITIES

For the past twenty-five years or so SLE and other rheumatic diseases have been considered to have a basis in hypersensitivity. This is due to the characteristic hypergammaglobulinemia and the similarities between SLE and the clinical and serological pictures of serum sickness and hypersensitivity states provoked in experimental animals with chemicals. In recent years, objective evidence of immunological abnormalities in patients has been obtained: (1) identification of many different types of autoantibodies in the sera and of γ-globulin localized on the glomerular basement membrane; (2) a curious skin reactivity to autologous tissue constituents; (3) low levels of circulating complement; and (4) the presence of immunological abnormalities and clinical rheumatic disease in the relatives of patients with SLE. Particularly through studies of relatives, relationships between the rheumatic diseases on the one hand and lymphomatous or granulomatous diseases on the other have emerged. The immunological and clinical abnormalities in the families imply a genetic predisposition to rheumatic disease.

SEROLOGICAL AUTOREACTIVITY

More so than any other disease, SLE is characterized by circulating serum factors capable of reacting with many different autologous tissue constituents *in vitro* [4, 8]. Certain of them are readily identifiable in the clinical laboratory, such as the LE cell factor responsible for the formation of LE cells, the γ-globulin which causes a positive Coombs reaction, the γ-globulin which reacts with thromboplastin or thrombin and leads to prolonged clotting time, and the Wassermann reagin responsible for a false positive reaction. Studies on the mechanism of formation of LE cells has led to identification of the LE cell factor as an antibody capable of reacting with the desoxyribonucleohistone of the cell nucleus (Fig. 66-1). It is one of a group of antinuclear and anticytoplasmic antibodies which may be identified through complement fixation, immunofluorescence, hemagglutination, flocculation, passive cutaneous anaphylaxis, and occasionally precipitin reactions (Table 66-1). An individual antitissue antibody will enter into one or more, but usually not all, of these types of reaction. Proof that the circulating autoreactive serum factors are antibodies has been rigorous in only two instances: the LE cell factor, and the antibody which reacts with purified desoxyribonucleic acid (DNA). Characteristically, the antitissue autoantibodies lack species or organ specificity.

Available evidence also suggests that the autoantibodies are not directly harmful to normal tissues *in vivo*. Although they pass the placenta, they have not been shown to harm the infant. In tissue culture, they do not appear to be damaging to cells. Despite their presence in abundance before death, they are not found localized on or within most cells at postmortem examination [5, 6]. Indeed, these antibodies are not restricted to abnormal states. Certain of them can be found in some apparently normal individuals; in the chicken

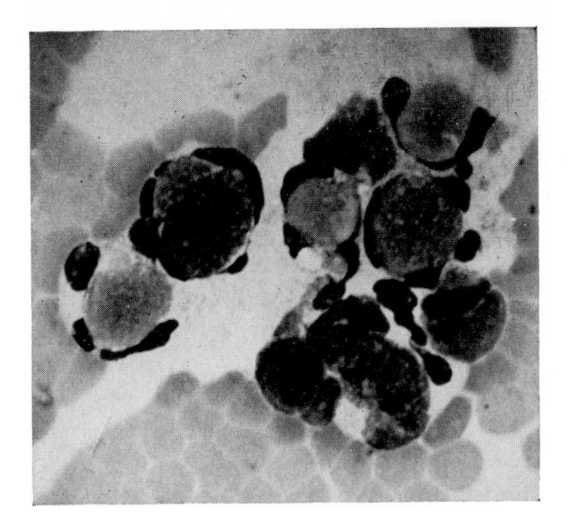

Fig. 66-1. Cluster of LE cells. Free nuclear material at lower right is swollen and less basophilic than the normal nucleus. Swelling and extrusion of altered nuclei from the cell are result of a reaction between the desoxyribonucleohistone and an autoantibody. Altered nuclei have been phagocytized by other white blood cells, resulting in LE cell formation.

and the rabbit autoreactive serum factors are found uniformly [9]. In the latter species, the titers of autoreactive serum factors rise during an immune response to a foreign antigen; this has not yet been shown to be true in man. Thus both the origin and the biological and clinical significance of autoantibodies remain unknown.

The initial impression that autoantibodies are specific for a given disease and therefore of decisive diagnostic value has proved to be erroneous. The more autoantibodies have been sought in different diseases, the more they have been found. The LE cell factor has been identified in patients with different rheumatic diseases as well as with such illnesses as chronic relapsing hepatitis and ulcerative colitis. Antinuclear and anticytoplasmic antibodies have been demonstrated by complement fixation and immunofluorescence in an even broader range of illnesses. Antibodies to thyroglobulin are found frequently in all clinical states of thyroid abnormality, to a lesser extent in most rheumatic diseases, and perhaps also in a significant segment of the population at random. It is generally true, however, that the highest titers of these antibodies are found in the classic disease states with which they were first identified. Thus the LE cell factor is more abundant in SLE, the thyroid antibody in thyroiditis,

TABLE 66-1. Complement Fixation Reactions between SLE Serum and Cell Constituents[a]

Pt.	LE Cells	Antigen Used in Comp. Fix.	Serum Dilution									
			2	4	8	16	32	64	128	256	512	1,024
		Whole cytoplasm	4	4	4	4	4	4	3	0	0	0
		Cyto. mitochondria	4	4	4	4	4	4	3	0	0	0
		Cyto. microsomes	4	4	4	4	4	4	4	4	0	0
		Soluble residue	4	4	4	4	4	4	4	4	0	0
Ah.	++++	Whole nuclei	4	4	4	4	4	3	0	0	0	0
		Nuclear extract	4	4	4	4	4	4	3	0	0	0
		Nucleoprotein	4	4	4	4	4	0	0	0	0	0
		DNA	4	4	4	4	4	0	0	0	0	0
		Histone	4	4	4	0	0	0	0	0	0	0
		Whole cytoplasm	4	4	4	4	4	4	4	4	2	0
		Cyto. mitochondria	4	4	4	4	4	3	0	0	0	0
		Cyto. microsomes	4	4	4	4	4	4	0	0	0	0
		Soluble residue	4	4	4	4	4	4	4	4	3	0
Be.	++	Whole nuclei	4	3	2	0	0	0	0	0	0	0
		Nuclear extract	4	4	4	4	4	4	4	4	0	0
		Nucleoprotein	0	0	0	0	0	0	0	0	0	0
		DNA	0	0	0	0	0	0	0	0	0	0
		Histone	0	0	0	0	0	0	0	0	0	0
		Whole cytoplasm	0	0	0	0	0	0	0	0	0	0
		Cyto. mitochondria	0	0	0	0	0	0	0	0	0	0
		Cyto. microsomes	0	0	0	0	0	0	0	0	0	0
		Soluble residue	0	0	0	0	0	0	0	0	0	0
Fr.	++++	Whole nuclei	0	0	0	0	0	0	0	0	0	0
		Nuclear extract	0	0	0	0	0	0	0	0	0	0
		Nucleoprotein	0	0	0	0	0	0	0	0	0	0
		DNA	0	0	0	0	0	0	0	0	0	0
		Histone	0	0	0	0	0	0	0	0	0	0

[a] An individual serum may react with all, some, or none of the various cell constituents used as antigens. Certain sera will react with only nuclear constituents. The LE cell factor apparently does not fix complement when reacting with desoxyribonucleohistone.

and the rheumatoid factor in rheumatoid arthritis. Clarification of the true incidence of autoantibodies in various disease states is hampered by the variability and sensitivity of the methods used to detect them. Immunofluorescence techniques often disclose antibodies difficult to detect by other measures. An example of this has been the recent demonstration of localization of γ-globulin on heart muscle in rheumatic fever and on skeletal muscle in myasthenia gravis, suggesting the existence in these states of autoreactive serum factors.

SKIN REACTIVITY TO AUTOLOGOUS CELL CONSTITUENTS

A peculiar skin reactivity to autologous tissue constituents is also present in SLE [10–12]. On intradermal injection of a suspension of autologous leukocytes or homogenates of leukocytes, the patients respond with an indurated and erythematous reaction which begins about 8 hours after inoculation and usually achieves its maximum between 18 and 24 hours. In appearance, this response is indistinguishable from a tuberculin reaction despite the difference in timing. Its development is not conditioned by the degree of disease activity or the existence of circulating antitissue antibodies. In these respects it resembles a delayed hypersensitivity reaction.

On the other hand, the reaction is not unique for SLE. It has been found in rheumatoid arthritis, rheumatic fever, dermatomyositis, and even in certain cases of such tissue damage as that which accompanies myocardial infarction. Although a positive reaction rarely occurs on the first test in normal individuals, after one or two inoculations with autologous leukocytes most normal individuals develop a positive reaction. Thus the diseases in which this reaction appears differ from normal only in the appearance of a positive reaction on the first inoculation. The development of a positive response after one or more tests precludes sequential study of the reaction in a single individual.

An analogous kind of skin response has been reported in other situations. In thyroiditis, there is a similar responsiveness to thyroid extract, and after an individual has rejected a homograft, an intradermal inoculation of donor white blood cells provokes such a reaction. The timing of these reactions is the same as in SLE.

DECREASED SERUM COMPLEMENT LEVELS

Serum complement levels are often depressed in SLE with or without nephropathy [13]. They are also depressed in acute glomerulonephritis but not in rheumatoid arthritis, dermatomyositis, or scleroderma. All four components of complement are reduced. Fluorescent antibody to the β_{1C}-globulin which is a component of complement has been used to demonstrate localization of this component in the glomerular and splenic periarteriolar depositions of γ-globulin. Taken together, these data suggest that *in vivo* utilization of complement occurs, presumably by immunological reaction, and are compatible with the possibility that these reactions may be harmful to tissues.

CERTAIN OTHER RELEVANT IMMUNOLOGICAL CONSIDERATIONS

The existence of hypergammaglobulinemia, of circulating autoantibodies, and of the peculiar skin reactivity to autologous tissue constituents all suggest a general immunological hyperresponsiveness in patients with SLE, but the data are not decisive. No clear evidence has emerged from numerous studies to suggest that the antibody response to common exogenous antigens in patients with SLE is greater than that in normal individuals. Likewise, the ability to develop delayed hypersensitivity reactions to various foreign antigens has not been proved abnormal. Furthermore, in limited studies, patients with SLE have retained autologous skin grafts and rejected unrelated and maternal skin in a normal manner. Untreated patients with SLE are not more susceptible to infection, nor do they appear to be more resistant to it. Although not all of these possibilities have been exhaustively explored, at present there does not appear to be a generalized unrestricted increase in the immunological responsiveness.

Despite the abundance of autoimmune reactions in SLE, often involving crucial cell constituents such as chromosomal and genetic materials, not a single type of tissue damage has been identified which can be ascribed to these reactions. Indeed, preliminary evidence suggests that in certain circumstances antitissue antibodies, whether autoantibodies or not, may be protective rather than harmful [14, 15]. Pending clarification of the biological role of autoantibodies and the elucidation of pathogenic mechanisms, the term "autoimmune disease" should either be used with qualification or be avoided. The presence of autoantibodies, even if they are regarded as by-products of the pathogenic mechanism, suggests that immunological phenomena might play a role in pathogenesis, but our inadequate understanding of human immunological responses makes its unwise to convert the suggestion into an assumption.

Dixon *et al.* [16] have developed experimental observations in rabbits which are interesting. When rabbits are immunized with a foreign protein such as bovine serum albumin, they respond in one of three general patterns. A significant number produce large amounts of antibody and often develop limited acute glomerulitis, following which they remain healthy. These animals continue to produce large amounts of antibody after subsequent injections of bovine serum albumin and appear to be able to remove the bovine protein from the circulation. A second group of animals responds to the provocative immunization less vigorously and produces less antibody. The intensity of their immune response is such that, following immunization with bovine serum albumin, they produce only enough antibody to place the plasma antigen-antibody ratio in the region of antigen excess. As a result, they have circulating soluble antigen-antibody complexes. In time, a nephropathy develops that is indistinguishable on light and electron miscroscopy from membranous glomerulonephritis in man. The antigen-antibody complexes are found localized at the glomerular membrane on immunofluorescent microscopy. The third group of animals, by far the smallest, does not produce antibody and does not develop visible disease.

These studies raise the possibility that circulating soluble antigen-antibody complexes may be harmful to tissues, even though the antibody of the complex is not directed against a specific constituent of the tissue which is damaged. Second, the observations are compatible with the possibility that a wide range of infectious agents and other foreign materials may initiate an immune response which eventually results in formation of harmful complexes. Third, the results suggest that the appearance of pathological lesions may be directly related to the intensity and quality of the immune response of the recipient; hereditary variations in the nature of the immune response could lead to a predisposition to the development of circulating antigen-antibody complexes and thereby to certain types of tissue lesions.

An inbred strain of mice (NZB) has been discovered in New Zealand which spontaneously develops hemolytic anemia and thymic lesions. In the F_1 hybrid generation from mating of this strain with another strain (NZW), a nephropathy similar to that seen in SLE develops, and serum from these mice is able to induce LE cell formation [17]. Aleutian disease of mink, to which there is a genetic susceptibility and which is characterized by increased γ-globulin levels, resembles polyarteritis nodosa pathologically and has been shown to be devoid of autoimmune reactions and to be probably of viral origin [18]. States resembling human disease accompanied by autoimmune reactions have also been described in the dog. The former two diseases combine a genetic predisposition with immunological abnormalities; Aleutian disease may result from the influence of an environmental factor (virus) on a particular immunological constitution.

Multiple efforts have been made to provoke autoimmunity in normal experimental animals by immunization with autologous cell constituents. They have had only qualified success. Thyroiditis and demyelinating disease of the nervous system can be achieved through autoimmunization with thyroid or brain tissues, respectively, but it has not been possible to attain experimental states analogous to the various rheumatic diseases. In view of the evidence of a genetic predisposition to rheumatic disease in man, it has been reasonable to assume that experimental autoimmunization would be unlikely to produce a comparable disease state in animals unless the proper predisposition existed. The diseases of mice and mink described above support this contention.

The important role of the thymus in the maturation of immunological responsiveness has been established (Chap. 4 and Ref. 19). It has not been demonstrated, however, whether the thymus is the site of formation of the first immunologically competent cells which then populate other sites in the body, is the source of a "hormone" essential for cell maturation, or has a combination of these functions. The correlation of thymoma with certain types of myasthenia gravis, the finding of thymoma or thymic lesions in occasional cases of SLE, and the identification of serological autoimmune reactions in certain patients with myasthenia gravis have all led to the suggestion that a thymic lesion might be primarily responsible for the development of a disease such as SLE. To date, no evidence supporting this contention has been forthcoming.

ETIOLOGY

The etiology of SLE remains unknown. There is no correlation epidemiologically or serologically with streptococcal infections. The discovery of autoimmunity has provided an important clue, and recent clinical and immunological evidence suggests the existence of a familial predisposition [20].

For many years a genetic predisposition to rheumatic fever was suspected but not established. Epidemiological and serological studies in rheumatoid arthritis suggest a familial predisposition to at least certain forms of the disease. Now family studies in SLE have yielded much additional information. Relatives of patients with SLE have been found to have a higher incidence of rheumatic disease, hypergammaglobulinemia and autoantibodies than the general population. Within a given family, the propositus of the study may have SLE while close relatives may have rheumatoid arthritis, SLE, dermatomyositis, or rheumatic fever or may have immunological abnormalities without clinical disease (Figs. 66-2 and 66-3). Among the abnormal relatives, the latter are the most common. Immunological abnormalities include elevated serum γ-globulin levels, significant titers of rheumatoid factor, antitissue antibodies, or false positive Wassermann reactions. The rheumatic disease

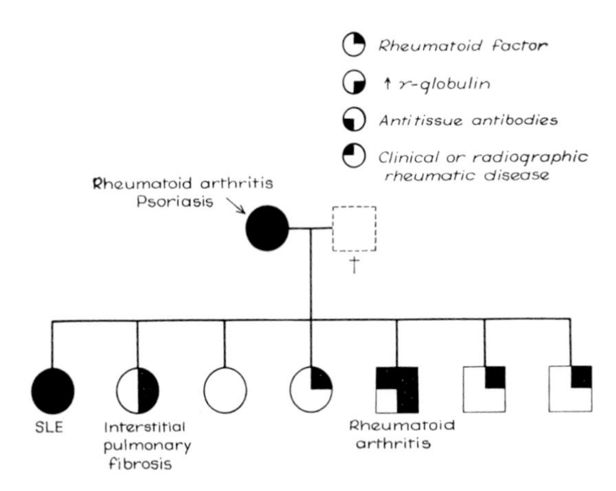

Fig. 66-2. Family pedigree. Mother of the proband had extensive serological abnormalities and clinical rheumatoid arthritis. Five of six siblings are abnormal. Two siblings have clinical disease; one, pulmonary fibrosis which may be a part of the rheumatic disease picture. Individual indicated by broken line was not studied. (Figs. 66-2 and 66-3 from Holman, H. R., in *Progress in Medical Genetics* [New York: Grune & Stratton, Inc., 1962], Vol. 2, p. 210; by permission.)

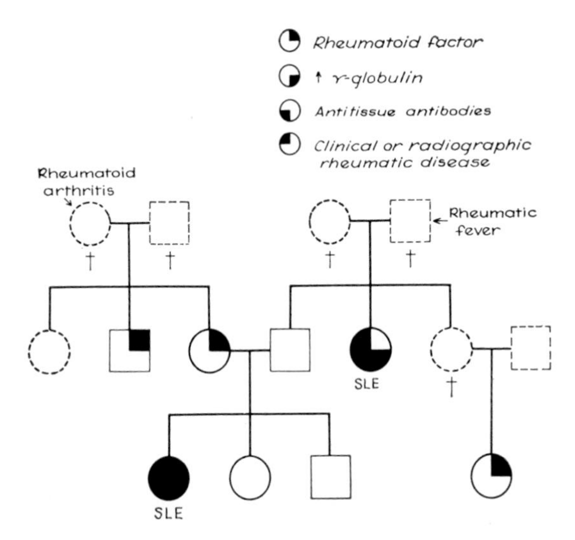

Fig. 66-3. Family pedigree. Father of the proband has borderline elevation of serum γ-globulin, not indicated in pedigree. One paternal aunt has SLE; the other paternal aunt died of unexplained renal disease. Daughter of the paternal aunt was considered to have SLE by other physicians, but had only a circulating rheumatoid factor at the time of testing. Paternal grandfather was alleged to have had rheumatic heart disease. Mother of the proband has morning stiffness and arthralgia in addition to a circulating rheumatoid factor. Maternal grandmother was alleged to have had typical rheumatoid arthritis. Individuals indicated by broken line were not studied.

found most frequently in the families of patients with SLE is rheumatoid arthritis, emphasizing again the relationships between the various illnesses in the rheumatic category. A similar situation obtains among relatives of patients with scleroderma; comparable studies have not been made in other so-called connective tissue diseases.*

It is possible that individuals with serological abnormalities but without clinical disease are predisposed to rheumatic disease. An illuminating and relevant study was initiated by Moore and his colleagues three decades ago [21]. Their results indicate that individuals with biologically false positive reactions for syphilis develop rheumatoid arthritis or a related disease more frequently than other illnesses in later life.

Cumulative evidence therefore indicates but does not prove an inherited predisposition to rheumatic diseases. Equally important has been the appearance within these families of disease not hitherto considered related to rheumatic diseases. Various types of lymphoma, macroglobulinemia, myeloma, and agammaglobulinemia have been identified [22–24]. These interrelationships now involve most of the disease states accompanied by abnormalities in serum γ-globulins. Thus the electrophoretically broad-based hypergammaglobulinemia of rheumatic diseases appears to be related to the selective narrow-based hypergammaglobulinemia of myeloma and macroglobulinemia, to the mild hypogammaglobulinemia of lymphoma, and even to the severe hypogammaglobulinemia wherein susceptibility to infection develops.

The precise meaning of these interrelationships in terms of pathogenesis is not clear. They strengthen the view, however, that immunological abnormalities play a role in these illnesses and that the abnormalities are at least partially under genetic influence.

Certain clinical observations provide clues to the etiology of SLE. For example, intercurrent infections, usually bacterial, can cause an exacerbation of quiescent SLE. Treatment of the infection alone will sometimes result in

* *Editor's comment:* It has been difficult for me to feel convinced by most of the studies that have alleged an increased predisposition to immunological disease in families of patients with lupus. However, a recent report by Leonhardt (*Acta Med. Scand.*, 176:5, 1964) was extensive and remarkably well conducted, and it is hard to ignore.—J. H. V.

disappearance of the activity of SLE. However, there has been no correlation between the *initial* appearance of SLE and identifiable bacterial or viral infection. Thus the possible relationship of infection to SLE is not clearly analogous to that of streptococcal infection to the appearance of rheumatic fever. Nonetheless infection might provide a primary or secondary stimulus resulting in cell damage and, by inducing certain antigenic changes in cell constituents, might lead to initiation of autoimmune reactions. If so, the persistence of the infective agent or possibly of the autoantibodies themselves might perpetuate tissue damage.

Other precipitating factors exist. Some patients become worse on exposure to sunlight, with subsidence of disease activity when sunlight is avoided. Ingestion of certain drugs, most notably sulfonamides, hydantoins, and hydralazine, has been correlated with acute attacks of SLE. With hydralazine, the clinical symptoms resembling SLE subside when the drug is withdrawn. Although none of these drugs is established as a primary causative agent of SLE, it is possible that a drug hypersensitivity could initiate the disease, particularly in a susceptible person. In other instances, it may be that the drug is used to treat clinical disorders such as seizure patterns which are manifestations of SLE itself.

CLINICAL DIAGNOSIS

It might be inferred that there is such fluctuation in the clinical course of SLE, such variation in the organs involved, and so minimal morphological change in the tissues, that diagnosis would be extremely difficult. In fact, this is not the case. Certain clinical patterns emerge which are characteristic even though not diagnostic in themselves. The skin rash is usually limited to the upper portion of the body and consists typically of raised, erythematous, scaling, nonfriable lesions which are often aggravated by exposure to sun. At times, it is mixed with the characteristic atrophic, depressed, hyperpigmented or depigmented lesions of discoid lupus erythematosus. The arthritis is characteristically migratory and only rarely leads to joint destruction and deformity. The hematological picture is one of mild to moderate anemia, with or without leukopenia and thrombocytopenia and with a normal or slightly hypercellular bone marrow. The renal lesion is usually a mixed one, both functionally and morphologically, with elements of acute and membranous glomerulonephritis. Effusions may occur over any serous surface and present as pleuritis, pericarditis, or peritonitis. The central nervous system manifestations are usually those of an idiopathic grand mal seizure pattern but may present with any degree or pattern of organic defect, mental aberration, or frank psychosis.

Abnormalities which are detectable on physical examination are varied and depend on the organ systems involved. The rash may be typical, as described above, or may simply have a nondescript erythematous appearance. Other physical findings which are particularly useful in establishing the diagnosis are generalized alopecia, discrete retinal exudates (cytoid bodies) without accompanying hemorrhage, photophobia, Raynaud's phenomenon, superficial bruising, diffuse adenopathy, hepatosplenomegaly, acute effusive arthritis, mild muscle tenderness, and peripheral neuropathy. If the patient has thrombocytopenia, purpura may be present. If the patient has pleuropericardial effusions, interstitial pneumonitis, and/or myocarditis, respiratory and cardiac symptoms may predominate. At times, a nonbacterial, verrucous endocarditis, often called Libman-Sacks endocarditis, may be present and result in cardiac murmurs of a valvular origin. If the patient has an isolated peritoneal effusion or mesenteric vasculitis, the appearance may be that of an acute abdominal crisis.

Usually there is not a predominant clinical involvement of one organ system, such as the heart in rheumatic fever, the joint in rheumatoid arthritis, the peripheral artery in polyarteritis, the skin in scleroderma, or the muscle in dermatomyositis. Instead, the hallmark of SLE is involvement of many organs often simulating any one of the foregoing diseases and, with the exception of the kidney, usually not characterized by a relentless course leading to tissue destruction. The diagnosis is made through the finding of the salient clinical features together with certain laboratory abnormalities. The crucial consideration for the clinician is recognition of the multiple ways in which the disease may present itself and the changing patterns which may evolve.

The most useful laboratory abnormalities fall into four general categories: hematological, serological, renal, and neurological. The commonest hematological changes are elevated sedimentation rate, hemolytic anemia with or without a positive Coombs reaction, leukopenia with relative lymphocytosis or a normal differential count, and perhaps thrombocytopenia. The common serological changes include hypergammaglobulinemia of the broad-base type and multiple circulating autoantibodies capable of reacting with red blood cells, white blood cells, many different nuclear and cytoplasmic constituents, thromboplastin, occasionally thrombin, and the Wassermann reagin. The rheumatoid factor is often present. Renal abnormalities consist of hematuria, proteinuria, decreased glomerular filtration, and azotemia. Neurological abnormalities include peripheral neuropathy with decreased nerve conduction time, an abnormal electroencephalogram, and an elevated cerebrospinal fluid protein level. Electromyography may reveal evidence of myositis.

Clearly, none of these abnormalities is specific for SLE. Many are present individually or in groups in a variety of other illnesses, particularly other rheumatic illnesses. It is the presence of a representative group of abnormalities which is helpful in diagnosis. Furthermore, certain distinctions between SLE and these other diseases can be made. For example, polyarteritis nodosa is characterized by leukocytosis and occasional eosinophilia, with infrequent hypergammaglobulinemia or circulating autoantibodies. Rheumatic fever is rarely accompanied by hypergammaglobulinemia or abnormal autoantibodies but is characterized by antibodies to streptococcal products. Rheumatoid arthritis usually presents a normal or slightly elevated white blood cell count with a normal differential count, a greater incidence of rheumatoid factor, and a correspondingly lesser incidence of antitissue antibodies. The serological and hematological abnormalities in dermatomyositis and scleroderma tend to resemble those in SLE. Differentiation of SLE from thrombotic thrombocytopenic purpura, subacute bacterial endocarditis (particularly when verrucous endocarditis is present), and various types of lymphoma is sometimes difficult and must be based on tissue biopsy, bacteriological studies, and observation of the course of the disease.

At times, there is an inadequate number of clinical and laboratory abnormalities to permit a confident diagnosis. At other times, an abundance of abnormalities provides evidence of many different rheumatic diseases. When typical manifestations of the disease are not apparent or when a patient presents features common to SLE and other rheumatic disorders at the same time, diagnosis is usually provisional and should be based on the relative similarity of clinical and laboratory findings to the various alternative possibilities. Treatment should be governed by an assessment of the state and course of the illness.

TREATMENT

Despite its pragmatic origins, the current treatment of SLE is reasonably effective. Among the so-called connective tissue diseases, the best results are obtained in SLE and dermatomyositis. Prolonged remissions often occur.

Historically, the management of SLE has involved use of symptomatic measures and anti-inflammatory agents. Salicylates and later corticosteroids were given. More recently, as the probable immunological nature of this disease has become apparent and the immunosuppressive effects of corticosteroids have been recognized, other immunosuppressive agents have been tried. Experience with the latter is recent and limited and is inadequate for detailed evaluation at this time. On the basis of chance observation, antimalarial agents have been found to be effective at times, although the mechanism of their action is unknown.

A decisive improvement in management followed the introduction of corticosteroids. These drugs were found to suppress acute episodes and to prolong life. Because of the potentially devastating character of the disease, physicians have been unwilling to deny treatment to patients, so that adequately controlled studies have not been made to establish with precision the benefits of corticosteroid therapy. For the severely ill patient, however, retrospective studies suggest that the average duration of life from diagnosis to death without the use of corticosteroids, including spontaneous periods of remission, was not more than two years. Even the use of cortisone in the early 1950's in comparatively small doses resulted in at least a doubling of survival time [1]. Current usage appears to result, in the majority of instances, in a great prolongation of life and many years of nearly normal existence for most patients.

The most striking consequence of the use of corticosteroids, aside from the prolongation of life, has been the change in the course of the illness. The old lupus crisis, an acute, effusive, frequently fatal episode, has virtually disappeared because of the responsiveness of the skin rash, fever, arthritis, and serositis to steroid therapy. Verrucous endocarditis is now rarely seen. As these aspects of the disease have been brought under control, other elements have come to the fore as the most resistant to management and the most likely to cause death. Particularly notable are the mixed nephropathy leading to renal failure and the various forms of encephalopathy.

Three stages may be identified in the response to corticosteroid treatment when a dose equivalent to about 60 mg. of prednisone is employed in the average 70-kg. adult. The first is disappearance of acute symptoms such as fever, rash, arthritis, and serositis. This may occur within hours or days. The second stage involves correction of the hematological and serological abnormalities, with disappearance of the anemia, hypergammaglobulinemia, and abnormal antibodies and a return of the sedimentation rate to normal. Usually these improvements will not have begun at the time symptoms disappear. Treatment must be continued for an average of 3 to 4 weeks for them to occur. The third stage, the disappearance of renal disease when present, usually takes 6 to 10 weeks of treatment with 60 mg. of prednisone daily. The endpoint of improvement is considered to be a disappearance of hematuria and azotemia and a significant diminution of proteinuria. If treatment is discontinued at the time of symptomatic response, while serological and renal abnormalities persist, it is almost predictable that the disease process will smolder and that exacerbation will occur. If, however, the intensive therapy is continued until all abnormalities have either disappeared or greatly improved and become stabilized, the chances of withdrawing the drug without exacerbation are much better. Whether or not corticosteroids should ever be used exclusively in low doses in milder forms of the disease is a debatable point. It seems preferable, once the decision has been made to use corticosteriods, to give them in high enough doses to obtain the effects mentioned. When only an incomplete remission is obtained by high-dose treatment, low-dose maintenance therapy may subsequently be necessary.*

Clinical and morphological data now at hand demonstrate that a sizable percentage of patients with lupus nephropathy will improve if appropriate corticosteroid therapy is employed [10, 25]. Not only is there measurable improvement in kidney function but there is also improvement in the morphological picture in the kidney on biopsy when studied by light or immunofluorescent microscopy. The types of nephropathy that respond are acute nephritis or the nephrotic syndrome with proteinuria and hematuria. Apparently the more acute the glomerulitis, the more responsive the lesion. No evidence of improvement has been obtained when the nephritis has reached the point of universal glomerular scarring, with small shrunken kidneys and the clinical syndrome of chronic glomerulonephritis. It is also probable that an advanced stage of membranous glomerulonephritis is not responsive. Fortunately, the most common form of the illness is acute glomerulitis without severe widespread damage to the basement membrane. When diagnosed early and treated properly, this type is likely to respond.

The mechanism of the steroid-induced improvement in SLE is unknown. Not only are the peripheral inflammatory manifestations suppressed, but the lymph node hypertrophy and splenomegaly are diminished. In the dose range of 60 mg. of prednisone per day, there are heightened susceptibility to infection and suppression of the immune response to antigenic stimulus. A distinct drop in serum γ-globulin level and abnormal antibody titers is usually observed in the patient. Presumably, therefore, immunosuppression plays a role in

* *Editor's comment:* Clinicians charged with the care of patients with lupus nephropathy would be well advised to read the report by Rothfield *et al.* (*New Eng. J. Med.* 269:537, 1963). In many respects their experience agrees with Holman's; but they make a plea for a somewhat more conservative program of steroid management than Holman seems to espouse, and certainly more conservative than Pollak's program [25]. Until more definitive data are available, it would seem to me best to treat patients with lupus nephropathy with as vigorous a steroid program as is needed to bring systemic signs of activity under control, the steroid dosage being dropped as indicated by the general clinical picture. According to Rothfield, the activity of the kidney disease can be expected to follow the pattern exhibited by the systemic activities. Others (quoted by Rothfield *et al.*) do not agree with this, however.—J. H. V.

inducing improvement. Why the improvement should remain in many instances after the higher dose of corticosteroids is discontinued is unknown.

The mechanism of renal improvement is also unknown. However, the studies of Farquhar and Palade [26] have demonstrated a dynamic state within the glomerulus involving phagocytosis of damaged glomerular membrane by deep endothelial cells and actual replacement of the membrane. This suggests that if the initial, presumably immunological, insult is terminated and an adequate period of time given for the kidney to repair itself, healing could occur.

Lupus encephalopathy is not so responsive to corticosteroids. Nevertheless central and peripheral neurological lesions will improve in many cases and seizure patterns often cease. The mechanism of this improvement is also obscure.

In addition to corticosteroids, antimalarials such as chloroquine and related compounds have been used. Their value in discoid lupus erythematosus has been established by comparative studies. It appears that the antimalarials are also beneficial for the skin lesions of SLE and that, when used in conjunction with corticosteroids, they may permit a more rapid and earlier reduction of steroid dose.

The mechanism of action of antimalarials is unknown. They appear to protect the skin against the harmful effects of ultraviolet light. This may in some way contribute to their usefulness. They are basic compounds which combine with acidic materials in the cell, including DNA. When they have combined with the nucleic acids of cells, they prevent the autoantibodies from subsequently uniting with these nucleic acids. There is no evidence, however, that this interference with an antigen-antibody interaction is pertinent to the therapeutic benefit, because there is no evidence that this reaction itself is involved in pathogenesis. Many of the different antimalarial compounds have been used with approximately equal success.

Because of the mild forms of the disease which occur and the spontaneous remissions which may characterize even an active case, vigorous treatment with corticosteroids may not always be necessary. When no crucial organ is involved and the patient's discomfort is minimal, management may be attempted at least for a time with salicylates and antimalarials alone, as long as the patient is carefully observed and more active treatment is used if there is evidence of disease progression.

There are other helpful means of management. It seems true that the presence of a bacterial and possibly a viral infection will make SLE resistant to therapy or even precipitate an acute flare in a patient in remission. The eradication of infection is therefore of great importance. Urinary tract infections, particularly cystitis, are very common in patients with SLE, especially when they have been receiving corticosteroids. The treatment of an infection alone may lead to a dramatic remission in SLE.

Avoidance of the use of certain drugs is occasionally decisive. The sulfonamides and antibiotics such as penicillin can provoke acute attacks of the disease in some patients. This is also true of the hydantoin drugs used in the management of seizures. When they must be used, careful scrutiny and control are essential.

Recently, other immunosuppressive agents such as radiomimetic drugs and purine antagonists have been studied. Initial reports are encouraging, particularly for the use of nitrogen mustards in the treatment of steroid-resistant lupus nephropathy. Preliminary studies suggest that 6-mercaptopurine and 6-thioguanine may have limited usefulness in hemolytic anemia and steroid-resistant nephrosis respectively. The data are too fragmentary to confirm the benefit of these drugs, but they should probably be tried in patients whose condition is deteriorating despite apparently adequate doses of corticosteroids. Such efforts should be made only under careful supervision, for they are still experimental.

REFERENCES

1. Harvey, A. M., Shulman, L. E., Tumulty, P. A., Conley, C. L., and Schoenrich, E. H. *Systemic Lupus Erythematosus: Review of the Literature and Clinical Analysis of 138 Cases.* Baltimore: Williams & Wilkins Company, 1955.
2. Talbott, J., and Ferrandis, R. *Collagen Diseases.* New York: Grune & Stratton, Inc., 1956.
3. Symposium on systemic lupus erythematosus. *J. Mount Sinai Hosp. N.Y.* 24:233, 1959.
4. Symposium on immunologic aspects of rheu-

matoid arthritis and systemic lupus erythematosus. *Arthritis Rheum.* 6:402, 1963.

5. Mellors, R. C., Ortega, L. G., and Holman, H. R. Role of gamma globulins in pathogenesis of renal lesions in systemic lupus erythematosus and chronic membranous glomerulonephritis, with an observation on the lupus erythematosus cell reaction. *J. Exp. Med.* 106:191, 1957.
6. Vazquez, J. J., and Dixon, F. J. Immunohistochemical study of lesions in rheumatic fever, systemic lupus erythematosus, and rheumatoid arthritis. *Lab. Invest.* 6:205, 1957.
7. Freedman, P., and Markowitz, A. S. Isolation of antibody-like gamma globulin from lupus glomeruli. *Brit. Med. J.* 1:1175, 1962.
8. Holman, H. R. The L. E. cell phenomenon. *Ann. Rev. Med.* 11:231, 1960.
9. Asherson, G. L., and Demonde, D. C. Autoantibody production in rabbits. *Immunology* 6:19, 1963.
10. Holman, H. R. Systemic lupus erythematosus. *J. Pediat.* 56:109, 1960.
11. Friedman, E. A., Bardawil, J. P., and Hanau, C. "Delayed" cutaneous hypersensitivity to leukocytes in disseminated lupus erythematosus. *New Eng. J. Med.* 262:486, 1960.
12. Bennett, J. C., and Holley, H. L. Intradermal hypersensitivity in systemic lupus erythematosus *Arthritis Rheum.* 4:64, 1961.
13. Morse, J. H., Muller-Eberhard, H. J., and Kunkel, H. G. Antinuclear factors and serum complement in systemic lupus erythematosus. *Bull. N.Y. Acad. Med.* 38:642, 1962.
14. Paterson, P. Y., and Harwin, S. M. Suppression of allergic encephalomyelitis in rats by means of antibrain serum. *J. Exp. Med.* 117: 755, 1963.
15. Snell, G. D., Winn, H. J., Stimpfling, J. H., and Parker, S. J. Depression by antibody of the immune response to homografts and its role in immunological enhancement. *J. Exp. Med.* 112:293, 1960.
16. Dixon, F. J., Feldman, J., and Vazquez, J. Experimental glomerulonephritis. *J. Exp. Med.* 113:899, 1961.
17. Helyer, B. J., and Howie, J. B. Renal disease associated with positive lupus erythematosus tests in a crossbred strain of mice. *Nature* (London) 197:197, 1963.
18. Henson, J. B., Gorham, J. R., Leader, R. W., and Wagner, B. M. Experimental hypergammaglobulinemia in mink. *J. Exp. Med.* 116: 357, 1962.
19. Miller, J. F. A. P. Role of the thymus in immunity. *Brit. Med. J.* 2:459, 1963.
20. Holman, H. R. Clinical and immunologic evidence for a predisposition to rheumatic disease in certain families. *Progr. Med. Genet.* 2:210, 1962.
21. Moore, J. E., and Lutz, W. Natural history of systemic lupus erythematosus: An approach to its study through chronic biologic false positive reactors. *J. Chron. Dis.* 1:297, 1955.
22. Waldenström, J. Studies on conditions associated with disturbed gamma globulin formation (gammopathies). Harvey Lect. 56:211, 1960–61.
23. Fudenberg, H., German, J. L., and Kunkel, H. G. The occurrence of rheumatoid factor and other gamma globulin abnormalities in the families of patients with agammaglobulinemia. *Arthritis Rheum.* 5:565, 1962.
24. Wolf, J. K. Primary acquired agammaglobulinemia, with a family history of collagen disease and hematologic disorders. *New Eng. J. Med.* 266:473, 1962.
25. Pollak, V. E., Pirani, C. L., and Kark, R. M. Effect of large doses of prednisone on the renal lesions and life span of patients with lupus glomerulonephritis. *J. Lab. Clin. Med.* 57:495, 1961.
26. Farquhar, M. G., and Palade, G. E. Functional evidence for the existence of a third cell type in renal glomerulus: Phagocytosis of filtration residues by a distinctive "third" cell. *J. Cell. Biol.* 13:55, 1962.

67. Polyarteritis Nodosa

GEOFFREY A. ROSE

DEFINITION AND CLASSIFICATION

Polyarteritis nodosa is a disease characterized by numerous foci of arterial necrosis and inflammation. These may affect almost any organ, or combination of organs, in the body. The manifestations of the disease are mainly due to obstruction of blood flow through affected vessels, leading to infarction and scarring. Nearly all cases diagnosed in life prove fatal. Perhaps this only reflects the difficulty of clinical diagnosis: it is quite possible that milder forms of the disease occur but escape detection.

Certain groups of cases which show acceptable histological changes are nevertheless usually not included as "polyarteritis nodosa." (1) Some tissue injuries produce *secondary arteritis*. For example, in tuberculous meningitis, or on the borders of a pulmonary infarct, there may be seen foci of necrotizing arteritis which, viewed in isolation, are indistinguishable from polyarteritis nodosa; yet clearly they should not be so diagnosed. Such cases illustrate how a variety of mechanisms may ultimately produce the same histological changes. They serve as a warning, often ignored, against assuming that the lesion makes the disease. The production of arteritis in animals, for example, by hypersensitivity or hypertension, does not prove that these mechanisms are involved in polyarteritis nodosa. (2) *Giant cell arteritis,* though sharing some features with polyarteritis nodosa, is so distinctive in its age restriction and pathology as to justify its separate classification. (3) Similarly, *thromboangiitis obliterans* can be excluded, despite the fact that occasional lesions resemble polyarteritis nodosa.

From this it can be seen that polyarteritis nodosa is really a diagnosis by exclusion: the label covers all cases of necrotizing arteritis that remain after more specific groups have been split off. Do the remaining cases, in fact, represent a single disease, or are there still various diseases sharing a common lesion? The type of case originally described by Kussmaul and Maier [1], with nodes and aneurysms on medium-sized arteries, seemed a well-defined entity. Nowadays, however, most cases diagnosed as polyarteritis nodosa are very different, with a majority of lesions affecting small vessels which do not form aneurysms. This type of case may well have become much commoner in recent years, whereas "classic" polyarteritis nodosa remains, as it always was, a rarity. This naturally provokes the suggestion [2] that there are two forms of the disease: "classic" and "microscopic." But although these extremes may be clearly different, unfortunately it is common to find intermediate and mixed forms.

Wegener [3] described a syndrome, known since by his name, of granulomatous arteritis and glomerulonephritis, combined with destructive granulomata unrelated to arteries. Others [4–6] described a syndrome of asthma, eosinophilia, arteritis, and, again, nonarterial granulomata. Rose and Spencer [7] showed that these two syndromes are variants of a single type, which they called "polyarteritis with lung involvement." Such cases tend to show a number of features which do not occur (or occur very rarely) in cases of polyarteritis nodosa without lung involvement. These features are: (1) a specific respiratory illness preceding systemic polyarteritis [8]; (2) blood eosinophil level of 1,500 or more per cu. mm.; (3) destructive granulomata in the upper respiratory tract and elsewhere, and (4) eosinophilic arteritis in early lesions, progressing to granulomatous arteritis with giant cells.

Not all cases with lung involvement show all of these features. Some resemble Wegener's syndrome, and lack eosinophilia; others are of the asthma/eosinophilia type; others are mixed. But taken as a whole, the cases can be clearly distinguished from the group without lung involvement, indicating that the lungs have some special role, at present unknown, in relation to the pattern of the disease. It is very rare to find an exception to the rule that, in polyarteritis nodosa, if the lungs are spared at the start they will not be involved later. This is not true of any other organ. Indeed, in some florid cases without lung involvement, it is most remarkable how almost every other organ in the body may be full of arteritis, which extends even to bronchial arteries, and yet the pulmonary vessels are completely spared.

Zeek's classification [9] includes a group (allergic granulomatous angiitis) which corresponds in part to "polyarteritis nodosa with lung involvement." She subdivides the remaining cases into "periarteritis nodosa," which she believes to be due to hypertension, and "hypersensitivity angiitis," attributed to drug sensitization. This scheme is unsatisfactory in two ways: (1) the pathological criteria proposed do not in practice yield two distinct groups, and (2) the reasoning on etiology is unsound, particularly in dealing with the "hypertensive" group. It is true that hypertensive rats often develop necrotizing mesenteric arteritis [10–12], but this is a species peculiarity of the rat. In man, polyarteritis nodosa seems to be neither caused nor aggravated by high blood pressure [7]. The only human analogy to the hypertensive arteritis of rats is in the rare development of arteritis confined to the pulmonary tree in cases of pulmonary hypertension [13].

In the type of case considered so far, necrotizing arteritis has been a dominant and usually lethal feature. Similar lesions, but few in number, have also been noted as an incidental finding in some other diseases, particularly rheumatoid arthritis [14, 15] and rheumatic fever with rheumatic heart disease [16]. These same diseases have another link with polyarteritis nodosa, in that their prevalence among cases of polyarteritis nodosa is unduly high (see under Clinical and Laboratory Observations). It is tempting to suppose that individuals with these rheumatic diseases have a general tendency to polyarteritis, which may range from a few minor lesions to major polyarteritis nodosa. This supposes that a whole spectrum of severity of arteritis exists between these extremes [17]. But at present it is only the extremes that have been identified, and judgment on this interesting point must be suspended.

PATHOLOGY

Six distinct types of lesion occur in polyarteritis nodosa, although two of them are rare.

ARTERITIS

As the name of the disease implies, this is a focal lesion. It affects short lengths of vessel wall, and often only a segment of the circumference. Most lesions involve vessels of 200 to 500 μ external diameter, but larger or (more often) smaller arteries may also be affected. Cases with lesions of the small arteries often have similar changes in small veins.

The earliest lesion is necrosis and fibrinoid change, beginning in the inner part of the media and extending to interrupt both media and internal elastic lamina. Studies with fluorescein-labeled rabbit antihuman fibrin [18] suggest that the hyaline material is actual fibrin; γ-globulin and albumin are also present [19, 20]. Mellors and Ortega [20] believe that this γ-globulin is, at least in part, antibody attached to a vascular antigen. But Paronetto and Strauss [19] regard its appearance as secondary. They failed to demonstrate precipitation of soluble human vessel antigen by serum from a patient with polyarteritis nodosa (using the agar double-diffusion technique); and the patient's fluorescein-labeled serum γ-globulin did not bind to either normal or polyarteritic segments of his blood vessels. They concluded that this ruled out an autospecific antigen-antibody interaction in the vessel wall. This seems, however, an unjustified conclusion to draw from negative results.*

Within the affected segments, intimal thickening and thrombosis obstruct the blood flow and lead to infarction distally. Inflammatory cells accumulate, neutrophils and eosinophils later giving place to mononuclears (including plasma cells) and fibroblasts. In cases with lung involvement, a proliferative granulomatous reaction may occur, with giant cells of either Langhans or foreign body type. The lesion progresses to a scar, although in time

* *Editor's comment:* On the other hand, it is fuel for those who advocate that polyarteritis in man may, like serum sickness in rabbits (Dixon *et al.*, in Lawrence, H. S. [Ed.], *Cellular and Humoral Aspects of the Hypersensitive States* [New York: Paul B. Hoeber, Inc., 1959], Chap. 9), be due to vascular damage from circulating antigen-antibody complexes.—J. H. V.

even this seems able to disappear: at necropsy no evidence of arteritis may be found in an organ which was certainly affected earlier by extensive polyarteritis.

Although typical lesions involve necrosis, many others show only inflammatory change. In one of our cases, serial biopsy of skin lesions showed that the entire cycle of development and resolution occurred without any demonstrable necrosis: by light microscopy, at any rate, the lesions were purely inflammatory. Conversely, cases partially controlled by steroid therapy may show necrosis without inflammation, giving lesions like those of malignant hypertension.

GLOMERULITIS

Focal fibrinoid change may occur in the glomerular tufts, accompanied by early and striking capsular proliferation [21]. This combination distinguishes the lesion from ordinary acute glomerulonephritis. Affected glomeruli may contain γ-globulin [19, 20] and possibly complement [22]. Glomerular disorganization is often severe. If the patient survives (which is unusual), the final picture is of nonspecific chronic nephritis.

A most interesting case was reported by Hume *et al.* [23]. A cadaver kidney was grafted into a woman with severe polyarteritic glomerulitis. The donor kidney never functioned, despite an adequate blood supply. At necropsy 38 days after operation, it showed proliferative glomerulitis resembling that seen in the host's own kidneys and quite different from the changes which ordinarily accompany graft rejection at that stage. The evidence is strong that this patient had a circulating factor capable of damaging the donated kidney, possibly an antikidney antibody.* Necrotizing renal arterial lesions have also been observed as part of the homograft rejection reaction [24], and glomerulitis may occur in homografts when the recipient has glomerulonephritis.

NONARTERIAL GRANULOMATA

These lesions, restricted to patients with lung involvement, may affect both upper and lower respiratory tracts and also other organs (principally spleen and kidney). Possibly the earliest change is capillaritis, but it is hard to be sure. The lesions evolve like those of tuberculosis, for which they may be mistaken; miliary granulomata coalesce, invade and destroy local tissues, and may develop central necrosis. They produce nasal lesions ("midline granuloma," etc.) and serious disorganization of lungs and of bronchial walls; elsewhere they cause little trouble.

PLASMA CELLS

These are common in the inflammatory exudate of healing polyarteritis. They may also be numerous throughout the reticuloendothelial system [25] and may contain γ-globulin [19]. In one case, the latter fluoresced with an antihuman 19S macroglobulin. In view of the role of plasma cells in antibody production, these observations are relevant to the question of a hypersensitivity state in polyarteritis nodosa.

HEPATITIS AND MYOCARDITIS

Diffuse interstitial infiltration by round cells is seen occasionally in the liver and heart, although hepatitis is less frequent than in systemic lupus erythematosus.

COLLAGEN LESIONS

Although often referred to as a collagen disease, polyarteritis nodosa as a rule shows no sign of any primary collagen disorder. Very rarely, however, foci of collagen degeneration may occur in splenic capsule, endocardium, or elsewhere, as in systemic lupus erythematosus.

CLINICAL AND LABORATORY OBSERVATIONS

Polyarteritis nodosa occurs at all ages. Although clinical diagnosis is commonest in young adults, the disease is actually most frequent in the elderly [26]; this rising age incidence is the reverse of what happens in rheumatic fever and acute glomerulonephritis. The occurrence and course of disease in women seem unrelated to puberty, pregnancy, and the menopause. Geographic, racial, hereditary, and occupational factors, and smoking habits, appear to be unimportant, but disease begins most often in the winter [27].

* *Editor's comment:* See my comment in footnote on page 750. If one were to accept that polyarteritis may be due to circulating antigen-antibody complexes without any specific antikidney antibody being present, glomerulonephritis in the transplanted kidney may likewise be due to such complexes.—J. H. V.

ONSET

Sometimes a completely fit person falls ill with polyarteritis nodosa; but in about one half of the cases there are antecedents [7]. About 25 percent of cases have preceding chronic respiratory infection, often bronchiectasis. Others have had recent acute hemolytic streptococcal infection, most commonly about two weeks before the onset of polyarteritis. The antistreptolysin 0 titer may be high. About 8 percent of patients have active or quiescent rheumatoid arthritis [26, 28]. Patients with rheumatoid arthritis have an increased risk of polyarteritis nodosa even if they have not received steroids. Some patients have rheumatic heart disease or a history of rheumatic fever; in others, polyarteritis nodosa is accompanied by apparently typical active rheumatic fever, sometimes with Aschoff bodies in the myocardium [29–32, 7]; the arthritis responds to salicylates, the true arthritis of polyarteritis nodosa does not.

Polyarteritis nodosa is sometimes associated with one of the other connective tissue diseases, including systemic lupus erythematosus, scleroderma, dermatomyositis, and Sjögren's syndrome. These are probably instances of simultaneous occurrence of two diseases, rather than mixed intermediate forms; a patient with any one of the group has a heightened susceptibility to the others.

CLINICAL MANIFESTATIONS

There is nearly always a general illness, and this may be severe, with fever, tachycardia, sweating, weight loss, and diffuse aching. It is not known whether this illness is simply a result of extensive inflammatory and ischemic injury or whether it is part of the primary disease disturbance. Local manifestations almost all result from ischemia. For each individual organ they mostly follow a characteristic course: the complexity of the complete clinical picture results from the variety of possible organ involvements. Full information is available in many reviews [33–35].

A striking characteristic is the way that at different, and largely unpredictable, stages different systems become vulnerable. For example, a patient who has had the disease in skin and joints for some months may then over a short period develop extensive peripheral nerve involvement; this may later fail to recur despite continued activity of the disease elsewhere. Evidently at that particular stage the vasa nervorum, behaving as a distinct system, became temporary targets of injury. A full immunological account of polyarteritis nodosa would have to explain not only why some people get it but also why those who have it evince this curious timing of individual organ and system vulnerability.

Joint involvement usually causes episodes of acute or subacute arthritis, followed within a few days or weeks by full recovery; synovial arteritis has been demonstrated. Occasionally arthritis is more chronic and deforming (? atypical rheumatoid). The muscles are often painful and tender; nodules may be felt, either in muscle or beneath the skin. Arteritis in the *skin* produces maculopapular foci, often hemorrhagic or necrotic. Biopsy of an early lesion may clinch the diagnosis. In the absence of suitable skin lesions, a "blind" muscle biopsy has a reasonable chance of including a focus of arteritis.* *Alimentary* involvement causes abdominal pain and attacks of diarrhea, often blood-stained; physical signs are usually vague. *Coronary* lesions lead to cardiac enlargement and failure and nonspecific changes in the electrocardiogram; the typical picture of infarction is surprisingly rare. Arteritis of *vasa nervorum* causes peripheral neuropathy, usually asymmetrical and ranging from mere paresthesiae to profound paralysis and wasting. The *central nervous system* is rarely affected.

In terms of prognosis, the *kidney* is the key organ: renal lesions are the commonest cause of death, and spontaneous recovery from renal involvement is extremely rare. There are two distinct lesions. Polyarteritis of renal arteries causes cortical infarction, with proteinuria, slight microscopic hematuria, and often renal failure. There may also arise a characteristic glomerulitis [21], with heavy hematuria, oliguria, and renal failure but, curiously, a normal blood pressure. Why the pressure should remain normal in the presence of profound obstruction to renal blood flow has never been explained. If the patient survives the acute phase of renal polyarteritis or glomerulitis, healing and fibrosis tend to be accompanied by progressive hypertension [7]. This hypertension does not activate the arteri-

* *Editor's comment:* In our experience, the term "reasonable chance" suggests, we are afraid, an unduly hopeful estimate.—M. S.

tis, contrary to the theory of Zeek [9], who has postulated on the basis of experience with rats that human polyarteritis nodosa must often be due to high blood pressure.

The *lungs,* as mentioned earlier, are often affected by pre-existing infections, sometimes dating back to childhood. In about one third of cases, they are also affected by specific polyarteritic lesions (arteritis and granulomata) [36]. The accompanying clinical illness may be asthmatic, pneumonic, or bronchitic [8]. The *asthma* of polyarteritis nodosa is not ordinary bronchial asthma: it is distinct in its age distribution, the absence as a rule of a personal or family history of allergy, the presence from the start of specific pathological changes in the lungs and bronchi, and the frequency of high blood eosinophilia. *Pneumonic* cases tend to follow a course intermediate between acute bacterial pneumonia and tuberculosis. Antibiotics are ineffective. *Bronchitic* cases have productive cough, often with hemoptysis and wheezy dyspnea.

Radiological changes are varied, and include miliary shadows, larger infiltrations (sometimes transitory or migratory), abscesses and fibrosis.

For a period which may range from days to years, the disease remains confined to the lungs. Systemic generalization usually occurs acutely and severely, and few patients survive the next six months. This characteristic pattern of illness must have some meaning in relation to pathogenesis. Possibly a bacterial or parasitic antigen gains entry through the respiratory tract; but this, although accounting for bronchial lesions, would hardly explain the early involvement of pulmonary arteries.

LABORATORY FINDINGS

Neutrophil leukocytosis is common, presumably as a consequence of inflammatory lesions and ischemic necrosis. Patients with lung involvement may have high eosinophilia, often curiously intermittent. Sputum culture may yield β-hemolytic streptococci, which are rarely found in other chest diseases. Most patients have normo- or hypochromic anemia; excessive hemolysis or a positive reaction to the Coombs test is uncommon [37].

In active disease, the erythrocyte sedimentation rate is almost invariably raised, and provides an efficient guide to treatment. Serum electrophoresis shows an increase in γ- and often also in α_2-globulin, with reciprocal lowering of albumin. The sensitized sheep cell agglutinin titer is positive in a minority of cases. Macroglobulins have occasionally been reported [38], and a few patients have cold agglutinins.

COURSE

Sometimes polyarteritis nodosa is an acute illness which subsides within a few weeks or months. Much more often, if the patient survives, active disease persists; and the longer it lasts, the less likely it is ever to remit. Presumably in the acute type of illness either the patient is only transiently exposed to the cause of the disease, or else he develops resistance to it. In the more usual persistent case, either exposure to the cause persists or else the disease process, once initiated, is self-perpetuating. Most of the chronic cases show unpredictable variations in activity. Exceptionally, complete remission occurs. This may be permanent, or, perhaps after years, there may be relapse.

TREATMENT

The only drugs known to affect the disease are glucocorticoids. In a small personal experience, antimalarials, nitrogen mustard, and long-term penicillin administration were all without apparent effect.

In adequate dosage, which may need to be high, steroids prevent new arteritis and relieve the constitutional illness. There is no evidence that they promote healing—arteritis heals anyway; nor do they shorten the duration of the disease. Indeed, there is an impression that if treatment is reduced or withdrawn, the patient may sometimes become worse than if steroids had never been started. Similarly, the period following steroid withdrawal in rheumatoid arthritis seems to be particularly associated with a risk of manifest polyarteritis [39]. The effect of treatment on granulomata is less than the effect on arteritis.

The immediate response to treatment is usually dramatic, but the long-term outcome is disappointing. The large doses usually needed are toxic and may compel reduction to an inadequate level. In addition, the late effects of the disease (especially hypertension) may prove fatal even in the absence of active arteritis. The British Medical Research Council [40] carried out a trial based on 21 treated cases and 19 controls; all cases were proved by biopsy. Regrettably, but inevitably, the latter were studied retrospectively. The results are summarized in Table 67-1. They suggest, unfortunately, only a postponement of death.

TABLE 67-1. Survival among 21 Cortisone-treated Patients and 19 Retrospectively Studied Controls[a]

Interval from Biopsy Diagnosis	*% Alive*	
	Treated	*Control*
0 months	100	100
3 months	95	58
6 months	90	47
9 months	86	37
12 months	71	37
2 years	71	37
3 years	62	37
4 years	43	39
5 years	40	39

[a] Results of British Medical Research Council trials [40]. Follow-up not complete after three years.

ETIOLOGY

The causes of polyarteritis nodosa are unknown, but an immunological abnormality has been widely suspected. The absence of any alternative hypothesis and the premature labeling of syndromes as "allergic" have encouraged easy acceptance of the idea. Critical re-examination of the evidence is needed.

EVIDENCE FROM ANIMALS

Arteritis occurs in animals in a wide variety of circumstances, some of which are of very doubtful relevance to polyarteritis nodosa in man. These include spontaneously occurring arteritis [41, 11], hypertensive arteritis in rats and occasionally in dogs [11], pulmonary arteritis in rats produced by 4′-fluoro-10-methyl-1,2-benzanthracene [42], and a curious syndrome of malignant nephrosclerosis, arteritis, and degeneration of islets of Langerhans produced in monkeys by unilateral nephrectomy and administration of sodium and a potent mineralocorticoid [43].*

More relevant is the demonstration of arteritis in animals sensitized to foreign proteins [44]. Most of the numerous experiments of this type have followed the techniques of Rich and Gregory [45], who induced a high level of sensitivity to horse serum in rabbits, most of which developed a single crop of glomerulitis, with necrotizing arteritis in small visceral arteries. In Rich's view, "these experiments demonstrate that periarteritis nodosa is one manifestation of the anaphylactic type of hypersensitivity." But this seems a deduction that cannot be warranted by animal experiments, which can only demonstrate that in certain circumstances protein hypersensitivity can cause a form of arteritis.

Glaser and his colleagues [46] studied the effects of repeated streptococcal infection in rats. A suspension of streptococci, derived from a case of rheumatic fever, was injected into the lungs at intervals of two to three weeks; each infection was controlled by penicillin. The animals were killed after two to seven injections, when 29 percent of them were found to have segmental necrotizing coronary arteritis. Similar lesions were seen occasionally in control animals. If these lesions are analogous to those of serum-sensitized rabbits, it suggests that bacterial antigens also may cause lesions of polyarteritic type. This could be relevant to the association in man between respiratory infections (especially streptococcal) and polyarteritis nodosa.

EVIDENCE FROM MAN

A number of characteristics of the disease suggest, or are consistent with, an immunological basis. (1) The lesions are of the disseminated focal pattern typical of hypersensitivity; and often (e.g., neuropathy, glomerulitis) they show striking organ or tissue specificity. (2) Other features characteristic of immunological abnormality are common in polyarteritis nodosa, including raised serum γ-globulin, abnormal serum proteins [38], and response of the disease to glucocorticoids. Asthma and eosinophilia are also often instanced as evidence of hypersensitivity. (3) The frequency of glomerulitis suggests an analogy with acute glomerulonephritis, which is known to be linked with sensitivity to hemolytic streptococci. (4) The disease may follow hemolytic streptococcal infections, including some that have not received drug therapy [7]. Many other patients have preceding chronic respiratory infections. Bacterial

* *Editor's comment:* Polyarteritic disease also has been described both in horses (*Cornell Vet.* 47:52, 1957) and in mink (*Arthritis Rheum.* 6:386, 1963). In each of these species the disease apparently has a viral etiology.—J. H. V.

hypersensitivity is a possibility in these cases. (5) The disease may be associated with other conditions in which immunological abnormality is present or suspected, including rheumatic fever [16], rheumatoid arthritis [26, 28], systemic lupus erythematosus [26], and Coombs-positive hemolytic anemia [37]. (6) In the case reported by Hume *et al.* [23], mentioned earlier, there was almost certainly a circulating antibody against a component of renal glomeruli.* (7) The literature abounds with reports of polyarteritis nodosa allegedly following, and due to, drug administration. These originated with the observations of Clark and Kaplan [47], and later of Rich [48], of arteritis in cases of fatal serum sickness. Clark and Kaplan concluded that "inferences concerning the pathogenesis of periarteritis nodosa which are based only on morphologic resemblance are of dubious value"; and, in addition, the histology in their two cases was not typical of polyarteritis nodosa. Nevertheless these observations extend to man the findings in serum-sensitized rabbits. They show that hypersensitivity can cause arteritis; but they do not tell us whether most cases of polyarteritis nodosa are caused by hypersensitivity.

There have since been many other reports of polyarteritis nodosa linked with drug administration. In many of them it is, in fact, likely that polyarteritis nodosa was already established, though undiagnosed, before the drug was given. Evidence from the remainder is of three types. The first is based on an impression that polyarteritis nodosa arises with undue frequency in patients who have recently received drugs. Uncontrolled information of this kind is hard to interpret; and in most instances, the drug in question was given for a respiratory infection, so that it is impossible to know whether the drug or the infection, if either, was responsible.

In the second group of cases it is claimed that there was specific evidence of a drug reaction (as in the serum sickness cases already discussed). Although positive Prausnitz-Küstner reactions have been reported [49, 50], isolated case reports may give a misleading impression of frequency. In the largest consecutive series [7], manifestations of histamine-type hypersensitivity were rare, especially considering how many and various were the drugs these patients had received.

In the third type of report, it is claimed that separate episodes of drug administration each provoked an episode of active polyarteritis nodosa. Such cases are very rare, but a few are convincing. In McCormick's [51] case, exacerbations closely followed four separate courses of thiouracil, occurring in one instance twelve hours after a test dose of the drug. Others have also reported polyarteritis nodosa arising during treatment with thiourea derivatives [52–57, 7]. Another report strongly incriminates neoarsphenamine bromide [34]. It should be noted that in several of these drug cases the pathological appearances were unusual. In all of them illness occurred, as one would expect of a drug reaction, in the form of an acute episode. By contrast, most cases of polyarteritis nodosa follow a prolonged course of exacerbations and remissions quite unrelated to drug administration. It has to be remembered also that most patients who have polyarteritis nodosa have not recently taken any drugs.

* *Editor's comment:* And see my comment on this case in footnote on page 750.—J. H. V.

REFERENCES

1. Kussmaul, A., and Maier, R. Ueber eine bisher nicht beschriebene eigenthümliche Arterienerkrankung (Periarteritis nodosa), die mit Morbus Brightii und rapid fortschreitender allgemeiner Muskellähmung einhergeht. *Deutsch. Arch. Klin. Med.* 1:484, 1866.
2. Wainwright, J., and Davson, J. The renal appearances in the microscopic form of periarteritis nodosa. *J. Path. Bact.* 62:189, 1950.
3. Wegener, F. Ueber eine eigenartige rhinogene Granulomatose mit besondere Beteiligung des Arteriensystems und der Nieren. *Beitr. Path. Anat.* 102:36, 1939.
4. Rackemann, F. M., and Greene, J. E. Periarteritis nodosa and asthma. *Trans. Ass. Amer. Physicians* 54:112, 1939.
5. Harkavy, J. Vascular allergy: Pathogenesis of bronchial asthma with recurrent pulmonary infiltrations and eosinophilic polyserositis. *Arch. Intern. Med.* 67:709, 1941.
6. Churg, J., and Strauss, L. Allergic granulomatosis, allergic angiitis, and periarteritis nodosa. *Amer. J. Path.* 27:277, 1951.
7. Rose, G. A., and Spencer, H. Polyarteritis nodosa. *Quart. J. Med.* 26:43, 1957.
8. Rose, G. A. Clinical features of polyarteritis

nodosa with lung involvement. *Brit. J. Dis. Chest* 51:113, 1957.
9. Knowles, H. C., Zeek, P. M., and Blankenhorn, M. A. Studies on necrotizing angiitis: IV. Periarteritis nodosa and hypersensitivity angiitis. *Arch. Intern. Med.* 92:789, 1953.
10. Wilson, C., and Byrom, F. B. Renal changes in malignant hypertension. *Lancet* 1:136, 1939.
11. Smith, C. C., Zeek, P. M., and McGuire, J. Periarteritis nodosa in experimental hypertensive rats and dogs. *Amer. J. Path.* 20:721, 1944.
12. Selye, H., and Pentz, E. I. Pathogenetical correlations between periarteritis nodosa, renal hypertension, and rheumatic lesions. *Canad. Med. Ass. J.* 49:264, 1943.
13. Symmers, W. St. C. Necrotizing pulmonary arteriopathy associated with pulmonary hypertension. *J. Clin. Path.* 5:36, 1952.
14. Sokoloff, L., Wilens, S. L., and Bunim, J. J. Arteritis of striated muscle in rheumatoid arthritis. *Amer. J. Path.* 27:157, 1951.
15. Cruickshank, B. The arteritis of rheumatoid arthritis. *Ann. Rheum. Dis.* 13:136, 1954.
16. VonGlahn, W. C., and Pappenheimer, A. M. Specific lesions of peripheral blood vessels in rheumatism. *Amer. J. Path.* 2:235, 1926.
17. Sokoloff, L., and Bunim, J. J. Vascular lesions in rheumatoid arthritis. *J. Chron. Dis.* 5:668, 1957.
18. Gitlin, D., Craig, J. M., and Janeway, C. A. Studies on the nature of fibrinoid in the collagen diseases. *Amer. J. Path.* 33:55, 1957.
19. Paronetto, F., and Strauss, L. Immunocytochemical observations in periarteritis nodosa. *Ann. Intern. Med.* 56:289, 1962.
20. Mellors, R. C., and Ortega, L. G. III. New observations on the pathogenesis of glomerulonephritis, lipid nephrosis, periarteritis nodosa, and secondary amyloidosis in man. *Amer. J. Path.* 32:455, 1956.
21. Davson, J., Ball, J., and Platt, R. The kidney in periarteritis nodosa. *Quart. J. Med.* 17:175, 1948.
22. Lachmann, P. J., Müller-Eberhard, H. J., Kunkel, H. G., and Paronetto, F. The localization of *in vivo* bound complement in tissue sections. *J. Exp. Med.* 115:63, 1962.
23. Hume, D. M., Merrill, J. P., Miller, B. F., and Thorn, G. W. Experiences with renal homotransplantation in the human: Report of 9 cases. *J. Clin. Invest.* 34:327, 1955.
24. Porter, K. A., Thomson, W. B., Owen, K., Kenyon, J. R., Mowbray, J. F, and Peart, W. S. Obliterative vascular changes in 4 human kidney homotransplants. *Brit. Med. J.* 2:639, 1963.
25. More, R. H., and Movat, H. Z. The significance of plasma cells in the lesions of acute polyarteritis. *J. Path. Bact.* 75:127, 1958.
26. Rose, G. A. The natural history of polyarteritis. *Brit. Med. J.* 2:1148, 1957.
27. Rose, G. A. The Natural Course of Polyarteritis Nodosa, with Special Reference to the Respiratory Tract. In Mills, L. C., and Moyer, J. H. (Eds.), *Inflammation and Diseases of Connective Tissue.* Philadelphia: W. B. Saunders Company, 1961.
28. Ball, J. Rheumatoid arthritis and polyarteritis nodosa. *Ann. Rheum. Dis.* 13:277, 1954.
29. Rothstein, J. L., and Welt, S. Periarteritis nodosa in infancy and childhood. *Amer. J. Dis. Child.* 45:1277, 1933.
30. Spiegel, R. Clinical aspects of periarteritis nodosa. *Arch. Intern. Med.* 58:993, 1936.
31. Rose, M. H., Littmann, D., and Houghton, J. Polyarteritis nodosa: A clinical and pathological study and report of 6 cases. *Ann. Intern. Med.* 32:1114, 1950.
32. Pagel, W. Polyarteritis nodosa and the "rheumatic" diseases. *J. Clin. Path.* 4:137, 1951.
33. Grant, R. T. Polyarteritis nodosa. *Clin. Sci.* 4:245, 1940.
34. Miller, H. G., and Daley, R. Clinical aspects of polyarteritis nodosa. *Quart. J. Med.* 15:255, 1946.
35. Zeek, P. M. Periarteritis nodosa: A critical review. *Amer. J. Clin. Path.* 22:777, 1952.
36. Spencer, H. Pulmonary lesions in polyarteritis nodosa. *Brit. J. Dis. Chest* 51:123, 1957.
37. Illis, L. Association of peripheral neuritis with "autoimmune disease." *Brit. Med. J.* 2:835, 1962.
38. Svartz, N., and Hedman, S. Are the macroglobulins giving rise to a positive sheep cell test in different diseases identical? *Acta Med. Scand.* 173:249, 1963.
39. Slocumb, C. H. Rheumatic complaints during chronic hypercortisonism and syndromes during withdrawal of cortisone in rheumatic patients. *Proc. Mayo Clin.* 28:655, 1953.
40. Medical Research Council. Treatment of polyarteritis nodosa with cortisone: Results after 3 years. *Brit. Med. J.* 1:1399, 1960.
41. Wilens, S. L., and Sproul, E. E. Spontaneous cardiovascular disease in the rat: II. Lesions of the vascular system. *Amer. J. Path.* 14:201, 1938.
42. Hartmann, H. A., Miller, E. C., and Miller, J. A. Periarteritis in rats given single injection of 4′-fluoro-10-methyl-1,2-benzanthracene. *Proc. Soc. Exp. Biol. Med.* 101:626, 1959.
43. Selye, H., and Bois, P. The hormonal production of nephrosclerosis and periarteritis nodosa in the primate. *Brit. Med. J.* 1:183, 1957.
44. Boughton, T. H. Studies in protein intoxication: II. Vascular lesions in chronic protein intoxication. *J. Immun.* 2:501, 1917.
45. Rich, A. R., and Gregory, J. E. The experimental demonstration that periarteritis nodosa is a manifestation of hypersensitivity. *Bull. Hopkins Hosp.* 72:65, 1943.
46. Glaser, R. J., Dammin, G. J., and Wood, W. B.

Effect of repeated streptococcal pulmonary infections on the cardiovascular system in rats. *Arch. Path.* 52:253, 1951.

47. Clark, E., and Kaplan, B. I. Endocardial, arterial, and other mesenchymal alterations associated with serum disease in man. *Arch. Path.* 24:458, 1937.
48. Rich, A. R. The role of hypersensitivity in periarteritis nodosa. *Bull. Hopkins Hosp.* 71: 123, 1942.
49. Rasmussen, H. Iodide hypersensitivity in the etiology of periarteritis nodosa. *J. Allerg.* 26: 394, 1955.
50. McLetchie, N. G. B., MacDonald, R. M., and Cutts, J. H. Polyarteritis nodosa: Report of a case with proof of drug allergy. *Canad. Med. Ass. J.* 76:213, 1957.
51. McCormick, R. V. Periarteritis occurring during propylthiouracil therapy. *J.A.M.A.* 144: 1453, 1950.
52. Gibson, P. C., and Quinlan, J. T. Periarteritis nodosa in thiourea therapy. *Lancet* 2:108, 1945.
53. Moore, F. D. Toxic manifestations of thiouracil therapy. *J.A.M.A.* 130:315, 1946.
54. Foss, G. L. Treatment of thyrotoxicosis with 2-mercaptoimidazole. *Brit. Med. J.* 2:1252, 1950.
55. Barnum, D. R., de Takats, G., Dolkart, R. E. Periarteritis nodosa following thiouracil therapy of hyperthyroidism: Resultant hypertension benefited by sympathectomy. *Angiology* 2:256, 1951.
56. Dalgleish, P. G. Polyarteritis nodosa after thiouracil. *Lancet* 2:319, 1952.
57. Hicks, J. D., and Cowling, D. C. A review of cases of polyarteritis nodosa: With special reference to the pathology. *Aust. Ann. Med.* 1:125, 1952.

68. *Polymyositis and Dermatomyositis**

CARL M. PEARSON

POLYMYOSITIS AND DERMATOMYOSITIS are members of a general class of primary myopathies in which muscular weakness is the chief clinical symptom. Pathologically, the principal lesions are degeneration of muscle fibers and infiltration by chronic inflammatory cells. These conditions may be related to the various "collagen" or connective tissue diseases, since a number of them show clinical and pathological overlaps, especially with scleroderma and rheumatoid arthritis. Certain of the cases are also associated with a visceral malignancy, especially in persons beyond middle age. The association of myositis with malignancy suggests some type of interrelationship. It is most likely, although far from proved, that this is due to an immunological cross-reaction.

Dermatomyositis has been recognized as a clinical entity since its first description by Unverricht [1] in 1887. The inflammatory skin lesions in combination with muscular weakness and pain are hallmarks of that syndrome, which was generally considered to be a rarity. Only within the past decade has it been realized that the large majority of patients with the myositides do not have dermal lesions, or at best they appear in unusual forms. These are cases of pure polymyositis. In this review, polymyositis will encompass all cases of the inflammatory nonsuppurative myositides, and dermatomyositis will form but one subgroup in this general category.

CLASSIFICATION

The classification of cases of polymyositis is both difficult and somewhat controversial because of lack of information about the etiology, the pleomorphism of clinical features, and the variability of pathological findings. On the one hand, Shy [2] proposes that the myopathies of late life should simply be referred to as polymyopathies and should be identified as separate entities only when the underlying etiological factors in any particular case are known. Denny-Brown [3], on the other hand, prefers a classification which is essentially pathological. He suggests that only when there is evidence of inflammatory reaction in muscle should a case be called polymyositis. He would classify other cases as necrotizing myopathy (with or without myoglobinuria), chronic progressive vacuolar myopathy, and progressive granular degeneration of muscle. Neither of these suggestions seems wholly satisfactory. Walton and Adams [4] have proposed a classification based primarily on clinical characteristics and associated features. I have modified this classification slightly, based on experience with nearly 60 cases in the past six years, and suggest the following six subdivisions for cases of polymyositis:

Type I: Polymyositis in Adults. This is the most common type of myositis and occurs mostly in females, especially in the third through the fifth decades. It usually has an insidious onset and may be accompanied by an atypical skin rash, the Raynaud phenomenon, mild arthritis, and certain other features which also often occur in other connective tissue diseases.

Type II: Typical Dermatomyositis. This form occurs only from the second to the seventh decades. The skin rash is erythematous and appears on the face, in the periorbital areas, on the neck and shoulders (Fig. 68-1), and occasionally more diffusely in conjunction with linear erythematous streaks on the knuckles, elbows, and sometimes on the knees and medial malleoli. These dermal lesions appear in conjunction with progressive muscular weakness and sometimes with muscular pain and tenderness. The onset may be either

* This study was supported in part by grants from the Muscular Dystrophy Associations of America, Inc.

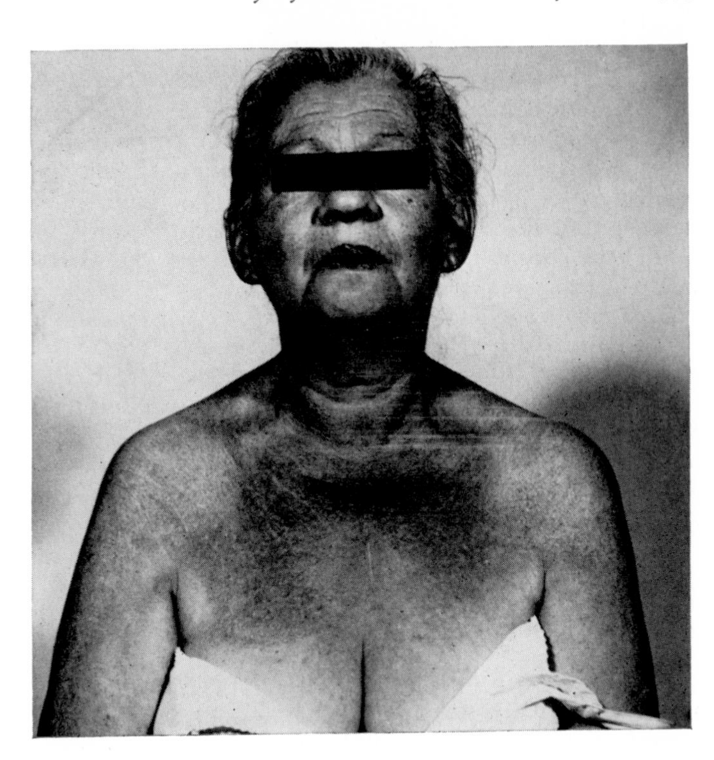

Fig. 68-1. Typical eruption of dermatomyositis in a 58-year-old woman. There is diffuse, slightly scaly erythema of the face, neck, anterior chest, shoulders, and outer arms.

acute or subacute. It is more common in women than in men. It may be associated with articular symptoms which resemble moderate rheumatoid arthritis.

Type III: Typical Dermatomyositis, or Polymyositis, with Malignant Tumor. These forms occur more commonly in males (3 : 1) in the tumor-bearing age from the fourth decade onward. A skin rash typical of dermatomyositis occurs in the majority.

Type IV: Childhood Dermatomyositis. This type presents either as an acute intermittent or as a chronic disease, more often the latter. It may cause severe contractures, skin ulcerations, and calcifications in the affected muscles late in the disease. The underlying pathology is vasculitis with ischemic necrosis of segments of muscle. It is never associated with malignancy.

Type V: Acute Intermittent Myolysis. This type, as implied in the title, is always acute and devastating. Myoglobinuria is common. It is somewhat difficult to distinguish from paroxysmal myoglobinuria, but in myolysis the attacks are sporadic and not initiated by exercise, as is usual in paroxysmal myoglobinuria. This form seems to be initiated in some instances by a viral infection.

Type VI: Polymyositis in Sjögren's Syndrome. The myopathy in this condition is proximal in distribution, chronic, and relentlessly progressive. The muscle tissue is massively invaded by plasma cells and lymphocytes. Other features of Sjögren's syndrome are commonly present, and the serum globulin levels in the two cases in my series have been remarkably elevated.

One advantage of this classification is that the various types respond somewhat differently to corticosteroid therapy, as will be related later. Therefore, if one can satisfactorily classify a case early, a reasonably accurate prediction may be made about ultimate prognosis and response to therapy.

INCIDENCE

Polymyositis and dermatomyositis may occur at any age from infancy to late adult life [5]. The largest proportion, however, arises in the fifth and sixth decades. Females are affected twice as commonly as are males. In a composite of 414 cases from several large series [5], 279 (67 percent) were in females and 137 (33 percent) were in males. It appears that no race is particularly prone to develop these conditions, or to be immune to them [6], nor is geographic area significant. The myopathic condition that polymyositis must be most carefully differentiated from is progressive muscular dystrophy. In the experience of nearly everyone, polymyositis is somewhat more common than dystrophy in adults, but dystrophy is much more frequent in childhood.

An appraisal of the frequency of polymyositis in comparison to other medical diseases was made from our clinic and hospital population. It was found, for instance, that each year we see about 80 new cases of rheumatoid arthritis, 25 cases of lupus erythematosus, 15 of scleroderma, 10 of polymyositis (and dermatomyositis), 3 of polyarteritis nodosa, 4 of endogenous Cushing's disease, and 12 cases of gout.

CLINICAL MANIFESTATIONS

ONSET

The characteristic early symptom of polymyositis is muscular weakness. This is most frequently manifested by an inability to perform certain activities handled by the proximal limb and girdle muscles, especially those of the lower extremities. Systemic signs and symptoms are rarely present early, or in fact in any stage of the disease, except in the childhood form and in the infrequent cases of acute dermatomyositis or acute intermittent myolysis. Some cases of dermatomyositis may have a rather rapid onset, so that dysphagia and proximal muscular weakness develop within two to three weeks. Typically, the onset is insidious, with weakness of the proximal muscles of the lower and upper limbs and of the swallowing mechanisms gradually appearing over weeks to months. Moderate fluctuations in intensity of the clinical disease are characteristic.

MUSCULAR SIGNS AND SYMPTOMS

Weakness of the striated musculature of the body is present in *all* cases of polymyositis and dermatomyositis (Fig. 68-2), and this diagnosis can hardly be made in its absence. With an *acute* onset, the generalized muscular weakness, most pronounced in the proximal muscles, may develop in two to three weeks, with pain on movement of the limbs and tenderness to pressure of the muscles. Dysphagia, a nasal voice, and shallowness of the respiration with diminished vital capacity may all be features of this type of disease.

In *subacute* or *chronic* cases, the weakness

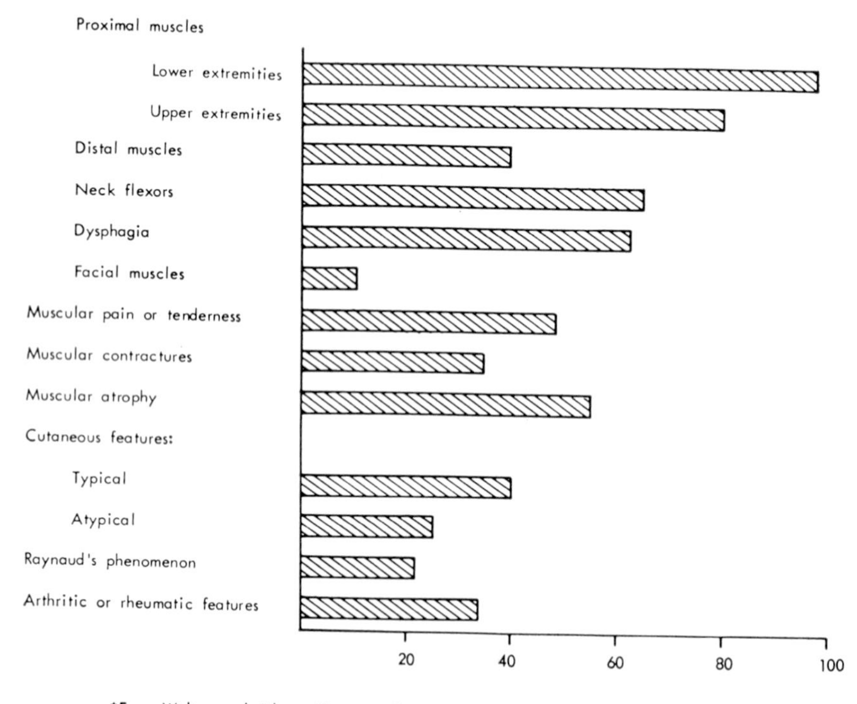

Fig. 68-2. Percentage of clinical signs and symptoms in 116 cases of polymyositis. (From Pearson [5]; courtesy *Postgrad. Med.*)

comes on more slowly. It first affects the lower limbs and at that time closely resembles muscular dystrophy. Muscular pain and tenderness are much less common in this type, and dysphagia is usually mild. When the disorder has persisted for months or longer, considerable weakness may have developed in the proximal musculature. It may then be impossible to arise from a low lounge chair or even from a regular bed, and turning in bed is very difficult. Stairs can be ascended only with the assistance of a hand railing, and the gait may be clumsy and waddling, again as in muscular dystrophy. There is, at this time, a tendency to fall, with inability to arise without assistance.

At some point, usually after the appearance of pelvic girdle and proximal leg weakness, diminution in strength of the shoulder girdle muscles also becomes clinically evident. Raising the arms above the head and especially maintaining them in the overhead position, as in combing the hair, then becomes impossible. At this time, also, weakness of the anterior neck muscles is demonstrated by inability to elevate the head from the pillow when reclining. Involvement of the posterior phalangeal muscles may cause the picture of pseudobulbar palsy with dysphagia, dysphonia, and occasionally dysarthria.

In *severe* or *advanced* cases, the weakness may be extreme and the patient is then bedridden or at best confined to a wheelchair. Such patients are fortunately uncommon. In most cases of type III disease in which a malignancy coexists, the muscular weakness is refractory to corticosteroid therapy, so that this type is usually progressive and devastating. Contractures or shortening of muscles rarely occur early; these are features of longstanding disease. Atrophy of muscles is also a late event. Calcinosis of muscles and adjacent connective tissues may occasionally result from a severe episode of acute myolysis (type V), or it may occur in type IV disease in children.

DERMATOLOGICAL FEATURES

The typical skin rash of dermatomyositis occurs in about 40 percent of all patients with polymyositis (Fig. 68-2). In another 25 percent, dermal changes may vary from the hidebound thickening of scleroderma or widespread dermal atrophy (poikiloderma) to transitory erythema or a scaling eruption.

The typical rash consists of a dusky erythematous eruption on the face, especially in "butterfly" distribution. It also may appear on the forehead, neck, shoulders, front and back of the upper chest, and proximal or distal portions of the arms (Fig. 68-1). A peculiar dusky lilac suffusion may occur on the upper eyelids. It has been called the "heliotrope rash" and is said to be pathognomonic for dermatomyositis. In dermatomyositis, and also in other types of polymyositis, it is quite common to find red, slightly elevated, smooth or scaly patches on the elbows, knuckles, knees, and medial malleoli at the ankles. In conjunction, there is usually hyperemia at the base of the fingernails, along the sides of the nails, and on the finger pads. The pads may become shiny, red, and atrophic and are constantly flaking or peeling. Raynaud's phenomenon occurs in about one third of patients with polymyositis. It is usually not severe and never proceeds to necrosis or permanent and serious change. Typically, it is brought on by cold or emotional stress.

OTHER FEATURES

The link between polymyositis and certain of the "collagen" diseases can be observed not only by similarities in the skin manifestations between lupus erythematosus or scleroderma and polymyositis but also by the presence of certain other features. Thus mild or transitory arthritis or rheumatic symptoms occur in about one third to one half of all cases [7]. Polymyositis of any type may be heralded by acute arthralgias or arthritis with effusions, especially in the joints of the fingers and wrists. These articular manifestations are usually very mild, but in other respects they closely resemble rheumatoid arthritis and have been diagnosed as such in some patients. The articular and rheumatic manifestations always respond promptly to corticosteroid therapy, and permanent articular alterations rarely occur.

The dysphagia in polymyositis is due principally to weakness of the striated muscle of the posterior pharynx so that a bolus of food cannot be propelled from the mouth down into the esophagus, or can be propelled only with great effort. This is easily demonstrated fluoroscopically, by using a swallow of thick barium.

Visceral manifestations are uncommon in polymyositis, in contrast to the internal changes in a number of connective tissue diseases. However, x-ray studies with barium will demonstrate a hypotonicity of the esophagus in about 30 percent of cases, which is similar or identical to that observed in scleroderma [8]. This defect is rarely apparent clinically and usually does not contribute materially to the dysphagia. Two of our patients have also had x-ray evidence of disease of the small intestine, again similar to that observed in scleroderma. These features consisted of severe hypomotility and poor absorption through the small intestine. Both patients had chronic polymyositis and only minimal cutaneous features of scleroderma. Other visceral or neurological manifestations in polymyositis are extremely rare, clinically insignificant, or coincidental [4].

LABORATORY INVESTIGATIONS

The most helpful clinical and laboratory tests for the diagnosis of polymyositis are (1) measurement of serum enzymes, (2) electromyography, and (3) the histopathological study of a muscle biopsy.

An increase in level of activity of certain serum enzymes is of great assistance in diagnosing polymyositis. The serum glutamic oxaloacetic transaminase and serum aldolase are the most significant, although the levels of other enzymes are also elevated. These enzymes normally are in muscle tissue and apparently are released as a result of the destructive myopathy. Almost invariably in the acute or subacute stages of the disease, the enzyme levels are elevated, whereas in clinically inactive cases or those in remission they are normal. Serial determination of the levels of these enzymes is the best laboratory guide to the status of the illness as well as to its treatment. These studies are particularly useful in differentiating myopathy from the muscular weakness and wasting due to primary neurological disease [9].

Electromyographic findings in polymyositis have been reviewed in detail elsewhere [4, 10]. Briefly, abnormal electrical potentials may be found in nearly all stages of the disease. They are most prominent in the proximal musculature of the lower and upper limbs. The changes are as follows: (1) at rest, small potentials are noted that are indistinguishable from those of spontaneous fibrillation; (2) on voluntary activity, a complex polyphasic pattern of motor unit action potentials is observed, and (3) short bursts of rapidly repeating action potentials that fade away after a brief initial period have been described as "pseudomyotonia." These three findings are not specific for polymyositis but strongly suggest its presence. A reduction of mean duration and amplitude of motor unit potentials is seen in any myopathy, including muscular dystrophy; it is the presence of abnormal activity at rest and the initiation of pseudomyotonic discharges on movement of the needle electrode that is most suggestive of polymyositis.

Muscle biopsy will ordinarily disclose pathological changes if the muscle which is sampled is carefully selected. In general, a proximal muscle that is partially, but not completely, weakened is the best choice. If an initial biopsy specimen does not reveal abnormalities, and the diagnosis is still strongly considered, it is wise to repeat the biopsy in another area. Often, an electromyographic study assists in reaching a decision about a site for biopsy, since in an area where one observes significant abnormal electrical activities the biopsy is most likely to show abnormalities. One must, however, keep in mind that insertion of the biopsy needle may induce small focal areas of muscle fiber damage, so that it is best to avoid the precise spot where the needle was inserted when performing the biopsy.

The most characteristic and constant features found on muscle biopsy in polymyositis include, in general order of frequency: (1) primary focal or extensive degeneration of muscle fibers, sometimes with vacuolation (Fig. 68-3); (2) evidence of regeneration, as demonstrated by sarcoplasmic basophilia and the presence of large vesicular nuclei and prominent nucleoli (Fig. 68-4); (3) necrosis of a part or the whole of one or more fibers, with phagocytosis of their substance; (4) interstitial infiltrates of chronic inflammatory cells, sometimes focal (Fig. 68-5) and sometimes diffuse (Fig. 68-3), and often with a perivascular component (Fig. 68-4); (5) significant variation in individual fiber size, as viewed in cross-section (Figs. 68-4 and 68-5), especially in cases of several months' duration, and (6) interstitial fibrosis. These changes have been described and illustrated in detail elsewhere [4, 11, 12].

Certain other laboratory abnormalities which are much less specific and helpful are noted in some cases. For example, the eryth-

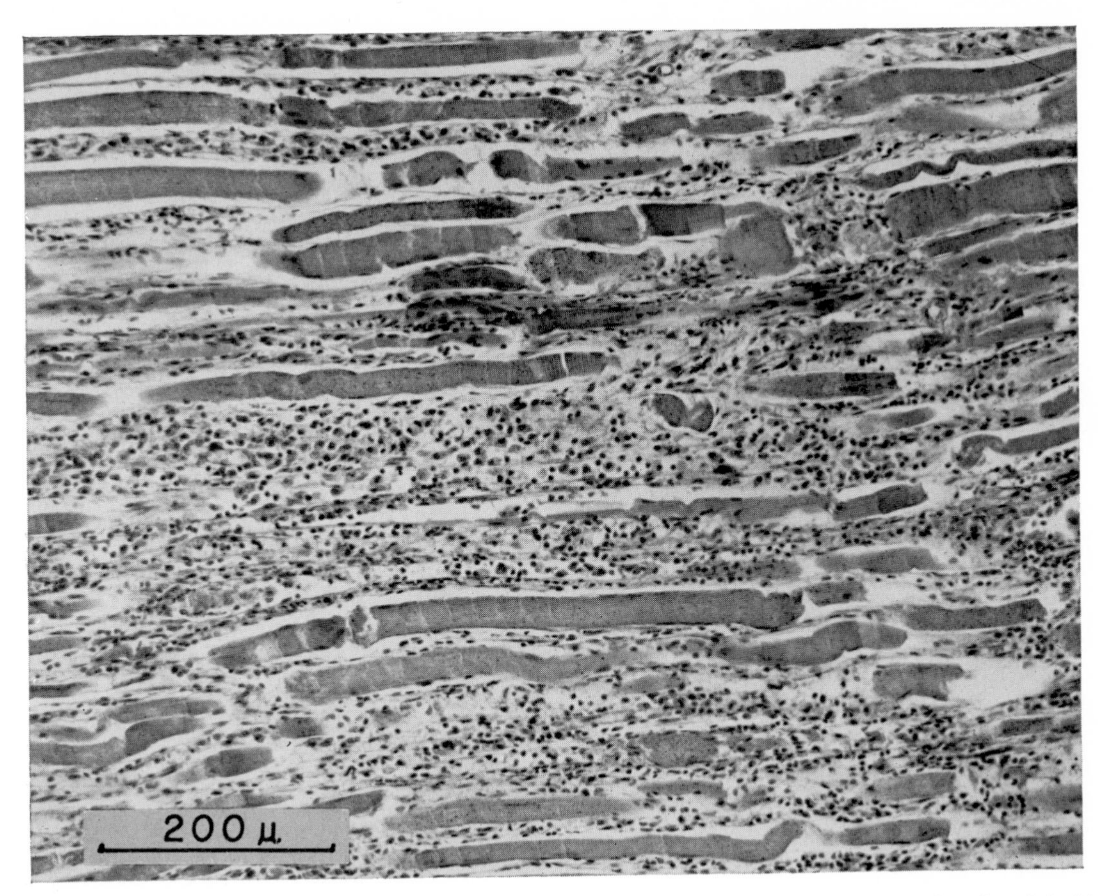

Fig. 68-3. Extensive inflammatory infiltration by lymphocytes and plasma cells in the deltoid muscle of a 54-year-old woman with coexistent features of Sjögren's syndrome. There is hyaline necrosis of most of the remaining muscle fibers.

rocyte sedimentation rate may be elevated in about 60 percent of patients during the active stages of disease. The serum protein electrophoretic pattern may be abnormal, especially with elevation of the α_2- and γ-globulins [13] in about 50 percent of cases. A positive reaction to the latex fixation or Rose-Waaler test for rheumatoid factor was obtained in approximately 50 percent of our cases [7], but in less than 10 percent of those studied by Barwick and Walton [6]. Mild anemia is found in a few cases. Electrocardiographically "nonspecific" T-wave changes are noted in about 20 percent of the cases during the acute or subacute stages of polymyositis. However, clinical signs of cardiac disease rarely develop.

ETIOLOGY

Although this discussion on polymyositis is included in a book on immunological diseases, there is no definite proof, only reasonable suspicion, that these myopathies are mediated through hypersensitivity mechanisms. With this thought in mind, it is appropriate to consider various etiological suggestions which have been made in the past.

Since the histopathological evidence of an inflammatory reaction is quite striking in many cases of polymyositis, it is not surprising that extensive searches have been made for an infective agent. Garcin *et al.* [14] mentioned a long list of possible causes, as considered by others in individual cases. These include tuberculosis, scarlet fever, and prostatitis, among others. Van Bogaert *et al.* [15] discussed the possibility of a viral etiology but came to no definite conclusions. Although in many of these reports there are suggestions of an infective etiology in isolated instances, no single thread of continuity prevails among them. Moreover, in a much greater number of cases, there is no suggestion at all of the

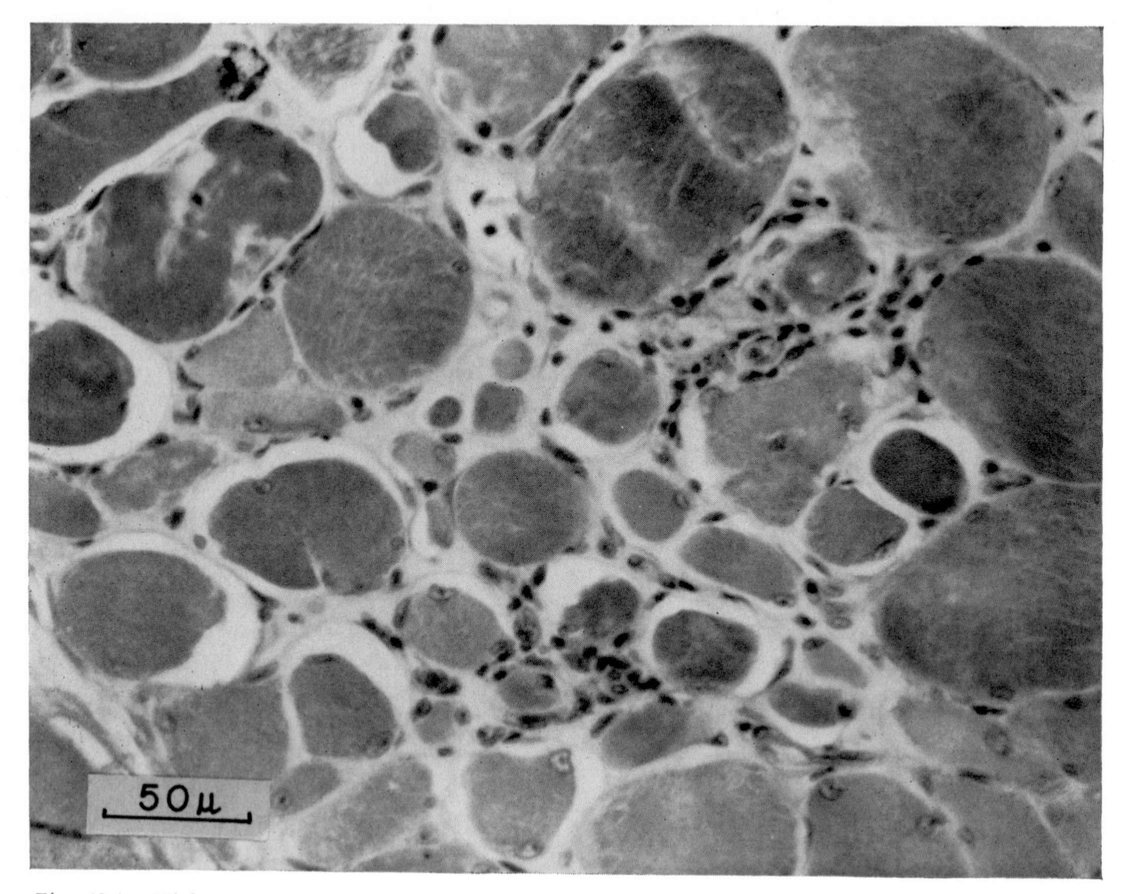

Fig. 68-4. High magnification of muscle fibers in type I polymyositis in a woman aged 39. Note the great variability in cross-sectional size, prominent nuclei in the smaller fibers which indicate that they are regenerating, and sparse perivascular and interstitial inflammatory infiltrates.

presence of an active infection. The possibility remains that in some individuals an infective agent of some type or other can initiate a hypersensitivity response which for unknown reasons becomes focused on the skeletal muscle fibers and their supporting tissues. Such a mechanism could explain certain cases which seem to have been initiated by a drug sensitivity reaction, such as to sulfonamides [16] or penicillin [17]. If any of these are inciting factors, they may be so because of some fundamental derangement in the immune mechanism itself. At this point, it might be mentioned that in polymyositis no prior history of common allergic disease can, as a rule, be uncovered.

The frequent interrelationships of polymyositis and the various "collagen" or connective tissue diseases have been stressed elsewhere in this chapter. Since all of the other members of this group are under suspicion as "hypersensitivity" diseases, caused either by an external allergen or by an autoallergen, one can equally consider the myositides in this light.

Histopathologically, skeletal muscle lesions are common in all of the "collagen" diseases, but the muscles are usually clinically affected only in myositis. In the other conditions, the microscopic involvement is predominantly an interstitial inflammation in the muscular connective tissues or in and around the small blood vessels, and only rarely does one find damage to an isolated muscle fiber. Thus in systemic lupus erythematosus, rheumatoid arthritis, scleroderma, and rheumatic fever, the pathology is essentially an *interstitial* polymyositis, and it is not possible on biopsy to differentiate between these various conditions [12]. In polyarteritis nodosa, on the other hand, the vascular element is prominent and may cause secondary changes in the muscle fibers due to ischemia or denervation. In polymyositis and dermatomyositis, the in-

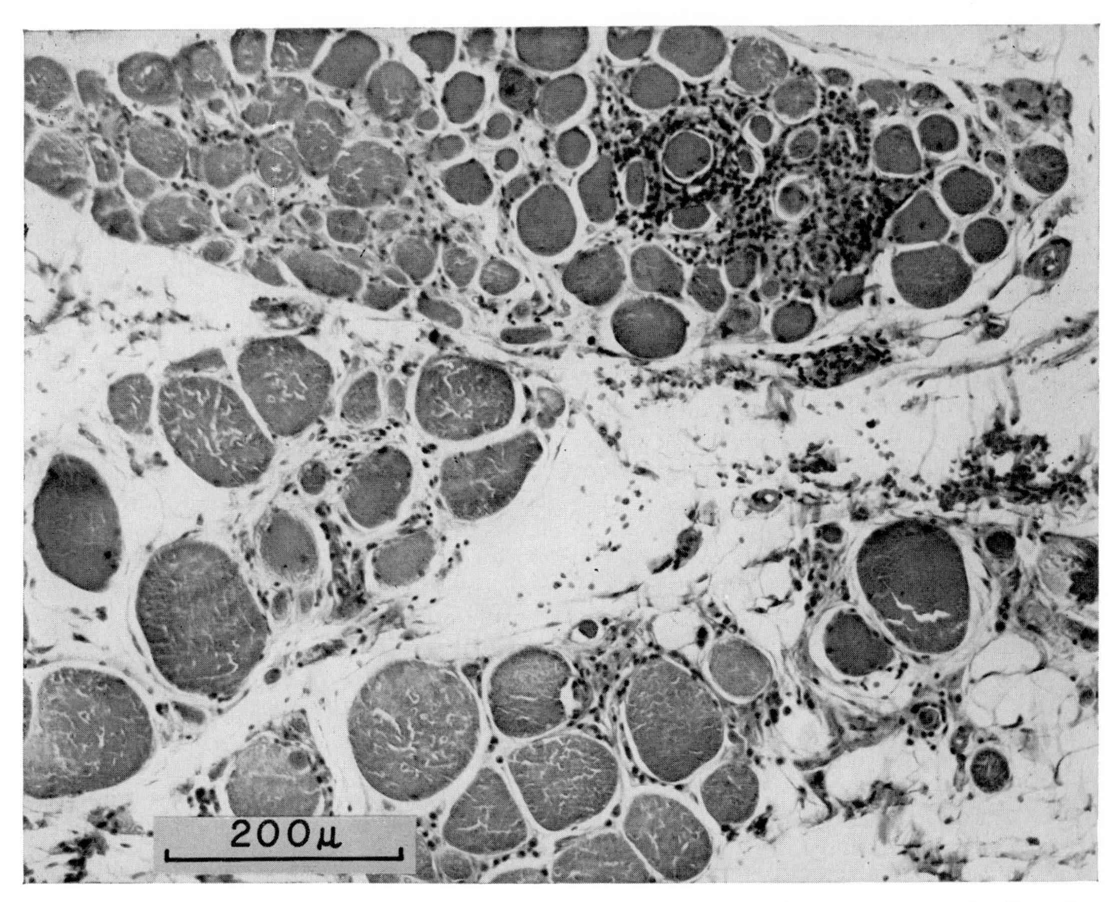

Fig. 68-5. Chronic polymyositis of at least six years' duration. Note great variation in fiber size, the one large and several small foci of inflammation, and some interstitial fibrosis.

terstitial and perivascular features are both common, but there is additional involvement of the muscle fibers, the myopathy of which is proportionately greater than the stromal involvement (Figs. 68-3 to 68-5). This finding indicates the presence of a process which has something in common with the other "collagen" diseases and yet has a more specific component which seems to be directed at the muscle fiber or some segment of it.

Since muscle tissue can be accessible in relatively generous amounts in polymyositis, it should be investigated more extensively by the same approaches that have been applied to the renal and vascular lesions in systemic lupus erythematosus, scleroderma, and so on, since a single unequivocal finding in any one of these conditions could open the door to more positively directed researches in all of the others.

The principal clue to the etiology of poly- and dermatomyositis is the unequivocal association of certain of these cases and neoplastic disease. One could consider three possible explanations for this combination: (1) that the myopathy is due to a direct toxic effect of a substance released from the tumor cells; (2) that it is the result of a hypersensitivity response due either to an error in the immune mechanism which has misdirected the response or to the presence of a similar antigen in the tumor cells and the muscle fibers so that a single immune response affects both cells; or (3) that both the malignancy and the myositis are independent effects of a single causative agent.

From among these possibilities, the hypersensitivity response seems to be the most likely, but data to support it are meager. Of interest in this respect are the studies of two groups [18, 19] on possible autosensitization in the presence of myositis and tumor. In one patient with dermatomyositis and cancer of the breast [18], an immediate skin reaction developed to intracutaneous inoculation of an extract of her own tumor, and a positive passive transfer reaction also occurred. Similar findings were noted in another woman with dermatomyositis and bronchogenic carcinoma [19]. In a very preliminary study, we have sought antimuscle antibodies in the serum of ten patients with various types of myositis, both acute and chronic, by using the agar gel diffusion technique. Three different "antigens" were prepared from relatively fresh human autopsy muscle by extraction with water, KOH, or 95 percent alcohol. All results have so far been negative. Similar preliminary negative results were reported by Barwick and Walton [6], who searched for circulating antibodies against muscle and connective tissue by using the tanned red cell agglutination method.

In certain cases of myasthenia gravis, a serum globulin has been found which fixes complement and has an affinity for muscle fibers when the fluorescent antibody technique is applied to fresh muscle tissue [20, 21]. Similar studies on serum of five of our patients with myositis (two, acute type II; three, chronic type I), using fresh-frozen human muscle as substrate, failed to disclose muscle antibodies, although in one of the acute cases, antinuclear antibody was noted. This antibody fixed to all nuclei, including those in the muscle fibers.

It is not possible at this time to reach any firm conclusions on the etiology of polymyositis and dermatomyositis. Clinically and pathologically, there are possiblities that some, if not all, cases result from a hypersensitivity reaction. However, there is no experimental evidence that this is the case. It is quite clear, however, that a thorough investigation, using many immunological techniques, has not been conducted. The few negative results which have been obtained may be due to the improper selection of investigative methods or of preparation of the muscle "antigen." Since there is a reasonable suspicion that these diseases are related to an antigen located somewhere in muscle fibers or their connective tissues, further careful immunological studies are urgently needed.

TREATMENT

Until ACTH and the corticosteroids were discovered, there was no satisfactory treatment for polymyositis or dermatomyositis. As already mentioned, spontaneous remissions and exacerbations are noted in some of the more chronic cases, but the natural course is almost invariably progressive.

We have used prednisone almost exclusively, having chosen it over the fluorinated steroids such as dexamethasone and triamcinolone because the latter compounds have themselves the ability to induce muscular weakness, producing the so-called "steroid myopathy" in normal individuals [22, 23]. If this should occur in an individual with polymyositis, it would make evaluation of the response to treatment almost impossible.

Serial analyses of one or more serum enzyme levels will provide the best guide and prognostic tool for conducting therapy. If enzyme levels return toward normal, even though clinical weakness is still severe or increasing, it is possible to predict that a reversal of the underlying myopathy has been achieved and that recovery of strength will soon occur. This was noted clinically in nearly all of our cases within four to six weeks at most.

In acute disease, the prednisone dosage should be 50 to 70 mg. daily, given in divided doses every six to eight hours. Once the serum enzyme levels have returned to, or toward, normal, a lowering of the dosage can be attempted. This should, however, be done very slowly. A reduction of 5 mg. every two or three weeks is all that can be safely recommended. When a dose of 25 to 30 mg. per day is reached, one should hesitate in the reduction program for several weeks in order to evaluate the situation fully. If, following any increment of reduction, the enzyme levels rise, the dose should immediately be increased by 10 to 15 mg. daily over the present dosage and the reduction program followed more slowly thereafter. Rapid lowering of dosage, or attempts to discontinue therapy completely, have almost invariably been met with recurrent elevation of serum enzyme levels and reappearance of clinical weakness several weeks later.

Maintenance therapy should be continued for months or years with a prednisone dosage ranging from 7.5 to 20 mg. daily (average, 12.5 mg.). Since maintenance therapy seems to be necessary in most cases, one can conclude that this treatment is not curative, merely suppressive. This fact has been further borne out by mild biochemical and clinical relapses in several of our cases. These relapses have occurred up to four or five years after the onset of acute disease if, at that time, the prednisone dosage was decreased further or if some stressful factor such as an infection incited a flare-up of the disease.

In general, in types I and II polymyositis, if the treatment is begun within two months of the clinical onset of disease, improvement on prednisone therapy will nearly always occur. The restoration of almost normal strength can be expected in nearly all cases [5, 24].

In chronic myositis of either types I or II which has existed for several months or years, the serum enzyme levels return to normal more slowly on corticosteroid treatment and strength is not fully regained. This, no doubt, is explainable by some irreversible damage to the muscle which occurred prior to the initiation of prednisone therapy.

In the other types of myositis, prednisone therapy is much less beneficial [24] or to no avail. In the cases associated with a malignancy, initial transitory improvement in strength may be observed and the serum enzyme levels may temporarily return to, or toward, normal. These benefits are, however, soon reversed, so that within three to six months, progressive clinical weakness and moderate elevation of serum enzyme levels reappear. At this time, the patient seems refractory to even large amounts of prednisone, so that severe dysphagia, dyspnea, and diminished respiratory excursions develop. Death then ensues from anoxia or complicating infection.

All patients receiving prednisone in dosage above 15 mg. daily should be given antacids several times a day as well as potassium supplementation. Complications from high dosage therapy have been remarkably few in our series. However, one acute steroid induced ulcer and one overwhelming infection were observed. Bed rest is imperative during the acute or subacute stages of the disease. The need for a specific program of physical therapy or exercise is not critical in most cases, but it may be of some supportive and stimulatory benefit in the later stages during recovery from an episode of acute and extensive myositis.

Acknowledgments: Appreciation is expressed to Mrs. Rosemarie Shaw and Mr. Philip Bleicher for their technical assistance and to Mrs. Jackie Brunke for help with this manuscript.

REFERENCES

1. Unverricht, H. Polymyositis acuta progressiva. *Z. Klin. Med.* 12:533, 1887.
2. Shy, G. M. The late onset myopathy. *World Neurol.* 3:149, 1962.
3. Denny-Brown, D. The nature of polymyositis and related muscular diseases. *Trans. Coll. Physicians Philadelphia* 28:14, 1960.
4. Walton, J. N., and Adams, R. D. *Polymyositis.* Edinburgh: E. & S. Livingstone, Ltd., 1958.
5. Pearson, C. M. Polymyositis: Clinical forms, diagnosis and therapy. *Postgrad. Med.* 31:450, 1962.
6. Barwick, D. D., and Walton, J. N. Polymyositis. *Amer. J. Med.* 35:646, 1963.
7. Pearson, C. M. Rheumatic manifestations of polymyositis and dermatomyositis. *Arthritis Rheum.* 2:127, 1959.
8. Donoghue, F. D., Winkelmann, R. K., and Moersch, H. J. Esophageal defects in dermatomyositis. *Ann. Otol.* 69:1139, 1960.
9. Pearson, C. M. Serum enzymes in muscular dystrophy and certain other muscular and neuromuscular diseases: I. Serum glutamic oxalacetic transaminase. *New Eng. J. Med.* 256:1069, 1957.
10. Buchthal, F., and Pinelli, P. Muscle action potentials in polymyositis. *Neurology* 3:424, 1953.
11. Pearson, C. M. Polymyositis and Related Disorders. In Walton, J. N. (Ed.), *Disorders of Voluntary Muscle.* Boston: Little, Brown, 1964.
12. Adams, R. D., Denny-Brown, D., and Pearson, C. M. *Diseases of Muscle: A Study in Pathology* (2nd ed.). New York: Paul B. Hoeber, Inc., 1962.
13. Sande, M. Applications de l'électrophorèse sur papier à l'étude des protéines sériques chez des sujets atteints de polymyosite. *Acta Neurol. Belg.* 54:78, 1954.
14. Garcin, R., Lapresle, J., Gruner, J., and Scherrer, J. Les polymyosites. *Rev. Neurol.* (Paris) 92:465, 1955.
15. Van Bogaert, L., Radermecker, M. A., Löwenthal, A., and Ketelaer, C. J. Les polymyosities chroniques (essais avec la cortisone). *Acta Neurol. Belg.* 11:869, 1955.
16. Sheard, C. Dermatomyositis, *Arch. Intern. Med.* 88:640, 1951.
17. Hyman, I., Arbesman, C. E., and Terplan, K. L. Dermatomyositis following penicillin injections. *Neurology* (Minneap.) 6:63, 1956.

18. Grace, J. T., and Dao, T. L. Dermatomyositis in cancer: A possible etiological mechanism. *Cancer* 12:648, 1959.
19. Curtis, A. C., Heckaman, J. H., and Wheeler, A. H. Study of the autoimmune reaction in dermatomyositis. *J.A.M.A.* 178:571, 1961.
20. Strauss, A. J. L., *et al.* Immunofluorescence demonstration of muscle binding complement-fixing serum globulin fraction in myasthenia gravis. *Proc. Soc. Exp. Biol. Med.* 105:184, 1960.
21. Beutner, E. H., Witebsky, E., Ricken, D., and Adler, R. H. Studies on autoantibodies in myasthenia gravis. *J.A.M.A.* 182:46, 1962.
22. Perkoff, G. T., Silber, R., Tyler, F. H., Cartwright, G. E., and Wintrobe, M. M. Myopathy due to administration of therapeutic amounts of 17-hydrocorticosteroids. *Amer. J. Med.* 26:891, 1959.
23. Golding, D. N., and Begg, T. B. Dexamethasone myopathy. *Brit. Med. J.* 2:1129, 1960.
24. Pearson, C. M. Patterns of polymyositis and their responses to treatment. *Ann. Intern. Med.* 59:827, 1963.

*69. Progressive Systemic Sclerosis (Diffuse Scleroderma)**

GERALD P. RODNAN

PROGRESSIVE SYSTEMIC SCLEROSIS (PSS) is a systemic disorder of connective tissue characterized by inflammatory, fibrotic, and degenerative changes in the skin (scleroderma), synovium, and certain internal organs, notably the gastrointestinal tract, heart, lung, and kidney [1–13]. Although the disease often appears to remain confined to the integument for many months or years, in most cases there is evidence of steadily, and at times rapidly, progressive visceral involvement, which may cause death from myocardial failure or renal insufficiency [14, 15].

There is an abundance of theories concerning etiology and pathogenesis, but the fundamental nature of PSS remains obscure. In recent years, however, there has been an impressive accumulation of clinical and serological evidence of immunological abnormalities in a high percentage of patients with this disorder [15–17].

Historical Note. Descriptions of skin conditions *compatible* with scleroderma may be found in the writings of the ancients, but the first convincing account is generally credited to Carlo Curzio, a physician of Naples, in 1753 [18]. The disease was rediscovered by Grisolle and by Forget in 1847, and quickly designated *sclérodermie* by Gintrac. Despite the fact that scleroderma was widely recognized and that many patients were known to have serious visceral disturbances soon after the development of cutaneous changes, the systemic nature of this disease was not clearly appreciated until well into this century [18]. Gradually increasing awareness that scleroderma is the external manifestation of a truly generalized disorder was crystallized in 1945, when Goetz [1] proposed that the disease be renamed progressive systemic sclerosis.

The possibility of a relation or "common denominator" between scleroderma and dermatomyositis, disseminated lupus erythematosus, and certain other disorders was raised in 1941 by Banks [19], who was impressed by similarities in their clinical and pathological features and, in particular, by the evidence of widespread lesions of small blood vessels. The following year Klemperer, *et al.* [20] grouped scleroderma with acute disseminated lupus erythematosus and rheumatic fever in a new category of "diffuse collagen disease" or "systemic disease of the connective tissues."

CLINICAL FEATURES

GENERAL CONSIDERATIONS

Women are affected by PSS approximately twice as often as men. The vast majority of patients described to date have been whites, but the disease is now frequently recognized in Negroes. Initial symptoms usually appear between age 30 and 50 years, but many patients first become ill after 60. The disease is relatively uncommon in childhood [21].

OCCUPATIONAL HISTORY

Typical PSS has been described in patients in a wide variety of occupations. Of interest, however, are recent reports of the frequent occurrence of a peculiarly fulminant form of the disease among goldminers, coalminers, and workers in certain other jobs marked by heavy exposure to silica dust [22, 23].

* Supported by a Graduate Training Grant in Arthritis and Rheumatism (2A-5031), USPHS Grant 5 MO1 FR-00056, and research grants from the Western Pennsylvania Chapter, Arthritis and Rheumatism Foundation, and the Health Research and Services Foundation.

INITIAL SYMPTOMS*

In most cases the patient's first complaint is either digital Raynaud's phenomenon or painless swelling or thickening of the skin of the hands and fingers [14, 15]. Nearly one third of the patients whom we have seen have been troubled initially by rheumatic symptoms, most commonly pain and stiffness of the finger joints and knees and less often of the other peripheral articulations [12]. A number of these patients have true polyarthritis, which may be migratory, and are at first thought to have rheumatoid arthritis. In a small proportion of cases, presenting symptoms are referable to neither the skin nor joints but to visceral involvement. Patients may have exertional dyspnea, for example, as a result of myocardial or pulmonary disease, or be troubled by dysphagia or disturbances in intestinal motility.

Early in the course of the disease there may be spontaneous improvement after a period of several weeks or months. More often, the symptoms persist and remain confined to the skin and joints for a variable time, sometimes as long as several years. In most cases, however, there is a gradual worsening in the condition of the skin and the insidious development of symptoms indicative of involvement of the esophagus, intestinal tract, lung, and heart.

CLINICAL AND PATHOLOGICAL FINDINGS IN SYSTEMIC INVOLVEMENT

Skin. The majority of patients have diffuse scleroderma which, in all but rare instances, affects first the skin of the fingers and distal portions of the upper extremities, spreading in varying degree to the forearms, face, neck, upper anterior chest, abdomen, and back. In the early stages, the fingers tend to be tightly swollen and have often been compared to sausages in their appearance. The sparing of the lower extremities in many patients with severe involvement of the arms is notable. Many patients have flexion contractures of the fingers and are troubled by recurrent ulcerations and infections of the fingertips which prove extremely refractory to treatment. As a result of such recurrent infections, and on occasion in the absence of this complication, there tends to be a progressive loss of the soft tissue and bony substance of the fingertips which may result in eventual dissolution of one or more terminal phalanges. Roentgenograms of the hands frequently disclose subcutaneous calcinosis, and patients may note the drainage of calcific matter from the fingertips and from areas of intracutaneous nodulation on the elbows and knees. Thickening of the skin of the face leads to difficulty with ingestion and with dental repairs. We have seen a number of women who have had the latter problem for years before the recognition of changes in the skin of their fingers.

Examination of biopsies obtained from areas of skin with more advanced scleroderma discloses a marked increase in dermal collagen and such other classic histopathological changes as thinning of the epidermis with loss of rete pegs, atrophy of dermal appendages, and hyalinization of arterioles (Fig. 69-1) [24, 25]. In cases considered clinically to be "early" scleroderma, however, there may be only minimal homogenization of collagen, so that diagnosis at this stage by means of skin biopsy has proved difficult.

Joints. Involvement of the joints is usually marked by polyarthralgia, swelling and stiffness of the fingers, wrists, and knees, as well as other peripheral articulations, and less commonly by signs of frank arthritis, including swelling, redness, warmth, and synovial effusion [12]. Some patients exhibit a peculiar leathery crepitus on flexion of their knees or wrists. Similar grating sensations and leathery friction rubs, accompanied at times by audible creaking, have been noted over the distal part of the forearms, legs, and other tendinous areas and have been related to fibrous proliferation of peritendinous connective tissue and fibrinoid deposits on the surfaces of the tendon sheaths and overlying fascia [26]. Roentgenographic changes in and around the joints are limited, for the most part, to narrowing of the cartilage space, juxta-articular osteoporosis, thickening of the soft tissues, and subcutaneous calcinosis. There is little tendency to subchondral bone destruction.

Specimens of synovium taken from patients with clinical evidence of acute inflammation have shown synovitis marked by infiltrations of lymphocytes and plasma cells, present in focal aggregates or scattered diffusely throughout the tissue (Fig. 69-2, *a*) [12]. Morphologically, the synovitis is not unlike that encount-

* *Editor's comment:* We have observed two patients in whom the initial presentation was generalized pitting edema, which progressed insidiously to scleroderma. There was no renal, cardiac, or venous disease in these patients.—J. H. V.

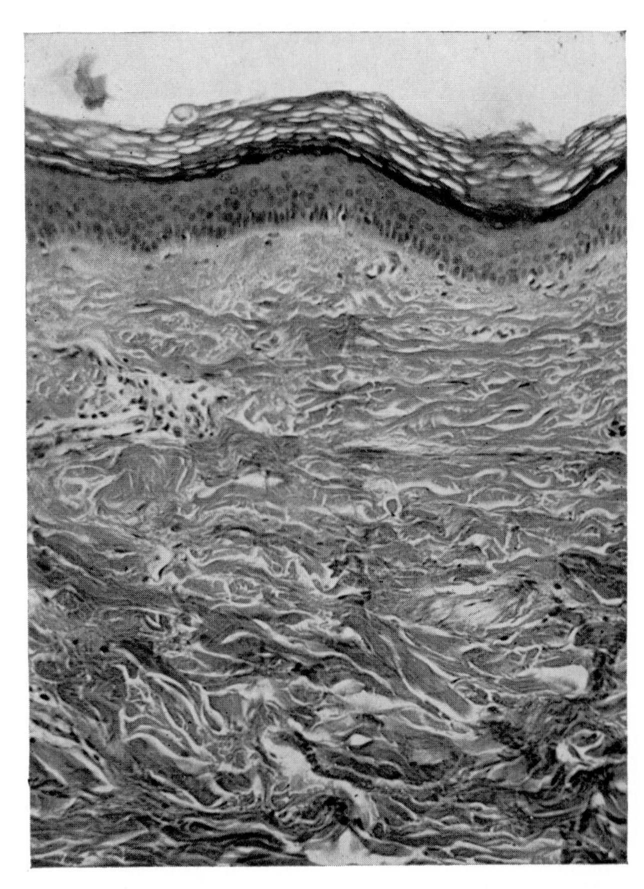

Fig. 69-1. Skin biopsy of woman with severe scleroderma, illustrating thinning of epidermis and increase in dermal collagen, which is homogenized and appears to be arranged in bundles parallel to the epidermal surface.

ered in mild cases of rheumatoid arthritis [27, 28]. Later in the course, sections show intense fibrosis of the synovium. In some instances, only the more superficial portions of the synovium are involved, with loss of the normal villous folds. In other cases, the entire membrane consists of dense, homogeneous, hypocellular collagenous tissue which encompasses and obliterates the vascular structures (Fig. 69-2, *b*).

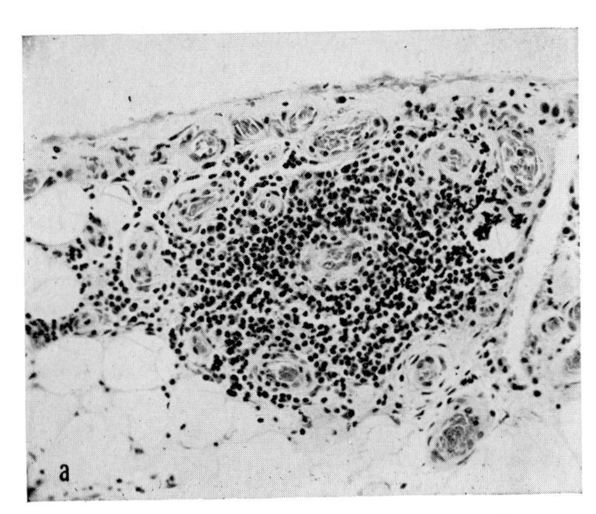

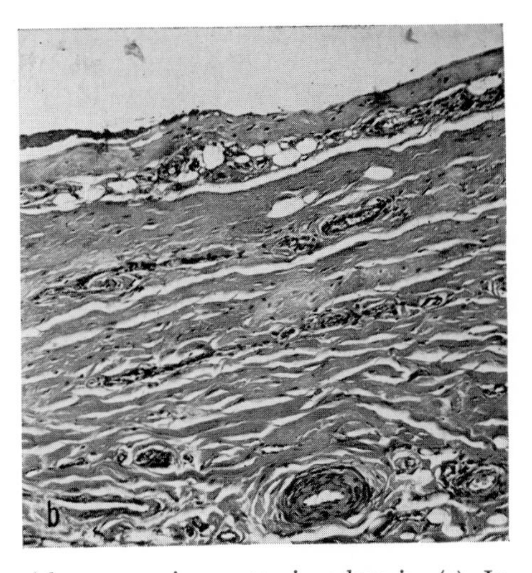

Fig. 69-2. Synovium (suprapatellar bursa) of two men with progressive systemic sclerosis. (*a*) Inflammation with focal infiltration of lymphocytes and thickening of small blood vessels. (*b*) Dense fibrosis of the entire synovium with obliteration of blood vessels.

Esophagus. Dysfunction of the esophagus occurs in over one half of the patients and it is so distinctive as to constitute a clinical hallmark of PSS [14, 15]. Dysphagia is, in fact, the most common manifestation of visceral involvement and often proves to be the dominant feature in the patient's illness. There are a number of cases in which a disturbance in swallowing has occurred in the absence of any cutaneous disease, giving rise, as it were, to a form of PSS *sine* scleroderma [29]. Early in the course, the patient may note only retrosternal burning pain or unusual fullness after completion of a meal. Later, there is difficulty in the passage of solids, which may become impacted in the esophagus and require instrumental removal.

Fluoroscopic examination characteristically reveals a diminution to total absence of peristaltic activity of the esophagus and, later, dilatation (less often, narrowing) of the lower one half or two thirds of the organ [30, 31].* In addition, a number of patients are found to have hiatal hernia. Manometric studies have confirmed the loss of contractile power (motor failure) of the lower two thirds of the body of the esophagus and have revealed a reduction in tone of the gastroesophageal sphincter, which permits the reflux of gastric juice and accounts for the frequent occurrence of peptic esophagitis and ulceration [32, 33].

The histological changes found in the esophagus are most marked in the lower two thirds [3, 8, 13]. There is thinning of the mucosa, which is often ulcerated. The lamina propria and submucosa tend to be thickened by dense collagen, and there is a variable degree of atrophy of the muscularis, which may be almost totally replaced by scar tissue. There is a notable sparing of the striated muscle in the upper portion of the esophagus. The walls of smaller arteries and arterioles are thickened and often surrounded by periadventitial deposits of collagen. Cellular infiltrates have been noted in the submucosa and may occur around the myenteric plexuses of Auerbach, which otherwise do not appear abnormal [33].

Lungs. Pulmonary involvement is recognized to be a frequent and important feature of PSS [3, 4]. Clinical and/or roentgenographic evidence of pulmonary fibrosis is noted in most patients, and interstitial and alveolar fibrosis are found in the great majority of cases at postmortem examination [3, 15]. The most prominent symptom resulting from pulmonary fibrosis (and complicating infection) is exertional dyspnea. Less commonly, there is a chronic cough, which may be productive. Many patients remain free from any complaints, however, despite roentgenological or histological evidence of severe fibrosis. Physical examination of the lungs of those who do have symptoms may reveal tachypnea and basilar rales, but more often proves quite unremarkable. The occurrence of pneumothorax has been reported [34]. In most, but not all, of these patients, roentgenographic study reveals a pattern of interlacing linear densities which are most pronounced in the lower two thirds of the lung fields and which in some cases assume the appearance of diffuse mottling or honeycombing, indicative of cystic lesions [4, 35].

Recent studies have revealed that the earliest and dominant disturbance in pulmonary function is in gas exchange [36–39]. Low diffusing capacities have been found frequently in the absence of any significant alteration in ventilation or any roentgenographic evidence of fibrosis. Electron microscopic examination of the lung of one patient with such a disturbance in pulmonary gas exchange revealed widening of the basement membranes of alveolar lining cells and the endothelium of small blood vessels (Fig. 69-3) [39]. In addition to the disturbance in diffusion, there has been evidence in some cases of restrictive ventilatory disease, indicated by reduction in vital capacity and total lung capacity (which may be ascribed to impairment of chest motion and diffuse peribronchial fibrosis), and of obstructive disease, manifested by a reduction in maximal breathing capacity and increased residual volume. Despite these disturbances, however, impairment of pulmonary function is rarely sufficiently severe to dominate the clinical picture, except in the event of complicating infection.

The predominant histological changes in the lungs consist of diffuse interstitial and alveolar fibrosis together with variable sclerosis of the smaller pulmonary vessels. In many cases, the alveolar walls are simply thickened,

* *Editor's comment:* Stevens *et al.* (*Arthritis Rheum.* 6:301, 1963) believe that there is a strong correlation between the defective peristaltic activity and presence of Raynaud's phenomenon. These symptoms may, indeed, antedate the onset of detectable scleroderma by months or years.—J. H. V.

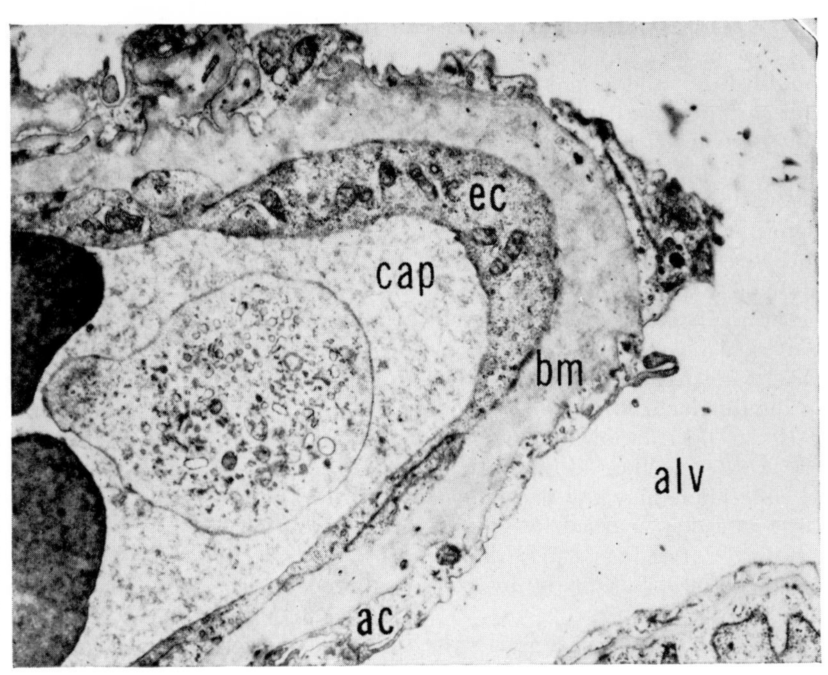

Fig. 69-3. Electron photomicrograph of lung of woman with PSS who had abnormally low pulmonary diffusing capacity. There is thickening of the basement membrane between the cytoplasm of the alveolar lining cell and the cytoplasm of the endothelium of a small blood vessel. *ac* = alveolar lining cell cytoplasm; *alv* = alveolar space; *bm* = basement membrane; *cap* = capillary lumen; *ec* = endothelial cell cytoplasm.

while in others, there are degeneration and rupture of septa leading to the formation of cystlike cavities and small areas of bullous emphysema [4, 35]. There may also be inflammation and fibrosis of the pleura, rarely accompanied by effusion. Malignant alveolar or bronchiolar cell neoplasms have been observed in a number of patients with severe pulmonary fibrosis, either of the diffuse interstitial or compact cystic (honeycomb lung) variety, and are believed to arise as a complication of intense bronchiolar epithelial proliferation which accompanies this fibrosis [40, 41].

Heart. The nature and severity of cardiac disease depend in part on the degree of underlying myocardial fibrosis and in part on the extent to which concurrent pulmonary involvement places an added burden on the circulation [42]. Many patients whose hearts are otherwise normal on physical examination have an accentuation of the pulmonic second sound, and recent studies have disclosed a remarkably high frequency of pulmonary hypertension [17, 42, 43], even in patients with little or no evidence of pulmonary fibrosis. Despite this, the number in whom cor pulmonale develops appears to be less than those who have prime difficulty with left ventricular function. In addition to the symptoms of myocardial insufficiency, which, as a rule, do not appear until late in the course, a number of patients have chest pain which is not unlike angina [10]. Supraventricular arrhythmias occur, and abnormal electrocardiograms are noted in a high percentage of cases [14, 15, 44, 45]. The more frequent findings include low voltage, complete or incomplete right bundle-branch block, numerous premature ventricular contractions, and ST-T wave changes. Pericardial effusion has been described [46, 47], but this is uncommon. Patients who are treated with digitalis for cardiac failure often respond poorly and tend to become intoxicated with its continued administration. Many die after a protracted period of circulatory shock; others die suddenly, presumably as a result of an arrhythmia.

Small irregular patches of interstitial myocardial fibrosis prominent in, but not limited to, perivascular areas are found at postmortem examination in a majority of cases [3, 15]. In patients with more serious heart disease, there may be extensive replacement of myocardial fibers. In addition, there may be focal infiltrations by inflammatory cells and thickening of smaller coronary vessels.*

Intestinal Tract. The percentage of patients who have symptoms referable to intes-

* There has been a recent case report of the association of progressive systemic sclerosis with nonsyphilitic panaortitis and aortic valvulitis (Roth and Kissane, *Amer J. Clin. Path.* 41:287, 1964).

tinal disease appears to be relatively small [14, 15]. There are, however, a number who are troubled by abdominal bloating, vomiting, and chronic constipation interrupted by periodic diarrhea [13, 31, 48]. These patients may become badly malnourished as a result of a disturbance in absorption [48]. It may be of significance that cutaneous changes in patients with severe intestinal involvement are often minimal or absent [29].

Roentgenographic study frequently discloses a marked delay in the transit of the barium meal, with dilatation and retention of barium in the duodenal bulb or loop (loop sign) and irregular flocculation and hypersegmentation of the other portions of the small intestine [13, 31, 49]. There may also be involvement of the large intestine, marked by sacculation (wide-mouthed false diverticula) due to muscular atrophy and occasionally by colonic dilatation [50].

The pathological changes in the intestinal tract are similar to those noted in the esophagus, discussed earlier.

Kidneys. There appears to have been little awareness of kidney disease in PSS until 1952, when Moore and Sheehan [51] described three patients who died of renal insufficiency and were found to have certain unusual histological changes. Since then, it has become clear that renal involvement is of frequent occurrence and is almost always associated with a form of highly malignant arterial hypertension [7, 52] which, in at least one large series of patients, has accounted for nearly one half of the deaths in the disease [15]. Most patients with this disturbance have had scleroderma for two years or less before the development of hypertension, which is characteristically abrupt in onset and often marked by a sudden disturbance of vision and the appearance of malignant hypertensive retinopathy. Within several days or weeks, there is evidence of rapidly progressive renal disease, indicated at first by azotemia and proteinuria and later by oliguria and uremia. These patients have died of renal insufficiency, cardiac failure, or cerebral hemorrhage, despite treatment with a variety of antihypertensive medications. Several reports have suggested that the development of hypertension and renal lesions may have been related to treatment with corticotropin (ACTH) or cortisone and related steroids [7]. There have been a number of patients, however, who received none of these medications, and there are several cases which antedate the steroid era. It is not clear, therefore, whether these agents truly induce the hypertension or simply accelerate the progression of already existing renal disease.

It has been suggested that the renal lesions in PSS may be produced by localized abnormal vasomotor activity in the small renal vessels, akin to Raynaud's phenomenon in the digital circulation [7], but it appears possible that these lesions may be the result rather than the cause of the malignant systemic hypertension.* Study of the pressor responses of patients with PSS in the normotensive state has revealed hyperreactivity to angiotensin and normal cold pressor reactions, which suggest the presence of an intrinsic arteriolar disturbance [53]. Urai *et al.* [54] reported that effective renal plasma flow was reduced in most patients with PSS, while glomerular filtration rate was normal in all but 2 of 25 cases, and they considered this indicative of efferent arteriolar constriction.

The kidneys of patients dying of malignant hypertension and renal insufficiency are often larger than normal and usually contain a number of small infarcts [7, 51, 52, 55]. The lesions found on microscopic examination are predominantly focal in distribution and include such changes as localized or diffuse thickening of glomerular basement membranes (with occasional instances of wireloop changes indistinguishable from those seen in lupus erythematosus), fibrinoid necrosis of the walls of afferent arterioles and glomerular tufts, and hyperplasia of interlobular and smaller arteries, the intimas of which contain large deposits of acellular material rich in acid mucopolysaccharides (Fig. 69-4) [55]. Examination of a corrosion preparation of a kidney revealed obstruction of a majority of the interlobular arteries and arterioles, a sharp decrease in glomerular filling, and a considerable increase in the number of aglomerular arterioles [56]. The appearance of the kidney in these cases is indistinguishable from that encountered in "ordinary" malignant nephrosclerosis [55], and it is of interest that in both conditions immunohistochemical analysis of

* We have recently observed a woman with PSS who died in uremia after a three-week period of anuria and who did not develop hypertension. Renal angiograms and injection study of the kidneys *post mortem* revealed striking constriction of the intralobular vessels.—G. P. R.

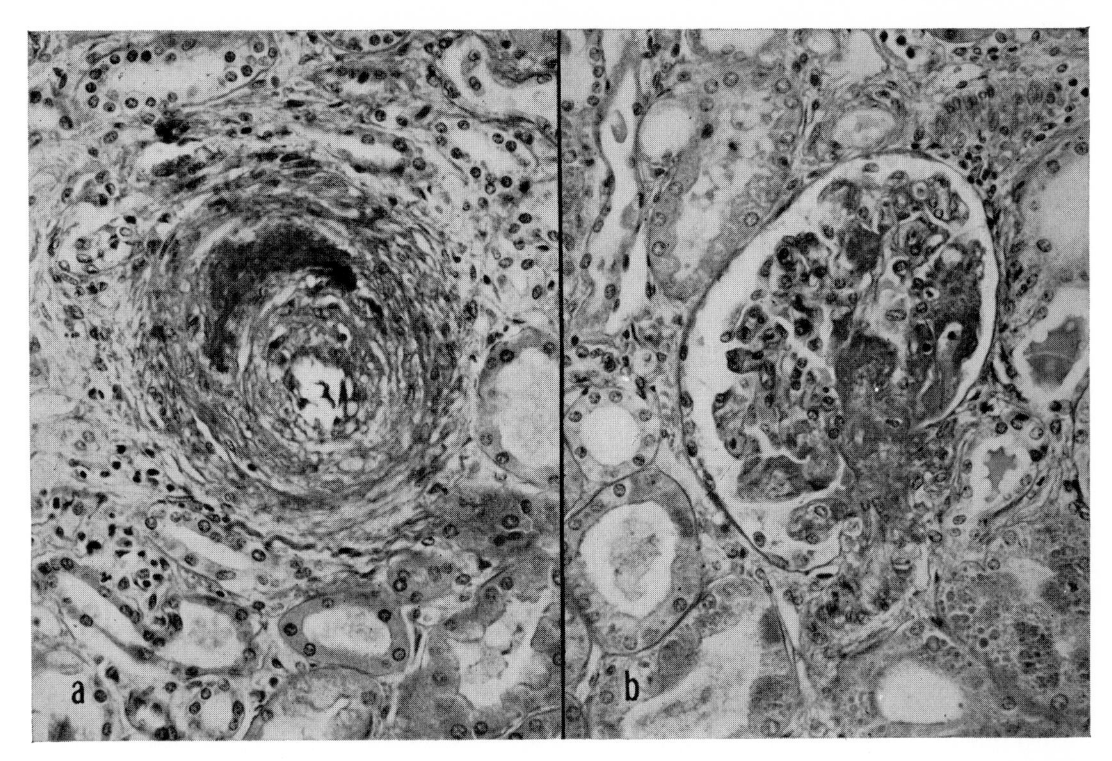

Fig. 69-4. Kidney of woman with progressive systemic sclerosis who died of malignant hypertension and renal insufficiency. (*a*) Thickening and fibrinoid necrosis of wall of small artery. (*b*) Fibrinoid necrosis of glomerular capillaries.

fibrinoid vascular lesions has shown a preferential concentration of fibrinogen and not of γ-globulin [57].

Miscellaneous. A few patients with PSS have had mono- or polyneuropathy [58, 59]. Histological examination in one case revealed increased thickness of the connective tissue sheaths of the nerve, deposition of mucoid material around the nerve fibers, and thickening of the arteriae nervorum [58]. However, weakness of the extremities can usually be ascribed to muscle atrophy which results from disuse of the parts. In addition, there may be an inflammatory reaction in skeletal muscle, characterized by cellular infiltrations (chiefly lymphocytes) in the endomysium and around small blood vessels in the perimysium [60, 61]. This lesion—interstitial (nodular) polymyositis—is similar to that observed in patients with rheumatoid arthritis and systemic lupus erythematosus (SLE).

Dental roentgenograms of patients with PSS often show widening of the periodontal membrane and dissolution of the lamina dura [14, 62]. The teeth most frequently affected are the bicuspids and molars. Histological examination has revealed an increase in the number of collagenous fibers in the periodontal membrane [62, 63].

COURSE OF THE DISEASE

It seems clear that most, if not all, patients with scleroderma will develop evidence of visceral sclerosis if followed long enough [14, 15]. The determination of prognosis with respect to both disability and death is difficult. In general, the outlook is poor in cases marked by rapid progression of dermal disease, severe malabsorption, or cardiac failure and is particularly bad in patients who develop malignant hypertension with renal involvement [15]. In many cases, however, the limitation of activity incident to cutaneous and internal disease may be only moderate and not necessarily threatening to life.

METABOLISM OF CONNECTIVE TISSUE IN PSS

It has generally been presumed that the fibrosis of the skin and certain internal organs of patients with PSS is due to an overproduction of collagen, a fibrous protein which, in the normal adult, is relatively metabolically inert [64]. There is, however, little or no information concerning quantitative composition of the skin and other tissues in this disease or of the physical and chemical characteristics of the collagen, save for certain histochemical and electron microscopic studies of the skin [24, 25, 65].* These have shown no abnormalities of the collagen fibrils other than occasional fraying and shortening of their ends [65]. Most patients with diffuse scleroderma appear to excrete a normal amount of urinary hydroxyproline, although a moderate increase has been found in a few patients early in the disease [66].

There is histological evidence of an increase in acid mucopolysaccharides in the initial stage of diffuse scleroderma [65], and the abnormally high uptake of radioactivity in the skin of patients given an intravenous injection of $Na_2[^{35}S]0_4$ [67] and the high concentration of acid mucopolysaccharide in the serum [17] may be interpreted as indicative of an increased rate of synthesis of sulfated mucopolysaccharides. Later in the course of the disease, however, there is a notable diminution or absence of these materials in the skin [24, 25].

IMMUNOLOGICAL ABNORMALITIES

Progressive systemic sclerosis was originally linked with rheumatoid arthritis, SLE, and certain other rheumatic diseases because of a number of clinical and morphological similarities which suggested that these conditions might represent disturbances of (or in) a single system, namely, the collagen-vascular or connective tissue system [20]. Early support for the role of an immunological mechanism as the common denominator in the pathogenesis of these conditions was derived from certain morphological similarities with the lesions of experimental and human serum sickness, polyarteritis, and drug hypersensitivity [68]. These concepts have been strengthened over the past few years by evidence from a number of different lines of clinical and laboratory investigation.

* Recent chemical analysis of dermis from patients with scleroderma has shown a normal concentration of water and hydroxyproline; amino acid and x-ray diffraction patterns of the collagen were normal (Fleischmajer, *Arch. Derm.* 89:437, 1964).

MORPHOLOGICAL FINDINGS

Although the distinctive and most widely appreciated pathological change in PSS is hyperplasia of the collagenous connective tissue, there are two other findings, *inflammation* and *vascular lesions,* which bear a similarity to changes observed in rheumatoid arthritis and SLE. The most convincing example of inflammation in PSS occurs in the form of synovitis (discussed earlier), but infiltrations by lymphocytes and other cells have also been observed during the early stages of disease in the gastrointestinal tract, skin, and other locations [17]. Vascular lesions were first emphasized by Matsui [69] and have been described in a number of organs, including the lung, heart, gastrointestinal tract, and, most impressively, the kidney (reviewed earlier). Although, with the exception of the kidney, the changes in the vessels become relatively inconspicuous later in the course of the disease, they may well be of significance in pathogenesis, albeit the manner in which they lead to fibrosis of the tissues is poorly understood.

ASSOCIATION OF PSS WITH DISORDERS OF KNOWN OR STRONGLY SUSPECTED IMMUNOLOGICAL ORIGIN

Like rheumatoid arthritis and SLE, PSS has been found in a number of patients with Sjögren's syndrome, Hashimoto's thyroiditis, and at least two patients with hypogammaglobulinemia [16, 17, 70–72]. The patients who have PSS and Sjögren's syndrome tend to be anemic, and some have clinical evidence of SLE or polymyositis and positive LE cell reactions [16]. These associations are clearly not a matter of chance alone and appear to provide strong support for the concept of a close relationship among these various disorders.

SEROLOGICAL ABNORMALITIES

Serum Proteins. Approximately one half of the patients with PSS have hypergammaglobulinemia [17, 73]. In most cases, the increase is only moderate in degree (1.4 to 2.0 gm. per 100 ml.), and values greater than 3.0 gm. are unusual. Immunoelectrophoresis of serum has shown increases in α_1-globulin, α_2-macroglobulin, and β_2-macroglobulin and a peculiar increase and splitting of the γ-globulin arc [74].

Hemagglutination and Latex Agglutination Reactions. Positive reactions with γ-globulin-coated particles have been noted in 22 to 41 percent of patients with PSS [15, 75, 76]. In most cases, the serum titers have been 1:160 or less [15]. There appears to be no particular correlation between a positive agglutination reaction and the presence of joint involvement [12].

LE Cell Reaction. There have been a number of reports of positive LE cell reactions in patients with PSS [16, 17, 77]. We have encountered three such individuals, none of whom presented clinical findings particularly indicative of lupus erythematosus. There are, however, other patients with PSS and positive LE cell reactions who have also had evidence of SLE and of Sjögren's syndrome [16]. In addition, a few patients with typical PSS have had chronic biological false positive serological reactions for syphilis [16, 17].

Antinuclear and Other Tissue Antibodies. Immunohistochemical studies of the sera of patients with PSS have revealed antinuclear globulins in a high percentage of cases [17, 78–80]. Beck *et al.* [80] detected antinuclear antibodies, often of high titer, in 25 (78 percent) of 32 patients. The relative prevalence of "homogeneous" and of "speckled" staining patterns (Fig. 69-5), indicative, respectively, of reactions with nucleohistone and with a small saline-soluble nuclear protein [81], was similar to that observed in the sera of patients with SLE. Bardawil *et al.* [78] found that the sera of patients with SLE failed to inhibit (block) the tissue binding of γ-globulin from patients with PSS, while Fennell *et al.* [79] noted that certain of the sera of patients with PSS which stained nuclear membrane and chromatin exerted partial inhibition of staining by both SLE and certain PSS sera.

Fennell *et al.* also found that sera of three patients with PSS (one of whom had Sjögren's syndrome) displayed nucleolar staining (Fig. 69-6) [79]. These sera produced cross-inhibition but had no effect on staining by sera of patients with SLE or of other patients with PSS. Beck *et al.* [82] detected antinucleolar antibodies in 11 of 358 sera from patients with various connective tissue diseases. These antibodies were found most commonly in patients with PSS (6 of 32 tested) and Sjögren's disease (2 of 43), and in all cases were associated with antibodies to other nuclear constituents [80]. Blocking experiments suggested that the antinuclear antibodies all reacted with the same antigenic component of nucleoli, which was neither organ- nor species-specific.

Serum Complement. Although the level of serum complement in patients with PSS has been found to be normal [83], it has been reported that the sera of certain patients with PSS, rheumatoid arthritis, and SLE exert an inhibitory effect on complement fixation reac-

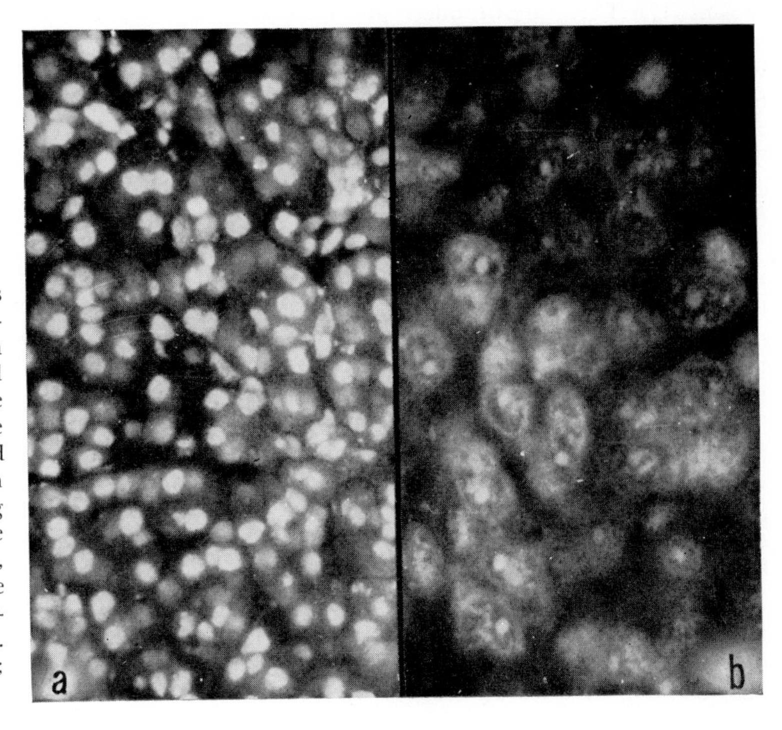

Fig. 69-5. Human pancreas stained with fluorescein-conjugated whole human serum of (*a*) a patient with SLE and (*b*) a patient with PSS. In the case of SLE, the nuclei are bright and uniformly stained except for occasional cells in which there is a nonstaining area which represents the nucleolus. In the case of PSS, there is staining of the nuclear membrane and irregular areas of chromatin. (From Fennell *et al.* [79]; courtesy *Lab. Invest.*)

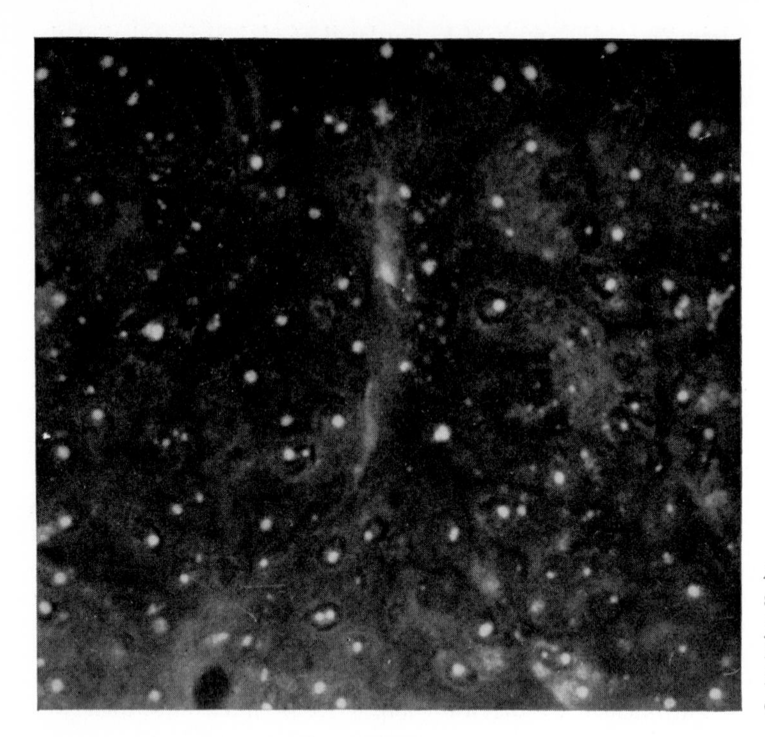

Fig. 69-6. Human pancreas stained with fluorescein-conjugated serum of a patient with PSS, illustrating nucleolar staining. (From Fennell *et al.* [79]; courtesy *Lab. Invest.*)

tions [84]. The factor responsible for the effect appears to be absorbed by antigen-antibody complexes but is separable and distinct from rheumatoid factor.

Family Studies. The occurrence of PSS on a familial basis seems to be rare, although the disease has been reported in sisters and in first cousins [17]. There are instances, also uncommon, in which a sibling or child of a patient with PSS has developed one or another systemic rheumatic disease, including rheumatoid arthritis, SLE, and dermatomyositis [85, 86]. These observations are much too scant, however, to indicate a familial or heritable predisposition to the disease.

Study of the serum proteins and serological reactions in the first-degree relatives of patients with PSS has disclosed the occasional presence of unexplained hypergammaglobulinemia and a very high incidence of antinuclear factors [87–89]. Thus Fennell *et al.* [89] noted positive reactions with the sera of 29 of 50 relatives in 12 families. In some instances, the sera of both parents and siblings gave positive reactions.

HOMOLOGOUS DISEASE

Stastny *et al.* [90] have reported the development of skin lesions closely resembling those of scleroderma in Sprague-Dawley rats which had homologous disease produced by the injection of large numbers of lymphoid cells from an unrelated strain of donor animals. The changes in the skin included atrophy of the epidermis, thickening and collagenous hyperplasia of the dermis, and atrophy of dermal appendages. Many of these animals developed synovitis and some showed inflammatory and degenerative changes in the heart valves and myocardium. Collagenous thickening of the dermis was also noted in autografts undergoing chronic rejection, and this, too, was considered suggestive of an immunological basis for the skin lesions of scleroderma. Whether or not the skin changes seen in homologous disease involve an antibody to collagen is not known. Although most attempts to induce antibody to purified collagen have proved unsuccessful, Rothbard and Watson [91] reported evidence that rabbit antirat collagen antibody produces renal glomerular lesions in rats prepared by the injection of adjuvant. The histological changes differed from those found following administration of antikidney serum, and it was suggested that tissue damage resulted from the interaction of rat antibody with rabbit antiglobulin bound to its antigen (collagen) in the kidney.

The means by which immunological reactions may lead to the deposition of increased amounts of collagen is not clear. Zarafonetis *et al.* [92] noted scleroderma-like changes in the legs of a patient with carcinoid syndrome and suggested that the fibrosis might have resulted from a derangement in serotonin metabolism in the tissues. Support for this concept can be derived from observations on the extreme sensitivity of patients with PSS to minute quantities of serotonin [93] and a report that the subcutaneous injection of serotonin in experimental animals leads to pronounced local fibrosis [94]. Further, serotonin has been found to be released in response to antigen-antibody interactions and may play a role in anaphylaxis [95].*

TREATMENT

The treatment of the patient with PSS consists of supportive measures designed to limit or compensate for the damage wrought to skin, joints, and internal organs and of empiric remedies which may inhibit the underlying pathological process(es) which gives rise to progressive fibrosis of connective tissue. Evaluation of the effectiveness of treatment is difficult because of the slowly progressive nature of PSS, the tendency to spontaneous variation or remission, the potent influence of psychophysiological factors on many of the symptoms, and the limitations in objective criteria for ascertaining improvement (or deterioration) of both the cutaneous and the visceral manifestations of the disease.

An impressively long list of vitamins, hormones, drugs, and surgical procedures has been used in PSS [2, 5, 96, 97]; nearly all of these have been abandoned more or less completely, after varying periods of, at first, enthusiastic and, later, more critical trial. There is no single drug or combination of drugs which has been adequately proved to be effective in controlled studies or which is generally accepted in treatment. Although corticotropin (ACTH) and cortisone and related steroids have been shown to cause atrophy of dermal collagen bundles and disappearance of mucopolysaccharides [98], and may be effective temporarily in the control of cutaneous and articular manifestations in early cases [99], their influence on visceral disease has proved disappointing. In view of the many problems involved in their administration for prolonged periods and the possible special hazard to the kidney, their use cannot be recommended. Relaxin, an ovarian polypeptide which affects the ground substance of the pelvic connective tissues and may play an important role in normal parturition, has been reported of worth in the relief of digital vasospasm, healing of ulcerations, and decrease of skin tightness [100]; others have found this costly hormone to be of no value [101].

Demonstration of a diminution in subcutaneous calcinosis in a patient following intensive treatment with sodium versenate (disodium-ethylenediaminetetraacetate) [102] has led to widespread use of this agent in PSS [97, 103, 104]. Initial enthusiasm has not been sustained, however [105]. Zarafonetis [106] reported moderate to considerable improvement in the skin of 97 of 104 consecutive, unselected patients with scleroderma who were treated by the prolonged (longer than three months) administration of 12 gm. daily of potassium para-aminobenzoate, combined with physiotherapy and dynamic traction splints. The effects, if any, on visceral disease, and the mechanism of action of this drug are not clear. Zarafonetis has suggested that it increases oxygen uptake in the tissues and may promote the action of monoamine oxidase, thus decreasing the level of serotonin (discussed earlier). In the recommended dose, potassium para-aminobenzoate is often nauseating and may occasionally produce drug fever and rash. Despite these difficulties and the danger of severe hypoglycemia in case it is continued during a period of inadequate food intake, the drug is now receiving extensive trial.

Thoracic sympathectomy may be followed by transitory improvement in digital vasospasm, but appears to have no significant or ultimate effect on the visceral disturbances or the course of the cutaneous involvement [5].

SUPPORTIVE MEASURES

Careful discussion with the patient and family concerning the nature of PSS is the first step in supportive management. Nearly all patients are troubled by Raynaud's phe-

* *Editor's comment:* The demonstration that an abnormal tissue, i.e., that of patients with connective tissue disease, is more sensitive to serotonin than normal tissues does not necessarily support the hypothesis that serotonin is implicated in the etiology of the disease. The release of serotonin by antigen-antibody interactions may have no meaning in the context of systemic sclerosis, even though apposition of these two observations may be superficially attractive.—J. H. V.

nomenon, and, to the extent that it is precipitated by low temperatures rather than emotional upset, this difficulty may be prevented by avoidance of exposure to cold environment. Many patients feel better during the summer but tend to sun-burn easily. Vasodilating drugs have been disappointing, doing little, if any, more good than socks and mittens. Special lotions, soaps, and bath oils should be used because of the excessive dryness of the skin, and household detergents should be avoided. If ulcerations of the fingertips become infected, healing may be assisted by the use of bactericidal antibiotic ointment, preceded in some cases by soaking with hyaluronidase to promote penetration of fibrinous exudate. Articular complaints may be helped by simple analgesics and the cautious use of moist heat and other forms of physical therapy, including traction splints [106].

Patients with difficulty in swallowing usually learn to masticate fully and to avoid foods such as meat and dry bread that are likely to cause dysphagia. Bethanechol chloride, a 5 or 10 mg. tablet crushed and swallowed before meals [106], and tincture of belladonna have been recommended but appear to be of little value [13]. The development of esophageal stricture may require periodic dilatation with sounds; esophageal hiatal hernia and peptic esophagitis call for additional appropriate measures. Patients with pulmonary fibrosis who have pneumonia or other infections require prompt treatment with appropriate antibiotics and oxygen and vigorous efforts to maintain ventilation. Those in whom pulmonary infection precipitates or is associated with heart failure often respond poorly to digitalis and easily become intoxicated, as has been mentioned. The treatment of patients with hypertension and renal insufficiency with a wide variety of antihypertensive agents has proved ineffective [15].

REFERENCES

1. Goetz, R. H. The pathology of progressive systemic sclerosis (generalized scleroderma). *Clin. Proc.* (Cape Town) 4:337, 1945.
2. Leinwand, I., Duryee, A. W., and Richter, M. N. Scleroderma: Based on a study of over 150 cases. *Ann. Intern. Med.* 41:1003, 1954.
3. Piper, W. N., and Helwig, E. B. Progressive systemic sclerosis: Visceral manifestations in generalized scleroderma. *Arch. Derm.* 72:735, 1955.
4. Opie, L. H. Pulmonary manifestations of generalized scleroderma (progressive systemic sclerosis). *Dis. Chest* 28:655, 1955.
5. Talbott, J. H., and Ferrandis, R. M. *Collagen Diseases.* New York: Grune & Stratton, Inc., 1956. P. 137.
6. Orabona, M. L., and Albano, O. Systemic progressive sclerosis (or visceral scleroderma): Review of the literature and report of cases. *Acta Med. Scand.,* vol. 160, supp. 333, 1957.
7. Rodnan, G. P., Schreiner, G. E., and Black, R. L. Renal involvement in progressive systemic sclerosis (generalized scleroderma). *Amer. J. Med.* 23:445, 1957.
8. Goldgraber, M. B., and Kirsner, J. B. Scleroderma of the gastrointestinal tract: A review. *Arch. Path.* 64:255, 1957.
9. Stava, Z. Diffuse scleroderma: A clinical study of sixty-five cases. *Dermatologica* 117:135, 1958.
10. Oram, S., and Stokes, W. The heart in scleroderma. *Brit. Heart J.* 23:243, 1961.
11. Tuffanelli, D. L., and Winkelmann, R. K. Systemic scleroderma: A clinical study of 727 cases. *Arch. Derm.* 84:359, 1961.
12. Rodnan, G. P. The nature of joint involvement in progressive systemic sclerosis (diffuse scleroderma): Clinical study and pathologic examination of synovium in 29 patients. *Ann. Intern. Med.* 56:422, 1962.
13. Hoskins, L. C., Norris, H. T., Gottlieb, L. S., and Zamcheck, N. Functional and morphologic alterations of the gastrointestinal tract in progressive systemic sclerosis (scleroderma). *Amer. J. Med.* 33:459, 1962.
14. Farmer, R. G., Gifford, R. W., Jr., and Hines, E. A., Jr. Prognostic significance of Raynaud's phenomenon and other clinical characteristics of systemic scleroderma: A study of 271 cases. *Circulation* 21:1088, 1960.
15. Rodnan, G. P. The natural history of progressive systemic sclerosis (diffuse scleroderma). *Bull. Rheum. Dis.* 13:301, 1963.
16. Tuffanelli, D. L., and Winkelmann, R. K. Scleroderma and its relationship to the "collagenoses": dermatomyositis, lupus erythematosus, rheumatoid arthritis and Sjögren's syndrome. *Amer. J. Med. Sci.* 243:133, 1962.
17. Rodnan, G. P. A review of recent observations and current theories on the etiology and pathogenesis of progressive systemic sclerosis (diffuse scleroderma). *J. Chron. Dis.* 16:929, 1963.
18. Rodnan, G. P., and Benedek, T. G. An historical account of the study of progressive

systemic sclerosis (diffuse scleroderma). *Ann. Intern. Med.* 57:305, 1962.

19. Banks, B. M. Is there a common denominator in scleroderma, dermatomyositis, disseminated lupus erythematosus, the Libman-Sacks syndrome and polyarteritis nodosa? *New Eng. J. Med.* 225:433, 1941.
20. Klemperer, P., Pollack, A. S., and Baehr, G. Diffuse collagen disease: Acute disseminated lupus erythematosus and diffuse scleroderma. *J.A.M.A.* 119:331, 1942.
21. Jaffe, M. O., and Winkelmann, R. K. Generalized scleroderma in children: Acrosclerotic type. *Arch. Derm.* 83:402, 1961.
22. Erasmus, L. D. Scleroderma in gold-miners on the Witwatersrand with particular reference to pulmonary manifestations. *S. Afr. J. Lab. Clin. Med.* 3:209, 1957.
23. Rodnan, G. P., and Cammarata, R. J. The association of progressive systemic sclerosis (diffuse scleroderma) with coal-miners' and other forms of pneumoconiosis. *Arthritis Rheum.* 6:294, 1963 (abst.).
24. O'Leary, P. A., Montgomery, H., and Ragsdale, W. E., Jr. Dermatohistopathology of various types of scleroderma. *Arch. Derm.* 75:78, 1957.
25. Fisher, E. R., and Rodnan, G. P. Pathologic observations concerning the cutaneous lesion of progressive systemic sclerosis: An electron microscopic, histochemical, and immunohistochemical study. *Arthritis Rheum.* 3:536, 1960.
26. Shulman, L., Kurban, A. K., and Harvey, A. M. Tendon friction rubs in progressive systemic sclerosis (scleroderma). *Trans. Ass. Amer. Physicians* 74:378, 1961.
27. Kulka, J. P., Bocking, D., Ropes, M. W., and Bauer, W. Early joint lesions of rheumatoid arthritis. *Arch. Path.* 59:129, 1955.
28. Rodnan, G. P., Yunis, E. J., and Totten, R. S. Experience with punch biopsy of synovium in the study of joint disease. *Ann. Intern. Med.* 53:319, 1960.
29. Rodnan, G. P., and Fennell, R. H., Jr. Progressive systemic sclerosis *sine* scleroderma. *J.A.M.A.* 180:665, 1962.
30. Harper, R. A. K. The radiological manifestations of diffuse systemic sclerosis (scleroderma). *Proc. Roy. Soc. Med.* 46:512, 1953.
31. Abrams, H. L., Carnes, W. H., and Eaton, J. Alimentary tract in disseminated scleroderma with emphasis on small bowel. *Arch. Intern. Med.* 94:61, 1954.
32. Creamer, B., Andersen, H. A., and Code, C. F. Esophageal motility in patients with scleroderma and related diseases. *Gastroenterologia* 86:763, 1956.
33. Treacy, W. L., Baggenstoss, A. H., Slocumb, C. H., and Code, C. F. Scleroderma of the esophagus: A correlation of histologic and physiologic findings. *Ann. Intern. Med.* 59:351, 1963.
34. Israel, M. S., and Harley, B. J. S. Spontaneous pneumothorax in scleroderma. *Thorax* 11:113, 1956.
35. Mahrer, P. R., Evans, J. A., and Steinberg, I. Scleroderma: Relation of pulmonary changes to esophageal disease. *Ann. Intern. Med.* 40:92, 1954.
36. Adhikari, P. K., Bianchi, F. A., Boushy, S. F., Sakamoto, A., and Lewis, B. M. Pulmonary function in scleroderma. *Amer. Rev. Resp. Dis.* 86:823, 1962.
37. Catterall, M., and Rowell, N. R. Respiratory function in progressive systemic sclerosis. *Thorax* 18:10, 1963.
38. Hughes, D. T. D., and Lee, F. I. Lung function in patients with systemic sclerosis. *Ibid.,* p. 16.
39. Wilson, R. J., Rodnan, G. P., and Robin, E. D. An early pulmonary physiologic abnormality in progressive systemic sclerosis (diffuse scleroderma). *Amer. J. Med.* 36:361, 1964.
40. Zatuchni, J., Campbell, W. N., and Zarafonetis, C. J. D. Pulmonary fibrosis and terminal bronchiolar ("alveolar-cell") carcinoma in scleroderma. *Cancer* 6:1147, 1953.
41. Collins, D. H., Darke, C. S., and Dodge, O. G. Scleroderma with honeycomb lungs and bronchiolar carcinoma. *J. Path. Bact.* 76:531, 1958.
42. Conner, P. K., and Bashour, F. A. Cardiopulmonary changes in scleroderma: A physiologic study. *Amer. Heart J.* 61:494, 1961.
43. Sackner, M. A., Akgun, N., Kimbel, P., and Lewis, D. H. The pathophysiology of scleroderma involving the heart and respiratory system. *Ann. Intern. Med.* 60:611, 1964.
44. Escudero, J., and McDevitt, E. The electrocardiogram in scleroderma: Analysis of 60 cases and review of the literature. *Amer. Heart J.* 56:846, 1958.
45. Windesheim, J. H., and Parkin, T. W. Electrocardiograms of ninety patients with acrosclerosis and progressive diffuse sclerosis (scleroderma). *Circulation* 17:874, 1958.
46. Meltzer, J. I. Pericardial effusion in generalized scleroderma. *Amer. J. Med.* 20:638, 1956.
47. Steinberg, I., and Rothbard, S. Pericardial effusion and cor pulmonale in progressive systemic sclerosis (scleroderma): Role of angiocardiography in diagnosis in two cases. *Amer. J. Cardiol.* 9:953, 1962.
48. Rosenthal, F. D. Small intestinal lesions with steatorrhea in diffuse systemic sclerosis (scleroderma). *Gastroenterology* 32:332, 1957.
49. Reinhardt, J. F., and Barry, W. F., Jr. Scleroderma of the small bowel. *Amer. J. Roent., Rad. Ther.* 88:687, 1962.

50. Meszaros, W. T. The colon in systemic sclerosis (scleroderma). *Amer. J. Roent., Rad. Ther.* 82:1000, 1959.
51. Moore, H. C., and Sheehan, H. L. The kidney of scleroderma. *Lancet* 1:68, 1952.
52. Levine, R. J., and Boshell, B. R. Renal involvement in progressive systemic sclerosis (scleroderma). *Ann. Intern. Med.* 52:517, 1960.
53. Rodnan, G. P., Shapiro, A. P., and Krifcher, E. The occurrence of malignant hypertension and renal insufficiency in progressive systemic sclerosis (diffuse scleroderma). *Ann. Intern. Med.* 60:737, 1964 (abst.).
54. Urai, L., Nagy, Z., Szinay, G., and Wiltner, W. Renal function in scleroderma. *Brit. Med. J.* 2:1264, 1958.
55. Fisher, E. R., and Rodnan, G. P. Pathologic observations concerning the kidney in progressive systemic sclerosis. *Arch. Path.* 65:29, 1958.
56. Urai, L., Munkacsi, I., and Szinay, G. New data on the pathology of "true scleroderma kidney." *Brit. Med. J.* 1:713, 1961.
57. Fennell, R. H., Jr., Reddy, C. R. R. M., and Vazquez, J. J. Progressive systemic sclerosis and malignant hypertension: Immunohistochemical study of renal lesions. *Arch. Path.* 72:209, 1961.
58. Richter, R. B. Peripheral neuropathy and connective tissue disease. *J. Neuropath. Exp. Neurol.* 13:168, 1954.
59. Kibler, R. F., and Rose, C. F. Peripheral neuropathy in the "collagen diseases." *Brit. Med. J.* 1:1781, 1960.
60. LeCoulant, P., and Texier, L. Histological lesions of muscle in dermatomyositis, differentiation from related musculo-cutaneous syndrome. *Brit. J. Derm.* 69:299, 1957.
61. Adams, R. D., Denny-Brown, D., and Pearson, C. M. *Diseases of Muscle: A Study in Pathology* (2nd ed.). New York: Hoeber Med. Div., Harper & Row, 1962. P. 436.
62. Stafne, E. C. Roentgenologic manifestations of systemic disease in dentistry. *Oral Surg.* 6:483, 1953.
63. Fullmer, H. M. and Witte, W. E. Periodontal membrane affected by scleroderma: A histochemical study. *Arch. Path.* 73:184, 1962.
64. Neuberger, A. The proteins of connective tissue and their metabolism. *Ann. Rheum. Dis.* 19:1, 1960.
65. Keech, M. A. The effect of collagenase on the fixed and unfixed skin lesions of morphea: an electron-miscroscope study. *J. Path. Bact.* 77:351, 1959.
66. Rodnan, G. P., and Cammarata, R. J. Urinary excretion of hydroxyproline in progressive systemic sclerosis (diffuse scleroderma). *Arthritis Rheum.* 6:294, 1963 (abst.).
67. Denko, C. W., and Stoughton, R. B. Fixation of S^{35} in the skin of patients with progressive systemic sclerosis. *Arthritis Rheum.* 1:77, 1958.
68. Rich, A. R. Hypersensitivity in disease, with special reference to periarteritis nodosa, rheumatic fever, disseminated lupus erythematosus and rheumatoid arthritis. *Harvey Lect.* 42:106, 1946–47.
69. Matsui, S. Ueber die Pathologie und Pathogenese von Sklerodermie universalis. *Mitt. Med. Fak. Tokyo* 31:55, 1924.
70. Shearn, M. A. Sjögren's syndrome in association with scleroderma. *Ann. Intern. Med.* 52:1352, 1960.
71. Stoltze, C. A., Hanlon, D. G., Pease, G. L., and Henderson, J. W. Keratoconjunctivitis sicca and Sjögren's syndrome. *Arch. Intern. Med.* 106:513, 1960.
72. Bunim, J. J. A broader spectrum of Sjögren's syndrome and its pathogenetic implications. *Ann. Rheum. Dis.* 20:1, 1961.
73. Stava, Z. Serum proteins in scleroderma. *Dermatologica* 117:147, 1958.
74. Zlotnick, A. and Rodnan, G. P. Immunoelectrophoresis of serum in progressive systemic sclerosis (diffuse scleroderma). *Proc. Soc. Exper. Biol. Med.* 107:112, 1961.
75. Ziff, M. The agglutination reaction in rheumatoid arthritis. *J. Chron. Dis.* 5:644, 1957.
76. Kellgren, J. H., and Ball, J. Clinical significance of the rheumatoid serum factor. *Brit. Med. J.* 1:523, 1959.
77. Rowell, N. R. Lupus erythematosus cells in systemic sclerosis. *Ann. Rheum. Dis.* 21:70, 1962.
78. Bardawil, W. A., Toy, B. L., Galins, N., and Bayles, T. B. Disseminated lupus erythematosus, scleroderma, and dermatomyositis as manifestations of sensitization to DNA-protein: I. An immunohistochemical approach. *Amer. J. Path.* 34:607, 1958.
79. Fennell, R. H., Jr., Rodnan, G. P., and Vazquez, J. J. Variability of tissue-localizing properties of serum from patients with different disease states. *Lab. Invest.* 11:24, 1962.
80. Beck, J. S., Anderson, J. R., Gray, K. G., and Rowell, N. R. Antinuclear and precipitating autoantibodies in progressive systemic sclerosis. *Lancet* 2:1088, 1963.
81. Beck, J. S. Variations in the morphological patterns of "autoimmune" nuclear fluorescence. *Lancet* 1:1203, 1961.
82. Beck, J. S., Anderson, J. R., McElhinney, A. J., and Rowell, N. R. Antinucleolar antibodies. *Lancet* 2:575, 1962.
83. Williams, R. C., and Law, D. H. Serum complement in connective tissue disorders. *J. Lab. Clin. Med.* 52:273, 1958.
84. Heimer, R., Levin, F. M., Primack, A., Corcos, J. M., and Nosenzo, C. Inhibition of complement fixation by human serum. *J. Immun.* 89:382, 1962; and *Arthritis Rheum.* 4:112, 1961 (abst.).
85. Hagberg, B., Leonhardt, T., and Skogh, M.

Familial occurrence of collagen diseases: I. Progressive systemic sclerosis and systemic lupus erythematosus. *Acta Med. Scand.* 169:727, 1961.
86. Leonhardt, T. Familial occurrence of collagen disease: II. Progressive systemic sclerosis and dermatomyositis. *Ibid.*, p. 735.
87. Corcos, J. M., Robbins, W. C., Rogoff, B., and Heimer, R. Some serum protein abnormalities in patients with progressive systemic sclerosis and their relatives. *Arthritis Rheum.* 4:107, 1961 (abst.).
88. Rodnan, G. P., Maclachlan, M. J., Fisher, E. R., Zlotnick, A., and Creighton, A. Serum proteins and serological reactions in patients with progressive systemic sclerosis (diffuse scleroderma) and their families. *Clin. Res.* 9:149, 1961 (abst.).
89. Fennell, R. H., Jr., Maclachlan, M. J., and Rodnan, G. P. The occurrence of antinuclear factors in the sera of relatives of patients with systemic rheumatic disease. *Arthritis Rheum.* 5:296, 1962 (abst.).
90. Stastny, P., Stembridge, V. A., and Ziff, M. Homologous disease in the adult rat, a model for autoimmune disease. I. General features and cutaneous lesions. *J. Exp. Med.* 118:635, 1963.
91. Rothbard, S., and Watson, R. F. Renal glomerular lesions induced by rabbit anti-rat collagen serum in rats prepared with adjuvant. *J. Exp. Med.* 109:633, 1959.
92. Zarafonetis, C. J. D., Lorber, S. H., and Hanson, S. M. Association of functioning carcinoid syndrome and scleroderma: I. Case report. *Amer. J. Med. Sci.* 236:1, 1958.
93. Scherbel, A. L. The Possible Role of Serotonin in Rheumatoid Arthritis and Other Collagen Diseases. In Mills, L. C., and Moyer, J. H. (Eds.), *Inflammation and Diseases of Connective Tissue.* Philadelphia: W. B. Saunders Company, 1961. P. 152.
94. MacDonald, R. A., Robbins, S. L., and Mallory, G. K. Dermal fibrosis following subcutaneous injections of serotonin creatinine sulfate. *Proc. Soc. Exp. Biol. Med.* 97:334, 1958.
95. Udenfriend, S., and Waalkes, T. P. On the Role of Serotonin in Anaphylaxis. In Shaffer, J. M., LoGrippo, G. A., and Chase, M. W. (Eds.), *Mechanisms of Hypersensitivity.* Boston: Little, Brown, 1959. P. 219.
96. Evans, J. A., Rubitsky, H. J., and Perry, A. W. Treatment of diffuse scleroderma. *J.A.M.A.* 151:891, 1953.
97. Perry, H. O. Recent treatment programs for generalized scleroderma. *Arch. Derm.* 83:300, 1961.
98. Mancini, R. E., Stringa, S. G., and Canepa, L. The action of ACTH, cortisone and prednisone on the connective tissue of normal and sclerodermic human skin. *J. Invest. Derm.* 34:393, 1960.
99. Zion, M. M., Goldberg, B., and Suzmann, M. M. Corticotrophin and cortisone in the therapy of scleroderma. *Quart. J. Med.* 24:215, 1955.
100. Casten, G. G., and Boucek, R. J. Use of relaxin in the treatment of scleroderma. *J.A.M.A.* 166:319, 1958.
101. Jefferis, J. E., and Dixon, A. St. J. Failure of relaxin in the treatment of scleroderma. *Ann. Rheum. Dis.* 21:295, 1962.
102. Klein, R., and Harris, S. B. Treatment of scleroderma, sclerodactylia and calcinosis by chelation (EDTA). *Amer. J. Med.* 19:798, 1955.
103. Muller, S. A., Brunsting, L. A., and Winkelmann, R. K. The treatment of scleroderma with the new chelating agent, Edathamil. *Arch. Derm.* 80:187, 1959.
104. Winder, P. R., and Curtis, A. C. Edathamil in the treatment of scleroderma and calcinosis cutis. *Arch. Derm.* 82:732, 1960.
105. Neldner, K. H., Winkelmann, R. K., and Perry, H. O. Scleroderma: An evaluation of treatment with disodium edetate. *Arch. Derm.* 86:305, 1962.
106. Zarafonetis, C. J. D. The Treatment of Scleroderma: Results of Potassium Para-aminobenzoate Therapy in 104 Cases. Ref. 93, p. 688.

70. Sjögren's Syndrome

RICHARD F. BAKEMEIER AND JOHN P. LEDDY

THE TRIAD OF KERATOCONJUNCTIVITIS sicca, xerostomia, and a "connective tissue disorder" has been termed Sjögren's syndrome. Synonyms occasionally applied to this condition are the sicca syndrome and the Sjögren-Mikulicz syndrome.

The connective tissue disorder involved is most commonly rheumatoid arthritis (RA) (41 percent of 261 patients in four large recent series) [1–4]. However, the ocular and oral features of the triad also may occur alone, or in association with myopathy, scleroderma, systemic lupus erythematosus (SLE), or periarteritis nodosa. The diagnosis is often considered established in the presence of any two of the features in the triad [3].

It is uncertain whether this syndrome represents a distinct disease, a variant of a generalized connective tissue disorder such as RA, or a combination of two or more causally unrelated pathological processes.

CLINICAL MANIFESTATIONS

A large number of patients appear to have relatively long histories of typical RA of varying severity and the added complaints of dry mouth, with or without salivary gland enlargement, and recurrent redness, burning, and dryness of the eyes. Other patients, however, may have more rapidly progressive generalized disease, with clinical manifestations of scleroderma, myopathy (sometimes termed polymyositis) [2], or SLE [1, 5].

In Sjögren's syndrome, the incidence in women exceeds that in men by about 9 : 1 [1–4]. In one reported group [3], the first symptom often occurred before age 40. This is somewhat contrary to the concept of many earlier observers that Sjögren's syndrome occurs predominantly in women in the middle and older age groups. The earliest symptom may be arthralgia or arthritis, preceding other features of the syndrome by several years in many [3, 4]. This arthritis does not differ appreciably from uncomplicated RA.

Keratoconjunctivitis sicca was the initial symptom in almost half of one series [4]. This condition is best diagnosed by slit lamp examination to detect minute breaks in the cornea, which stain with fluorescein, and by the observation of grossly apparent conjunctival staining with rose bengal dye. The Schirmer filter paper test may also be used for confirmation. The result is considered positive if lacrimal secretions fail to wet a specified segment of the paper, inserted inside the lower eyelid near the external canthus [6]. False positive results may be obtained in elderly patients. Many patients with the diagnosis keratoconjunctivitis sicca never exhibit other features of Sjögren's syndrome, and thus may represent examples of an unrelated pathological process [3].

Salivary gland swelling may be the initial complaint. This may recur intermittently for many years, with somewhat painful episodes of either unilateral or bilateral swelling of the parotids, or, less commonly, the submaxillary glands. Over half of reported patients with Sjögren's syndrome have given a history of dry mouth, and if salivary flow studies have been made, almost all patients have shown objective evidence of xerostomia [2, 7]. Abnormal sialograms have usually been observed when included in diagnostic studies [2]. Eventual atrophy of the involved gland may occur. Histological studies of the salivary and lacrimal glands disclose lymphocyte and plasma cell infiltrations, increased fibrous tissue, acinar atrophy, and occlusion of the ducts [8]. Similar infiltrative changes may be found in the mucous glands of the pharynx and larynx and in the submucous glands of the esophagus, trachea, and bronchi. The latter lesions have been implicated as causes of dysphagia and recurrent bronchitis in occasional patients [9].

Lymphocytic infiltration of the thyroid may also occur. In one series of 40 patients, 6 had either nodular goiter or diffuse enlargement of the thyroid, with 2 of them having a histological diagnosis of Hashimoto's thyroiditis [2].

Skeletal muscle involvement has been demonstrated, and proximal muscle weakness without tenderness may be a prominent clinical feature [2].

Hematological findings include mild to moderate anemia in up to 41 percent of patients [1]; this is usually normocytic and either normochromic or hypochromic. Leukopenia has been observed in 10 to 33 percent of various series, and mild eosinophilia has been reported with variable frequency.

The development of malignant lymphoma in at least four patients with Sjögren's syndrome has been described [10]. Two of these patients had received radiation therapy to enlarged parotid glands. Hodgkin's disease (one case cited in Ref. 10), Waldenström's macroglobulinemia (nine cases) [1], and sarcoidosis [11] have also been reported in association with Sjögren's syndrome.

SEROLOGICAL FINDINGS

Hypergammaglobulinemia, usually moderate but sometimes marked, has been a very common but not invariable finding. The increased γ-globulin concentration involves chiefly the more slowly migrating γ-globulins on paper electrophoresis [12] and 7S components on analytical ultracentrifugation [4, 12]. The 22S complexes have been noted in some cases [12].

Associated with this apparently exaggerated γ-globulin production, antibody-like serological activities have been described in such variety as to rival SLE in this respect. Rheumatoid factor (Chap. 65) has been detected in 75 to 100 percent of cases [2–4]. This serological activity was not confined to patients with RA, although in one series [4], the highest titers in the Rose-Waaler test were among patients with severe arthritis. Antinuclear factors (ANF) have been reported in 50 to 75 percent of patients, including those without clinical features of SLE [2, 3]. Of interest is the observation [2] that patients with RA occurring in the context of Sjögren's syndrome had a four times higher incidence of ANF than did RA patients without the Sjögren features. The LE cell phenomenon was encountered infrequently in two recent series [2, 3], and then only in patients having frank SLE or severe RA. On the other hand, an earlier study [5] reported LE cells in more than one third of patients; at least some of these had certain clinical features suggesting SLE. Thus the extent to which an associated disorder like SLE accompanies the distinctive Sjögren features in a given series might be expected to affect the incidence of various serological findings such as LE cells, positive results of direct antiglobulin tests, and false positive Wassermann reactions. Responses to the latter two tests, although more often negative, have been positive in a number of patients with Sjögren's syndrome in the absence of clinical SLE [3, 12].*

The precipitin or complement (C′)-fixation reactions (Chap. 14) between the sera of patients with Sjögren's syndrome and antigens derived from human salivary or lacrimal glands appear to have no organ or even species specificity [13–16]. With one or more human tissue antigens, C′ fixation is produced by the sera of 25 to 50 percent of patients with Sjögren's syndrome. Precipitin reactions are less frequent. More than one tissue antigen appears to be involved, but they have not yet been clearly characterized [14]. The serum factors responsible for such precipitin or C′ fixation reactions have been shown to migrate as γ-globulins electrophoretically [14, 16], and their true autoreactivity has been demonstrated in some instances [14]. These antitissue reactions lacking organ or species specificity thus resemble similar reactions encountered in SLE and certain other chronic diseases [16–19]. The patient's clinical status is apparently not related to the presence or titer of such antibodies [14]. Skin testing with tissue extracts, as a test of delayed hypersensitivity, seems not to have been described.

Specific antibodies against human thyroglobulin apparently have been demonstrated by the hemagglutination technique in 33 to 50 percent of patients with Sjögren's syndrome with or without attendant thyroid disease [2, 4, 15]. This reaction also occurs in a variety of other clinical states without recognized thyroid disease [20]. Precipitin reactions

* Whether the red cells giving positive reactions to direct antiglobulin tests were sensitized with γ-globulin or complement was not specifically determined. The failure to recover serologically active eluates from such cells [12] suggests the probability of "non-γ" or complement sensitization.

against thyroglobulin have also been described in Sjögren's syndrome [14].

Attempts to produce an experimental version of Sjögren's syndrome by inoculating animals with homologous salivary or lacrimal gland in adjuvant have failed [21].

Sjögren's syndrome thus shows a strong similarity to SLE and RA in its serological manifestations. There appear to be no distinguishing serological tests on which the clinician can rely in seeking a diagnosis.* It seems difficult at this time to assign a pathogenetic role to any of these serological reactions, despite their apparent autoreactive nature.

TREATMENT

The two primary objectives in the treatment of Sjögren's syndrome are the relief of the ocular and oral symptoms and the amelioration of any associated connective tissue disorder. Therapy for the latter is described elsewhere in this volume under the specific clinical entity.

Local treatment of the eyes to relieve dryness, thereby preventing mechanical damage and infection, includes drops of 1 percent methylcellulose in saline, or artificial tears. Corticosteroid drops have been used with variable success [22], although some authors have avoided them to minimize the risk of infection [4]. Severe keratoconjunctivitis sicca has been treated by electrocoagulative closure of the lacrimal puncta. Lozenges containing glycerin and gelatin may relieve the oral dryness [4].

Systemic therapy to improve parotid and lacrimal gland function has included a wide variety of agents, but none has been uniformly successful [1, 22]. Treatment with a combination of prednisone and desiccated thyroid substance seemed to give considerable improvement in 4 patients of one series, although no clinical evidence of thyroid disease had been evident [7]. Recently, the use of the antimalarial drug hydroxychloroquine has been accompanied by symptomatic improvement in 12 of 15 patients with Sjögren's syndrome [23].

REFERENCES

1. Stoltze, C. A., Hanlon, D. G., Pease, G. L., and Henderson, J. W. Keratoconjunctivitis sicca with Sjögren's syndrome: Systemic manifestations and hematologic and protein manifestations. *Arch. Intern. Med.* 106:513, 1960.
2. Bunim, J. J. A broader spectrum of Sjögren's syndrome and its pathogenetic implications. *Ann. Rheum. Dis.* 20:1, 1961.
3. Vanselow, N. A., Dodson, V. N., Angell, D. C., and Duff, I. F. A clinical study of Sjögren's syndrome. *Ann. Intern. Med.* 58:124, 1963.
4. Crews, S. J., and Whitfield, A. G. Sjögren's syndrome. *Postgrad. Med. J.* 39:324, 1963.
5. Heaton, J. M. Sjögren's syndrome and systemic lupus erythematosus. *Brit. Med. J.* 1:466, 1959.
6. Henderson, J. W. Keratoconjunctivitis sicca: A review with a survey of 121 additional cases. *Amer. J. Ophthal.* 33:197, 1950.

* *Editor's comment:* The claim that a "speckled" pattern of immunofluorescent antinuclear staining is characteristic of Sjögren's syndrome is tempered by similar staining patterns encountered in both SLE and RA without the sicca manifestations. Bunim (Conference on Autoimmunity, New York Academy of Sciences, February, 1964) reported that the rheumatoid factor-like activity in Sjögren's syndrome tends to have much less anti Gm activity than does the rheumatoid factor activity in RA alone.—J. H. V.

7. Denko, C. W., and Bergenstal, D. M. The sicca syndrome (Sjögren's syndrome): A study of 16 cases. *Arch. Intern. Med.* 105:849, 1960.
8. Cardell, B. S., and Gurling, K. J. Observations on the pathology of Sjögren's syndrome. *J. Path. Bact.* 68:137, 1954.
9. Bucher, U. G., and Reid, L. Sjögren's syndrome: Report of a fatal case with pulmonary and renal lesions. *Brit. J. Dis. Chest* 53:237, 1959.
10. Talal, N., and Bunim, J. J. The development of malignant lymphoma in the course of Sjögren's syndrome. *Amer. J. Med.* 36:529, 1964.
11. Gruber, E. Sarcoidosis of the lacrymal glands associated with Sjögren's syndrome. *Arch. Ophthal.* 55:42, 1956.
12. Bloch, K. J., Wohl, M. J., Ship, I. I., Oglesby, R. B., and Bunim, J. J. Sjögren's syndrome: I. Serologic reactions in patients with Sjögren's syndrome with or without rheumatoid arthritis. *Arthritis Rheum.* 3:287, 1960.
13. Jones, B. R. Lacrimal and salivary precipitating antibodies in Sjögren's syndrome. *Lancet* 2:773, 1958.
14. Anderson, J. R., Gray, K. G., Beck, J. S., and Kinnear, W. F. Precipitating autoantibodies in Sjögren's syndrome. *Lancet* 2:456, 1961.
15. Bloch, K. J., Bunim, J. J., Wohl, M. J., and

Zvaifler, N. J. Unusual occurrence of multiple tissue component antibodies in Sjögren's syndrome. *Trans. Ass. Amer. Physicians* 73:166, 1960.
16. Deicher, H. R. G., Holman, H. R., and Kunkel, H. G. Anti-cytoplasmic factors in the sera of patients with systemic lupus erythematosus and certain other diseases. *Arthritis Rheum.* 3:1, 1960.
17. Gajdusek, D. C. An "autoimmune" reaction against human tissue antigens in certain acute and chronic diseases. *Arch. Intern. Med.* 101:9, 1958.
18. Asherson, G. L. Antibodies against nuclear and cytoplasmic cell constituents in systemic lupus erythematosus and other diseases. *Brit. J. Exp. Path.* 40:209, 1959.
19. Anderson, J. R., Gray, K. G., Beck, J. S., Buchanan, W. W., and McElhinney, A. J. Precipitating auto-antibodies in the connective tissue diseases. *Ann. Rheum. Dis.* 21:360, 1962.
20. Hackett, E., Beech, M., and Forbes, I. J. Autoimmune complement-fixation reaction in 1,014 patients. *Brit. Med. J.* 2:17, 1960.
21. Bloch, K. J., and McMaster, P., Jr. Unpublished observations, 1960 (cited in Ref. 2).
22. Eadie, S., and Thompson, M. Kerato-conjunctivitis sicca treated with cortisone and ACTH. *Brit. J. Ophthal.* 39:90, 1955.
23. Heaton, J. M. The treatment of Sjögren's syndrome with hydroxychloroquine. *Amer. J. Ophthal.* 55:983, 1963.

71. The Demyelinating Diseases*

PHILIP Y. PATERSON

PREVAILING OPINION HOLDS THAT the demyelinating diseases of man may have an immunological basis. The total evidence for this view is impressive and persuasive, but unhappily it is largely indirect and does not alter the fact that the pathogenesis of demyelinating disease remains an enigma.

One purpose of this chapter is to summarize the clinical features and pathological aspects of the demyelinative diseases from the viewpoint of an internist. Another purpose is to examine, as an immunologist, the evidence suggesting that the demyelinative disorders have an immunological basis.† What emerges is a spectrum of demyelinative diseases ranging from hyperacute to chronic and held together by key clinical, pathological, and immunological characteristics. This spectrum and the hard core of supporting immunological evidence are set out here for purposes of introduction and orientation, since they form the axis around which this chapter will turn.

SPECTRUM AND INTERRELATIONSHIPS OF THE DEMYELINATING DISEASES

As shown in Figure 71-1, at one end of the spectrum is an explosive disease called acute hemorrhagic encephalopathy characterized by extremely acute focal perivascular lesions. There is little destruction of myelin, probably because death so often occurs before this change can become conspicuous. Acute disseminated encephalomyelitis (ADE) occupies an intermediate position. Although it is an acute disease and, again, characterized by focal, disseminated lesions having a perivascular and periventricular orientation, the tempo is slower and there is time for appreciable myelin destruction and astrocytic activation to occur. At the other end of the spectrum is the prototype demyelinating disease—multiple sclerosis.‡ This is a subacute or chronic remitting disorder in which demyelination and astrocytic proliferation are outstanding and culminate in firm plaquelike lesions. Inflammatory changes are inconspicuous, in keeping with the relatively slow and almost imperceptible march of events.

Although each of the demyelinative diseases tends to follow a pattern or course of its own (large vertical arrows, Fig. 71-1) there are instances in which one disease appears to merge with another (small horizontal arrows). For example, Adams [1, 2] and van Bogaert [3] cite transitions between acute hemorrhagic encephalopathy and ADE and between ADE and less acute forms of demyelinating disease. Occurrence of a form of encephalomyelitis resembling multiple sclerosis after injections of rabies vaccine, rather than the usual ADE, has

* Studies carried out by the author and referred to in this chapter were supported in part by Research Grants from the National Institute of Allergy and Infectious Diseases and the National Institute of Neurological Diseases and Blindness, U.S. Public Health Service, and in part by an Award (Established Investigatorship) of the American Heart Association, Inc.

† Limitations of space preclude a complete review. Studies cited represent important landmarks, have special interest or meaning to this writer, or point to promising paths of investigation.

‡ A qualifying statement is required concerning multiple sclerosis. This disease is considered by many to be a "prototypic" demyelinating diease. Several other demyelinating diseases might have been included for discussion here, e.g., diffuse leukodystrophy, Schilder's encephalitis periaxialis diffusa, Balo's concentric sclerosis, and neuromyelitis optica (Devic's disease). Although these are often treated as distinct entities, as their descriptive labels imply, there is no serious reason for believing that they represent disorders etiologically distinct from multiple sclerosis.

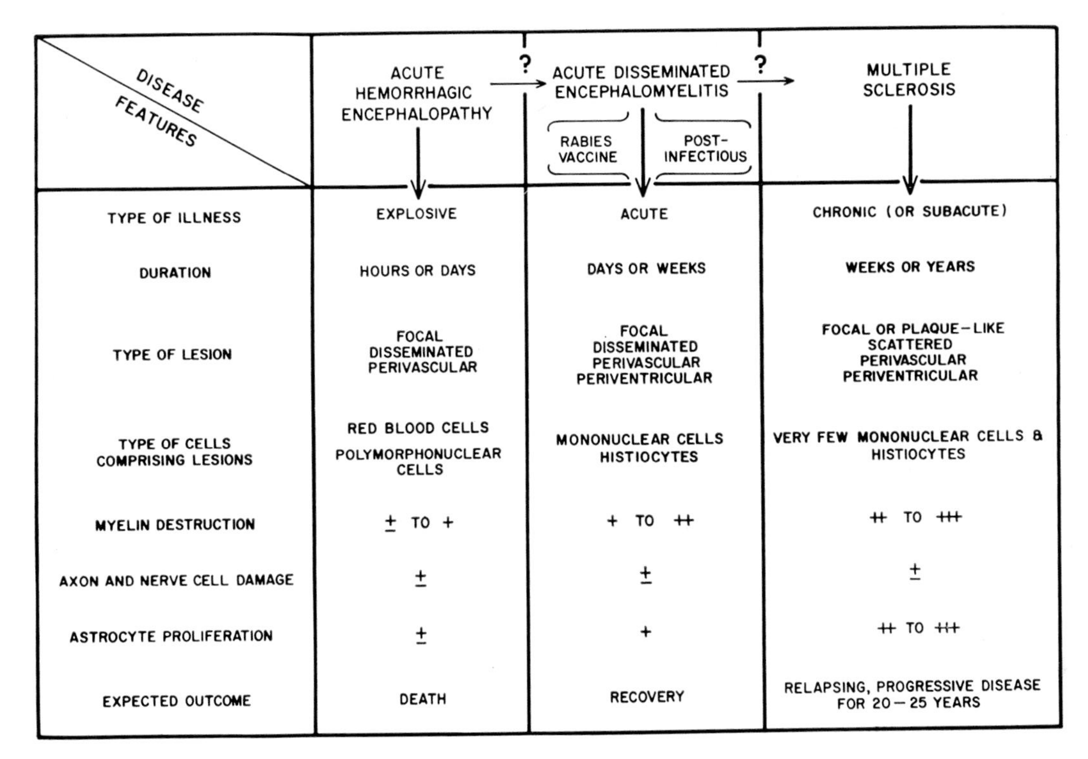

Fig. 71-1. Spectrum and interrelationships of the demyelinating diseases.

been reported by Shiraki *et al.* [4, 5]. How often such merging occurs and how long it takes is unknown (represented by question marks over the small arrows, Fig. 71-1). But the overlappings do occur and emphasize how much the tempo at which the individual diseases unfold influences the pathological changes used to identify them.

HARD-CORE IMMUNOLOGICAL EVIDENCE

It has been known for decades that mammalian nervous tissue is antigenic and when injected into animals calls forth complement-fixing antibodies directed specifically against nervous tissue [6, 7]. About 30 years ago, Rivers *et al.* [8, 9] found that repeated injections of nervous tissue induced an acute encephalomyelitis in monkeys which resembled the ADE seen in man after injections of rabies vaccine or other provoking events (Fig. 71-1). In 1947, it was discovered that an accelerated form of ADE, now known as experimental allergic encephalomyelitis (AE), could be produced within two to three weeks in a variety of laboratory animals by a single injection of nervous tissue emulsified in Freund's adjuvant [10–13]. Allergic encephalomyelitis represents at present the strongest experimental evidence favoring the immune concept of demyelinating disease.

Bornstein and Appel [14] and more recently Koprowski and Fernandes [15] and Berg and Källén [16] have reported that sera of animals with AE cause dissolution of myelin and swelling or disruption of brain glial cells. The serum factors are believed to be antibodies directed specifically against these constituents of nervous tissue. An exciting development is the finding of Bornstein [17] and his group and Berg and Källén [18] that these same myelinotoxic and glial-toxic serum factors occur in multiple sclerosis. This evidence, coming directly from patients, is vital, for it indicates that the immune responses found in AE of animals are also found in demyelinative disorders of man and that AE and the demyelinating diseases may have common underlying pathogenic mechanisms.

ACUTE HEMORRHAGIC ENCEPHALOPATHY

This is a rare disease, largely affecting adults and recognized as a distinct entity only during the past two decades [19, 20]. Cases of survival for longer than a few days are of special interest because they emphasize how this disease may merge with less acute forms of demyelinating disease. Adams *et al.* [20] described one case characterized by clearcut relapses and which resulted in death three to fourth months after onset. Here the clinical course and histological findings resembled a subacute form of multiple sclerosis. Russell [21] described two cases with extensive perivascular demyelination and round cell infiltration of the type characterizing ADE. In one of these cases, striking perivascular demyelination was found in the spinal cord, which is ordinarily relatively spared in acute hemorrhagic encephalopathy.

Clinical Features. There is often a prodrome of several days consistent with undifferentiated acute respiratory disease, influenza, or the common cold. Either immediately following these vague complaints or after return to good health for a few days, neurological manifestations break forth with explosive force. There are an abrupt rise of fever (101 to 105° F.), headache, prostration and, occasionally, nuchal rigidity. Cerebral and brain stem signs then follow: lethargy yielding to stupor or coma, hemiplegia, convulsions, and the ominous signs of medullary failure (respiratory and cardiovascular collapse). The disease usually terminates fatally within a matter of hours to approximately one week.

Laboratory Findings. The peripheral blood examination reveals polymorphonuclear leukocytosis. The spinal fluid is usually under increased pressure and exhibits intense pleocytosis (with cell counts up to 3,000 to 5,000 per $mm.^3$, with almost all cells polymorphonuclear), elevated protein and normal or somewhat decreased glucose concentrations. An early clue attracting attention away from bacterial meningitis, which this disease mimics in many respects, is the absence of demonstrable bacteria in spinal fluid smears and consistent sterility of spinal fluid cultures.

Pathological Features. The identifying histological changes of acute hemorrhagic encephalopathy are noteworthy not only because they assume a pattern similar to that associated with other demyelinating diseases but because virtually identical lesions may be found in AE induced in animals by sensitization to nervous tissue. The lesions are apt to be mainly confined to cortical and subcortical white matter, corpus callosum, cerebral and cerebellar pednucles, and the brain stem (usually the pons). The individual lesions usually range in size from 0.1 to 1 mm.; rarely, they may attain a size of 1 to 2 cm. The orientation of lesions around vessels, especially small veins, is a conspicuous feature. Major changes consist of necrosis and fibrin deposits within the vessel walls and just beyond. Fresh hemorrhages through the vessel walls and into the immediate perivascular spaces are an identifying feature. With these changes are found perivascular demyelination and intense inflammatory (polymorphonuclear cell) infiltrates. Axon fibers within the areas of most intense damage may exhibit injury varying from clubbing to frank destruction. The response of microglial or histiocytic cells in the affected areas is usually inconspicuous, probably because of the rapid tempo of the disease.

ACUTE DISSEMINATED ENCEPHALOMYELITIS (ADE)

INDUCED BY RABIES VACCINE

Reasons for Special Consideration. This disease, when associated with injections of rabies vaccine, is virtually indistinguishable from that following certain viral diseases but warrants separate discussion here. First, it is a man-made disease, the result of injection of mammalian nervous tissue containing attenuated or killed rabies virus. Second, with respect to *all* of its features (mode of induction, clinical neurological signs, identifying pathological changes, and course), it is essentially identical to AE in laboratory animals. This fact is vital. It represents a cornerstone supporting the widely held view that AE is a meaningful and valid laboratory model for the demyelinating diseases of man. And because immunological mechanisms are clearly implicated in the experimental disease, it is commonly assumed that the demyelinating diseases as a group may have an "allergic" basis. Third, within the past few years an efficacious rabies vaccine prepared from duck embryo has widely replaced the Semple type of vaccine derived from rabbit nervous tissue [22]. Duck embryo has much less paralytogenic activity, i.e., capacity to induce AE in experimental animals [23]. As far as I am aware, only one report [24] has appeared of acute neurological disease associated with use of duck-embryo rabies vaccine.* The proved effectiveness of hyperimmune rabies antiserum offers a means for ultimately dispensing with the need for injection of any nervous tissue in rabies prophylaxis. Thus it is likely that rabies-vaccine ADE will be of decreasing practical concern in the future, in contrast to the other demyelinating diseases under discussion.

Like the AE which serves as its experimental counterpart, the disease induced in man by rabies vaccine may range from an extremely transitory affair with almost evanescent clinical signs to a devastating and fulminating disease. Worthy of emphasis is the expected complete and almost invariably sustained recovery of those patients who survive the acute neurological episode. This point, and the lack of any strong tendency to follow a progressive or relapsing type of course, resemble the features characteristic of AE in experimental animals sensitized to nervous tissue.

Historical Background. Details concerning emergence of this disease as an entity soon after introduction of the Pasteur vaccine for rabies in 1885 may be found elsewhere [25, 26]. Briefly, the vaccine devised by Pasteur consisted of dried rabbit spinal cord containing rabies virus which had lost its pathogenicity for dogs by virtue of more than one hundred serial passages through rabbits. This was a live vaccine containing attenuated virus. A series of ten to fourteen subcutaneous injections of graded infectivity (as determined in rabbits) was found to protect dogs against naturally occurring "street" rabies virus. Paralysis associated with use of the vaccine in man was described as early as 1888. Controversy immediately arose as to the cause of these neurological "accidents." Were they due to infection with the "attenuated" rabies virus in the vaccine? Did they represent natural rabies infection which had been modified in some way by injections of the vaccine? Or were they caused by the injection of the large amounts of nervous tissue comprising the vaccine? Continued occurrence of "paralytic accidents" despite use of phenol-treated, killed rabies virus vaccine (introduced by Semple in 1919) and occurrence of paralytic signs in individuals bitten by obviously nonrabid animals strongly suggested that the paralytogenic activity of rabies vaccines resided in the nervous tissue.

This view gained support from two sources. By the early 1930's, mammalian nervous tissue had been shown to be antigenic and, when injected into animals, capable of eliciting antibodies which fix complement specifically with brain extracts *in vitro* [6, 7]. Second, often-repeated injections of presumably normal nervous tissue into monkeys and other laboratory animals were found to induce an acute disseminated encephalomyelitis essentially identical to that seen in man [8, 9]. These facts led to acceptance of the view that the encephalomyelitis associated with rabies vaccine has an immunological pathogenesis related to injection of mammalian brain tissue as the antigen(s).

Incidence. In 1927 Remlinger [27] reported a rate of 0.28 per 1,000 based on extensive experience with attenuated rabies vaccine. Since 1930, phenol-killed (Semple type) vaccine has been used in most parts of the world, and with this type of vaccine (used as described below) the incidence of ADE has ranged from 1 per 1,000 to 1 per 4,000.

Clinical Aspects. In Europe, the United States, and many other parts of the world, a course of rabies vaccination consists of fourteen or more daily subcutaneous injections of killed (Semple type) vaccine. The injections, of about 2 ml. each, are usually made in the periumbilical region of the abdomen. Clinical neurological signs most often appear 4 to 15 days after the first injection, i.e., during the two-week course of vaccination [28]. Although adults were once believed solely affected, cases do occur in children, without question. Local signs such as pain, redness, induration, or urticaria at one or more of the subcutaneous injection sites or transitory waves of "hives" and generalized pruritus may herald the onset of clinical neurological signs. These local signs

* In this case, the classic picture of transverse myelitis with a level at L_2 occurred abruptly in a 33-year-old man 48 hours after the fourteenth and last daily subcutaneous injection of duck-embryo rabies vaccine. Spinal fluid was unremarkable. The patient made a complete recovery within 2 months. The pathogenesis of this acute episode is not clear. Negative viral studies and the temporal relationship between the myelitis and the vaccine implies that the myelitis was the result of duck-embryo vaccine injection rather than some coincidental spontaneous viral infection. The neurological picture may have represented a marked exaggerated response to minute amounts of some paralytogenic constituent of the vaccine. Alternatively, nonparalytogenic protein antigens in the duck-embryo vaccine may have induced an acute allergic response manifested as acute angioneurotic edema of the spinal cord.

clearly reflect heightened immunological reactivity of an immediate or Arthus type directed against the heterologous rabbit protein antigens contained in the vaccine. It is not known whether they have any direct bearing on the occurrence of neurological manifestations or merely represent parallel and independent events.*

The clinical neurological picture usually consists of signs of meningeal inflammation (headache, backache, stiff neck), peripheral nerve involvement or/and spinal cord disease (weakness or paralysis of one or more extremities, deep tendon reflex changes, transverse myelitis with a distinct "level") [28].† Uncommon are signs of serious cerebral involvement (lethargy, confusion, excitement, stupor, or coma). Since low-grade fever accompanied by myalgia and general malaise occur, the picture may simulate aseptic meningitis or meningoencephalomyelitis of viral origin. In as many as perhaps one quarter to one third of cases, the syndrome known as Landry's ascending paralysis (unaccompanied by sensory or sphincter disturbances) occurs. The course is rapid and leads to fatal medullary failure in one third of the patients. Mortality associated with the other more common clinical patterns is low, probably less than 5 percent. In the four cases followed by the author, a mixed picture with meningeal and spinal cord signs was observed; all patients recovered completely within a fortnight.

Laboratory Findings. There are no characteristic changes in the peripheral blood. The spinal fluid pressure is usually normal. There is pleocytosis in most cases, consisting largely of mononuclear cells (with cell counts as high as 500 per mm^3). Spinal fluid protein may be increased; sugar content is rarely abnormal. Cultures of the blood and spinal fluid are invariably sterile.

Pathological Features of Rabies-Vaccine ADE in Man. Classically, one expects to find only microscopic lesions consisting of focal areas of vasculitis largely confined to the spinal cord and brain stem [1, 2]. The meninges may show a spotty or, rarely, diffuse infiltration by mononuclear cells. The focal lesions consist of vascular-perivascular accumulations of inflammatory cells and associated perivascular demyelination. The cellular infiltrates consist of small numbers of polymorphonuclear cells (unless death occurs rapidly, when such cells may clearly predominate), large numbers of histiocytes and lymphocytes, and a fair number of plasma cells. There is a distinct and characteristic orientation of these lesions around small veins or venules within the gray or white matter, with some predilection for the latter. The areas of perivascular demyelination may be striking and reach appreciable size due to confluence of several small focal areas of myelin loss. Some damage to axon fibers may occur, and subtle changes in the nerve cell bodies may be noted. Activity of astrocytes within or around the areas of myelin damage and cellular infiltrations is not an outstanding feature. Gliosis is therefore not a hallmark, and the glial plaques of multiple sclerosis are not found. This last point constitutes an important argument that ADE associated with rabies vaccine and multiple sclerosis are distinct diseases (see below).

* It is worth emphasizing that occurrence of a local or generalized urticarial eruption may represent serum sickness caused by antitetanus toxin (horse) serum commonly used in general treatment of the wound and thus have no relationship whatever to administered rabies vaccine.

† Occurrence of peripheral nervous system lesions after injection of rabies vaccine prepared from central nervous system tissue might be anticipated, since peripheral nerves and spinal ganglia share antigenic constituents found in brain and spinal cord.

POSTVACCINIAL AND POSTINFECTIOUS ADE

In 1926 Turnbull and McIntosh [29] described the morphological changes in seven fatal cases of acute encephalitis which followed what were otherwise routine smallpox vaccinations. During the next few years, evidence from several quarters indicated that ADE may follow spontaneously occurring smallpox and several other viral diseases, e.g., measles (both rubeola and rubella) and chickenpox.

Incidence. Probably the only definite statement that can be made is that there is an unpredictability and variability in occurrence of ADE after viral infection. For example, in a single year of intensive smallpox vaccination, incidence rates were reported of 1 per 21,000 in Edinburgh and 1 per 70,000 in Glasgow. A unique opportunity of accurately determining the incidence rate was the mass vaccination of 5 million people in New York City over a two month period in 1947. According to Greenberg [30], 49 cases of encephalitis believed related to use of smallpox vaccine were reported. Based on these figures, the incidence of this neurological complication was about 1 per 100,000. The actual occurrence rate may well have been lower, since 4 of the 49 cases were fatal and at autopsy were found to lack the essential changes of postvaccinial encephalomyelitis and death was due to other causes. The incidence of encephalitis associated with rubeola appears to be much higher, in the range of approximately 1 per 1,000, based on several reported series reviewed by Miller *et al.* [31]. Occurrence rates of encephalitis associated with rubella, varicella, and smallpox (variola) are not accurately established.

Clinical and Laboratory Findings. Of diagnostic importance is the relatively characteristic latent period between virus infection and occurrence of the encephalomyelitis. In postvaccinial encephalitis, neurological signs almost invariably make their first appearance 10 to 13 days after vaccination, with the greatest number of cases occurring on the eleventh day after vaccination. In the case of rubeola (and probably varicella), neurological signs usually appear 2 to 6 days after onset of the cutaneous eruption, and perhaps even earlier in association with rubella, i.e., 1 to 2 days after the eruption.

Clinical manifestations appear abruptly. There is a short prodrome consisting of headache, vomiting, and sharp rise in temperature. Alarming changes in the sensorium occur which may rapidly lead to coma and convulsions. Patients who do not succumb rapidly may exhibit weakness or frank paralysis of one or more extremities and/or cranial nerve involvement. There may be autonomic nervous system dysfunction (bladder and bowel), and evidence of meningitis may be conspicuous. In a very small proportion of cases (perhaps less than 5 percent), the clinical picture may be predominantly that of myelitis or even polyradiculitis. Pyramidal tract signs are uncommon. Death may occur in two to four days in fulminating cases. Mortality rates remain alarmingly high, that for ADE associated with measles being in the vicinity of 20 percent and that for postvaccinial encephalitis being reported to run as high as 50 percent (in contrast to less than 10 percent in the New York City study reported by Greenberg [30]).

The spinal fluid is usually under increased pressure, and there is some increase in the number of white cells (usually less than 100 per mm^3). in the majority of cases. Although lymphocytes often predominate, a high percentage of polymorphonuclear cells may be found in fluids examined very soon after onset. There may be an increase in protein content. The sugar level is usually normal or elevated. Smears and cultures fail to reveal microorganisms.

Pathological Features. Although the duration of illness before death (which is a direct reflection of the tempo of the disease) may influence certain details of the pathological picture, it should be emphasized that the general picture which does emerge is very similar to that of ADE induced by rabies vaccine injections and the AE induced in animals by brain sensitization. In addition, there are histological changes which seem noteworthy because they serve as morphological links between ADE and acute hemorrhagic encephalopathy on the one hand and ADE and subacute forms of multiple sclerosis on the other (see Fig. 71-1 and Ref. 1–3, 32).

The initial changes consist of infiltration of small vessel walls by mononuclear cells, perhaps some polymorphonuclear cells, and small hemorrhages may be present. With the passage of time there is an intense perivascular infiltrative process, the inflammatory cells being mainly histiocytic or lymphocytic. Accompanying the cellular infiltration, but rarely if ever preceding it, are conspicuous areas of perivascular demyelination. Marked demyelination is usually seen only in cases of death three or four days or longer after onset [33]. There is a variable astrocytic reaction with some gliosis. Degenerative changes involving the neurons as well as the nerve tract are not features. Disseminated focal lesions are found scattered throughout the neuraxis, with perhaps a predilection for ventral portions of the pons, areas adjacent to the lateral ventricles, and subpial areas over the ventral and lateral aspects of the cord. In very acute cases, necrotic changes in small vessel walls may be present, and hemorrhagic changes may be extensive.

Clinical Course. Although patients who survive the acute neurological episode generally have a relatively complete and sustained recovery, occasional cases follow a different pattern. These may show relapses at a later date and assume the course of a remitting, subacute type of illness covering a period of weeks or months [3]. These cases have special significance because they suggest merging of

ADE with subacute forms of multiple sclerosis, and this view receives support from the pathological changes which may be found at autopsy. In addition, the fact that ADE associated with viral infection is not always a monophasic illness raises the important question of whether it may in some obscure way be a harbinger of chronic multiple sclerosis which does not make its appearance until years later.

MULTIPLE SCLEROSIS

General Aspects. Detailed accounts of the many facets of this old and important disease may be found in well-known monographs [34, 35]. Classically, multiple sclerosis affects males and females between about 20 and 40 years of age. This is so true that for patients much outside these two decades, a diagnosis of the disease is in jeopardy. There are no accurate figures concerning general incidence and prevalence.* There is widespread feeling that the disease is more frequent in temperate regions than in subtropical or tropical areas, and several studies seem convincing along this line. For example, the study by Alter *et al.* [36] carried out in comparable communities in Nova Scotia and South Carolina, which are separated by about 1,200 miles, showed the incidence of multiple sclerosis to be 2.4 times greater in the more northern, Nova Scotia community.

The disease has a familial tendency but does not follow any common genetic pattern. More than one case within a family thus serves to strengthen rather than weaken the diagnosis. Dreary lists can be found of the "specific factors or events" believed to precipitate attacks, including such things as infection, emotional upheaval, trauma, physical exertion, allergy, and pregnancy. Virtually the same list appears for a variety of chronic diseases which, like multiple sclerosis, are of unknown etiology and wax and wane over the years. Perhaps trauma and physical exertion may be real factors, at least in terms of enhanced passage of a neurotropic factor causing the disease into a selected portion of the neuraxis (as discussed below). While multiple sclerosis is believed to have an allergic basis, it is worth noting that no convincing evidence exists that patients with the disease are particularly apt to have an allergic diathesis. Pregnancy appears to have no beneficial influence, nor is any clear-cut beneficial effect exerted by adrenocorticotropic hormone or the adrenal corticoids on chronic forms of the disease (see later discussion of Treatment).

Clinical Picture. The clinical manifestations are extremely varied. In some patients, the disease begins in an insidious way. In others, symptoms may appear and become alarming in minutes or hours. Irrespective of the type of onset, the disease tends to follow an undulating, remitting and relapsing course. This feature is so common that competent neurologists are reluctant to make the diagnosis in its absence. In about one half of the cases, initial symptoms are referable to the motor system (e.g., loss of abdominal reflexes, increased deep tendon reflexes, and Babinski sign). In others, the symptoms are referable to the visual tracts, the sensory tracts, or rarely the autonomic system. Common sensory complaints include tingling, numbness, or such unusual sensations as "bands" or "wetness." With time, abnormalities of touch, vibration, and position sense appear. Lhermitte's sign, which consists of tingling or an "electric shock" running down the spine after brisk dorsiflection of the head or neck, is often present. This symptom is *not* diagnostic of multiple sclerosis and may occur in a number of spinal cord diseases (e.g., arachnoiditis, tumors, and subacute combined degeneration), some of which are specifically treatable.

Involvement of the optic nerve tracts or chiasma is frequent and leads to retrobulbar neuritis with blurring of vision or loss of sight. This is often transitory, lasting a few hours to several weeks and disappearing as abruptly as it appeared, only to reappear at a later date. Congestion of the optic discs may eventually be observed and lead to nerve head pallor. Brain stem signs encountered often are those referable to one or more of the cranial nerve nuclei (diplopia, oculomotor paralysis, trigeminal type pain, facial weakness, and vertigo are common).

Clinical Course. Although this may be rapidly progressive and culminate in death within a relatively short time, multiple sclerosis is classically a subacute or chronic disease spanning a period of years. At least one fourth of patients recover from the initial

* According to estimates by the National Multiple Sclerosis Society, there are about 250,000 active cases in the United States alone.

neurological episode and suffer a relapse within 1 year. Three fourths relapse within 5 years. Despite the trend of relapses to occur more often and remit less completely with passage of time, the average duration of life from onset is of the order of 20 to 25 years.

Cerebrospinal Fluid Abnormalities. In about one third of patients, the cerebrospinal fluid contains an abnormal number of cells (6 to 70 per mm^3), predominantly lymphocytes of the small variety. Although polymorphonuclear cells are rare, the author has seen them in two cases of multiple sclerosis with acute onset.

An increase in spinal fluid γ-globulin of more than 14 percent of the total protein, as determined by immunochemical means, is found in up to 80 percent or even more of patients [37]. The increase in γ-globulin does not necessarily accompany an increase of globulin in the peripheral blood, a point which prompted Kabat *et al.* [37] to suggest that the spinal fluid γ-globulin level may arise, at least in part, from synthesis of the protein within the central nervous system. The apparent lack of any great hindrance to rapid movement of relatively small molecular weight protein from the spinal fluid into the blood [38], in contrast to the well known "barrier" restricting passage in the opposite direction, further supports this view. Perhaps the focal meningeal infiltrates of lymphocytes and plasma cells which may be found in cases of multiple sclerosis provide an explanation not only for increased numbers of cells but for the increased γ-globulin in the spinal fluid. Important is the question whether the γ-globulin is antibody and, if antibody, whether it is directed against constituents of nervous tissue. Field and Ridley [39] obtained indirect evidence that the bulk of the γ-globulin in spinal fluid is probably not antibrain antibody, but their study does not exclude a small fraction of the total γ-globulin being immunologically configured and directed against nervous tissue. These questions need further study because they have direct bearing on matters of pathogenesis.

Pathological Features. The characteristic finding in multiple sclerosis is multiple, sharply defined, grayish plaques which may range up to several centimeters in size [34, 35, 40]. These are the "islands of hardness" (sclérose en îles) noted by Cruveilhier more than a century ago. Although these plaques may occur anywhere in the central neuraxis, they tend to arise around the ventricular system (close to the ependymal lining), within the subcortical white matter and cerebellum, and within the cervical and lumbar portions of the spinal cord. They do not occur in the peripheral nervous system (nerves and spinal ganglia).* Insufficiently stressed is the occurrence of small and presumably recent plaques alongside or around small veins or venules. With larger plaques, which may well form by fusion of small ones, this relationship to blood vessels is difficult or impossible to appreciate. Microglial cells, lymphocytes, and perhaps some plasma cells may accumulate around vessels in the vicinity of active plaques, but perivascular inflammation is in no sense a major feature of multiple sclerosis. This is in contrast to the other demyelinating diseases under discussion in this chapter. Microscopically, the plaques consist of disintegrating or destroyed myelin and gliosis. Only in about 10 percent of cases can appreciable axon damage be found. The plaque spreads across as well as down the axis of nerve fibers and always outward or centrifugally with a fairly sharp advancing peripheral border. Astrocytes in the vicinity of plaques become enlarged, proliferate, and put out fibrillary processes or glial fibers. These account for the firmness of the plaque.

Oligodendrocytes and myelin synthesis. A feature of potentially great importance is the relative lack of oligodendrocytes within the plaques, especially those of any size. These cells become less and less numerous toward the peripheral portions of the plaques and virtually disappear at the edge. McAlpine *et al.* [35] consider the striking disappearance of oligodendroglia to be a key finding because of the evidence that these cells may have a definite role in myelin synthesis. There are two ramifications to this view. First, it will be important to learn whether the cytotoxic factors in sera of multiple sclerosis patients described by Bornstein [17] and Berg and Källén [18] are directed specifically against oligodendroglia. If these cells are indeed in-

* The virtual absence of peripheral nerve and spinal ganglion lesions speaks against multiple sclerosis's having an immune basis like that postulated for AE in view of the known sharing of antigenic constituents by the peripheral and central nervous systems (see earlier discussion of rabies vaccine-induced ADE, clinical aspects).

jured by cytotoxic antibody, a readily available mechanism exists to account for subsequent demyelination. Second, if myelin synthesis is dependent on cell function, then demyelination becomes a reflection of cellular disease rather than some injury affecting myelin per se. This line of thinking is important in considering viral agents as etiological agents in multiple sclerosis. Since viral agents are obligate intracellular parasites, they would not be likely to infect and damage myelin fibers directly. But they could well parasitize oligodendrocytes, and by injuring these cells or others shown to be important in myelin synthesis, they ultimately could lead to a demyelinating disease such as multiple sclerosis.

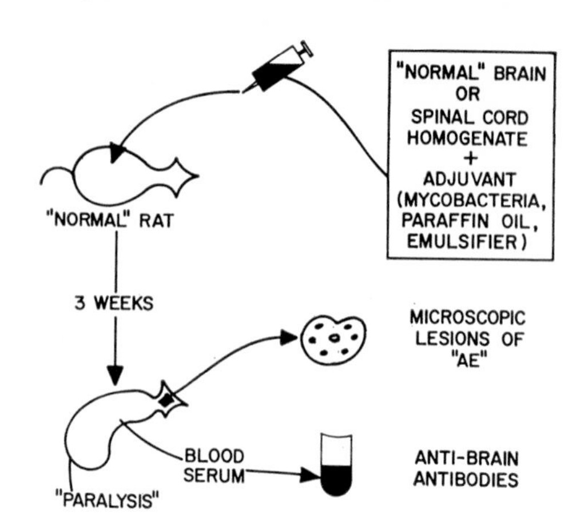

Fig. 71-2. Induction of allergic encephalomyelitis (AE) in the rat.

PATHOGENESIS OF THE DEMYELINATING DISEASES

HYPERSENSITIVITY TO NERVOUS TISSUE

The generally held view at present is that immunological forces are in some way implicated in the pathogenesis of the demyelinating diseases. The hard-core evidence for this view was presented earlier and here will be dealt with in detail. The cornerstone of evidence is the fact that injections of nervous tissue into man or animals may induce an acute encephalomyelitis characterized by perivascular demyelination and associated with circulating antibrain antibodies [41]. The recent finding of serum factors directed against myelin and glial cells in the sera of patients with multiple sclerosis has given additional support to the belief that immunological factors might induce demyelinating disease. It should be emphasized, however, that the *in vitro* demonstration of antibody cannot be equated to what may occur in an intact animal or intact nervous system. And a more pressing problem is whether any of the antibodies uncovered so far have a role in initiating neurological disease or merely represent parallel and unrelated immunological responses.

Experimental Allergic Encephalomyelitis (AE)

Induction of AE. For purposes of reference, the method used in our laboratory for induction and study of AE is shown schematically in Figure 71-2. Brain or spinal cord homogenate and complete Freund's adjuvant are mixed to form the emulsion for sensitization. This emulsion is usually injected intracutaneously (in one or several sites) into a suitable laboratory animal. Clinically, AE is recognized by the appearance of hindleg paralysis (or other neurological signs) two to three weeks after sensitization. Microscopic examination of the brain and spinal cord of the sensitized animals usually reveals the disseminated focal lesions identifying AE. Some animals develop peripheral nerve lesions. Blood serum collected at this time or later may contain antibrain antibodies which fix complement *in vitro.*

The characteristic tissue damage of AE is highly organ-specific, being confined to the nervous system and being induced regularly only by nervous tissue. Either heterologous or homologous brain or spinal cord plus adjuvant induces the disease. It is of great interest that an animal's own (autologous) brain is capable of inducing AE [42]. In addition, animals given injections of heterologous nervous tissue produce complement-fixing (CF) antibrain antibodies that react with their own brain [43]. These observations imply that the components responsible for AE exist as antigenic constituents within intact, living nervous tissue.

Identifying Pathological Features. The identifying pathological feature of AE is an acute vasculitis accompanied by variable perivascular myelin damage [41]. The individual lesions most often involve small veins or venules. Although they are scattered throughout the neuraxis, they have a propensity for arising near the ventricular system (often just beneath the ependymal lining or within the choroid plexus), in the subcortical white matter, and in the pons and long tracts of the spinal cord. Inflammatory cells accumulate within the vessel wall and just beyond, in the so-called perivascular space. In extremely acute-appearing and early lesions of AE, the infiltrating cells may be mostly polymorphonuclear, and conspicuous hemorrhagic and necrotic changes may involve the vessel wall and surrounding nervous tissue parenchyma. Such lesions are most apt to be seen in the monkey, dog, and cat. More commonly, the cellular infiltrate is mononuclear, being comprised of lymphocytes, histiocytes, and, with time, some plasma cells. Comparable cellular infiltrates may often be found in the meninges, similarily oriented around vessels. Whether these infiltrates are focal or diffuse and contain many or few polymorphonuclear cells appears to be a reflection of the tempo or rate of progression of AE in individual animals. The meningeal inflammation readily accounts for spinal fluid changes (pleocytosis and increased protein) similar to those already described for acute hemorrhagic encephalopathy, ADE and multiple sclerosis. Depending on the species of animal and the time after onset of clinical signs of AE, demyelination of variable intensity will be found in intimate association with the focal vasculitis. All evidence indicates that the demyelination follows or lags behind the vasculitis, thereby suggesting that the myelin damage is secondary in nature. Although perivascular demyelination may be striking due to coalescence of several small focal areas and although astrocytic activity may result in formation of numerous glial fibers, the plaque lesions of MS do not occur.

Comparisons with the Demyelinating Diseases. Many comparisons have been made of AE and the demyelinating diseases of man [1, 4, 28]. Almost certainly, the ADE associated with injections of killed rabies vaccine and AE are identical diseases, both induced by deliberate injections of nervous tissue. If sufficient attention is devoted to the particular species of animal used to study AE, the time elapsing between sensitization to nervous tissue and pathological examination and the tempo at which AE tends to progress in a given sensitized animal, extraordinary parallels may be found between the pathological changes of AE and those characterizing acute hemorrhagic encephalopathy, ADE and subacute multiple sclerosis. Wolf [44] published a beautifully illustrated review of these morphological similarities.

There are clinical similarities as well as these morphological ones. In most animals, AE is a monophasic, often transitory type of disease. If animals survive the acute episode, they usually show sustained and complete recovery. In the monkey, and perhaps the dog and cat, AE may follow a remitting clinical course, with striking remissions and exacerbations [41]. Such a course may resemble multiple sclerosis in several respects. However, these animals tend to be exceptions, and from a pathological standpoint it is clear that a crisp distinction exists between the two diseases. The most conspicuous difference is the lack of demonstrable plaques of demyelination of the kind characterizing multiple sclerosis in the nervous system of animals with AE. This may be explained by the relatively short-term observations made of animals with AE, in contrast to the many years which may be required for plaque formation. It is noteworthy, however, that although a few monkeys with AE observed for about two years had a patchy gliosis, plaques of myelin damage were conspicuously absent [45].

AE as an Immunological Disease. The evidence that AE has an immunological mechanism is compelling. There is the usual or required latent period between injection of nervous tissue (the antigen) and development of the disseminated encephalomyelitis. Specific antibodies which fix complement with nervous tissue extracts may be demonstrated in the sera of a high proportion of sensitized animals [41, 46]. Whole body x-radiation inhibits CF antibrain antibody production and suppresses or prevents AE in rats [47]. A single injection of a relatively large amount of nervous tissue homogenate into neonatal rats induces immunological unresponsiveness or tolerance in the sense that the majority of such rats fail to develop AE when challenged some eight to ten weeks later with standard spinal cord-adjuvant emulsion [48]. It has been reported that rabbits exhibit cutaneous hypersensitivity to nervous tissue of the tuberculin type and that such cutaneous reactivity may be related to development of AE [12, 49, 50]. Freund's adjuvant, known to enhance immune responses of both the immediate and delayed type to a variety of antigens, exerts a striking potentiating effect on induction of AE. This potentiating effect appears to reside in the mineral oil rather than the killed mycobacteria, at least as far as production of AE in the rat is concerned [51, 52]. It is clear that lymph nodes draining the sensitization sites produce the factor causing AE. Early extirpation of the nodes or their exposure to x-radiation suppresses or completely prevents AE [26]. Finally, the disease has been transferred in rats with living lymph node cells derived from donors sensitized to nervous tissue [53–56]. More recently, lymph node cell transfers have also been reported, using rabbits and guinea pigs [57, 58].

The Nervous Tissue Antigens. A major problem is the nervous tissue constituents against which the immune responses causing AE are directed. Their nature and their location within nervous tissue remain virtually undefined [41]. There is a wide feeling that they are natural or normal constituents of brain and spinal cord. There have been claims over the years that the antigen is a proteolipid, a glycoprotein, a protein, or a lipid. This diversity of claims suggests that the antigen awaits precise identification. Although it is generally accepted that myelin contains the antigenic activity associated with nervous tissue, there is no compelling or final evidence for this point.

Too little attention has been paid to the possibility that the antigenic determinants in question are not normal constituents in the usual sense but, rather, are associated with intact viral particles or microbial fragments of one kind or another. Although there is no evidence to support such a view, it should be stressed that there is none to exclude it. It would therefore seem wise for any thesis concerning the pathogenesis of AE and the demyelinating diseases of man to include the possibility that infectious agents may play a role.

Nature of the Immune Response Responsible for AE. (*a*) *Delayed type hypersensitivity to brain.* Another problem, and one equally unsettled, is the nature of the immune mechanism responsible for AE. One school of thought views AE as resulting from a direct interaction between antigenic constituents in nervous tissue and living lymphoid cells. It is postulated that the lymphoid cells carry a stereospecific configuration on their surface of the kind responsible for the delayed or tuberculin type allergy [59]. Data often cited as favoring "sensitized" cells as immune agents are: the histological changes of AE, which resemble those associated with delayed type reactions; the demonstration of delayed type cutaneous hypersensitivity to brain in sensitized animals; and the transfer of AE with lymph node cells as used for transferring tuberculin hypersensitivity within guinea pigs. According to this view, conventional antibodies play no role in the disease and represent irrelevant responses to nervous tissue sensitization.

Another view, shared by the writer, is that the precise mechanism of AE is still unknown and that, in continued attempts to define it, attention must be given not only to cellular factors but to conventional circulating antibodies [55, 60].

(*b*) *Role of serum antibody in AE.* Evidence favoring AE as an antibody-mediated disease can be found at both the histological and the immunological level. For example, in some lesions of AE there can be found considerable numbers of plasma cells. In others, such changes as necrosis, heavy infiltration by polymorphonuclear cells, and even hemorrhage may be observed. These changes speak for an Arthus type of immune reaction more than they do for one of the tuberculin or delayed type. The direct relationship between dose of whole body x-radiation and suppression of both AE and CF antibrain antibody production in the rat is suggestive of an antibody-mediated condition [47]. In our study of transfer of AE with lymph node cells in rats [53, 54], it was stressed that while the data provided direct evidence that AE has an immune mechanism, the transfer of the disease with cells did not clarify whether antibody or sensitized cells represented the immune response or agents responsible for causing the disease. It was impossible to determine whether the lesions of AE in the recipients resulted from antibody produced by the cells after their transfer or resulted from an interaction between the brain of the recipients and the transferred cells themselves.

Until recently, the only serum antibrain antibodies demonstrable were those which fixed complement *in vitro* with brain extracts. Detailed study of these CF antibrain antibodies several years ago revealed no direct relationship between their presence or titer and occurrence or severity of AE in individual sensitized animals [46]. In later work, these antibodies appeared to be directed against antigens other than those responsible for causing AE [61]. Thus the available evidence has consistently indicated that the CF antibrain antibodies do not initiate the disease.

A major development has been the demonstration of cytotoxic factors directed against myelin and glial cells in the sera of animals with AE. The cytotoxic factor described by Bornstein and Appel [14] appears to have the properties of antibody and to be directed against antigenic determinants which reside in both myelin and glial cells. Its presence appears to be related to development of AE in individual sensitized rabbits. The serum and leukocyte factors reported by Koprowski and Fernandes [15] and by Berg and Källén [16] to be cytotoxic for glial cells are perhaps antibodies, but the point is not clear. Whether they are similar or identical to the serum factor described by Bornstein [14, 17] is not known. It should be noted that the cytotoxic factors reported by all three groups of investigators had eluded detection for years. It was only after use of a tissue culture system containing "targets" (myelin and glial cells) that presence of such factors was readily uncovered.

An important question is whether cytotoxic antibody plays a role in the transfer of AE in rats. To answer this question, Dr. Bornstein's laboratory and ours joined forces. Lymph node cell transfers were carried out in rats, using the techniques we had previously described. The recipients were killed six or nine days after cell transfer and their brains and spinal cords were examined microscopically for lesions of AE. Sera were obtained from the recipients when they were killed, and these sera were assayed for cytotoxic antibody by Dr. Bornstein's laboratory. So far, in two preliminary experiments, only those recipients with cytotoxic antibody in their sera when killed have been found to have lesions of AE [60]. These data indicate that sensitized rat lymph node cells represent at least one site for production of cytotoxic antibody. The parallel occurrence of AE lesions and cytotoxic antibody in the rat-transfer model constitutes the strongest evidence obtained so far that cytotoxic antibody may play a direct role in causing AE rather than represent a parallel and unrelated event.

Another question which arose was whether cytotoxic antibody could be shown to be distinct from the CF antibodies known to appear in animals with AE but have little to do with initiation of the disease. This question was answered by the following means. Dr. Bornstein's laboratory provided us with rabbit immune sera which had previously been assayed for cytotoxic activity in the rat brain culture system. We assayed the sera for their content of CF antibrain antibodies against rat brain, using a precise, quantitative technique. The results, based on 15 sera so assayed, were clear-cut and showed that cytotoxic antibody and CF antibody represent independent immunological responses to nervous tissue [62]. For example, some rabbit sera had exerted a striking demyelinating effect on rat brain cultures but had no demonstrable CF antibody in the presence of either rat or rabbit brain extracts used as sources of antigen. Other sera which contained high-titer CF antibody were devoid of cytotoxic activity.

The strongest argument against cytotoxic antibody or any serum factor causing AE and, by implication, being of importance in demyelinating diseases of man, is the failure so far to transfer AE passively by injections of serum into recipients. Transfer of AE with living lymph node cells, in contrast to serum, may hold a definite advantage in that the transferred cells contain the machinery for continued synthesis of the factor causing the disease, e.g., cytotoxic antibody or some as yet undetected factor. With continued synthesis and release of the factor, higher blood levels are achieved and greater penetration of the antibody into the nervous system is assured. Alternatively, the transferred lymphoid cells may cross the blood-brain-barrier of the recipient by an active process, in contrast to diffusion of antibody by a passive one. By coming directly into contact with glial cells and myelin fibers, even minute amounts of cytotoxic antibody on the surface of cells or released into the immediate vicinity would be able to cause appreciable damage. Although these statements may be valid and serve to emphasize technical difficulties, they do not minimize the hard fact that the disease, AE, has not yet been transferred with any serum. This is a conspicuous break in the chain of evidence used to support the role of a humoral immune factor.

CF Antibrain Antibodies as a Protective Response. The question might be raised, if a case is made for cytotoxic antibody, what role may be assigned to the CF antibrain antibodies known to appear in animals sensitized to nervous tissue? Evidence that these CF antibodies in all probability do not cause AE has already been cited. Recent work in our laboratory has suggested that the CF antibrain antibodies may have a protective function or role. Briefly, some of the observations leading to this impression were as follows. In earlier studies [46], AE tended to occur more often in dogs *without* CF antibody. Dogs with high-titer CF antibody tended to have mild disease or more often remained well. In guinea pigs, a fulminating, usually lethal form of AE developed, and CF antibodies could rarely be detected. More recently, rats were found to develop a mild and transitory form of AE and usually appear clinically well four to six weeks after initial sensitization to spinal cord plus adjuvant [63]; during the recovery period, CF antibrain antibodies were most apt to be found [64].

Finally, repeated injections of pooled rat immune serum containing CF antibrain antibody conferred protection against AE upon rats actively sensitized to nervous tissue-adjuvant and otherwise destined to develop the disease [63]. Clinical signs of AE were rare among the serum-treated rats, and the lesions of AE that did occur were often mild and sparse. Up to one half of the serum-treated animals failed to show either clinical or pathological evidence of AE. Serum pools containing CF antibrain antibody consistently transferred protection, although the degree of protection was not always related to the level of CF antibody in the serum pool employed for treatment. Pools devoid of CF antibody gave no protection. Although the evidence is consistent with the concept that the CF antibodies account for the serum protective effect, it should be emphasized that the only antibodies detectable by current methods in our laboratory are the CF antibodies, and they may merely parallel the protective effect of immune serum rather than be responsible for it.

Although the protective effect of immune serum is clear cut, its mechanism is not. It is conceivable that passively administered CF antibrain antibody may protect by suppressing active production of another immune response causing AE, e.g., cytotoxic antibody. It is also possible that the CF antibodies act as "blocking antibodies." By harmlessly combining with antigenic sites in the brain and spinal cord of the serum-treated and actively sensitized rat, they may "block" or prevent sensitized cells or cytotoxic antibody from interacting with these sites. The fact that serum containing high-titer CF antibrain antibody may exert no cytotoxic effect on brain cultures [62] is consistent with this hypothesis.* How soon CF antibody is produced after exposure to brain antigen, especially in relation to appearance of other immune responses, may be a factor influencing whether AE will or will not occur. For example, CF antibody produced early (i.e., within a few days) after brain sensitization might exert an effect comparable to that of passively administered CF antibody, viz., protection against AE. Relatively late production of the antibody or complete failure of its production might facilitate production of AE and increase its severity. Support for both possibilities has been found in current studies in our laboratory in rats of different lines, including one that appears to lack the capacity for CF antibrain antibody production after years of inbreeding.

Immunological Responses in Demyelinating Diseases of Man

Cutaneous Reactivity to Nervous Tissue. There are relatively few studies of this point. One reason probably lies in the lack of available defined antigenic preparations for skin testing. With the relatively crude preparations now at hand, it might well be hazardous to proceed with extensive skin testing programs. The intracutaneous route is noted as a highly effective route for sensitization. An intracutaneous injection of even minute amounts of

* An important experiment yet to be carried out consists of exposing brain cultures for several hours to serum containing CF antibrain antibody and then exposing the cultures to serum known to contain cytotoxic activity. Prevention of the usual cytotoxic effects by prior exposure to serum containing CF antibody would be directly in line with the postulated "blocking action" of the CF antibodies.

Editor's comment: Two major uncertainties limit our ability to interpret the meaning of the CF data. (1) We do not know whether one or more nervous tissue antigens are detected by the CF test. (2) We do not know whether the CF antigen(s) is on the surface or within the nervous tissue cells. If the latter, the antigen would not be available to react with the CF antibody. Experiments such as that proposed by Dr. Paterson may help decide this latter. These experiments are, however, no substitute for the ultimate need to identify chemically and localize precisely the tissue antigen(s) involved. It can reasonably be assumed, from what is revealed in Dr. Paterson's text, that the findings on the nature of the antigen(s) in AE will be directly useful in exploring ADE and multiple sclerosis in man.—J. H. V.

nervous tissue extracts or fractions could lead to active sensitization to paralytogenic antigens with consequent risk of induction of acute encephalomyelitis equivalent to AE induced in animals.

In several reported studies [65–67], multiple sclerosis patients were given skin tests with nervous tissue homogenates or proteolipid fractions prepared therefrom. Cutaneous reactions to these materials were either absent or no greater than those found in similarly tested control patients. With the full realization that the test reagents used may not have been optimal, it is important to note that so far delayed hypersensitivity to nervous tissue has not been shown to exist in association with the demyelinating diseases.

Cytotoxic Antibrain Antibodies in Multiple Sclerosis. Bornstein [17] demonstrated a cytotoxic factor in the serum of patients with multiple sclerosis, but the factor is not present in the serum of all patients with the disease and is virtually absent from serum of healthy individuals and patients with other forms of neurological disease. Serum from one patient with postinfectious ADE was found to be cytotoxic, whereas that from another patient during the recovery period was devoid of any myelinotoxic effect.

The cytotoxic serum factor appears to be an antibody which is specifically directed against antigenic determinants in myelin and glial cells. If the antibody can be shown to react with oligodendroglial cells, some of the myelin dissolution seen in the brain cultures may be a secondary effect, since these cells are believed to be important in the synthesis of myelin. This sequence of events would agree with the striking absence of oligodendroglia in the peripheral and advancing edges of the plaque lesions of multiple sclerosis. It is of considerable interest that the cytotoxic antibody can be washed away after causing destruction of myelin in culture, and remyelination is then demonstrable within several days [17]. This finding illustrates the reality of myelin resynthesis and may have meaning in terms of the characteristic relapsing and remitting course of multiple sclerosis.

Cytotoxic factors in multiple sclerosis, in ADE of the postinfectious type, and in animals with AE are as yet indistinguishable. Although it is not yet established that the two cytotoxic activities described in serum from patients with multiple sclerosis by Bornstein [17] and Berg and Källén [18] are identical, it seems clear that there are immunological responses common to demyelinating disease of man and AE of animals which suggest potential pathogenic interrelationships. As already stated, the major question to be answered is whether any of the serum factors have a primary role in causing disease.

CF Antibrain Antibodies in Demyelinating Disease. (*a*) *In multiple sclerosis.* Before the introduction of tissue culture techniques led to the finding of cytotoxic antibodies, several laboratories had searched for conventional CF antibrain antibodies in the sera of patients with multiple sclerosis. Sachs and Steiner [68] and Raskin [69] reported a high incidence of CF antibody in the sera of such patients. The specificity of the serological reactions reported is questionable, and it is noteworthy that a high proportion of the controls were found to have CF antibrain antibody. In contrast to these reports are others [25, 65, 66, 70–73] that contain sufficient details to allow critical evaluation. Without exception, these studies indicate that circulating CF antibrain antibodies either do not occur at all in multiple sclerosis or occur no more often than in control patients.

(*b*) *In ADE induced by rabies vaccine.* In view of the experimental studies establishing the antigenicity of mammalian nervous tissue, it is not surprising that patients receiving injections of rabies vaccine prepared from rabbit brain or spinal cord produce CF antibrain antibody identical to that found in the sera of animals with AE. As in the case for the CF antibodies in AE, these antibodies are organ-specific but not species-specific. Thus, although produced in response to injection of rabies vaccine prepared from rabbit or guinea pig brain, the CF antibrain antibodies react with these and other species of mammalian brain extracts, including human brain.

A careful study of CF antibrain antibody production following administration of rabies vaccine was carried out several years ago by Koprowski and LeBell [74]. They found that none of 16 patients receiving 7 injections or less of vaccine (of the killed or Semple type prepared from rabbit tissue) produced CF antibody. In contrast, among 34 patients receiving a full course of 14 injections of vaccine, CF antibrain antibodies could be demonstrated in 17. Once present, the antibodies persisted for as long as 227 days. Thus the occurrence of CF antibody appears to be directly related to the antigenic mass of vaccine (nervous tissue) injected. These findings parallel those of Appelbaum *et al.* [75] showing that the rate of occurrence of ADE after rabies vaccination is fivefold greater in patients receiving a full course of 14 injections than in those receiving a shorter course of 7 injections or less. With these facts, it is not a surprise that presence of CF antibrain antibodies is associated with the occurrence of ADE induced by rabies vaccine. In each of the 3 cases of AE studied by Koprowski and LeBell [74] and in the 1 case reported by Kirk and Ecker [76], CF antibrain antibodies were present in high titer.

Although studies such as these might imply that the CF antibrain antibodies bear a causal relationship to the development of ADE, all evidence is to the contrary. The overwhelming majority of patients who do develop CF antibody after injections of rabies vaccine, as do animals in the AE model, do not develop clinically apparent ADE [74]. Thus the question is again raised whether the CF antibrain antibodies may have a protective function. It becomes crucial to know how soon after the start of a course of rabies vaccine the CF antibrain antibodies appear. If the antibodies are protective, appreciable delay in their production in certain patients might favor development of ADE.

"Multiple Sclerosis" Induced by Rabies Vaccine. In 1957, Shiraki *et al.* [4, 5] reported some remarkable observations on reactions to various types of rabies vaccine among the Japanese. A high proportion were observed to develop what was termed "a cerebral form" of disseminated encephalomyelitis. This form obviously deserved to be singled out for special consideration because it differed in several respects from the predominantly spinal form so well known elsewhere. It had a latent period of usually 35 to 56 days after initial injection of rabies vaccine, with periods as long as 80 to 100 days being noted in some instances. Conspicuous clinical features included a high incidence of visual field defects, pupillary and cranial nerve abnormalities, ataxia, lack of cremasteric and abdominal reflexes, and mental changes. Although the cerebral form in many patients followed a course lasting about 2 weeks, in some patients signs of active disease persisted over a span of 41 to 131 days. The mortality rate was about 20 percent. Many of the surviving patients failed to recover completely and showed residual neurological and personality defects. Most arresting were the histological changes associated with the cerebral form, because in their distribution and morphological details they bore a striking similarity to the lesions of multiple sclerosis.

There was considerable debate about the meaning of the data reported by Shiraki and co-workers. Some intimated that he had inadvertently included patients with multiple sclerosis who, because they had received injections of rabies vaccine, suffered clinical relapses. The very fact that this question was seriously considered indicates how much the lesions described by Shiraki resembled those considered characteristic of multiple sclerosis. The high incidence of encephalomyelitis in general and occurrence of the cerebral form in particular were puzzling but accepted as evidence that Japanese react differently to rabies vaccine. Despite these problems in interpretation, Shiraki's findings were generally believed to constitute major evidence of a close interrelationship of AE, ADE (induced by rabies vaccine), and multiple sclerosis. The feeling grew that these three entities could now be considered a trilogy, with sensitivity to nervous tissue being the basic theme.

TABLE 71-1. Occurrence Rate and Clinical Forms of ADE Following Use of Live or Killed Rabies Vaccine[a]

Rabies Vaccine Employed[b]			No. of Individuals Vaccinated	No. of Individuals with ADE		Occurrence Rate of ADE (per 1,000)
Type	Total Dose (mg.)	Route		Spinal Form	Cerebral Form	
Live	80–120	Subcut.	6,367	17	19	5.7
Killed	70–100	Subcut.	970	2	1	3.0
Killed	5–10	Intracut.	3,869	3	0	0.8

[a] Data reported by Shiraki *et al.* [4, 77].

[b] Killed vaccine injected subcutaneously had been inactivated by ultraviolet light only, whereas that injected intracutaneously had been treated with ultraviolet, formol or merthiolate. Figures for total dose are those given by the authors and represent milligrams of dry nervous tissue per vaccination course.

Data from papers by Shiraki *et al.* [4, 77] are presented in Table 71-1. Factors to keep in mind in interpreting these data are type of vaccine, total dose of vaccine (nervous tissue) injected, and the route of injection. The highest paralytic rate observed was 5.7 per 1,000 and is accounted for in large part by occurrence of the cerebral form (a rate of 3.0 per 1,000 being observed for this form of encephalomyelitis by itself). These high rates were directly associated with the use of live, attenuated rabies vaccine. Use of inactivated or killed vaccines in comparable doses resulted in a marked reduction in the paralytic rate due to virtual disappearance of the cerebral form. The single instance of the cerebral form associated with killed vaccine may be due to use of one minute of ultraviolet light for "killing" the virus, raising some question as to whether the vaccine was, in fact, totally inactivated. The lowest paralytic rate was observed with killed vaccine used in the smallest dose, in agreement with findings of others that a direct relationship exists between total dose of vaccine and incidence of ADE.

It is clear that occurrence of the cerebral form of ADE reported by Shiraki was intimately associated with injection of rabies vaccine containing attenuated rabies virus. It seems likely that living rabies virus was of major importance in its pathogenesis. A major objection to this conclusion is the apparent lack of the cerebral form in other parts of the world despite use of the same type of vaccine on a wide scale until about 1930, when it was replaced by killed vaccine of the Semple type. The attenuated strain used in Japan may have been less attenuated than those used elsewhere. Data concerning rabbit or mouse infectivity assays are not available in order to answer this question. However, another explanation can be offered, based on the method of injecting attenuated rabies vaccine. In Japan, the numerous injections are given in the interscapular region, whereas elsewhere they are given usually in the periumbilical region. This difference in injection sites may be important. Clinical manifestations of neurotropic virus infections may be influenced by specific sites of trauma or injections. The increased incidence of bulbar poliomyelitis associated with tonsillectomy and the increased incidence of paralytic poliomyelitis in an extremity previously inoculated for one reason or another (the "provoking effect") are familiar examples [78, 79]. Trueta [80] showed that injection of an irritant into an extremity decreases the blood-brain-barrier in that portion of the neuraxis corresponding to the dermatome in question. The implication is that an injection may lead to a local decrease in the vascular barrier and by so doing facilitate passage of a neurotropic agent such as poliomyelitis virus into a select portion of the neuraxis during the time the virus circulates in the blood. It is conceivable that injection of living rabies vaccine into the interscapular region in some fashion facilitates passage of attenuated rabies virus into the cerebrum, for which it has greater affinity than the spinal cord.

Whatever the explanation may be for occurrence of the "multiple sclerosis-like" form of ADE in Japan, the facts are that it is intimately associated with injection of living, attenuated rabies virus. Moreover, if it is accepted that the lesions observed closely simulate those of multiple sclerosis, compelling reasons exist for leaving open the possibility that a viral agent may be implicated in the pathogenesis of demyelinating diseases. In this regard, the claim by Russian investigators that a virus antigenically related to rabies may be isolated from brain tissues of patients with disseminated encephalomyelitis has relevance.

MICROBIAL AGENTS AND THE ROLE OF INFECTION

For many decades, infectious agents have received attention as possible etiological factors in demyelinating diseases. The intimate association between ADE and certain viral diseases (e.g., measles, chickenpox) has pointed in this direction. Moreover, the immunological and morphological relationships between ADE and multiple sclerosis have prompted a continuing search for a viral agent in the latter disease.

Bacteria and Spirochetes

Classic bacteria have been virtually excluded, at least in their usual form. The existence of bacteria as spheroplasts or protoplasts without cell walls is another matter and one that has received virtually no attention. The recent results of search for protoplasts in renal disease demonstrate how productive this approach can be [81]. For a long time, structures resembling spirochetes have been periodically reported to be present in the spinal fluid and brain tissue of patients with multiple sclerosis. Steiner [82] has been the most enthusiastic long-term proponent of the spirochetal etiology and has attempted to build a case for *Spirochaeta myelophthora* as the responsible agent. Ichelson [83] has more recently reported isolation of spirochetes from spinal fluids of a fairly high proportion of patients with multiple sclerosis. This work has not been confirmed in other laboratories, and it is disturbing that a later report by Ichelson's group [84] states that viable spirochetes may be found in the spinal fluid of control patients as well as of those with demyelinating disease. At present, whatever spirochetes have to do with demyelinating diseases, if anything, is no more settled than it was in the early 1900's.

Viruses

Viral Agents in ADE. The most likely place to look for a virus would be in the fatal cases of ADE following smallpox vaccination or associated with measles or chickenpox. Attempts to isolate the virus in question have usually proved unsuccessful. It may be argued that sensitive tissue culture methods essential for detection of relatively small amounts of measles and chickenpox viruses have been available only recently and that this may account, at least in part, for the general inability to isolate these viruses in the past.* This argument does not hold for smallpox virus, since this virus may be grown in embryonated eggs or the skin of a rabbit with relative ease. Although Turnbull and McIntosh [29] were able to isolate vaccinia virus from the brain of some patients with fatal ADE following smallpox vaccination, attempts by other workers during subsequent decades more often than not were unsuccessful. The relative lack of success in isolating these viruses may be related to the fact that antiviral neutralizing antibody occurs in the serum at about the time the characteristic exanthema indicates presence of the viral diseases in question. Presence of neutralizing antibody and other antiviral responses (including interferon production) may adequately explain the absence of virus a few days later when ADE appears, or later when death occurs. Whatever further might be said, there is no convincing evidence that these viruses directly cause ADE.

The "Multiple Sclerosis Virus." In 1946, Margulis *et al.* [85] reported isolation of a neurotropic virus in laboratory animals from the blood and cerebral tissue of 2 patients with ADE and a remitting type of disease suggestive of multiple sclerosis, respectively. Both strains of virus were neutralized by sera from a high proportion of patients with either acute encephalitis or chronic multiple sclerosis. The neutralizing activity was believed to be due to specific antibody. The implications of this study were clear. Little more was heard until 1958, when Dick *et al.* [86] reported their studies with the SV strain of neurotropic virus supplied by the Russian investigators. In confirmation of the Russian claim, the virus was found to have all the properties of rabies virus. This point is of particular interest since it was suggested earlier (see earlier discussion of rabies-vaccine ADE) that rabies virus may be implicated in the production of disease resembling subacute multiple sclerosis in patients receiving live, attenuated rabies vaccine. But Dick *et al.* [86] found that sera from 50 patients with multiple sclerosis gave no consistent, convincing neutralization of the SV strain of virus. Whereas a few of the sera neutralized up to 1 log of virus when first tested, this weak neutralizing activity disappeared after mild heating (inactivation) of the sera. To this writer's knowledge, no further published accounts are available concerning the Russian virus and its relationship to demyelinating disease.

The Continuing Search for Viruses. The foregoing stands as a marked exception to the otherwise unsuccessful attempts of a large number of investigators to obtain any evidence that multiple sclerosis has a viral etiology. A variety of techniques have been employed. For example, Lumsden [87] tried to "unmask" a virus by maintaining freshly collected multiple sclerosis plaque-lesions in tissue culture and searching for cytopathogenic effects in the explanted cells emerging from the edges of the plaques. This technique, it may be recalled, proved highly successful in "unmasking" adenoviruses in tonsillar and adenoid tissues by investigators in the field of respiratory diseases a decade ago.

* The old report of isolation in monkeys of rubeola virus from brain tissue of a fatal case of post-measles encephalomyelitis (Shaffer, M. F., Rake, G., and Hodes, H. L., *Amer. J. Dis. Child.* 64:815, 1942) suggests that paucity of fatal cases and lack of attempts to perform viral studies with material available may be more important than methodology in explaining the widespread view that virus does not exist in the neuraxis where clinical signs of ADE are manifest.

Possible Roles of Viral Agents in Demyelinating Disease

Alteration of Host Tissues. Because of their obligate intracellular existence, viruses are in an excellent position to alter host cells and render them "foreign" or potentially antigenic in terms of the immunological self-recognition system. Possibilities include formation of virus-host cell complexes, along the lines of the "self plus X" theory proposed by Lawrence [88], or abnormal products synthesized by the host cells because of the infecting virus. Support for these thoughts may be found in the early studies of Schwentker and Rivers [89]. In their attempts to produce ADE in rabbits, they found that injections of homologous brain altered by autolysis or brain infected with vaccinia virus was more antigenic than were fresh brain homogenates, as judged by production of circulating antibrain antibody.

*Persistence of Virus.** Although the ADE following acute viral infections is usually a self-limiting or monophasic type of illness, as already emphasized, there are exceptions. These exceptions have particular significance for they raise the question whether those viruses (e.g., measles virus) intimately associated with ADE may persist in host tissues and in some way be a harbinger for chronic demyelinating disease. An attempt to gather evidence bearing on this point was made by van Bogaert [3], and from the data he presented, there is a strong hint that a high proportion of patients with ADE may turn up years later with neurological disease resembling multiple sclerosis. Adams and Imagawa [90] recently examined the possibility that persistence of measles virus may be a factor in multiple sclerosis by testing serum and spinal fluid for antibodies to the virus. Multiple sclerosis sera had only slightly higher titers of antibody than did control sera. In contrast, more than 75 percent of the multiple sclerosis spinal fluids contained antibody, whereas none was found in the spinal fluids from the control group, which included other inflammatory central nervous system diseases.

At the experimental level, Herpes simplex virus is known to persist for extended periods in the brains of rabbits during adult life [91]. A striking example of long persistence (perhaps "life-long") is that of lymphocytic choriomeningitis (LCM) virus in mice immunologically tolerant of the virus because of infection with it at the time of birth or during early neonatal life (see review by Hotchin [92]). Only after the "LCM-tolerant" mice are provided with lymphoid cells from other mice which are immunologically competent and are actively making an immune response to LCM virus, do the "tolerant" mice develop neurological disease and die. From a theoretical standpoint, persistent virus may exert direct cytotoxic effects or it may be pathogenic only by way of the host's immune response to it alone or to the product of some virus-central nervous system interaction.

Two Lessons from Virology

Problem of Host Specificity. If a virus is implicated in the demyelinating diseases, it does not necessarily follow that it could be detected or cultivated in any host other than man. For example, there are yet no convincing demonstrations of growth of the hepatitis virus outside its natural host, i.e., man. As far as is known, there are no published accounts concerning transmission of multiple sclerosis in man.

The Scrapie Example. New knowledge of viruses, their properties and their behavior in their respective hosts is accumulating at a rapid rate. It seems certain that, with more information, many events which today seem inexplicable in terms of a self-replicating agent or virus will eventually be shown to have an infectious basis.

Scrapie is a disease of sheep known to occur in Great Britain and other parts of the world. It is transmissible from sheep to sheep and from sheep to goats by injection of brain extracts containing the responsible agent [93]. Two other neurological diseases of sheep which are similarly transmissible by means of brain extracts are visna and rida [94, 95]. Although rida may in fact be scrapie, visna is clearly a distinct disease. As a group, these diseases are of interest because unusual histological changes develop in the neuraxis of infected sheep. These include proliferation of

* Brill-Zinsser disease is an outstanding example. This disease was believed on epidemiological, clinical, and other grounds to be a distinct entity. It is now known that it represents a recrudescence of epidemic or louse-borne typhus. Up to 20 or more years may elapse between the original typhus infection and appearance of the recrudescence, i.e., Brill-Zinsser disease. During the intervening period, the causative agent (*Rickettsia prowazeki*) silently parasitizes its original host.

astrocytes and gliosis (scrapie) and patchy areas of demyelination (visna) in addition to neuronal degeneration and variable inflammatory changes. Of greater interest is the fact that all three diseases are caused by filtrable agents having most unusual properties. Scrapie brain extracts retain their infectivity after treatment with organic solvents, boiling, and even short periods of autoclaving. The incubation periods for all three sheep diseases are exceptionally long, ranging from seven months to two years or longer. The scrapie agent has recently been adapted to mice [96], and from study of such mice in our laboratory [97] there appears to be no direct relationship between lesions produced by the scrapie virus and the lesions of AE.

Some meager evidence has accrued to suggest a relationship between scrapie and visna and the demyelinating diseases of man. For example, Campbell *et al.* [98] reported several years ago that four of seven members of a research team in Great Britain, which during the 1930's was investigating "swayback" in sheep (a demyelinating disease in this species related to copper deficiency), developed neurological manifestations consistent with multiple sclerosis. The illness in each followed a remitting, nonfatal course. Three of the four patients had had contact with ewes and lambs or with blood, tissue, and soil samples under study in the project. It is conceivable that some of the sheep under study were latently infected with scrapie, in addition to having "swayback," and that the neurological disease among the laboratory workers was related to this viral agent.

Direct support for this thesis has been provided by the recent reports by Field *et al.* [99] and Campbell *et al.* [100] that brain tissue from two patients with disseminated sclerosis (multiple sclerosis) and subacute encephalitis, respectively, after injection into sheep produced the clinicopathological picture of scrapie. Unresolved yet is the pressing question whether the scrapie agent resided latently in the sheep before they were used for the isolation studies or whether it resided in the human brain inocula. It will be important to learn whether sera from patients with neurological diseases contain antibody directed against scrapie (or visna) agents, e.g., by means of serum neutralization experiments carried out in sheep.

TREATMENT

There is no specific therapy, and this brief discussion is included only for the sake of completeness. Although many drugs and procedures have been thought at one time or another to influence the course of multiple sclerosis favorably, the impressive length of the list in itself suggests a lack of specificity. Above all is the ever-important problem of general management [35].

There is some enthusiasm for the use of ACTH and corticosteroids in the treatment of ADE and acute, life-threatening exacerbations of multiple sclerosis. The basis for such therapy is the capacity of these hormones to suppress inflammation and some reports that they may suppress development of AE in experimental animals. Best results in AE have been obtained if these drugs are administered either at the very onset of neurological signs or, better still, at the time of nervous tissue sensitization [41]. Although some favorable results may be expected following use of ACTH or cortisone in ADE, the efficacy of these hormones in chronic progressive multiple sclerosis is debatable at best [101].

REFERENCES

1. Adams, R. D., and Kubik, C. S. The morbid anatomy of the demyelinative diseases. *Amer. J. Med.* 12:510, 1952.
2. Adams, R. D. A Comparison of the Morphology of the Human Demyelinative Diseases and Experimental "Allergic" Encephalomyelitis. In Kies, M. W., and Alvord, E. C., Jr. (Eds.), *"Allergic" Encephalomyelitis.* Springfield, Ill.: Charles C Thomas, Publisher, 1959. P. 183.
3. Van Bogaert, L. Post-infectious encephalomyelitis and multiple sclerosis: The significance of perivenous encephalomyelitis. *J. Neuropath. Exp. Neurol.* 9:219, 1950.
4. Shiraki, H., and Otani, S. Clinical and Pathological Features of Rabies Post-Vaccinal Encephalomyelitis in Man. Ref. 2, p. 58.
5. Uchimura, I., and Shiraki, H. A contribution to the classification and the pathogenesis of demyelinating encephalomyelitis. *J. Neuropath. Exp. Neurol.* 16:139, 1957.
6. Witebsky, E., and Steinfeld, J. Untersuch-

ungen über spezifische Antigen Funktionen von Organen. *Z. Immunitaetsforsch.* 58:271, 1928.
7. Lewis, J. H. The immunologic specificity of brain tissue. *J. Immun.* 24:193, 1933.
8. Rivers, T. M., Sprunt, D. H., and Berry, G. P. Observations on attempts to produce acute disseminated encephalomyelitis in monkeys. *J. Exp. Med.* 58:39, 1933.
9. Rivers, T. M., and Schwentker, F. F. Encephalomyelitis accompanied by myelin destruction experimentally produced in monkeys. *J. Exp. Med.* 61:689, 1935.
10. Morgan, I. M. Allergic encephalomyelitis in monkeys in response to injection of normal monkey nervous tissue. *J. Exp. Med.* 85:131, 1947.
11. Kabat, E. A., Wolf, A., and Bezer, A. E. The rapid production of acute disseminated encephalomyelitis in rhesus monkeys by injection of heterologous and homologous brain tissue with adjuvants. *Ibid.*, p. 117.
12. Freund, J., Stern, E. R., and Pisani, T. M. Isoallergic encephalomyelitis and radiculitis in guinea pigs after one injection of brain and mycobacteria in water-in-oil emulsion. *J. Immun.* 57:179, 1947.
13. Morrison, L. R. Disseminated encephalomyelitis experimentally produced by the use of homologous antigen. *Arch. Neurol. Psychiat.* 58:391, 1947.
14. Bornstein, M. B., and Appel, S. H. The application of tissue culture to the study of experimental "allergic" encephalomyelitis: I. Patterns of demyelination. *J. Neuropath. Exp. Neurol.* 20:141, 1961.
15. Koprowski, H., and Fernandes, M. V. Autosensitization reaction *in vitro:* Contactual agglutination of sensitized lymph node cells in brain tissue culture accompanied by destruction of glial elements. *J. Exp. Med.* 116:467, 1962.
16. Berg, O., and Källén, B. An *in vitro* gliotoxic effect of serum from animals with experimental allergic encephalomyelitis. *Acta Path. Microbiol. Scand.* 54:425, 1962.
17. Bornstein, M. B. A tissue-culture approach to demyelinative disorders. *Nat. Cancer Inst. Monogr.* 11:197, 1963.
18. Berg, O., and Källén, B. Gliotoxic effect of serum from patients with neurological diseases. *Lancet* 1:1051, 1962.
19. Hurst, E. W. Acute haemorrhagic leucoencephalitis: A previously undefined entity. *Med. J. Aust.* 2:1, 1941.
20. Adams, R. D., Cammermeyer, J., and Denny-Brown, D. Acute necrotizing hemorrhagic encephalopathy. *J. Neuropath. Exp. Neurol.* 8:1, 1949.
21. Russell, D. S. The nosological unity of acute haemorrhagic leucoencephalitis and acute disseminated encephalomyelitis. *Brain* 78:369, 1955.
22. Peck, F. B., Powell, H. M., and Culbertson, C. G. A new antirabies vaccine for human use. *J. Lab. Clin. Med.* 45:679, 1955.
23. MacFarlane, J. O., and Culbertson, C. G. Attempted production of allergic encephalomyelitis with duck embryo suspensions and vaccines. *Canad. J. Public Health* 45:28, 1954.
24. Fuerst, H. T. Central nervous system disease following duck embryo rabies vaccine injection. *Morbid. Mortal.* 11:362, 1962.
25. Kolb, L. C. The relationship of the demyelinating diseases to allergic encephalomyelitis. *Medicine* 29:99, 1950.
26. Condie, R. M., and Good, R. A. Experimental Allergic Encephalomyelitis: Its Production, Prevention, and Pathology as Studied by Light and Electron Microscopy. In Korey, S. R. (Ed.), *The Biology of Myelin.* New York: Paul B. Hoeber, Inc., 1959. P. 321.
27. Remlinger, P. Paralyses of Anti-rabies Treatment. *League of Nations International Rabies Conference.* Geneva: 1927. P. 70.
28. Stuart, G., and Krikorian, K. S. The neuroparalytic accidents of anti-rabies treatment. *Ann. Trop. Med.* 22:327, 1928.
29. Turnbull, H. M., and McIntosh, J. Encephalo-myelitis following vaccination. *Brit. J. Exp. Path.* 7:181, 1926.
30. Greenberg, M. Complications of vaccination against smallpox. *Amer. J. Dis. Child.* 76:492, 1948.
31. Miller, H. G., Stanton, J. B., and Gibbons, J. L. Para-infectious encephalomyelitis and related syndromes. *Quart. J. Med.* 25:427, 1956.
32. Perdrau, J. R. The histology of post-vaccinal encephalitis. *J. Path. Bact.* 31:17, 1928.
33. Appelbaum, E., Dolgopol, V. B., and Dolgin, J. Measles encephalitis. *Amer. J. Dis. Child.* 77:25, 1949.
34. *Multiple Sclerosis and the Demyelinating Diseases* (Proceedings of Association for Research in Nervous and Mental Disease, Vol. 28). Baltimore: Williams & Wilkins Company, 1950.
35. McAlpine, D., Compston, N. D., and Lumsden, C. E. *Multiple Sclerosis.* London: E. & S. Livingstone, Ltd., 1955.
36. Alter, M., Allison, R. S., Talbert, O. R., and Kurland, L. T. Geographic distribution of multiple sclerosis. *World Neurol.* 1:55, 1960.
37. Kabat, E. A., Freedman, D. A., Murray, J. P., and Knaub, V. A study of the crystalline albumin, gamma globulin and total protein in the cerebrospinal fluid of one hundred cases of multiple sclerosis and in other diseases. *Amer. J. Med. Sci.* 219:55, 1950.
38. Sherwin, A. L., O'Brien, G. J., Richter, M., Cosgrove, J. B. R., and Rose, B. Antibody

formation following injection of antigen into the subarachnoid space. *Neurology* (Minneap.) 13:703, 1963.
39. Field, E. J., and Ridley, A. Cerebrospinal fluid gamma globulin in multiple sclerosis. *Brit. Med. J.* 2:1053, 1960.
40. Greenfield, J. G., Blackwood, W., Meyer, A., McMenemey, W. H., and Norman, R. M. *Neuropathology.* London: Edward Arnold, Ltd., 1958.
41. Paterson, P. Y. Organ-Specific Tissue Damage Induced by Mammalian Tissue-Adjuvant Emulsions. In Lawrence, H. S. (Ed.), *Cellular and Humoral Aspects of the Hypersensitive States.* New York: Paul B. Hoeber, Inc., 1959. P. 469.
42. Kabat, E. A., Wolf, A., and Bezer, A. E. Studies on acute disseminated encephalomyelitis produced experimentally in rhesus monkeys: IV. Disseminated encephalomyelitis produced in monkeys with their own brain tissue. *J. Exp. Med.* 89:395, 1949.
43. Harwin, S. M., Paterson, P. Y., and Didakow, N. C. Antibodies against autologous brain in rats with allergic encephalomyelitis. *Nature* (London) 189:322, 1961.
44. Wolf, A. Spontaneous Human and Experimental Simian Demyelinating Disease. In Rose, A. S., and Pearson, C. M. (Eds.), *Mechanisms of Demyelination.* New York: Blakiston Division, McGraw-Hill Book Company, Inc., 1963. P. 72.
45. Roizin, L., and Kolb, L. C. Neuropathologic Relationship of Multiple Sclerosis to the Experimental Allergic Encephalomyelitides (Comparative Histologic and Some Histochemical Studies). In *III Congrès International de Neuropathologie: Rapports et Discussions.* Bruxelles; *Acta Medica Belgica,* 1957. P. 57.
46. Thomas, L., Paterson, P. Y., and Smithwick, B. Acute disseminated encephalomyelitis following immunization with homologous brain extracts: I. Studies on the role of a circulating antibody in the production of the condition in dogs. *J. Exp. Med.* 92:133, 1950.
47. Paterson, P. Y., and Beisaw, N. E. Effect of whole body x-irradiation on induction of allergic encephalomyelitis in rats. *J. Immun.* 90:532, 1963.
48. Paterson, P. Y. Studies of immunological tolerance to nervous tissue in rats. *Ann. N.Y. Acad. Sci.* 73:811, 1958.
49. Waksman, B. H., and Morrison, L. R. Tuberculin type sensitivity to spinal cord antigen in rabbits with isoallergic encephalomyelitis. *J. Immun.* 66:421, 1951.
50. Waksman, B. H. Further study of skin reactions in rabbits with experimental allergic encephalomyelitis. *J. Infect. Dis.* 99:258, 1956.
51. Bell, J., and Paterson, P. Y. Rapid induction of allergic encephalomyelitis in rats without the use of mycobacteria. *Science* 131:1448, 1960.
52. Paterson, P. Y., and Bell, J. Studies of induction of allergic encephalomyelitis in rats and guinea pigs without the use of mycobacteria. *J. Immun.* 89:72, 1962.
53. Paterson, P. Y. Transfer of allergic encephalomyelitis in rats by means of lymph node cells. *J. Exp. Med.* 111:119, 1960.
54. Paterson, P. Y., and Didakow, N. C. Transfer of allergic encephalomyelitis using splenectomized albino rats. *Proc. Soc. Exp. Biol. Med.* 108:768, 1961.
55. Paterson, P. Y. Cellular and Humoral Immune Factors in Allergic Encephalomyelitis. In Grabar, P., and Miescher, P. A. (Eds.), *Immunopathology* (2nd International Symposium). Basel: Benno Schwabe & Co., 1962, p. 184.
56. Koprowski, H. The role of hyperergy in measles encephalitis. *Amer. J. Dis. Child.* 103: 273, 1962.
57. Astrom, K., and Waksman, B. H. The passive transfer of experimental allergic encephalomyelitis and neuritis with living lymphoid cells. *J. Path. Bact.* 83:89, 1962.
58. Stone, S. H. Transfer of allergic encephalomyelitis by lymph node cells in inbred guinea pigs. *Science* 134:619, 1961.
59. Waksman, B. H. Auto-immunization and the lesions of auto-immunity. *Medicine* 41:93, 1962.
60. Paterson, P. Y. Cells, Antibodies and Autoimmune Disease. In Amos, B., and Koprowski, H. (Eds.), *Cell-bound Antibodies.* Philadelphia: Wistar Institute Press, 1963. P. 101.
61. Paterson, P. Y. A study of experimental encephalomyelitis employing mammalian and nonmammalian nervous tissues. *J. Immun.* 78:472, 1957.
62. Paterson, P. Y. Serum factors in experimental allergic encephalomyelitis and neurological diseases of man (designated discussion). *Nat. Cancer Inst. Monogr.* 11:212, 1963.
63. Paterson, P. Y., and Harwin, S. M. Suppression of allergic encephalomyelitis in rats by means of antibrain serum. *J. Exp. Med.* 117: 755, 1963.
64. Paterson, P. Y., Harwin, S. M., and Didakow, N. C. Acquired resistance to allergic encephalomyelitis and the role of a serum factor. *J. Clin. Invest.* 40:1069, 1961 (abst.).
65. Stauffer, R. E., and Waksman, B. H. Dermal and serological reactions to nervous tissue antigens in multiple sclerosis. *Ann. N.Y. Acad. Sci.* 58:570, 1954.
66. Broman, T., Lidvall, H., Lind, A., and Meyer, P. Investigations of multiple sclerosis patients concerning skin and serological reactions to injections with brain tissue. *Acta Psychiat. Neurol. Scand.* 35:403, 1960.
67. Böhme, D., Paal, G., Kersten, W., and Kersten, H. Skin reactions in neurological pa-

tients after intracutaneous administration of proteolipid A extracted from human brain. *Nature* (London) 197:609, 1963.
68. Sachs, H., and Steiner, G. Serologische Untersuchungen bei Multipler Sklerose. *Klin. Wschr.* 13:1714, 1934.
69. Raskin, N. Antibrain antibodies in multiple sclerosis: Study of the antibrain antibodies in the blood of multiple sclerosis patients by complement fixation tests. *Arch. Neurol. Psychiat.* 73:645, 1955.
70. Lumsden, C. E., Kabat, E. A., Wolf, A., and Bezer, A. E. Studies on acute disseminated encephalomyelitis produced experimentally in rhesus monkeys: V. Complement-fixing antibodies. *J. Exp. Med.* 92:253, 1950.
71. Berg, O., and Dencker, S. J. Studies on sera of animals with experimental allergic encephalomyelitis and patients with multiple sclerosis using immune precipitation in agar gel and immuno-electrophoresis. *Acta Path. Microbiol. Scand.* 54:434, 1962.
72. Ahrengot, V. Examinations for myelin autoantibodies in patients with multiple sclerosis: Demyelination experiments in guinea-pigs by treatment with antimyelin serum. *Acta Psychiat. Neurol. Scand.* 32:192, 1957.
73. MacLeod, I., Ridley, A. R., Smith, C., and Field, E. J. Failure to demonstrate circulating antibody to alcoholic brain extracts in multiple sclerosis. *Brit. Med. J.* 1:1525, 1962.
74. Koprowski, H., and LeBell, I. The presence of complement-fixing antibodies against brain tissue in sera of persons who had received antirabies vaccine treatment. *Amer. J. Hyg.* 51: 292, 1950.
75. Appelbaum, E., Greenberg, M., and Nelson, J. Neurological complications following antirabies vaccination. *J.A.M.A.* 151:188, 1953.
76. Kirk, R. C., and Ecker, E. E. Time of appearance of antibodies to brain in the human receiving anti-rabies vaccine. *Proc. Soc. Exp. Biol. Med.* 70:734, 1949.
77. Shiraki, H., Otani, S., Tamthai, B., Chamuni, A., Chitanondh, H., and Charuchinda, S. Rabies postvaccinal encephalomyelitis and genuine rabies in human beings. *World Neurol.* 3:125, 1962.
78. Rosen, L., and Thooris, G. Poliomyelitis in French Oceania: Epidemiologic observations on an outbreak with notes on the incidence of paralysis following intramuscular injections. *Amer. J. Hyg.* 57:237, 1953.
79. Bodian, D. Viremia in experimental poliomyelitis: II. Viremia and the mechanism of the "provoking" effect of injections or trauma. *Amer. J. Hyg.* 60:358, 1954.
80. Trueta, J., and Hodes, R. Provoking and localising factors in poliomyelitis: An experimental study. *Lancet* 1:998, 1954.
81. Braude, A. I., Siemienski, J., and Jacobs, I. Protoplast formation in human urine. *Trans. Ass. Amer. Physicians* 74:234, 1961.
82. Steiner, G. Morphology of spirochaeta myelophthora in multiple sclerosis. *J. Neuropath.* 13:221, 1954.
83. Ichelson, R. R. Cultivation of spirochaetes from spinal fluids of multiple sclerosis cases and negative controls. *Proc. Soc. Exp. Biol. Med.* 95:57, 1957.
84. Roach, L. L., Rosenberg, S., and Ichelson, R. R. Immunological considerations of an antigenic fraction from cultures of spirochetes isolated from cerebrospinal fluid of multiple sclerosis cases: Preliminary report. *Amer. J. Med. Sci.* 237:8, 1959.
85. Margulis, M. S., Soloviev, V. D., and Shubladze, A. K. Aetiology and pathogenesis of acute sporadic disseminated encephalomyelitis and multiple sclerosis. *J. Neurol., Neurosurg. Psychiat.* 9:63, 1946.
86. Dick, G. W. A., McKeown, F., and Wilson, D. C. Virus of acute encephalomyelitis of man and multiple sclerosis. *Brit. Med. J.* 1:7, 1958.
87. Lumsden, C. E. Multiple Sclerosis: A report of some recent laboratory investigations. In *Proceedings, II International Congress of Neuropathology*. Amsterdam: Excerpta medica, 1955, p. 429.
88. Lawrence, H. S. Homograft sensitivity: An expression of the immunologic origins and consequences of individuality. *Physiol. Rev.* 39:811, 1959.
89. Schwentker, F. F., and Rivers, T. M. The antibody response of rabbits to injections of emulsions and extracts of homologous brain. *J. Exp. Med.* 60:559, 1934.
90. Adams, J. M., and Imagawa, D. T. Measles antibodies in multiple sclerosis. *Proc. Soc. Exp. Biol. Med.* 111:562, 1962.
91. Good, R. A., and Campbell, B. The precipitation of latent herpes simplex encephalitis by anaphylactic shock. *Proc. Soc. Exp. Biol. Med.* 68:82, 1948.
92. Hotchin, J. The biology of lymphocytic choriomeningitis infection: Virus induced immune disease. *Cold Spring Harbor Sympos.* 27:479, 1962.
93. Hadlow, W. J. The pathology of experimental scrapie in the dairy goat. *Res. Vet. Sci.* 2:289, 1961.
94. Sigurdsson, B., Palsson, P. A., and Grimsson, H. Visna, a demyelinating transmissible disease of sheep. *J. Neuropath. Exp. Neurol.* 16:389, 1957.
95. Sigurdsson, B. Rida, a chronic encephalitis in sheep: With general remarks on infections which develop slowly and some of their special characteristics. *Brit. Vet. J.* 110:341, 1954.
96. Morris, J. A., and Gajdusek, D. C. Encephalopathy in mice following inoculation of scrapie

sheep brain. *Nature* (London) 197:1084, 1963.

97. Paterson, P. Y., Coia, E. M., and Fox, A. M. Unpublished data, 1962.
98. Campbell, A. M. G., Daniel, P., Porter, R. J., Russell, W. R., Smith, H. V., and Innes, J. R. M. Disease of the nervous system occurring among research workers on swayback in lambs. *Brain* 70:50, 1947.
99. Field, E. J., Miller, H., and Russell, D. S. Observations on glial inclusion bodies in a case of acute disseminated sclerosis. *Brit. J. Clin. Path.* 15:278, 1962.
100. Campbell, A. M. G., Norman, R. M., and Sandry, R. J. Subacute encephalitis in an adult associated with necrotising myelitis and results of animal inoculation experiments. *J. Neurol., Neurosurg., Psychiat.* 26:439, 1963.
101. Editorial (Leading Article). Steroid treatment in disseminated sclerosis. *Brit. Med. J.* 2:513, 1963.

72. Endogenous Uveitis

A. EDWARD MAUMENEE

INTRAOCULAR INFLAMMATION MAY be divided into two general types. The first, frequently termed panophthalmitis, is characterized in most cases by a suppurative inflammation. This usually results from the introduction of an organism or foreign body into the eye at the time of surgery or an injury. The organisms may enter the eye, however, by blood-borne metastasis, or by invasion of the optic nerve in meningitis, or through the cornea during ulceration. On occasions, inflammations of this type do not involve the sclera and tissues immediately adjacent to the globe, and are then termed endophthalmitis. The first category of intraocular inflammations also includes reactions to chemical and blunt injuries. Although the eye may be destroyed and require enucleation as a result of an acute or chronic response, inflammations of this type usually do not have repeated exacerbations and remissions.

The second type of intraocular inflammation is often called endogenous uveitis. In contrast to the first type, it is usually nonsuppurative, but may be so. The etiological factor is frequently unknown: a systemic infection may involve the eye via the blood stream or, on rare occasions, a virus may pass through the cornea. Allergic factors are thought to contribute significantly to the pathogenesis. The reaction is characterized by exacerbations or remissions over a period of years. Although this response is usually called uveitis, the causative organisms are often in the retina or vitreous.

PATHOGENESIS OF ENDOGENOUS UVEITIS

The pathogenesis of uveitis is usually not known, due to two factors. First, biopsy carries a risk of damaging the vision. Aqueous humor from the anterior chamber or a piece of iris can be obtained with relatively little risk; however, patients are usually reluctant to undergo even this small chance of loss of vision during the first few days of an attack of iritis. Biopsies taken during the chronic stage have failed to reveal causative organisms. Examination of the aqueous for antibodies has proved to be of value (discussed later). Biopsies of the ciliary body, choroid, or retina would entail great danger to vision and are not warranted. When the inflammatory processes lead to blindness and enucleation is required because of pain, examination of these specimens has occasionally revealed an etiological agent. All too frequently, however, all that remains in such specimens are the nonspecific sequelae of a chronic inflammatory process.

The second problem that has limited our knowledge of uveal inflammation is the lack of a satisfactory experimental model for the disease. Ocular inflammation can be induced in experimental animals by various methods, such as systemic or intraocular inoculation of organisms, intraocular inoculation of antigens, and so on. Some of these procedures cause a chronic inflammation of the eye, but they do not result in a chronic, spontaneously recurring process, as occurs in man.

Spontaneous intraocular infections are known to occur in animals, but few of them have been studied extensively with a view to relating them to uveitis in man. An exception is periodic ophthalmia in horses. This uveal inflammation is thought to be due to leptospirosis [1], but the organism has not been isolated from the eye. Witmer [2] titrated the antibody content in the aqueous and compared this with the serum of affected animals. When the titers were adjusted to the protein content in the two fluids, he found a higher content of *Leptospira* antibodies in the aqueous of some eyes with uveitis than in the blood. This suggested an ocular inflammation with this organism and the local production of antibodies.

Uveal inflammation has been found in chickens as a manifestation of avian lymphomatosis. The virus which produces the systemic lesions has not been isolated from the eye [3]. A granulomatous chorioretinitis has been noted in turkeys [4], and retinal inflammation has been observed in canine distemper [5] and hog cholera [6].

On the basis of clinical and experimental observations, Woods [7] has suggested that there are two general types of inflammatory reactions in the uveal tissue. The first of these, nongranulomatous uveitis, is caused by a sterile insult by antigen, usually bacterial, or occasionally viral. The second, granulomatous uveitis, is caused by actual invasion of the uveal tract by the pathogenic agent. These two types of lesions can be clearly differentiated when they involve the anterior segment of the eye. They are more difficult to distinguish when they involve the posterior segment.

In man, the onset of nongranulomatous uveitis of the anterior segment is usually acute, rather than insidious. Inflammatory reaction in the iris is usually slight and limited to loss of luster, blurring of the iris pattern, and dilatation of the capillaries. There are no nodules and but little tendency to the formation of posterior synechiae, unless there are repeated recurrences. The aqueous ray is usually intense, due to outpouring of serum, and there may even be a heavy gelatinous or fibrous exudate in the anterior chamber. The deposits on the posterior surface of the cornea are small and pinpoint and are composed chiefly of lymphocytes. Heavy, greasy exudates do not occur, and there is little or no tendency to capsular clouding of the lens. Koeppe nodules are never observed. The course of nongranulomatous iritis is usually short, and the eyes usually recover with amazingly few residua. Only after repeated attacks is organic damage done to the eye. In the acute stage, the histological picture is predominantly that of nonspecific inflammation. In the advanced stages, both clinical and histological pictures may simulate those of granulomatous uveitis.

An almost identical type of uveal response, except for the spontaneous exacerbations and remissions, has been produced in experimental animals by intraocular injection of foreign proteins. Nicolle and Apt [8] in 1908 sensitized guinea pigs to horse sera by means of intraperitoneal injections. Once hypersensitivity was established, injections of the same antigen into the anterior chamber resulted in a picture of acute iritis. Sattler [9] in 1909 sensitized guinea pigs by intravitreal injection of horse serum in one eye and noted a delayed inflammation in these eyes eight to fourteen days later. Subsequent intravitreal injections of these or the fellow-eyes producd an immediate inflammatory reaction. These studies have recently been greatly amplified by Silverstein [10] and his co-workers, who have demonstrated an acute uveal inflammation to both humoral (immediate) and cell-bound (delayed) hypersensitivity when the exciting substance has been injected intravitreally. Subsequent injections of antigens intravenously have induced a focal reaction in the eye.

Silverstein [11] has also shown, in experimental animals, that persistence of local hypersensitivity in the eye beyond the time when circulating antibody can be detected in the blood is due to the persistence of plasma cells or other immunologically competent cells in the uveal tissue. He has demonstrated that ectopic antibody formation (the production of antibody outside the usual lymph organs) can and does take place in the eye and suggests that the mere process of the eye carrying out the function of the lymph nodes is sufficient to produce the clinical picture of nongranulomatous uveitis.

Woods [7] hypothesized that a second type, granulomatous uveitis, is caused by actual invasion of the uveal tract by the pathogenic agent. In this type of anterior uveal involvement, the onset is usually insidious. The cellular reaction in the tissue is greater than the vascular reaction, and the ciliary congestion is not as severe. Organic changes take place in the iris, with thickening of the stroma from cellular infiltration, with blurring of the iris pattern and loss of normal luster. Well-defined nodules (Busacca nodules) are present on the surface of the iris or in the iris stroma. There is a pronounced tendency to the formation of posterior synechiae, with greasy exudates on the anterior capsule of the lens and capsular clouding. The keratic precipitates are of the so-called mutton-fat variety. Histologically, these consist chiefly of epithelioid cells. Koeppe nodules, or accumulations of epithelioid cells, at the pupillary border of the iris are not uncommon. The aqueous ray may be intense but more often is rather mild. Woods cites the finding of organisms in histological sections of enucleated human material or their isolation in culture or experimental animals in support of his theory of the infectious nature of granulomatous uveitis. Those found were identified with syphilis, tuberculosis, leprosy, leptospirosis, trypanosomiasis, toxoplasmosis, and the nematodes *Onchocerca volvulus, Toxocara canis,* and *Cysticercus*. He also points out that sarcoidosis and sympathetic ophthalmia can produce granulomatous uveitis, but that a causative agent has not been found for these conditions. He further strengthens his argument by noting that granulomatous uveitis can be induced in experimental animals by inoculation with tubercle bacilli, *Toxoplasma gondii,* and *Histoplasma capsulatum*.

There is great merit in Woods's classification; but the fact that it is very difficult to differentiate granulomatous from nongranulomatous uveitis on a clinical basis in the posterior segment of the eye, the finding that in an occasional patient chronic nongranulomatous anterior uveitis will later become granulomatous, and the observation that some anterior uveal inflammations lie midway between the two responses have led some workers to revert to a simpler classification such as acute or chronic, anterior, posterior, or generalized uveitis. They are further subdivided according to a specific agent, if found, or into types associated with a systemic disease of unknown etiology. Finally, other cases have been subdivided because of the consistency of their clinical pictures.

TYPES OF UVEITIS

It is not appropriate here to give a detailed description of each type of uveal inflammation. Rather, a brief summary will be given of the uveal reactions most frequently seen in this country. The reader is referred to Woods's book [7] for a detailed description of these lesions and for a discussion of lesions associated with leptospirosis, onchocerciasis, cysticercosis, leprosy, and other conditions.

SYPHILIS

Formerly, many cases of uveal inflammation were attributed to tertiary syphilis because the patient had a positive Wassermann reaction. It is now known that a number of these gave false indications of syphilis. In some types of ocular inflammations, however, the incrimination of *Treponema pallidum* is on a firmer basis. These are diffusely distributed, circumscribed chorioretinal lesions, the salt-and-pepper chorioretinal changes, and pseudoretinitis pigmentosa fundal lesions of congenital syphilis. Chronic iridocyclitis and interstitial keratitis also may occur with congenital syphilis. *Treponema pallidum* has been found in the lesions just described without much difficulty, except in interstitial keratitis [12]. The failure to find the spirochete in the inflamed cornea of patients with congenital syphilis has led some workers to suggest that the corneal reaction was due to an allergic response to the spirochete rather than to toxic injury by this organism.

An unusual type of nodular iritis with necrosis of the tissue and many dilated vessels has been found in patients with early secondary syphilis. These lesions have been called iritis roseata, iritis papulosa, and iritis nodosa. A diffuse chorioretinitis with marked retinal edema and scattered perivascular retinal hemorrhages occurs in late secondary syphilis. Spirochetes have been found in a few eyes with lesions of this type. Other types of granulomatous chorioretinitis and generalized uveitis may be caused by late syphilis, but their failure to respond to antisyphilitic therapy and absence of spirochetes in the tissues of such enucleated eyes raise considerable doubt as to the syphilitic origin of the inflammatory response.

TUBERCULOSIS

Twenty years ago, the tubercle bacillus was frequently considered to be the etiological agent in granulomatous endogenous uveitis. However, failure of such lesions to respond to antituberculous therapy and absence of the tubercle bacillus in eyes with advanced changes weaken the importance of tuberculosis as a frequent cause of uveitis. The tubercle bacillus has been found, however, in lesions in the choroid and retina of patients who have died of miliary tuberculosis and tuberculous meningitis. Clinically, these appear as choroidal nodules with blurred margins and white areas of opacification in the retina. In patients who recover from disseminated tuberculosis, the choroidal lesions have been noted to clear with minimal residual scarring. In otherwise normal patients, the tubercle bacillus has been found in caseating necrosis of the ciliary body and in the retina of an eye with acute endophthalmitis [13].

TOXOPLASMOSIS

Toxoplasmosis has been considered a major cause of uveitis since 1952, when Wilder [14] reported organisms resembling *Toxoplasma* in fifty-two human eyes enucleated primarily because of ocular inflammation. In 1939, Wolf *et al.* [15] had discovered toxoplasmosis in man. They isolated the organisms from a 31-day-old infant in whom an acute fatal illness developed a few days after birth. Clinically, this infant had severe encephalomyelitis and bilateral retinochoroiditis. Since that time, the organism has been isolated from the eyes of several children and adults who had acute retinochoroiditis and subsequent destruction of the eye by inflammation.

The clinical picture in these severely infected eyes that have required enucleation suggests that some cases of milder retinochoroiditis may also be due to toxoplasmosis. The most important diagnostic feature of such lesions is a retinitis that produces a white opacification of the retina, obliterating both retinal and choroidal vessels. The vitreous immediately overlying the lesion in particular, and at times the entire vitreous, becomes quite cloudy due to infiltration by cells and leakage of proteinaceous material into the vitreous body. Such areas of inflammation are usually 1 disc diameter in size or larger and may be located in any portion of the ocular fundus. Not infrequently, and particularly in congenital toxoplasmosis, scars of previous chorioretinitis can be found adjacent to the area of active inflammation. If the retinochoroiditis is in the anterior portion of the retina, or if the lesion in the posterior fundus is quite large, the ciliary body and iris may become inflamed and mutton-fat deposits develop on the posterior surface of the cornea.

The duration of the inflammatory attacks is quite variable, but they usually persist for at least several weeks, and frequently for several months before spontaneous healing. The reaction may be so severe as to destroy the globe. In these eyes, the organisms are usually found in the retina, but the overlying vitreous and underlying choroid and sclera may be heavily infiltrated by inflammatory cells. The ciliary body and iris may also be inflamed, but the organisms are seldom found in these tissues.

Further evidence that the milder forms of retinochoroiditis just described are due to toxoplasmosis is found in a study by Van Metre and his co-workers [16]. Of 344 consecutively studied patients with uveal tract disease, 73 had focal exudative retinochoroiditis and 271 had other lesions. Delayed skin hypersensitivity to toxoplasmin was noted in 68 (94 percent) of the 72 satisfactorily tested patients* with focal exudative retinochoroiditis but in only 60 (23 percent) of the 266 tested patients with other types of lesions. Results of the Sabin dye test were positive in the titer of 1 : 8 or more in 67 (92 percent) of the 73 patients tested with focal exudative retinochoroiditis but in only 78 (33 percent) of the 237 tested patients with other lesions.

Hogan *et al.* [17] have classified ocular toxoplasmosis as follows: (1) retinitis of acute systemic toxoplasmosis; (2) acute recurrent retinitis without systemic disease; (3) acute endophthalmitis; and (4) late relapse of congenital toxoplasmic retinitis.

Daraprim and sulfadiazine are effective in the treatment of proliferating toxoplasmosis in both man and animals [18]. It was therefore thought that a therapeutic trial might be of value in establishing a diagnosis of toxoplasmosis; however, in a double blind study, Acers [19] has shown that Daraprim, sulfadiazine, and steroids were no more effective in the treatment of retinochoroiditis than were steroids alone. Somewhat similar results have been reported by Hogan and Leopold [18]. The failure of the ocular lesions to show a prompt response to this specific form of therapy for toxoplasmosis has led Frenkel [18] to suggest that the ocular inflammation may be in great part the result of an antigen-antibody interaction. This is supported by the scarcity or even lack of organisms in areas of pronounced inflammation in the choroid and sclera.

It is also known that the proliferative forms of toxoplasmosis are quite susceptible to chemotherapy, whereas the encysted forms are quite resistant. It has therefore been suggested that the encysted forms of the parasite remain in the retina at the margins of healed chorioretinal lesions and that rupture of these cysts at a later time causes a reactivation of the disease and accounts for the frequent daughter lesions or grouping of areas of chorioretinitis in toxoplasmosis.

NEMATODE ENDOPHTHALMITIS

It has long been known that the nematodes of onchocerciasis and cysticercosis produce ocular lesions [7]. These diseases were uncom-

* The seventy-third tested patient reacted to both toxoplasmin and toxoplasmin control.

mon in this country and Europe; therefore nematode endophthalmitis was of little interest to American and European clinicians until 1950, when Wilder [20] reported the finding of nematode larvae in 24 eyes of children and a characteristic reaction which justified a tentative diagnosis of nematode endophthalmitis in 22 other enucleated specimens. These organisms were first identified as the hookworm larva but were later found to be larva of *Toxocara canis* [21].

Two types of clinical lesions are now known to be caused by nematode larvae. The first is an inflammatory mass in the vitreous immediately adjacent to the retina. This somewhat resembles a retinoblastoma in that it is whitish with considerable reaction in the surrounding retina and underlying choroid. Histologically, the center of the lesion is an eosinophilic abscess surrounding the body of the worm. The process seldom causes a marked external inflammatory reaction of the eye, but the vitreous may become quite hazy so that details of the fundus cannot be seen. The lesion smolders for months to a year and then subsides, leaving a glial mass in the vitreous with either striking traction folds in the retina or total retinal detachment. Such eyes have frequently been enucleated because of suspected retinoblastoma.

A second type of lesion, reported by Ashton [22], consists of a subretinal or preretinal glial mass in the posterior pole of the fundus, not infrequently in the macular area.

Such lesions probably should not be included in a description of uveitis, for the primary site of the inflammatory response is frequently in the vitreous rather than in the retina and choroid, and the clinical course is one of a smoldering endophthalmitis rather than a recurrent one.

Diagnosis of this condition is based almost entirely on the ocular picture, for children with this type of infection seldom have eosinophilia and, since the organism does not run its normal life cycle in man, it is not found in the feces. It is possible that skin testing with an appropriate antigen might be diagnostically helpful. No specific therapy is known.

MISCELLANEOUS INFECTIONS

Cytomegalic inclusion disease produces a generalized infection involving the brain, liver, kidney, spleen, and eyes. On several occasions, the intranuclear inclusion bodies of the virus have been found in the retina [23]. The lesions in these eyes are not unlike those of toxoplasmosis, but they are usually smaller and are more disseminated than grouped, as in toxoplasmosis.

A chronic granulomatous uveitis is known to occur in patients with herpes zoster ophthalmicus when the nasociliary nerve is involved. Such patients usually have keratitis as well as involvement of the iris.

A low-grade inflammatory reaction in the iris is not uncommon in patients who have herpes simplex infections of the cornea. The uveal inflammation may recur on numerous occasions over a period of years in concurrence with repeated corneal infections. It has been difficult in such cases to isolate the herpes virus from the aqueous. On rare occasions, the virus may produce a mild dendritic lesion on the cornea which clears without scarring, but the individual will then have recurrent attacks of anterior uveitis. These have been thought to be due to the herpes simplex virus, but the organism has not been isolated in such eyes.

SARCOIDOSIS

The etiology of sarcoidosis is unknown. The eyes are frequently involved. Thus, Woods [7] reported 40 percent ocular involvement in 122 cases of sarcoidosis. Lesions of the globe include nummular keratitis, nodular scleritis, granulomatous iritis with Koeppe nodules at the periphery of the iris, and Busacca nodules in the iris stroma. Anterior uveal involvement in sarcoidosis is much more frequent than involvement of the posterior segment of the eye; however, probably the most specific lesions in sarcoidosis are snowball vitreous opacities that lie immediately in front of the retina in the inferior portion of the vitreous. In addition to these, perivasculitis, retinitis, choroiditis, and optic neuritis have been noted. Such ocular lesions are both chronic and recurrent and not infrequently lead to blindness and loss of the eye.

The early stages of the ocular reaction respond quite well to corticosteroid therapy, but once the lesion is well established and chronic, such treatment is of little value.

OCULAR LESIONS POSSIBLY DUE TO AUTOIMMUNITY

Two types of ocular inflammation are thought to be related to autoimmune disease. The first is phacoanaphylaxis or hypersensitivity to lens material. The second is sympathetic ophthalmia, which is thought to be due to hypersensitivity to uveal tissue.

Uhlenhuth [24] in 1903 was the first to demonstrate organ-specific antigens. He gave rabbits intravenous injections of saline homogenates of bovine lenses and produced antisera which precipitated lens homogenates but did not combine with other antigenic preparations of bovine origin. Interestingly, however, he was not able to stimulate antibodies in the rabbit with injections of rabbit lens. Apparently, organ-specific antigens act as haptens in their own species; i.e., they are capable of combining with antibodies that are already formed but fail to stimulate antibody formation. As with other haptens, the organ-specific haptens may be converted into antigens if injected with some kind of carrier or adjuvant. Halbert *et al.* [25] carried Uhlenhuth's work further and sensitized a number of species to their own lenses by incorporating the antigen into Freund's adjuvants.

Verhoeff and LeMoine [26] in 1922 suggested that a certain type of postoperative intraocular inflammation following cataract extraction might be due to a reaction between retained lens substance and ocular tissue hypersensitivity to lens substances. This was based on the fact that many of these patients reacted to intracutaneous injections of lens extract, whereas normal patients did not. On histological examination of the eyes removed after development of the inflammation, the lenses were found to have been invaded by leukocytes and macrophages, but no bacteria were demonstrated. These observations have been confirmd on both a clinical and a histological basis, and it is now well established that individuals may become sensitive to their own lens if the lens is ruptured by an injury or at the time of surgery. These patients have a rather violent granulomatous type of anterior uveitis that clears if the residual lenticular material is removed from the eye. It has also been noted that the second eye may develop an anterior uveal inflammation in a sensitized patient if the lens in the second eye becomes cataractous. This may occur when there is no obvious break in the capsule of the cataractous lens. Removal of the lens from these eyes leads to prompt subsidence of the inflammatory process [27].

There is little question that the lens contains organ-specific antigens and under proper conditions is capable of stimulating the production of circulating antibodies. Also, the clinical picture of hypersensitivity to lens proteins is a definite entity. However, the production of this type of ocular inflammation in experimental animals has been a most challenging and difficult problem. Burky [28] and Müller [29] have reported success in this matter, but others have been unable to repeat their experiments and have failed to produce lesions comparable to those that occur in man [30].

Hypersensitivity to uveal tissue has long been thought to be a factor in the inflammation of sympathetic ophthalmia. In this condition, a chronic inflammation follows a perforating injury or surgical procedure on one eye. Within nine days to a few months, the second, or sympathizing eye, also becomes inflamed. The interval between the initial injury and the time of involvement of the second eye is extremely variable, and instances have been reported in which the second eye did not become involved until twenty years* or more after the initial accident. The reaction is both chronic and recurrent and frequently leads to total loss of vision. In other instances, it may be milder and will finally "burn itself out," leaving the patient with varying degrees of visual loss.

When the lesion involves the anterior segment of the eye, it is granulomatous. There are many mutton-fat keratic precipitates and much destruction of the iris. When the posterior segment of the second eye is involved early in the disease, the lesion is almost entirely in the choroid, with slight involvement of the retina. After the inflammation has existed for a month or longer, the entire uveal tract becomes inflamed.

On histological examination, the uveal tissue is heavily infiltrated by inflammatory cells, consisting of nests of epithelioid cells which phagocytize the uveal pigment in small granules rather than in large clumps. Surrounding these are nests of lymphocytes and occasionally a rather marked infiltration by eosinophils. Epithelioid nodules may develop under the pigment epithelium, but the neuroretina usually shows very little inflammatory cell infiltration.

Since the work of Elschnig [31] in 1911,

**Editor's comment:* Postulation of a cause-effect relationship between events so distant in time would seem extreme except in those instances in which there was persistent or recurring inflammation in the initial eye throughout the intervening time interval.—J. H. V.

numerous attempts have been made to produce this type of uveal inflammation in animals. Collins [32] in 1953 reported a round cell infiltration in the uveal tissue of guinea pigs following intramuscular and intraperitoneal injections of uveal tissue combined with Freund's adjuvant. Aronson *et al.* [33] confirmed these experiments but pointed out that the ocular inflammatory reaction in animals differs in its chronicity and histological appearance from sympathetic ophthalmia in man.

Numerous attempts have been made to detect a circulating antibody to uveal tissue in patients with sympathetic ophthalmia, but all such studies have failed. Friedenwald [34], however, demonstrated histologically that bovine uveal pigment injected into the skin of individuals with sympathetic ophthalmia called forth an inflammatory response almost identical to that found in the uveal tissue in the eye. Such positive reaction sites contained a heavy infiltrate of epithelioid and giant cells which had engulfed the pigment granules in a fine suspension similar to that found in the uveal tract. Interspersed with and surrounding these cells were numerous lymphocytes. In patients with negative skin reactions, large amounts of free unphagocytized pigment remained and there was little inflammatory reaction at the time of skin biopsy fourteen days after the uveal pigment had been injected.

Thus there is strongly suggestive evidence that these two types of ocular inflammation in some way involve organ-specific antigens. However, Witebsky and Milgrom [35] warn against premature acceptance of the idea that a disease is caused by autosensitization and suggest criteria that should be fulfilled before considering a disease to be an autoimmune disorder (see Introduction, Part Four).

UVEITIS OF UNKNOWN ETIOLOGY

There are a number of patients with uveitis for which no etiological or inducing factor has been found. In some of these cases, the reaction is rather nonspecific and can only be classified as acute or chronic anterior or posterior uveitis. This probably comprises the minority of patients with uveal inflammation.

There are a number of other types of uveitis in which the etiology is either only suspected or unknown. In these, the ocular lesion follows a specific course and pattern so that the lesion may be described as a clinical entity. The first of this group of conditions is *hemorrhagic detachment of the macular area.* The condition occurs primarily in individuals below age 45 to 50 but usually over age 15 to 20. It is usually detected in the first eye when the macular area becomes involved with a small hemorrhage under the pigment epithelium. Clinically, this appears as a dark gray or greenish elevation which may have a small flare of hemorrhage at the margin in one area, or the lesion may be surrounded by a halo of hemorrhage. The red appearance of the blood at the margin of the lesion usually indicates that the red blood cells have broken through the pigment epithelium and lie under the retina. When the periphery of the fundus is examined carefully, clusters of isolated, small (0.2 to 0.1 disc diameter), punched-out lesions of chorioretinitis with minimal pigment can be found. Occasionally, such lesions may be noted at the margin of the optic disc and may even encircle the disc to form an atrophic halo. Strangely, hemorrhage does not accompany these peripheral lesions.

The hemorrhages in the macular area are recurrent. These are followed by fibroblasts, which form a connective tissue mass that appears as a whitish nodule in the macular region. Visual acuity is usually conspicuously impaired, occasionally to the level of counting fingers at 3 to 4 feet. Blindness never occurs in such patients, however.

Because these eyes do not become painful or totally blind, they are seldom removed for histological examination. The only specimens available for study are those in which a mistaken diagnosis of melanoma has been made. Thus the clinical descriptions of the cases available for histological study are usually inadequate. In a few cases, an inflammatory reaction in the choroid has been found, but in other eyes, the absence of inflammation calls forth the possibility that these lesions may be on a vascular rather than an inflammatory basis [36]. In support of the latter idea is the lack of inflammatory response in the vitreous overlying the macular hemorrhage.

In 1960, Woods and Wahlen [37] suggested the probable role of histoplasmosis in the etiology of this type of uveal lesion. Van Metre and Maumenee [38] have studied delayed hypersensitivity reactions in 61 patients with hemorrhagic macular detachment and peripheral areas of chorioretinitis. Fifty-seven (94%) of these had positive reactions to histoplasmin skin tests. Of 190 patients with other types of uveal disease, only 48 (25 percent) had a positive skin reaction. Complement fixation tests were positive in 16 percent of the former group and only 3 percent of the latter group. Fibrocalcific lesions in the lungs were found in 47 (90 percent) of 52 patients of the former group and 90 (54 percent) of 166 patients in the latter group. The evidence that histoplasmosis is the cause of the lesion just described is extremely weak. However, the high percentage of positive skin reactions to the histoplasmin antigen in these patients in contrast to the low incidence in patients with other types of uveitis does warrant further investigation of this problem.

Extensive therapeutic trials with amphotericin B are dangerous and probably not warranted because of the toxicity of the drug. However, in the few cases in which this medication has been used, the response of the lesion has not been dramatic.

Nongranulomatous iridocyclitis is a definite clinical entity that occurs in two general types. In the first, the patient has acute episodes in which there are marked vasodilatation of the conjunctiva and episclera and iris vessels and liberation of a great deal of protein and fibrin into the anterior chamber. A few cells become deposited on the posterior surface of the cornea and are arranged in fine dustlike deposits. The inflammatory reaction lasts for a week or two, then subsides spontaneously. Under intensive steroid therapy, the eye will clear in a day or two. Few sequelae result from this type of response, other than an occasional posterior synechia of the iris to the lens. Eyes have withstood as many as 15 to 20 attacks of uveitis of this type. The condition is usually bilateral, but one eye may be involved for several years before the second eye is affected. The lesion may then alternate from eye to eye, or may occur simultaneously in both eyes. During the active stage, a serous detachment of the macula may occur and the optic nerve and surrounding retina may become edematous.

A second form of nongranulomatous iridocyclitis is not entirely distinct from the first, but recurrent attacks may lead to a chronic, smoldering type of inflammation that never subsides completely. In other instances, particularly in children, the disease may begin in this fashion with very little external evidence of inflammation. The child is noted to have ocular difficulty only when his vision is checked in school or the parents note that he does not see well while playing. Various studies have linked this type of uveal inflammation to ankylosing spondylitis or to peripheral nonsuppurative arthritis in which the patients have a negative reaction to the test for the rheumatoid arthritis factor in serum [7].

Experimentally, an almost identical type of anterior uveal inflammation has been produced by Silverstein and Zimmerman [10] in animals by sensitizing the eye to a foreign protein and subsequently injecting the same antigen intravenously. As discussed earlier, intraocular antibody production is an important feature of this model. Thus it appears there is in animals a good experimental model for this type of uveal inflammation. However, the antigen which produces the uveal inflammation in man has not been detected, and therefore the pathogenesis for this condition remains unknown.

A slight variation of the entity is known as Reiter's syndrome. The ocular picture is that of acute nongranulomatous iridocyclitis, but associated with this are urethritis, prostatitis, polyarthritis, conjunctivitis, and, at times, a hyperkeratotic inflammation of the skin (keratodermia blennorrhagica).

A few other conditions should be mentioned merely by listing the clinical symptoms, for neither is the pathogenesis known nor has it been possible to produce similar lesions in experimental animals. The first of these has been called *pars planitis* for want of a better name [39]. The condition occurs primarily in individuals under age 40, is limited to the eye, and consists primarily of an exudative lesion in the retina or in the vitreous immediately overlying the retina in the far periphery of the fundus at about the level of the ora serrata. For some strange reason, the reaction always begins in the inferior portion of the eye, and only in very long-standing disease does it completely encircle the periphery of the globe. Edema of the optic nerve and surrounding retina with a serous detachment of the macular area may occur. External ocular signs of inflammation are almost never present and the iris is usually entirely normal. The condition is almost always bilateral, but occasional unilateral cases have been observed. No effective therapy is known.

Heterochromic iridocyclitis is typified by

the chronicity of the response. Again, there is no evidence of external congestion of the eye. The lesion is nearly always unilateral and is extremely chronic. Fine whitish keratic deposits develop on the posterior surface of the cornea. The iris gradually becomes depigmented and atrophic. Opacification of the lens with development of a mature cataract is a frequent complication. A few cells occur in the anterior vitreous, but otherwise the posterior segment of the eye remains relatively normal.

The *Vogt-Koyanagi-Harada syndrome* is quite similar to sympathetic ophthalmia in both clinical and histological appearance. The condition may begin either as anterior uveitis or, not infrequently, with posterior uveal involvement. In the very early stages, meningismus with increased cell and protein content of the spinal fluid has been reported. The patients then have an exudative retinal detachment that is quite similar to that which occurs in sympathetic ophthalmia. The lesion is usually bilateral and quite severe, reducing visual acuity to the level of about hand motions. About 30 percent of the patients recover with normal vision, however, but the prognosis is always serious and many patients become permanently blind. Dysacousia, vitiligo, poliosis, and alpecia may occur together or as isolated phenomena in conjunction with the uveitis.

Behçet's syndrome consists, in its full form, of uveitis with hypopyon iritis; ulcers on the mucous membranes of the mouth, tongue and genitalia; arthritis, erythema nodosum, thrombophlebitis, and hallucinations due to involvement of the brain. A viral etiology has been suspected but never proved. Histological examination of the eyes that have been removed has revealed necrotizing arteritis with destruction of the retina and choroid. This disease is rare but not unheard of in this country; it is much more prevalent in Egypt and the Near East.

REFERENCES

1. Roberts, S. R. Fundus lesions in equine periodic ophthalmia. *J. Amer. Vet. Ass.* 141: 229, 1962.
2. Witmer, R. Ocular Origin of Antibodies (Clinical). In Maumenee, A. E., and Silverstein, A. M. (Eds.), *The Immunopathology of Uveitis*. Baltimore: Williams & Wilkins Company, 1964.
3. Abrahams, I. W. Avian lymphomatosis and uveitis. *Amer. J. Ophthal.* 51:424, 1961.
4. Saunders, L. Z., and Moore, E. N. Blindness in turkeys due to granulomatous chorioretinitis. *Avian Dis.* 1:27, 1957.
5. Jubb, K. V., Saunders, L. Z., and Coates, H. V. The intraocular lesions of canine distemper. *J. Comp. Path. Ther.* 67:21, 1957.
6. Saunders, L. Z., Jubb, K. V., and Jones, L. D. The intraocular lesions of hog cholera. *J. Comp. Path. Ther.* 68:375, 1958.
7. Woods, A. C. *Endogenous Inflammations of the Uveal Tract*. Baltimore: Williams & Wilkins Company, 1961.
8. Nicolle, M., and Apt, G. Les anticorps des albuminoides et des cellules. *Ann. Inst. Pasteur* (Paris) 22:132, 1908.
9. Sattler, C. H. Untersuchungen über die Wirkung von Blutserum nach Einspritzung in's Auge. *Arch. Augenheilk.* 64:390, 1909.
10. Silverstein, A. M., and Zimmerman, L. E. Immunogenic endophthalmitis produced in the guinea pig by different pathogenetic mechanisms. *Amer. J. Ophthal.* 48:435, 1959.
11. Silverstein, A. M. Ectopic Antibody Formation in the Eye. Ref. 2.
12. Friedenwald, J. S. Ocular lesions in fetal syphilis. *Bull. Hopkins Hosp.* 46:185, 1930.
13. Theobald, G. D. Acute tuberculous endophthalmitis: Report of a case. *Trans. Amer. Ophthal. Soc.* 55:325, 1957.
14. Wilder, H. C. Toxoplasma chorioretinitis in adults. *Arch. Ophthal.* 48:127, 1952.
15. Wolf, A., Cowen, D., and Paige, B. H. Human toxoplasmosis: Occurrence in infants as an encephalomyelitis; Verification by transmission to animals. *Science* 89:226, 1939.
16. Van Metre, T. E., Knox, D. L., and Maumenee, A. E. The relation between toxoplasmosis and focal exudative retino-choroiditis. *Amer. J. Ophthal.* 58:6–21, 1964.
17. Hogan, M. J., Kimura, S. J., and O'Connor, G. R. Ocular toxoplasmosis. *Arch. Ophthal.* 72:592–600, 1964.
18. Maumenee, A. E. (Ed.) *Toxoplasmosis, with Special Reference to Uveitis*. Baltimore: Williams & Wilkins Company, 1962.
19. Acers, T. E. Toxoplasmic retinochoroiditis: A double blind therapeutic study. *Arch. Ophthal.* 71:58, 1964.
20. Wilder, H. C. Nematode endophthalmitis. *Trans. Amer. Acad. Ophthal. Otolaryng.* 54: 99, 1950.
21. Hogan, M. J., and Zimmerman, L. E. *Ophthalmic Pathology* (2nd ed.). Philadelphia: W. B. Saunders Company, 1962.

22. Ashton, N. Larval granulomatosis of the retina due to toxocara. *Brit. J. Ophthal.* 44: 129, 1960.
23. Christensen, L., Beeman, H. W., and Allen, A. Cytomegalic inclusion disease. *Arch. Ophthal.* 57:90, 1957.
24. Uhlenhuth, P. Zur Lehre von der Unterscheidung verschiedener Eiweissarte mit Hilfe spezifischer Sera. In *Festschrift zum 60. Geburtstage von Robert Koch.* Jena: Gustav Fischer, 1903. P. 49.
25. Halbert, S. P., Locatcher-Khorazo, D., Swick, L., Witmer, R., Seegal, B., and Fitzgerald, P. Homologous immunological studies of ocular lens: I. *In vitro* observations. *J. Exp. Med.* 105:439, 1957.
26. Lemoine, A. N., and Verhoeff, F. H. Hypersensitiveness to lens protein. *Amer. J. Ophthal.* 5:700–702, 1922.
27. Maumenee, A. E. The contributions of immunology to clinical ophthalmology. *Amer. J. Ophthal.* 58:230–238, 1964.
28. Burky, E. L. Experimental endophthalmitis phacoanaphylactica in rabbits. *Arch. Ophthal.* 12:536, 1934.
29. Müller, H. Tierexperimentelle Untersuchungen zur Ophthalmia phakogenetica. *Graefe Arch. Ophthal.* 153:1, 1952.
30. Goodner, E. K. Experimental Lens-Induced Uveitis. Ref. 2.
31. Elschnig, A. Studien zur sympathischen Ophthalmie: III. *Graefe Arch. Ophthal.* 78: 549, 1911.
32. Collins, R. C. Further experimental studies on sympathetic ophthalmia. *Amer. J. Ophthal.* 36:150, 1953.
33. Aronson, S. B., Hogan, M. J., and Zweigart, P. Homoimmune uveitis in the guinea pig: III. Histopathologic manifestations of the disease. *Arch. Ophthal.* 69:208, 1963.
34. Friedenwald, J. S. Notes on the allergy theory of sympathetic ophthalmia. *Amer. J. Ophthal.* 17:1008, 1934.
35. Witebsky, E., and Milgrom, F. The Nature of Autosensitization (with Particular Reference to the Eye). Ref. 2.
36. Maumenee, A. E. Serous and hemorrhagic disciform detachment of the macula. *Trans. Pacif. Coast Otoophthal. Soc.* 40:139, 1959.
37. Woods, A. C., and Wahlen, H. E. The probable role of benign histoplasmosis in the etiology of granulomatous uveitis. *Amer. J. Ophthal.* 49:205, 1960.
38. Van Metre, T. E., and Maumenee, A. E. Specific ocular uveal lesions in patients with evidence of histoplasmosis. *Arch. Ophthal.* 71: 314–24, 1964.
39. Welch, R. B., Maumenee, A. E., and Wahlen, H. E. Peripheral posterior segment inflammation, vitreous opacities, and edema of the posterior pole: Pars planitis. *Arch. Ophthal.* 64:540, 1960.

73. Thyroiditis*

NOEL R. ROSE, ERNEST WITEBSKY,
AND WILLIAM H. BEIERWALTES

TO THE MORPHOLOGIST, THE PHYSIOLOGIST, and the clinician, the thyroid gland has provided recurring problems of interest. Morphologically, the gland is essentially a collection of follicles filled with viscous colloid matter and lined by an active secretory epithelium. The interstitium is richly supplied with blood and lymphatic vessels which have no direct connection with the intrafollicular space. Functionally, thyroid cells have an extraordinary ability to collect iodide from circulating blood and to incorporate it into amino acids, eventually storing it in the form of thyroglobulin. This macromolecule makes up the bulk of the colloid. Thyroglobulin, in turn, is the source of active circulating thyroid hormone. To the clinician, aberrations in thyroid function are reflected in increased or decreased cellular activity in many parts of the body, creating a variety of disease signs frequently difficult to recognize. Often serious disturbance in thyroidal morphology or function seems to develop spontaneously with little being known about the underlying pathogenic mechanisms.

The immunologist has been attracted to the study of the thyroid gland because of its unusual serological properties. These include its pronounced organ specificity, the sequestered location of its chief component, thyroglobulin, and, finally, its autoantigenic potentiality. The first part of this chapter (N. R. R. and E. W.) describes current concepts of each of these aspects of thyroid immunology and the background of experimental evidence that has led to the present status of knowledge. In the second part (W. H. B.), immunological information is combined with clinical and morphological observations in an effort to elucidate the etiology and pathogenesis of one group of disorders of the thyroid gland.

SPECIFICITY OF THYROGLOBULIN

The earliest studies on the antigenic properties of the thyroid gland were initiated primarily by clinicians motivated by the hope that methods of serological therapy of thyroid disease could be developed. Typical of this era was the extensive report of Rogers and Beebe [1], who tested the effects of sheep and rabbit antisera to human thyroid proteins for the treatment of hyperthyroidism. Although convinced of the validity of this approach, they achieved but limited success and were unable to interest the medical community as a whole [2].

The modern immunological approach to the specificity of thyroid proteins opened with the work of Hektoen and Schulhof [3]. Using the method of Oswald [4], they isolated thyroglobulin from saline extract of thyroid tissue by ammonium sulfate precipitation. On injecting human thyroglobulin into rabbits, they obtained an antiserum that precipitated human thyroglobulin in high dilutions. The same antiserum reacted with thyroglobulin of bovine and porcine origin in lower dilutions. Absorption of the antiserum to remove antibodies to serum components in the thyroid extract was necessary in this study. Later, Hektoen *et al.* [5] extended these observations to show cross-reactions of thyroglobulin antisera with a variety of mammalian thyroglobulins, but there was no interaction of their rabbit antisera with extracts from chicken thyroid glands.

Working with an antiserum to human thyroglobulin, Hektoen *et al.* [5] found that its precipitins for beef and hog thyroglobulin could be removed by specific absorption with the respective heterologous preparation without observable loss of reaction with human

* The work of Dr. Rose and Dr. Witebsky was supported by U.S. Public Health Service Grant No. CA-02357, and that of Dr. Beierwaltes by Grant No. CA-05174-04.

thyroglobulin. This result pointed to the presence of a main thyroid-specific antigen that was species-limited, and to one or more antigens common to thyroglobulins of several species. Quantitative determinations of the extent of cross-reaction were undertaken by Stokinger and Heidelberger [6]. They found that heterologous thyroglobulins were able to precipitate only a portion of the total antibody to the homologous antigen; with sheep and beef thyroglobulins, 75 to 80 percent of the antibody cross-reacted, while with hog and human thyroglobulins, only 15 to 40 percent of the antibodies cross-reacted.

Witebsky [7] in 1929 used the method of complement fixation to demonstrate serological relationships among thyroglobulins of various species. However, on a quantitative basis, relatively little cross-reaction occurred between isolated thyroglobulin and crude thyroid extracts or suspensions of a particular species. For this reason, Witebsky felt that the purified thyroglobulin prepared by ordinary ammonium sulfate fractionation was sometimes partially altered in its serological specificity. Witebsky *et al.* [8] emphasized in further studies that thyroid tissue contains, in addition to blood serum antigens, antigenic components widely distributed among other tissues of the particular species. Antibodies to these species-specific tissue antigens, as well as antigens in blood, must be removed before an antiserum can be regarded as thyroid-specific.

The antigen primarily responsible for the thyroid specificity of these antisera was found to be a relatively heat-stable globulin which precipitated from crude extract between 33 and 50 percent saturation of ammonium sulfate [9]. The principal component, comprising about 80 percent of the extract, could be identified on the basis of its sedimentation and electrophoretic properties as the classic thyroglobulin [10]. More precise ammonium sulfate fractionation [11] separated almost all of the thyroid-specific antigen of crude thyroid extract in the narrow range of 1.60 to 1.70 M ammonium sulfate. By ultracentrifugal analysis, this fraction contained almost pure thyroglobulin. Small amounts of additional thyroid-specific antigens were brought down by higher levels of ammonium sulfate.

Antisera to thyroid crude extract cross-reacted with saline extracts of thyroid glands of many mammalian species, as do antisera to isolated thyroglobulin [12]. Quantitatively, the cross-reactions were minor as compared to the homologous reaction, and the cross-reacting antibodies could be separated by absorption. At least two types of thyroid-specific antibodies could be visualized in gel precipitation tests, one that interacts with thyroglobulins of certain foreign species and another that is species-limited [13]. However, it could not be stated with certainty whether one antigen or two were responsible for these two types of antibodies. If different kinds of molecules were involved, they could not be resolved by immunoelectrophoretic analysis. This suggested that thyroglobulin was the only antigen concerned, but that it exists in different configurations or carries more than one type of antigenic determinant. By means of partial papain digestion, it has been possible to separate human thyroglobulin into at least three subunits with differing serological specificities [14]. These experiences underline the hazards of considering even chemically purified thyroglobulin as a single antigen. Circulating antibody to thyroglobulin represents the sum total of several antibodies with specificities for various portions of the thyroglobulin molecule.

AUTOANTIBODIES TO THYROGLOBULIN

In connection with their studies on the serological specificity of thyroglobulin, Hektoen and Schulhof [15] prepared thyroglobulin from rabbits and injected it intravenously into other rabbits. Precipitins appeared which were capable of reacting with all preparations of rabbit thyroglobulin tested but not with thyroglobulin of other species. Later, they [5] found that sera of rabbits injected with certain foreign thyroglobulins, as from bear, zebra, and dog, precipitated rabbit thyroglobulin or even simple saline extracts of rabbit thyroid tissue. Some years later, Lerman [16] noticed that if he injected human thyroglobulin into rabbits, their sera precipitated rabbit as well as human and several heterologous preparations. Some of the injections were given into tuberculous nodules. Myxedema, evident from a decreasing basal metabolic rate, appeared in some of the rabbits after several months. The thyroid glands of the immunized animals showed no characteristic pathological change at the time

TABLE 73-1. Experimental Thyroiditis Following Auto-, Iso-, or Heteroimmunization

Antigen	Antibody (Tanned Cell Hemagglut.)	Path. Changes
In the Rabbit		
Autologous thyroid extract[a]	6/8[b]	4/8[b]
Pooled rabbit thyroid extract[a]	54/63	47/63
Alum precipitated	14/18	0/18
Alum and acid-fast bacilli	9/9	4/9
Alum precipitated[a]	30/30	18/30
Rabbit thyroglobulin[a]	6/6	6/6[c]
Hog thyroid extract[a]	14/14	6/14[c]
Dog thyroid extract[a]	3/7	2/7[c]
Beef thyroid extract[a]	6/6	2/6[c]
Human thyroid extract[a]	4/12	0/12
In the Guinea Pig		
Pooled guinea pig thyroid extract[a]	17/27	27/27
In the Dog		
Pooled dog thyroid extract[a]	12/20	15/20

[a] With complete Freund's adjuvant.
[b] Right-hand figure = no. of animals used; left-hand figure = no. of positive responses.
[c] Minimal changes.
SOURCE: Taken in part from Rose *et al.* [33a].

of sacrifice. Lerman was unable to immunize rabbits with thyroglobulin of the same species.

In 1956, Rose and Witebsky [17–19] reported on the production of rabbit thyroid antibodies in the rabbit (Table 73-1). In confirmation of the findings of Lerman (and in contradiction of those of Hektoen *et al.*), repeated intravenous or intradermal injection of rabbit thyroid crude extracts into rabbits did not elicit antibody formation. However, rabbits given intradermal injections of pooled rabbit thyroid crude extract emulsified with complete Freund's adjuvant developed circulating antibodies which reacted with rabbit thyroid extract, as demonstrated by complement fixation, precipitation, tanned cell hemagglutination, and passive cutaneous anaphylaxis. The antisera were specific for thyroid extract, not reacting with saline extracts of other rabbit organs or with rabbit erythrocytes. They cross-reacted with saline extracts of thyroid glands of certain other species, such as hog, dog, and horse [20], although absorption with these foreign thyroid extracts did not remove a measurable amount of rabbit antibody to rabbit thyroid extract (the homologous antigen). Thyroidectomized rabbits given injections of an extract of their own thyroid glands produced thyroid antibodies, and these antisera reacted with saline extracts of the rabbits' own thyroid glands. The serum factor had the usual characteristics of antibody. It migrated in the γ-globulin fraction in starch block electrophoresis [21] as well as in immunoelectrophoresis. It was stable when heated to 56° C. for 30 minutes, although it was destroyed by treatment at 65 to 70° C. for 30 minutes, in contrast to ordinary heteroantibody, which is more stable under these conditions. On the basis of this evidence, the antibodies seemed to fulfill the criteria of autoantibodies.

To determine the localization of the antigen, frozen sections of thyroid glands of normal rabbits were exposed to sera containing rabbit autoantibodies and stained with fluorescein-conjugated goat antisreum to rabbit globulin [22]. Fluorescence appeared in the colloid and extended into the adjoining portions of epithelial cells. By immunoelectrophoretic analysis of rabbit thyroid extract, the antigen responsible for precipitation was found to be an α-globulin immunochemically identical with thyroglobulin [14]. Finally, injection of partially purified rabbit thyroglobulin with Freund's adjuvant was even more potent on a weight basis in eliciting autoantibody formation than was whole thyroid extract [23].

In addition to producing circulating anti-

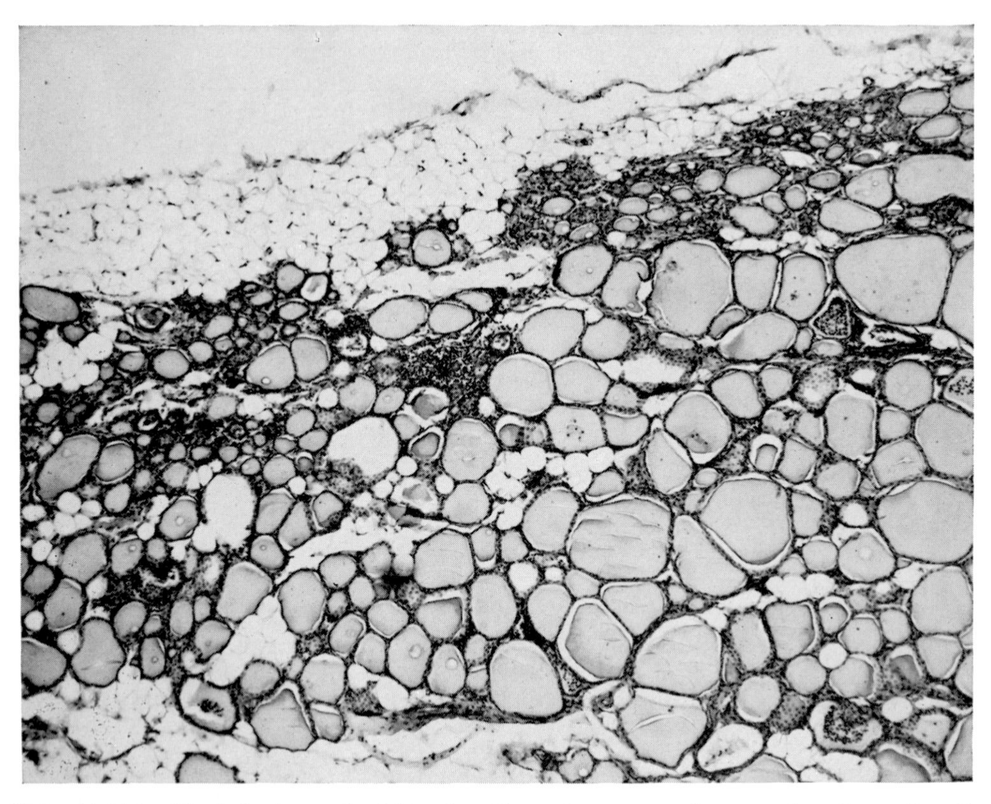

Fig. 73-1. Rabbit 879. Injections of rabbit thyroid crude extract plus complete Freund's adjuvant were given on three occasions in 20 weeks. At the time of sacrifice, it had a hemagglutination titer of 196,000 and positive skin reaction to rabbit thyroid extract. Inflammatory changes are especially pronounced close to the capsule of the thyroid. There are, however, a few cellular infiltrations within some colloid follicles. The rest of the thyroid gland appears normal. (Hematoxylin-eosin; ×73.) (We are indebted to Dr. K. Terplan, State University of New York at Buffalo, for histological interpretations of Figs. 73-1 to 73-4.)

body, the immunized rabbits gave direct skin reactions of the delayed type to thyroid extract or thyroglobulin, although the reaction did not necessarily correlate with the antibody titer of the serum [24]. After induction of autoantibody formation, the thyroid glands of the rabbits were examined immunologically and histologically [19]. A considerable reduction in content of available thyroid-specific antigen was found. From the histological point of view, obvious changes occurred in the thyroid glands of rabbits given injections of homologous thyroid extract. Areas of dense cellular inflammation were seen around the follicles, made up primarily of lymphoid cells and eosinophils. Sometimes desquamated epithelial cells and macrophages were present in the colloid itself. In extreme cases the follicular pattern was obscured, with great accumulations of large and small lymphocytes forming lymphoid follicles. The follicles themselves were occasionally disrupted, with inflammation in the interstitium. Focal fibrosis was also encountered (Figs. 73-1 to 73-4).*

The dog and the guinea pig, each immunized with homologous thyroid extract, showed similar immunological responses and histological evidence of thyroiditis of a similar pattern [25] (Table 73-1), occasionally even in the absence of demonstrable circulating antibody. In the rat, Jones and Roitt [26] observed basically the same process. Severely affected thyroids were greatly enlarged, and sometimes inflammation around the thyroid gland led to fusion of the gland with surrounding struc-

* *Editor's comment:* Hung *et al.* (*Acta Endocr.* 40: 297, 1962) studied the function of rabbit thyroid glands during experimentally induced thyroiditis. Radioiodine uptake was reduced in the thyroiditis animals, as was responsiveness to thyroid-stimulating hormone (TSH). Serum radioactivity was higher, and this was almost all in butanol-extractable form.—J. H. V.

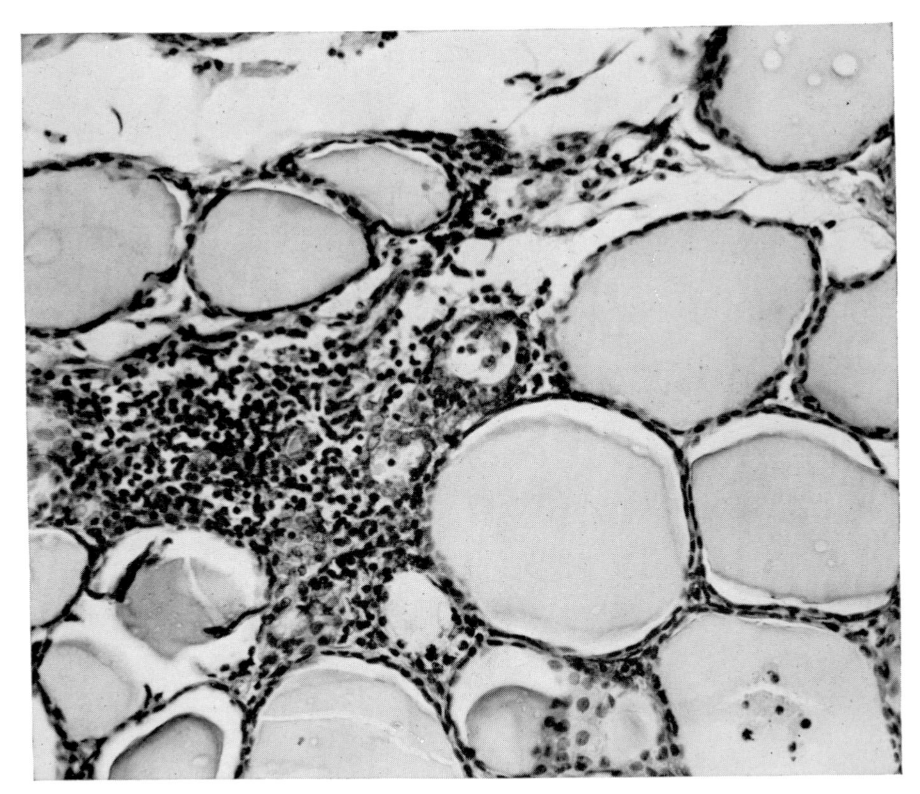

Fig. 73-2. Rabbit 879. Higher magnification shows dense focal lymphocytic infiltration and a few macrophages in the small colloid follicles at the upper border of the infiltrates. (×295)

tures. In some instances, thyroiditis was present in one lobe of the thyroid early in immunization, whereas the other lobe, removed several weeks later, was only slightly inflamed, suggesting that the process might be reversible. Metzgar and Grace [27] produced experimental thyroiditis by autoimmunization of mice. Since these original descriptions, several groups of investigators have reproduced these findings in experimental animals (Table 73-2).

Instead of homologous thyroid crude extract, extracts of beef, human, dog, and hog thyroid were injected into rabbits, using the Freund adjuvant method; these thyroids cross-reacted immunologically with the rabbit material [28]. Organ-specific thyroid antibodies appeared which were capable of reacting with rabbit thyroid extract, as demonstrated by tanned cell hemagglutination and precipitation. Quantitative absorption tests indicated that only a small amount of the total antibody to homologous thyroid antigen used for immunization could cross-react with rabbit thyroid extract. In Ouchterlony tests [21], a reaction of partial identity was obtained when antihog thyroid rabbit serum was tested simultaneously with hog thyroid and rabbit thyroid extracts, demonstrating that only a part of the antibody reacted with thyroid antigen prepared from the rabbit itself.

When these rabbit antisera to foreign thyroid extracts were tested with rabbit thyroid by complement fixation, no reaction was obtained [20], despite the presence of precipitins and hemagglutination antibodies, sometimes in high titers. The animals did not develop positive skin reactions to rabbit thyroglobulin, although they reacted strongly to the foreign thyroid extract used for immunization. Finally, there was no histological evidence of damage in the thyroids of the immunized animals. Other rabbits were given an intensive course of intravenous injections with hog thyroglobulin. After several months, some of these animals developed complement-fixing antibodies to rabbit thyroid extract but no demonstrable dermal sensitivity to this antigen. Minor focal areas of lymphoid infiltration developed in their thyroid glands [25] (Table 73-1).

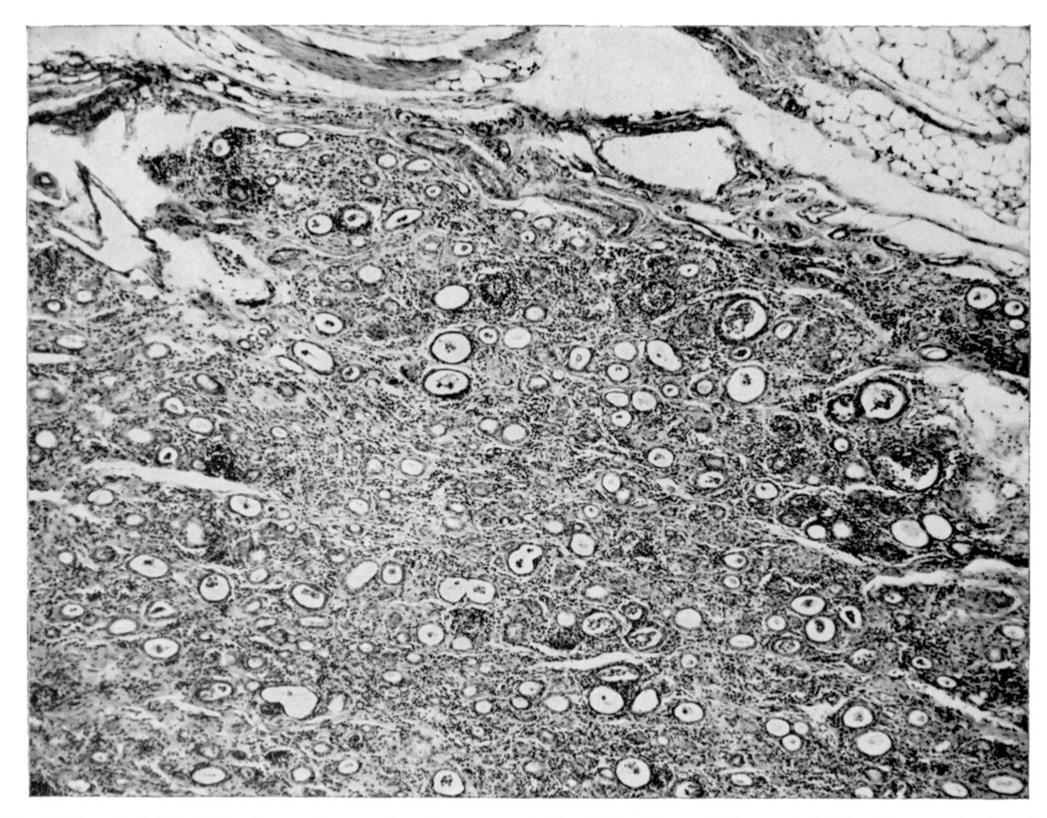

Fig. 73-3. Rabbit 878. Same immunizations as rabbit 879 (Figs. 73-1 and 73-2). Hemagglutination titer was also 196,000 and the skin reaction positive. Fairly uniform dense inflammatory infiltration with slight tendency to fibrosis is seen especially in the center of the picture. Cellular exudates occur in the lumina of several thyroid follicles. (×73)

Intravenous inoculation of rabbits with rabbit thyroid extract failed to elicit autoantibody production or thyroid inflammation. Simultaneous injection into the rabbit of bacterial lipopolysaccharide did not affect the outcome [24]. Neither surgical trauma nor administration of radioactive iodine was able to initiate an autoimmune reaction. Injection of rabbit thyroid extract mixed with complete Freund's adjuvant led to autoantibody formation and experimental thyroiditis in almost all rabbits tested. If acid-fast bacilli were omitted from the Freund mixture, titers of circulating antibody were significantly lower, and only occasionally did lesions develop in the animals' thyroids. Rabbits were also inoculated with alum-precipitated rabbit thyroid extract. Most of them developed complement-fixing and hemagglutinating antibodies in their sera. Skin test reactions were generally absent or very weak, and none showed evidence of thyroid damage. The circulating antibodies were sometimes present in high titers for long periods. Immunochemically, they seemed to be identical to antibodies produced by the intradermal-adjuvant method [14]. Addition of killed acid-fast bacilli to the alum-precipitated adjuvant increased strikingly the intensity of dermal hypersensitivity to thyroglobulin. About one half of the animals given such injections had typical lesions of thyroiditis (Table 73-1).

Using a strain of inbred guinea pigs to increase the uniformity of the response, McMaster *et al.* [29] noted evidence of thyroiditis as early as five days after injection of guinea pig thyroid extract and complete Freund's adjuvant. After seven weeks, severe thyroid damage was uniformly present, and the degree of thyroiditis correlated closely with titers of circulating antibody, as measured by a bentonite flocculation test. However, at later stages of immunization, a much closer correspondence was found between thyroid damage and delayed hypersensitivity to thyroid extract.

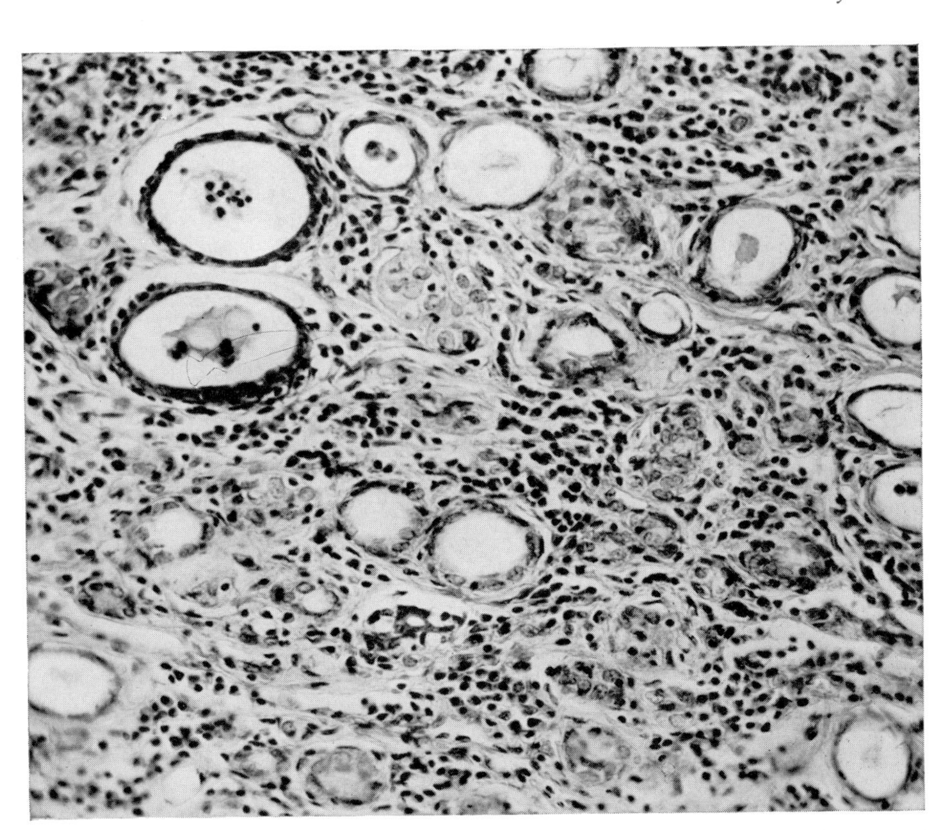

Fig. 73-4. Rabbit 878. Higher magnification shows uniform interstitial infiltration, consisting of numerous plasma cells. Outline of many of the small colloid follicles is obscured, being replaced by inflammatory infiltrations. There are vacuolization of colloid in several follicles and infiltration by leukocytes and macrophages. (×295)

Miescher *et al.* [30] compared responses of guinea pigs given injections of large and small amounts of picrylated guinea pig thyroglobulin plus Freund's adjuvant. They found no significant differences in skin test reactivity to thyroglobulin or in the incidence or intensity of thyroiditis in the two groups. However, circulating antibody titers, as measured by tanned cell hemagglutination, were markedly lower in animals receiving the smaller amounts of picryl-substituted antigen.

These experiments indicate that it is possible to dissociate the autoimmune response to thyroglobulin into hemagglutinating or precipitating antibody, complement-fixing antibody, specific delayed hypersensitivity, and thyroidal damage itself. By manipulation of the immunization procedures, one can favor one or another component of the response. By intravenous injection of 6-mercaptopurine as rabbits were receiving intradermal or intramuscular injections of rabbit thyroid extract in complete Freund's adjuvant, Rose *et al.* [30a] were able to suppress almost completely the development of thyroid lesions. Skin test reactions, however, were as strong as those in control animals, and circulating antibody titers only slightly lower. These results emphasize that the relationship among circulating antibody, delayed hypersensitivity, and immunopathological change is not necessarily simple or direct. Statistical comparisons have been made among these variables [24]. They reveal a high correlation coefficient of 0.76 between intensity of skin sensitivity and pathological alterations in the thyroid gland. A lower but still significant correlation was found between titers of complement fixation and pathology. Only slight correspondences emerged from comparisons of hemagglutination titers with pathological changes or skin test reactions.

Specific delayed hypersensitivity is closely associated with direct action of lymphoid cells rather than with circulating humoral antibody, due to the presence of so-called cell-

TABLE 73-2. Production of Experimental Autoimmune Thyroiditis

Rabbit		
Witebsky and Rose	1956	*J. Immun.* 76:408
Milcu *et al.*	1959	*Rumanian Med. Rev.* (Jan.–Mar.), p. 35
Beierwaltes *et al.*	1961	*Endocrinology* 69:863
David and Holborow	1961	*Lancet* 1:83
Porter and Fennell	1961	*New Eng. J. Med.* 265:830
Chandler *et al.*	1962	*Pediatrics* 29:961
Guinea pig		
Witebsky *et al.*	1957	*J.A.M.A.* 164:1439
Miescher *et al.*	1961	*Proc. Soc. Exp. Biol. Med.* 107:12
McMaster *et al.*	1961	*J. Exp. Med.* 113:611
Felix-Davies and Waksman	1961	*Arthritis Rheum.* 4:416
Sclare and Taylor	1961	*J. Path. Bact.* 82:29
Rat		
Jones and Roitt	1961	*Brit. J. Exp. Path.* 42:546
Metzgar and Grace	1961	*Fed. Proc.* 20:39
Mouse		
Metzgar and Grace	1961	*Fed. Proc.* 20:39
Dog		
Witebsky *et al.*	1957	*J.A.M.A.* 164:1439
Monkey		
Rose *et al.*	1965	*Ann. N.Y. Acad. Sci.* 124:201
Chicken		
Jankovic and Mitrovic	1963	*Nature* (London) 200:186

bound antibody. Passive transfer of even large amounts of antibody-containing serum and treatment of thyroid cell cultures have not produced visible cellular damage. Attention therefore has turned to the lymphoid cell itself as the pathogenic agent. In an effort to distinguish circulating from cell-bound antibody, Rose *et al.* [24, 31] constructed chambers of small pore-size molecular filters. One lobe of rabbit thyroid gland was removed, minced, and implanted in the chamber, the contralateral lobe being left untouched as control. The animals were then immunized with pooled rabbit thyroid extract and adjuvant until circulating antibodies appeared in their sera. The control lobe examined at this time showed typical changes of thyroiditis. In the chamber were seen a few thyroid follicles surrounded and invaded by lymphoid cells. It was not clear whether the cells passed through the membrane or differentiated *in situ.* In either case, they were strongly attracted to the target thyroid cells.

In preliminary communications, Felix-Davies and Waksman [32] and Goodman [33] reported that they were able to transfer experimental thyroiditis betwen inbred guinea pigs. They gave animals injections of homologous thyroid extract and adjuvant, then removed lymph nodes and spleen early in immunization before circulating antibody could be demonstrated by passive cutaneous anaphylaxis. Cell suspensions from these lymphoid tissues were inoculated intravenously into normal recipients of the same strain, in which slight to severe thyroid inflammation subsequently developed. These observations, which still need confirmation, assign to the lymphoid cells a crucial role in tissue damage. However, it must be remembered that the transferred cells may survive and proliferate in the histocompatible recipient, where they may form humoral as well as cell-bound factors.

To study the immunological capacities of lymph node cells from autosensitized rabbits, Rose *et al.* [24] cultured explanted cells *in vitro.* The explants formed specific autoantibody during growth over a period of two to three weeks. The production of antibody was stimulated by brief mixing of the cells with diluted thyroid extract before culture was initiated. Sometimes exposure to larger amounts of antigen *in vitro* actually inhibited antibody formation [33a]. A method for culturing follicular epithelial cells of the rabbit thyroid gland was developed by Kite [34]. Treatment of these cell cultures with serum of rabbits that had undergone active immunization to rabbit thyroid extract produced no visible cytotoxic reaction [31], thereby differentiating experimentally produced thyroiditis from human chronic thyroiditis in which cytotoxic antibody is frequently found. The thyroid cell cultures were then treated with suspensions of lymph node cells from autosensitized rabbits. Attachment of the lymphoid cells to thyroid cells was observed sometimes, followed by destruction of the thyroid monolayer. However, lymph node cells from rabbits inoculated with unrelated antigens such as bovine or human serum proteins produced similar effects, although quantitative comparison indicated that these control cells were less active. This quantitative difference was erased when cell-free extracts of the lymphoid cells were used. It was also found that radioisotope-labeled antigen was specifically taken up by lymph node cells from sensitized animals. This ability could be conferred on normal lymph node cells by previous treatment with serum of rabbits containing thyroid autoantibody, presumably due to the presence of a cytophilic antibody. One might conclude that "activated" lymphoid cells are capable of producing tissue destruction, but that the all-important factors responsible for the striking specificity of the inflammation must still be defined.

There are several important differences between chronic thyroiditis in man and thyroiditis as described thus far in the experimental animal. In the rabbit and most other animals, antibodies to thyroglobulin can be demonstrated by complement fixation as well as by precipitation or indirect agglutination methods. Thyroglobulin autoantibodies in man (discussed later in this chapter) fix complement very poorly, if at all. However, a second antibody can be found in certain human patients which reacts with microsomal particulates of human thyroid tissue. Circulating antibody is also found with direct cytotoxic effect on viable human thyroid cells in tissue culture.

When rhesus monkeys were given injections of homologous thyroid extract in complete Freund's adjuvant [30a], autoantibodies to monkey thyroglobulin developed, as demonstrated by the tanned cell hemagglutination test. No complement fixation was observed with this antibody. Later in the course of immunization, a second, distinct antibody directed to thyroid microsomes was detected by complement fixation tests. At the same time, cytotoxic effects could be produced by treating monkey thyroid cell cultures with the monkey antisera.

When thyroid tissue from these autosensitized monkeys was examined histologically, extremely severe inflammatory changes were observed. These experiments suggest that from both immunological and pathological points of view, experimental thyroiditis produced in the rhesus monkey resembles human chronic thyroiditis even more closely than does the experimentally induced disease in lower animals.

LOCALIZATION OF THYROGLOBULIN

Taking advantage of potent and specific antisera, Hektoen and Schulhof [15] observed that in the normal individual thyroglobulin is not present in the blood. For many years following this observation, the physiological significance of thyroglobulin as the actual thyroid hormone was debated. When radioactive iodine became generally available, it was possible to determine that iodide is taken up from the blood by thyroid epithelial cells where it is incorporated as organically bound iodine into thyroglobulin. It is deposited as such in the colloid of the thyroid follicles. Thyroglobulin is later hydrolyzed by proteolytic enzymes of the gland to yield free thyroxine. Thyroxine and similar iodinated amino acids are the forms of thyroid hormone released by the thyroid which actually circulate in the blood.

Hektoen and Schulhof [15] also examined the blood of patients with various thyroid diseases. In contrast to the findings with normal human sera, they demonstrated free thyroglobulin in the thyroid veins, using, as a test, precipitation with specific antihuman thyroglobulin rabbit serum. Of five patients with positive reactions, three had thyroid adenomas and two had hypertrophic glands. Lerman [16] also observed that thyroglobulin may leak into the circulation after surgery, but it rapidly disappeared from the bloodstream. Using the sensitive test of inhibition of tanned cell hemagglutination, Hjort [35] demonstrated leakage of thyroid antigen in many patients undergoing thyroidectomy.

More recently, the presence of an unusual iodinated protein was observed in the serum of many patients with thyroiditis by Owen and McConahey [36] and also by Stemmermann [37]. DeGroot *et al.* [38] extracted a low molecular weight iodoprotein from both thyroid tissue and serum of certain patients with thyroiditis. They suggested the possibility that it may represent a partial degradation product of thyroglobulin usually further metabolized in the thyroid gland.

Metzger *et al.* [39] treated beef thyroglobulin with trypsin. At its early stages, degradation produced three or four precipitating antigenic fragments. Further digestion led to smaller fragments which did not precipitate but which combined with antibody, as shown by inhibition of precipitation. Using rabbit antisera it was not possible to demonstrate antibody to "hidden determinants" uncovered during proteolysis. In this connection, it should be pointed out that Stokinger and Heidelberger [6] calculated for rabbit antiserum to human thyroglobulin a molecular ratio of antibody to antigen of 40 : 1 to 60 : 1. Similar measurements made by Shulman and Witebsky [40], using human autoantibodies to the same antigen, gave a ratio of about 2 : 1 to 6 : 1. These findings suggest that autoantibodies are directed to a more limited portion of the thyroglobulin molecule than are heteroantibodies.

The experiments described indicate that thyroglobulin as such does not normally occur in the bloodstream. Under abnormal conditions, however, the presence of thyroglobulin or antigenic fragments of thyroglobulin may be detected. The suggestion has been offered that the autoantigenic potentiality of thyroglobulin is due, in part at least, to its seclusion from antibody-forming centers. The possible significance of physiologically or genetically produced defects of thyroid integrity in initiating autoimmune responses in man is discussed later.

CLINICAL IMMUNOLOGY OF THYROID DISEASE IN MAN

After Witebsky and Rose [18] demonstrated changes similar to Hashimoto's disease in one lobe of the thyroid gland of a rabbit "immunized" with thyroglobulin from the opposite lobe, they searched for antibodies to thyroglobulin in patients with this disease. In 1957 they and their co-workers [23] reported that the sera of 12 of 18 patients had such antibodies.

In 1953, Fromm *et al.* [41] found significantly elevated values for serum γ-globulin. Others then noted this electrophoretic change in the serum and also demonstrated positive results of colloidal gold, thymol turbidity, and cephalin flocculation tests in thyroid disease.

In 1956, Roitt *et al.* [42] suggested that the serum abnormalities might represent an immunological response, having detected precipitin in the sera of seven of nine patients with Hashimoto's disease by layering human thyroglobulin over patient's serum [43]. In a relatively short time, various workers reported the detection of antithyroid antibodies (AAB) by the tanned red blood cell hemagglutination, complement fixation and precipitin tests.

It soon became evident that there is a discrepancy of results of the three most common methods of demonstrating AAB—the hemagglutination test using thyroglobulin-coated tanned cells, the complement fixation test, and the precipitin test. In general, the hemagglutination test proved to be the most sensitive, providing positive results in clinical testing in at least three times as many cases as did the precipitin test [44]. Early results in histologically proved cases of Hashimoto's disease suggested that precipitin tests were not commonly positive until the tanned cell titers were 1 : 250,000 or above [45], but our own experience indicates that sera with tanned cell titers as low as 1 : 1,000 or 1 : 2,000 are likely to give precipitation. Complement-fixing (CF) antibodies were not regularly present until the tanned cell titer reached a level of 1 : 2,500. At tanned cell titers of 1 : 2,500,000, both CF and precipitating antibodies were usually present, but it should be kept in mind that in human thyroiditis hemagglutination (or precipitation) and complement fixation are separate reactions caused by separate antigens and that, consequently, a true correlation cannot exist. Even so, in routine testing of sera of patients with Hashimoto's disease, the relative sensitivity of the three tests might loosely be stated to be: tanned cell, 1,000; CF, 100; and precipitin, 1.

ANTIBODIES

It was soon found that the discrepancies among the three tests were not simply a matter of their relative sensitivity, but that they varied in their ability to detect antibodies to different thyroid antigens. At present, three thyroid antigens have been fairly well defined: thyroglobulin, second antigen of colloid, and thyroid cell microsomes.

Thyroglobulin Antibodies. In most sera, thyroglobulin antibodies are of the normal 7S type, but some 19S precipitins have been reported. Thyroglobulin antibodies rarely fix complement and can produce passive cutaneous anaphylaxis in guinea pigs but not generalized anaphylaxis. Figure 73-5 shows the pattern of fluorescence when fluorescein-conjugated antibody to thyroglobulin from a patient reacts with the colloid of a normal thyroid.

Antibodies to Second Antigen of Thyroid Colloid. The sera of a small percentage of patients with Hashimoto's struma give negative results in the tanned cell and complement fixation tests but do stain the colloid of alcohol-fixed thyroid sections. The fluorescence antibody technique produces a pattern distinct from that obtained with thyroglobulin antibodies. The antigen has been shown to differ from thyroglobulin in its behavior in diethylaminoethanyl cellulose chromatography. It occurs in normal and pathological glands and contains no iodine [47]. Figure 73-6 shows the localization of fluorescence attached to this antibody in the colloid region.

Microsomal Antibodies. Most Hashimoto sera fix complement with extracts of thyroid glands from patients with Graves' disease. The antigen has been localized to the microsomal fraction of thyroid homogenates and appears to be intimately associated with the membranous component of the subcellular structures. Fluorescent complement-fixing antibodies to microsomes give diffuse staining to the epithelial cytoplasm of unfixed frozen thyroid sections (Fig. 73-7). Fluorescent cytoplasmic staining correlates well with the presence of the factor in Hashimoto serum previously shown to be cytotoxic to monolayer cultures of trypsinized human thyroid gland [48] (Fig. 73-8). The cytotoxic serum-factor has all the properties of immune cytolysin.

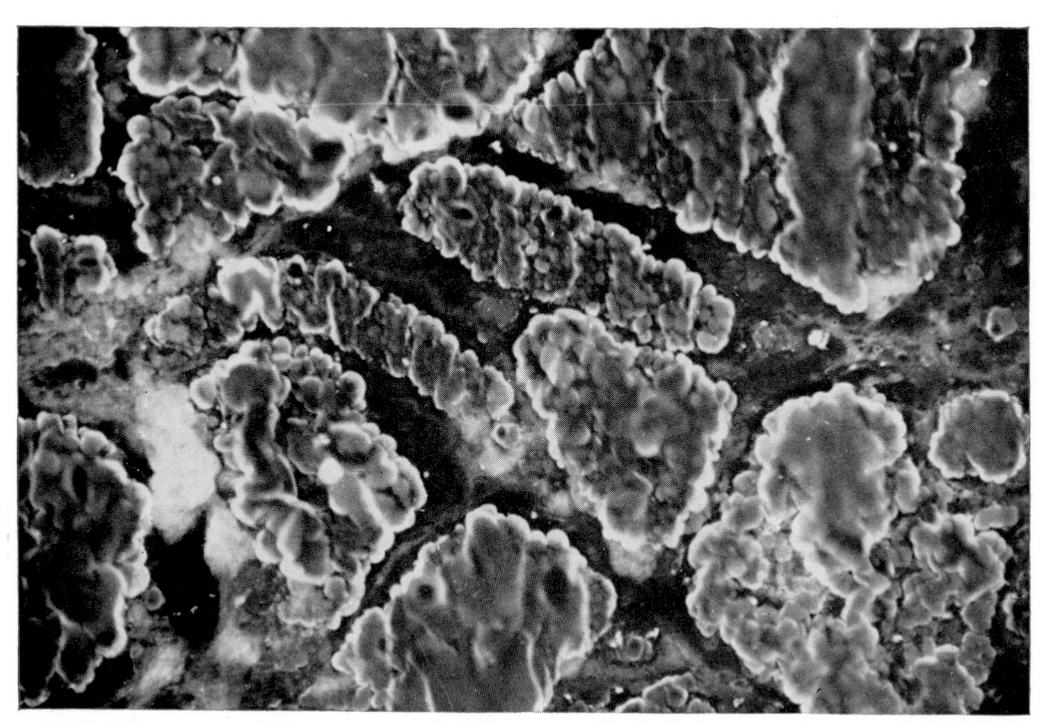

Fig. 73-5. Fluorescent staining with thyroglobulin precipitins. Frozen section of human thyroid fixed in alcohol and treated successively with serum from a Hashimoto patient followed by fluorescein-conjugated antihuman γ-globulin. A floccular pattern is seen in the colloid spaces. (Figs. 73-5 to 73-7, courtesy Drs. Doniach and Roitt, Middlesex Hospital Medical School, London.)

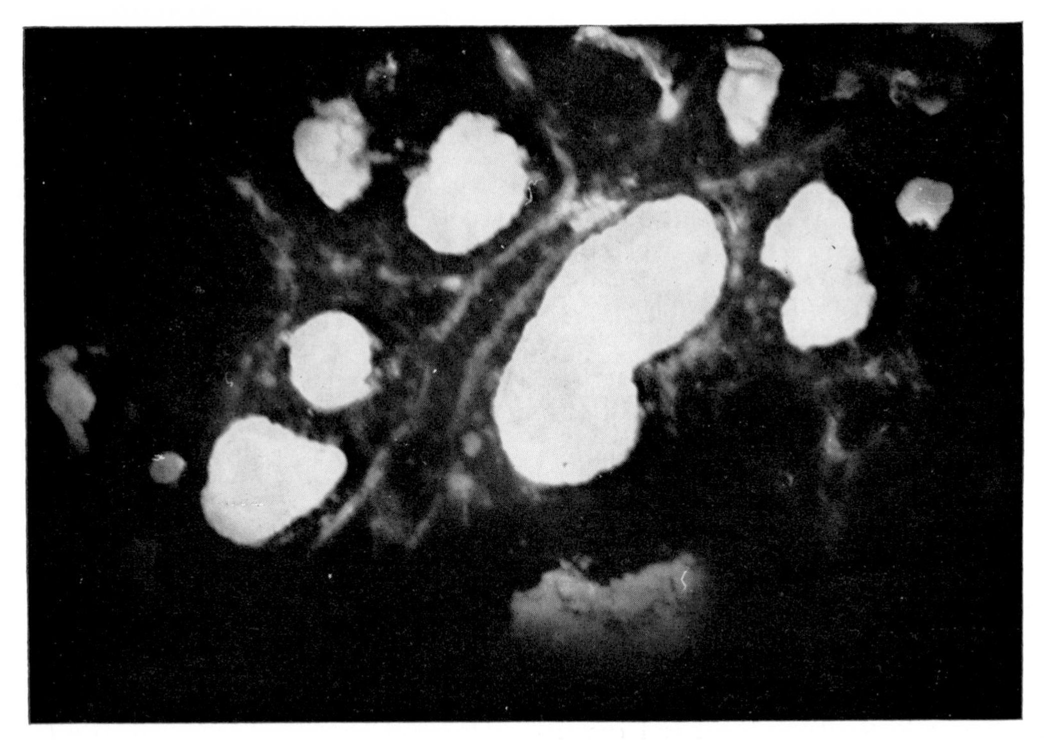

Fig. 73-6. Fluorescent staining with antibodies to the second colloid antigen. Fixed thyroid section treated as Figure 73-5. Colloid shows uniform staining, contrasting with that obtained with thyroglobulin precipitins.

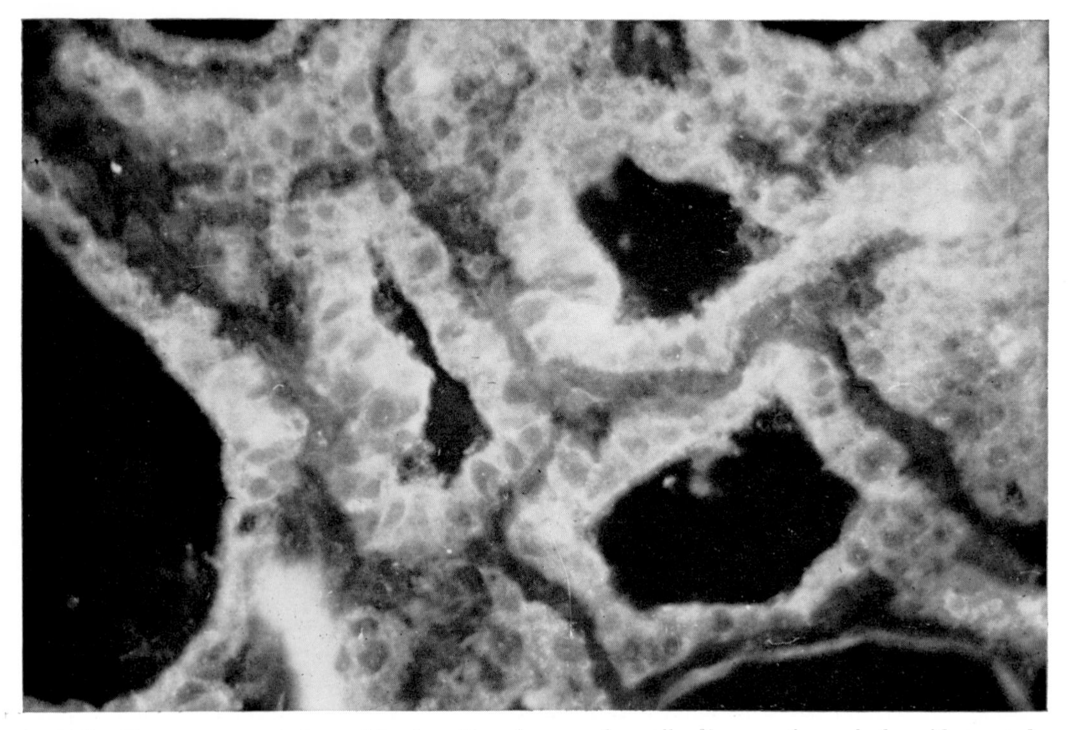

Fig. 73-7. Fluorescent staining with thyroid microsomal antibodies; section of thyroid treated as described for Figure 73-5. Fluorescence is localized to the cytoplasm of the acinar epithelial cells. Nuclei are unstained and colloid is leached out.

The antibody nature of the factor is shown by its localization in the γ-globulin fraction of the serum, its complement dependency, and its organ and species specificity. The cytotoxic phenomenon has been thought to involve the same microsomal immune system as the complement fixation test since most complement-fixing sera are cytotoxic and titers in both tests tend to parallel each other, but there are exceptions: sera which contain high titers of cytotoxic factors may contain little or no complement-fixing antibody, and vice versa. Microsomes from Graves' disease thyroid glands absorb out the cytotoxic activity of Hashimoto sera.

WORKING HYPOTHESIS OF ETIOLOGY AND PATHOGENESIS

It is generally believed that the development of antithyroid antibodies starts with the release of antigen from the thyroid gland that ordinarily is not found in the circulation. An "immune" response to this antigen results in a superimposed inflammatory infiltrate in the thyroid gland.

If the release of stored thyroid hormone, colloid or thyroglobulin, is sudden, a temporary reduction of thyroid function follows, as demonstrated by a diminished ability of the thyroid gland to concentrate I^{131}. This decrease of function of the gland may be caused directly by the damaging agent that produces the release of thyroid antigen or indirectly through inhibition of release of thyroid stimulating hormone (TSH) by the increased amounts of thyroid hormone appearing in the circulation.

When the phase of relatively acute inhibition of thyroid function ends, the pituitary responds to a subsequent insufficiency of normally iodinated, metabolically active thyroid hormone. Increased TSH production stimulates the thyroid gland to increased function and hyperplasia and the emptying of stored hormone from follicles. At this stage, the thyroidal radioactive iodine uptake may be increased and the gland may be hyperplastic at biopsy. The "defect" may persist permanently but be so mild that chronic hypertrophy, hyperplasia, and plasma cell and lymphocyte infiltration may be permanent but mild and nonprogressive. Or the defect may be severe enough, or become worse, so that all of the foregoing processes are progressive to the point of functional failure or "exhaustion" or "death" of the thyroid gland.

The initiating release of thyroid antigen may conceivably be caused by congenital thyroidal defects, by acute virus or irradiation thyroiditis, by various abnormalities associated with hyperplasia, or by thyroid surgery.

Congenital Defects. The initiating event could be an inherited or mutation-induced biochemical defect in the thyroid gland of the newborn. The familial occurrence of Hashimoto's disease was first described by Dunning in 1959. Hall *et al.* [49] demonstrated that the tendency to develop antibodies to thyroid is inherited as a codominant characteristic. The description of Hashimoto's disease in both members of two pairs of uniovular twins has been taken as further evidence of a genetic predisposition to this disease. DeGroot *et al.* [38] found goiter in 5 of 14 members of a family in which the histological picture of Hashimoto's disease was documented in 3 members and a butanol-insoluble iodinated protein was demonstrated in abnormally large amounts in 7 subjects tested. They found this abnormal iodoprotein not only in serum but also in thyroid gland and suggested that its increase in the thyroid gland in Hashimoto's disease could be a reflection of decreased thyroglobulin synthesis with iodination of an alternate protein. Its presence in the circulation might result from leakage through a fragmented thyroid cell basement membrane known to be present in thyroid autoimmune disease [50].

Acute Thyroiditis. The initiating event could also be a virus or irradiation thyroiditis with resultant necrosis and release of antigen or the persistence of a permanent biochemical defect after the acute virus infection had passed.

Hyperplasia. Any condition leading to increased function and hyperplasia of the thyroid gland could be considered an initiating event, since all the conditions in which the abnormal iodoprotein has been found in the serum have been associated with pronounced hyperplasia of the gland. Vickery and Hamlin [51] in 1961 found that hyperplasia of the thyroid seems to precede the development of Hashimoto's disease. Figure 73-9 shows the early hyperplasia and plasma cell and lymphoid infiltration in one of our patients who had a subtotal thyroidectomy in 1943 for suspected,

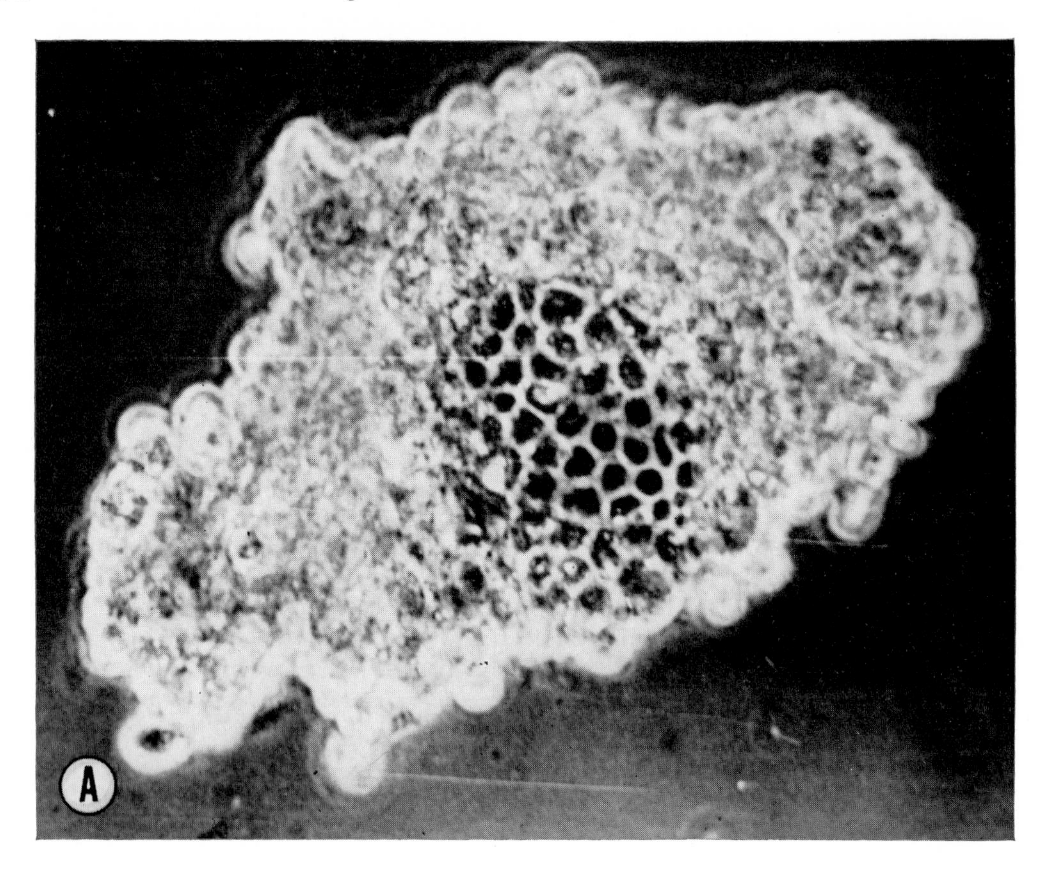
A

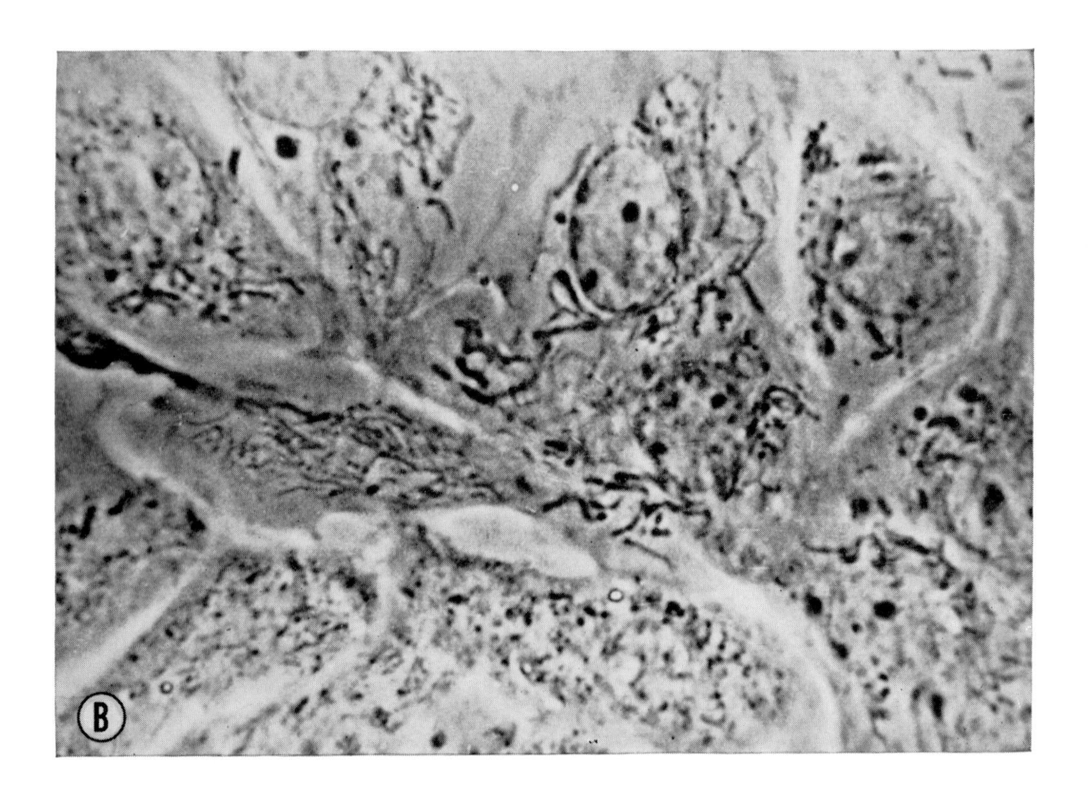
B

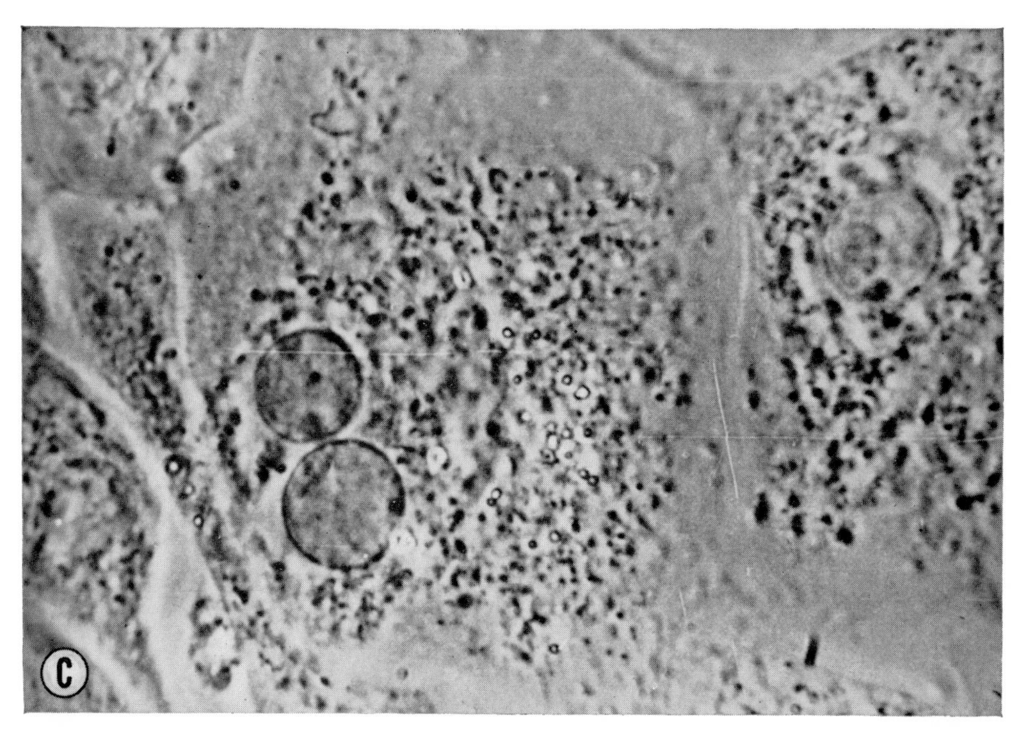

Fig. 73-8. (*A*) Clumps of thyroid cells after one hour of trypsinization. (*B*) Early stage of cytotoxic action of microsomal antibodies when mitochrondia are beginning to thicken. (*C*) Later stage, after exposure to cytotoxic serum, when mitochrondia have lost their filamentous shape and nuclear membrane has become opaque and nuclei have stopped rotating. The cells are not viable after the first half-hour of exposure.

but not documented, Graves' disease. In 1957 he was referred to us because he had a goiter, myxedema, serum protein-bound iodine (PBI) content of 2.9 μg. per 100 ml., and 24-hour thyroid I^{131} uptake of 11 percent. He had the typical clinical picture of Hashimoto's struma, with a tanned cell antithyroid antibody titer of 32,000. The myxedema and goiter disappeared on administration of 0.2 gm. of desiccated thyroid per day.

Common causes of hyperplasia of the thyroid gland include iodine deficiency, a biochemical defect in the manufacture of thyroid hormone, and Graves' disease.

Thyroid Surgery. The initiating event may be surgical thyroidectomy. If operations on the thyroid gland cause a leakage of thyroglobulin, autoimmunization might follow. Hjort [35] performed a hemagglutination-inhibition test for detection of thyroglobulin in the sera of 132 normal blood donors and found traces of thyroglobulin in only one serum. Thyroid surgery was followed by leakage of thyroglobulin into the circulation in 24 of 29 patients who had no thyroglobulin antibody in their sera before operation. Only 1 of these patients had traces of thyroglobulin antibody one month after surgery. We [52] were unable to demonstrate, by the tanned cell hemagglutination test, any significant change in antithyroid antibody titers over a period of months after thyroid surgery. Thus it seems unlikely that thyroid surgery is a common initial incident in the development of thyroid autoimmune disease.

THE CLINICAL DISEASE

ACUTE THYROIDITIS

De Quervain's thyroiditis (granulomatous thyroiditis, acute or subacute thyroiditis, virus thyroiditis) classically presents acutely, with diffuse rock-hard inflammatory swelling of the thyroid gland, 24-hour I^{131} uptake less than 5 percent, and increased serum concentration of PBI.

The patient may awaken with painful swelling and tenderness in the thyroid gland with radiation to the jaw or ears. Fever is the rule.

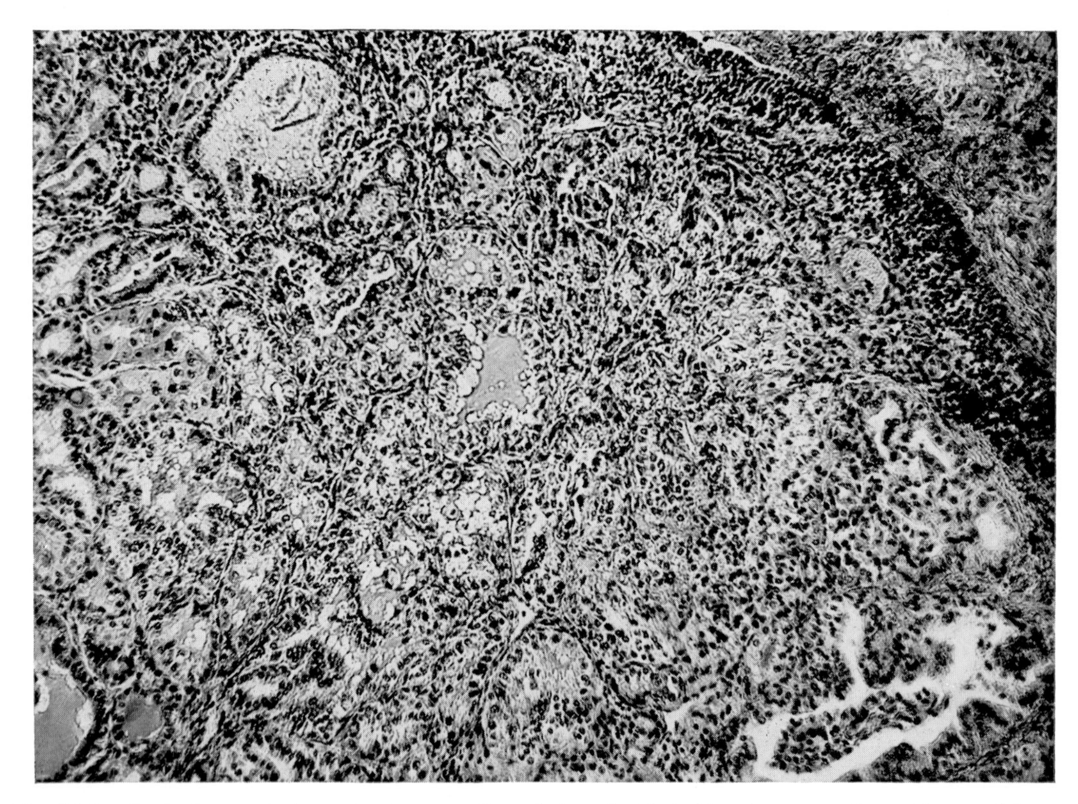

Fig. 73-9. Early hyperplasia and plasma cell and lymphoid infiltration seen in a 42-year-old man in 1943. In 1957, goiter recurred, with typical myxedema and tanned cell antithyroid antibody titer of 1:32,000. Myxedema and goiter disappeared on administration of 0.2 gm. of desiccated thyroid a day, characteristic of Hashimoto's struma.

With less acute onset, the patient may complain only of a sore throat that cannot be explained by examination of the oral pharynx. An "earache" associated with "sore throat" may represent referred pain from the thyroid gland. If the inflammation is severe, the discomfort may be accentuated by swallowing and by movements of the head. Usually the thyromegaly is discovered first in one lobe, more commonly the right than in the left. The clinically involved area of the gland may migrate elsewhere in the same lobe or to the opposite lobe within one day. When the inflammation begins to recede, resolution may be spotty at first, with the result that rock-hard nodules may now be seen and felt. One nodule may persist for months with no clinical signs of inflammation. Scintillation scanning with I^{131} will demonstrate that this nodule is radioactively "cold." Usually, the white blood cell count is normal but the sedimentation rate elevated during the acute stages. Cortisone administration results in a dramatic resolution of symptoms and signs within three days, but the dosage must be tapered off slowly over a period of three to four months if persistence or relapse of the disease is to be avoided.

Pathologically, there is disruption of normal follicular epithelium with residual colloid apparently undergoing progressive breakdown and phagocytosis surrounded by a zone of histiocytes and foreign-body giant cells [53]. The inflammatory cells which surround the colloid in some follicles may be partially or wholly composed of polymorphonuclear leukocytes, so that microabscesses are formed. Later, a fairly pronounced tuberculoid response occurs, with almost complete disappearance of colloid and somewhat more extensive inflammatory fibrosis. The pathological picture is compatible with the assumption that acute thyroiditis acts as an initiating event for the acute release of antigen. In the recovery stage of acute thyroiditis, I^{131} uptake commonly rises to supernormal levels; this functional change fits in with the morphological change of depletion of colloid and hyperplasia. Since several viruses have been proved to be associated with acute thyroiditis, it is logical to think that virus thyroiditis might be a common initiating event in the most classic thyroid autoimmune disease, Hashimoto's struma. Felix-Davies [54] in 1958 first observed that autoimmunization to purified human thyroglobulin took place after the acute stage of thyroiditis in a patient who had mumps thyroiditis, as demonstrated by hemagglutination tests for mumps virus antibody and biopsy of the thyroid gland.

We have observed acute thyroiditis in a group of patients seen within a period of a few months who complained only of an upper respiratory infection with "sore throat." In five families (27 individuals) in which at least 1 member eventually had classic "virus" thyroiditis—contrasted with 3 control families (18 individuals) in which at least 1 member of each family had a classic measles infection—the most notable findings were: (1) Only 1 member of each thyroiditis family had classic thyroiditis, yet 2 other members of the first family, 1 additional member of the second family, 3 additional members of the third family, and none of the fourth and fifth families developed signs of inflammatory swelling of the thyroid gland. (2) Demonstrable AAB appeared in the circulation of only 1 of these individuals (and 1 other subject seen at the same time, but whose family was not in the study). (3) The AAB disappeared from the circulation within two to five months in both cases. Although cortisone was given both of these individuals, antithyroid antibodies were not demonstrated after its withdrawal. (4) Thyroglobulin was not demonstrated in the serum of any of these individuals by the hemagglutination-inhibition technique. (5) No members of the control (measles) families had any evidence of thyroid disease or thyroid autoantibodies.

These observations suggest that the occurrence of thyroiditis may be difficult to elicit by a retrospect history. The data do not present evidence, however, to support the thesis that virus thyroiditis is the most common precursor of Hashimoto's struma.

HASHIMOTO'S STRUMA (LYMPHOMATOUS THYROIDITIS)

Hashimoto's struma is the commonest of the thyroiditides, being found about six times more often in surgical thyroid specimens than acute thyroiditis. The characteristic clinical picture is asymptomatic, diffuse, symmetrical, firm to rock-hard goiter in a woman 20 to 50 years of age. The goiter has been present for an average of 2.5 years when the diagnosis is made.

Usually, patients with Hashimoto's disease have a small amount of thyroid tissue functioning at an accelerated rate, synthesizing hormone inefficiently. One of the most characteristic sets of laboratory findings at this stage is a high normal to elevated 24-hour I^{131} uptake of 37 to 53 percent, not increased by stimulation with TSH, with normal PBI value and subnormal serum butanol-extractable iodine (BEI) concentration. Most of the PBI not accounted for by the BEI is probably the iodinated protein, mentioned before, that is not metabolically active. There is a defect in organic binding of iodine, demonstrated by prompt discharge of I^{131} after the administration of potassium thiocyanate.

Later in the disease, if the thyroid gland undergoes progressive destruction, both I^{131} uptake and serum PBI fall to subnormal values and clinical hypothyroidism develops. The simultaneous development of goiter and hypothyroidism in the adult warrants the diagnosis of Hashimoto's struma until proved otherwise. The clinical diagnosis of Hashimoto's struma without resort to surgical thyroidectomy is important, because these goiters commonly shrink or disappear completely on administration of desiccated thyroid in dosage of 0.2 gm. per day.

The circulating AAB were initially thought to cause the "inflammatory" histological alterations in the thyroid gland in this disease, but this now seems unlikely or is an oversimplification. The severity of histological change in the thyroiditides is not necessarily correlated with the level of AAB, and passive transfer by means of serum has failed to produce histological alteration of the thyroid gland of the guinea pig. The initial event in experimental thyroiditis in animals seems to be a reaction of the delayed hypersensitivity type. This has been substantiated by the production of thyroiditis in guinea pigs by transfer of lymphoid cells [32]. Evidence that a delayed hypersensitivity reaction is involved in human thyroiditis is incomplete, but the resemblance of the thyroid histology in Hashimoto's disease to that of experimental thyroiditis in animals and to the tuberculin reaction

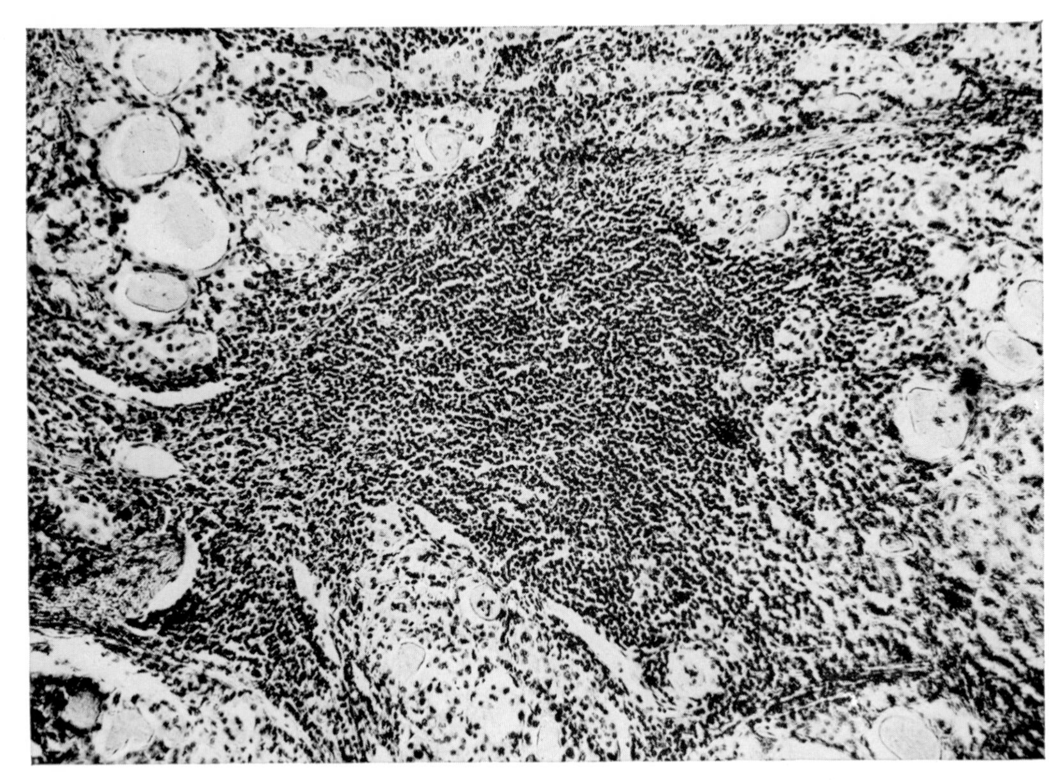

Fig. 73-10. Area of thyroiditis in a human thyroid gland affected by Hashimoto's struma.

is at least suggestive.* Figure 73-10 shows the resemblance of the histological appearance of a human thyroid gland in an early stage of Hashimoto's disease to that of experimental thyroiditis in rabbits (see Figs. 73-3 and 73-4). Skin reactions reaching a maximum of erythema and induration at 24 hours have been obtained after intradermal injections of human thyroid extracts in patients with Hashimoto's struma [33a, 46].

RIEDEL'S STRUMA (FIBROUS INVASIVE THYROIDITIS)

When Riedel's struma is carefully defined pathologically, it is the rarest of the thyroiditides, being one-thirtieth as common as Hashimoto's struma and one-fifth as common as acute thyroiditis [53]. Twenty cases were found by Woolner *et al.* [53] in a 36-year period during which approximately 42,000 thyroidectomies were performed at the Mayo Clinic, an incidence of 0.05 percent.

It has been emphasized that the goiter of Riedel's struma is usually of shorter duration at the time of diagnosis (average three to four months at the Mayo Clinic); is usually larger and harder than the goiter of Hashimoto's struma, although usually asymptomatic; occurs in females only four times more often than males whereas Hashimoto's struma occurs 56 times more commonly in females; and at operation is found to have invaded surrounding neck muscle, whereas Hashimoto's struma does not.

Rose and Royster, however, have reported a case of struma identical with Hashimoto's clinically, with demonstrable circulating AAB, which at operation was indistinguishable from Riedel's struma. We have observed an almost identical case, illustrated in Figure 73-11.

We have seen almost all gradations of adhesiveness or invasiveness of the fibrous variant of Hashimoto's struma up to and including invasion of muscle. We believe, therefore, that Riedel's struma is probably an unusual fibrous variant of Hashimoto's struma.

* *Editor's comment:* We continue to be plagued by uncertainty about the meaning of "delayed hypersensitivity," as the term is used here. As Mellors *et al.* have shown (*Amer. J. Path.*, 41:425, 1962), the round cells infiltrating the gland in chronic thyroiditis in man contain antibody to thyroglobulin, and spilled thyroglobulin is present in and around these cells in the interstitium. Delayed, or "cellular," hypersensitivity may, as Paterson notes (Chap. 71), be simply a more effective way to deliver antibodies to the target organ.—J. H. V.

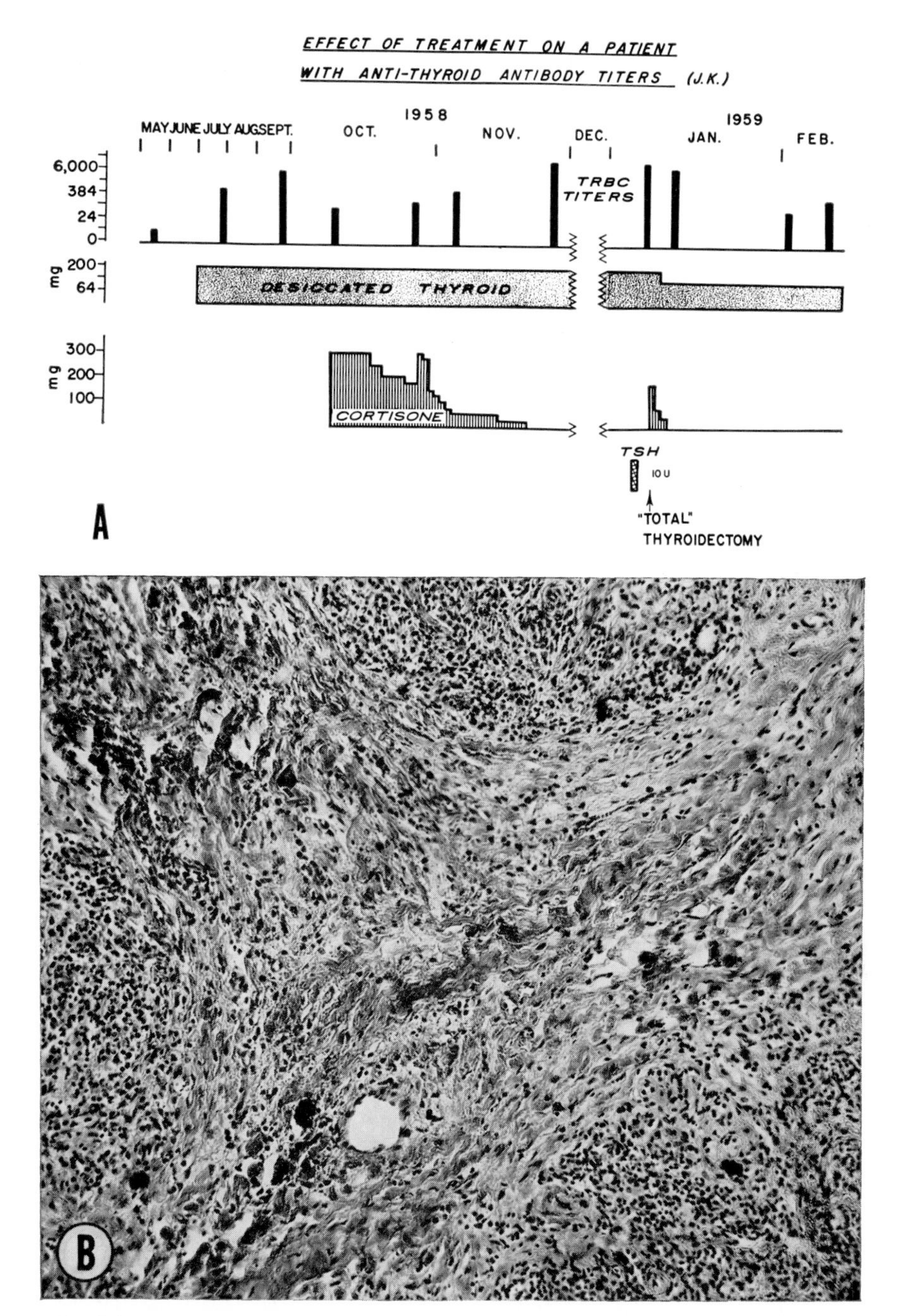

Fig. 73-11. (*A*) AAB titer (tanned cell) and goiter size in a patient thought to have rapidly progressive Hashimoto's struma. Goiter size and AAB titer failed to respond to desiccated thyroid, responded to 300 mg. per day of cortisone, increased again when steroid dosage was reduced, and required surgical thyroidectomy. Two pathologists interpreted the sections (see *B*) as compatible with Riedel's struma. Note replacement of thyroid tissue by heavy ligneous fibrous tissue.

MYXEDEMA

Mild forms of Hashimoto's disease are much more frequent than severe forms and in most cases are probably nonprogressive and do not lead to myxedema. Even when the gland is completely invaded, progression to destruction and fibrosis probably occurs only in about 50 percent of cases. However, almost all patients with "primary" myxedema are found to have circulating AAB when a wide variety of serological methods is used to search for them.

There is no doubt that Hashimoto's disease can end with the disappearance of goiter and appearance of myxedema. It is not clear, however, why Hashimoto's disease ends in "death" of the thyroid gland in some cases but not in others. It is also not known whether every occurrence of myxedema without obvious cause was preceded by the classic histological picture of Hashimoto's disease.

JUVENILE MYXEDEMA AND CRETINISM

An increased incidence of thyroid antibody titers has been found in juvenile myxedema and in euthyroid children with goiter but in less than 1 percent of children without thyroid disorders. An increased incidence has been

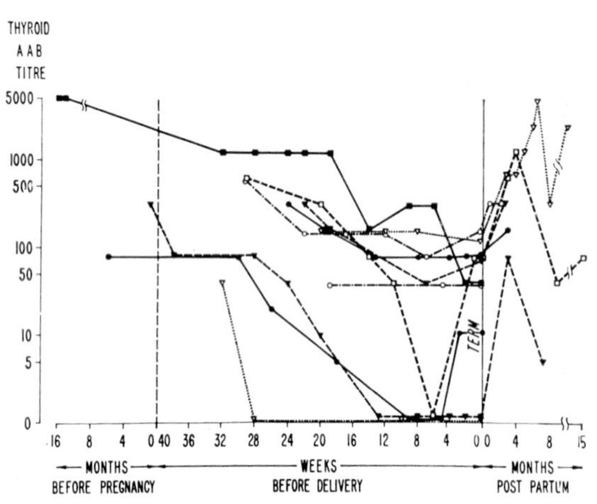

Fig. 73-12. Fall in AAB titers during pregnancy, and rise after termination of pregnancy.

reported in diabetic children. The hypothesis that athyreotic cretinism is due to placental transfer of thyroid antibodies has not been substantiated in recent studies [55, 56]. The tanned cell titers, when elevated at the onset of pregnancy, regularly fall during pregnancy and rise on its termination (Fig. 73-12). These antibodies are definitely transmitted transplacentally from mother to fetus in the human being [53] and in the rabbit [54].

THYROTOXICOSIS

Thyrotoxic patients with progressive exophthalmos tend to have higher antibody titers than do patients with uncomplicated thyrotoxicosis. Radioiodine treatment of hyperthyroidism does not seem to initiate the autoimmune process but does seem to be followed by an increase in existing AAB titers [47]. This increase in titer after relief from thyrotoxicosis may be related to a diminished degradation rate of γ-globulin with a decrease in general body metabolism.

THYROID CARCINOMA

In 605 cases of struma lymphomatosa [57], there were 18 instances of associated carcinoma (about 3 percent) and 12 of associated lymphosarcoma (about 2 percent). All of the carcinomas were papillary and of low malignancy but showed definite invasion of adjacent parenchyma. Obviously these figures represent the maximal incidence of carcinoma, since the physician elected to remove the goiter surgically, frequently because of a strong suspicion that carcinoma might be present. We have seen only 2 instances of severe generalized Hashimoto's struma with high AAB titers associated with carcinoma of the thyroid gland. Almost always, the AAB titer is relatively low and the lymphomatous infiltration focal (Fig. 73-13). Frequently the focal infiltration is near a necrotic papillary frond, as though it represented a local "immune" reaction to an altered or "new" antigen in the carcinoma.

We tested 116 patients with thyroid carcinoma who were treated by surgical extirpation of the thyroid gland as well as thyroid carcinoma, followed by I^{131} therapy (Table 73-3). Of 95 patients tested after apparent elimination of all thyroid tissue, 18 percent had demonstrable circulating AAB; and 14 percent of 21 patients with detectable residual thyroid tissue had circulating AAB. The in-

TABLE 73-3. Relation of Persistence of AAB to Remaining Thyroid Tissue after Surgery and Irradiation for Thyroid Carcinoma (116 Patients)

Remaining Thyroid Tissue	AAB	
	Pos.	Neg.
Detectable (21 patients)	3 (14%)	18 (86%)
Not detectable (95 patients)	13 (18%)	78 (82%)

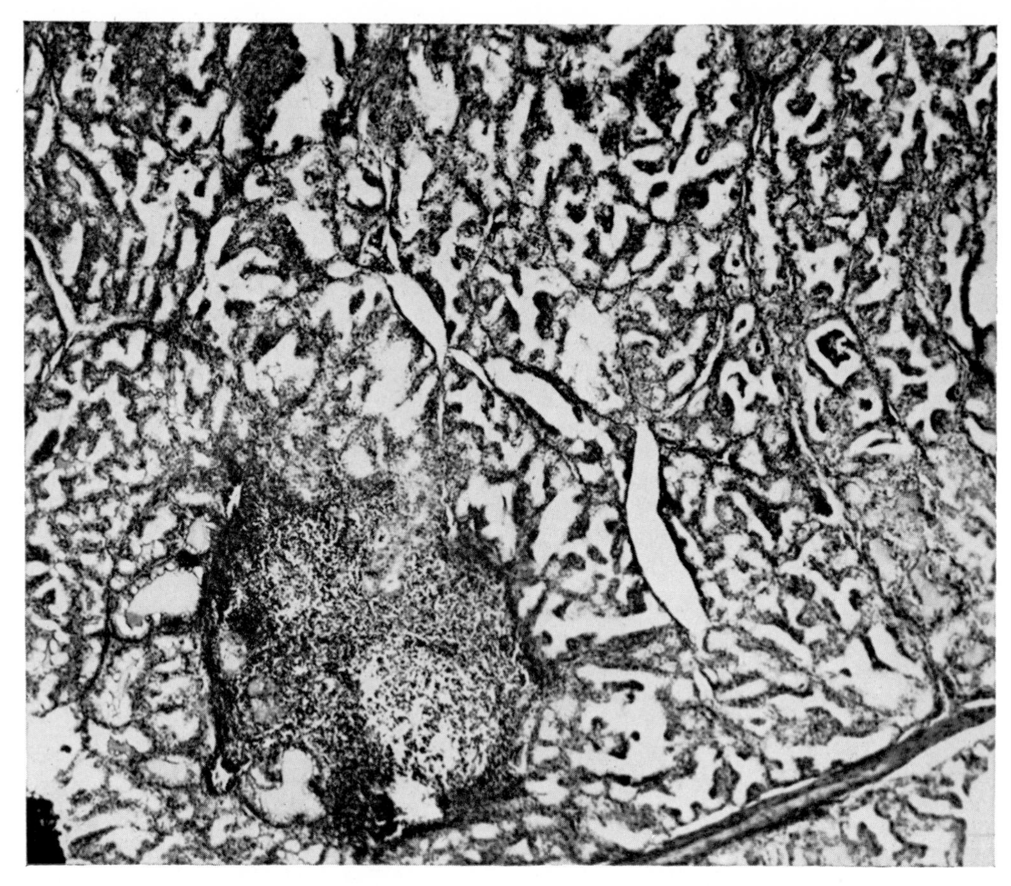

Fig. 73-13. Focal lymphomatous infiltration in a man with papillary carcinoma of the thyroid gland.

cidence of AAB in the serum of 100 women seen for any complaint in the Gynecology Clinic at the same hospital during the same period was 4 percent. The incidence of AAB in these patients tested after treatment did not differ significantly at any interval from the incidence in 29 patients tested before treatment. Circulating AAB were demonstrable through the 10 years of follow-up after treatment. The relationship between circulating AAB and papillary and follicular carcinoma is unknown. One possible, but unproved, reason for the persistence of AAB after apparent ablation of all thyroid tissue is that the tanned cell test is a more sensitive index of the persistence of functioning thyroid tissue than all other methods of testing in common use. Another possible explanation is that the papillary carcinoma may arise in a type of thyroid gland that is commonly associated with circulating AAB.

REFERENCES

1. Rogers, J., and Beebe, S. P. The treatment of thyroidism by a specific cytotoxic serum. *Arch. Intern. Med.* 2:297, 1908.
2. Rose, N. R., and Witebsky, E. Immunologische Untersuchungen bei Schilddrüsenerkrankungen. In Miescher, P., and Vorlaender, K. O. (Eds.), *Immunopathologie in Klinik und Forschung.* Stuttgart: Georg Thieme Verlag, 1960. P. 295.
3. Hektoen, L., and Schulhof, K. The precipitin reaction of thyroglobulin. *J.A.M.A.* 80:386, 1923.
4. Oswald, W. Die Eiweisskörper der Schilddrüse. *Z. Physiol. Chem.* 27:147, 1899.
5. Hektoen, L., Fox, H., and Schulhof, K. Specificness in the precipitin reaction of thyroglobulin. *J. Infect. Dis.* 40:641, 1927.
6. Stokinger, H. E., and Heidelberger, M. A quantitative theory of the precipitin reaction. *J. Exp. Med.* 66:251, 1937.

7. Witebsky, E. Die Serologische Analyse von Zellen und Geweben. *Naturwissenschaften* 40: 771, 1929.
8. Witebsky, E., Rose, N. R., and Shulman, S. Studies on organ specificity: I. The serological specificity of thyroid extracts. *J. Immun.* 75:269, 1955.
9. Rose, N. R., and Witebsky, E. Preliminary serological analysis of crude thyroid extracts. *Fed. Proc.* 14:476, 1955.
10. Shulman, S., Rose, N. R., and Witebsky, E. Studies on organ specificity: III. Ultracentrifugal and electrophoretic examination of thyroid extracts. *J. Immun.* 75:291, 1955.
11. Rose, N. R., Shulman, S., and Witebsky, E. Studies on organ specificity: XIII. Immunological analysis of thyroglobulin and thyralbumin. *J. Immun.* 88:229, 1962.
12. Rose, N. R., and Witebsky, E. Studies on organ specificity: II. Serological interrelationships among thyroid extracts of various species. *J. Immun.* 75:282, 1955.
13. Rose, N. R., Metzgar, R. S., and Isaacs, E. Studies on organ specificity: VIII. Serological interrelationships among thyroid extracts of various species revealed by gel diffusion precipitation techniques. *J. Immun.* 84:649, 1960.
14. Rose, N. R. Experimental Autoimmune Thyroiditis. In Metcoff, J. (Ed.), *Hereditary, Developmental, and Immunologic Aspects of Kidney Disease.* Chicago: Northwestern University Press, 1962. P. 90.
15. Hektoen, L., and Schulhof, K. The precipitin reaction of thyroglobulin. *Proc. Nat. Acad. Sci. U.S.A.* 11:481, 1925.
16. Lerman, J. Endocrine action of thyroglobulin antibodies. *Endocrinology* 31:558, 1942.
17. Rose, N. R., and Witebsky, E. Production of specific rabbit thyroid antibodies in the rabbit. *Fed. Proc.* 15:609, 1956.
18. Witebsky, E., and Rose, N. R. Studies on organ specificity: IV. Production of rabbit thyroid antibodies in the rabbit. *J. Immun.* 76:408, 1956.
19. Rose, N. R., and Witebsky, E. Studies on organ specificity: V. Changes in the thyroid glands of rabbits following active immunization with rabbit thyroid extracts. *Ibid.*, p. 417.
20. Rose, N. R., and Witebsky, E. Studies on organ specificity: VI. Cross-reaction of thyroid autoantibodies with thyroid of other species. *J. Immun.* 83:34, 1959.
21. Rose, N. R., and Witebsky, E. Experimental Immunological Thyroiditis. In Grabar, P., and Miescher, P. (Eds.), *Immunopathology* (1st International Symposium) Basel: Benno Schwabe & Co., 1959. P. 154.
22. Beutner, E. H., Witebsky, E., Rose, N. R., and Gerbasi, J. R. Localization of thyroid and spinal cord autoantibodies by fluorescent antibody technic. *Proc. Soc. Exp. Biol. Med.* 97:712, 1958.
23. Witebsky, E., Rose, N. R., Terplan, K., Paine, J. R., and Egan, R. W. Chronic thyroiditis and autoimmunization. *J.A.M.A.* 164:1439, 1957.
24. Rose, N. R., Kite, J. H., and Doebbler, T. K. Experimental Autoimmune Thyroiditis. In Miescher, P., and Grabar, P. (Eds.), *Mechanisms of Cell and Tissue Damage Produced by Immune Reactions.* Basel: Benno Schwabe & Co., 1962. P. 161.
25. Terplan, K. L., Witebsky, E., Rose, N. R., Paine, J. R., and Egan, R. W. Experimental thyroiditis in rabbits, guinea pigs and dogs, following immunization with thyroid extracts of their own and of heterologous species. *Amer. J. Path.* 39:213, 1960.
26. Jones, H. E. H., and Roitt, I. M. Experimental auto-immune thyroiditis in the rat. *Brit. J. Exp. Path.* 42:546, 1961.
27. Metzgar, R. S., and Grace, J. T. Production of experimental thyroiditis in rats and mice. *Fed. Proc.* 20:39, 1961.
28. Witebsky, E., and Rose, N. R. Studies on organ specificity: VII. Production of antibodies to rabbit thyroid by injection of foreign thyroid extracts. *J. Immun.* 83:41, 1959.
29. McMaster, P. R. B., Lerner, E. M., and Exum, E. D. The relationship of delayed hypersensitivity and circulating antibody to experimental allergic thyroiditis in inbred guinea pigs. *J. Exp. Med.* 113:611, 1961.
30. Miescher, P., Gorstein, F., Benacerraf, B., and Gell, P. G. H. Studies on the pathogenesis of experimental immune thyroiditis. *Proc. Soc. Exp. Biol. Med.* 107:12, 1961.

30a. Rose, N. R., Kite, J. H., Doebbler, T. K. Spier, R., Skelton, F. R., and Witebsky, E. Studies on experimental thyroiditis. *Ann. N.Y. Acad. Sci.* 124:201, 1965.

31. Rose, N. R., Kite, J. H., Doebbler, T. K., and Brown, R. C. *In vitro* Reactions of Lymphoid Cells with Thyroid Tissue. In Amos, B., and Koprowski, H. (Eds.), *Cell-bound Antibodies.* Philadelphia: Wistar Institute Press, 1963. P. 19.
32. Felix-Davies, D., and Waksman, B. H. Passive transfer of experimental immune thyroiditis in the guinea pig. *Arthritis Rheum.* 4:416, 1961.
33. Goodman, H. Discussion on Mechanisms of Tissue Damage in Experimental Autoimmune Disease. Ref. 24, p. 198.

33a. Rose, N. R., Kite, J. H., Doebbler, T. K., and Witebsky, E. Chronic Thyroiditis as an Autoimmune Disease. In Thomas, L. (Ed.), *Injury, Inflammation and Immunity.* Baltimore: Williams & Wilkins Company, 1964.

34. Kite, J. H. The cultivation of rabbit thyroid tissue *in vitro. Fed. Proc.* 21:158, 1962.

35. Hjort, T. Determination of serum thyroglobulin by a haemagglutination-inhibition test. *Lancet* 1:1262, 1961.
36. Owen, C. H., and McConahey, W. M. Unusual iodinated protein of serum in Hashimoto's thyroiditis. *J. Clin. Endocr.* 16:1570, 1956.
37. Stemmermann, G. N. Serum protein changes in subacute thyroiditis. *J.A.M.A.* 162:31, 1956.
38. DeGroot, L. J., Hall, R., McDermott, W. V., Jr., and Davis, A. M. Hashimoto's thyroiditis: A genetically conditioned disease. *New Eng. J. Med.* 267:267, 1962.
39. Metzger, H., Sharp, G. C., and Edelhoch, H. The properties of thyroglobulin: VII. The immunologic activity of thyroglobulin fragments. *Biochemistry* 1:205, 1962.
40. Shulman, S., and Witebsky, E. Studies on organ specificity: IX. Biophysical and immunochemical studies on human thyroid autoantibody. *J. Immun.* 85:559, 1960.
41. Fromm, G. A., Lascano, E. E., Bur, G. E., and Escalante, D. Tiroiditis cronica inespecifica: estruma linfoideo (Hashimoto), estruma granulomatoso (De Quervain), estruma fibroso (Riedel). *Rev. Asoc. Med. Argent.* 67:162, 1953.
42. Roitt, I. M., Doniach, D., and Campbell, P. N. The nature of the gamma globulins in lymphadenoid goitre. *Biochem. J.* 64:54P, 1956.
43. Roitt, I. M., Doniach, D., Campbell, P. N., and Hudson, R. V. Auto-antibodies in Hashimoto's disease (lymphadenoid goitre). *Lancet* 2:820, 1956.
44. Paine, J. R., Terplan, K., Rose, N. R., Witebsky, E., and Egan, R. W. A clinical study of chronic noninfectious thyroiditis and autoimmunization. *Surgery* 42:799, 1957.
45. Roitt, I. M., and Doniach, D. Human autoimmune thyroiditis: Serological studies. *Lancet* 2:1027, 1958.
46. Buchanan, W. W., Anderson, J. R., Goudie, R. B., and Gray, K. G. A skin test in thyroid disease. *Ibid.,* p. 928.
47. Doniach, D., and Roitt, I. M. Auto-antibodies in disease. *Ann. Rev. Med.* 13:213, 1962.
48. Forbes, I. J., Roitt, I. M., Doniach, D., and Solomon, I. L. The thyroid cytotoxic autoantibody. *J. Clin. Invest.* 41:996, 1962.
49. Hall, R., Owen, S. G., and Smart, G. A. Evidence for genetic predisposition to formation of thyroid autoantibodies. *Lancet* 2:187, 1960.
50. Sommers, S. C., and Meissner, W. A. Basement membrane changes in chronic thyroiditis and other thyroid diseases. *Amer. J. Clin. Path.* 24:434, 1954.
51. Vickery, A. L., and Hamlin, E., Jr. Struma Lymphomatosa (Hashimoto's thyroiditis). Observations on repeated biopsies in sixteen patients. *New Eng. J. Med.* 264:226, 1961.
52. Dodson, V. N., Haynie, T. P., III, Floyd, J. C., Jr., and Beierwaltes, W. H. Response of antithyroid antibody titers during treatment of goiter. *Univ. Mich. Med. Bull.* 25:333, 1959.
53. Woolner, L. B., McConahey, W. M., and Beahrs, O. H. Granulomatous thyroiditis (De Quervain's thyroiditis). *J. Clin. Endocr.* 17:1202, 1957.
54. Felix-Davies, D. Autoimmunization in subacute thyroiditis associated with evidence of infection by mumps virus. *Lancet* 1:880, 1958.
55. Parker, R. H. and Beierwaltes, W. H. Thyroid antibodies during pregnancy and in the newborn. *J. Clin. Endocr.* 21:792, 1961.
56. Beierwaltes, W. H., Elzinga, K. E., Schmidt, R. W., Dodson, V. N., Spafford, N. R., and Carr, E. A., Jr. Rabbit pregnancies after immunization with extract of thyroid gland. *Endocrinology* 69:863, 1961.
57. Woolner, L. B., McConahey, W. M., and Beahrs, O. H. Struma lymphomatosa (Hashimoto's thyroiditis) and related thyroidal disorders. *J. Clin. Endocr.* 19:53, 1959.

74. *Acquired Hemolytic Disease**

SCOTT N. SWISHER AND JOHN H. VAUGHAN

ACQUIRED HEMOLYTIC DISEASE [1, 2] was increasingly recognized in the early years of this century. The condition was clinically marked by acute onset of increased blood destruction, in contrast to the long chronic history of hemolysis and anemia characteristic of congenital hemolytic disorders. Nevertheless substantial confusion between acquired and congenital hemolytic disorders persisted over the years, for the acquired disease could become chronic, and then it was most difficult to distinguish it from, for example, hereditary spherocytosis.

These two major types of hemolytic diseases were first clearly separated by studies which employed measurements of red cell life span. It was found that the red cells of most patients with hereditary and congenital hemolytic disorders were intrinsically defective and incapable of surviving for a normal period in the circulations of either the patient or a normal recipient. On the other hand, patients with acquired hemolytic disorders had red cells which survived better when they were removed from the patient and transfused into a normal recipient. The terms "intracorpuscular defect" and "extracorpuscular hemolytic mechanism" were applied to the two contrasting processes of increased blood destruction.

The second major finding which served to sharpen the differentiation between acquired and congenital hemolytic disorders was the discovery of the antiglobulin test by Coombs *et al.* [3] and the application of this test to the red cells of patients with acquired types of hemolytic anemia by Boorman *et al.* [4]. It was found that the red cells of many of the patients with acquired hemolytic disease exhibited positive antiglobulin reactions, whereas only rarely was a positive reaction reported to occur in cases of congenital hemolytic disorders.

The possibility that an antibody-like substance was responsible for the increased blood destruction encountered in acquired hemolytic anemia had been suggested earlier. Analogies between acquired hemolytic anemia and experimental hemolytic disorders induced by the infusion of erythrocyte heteroantibodies into animals were also noted. However, it was the introduction of the antiglobulin test into immunohematology which clearly focused attention upon the possibility that immune mechanisms were involved in the pathogenesis of this disorder. During the era in which the serology and immunology of acquired hemolytic anemia has been elucidated, the concept of "autoimmunity" in general has also been developed. Although many lines of evidence remain incomplete in support of the general theory of diseases due to autosensitization, the concept that acquired hemolytic anemia is, in fact, a group of disorders characterized by an abnormal autoantibody response has gained increasing acceptance in recent years.† One of the principal lines of evidence supporting this view, as will be developed later, is the remarkable similarity between the substances coating the red cells of patients with acquired hemolytic anemia and typical erythrocyte isoantibodies. Although much of the past controversy about the nature of these substances has been settled by modern immunological and immunochemical techniques, the postulates proposed by Witebsky [5] for the rigorous demonstration of autosensitization processes have not been fulfilled in the case of acquired hemolytic disease. Nevertheless this

* Supported by grants from the National Foundation and the National Institutes of Health AM-00537 and AM-02443.

† There are other "acquired" hemolytic syndromes, for instance, those with glucose-6-phosphate dehydrogenase deficiency, in which immunological abnormalities are not involved. The present text has adopted the term "acquired hemolytic anemia," however, as that designating the syndromes characterizing "Coombs-positive disease."

chapter will take the view that the autosensitive etiology of this group of diseases presents far and away the most satisfactory theoretical explanation and understanding of the pathogenesis of the disorder.

Acquired hemolytic disease is unassociated with any demonstrable underlying disease process in from one half to two thirds of cases. This group has been termed "idiopathic." In the remaining cases, the acquired hemolytic disorder appears to be secondary to some underlying disease; this group has been termed "secondary" or "symptomatic" acquired hemolytic disease (AHD). The underlying diseases are, in general, malignant proliferative disorders of the lymphatic and reticuloendothelial apparatus, certain disorders of the "collagen-vascular" group, notably systemic lupus erythematosus (SLE) and, rarely, tumors, viral infections, or inflammatory diseases of a chronic nature such as ulcerative colitis, and sarcoidosis. In well over three quarters of the cases of secondary AHD, the underlying disorder is evident at the time the hemolytic process is first recognized, and becomes evident within one year in virtually all of the remaining cases. However, a small proportion of the patients, well less than 5 percent, may have long intervals between the onset of the hemolytic process and recognition of an underlying disorder. Thus it should be recognized that initial classification of a patient with idiopathic AHD (IAHD) must be somewhat tentative until sufficient time has passed to make unlikely the emergence of a secondary underlying disorder.

Cases of AHD may also be classified in another way: on the basis of the optimal temperature of interaction of the autoantibody and the patient's red cells. Two groups of cases again may be recognized: those in which the autoantibody is optimally active at body temperature, termed the "warm antibody" cases, and a smaller group of patients in which the autoantibody is optimally active at lower temperatures, i.e., at 4 to 10° C. The latter group is termed the "cold antibody" type. Idiopathic and symptomatic cases are recognized in both cold and warm autoantibody categories. Certain clinical differences are associated with the serological distinction in the thermal optimum of the autoantibody.

A small group of patients exhibiting essentially all of the clinical features of autosensitive acquired hemolytic anemia, but without serologically demonstrable evidence of an erythrocyte autoantibody, has been encountered. Many of these patients have well-defined major hemolytic processes associated with a malignant lymphoma or with chronic lymphocytic leukemia. Two views may be taken of this group of patients. They may have autosensitive hemolytic processes, but with autoantibodies or "cellular" autosensitivity which escape detection by current serological methods. Alternatively, the acquired hemolytic process in these cases may not involve autosensitive mechanisms. Further clarification of the mechanism of increased blood destruction in these patients is urgently needed.

HEMOLYTIC DISEASE ASSOCIATED WITH WARM-ACTIVE AUTOANTIBODIES

AHD of the "warm antibody" type occurs in both idiopathic and symptomatic forms at all ages. The disease is, however, relatively uncommon among children. The incidence of symptomatic AHD increases with age, reflecting the increasing number of malignant lymphatic disorders, particularly chronic lymphocytic leukemia, in older age groups. Among patients with IAHD, an excessive number of postmenopausal females have been encountered in several reported groups of cases. An over-all preponderance of women has been noted by several authors. There is no known racial propensity to AHD, although the bulk of the reported cases is in Caucasians. Similarly, genetic and epidemiological factors are not recognized to be of significance. It should be emphasized that AHD is a relatively rare disorder; the incidence of its recognition depends directly on the intensity with which it is sought, particularly among patients with primary disorders in which AHD is not uncommon. For example, evidences of erythrocyte autosensitization have been reported to occur at some time in the clinical course of approximately 20 percent of patients with chronic lymphocytic leukemia. In our own experience, the incidence of overt hemolytic anemia is substantially lower than this, less than 5 percent, although transiently positive results of antiglobulin tests unassociated with frank hemolysis have been found in additional patients. A much higher incidence of positive results of antiglobulin tests, associated with variable evidences of increased blood destruction, has been encountered in our experience in cases of SLE.

CLINICAL FEATURES

The clinical picture of AHD of the warm autoantibody type is extremely variable. In some cases, onset is slow and insidious over a period of months, with ultimate emergence of symptomatic anemia. In other cases, the onset is characterized by intermittent episodes of anemia and mild icterus over the course of many months, before an episode sufficiently severe to bring the patient to medical attention occurs. At the other end of this spectrum are patients with a sudden onset of violent hemolysis leading to acute anemia, prostration, and intense jaundice within a matter of a few days.

Physical findings are seldom remarkable in cases of AHD except for pallor, variable jaundice, hyperactive circulation in proportion to anemia, and slight to moderate splenomegaly. Massive splenomegaly is uncommon in IAHD, and its occurrence suggests an underlying neoplastic disorder of lymphoid tissue. In symptomatic cases, of course, the clinical picture may be dominated by the historical features and physical findings of the underlying disease.

The blood in cases of IAHD may show only minimal anemia and moderate but persistently elevated reticulocyte counts. In more active cases of hemolysis, anemia may be moderate to severe and the reticulocyte count markedly elevated to 50 percent or more. In these instances, some degree of spherocytosis of the red cells is usually seen on the blood smear, and distinct punctate basophilia and normoblastemia are common. Anticoagulated samples of blood examined in thin films streaming down the side of a bottle may show obvious autoagglutination. Agglutination may be prominent on blood smears. The leukocyte picture varies widely, from slight leukopenia and neutropenia to moderately elevated total leukocyte counts, in the range of 20,000 per mm^3., and relative neutrophilia. Erythrophagocytosis may be seen in the peripheral blood leukocytes, particularly the monocytes and polymorphonuclear neutrophils, in certain cases with particularly acute hemolysis. Platelets may be normal or decreased. As will be pointed out, a relationship may exist between the warm antibody type of AHD and idiopathic thrombocytopenic purpura (ITP).

Urinary findings are nonspecific, in that there may be some increase in urobilinogen and, in very severe disease, bile pigment. Hemoglobinuria is rarely encountered, although it is seen in occasional cases with intense hemolysis. Low levels of hemoglobinemia, and methemalbuminemia are somewhat more common.

Bone marrow examination usually discloses only marked normoblastic hyperplasia. Maximal compensatory increase in blood production usually lags three or four days behind the period of maximal anemia, as evidence from a rising reticulocyte count following the time of most severe anemia in many patients. If spherocytosis is present in the red cells of the blood smear, the red cell osmotic fragility and autohemolysis on incubation under sterile conditions at 37° C. for 48 hours will be increased almost invariably. Occasionally, small populations of osmotically fragile cells can be identified in the absence of clear-cut spherocytosis on the blood film. Autohemolysis tests, in which glucose has been added, may show no change or an increase in spontaneous red cell lysis over forty-eight hours of incubation. This contrasts with the uniform decrease in autohemolysis which is seen on the addition of glucose to the blood of patients with hereditary spherocytosis. Again, it should be pointed out that in cases of symptomatic AHD in which the underlying disease is a malignant disorder of lymphatic tissue, the laboratory findings may be primarily those of the underlying disorder or its treatment, with certain features attributable to AHD superimposed. If the bone marrow of the patient is infiltrated by malignant lymphoid tissue, or if the patient has received systemic alkylation or radiation therapy, the reticulocyte count may be much decreased in proportion to the severity of anemia.

Clinical measurements of red cell life span are seldom required to identify patients with overt hemolytic processes. On the other hand, this may be the only way to demonstrate relatively modest degrees of shortening of red cell life span. Chromium-51-labeled transfusions of small amounts of normal donor red cells to these patients may yield useful estimates of the patient's rate of red cell destruction. In cases in which the half-life ($T\frac{1}{2}$) of the Cr^{51}-labeled red cells is reduced to the neighborhood of 15 days (normal $T\frac{1}{2}$ of Cr^{51}-

labeled red cells is 27 to 35 days in various laboratories), there is commonly little or no anemia. The normal human bone marrow has the capacity to increase the production of red cells approximately sixfold. When the T½ of Cr^{51}-labeled red cells falls below about 5 days, this capacity to compensate is gradually exceeded. In cases of very acute hemolysis, the T½ for Cr^{51}-labeled normal red cells in the patient's circulation may be 1 day or less.

The clinical course of patients with the warm autoantibody type of AHD is as variable as the picture of the disorder at its onset. Frequently, in symptomatic cases, the clinical course is entirely dominated by the underlying disease. In idiopathic cases, a single short-lived episode of hemolysis may occur, with results of the antiglobulin test ultimately reverting to negative. More commonly, the initial episode may subside after a variable period of weeks to months, but the positive antiglobulin test may remain, sometimes for many years. During this interval, the patient may have recurrent episodes of active hemolysis, at times apparently precipitated by stressful situations such as infection, injury, surgery, or trauma. At other times, exacerbations of hemolytic activity appear to occur without precipitating cause. Pregnancy has been particularly provocative of exacerbations of hemolysis in our experience. It is of note that in three instances in which normal full-term infants were delivered by mothers with warm autoantibody AHD, there was no clinical or serological evidence of transplacental transmission of the disorder, although this has been claimed by others. Thrombophlebitis is a common complication of IAHD, and occasional cases are encountered in which widespread thromboses throughout the vascular tree occur in association with an acute hemolytic episode. These cases commonly have a fatal outcome.

GAMMA-GLOBULIN AUTOSENSITIZATION

In early studies of the antiglobulin reaction in patients with acquired hemolytic anemia, it was observed that the patients' red cells were agglutinated by antisera to human γ-globulins but not by antisera to albumin. The assumption that γ-globulins coat the red cells was easily confirmed by elution studies. Treatment of the sensitized red cells with heat, mild acid, or certain other solvents has yielded products which contain 7S γ-globulins* and also sensitize normal red cells to agglutination in the antiglobulin test. Nonhuman, mammalian red cells generally have failed to be sensitized by these eluates, although primate red cells sometimes are. Usually the eluates sensitize all the human red cells in the panels used by blood grouping laboratories for blood typing, and so the activity has been referred to as a panagglutinin or pan-antibody activity. Weiner and Vos [6] have recently shown that these eluates commonly fail to react with red cells congenitally deficient in antigens of the Rh group, suggesting that the activities may be due to antibodies to some fundamental structural unit held in common by red cells of several, or all, Rh types (see Ref. 7). Occasionally, eluates from AHD red cells, or less commonly their sera, may sensitize normal red cells belonging to one or another of the more commonly recognized human blood groups. In the majority of these latter instances, the specificities have been of an anti-Rh type, especially anti-e. The AHD red cells from which these eluates have been made have exhibited blood types corresponding to the specificities of their eluates. Anti-D and anti-Jk^a antibody activities have also been described in eluates.

There have been rare instances, however, in which the eluates from patients' red cells have shown homospecificity.† For example, anti-D activity has been eluted from cde/cde erythrocytes of a patient with AHD, anti-E has been recovered from CDe/CDe cells, and anti-C from cDE/cde cells (see p. 448 of Ref. 1). Those findings are confusing, but they may represent responses similar to the anti-D-like antibodies which can be elicited in guinea pigs given injections of extracts of human D-negative, as well as D-positive, erythrocytes [8]. Although this rather anomalous phenomenon emphasizes the inadequacy of our

* Leddy and Bakemeier (*J. Exp. Med.*, 121:1, 1965) have noted that the γ-globulin eluted from red cells in acquired hemolytic disease may be much more restricted in its electrophoretic and L chain distribution than was generally the case with Rh antibodies from patients sensitized by pregnancy or transfusion. Indeed, in one or two instances, the eluted γ-globulin in AHD very closely resembled myeloma proteins.

† This has commonly been referred to as "isospecificity" by blood bank serologists. The term is improper, however, for "isospecificity" refers to intrastrain (isologous) rather than intraspecies (homologous) specificity.

knowledge of erythrocyte serology, the interpretation that there are configurations in the Rh group of red cell antigens that are recognized in heterologous immunization (man to guinea pig) but rarely, if ever, in homologous immunization (man to man) seems possible. Overlapping of the configurations recognized in the heterologous system with those usually recognized in the homologous system could give the D-like antibody described in the guinea pig. Obviously, this explanation proposes a mechanism quite similar to that discussed above for Weiner and Vos's findings.

Much controversy has existed as to whether autoantibodies have a pathogenic role. As noted above, it has often been recognized that patients may remain "antiglobulin sensitive" for long periods during which their hemolytic disease is quiescent. Moreover, experiments have been cited in which Cr^{51}-labeled normal red cells sensitized *in vitro* with eluates from the red cells of patients with acute autoimmune hemolytic anemia have survived normally in normal volunteer recipients. Indeed, the patient's own red cells may survive well when transfused into normal recipients. Whether this improved survival is due to removal of the red cells from a hyperactive reticuloendothelial system in the patient, or to spontaneous elution and redistribution of antibody from the patient's transfused cells [9], or to other uncertain factors is not known. At any rate, the sensitizing proteins on the surfaces of the red cells in acquired hemolytic disease may have pathogenic meaning, only within certain limits.

Whatever these limits be, however, the serological specificities in AHD have clearly been shown to have pathogenic meaning in a few cases studied by selected transfusions (Ref. 1, p. 385). Normal red cells transfused into patients with acquired hemolytic anemia generally are rapidly destroyed. Prolonged survival of cde/cde cells and rapid elimination of CDe/cde cells was noted, however, in an AHD patient with anti-D autoantibody, while prolonged survival of cDE/cDE cells and rapid elimination of cde/cde cells was described in a patient with anti-e autoantibody. Similar studies have been reported by others. Since survival experiments like these were done at different times during the patient's illness and were, therefore, subject to uncontrolled variations in the hemolytic process with time, Mollison studied the survival of transfused e-negative cells in a patient with anti-e autoantibody by the Ashby technique of differential agglutination and, simultaneously, survival of the patient's autologous cells by Cr^{51} tagging. The transfused e-negative cells survived almost normally while the patient's own e-positive cells were being rapidly destroyed.

NON-GAMMA-GLOBULIN AUTOSENSITIZATION

Although there have been many descriptions of hemolytic disease with γ-globulin red cell sensitization, it has gradually become evident that the red cells in a number of patients are sensitized by globulins other than γ-globulins. Anti-"non-γ-globulin" rabbit sera have come to be used in the description of these cases. These sera have usually been antisera to whole human sera, absorbed exhaustively with human γ-globulins in the form of Cohn's fraction II. Studies with known blood group systems early gave some hint of what this "non-γ-globulin" material on sensitized red cells might be. Red cells mixed with complement-fixing blood group isoantibodies, or with cold agglutinins, develop "non-γ-globulin" sensitization in the presence of active serum complement but not in its absence.

This prompted the assumption that the non-γ-globulin sensitization of red cells in AHD may also be due to complement protein. More direct support for this, however, awaited the preparation of specific antisera against complement (β_{1A}-β_{1C} or β_{1E}) components, as well as antisera adequate to demonstrate that other human serum proteins did not contribute to the reactions. Such data are presented in Table 74-1 and Figure 74-1. Leddy *et al.* [10] found no evidence for γ_{1A} or γ_{1M} immunoglobulins participating in the positive antiglobulin tests (see also Ref. 11). The "non-γ" reaction was reproduced by an anticomplement serum, but not by an antiserum (anti-EE) to whole human serum from which antibodies to the immunoglobulins and complement had been removed (fondly and presumptuously referred to in our laboratories as anti-Everything Else!).

It has not been possible to elute and recover sensitizing activities from the "non-γ," complement-type sensitized red cells of patients with hemolytic disease. It has generally also been impossible to do so from control cells sensitized *in vitro* with complement-fixing isoantibody. Therefore little is known about the antibody specificities responsible for complement-type sensitization of red cells in AHD.

TABLE 74-1. Clinical and Laboratory Summary of Patients Studied

Patient	Age/Sex	Clinical Diagnosis	Hct/Retics. (%)	Direct Antiglobulin Pattern[a]	Serum Titer: Cold Agglut.	Serum Titer: Warm Auto-Aby	Serum Titer: Trypsin Factor	Serum Titer: Latex Agglut.	ANF: γ_2	ANF: γ_{1A}	ANF: γ_{1M}	Steroid Rx.
1	55/F	IAHD	43/8.4	γ_2	<10	—	1:8	—	—	—	1 : 16	Yes
2	58/F	IAHD	23/16.7	γ_2	<10	1:8	—	—	—	—	—	Yes
3	48/F	IAHD	41/0.9	$\gamma_2 + C'$	10	—	1:32	—	—	—	—	No
4	60/M	IAHD	40/1.7	$\gamma_2 + C'$	60	—	>1:512	1:40				No
5	67/F	IAHD	33/0.4	$\gamma_2 + C'$	<10	—	1:1	—	—	—	—	No
6	62/F	IAHD (?SLE)	29.5/0.4	$\gamma_2 + C'$	90	—	1:32	1:20–1:40	—	—	1 : 1	No
7	81/F	IAHD renal disease	23/1.7	$\gamma_2 + C'$	<10	—	—	—	—	—	—	No
8	56/M	IAHD	46/1.0	$\gamma_2 + C' +$ E.E.	<10	1:1	>1:512	—	+	+	+	Yes
9	38/F	IAHD	22/18.4	$C' +$ E.E.	<10	—	1:8	—	—	—	—	No
10	36/M	?IAHD	43.5/0.4	C'	20	—	1:128	—	—	—	—	No
11	63/F	IAHD	35.5/6.8	C'	180	—	1:512	—	1 : 1	—	1 : 256	Yes
12	75/F	IAHD	11/27	C'	640	—	>1:512	—				Yes
13	59/M	IAHD	40/0.8	C'	<10	—	—	—	—	—	—	No

[a] For titers, see Figure 74-1.

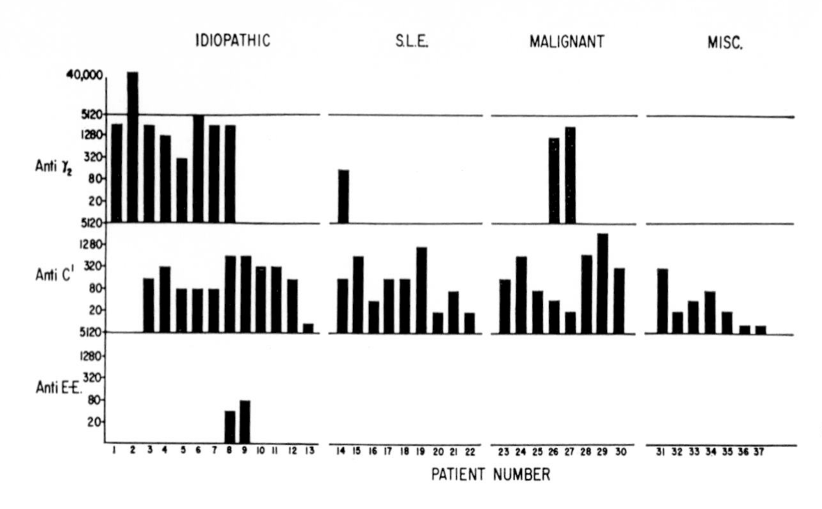

Fig. 74-1. Titers for antiglobulins in cases of IAHD, SLE, malignancy, and miscellaneous conditions [10].

Cold agglutinins and Donath-Landsteiner (D-L) antibodies are, however, exceptions (see later).

Complement-type sensitization of red cells may occur by means other than autoimmunization. Such sensitization may take place from an immunological event entirely unrelated to red cell antigenicity, one in which the red cell is merely an "innocent bystander" [12]. An example of this is the complement-type red cell sensitization and hemolysis that occurs occasionally in quinine or quinidine sensitivity. Normal red cells can be rendered "non-γ" positive, if mixed *in vitro* with quinine, quinine antibody, and complement. After this treatment, no γ-globulin is found on the red cell surfaces by anti-γ-globulin sera; the complement components so far identified are the β_{1A}-β_{1C} and β_{1E} globulins.

As seen in Figure 74-1, there is in our experience a great propensity for the Coombs-positive red cells in SLE and in lymphatic malignancy to be of the complement type; whether this means that the red cells in these diseases are more generally playing the role of "innocent bystanders" rather than acting as autoantigens is not known.

The possibility has long been considered that "non-γ" red cell sensitization in acquired hemolytic disease may be an entirely nonspecific adsorption of serum proteins onto damaged red cell surfaces. The data in Figure 74-1 suggest that, if this occurs, it is the exception rather than the rule. An intensive study of the nature of the serum proteins capable of coating red cells after various *in vitro* alterations of the surface membranes has been conducted by Leddy *et al.* [13]. The results support the opinion that nonimmunological binding of serum proteins to red cell surfaces probably has little to do with positive Coombs reactions in AHD.

The hemolytic process accompanying complement-type red cell sensitization may be mild or severe. Examples of the relation of the severity of disease to the strengths of the Coombs reactions can be seen in Table 74-1. Many of the patients with the "non-γ" sensitization were not anemic at the time of this study. Obviously such comparisons are superficial, limited as they are by the unknown specificities involved in the complement sensitizations and uncertainties of quantities involved.

SERUM ANTIBODIES

In the vast majority of cases of AHD of warm type, no serum antibody can be demonstrated with unmodified red cells. This has been assumed to mean that whatever antibody has been formed has not been in sufficient quantity to saturate all available combining sites on the red cells and then appear in excess in the serum. It may also sometimes mean, however, that the proper antigen (i.e., a drug, when the red cell is merely an "innocent bystander," or an enzyme-treated cell, if the antibody is reactive with a modified red cell) has not been chosen in the search for serum antibody.

Successful demonstration of serum antibodies has had to contend with the problem of differentiating the autoantibody which is part of the hemolytic disease process or antibodies which are part of an unrelated phenomenon. Isoantibodies from previous transfusions, from pregnancies, or from unknown sources (i.e., so-called "natural" antibodies) may confuse the serological findings on study of a patient's serum. It may be difficult or impossible to determine the presence or absence of certain antigens on the patient's erythrocytes, because the cells are already Coombs-positive. Antibody absorption techniques may be useful, unless the autoantibody already occupies all the antigen sites. As a result, it may be impossible to be sure that a given serological reactivity of an AHD patient's serum is an autoantibody or an isoantibody. There is some evidence that patients with AHD, particularly those with underlying lupus erythematosus, may be more likely to form isoantibodies to red cell antigens to which they are exposed by transfusions than are other groups of patients.

Allowing for these difficulties, however, serum autoantibodies reactive at 37° C. have occasionally been found. Special techniques are usually required for their demonstration. Performance of the agglutination test with red cells suspended in 20 percent serum albumin or in polyvinylpyrrolidone may bring out reactions not otherwise seen. Slight acidification of the serum to pH 6.8 to 7.0 has been used to reveal rare autohemolysins. Both of these procedures can be assumed to be simple maneuvers for enhancing secondary results (i.e., agglutination) of the antigen-antibody interaction without significantly changing the antigenic configurations on the red cell surfaces. The antibodies detected by these means are generally regarded as antibodies to normal red blood cell surface configurations. Successful demonstration of such serum antibodies is generally achieved only in very severe cases and often only during the acute hemolytic process.

Trypsinization of red cells to bring out agglutination reactions not otherwise seen may be a means of revealing antibody to "unnatural" surface antigens [1]. Although normal sera will sometimes agglutinate trypsinized red cells, the sera of patients with acquired hemolytic disease may do so in very high titer. In the presence of complement, hemolysis may be seen. The responsible serum factor has the electrophoretic migration characteristics of γ-globulins and is considered to be antibody reactive with trypsinized cells. It is not present in neonatal serum; it separates with the 19S globulins. The antibody is not absorbed from serum by untrypsinized erythrocytes but is taken up by trypsinized cells in the cold. The specificity of the antibody, therefore, is probably to a new configuration on the surface of the red cell consequent to the enzymatic action. Agglutinins for trypsinized cells in normal sera may be part of a natural antibody response to red cells damaged by tissue proteolytic activities essentially as a normal part of living. The enhanced titers of antibody activity seen in acquired hemolytic disease may well be a consequence of the disease rather than the cause. Proteolytic enzymes other than trypsin, such as bromelin, ficin, and papain, may also be used to modify red cells to bring out serum agglutinins similar to those found against trypsinized red cells.

If red cells are "lightly" treated with tryspin or bromelin, agglutination of the cells in serum does not occur. The cells become antiglobulin-positive, however, if the serum is fresh and the antiglobulin reagent is of the anticomplement type. This finding illustrates another possible mechanism for the production of antiglobulin-positive red cells in patients. It had been previously suspected that damaged red cell surfaces may somehow take on serum proteins to give "nonspecific" positive Coombs reactions. In fact, the Coombs test under these conditions is highly specific for complement. The sensitization appears to be due not to indiscriminate absorption of serum proteins but rather to complement fixation by serum antibody against "new" antigens on the damaged cell [13].

The possibility has been entertained that some of the agglutinating and other serological properties of eluates and sera in cases of acquired hemolytic disease are more lectin-like than antibody-like. Lectins are proteins found in certain plants which can cause highly specific red cell agglutination. Lectins are not γ-globulins and are not antibodies; they cannot be conceived of as existing in plants because of antigenic stimulation of the plants. Their prime functions in the plants are not known, and their abilities to react with red blood cells of specific antigenic content are probably happenstance. Although it is not possible categorically to deny that the serological entities in AHD are not also happenstance, data to support this interpretation are essentially nonexistent. It might be reasonable to consider the hypothesis of lectin-like autoreactivity more likely, however, if it could be shown that autoreactive γ-globulin in AHD attaches to red cell surfaces by a part of the molecule different from that by which ordinary antibodies attach to antigen. So far, no studies of this sort have been reported.

SERUM COMPLEMENT

Low serum complement titers have been reported in patients with "antiglobulin-positive" hemolytic disease. It has often been assumed that this is due to complement fixation by antibody combining with the red cell antigens. Adequate data have not always been given in these reports to rule out the possibility that the lowered complement titer was due to concomitant disease, such as lupus erythematosus, or to some other cause of low serum complement activity. Data adequate to permit correlation of serum complement titers with γ- or complement-type red cell sensitization are not available. Reduced serum complement has been more frequently found in cold autoantibody hemolytic disease than in the warm antibody type (see Ref. 1, p. 506).

PATHOLOGICAL PHYSIOLOGY

Red cell destruction in AHD proceeds by the so-called "extravascular" mechanism, in which preliminary sequestration of the sensitized red cells appears to occur in the sinusoidal portions of the circulation, primarily in the liver and spleen, before they are finally destroyed. The mechanism of injury and ultimate destruction of sequestered erythrocytes is not known. Their deprivation of important metabolites and *in vivo* repair processes may lead to their ultimate destruction. Although the spleen is probably an important site of red cell destruction in active AHD, it is not solely responsible for removal of the red cells. Following splenectomy, relapses of the hemolytic process can be observed which are indistinguishable from those attacks which occur before splenectomy.

Hemoglobinemia is usually associated with rapid *intravascular* hemolysis by a complement-fixing antibody, e.g., the destruction of A-positive erythrocytes erroneously transfused to a recipient who has anti-A in his plasma. Hemoglobinemia may also occur after incompatible transfusions involving anti-Rh; this isoantibody destroys red cells by an *extravascular* mechanism. The hemoglobinemia which is occasionally seen in cases of AHD exhibiting extremely rapid hemolysis is probably also the result of an "extravascular" hemolytic mechanism of red cell destruction comparable to that seen in cases of Rh-incompatible hemolytic transfusion reactions. It is probable that intravascular mechanisms of hemolysis are not responsible for red cell destruction in cases of warm autoantibody AHD.

The role of phagocytosis in the destruction of red cells in cases of AHD has been the subject of controversy. Prominent phagocytosis of red cells by the macrophages of the spleen, liver, bone marrow, and occasionally lymph nodes may be seen. As previously noted, it may also be observed *in vivo* in the peripheral blood leukocytes. These findings suggest that phagocytosis may be a significant mechanism of red cell destruction in this disorder. Unfortunately, there is no way to measure the number of red cells destroyed in this fashion *in vivo*. An opposing view holds that phagocytosis is only an end process which removes and digests red cells which have already been irreversibly injured by other processes. These two views of erythrophagocytosis as a mechanism of red cell destruction in AHD are not mutually exclusive, and both mechanisms may operate.

Factors which control the rate of red cell destruction, particularly those responsible for the sudden precipitation of acute hemolysis following long periods of quiescent disease, are essentially unknown. Tentative evidence has been brought forward to suggest that periods of rapid red cell destruction are associated with larger amounts of autoantibody bound to the red cell, as evident from some measure of the strength of the antiglobulin reactions. Whereas it is certainly true that the amount of sensitizing globulin on the surface of the red cells determines in some way the strength of the antiglobulin reaction, it has not been shown that a linear relationship exists between the two. Titrations of antiglobulin sera indeed measure more directly the characteristics of the antiglobulin reagent than the amount of the coating on the red cell surface. Evans and Weiser [9] suggested that the amount of antibody which can be transferred from the patient's red cells to normal red cells is a better measure of the amount of autoantibody the patient's cells carry, and they feel that this correlates better with the clinical course of the disease. Fudenberg *et al.* [14] have obtained similar data. These measurements are of great interest in that they demonstrate directly the *in vitro* transferability of warm autoantibodies from cell to cell and suggest the possibility that this occurs *in vivo* as well. The method does not apply, however, to cells sensitized to complement alone where no eluates with sensitizing activity can be obtained.

Other possible factors influencing the rate of red cell destruction which have been considered are: (1) expansion of or activation of the phagocytic capacity of the reticuloendothelial system; (2) a variety of hypothetical and undemonstrated humoral components which may interact in some unspecified way with the autoantibody-sensitized red cells to result in their removal and destruction, and (3) delayed hypersensitivity mechanisms. At the present time our knowledge in these areas must be regarded as quite incomplete.

Occasionally AHD is associated with persistent leukopenia and neutropenia or with persistent or recurrent thrombocytopenia. It has been suggested that these manifestations also have an autosensitive mechanism as their basis. Evans and Weiser have suggested that AHD and idiopathic thrombocytopenic purpura (ITP) represent ends of a spectrum of disorders. Certainly, occasional cases having intermediate clinical characteristics can be identified. In support of this concept are the observations that a small proportion of patients with otherwise typical ITP have positive red cell antiglobulin reactions and that occasionally there is evidence of increased blood destruction. Some patients with clear-cut AHD have had previous attacks of what was clinically typical ITP, and chronic or even recurrent acute and severe thrombocytopenia has been observed in the course of otherwise typical AHD. These apparent relationships cannot be unequivocally explained at present, and until improved serological methods for handling platelets and leukocytes are developed, it will be difficult to demonstrate serological and immunological relationships between these several processes of blood cell destruction.

Another interesting relationship appears to exist between AHD and thrombotic thrombocytopenic purpura (TTP), characterized by acute hemolytic anemia, thrombocytopenia, and vasculitis. Initially, it was reported that patients with TTP did not exhibit positive red cell antiglobulin reactions. In recent years, however, there are increasingly frequent reports of positive red cell antiglobulin reactions, primarily of the non-γ type in cases of typical TTP. The significance of this serological finding is unknown.

THERAPY

The introduction of corticosteroid hormone therapy for AHD must be regarded as a major therapeutic advance. These drugs may be dramatically effective in inducing prompt cessation or marked slowing of rapid blood destruction in approximately two thirds of patients with AHD so treated. Five to 10 percent of patients show essentially no response to corticosteroid therapy, and the remainder show variable minor degrees of improvement. Patients whose red cells give a negative reaction in the Coombs test seldom are strikingly improved by corticosteroid therapy, although 15 to 20 percent may show some evidence of slowing of blood destruction or improvement in hematocrit.

Relatively large doses of corticosteroid hormones are required initially to control acute hemolysis in patients with AHD. Doses equivalent to 40 to 80 mg. of prednisone daily administered to an adult may be needed for 10 to 14 days, with gradual decrease of this dosage to one quarter to one half of the starting dose after hemolysis has slowed. These dosages should then be administered for prolonged periods. After the patient has fully stabilized, with little or no evidence of hemolysis as shown by normal reticulocyte counts, the drug may be slowly withdrawn. Unless there are more specific contraindications, it is wise to treat these patients for a minimum of three or four months with low doses of corticosteroid hormones following subsidence of an acute episode of hemolysis. Critically ill patients with rapid hemolysis should be given hydrocortisone intravenously in doses of at least 100 mg. every six hours by infusion. Even larger doses of corticosteroid hormones have been recommended for patients who do not respond to the doses outlined, but this seems to be of doubtful value in our experience, although in desperately ill patients, it may be worth a trial. Similarly, administration of ACTH has been recommended for patients who do not respond to natural or synthetic corticosteroid drugs. There is no convincing evidence that this is effective in large groups of patients.

Splenectomy has been virtually abandoned

in this disorder. It may be warranted in patients who cannot be stabilized by any other means and in whom prominent sequestration of normal transfused red cells by the spleen can be shown by the use of Cr^{51}-labeled donor erythrocytes. When splenectomy was commonly carried out in this disorder, it was observed that some improvement commonly followed the operation. This was usually short-lived, and relapse commonly followed after a variable period of time.

Antimetabolites, such as 6-mercaptopurine and thioguanine, have been employed on the theory that these agents may in some way interfere with the synthesis of autoantibody. There is little direct clinical evidence in support of this hypothesis, although the theoretical basis of the use of these agents is well known. The use of alkylating agents for similar purposes has also been proposed. It is also difficult to assess the effectiveness of this approach in the treatment of AHD because of the great variability of the clinical course and because of the relatively small number of patients treated in this fashion that have been reported. It should be pointed out that both of these classes of cytotoxic agents have profound effects on cells other than those of the antibody-producing system. It may be that any favorable effects are not dependent on their influence on the rate of autoantibody synthesis. It is also noteworthy that initial attacks of acute AHD have been reported to follow alkylation therapy or x-ray treatment in cases of chronic lymphocytic leukemia or lymphosarcoma. The mechanism of this effect is also obscure.

Transfusion. It has long been recognized that transfusion of patients with AHD presents a serious clinical and serological problem. If the patient has autoantibody free in the serum, it may be impossible to find compatible donor blood. Even if *in vitro* serological compatibility between donor and patient can be demonstrated, the donor red cells may be destroyed rapidly *in vivo*. It is possible that donor red cells are more susceptible to the *in vivo* hemolytic mechanism operating in cases of AHD, presumably because they are all mature. The patient's own reticulocytes may enjoy a brief period of relative immunity from destruction. Transfusion of patients with AHD is usually followed by increasing signs of blood destruction with increase in jaundice, hemoglobinemia in some cases, and not infrequently a deteriorating clinical condition.

Because of these adverse clinical effects and serological difficulties, and because corticosteroid hormones have provided an effective approach to therapy, transfusion is infrequently employed at present. Rather, all possible supportive measures of the patient's circulation and oxygen transport should be undertaken and transfusion resorted to only when it is imperative as a life-saving measure.

Choice of a donor may be simplified if the autoantibody can be shown to have specificity. In this case, a donor lacking the antigen or antigens which interact with the patient's autoantibodies can be chosen. In cases in which there is no apparent specificity of the autoantibody, a donor compatible with the patient's own ABO and Rh blood group should be chosen and the result of the cross-match test examined carefully to be sure the donor's red cells react no more strongly with the patient's serum than do the patient's own red cells. These transfusions should be given as sedimented red cells, and at very slow rates of infusion, with careful observation of the patient. Repeated blood samples can be taken from the recipient and examined for hemoglobinemia. If hemoglobinemia appears, the transfusion should be discontinued promptly.

AHD OF WARM ANTIBODY TYPE OCCURRING AFTER INFECTION

Acute AHD is occasionally encountered in the course of illnesses that appear to be viral infections, particularly infectious mononucleosis. The patients may exhibit all of the clinical and serological findings of IAHD, although the rate of blood destruction is seldom extremely rapid. Similar cases of AHD are seen in the pediatric age group with a variety of ill-defined viral illnesses. These disorders differ from other types of idiopathic and symptomatic AHD in that the patient usually experiences only a single episode of hemolysis and, after a variable period of time in the convalescent phase of the infection, the antiglobulin test reverts to negative. The mechanism of induction of AHD in this interesting group of disorders is also unknown. It is of interest that the diseases with which it is associated, e.g., infectious mononucleosis, commonly induce hyperplasia of the reticuloendothelial and lymphatic apparatus.

HEMOLYTIC DISEASE ASSOCIATED WITH COLD-ACTIVE AUTOANTIBODIES

PAROXYSMAL COLD HEMOGLOBINURIA

The most dramatic form of acquired hemolytic disease is that characterized by acute intermittent massive hemolysis which follows exposure to cold; this disorder is frequently accompanied by hemoglobinuria, sometimes by severe acrocyanosis, and less commonly by cold urticaria. This form of disease was recognized in the latter part of the last century, but its relationship to autoantibodies was not then known. By 1884 a frequent identification with late syphilis had been noted, and in 1904, Donath and Landsteiner [15] described the complement-fixing autohemolytic serum antibody (D-L antibody) that is responsible for the hemolytic disease.

Clinical Features. Patients of any age can be affected, but the frequency of congenital syphilis in the Nineteenth and early Twentieth Centuries assured that many reported cases would be in children. Multiple cases within families have been seen. Typically, the attacks occur in cold seasons, but the degree of chilling required to induce hemolysis is highly variable from patient to patient. Constitutional symptoms begin minutes to hours after cold exposure, and the urine promptly becomes dark red. In the most acute cases, there may be aching pain in the back and extremities, acute abdominal cramps, and fever as high as 40° C. Generally, the symptoms abate in a few hours. The spleen may become transiently palpable. Raynaud's phenomenon of the hands, feet, ears, or nose may occur and lead to gangrene in extreme cases. Cold urticaria has been described. In abortive attacks, the constitutional symptoms without hemoglobinuria, or with only transitory albuminuria, may be seen.

The hemoglobin level can drop acutely by as much as 5 or 6 gm. per 100 ml. in severe attacks. Microspherocytosis may be seen on the blood smear. Direct Coombs tests on the patient's red cells may be positive during the attack. Serum complement titers are usually acutely depressed. Leukopenia during the paroxysm is followed by neutrophilic leukocytosis. Erythrophagocytosis by both neutrophils and monocytes has been seen on blood smears and has been readily induced by *in vitro* incubation of freshly drawn blood prior to smearing it on glass slides. Hemoglobinemia, of course, accompanies the hemoglobinuria and is easily demonstrated in the serum during the acute attack. Bilirubinemia follows in twenty-four to forty-eight hours.

Attacks can be avoided by guarding the patient from exposure to cold, and most patients survive long periods. Death from acute renal failure has been described rarely. In cases attributable to syphilis, effective treatment of the syphilis has often resulted in cure of the hemolytic disease. The disease has always been rare, but with the decreased incidence of syphilis, has become even more so. Today, most cases do not have evidences of syphilis and are termed "idiopathic," but time relationships in onset of measles, chickenpox, infectious mononucleosis, or upper respiratory infections have been noted in an acute transient form of the disease.

Serology. The D-L antibody is typically demonstrated by a two-phase test in which the patient's fresh serum is mixed with his own or another's erythrocytes at 4° C. and the mixture then warmed to 37° C. Intense or complete hemolysis of the red cells occurs. It has been shown that attachment of the antibody and complement occur in the cold [16], preparing the cell for lysis when the temperature is raised. In the absence of complement, the D-L antibody fails to attach or attaches weakly to the red cell, so that on subsequent exposure to complement at 37° C. there may be little hemolysis. The highest temperature at which effective sensitization of the red cells with antibody and complement takes place is generally below 20° C. and in some cases it may be as low as 10° C. Presumably this temperature dependence of the serological reaction is one of the major determinants of the severity of chilling needed to provoke an attack. Another important determinant undoubtedly is the titer of antibody.

It should be noted that the average temperature of the blood in the capillaries of the skin of the extremities is 28 to 30° C.; thus at any given time only a very small proportion of the total red cell mass can be in compartments of the intravascular space where the temperatures are low enough to bring about sensitization for subsequent lysis. Lysis may occur locally, but presumably much of the hemolysis takes place when the temperature of red cells and plasma is brought back to 37° C. on re-entry into the general circulation.

The titers of hemolysin demonstrated by the D-L test are moderate; activity in a dilution of 1 : 16 represents a strongly reactive serum. Little or no agglutination occurs unless special conditions are established to bring it out. The red cells may be rendered "non-γ" antiglobulin positive *in vitro,* attributable principally or entirely to the attachment of complement components. The antibody is a 7S γ-globulin [16]. It has recently been shown by Levine *et al.* [17] to have anti-Tja specificity in six successive instances. The Tja antigen is one of the so-called public antigens, being absent from less than 1 of every 10,000 persons' red cells. There is one report, however, of cold hemoglobinuria with a strictly autospecific antibody, thus not anti-Tja. It may be expected that other such cases will appear. Descriptions of reactivity of purified D-L antibody not only with human but also with certain heterologous erythrocytes indicate that the antigen may be widely distributed among animals. No information is available on the interesting question of whether D-L antibodies have the same specificities when the hemolytic process is associated with a given predisposing disease, such as syphilis, as when it occurs otherwise. D-L antibodies are distinct from the antibodies causing the Wassermann and Kahn reactions. Whether the D-L antibody is also responsible for the cold urticaria that occurs in some patients with paroxysmal cold hemoglobinuria is not known. Passive transfer of the cold urticaria to normal skin by a modified Prausnitz-Küstner technique has been effected successfully, but no test has been made of whether absorption of the D-L antibody from the serum would affect the transfer (Ref. 1, p. 550).

Treatment. In cases due to syphilis, treatment of the syphilis generally cures the hemolytic disease. Otherwise, only symptomatic therapy and preventive measures are indicated. A warm bed cannot be improved upon. Antihistaminic and sympathomimetic drugs may be of some benefit for the cold urticaria. Corticosteroid therapy has been disappointing, and splenectomy is not useful.

COLD AGGLUTININ DISEASE

During the first half of this century, cases of hemolytic disease having somewhat different clinical presentations from those due to the D-L antibody began to be recognized. The cardinal laboratory manifestation was intense autohemagglutination in the cold. Cold autohemagglutination had been noted before, but in 1925, Iwai and Mei-Sai [18] first showed that it could have clinical significance. When the conjunctivae or nailbeds of a patient with strong autohemagglutination were chilled, they observed arresting or sluggishness of the blood flow, with breaking of the blood columns in the fine vessels. This experiment was performed in a patient who had Raynaud's phenomenon, but apparently no hemoglobinuria.

Clinical Features. Subsequently, cases with hemoglobinuria as well as Raynaud's phenomenon were reported; others had no Raynaud's phenomenon at all. The variable clinical picture of cold agglutinin disease was thus established. At 4° C., serum cold agglutinin titers generally were 1,000 or more, sometimes over 1,000,000! The degree of anemia exhibited by patients with given titers of cold antibody is quite variable. This indicates that clinical manifestations depend also on other variables in the system, probably especially the function of the reticuloendothelial system.

Although cold agglutinin disease is distinctly more frequent than the paroxysmal cold hemoglobinuria due to D-L antibody, it is still a relatively uncommon entity. In two large series of reported cases of acquired hemolytic disease of all sorts, only 20 and 25 percent were due to cold agglutinins. Our own experience has given us a less frequent relative incidence.

Cold agglutinin disease may be acute or chronic. The acute form affects both sexes, and adults more than children. It develops as an infrequent complication of the elevated cold agglutinin titer which commonly follows Eaton agent pneumonia. In these cases, the onset is usually sudden, the patient developing pallor, jaundice, and weakness a week or two after having recovered from pneumonitis. Constitutional symptoms, like those accompanying the intense acute hemolysis due to D-L antibody, are rare, even though there may be hemoglobinuria in severe cases. Raynaud's symptoms may be present, and occasionally they may even be the only clinical manifestations. Gangrene has been described rarely. Phlebothrombosis with pulmonary emboli in the later part of the illness has been attributed to intravascular hemagglutination. The spleen may become palpable transiently. Red cell counts as low as 1,000,000 per mm^3 have been noted. There is generally leukocytosis, often very marked. Polychromasia, microspherocytosis, autoagglutination, erythrophagocytosis, and increased osmotic fragility are all characteristic hematological findings, as are hyperbilirubinemia and low or absent serum haptoglobins. The course of the acute postpneumonic disease is generally benign, and full recovery with fall in the cold agglutinin titer and loss of the complement-type antiglobulin reactivity of the red cells can be expected. Rarely, this sequence of events has been described in association with infectious mononucleosis. Here the process seems much the same, save for the interesting fact that the hemolytic anemia may occasionally develop simultaneously with the onset of symptoms of the infectious mononucleosis.

The chronic form of cold agglutinin disease is particularly seen in the elderly of both sexes. There is a correlation of severity of symptoms with cold weather; chronic anemia is present and is more severe in the winter. Raynaud's phenomenon frequently involves the fingers, toes, ears, or nose. Ulcerations and gangrene can be distressing complications. Hemoglobinuria may be experienced during hemolytic exacerbations in cold weather, but some patients never have this experience. Hemosiderinuria has been noted as a manifestation of lesser degrees of rapid hemolysis.

Physical examination of these patients typically reveals pallor and jaundice. Splenomegaly is occasionally seen. Marked autoagglutination and varying degrees of hemolysis may be seen in blood taken by ordinary venipuncture. This can be avoided if the collection is made entirely at 37° C. Anemia is usually moderate, but hemoglobin levels as low as 5 or 6 gm. per 100 ml. of blood are not rare. There is commonly mild microspherocytosis of the red cells, and the polychromasia is in keeping with the degree of anemia and associated normoblastic bone marrow hyperactivity. The direct antiglobulin test of the patient's red cells is positive, due to coating of the cells with complement components. Serum complement levels often are low. The white blood cell count is usually normal. Erythrophagocytosis is infrequently seen in direct smears of peripheral blood but may be present after *in vitro* incubation inhibition of a blood sample. Hyperbilirubinemia is variable, but usually mild.

Chronic cold agglutinin disease may be idiopathic, or it may accompany underlying neoplastic disease of the lymphoid or reticuloendothelial system. Its course may be extremely protracted and refractory to all therapy other than prophylaxis against exposure to cold. Under optimal care, 15- to 25-year survivals of patients have been reported. When secondary to neoplastic disease, the period of survival is generally dictated by the course of the neoplastic disease.

Serology. Cold agglutinins are 19S γ-globulins. As is typical of antibodies in general, cold agglutinins can be distinguished from other antibodies of their class only by their specific reactivities with the red cell antigens to which they are directed. It has recently been demonstrated that the majority of cold agglutinins in hemolytic disease have anti-I specificity. The I-antigen is found in almost all normal adult erythrocytes, but it is absent or poorly represented in neonatal erythrocytes. It is genetically absent in the red blood cells of about one of every four or five thousand adults. Specificities of pathological cold agglutinins for i-, H (O)-, M-, and B-antigens have also been described [19].

Pathological cold agglutinins also may cross-react with the red cells of various lower animals. Rabbit, pig, and primate red cells have been found to be especially reactive with cold agglutinins; guinea pig and rat red cells are less reactive, and erythrocytes of other species react poorly or not at all.

Anti-I specificity of the cold agglutinin has been seen in patients with AHD developing after primary atypical pneumonia due to the Eaton agent as well as in idiopathic cold agglutinin disease. The cold agglutinin has been found to be independent of Eaton agent antigens by cross-absorption tests.

Cold agglutinins are distinguished by reacting better at 4° than at 37° C. At intermediate temperatures, lesser titers are seen, and most sera are nonagglutinating at 30° C. At this temperature, however, they may nevertheless react with red cells to sensitize them to agglutination by antiglobulin reagents (see later). Hemolytic disease is especially seen in patients exhibiting high titered antibody which also has a high "thermal amplitude" (i.e., which still agglutinates red cells at room temperatures and above). The pH optimum for agglutination by cold agglutinins is broad, ranging from 6.0 to 8.5.

Lysis may occur with cold agglutinins if the sera are tested when fresh or with added complement. Some lysis occurs with almost all sera when the red cells are added to cold agglutinin in the presence of complement at room temperature, if the pH of the system is kept around or slightly below 7.0.

Attachment of complement components to normal red cells by cold agglutinins can be readily demonstrated by agglutinability of the cells with anticomplement sera. Both β_{1C}-β_{1A}(C′3a) and β_{1E}(C′4) components have been demonstrated on red cells; the attachment occurs even at 4° C. At this lower temperature no hemolysis occurs, since the final step in complement lysis of antibody-sensitized cells requires higher temperatures (Chap. 14). It is interesting that cold agglutinins cannot be demonstrated on the red cell surfaces after elution at 37° C., although complement components remain. Several laboratories [10] studied this with specific anti-19S γ-globulin sera. They found that the complement-coated red cells failed to be agglutinated by anti-19S γ-globulin sera. They noted the possibility that cold agglutinin can cause fixation of complement components to the red cell surface and then be free to move off the cell again, leaving the complement attached. Direct experimental support for this idea, using I^{131}-labeled cold agglutinin [20], has recently been offered.

The red cells of patients actively hemolyzing because of cold agglutinins frequently give positive reactions in direct antiglobulin tests. This is due to attachment of complement components. Negative antiglobulin reactions for residual 19S γ-globulins are also found. Thus the same type of red cell sensitization occurs *in vivo* in active disease as can be induced *in vitro*. Although it was at one time supposed that the "non-γ" sensitization of red cells by pathological cold agglutinin could be indicative of an "incomplete" cold-reactive antibody, the studies of Dacie *et al.* [21] and Leddy *et al.* [22] have made this postulation untenable.

Lowered serum complement titers during acute hemolytic episodes seem reasonably explained in most cases by fixation of complement components onto the circulating red cells by cold agglutinins. Other explanations are possible, however (as discussed on p. 852). The frequency of lowered serum complement titers in cases of cold agglutinin hemolytic anemia is significantly greater than in warm autoantibody hemolytic anemias.

Whether red cells are damaged by being coated with complement components or are made more susceptible to damage in the circulation is not entirely certain. Lewis *et al.* have shown that red cells reacted *in vitro* with complement and cold agglutinin may, on reinjection, be trapped in the liver and rapidly hemolyzed. Erythrocytes treated *in vitro* to allow less complement action survived better. In both instances, the cells were freely dispersed at 37° C. before being reinjected (see Ref. 1, p. 635).

On electrophoretic analysis, cold agglutinins usually are found broadly distributed among the 19S γ-globulins. When titers of cold agglutination of a serum exceeded 8,000, Christenson and Dacie [23] could generally demonstrate elevations in the amount of protein in the beta-gamma regions by paper electrophoresis. Absorption of the cold agglutinins from the serum reduced this electrophoretically separated component. Occasionally, cases have been described in which highly homogeneous proteins have been present in the gamma or beta-gamma regions; these proteins have been 19S in type and have had cold agglutinin activity in very high titer. On immunochemical analysis, slight differences have been detected between these cold agglutinin proteins and normal 19S γ-globulins. It is possible that cases such as these are examples of macroglobulinemia of the Waldenström type (Chap. 25), in which clones of abnormal lymphoid cells are synthesizing proteins which have this functional activity.

Occasionally, cryoprecipitation of cold agglutinins has been noted. The factors that determine whether or not cold agglutinins will precipitate from solution in the cold are not known. When this occurs, it seems that the patient may be rendered even more susceptible to Raynaud's phenomenon. Cases have also been described in which cryoglobulins and cold agglutinins coexist in the serum as separate entities.

Prognosis and Therapy. As has been noted, patients with cold agglutinin disease may survive many years, suffering minimal disability. In more severe cases, death may ensue, especially from infection, from the underlying neoplastic process, from severe anemia and its complications, or from complications of transfusion therapy, i.e., hepatitis or hemolytic transfusion reactions. Splenectomy and corticosteroid therapy have both been generally disappointing. Dacie [1] described "atypical" cases in which some improvement did follow splenectomy. As he suggests, splenectomy should be reserved for those infrequent cases of cold agglutinin disease in which *in vivo* studies with Cr^{51}-tagged red cells show predominant localization of radioactivity to the spleen rather than the liver. As Jandl *et al.* [24] have shown, strongly agglutinating cells are predominantly removed by the liver. Penicillamine given in the attempt to dissociate and thereby inactivate cold agglutinins has been claimed to have usefulness by some but has failed in other hands. The possible use of antimetabolite or alkylation therapy has not received much attention, probably because cold agglutinin disease commonly is relatively benign in relation to the hazards of these therapeutic agents. The mainstay of proper management of these patients is prophylaxis. A warm house and warm clothing should be assured. Transfusions should be administered only if clearly demanded. Most patients will tolerate their mild or moderate anemia quite well. Splenectomy should be performed only when Cr^{51}-labeled red cells show predominant localization to the spleen.

REFERENCES

1. Dacie, J. V. *The Hemolytic Anemias.* New York: Grune & Stratton, Inc., 1962.
2. Swisher, S. N. Autoimmune Hemolytic Disease. In Weinstein, I. M., and Beutler, E. (Eds.), *Mechanisms of Anemia.* New York: McGraw-Hill Book Company, Inc., 1962. P. 271.
3. Coombs, R. R. A., Mourant, A. E., and Race, R. R. A new test for the detection of weak and "incomplete" Rh agglutinins. *Brit. J. Exp. Path.* 26:255, 1945.
4. Boorman, K. E., Dodd, B. E., and Loutit, J. F. Haemolytic icterus (acholuric jaundice) congenital and acquired. *Lancet* 1:812, 1946.
5. Witebsky, E. The question of self-recognition by the host and problems of autoantibodies and their specificity. *Cancer Res.* 21:1216, 1961.
6. Weiner, W., and Vos, G. H. Serology of acquired hemolytic anemia. *Blood* 22:606, 1963.
7. Wiener, A. S., Gordon, E. B., and Gallop, C. Studies on autoantibodies in human sera. *J. Immun.* 71:58, 1953.
8. Levine, P., Celano, M. J., Wallace, J., and Sanger, R. A human "D-like" antibody. *Nature* (London) 198:596, 1963.
9. Evans, R. S., and Weiser, R. S. The serology of autoimmune hemolytic disease. *Arch. Intern. Med.* 100:371, 1957.
10. Leddy, J. P., Hill, R. W., Swisher, S. N., and Vaughan, J. H. Observations on the Immunochemical Nature of Red Cell Autosensitization. *Immunopathology* (3rd International Symposium). Basel: Benno Schwabe & Co., 1963.
11. Harboe, M., Müller-Eberhard, H. J., Fudenberg, H., Polley, M. J., and Mollison, P. L. Identification of the components of complement participating in the antiglobulin reaction. *Immunology* 6:412, 1963.
12. Shulman, N. R. Mechanism of blood cell destruction in individuals sensitized to foreign antigens. *Trans. Ass. Amer. Physician* 76:72, 1963.
13. Leddy, J. P., and Vaughan, J. H. Auto-sensitization of trypsin treated human red cells by complement. *Proc. Soc. Exp. Biol. Med.* 117: 734, 1964.
14. Fudenberg, H., Barry, I. and Dameshek, W. The erythrocyte coating substance in autoimmune hemolytic disease: Its nature and significance. *Blood* 13:201, 1958.
15. Donath, J., and Landsteiner, K. Ueber paroxysmale Hämoglobinurie. *München. Med. Wschr.* 51:1590, 1904.
16. Hinz, C. F., Jr. Serologic and physicochemical characterization of Donath-Landsteiner antibodies from six patients. *Blood* 22:600, 1963.
17. Levine, P., Celano, M. J., and Falkowski, F. The specificity of the antibody in paroxysmal cold hemoglobinemia (PCH). *Transfusion* 3: 278, 1963.
18. Iwai, S., and Mei-Sai, N. Etiology of Raynaud's disease (a preliminary report). *Jap. Med. World* 5:119, 1925.
19. Van Loghem, J. J., Pectoom, E., VanderHart, M., VanderVeer, M., Vander Giessen, M., Prins, H. K., Zurcher, C. and Engelfriel, C. P. Serological and immunochemical studies in haemolytic anemia with high titer cold agglutinins. *Vox Sang.* 8:33, 1963.
20. Personal communications. Evans, R. S., Harboe, M., and Boyer, J., have each independently performed such experiments.
21. Dacie, J. V., Crookston, J. H., and Christenson, W. N. "Incomplete" cold antibodies:

Role of complement in sensitization to antiglobulin serum by potentially haemolytic antibodies. *Brit. J. Haemat.* 3:77, 1957.

22. Leddy, J. P., Trabold, N. C., Vaughan, J. H., and Swisher, S. N. The unitary nature of "complete" and "incomplete" pathologic cold hemagglutinins. *Blood* 19:379, 1962.
23. Christenson, W. N., and Dacie, J. V. Serum proteins in acquired haemolytic anaemia (auto-antibody type). *Brit. J. Haemat.* 3:153, 1957. Christenson, W. N., Dacie, J. V., Croucher, B. E. E., and Charlwood, P. A. Electrophoretic studies on sera containing high-titre cold haemagglutinins: Identification of the antibody as the cause of an abnormal γ_1 peak. *Ibid.,* p. 262.
24. Jandl, J. H., Richardson-Jones, A., and Castle, W. B. The destruction of red cells by antibodies in man: I. Observations on the sequestration and lysis of red cells altered by immune mechanisms. *J. Clin. Invest.* 36:1428, 1957.

75. *Idiopathic Thrombocytopenic Purpura**

FRANK H. GARDNER

THE DIAGNOSIS OF IDIOPATHIC thrombocytopenic purpura (ITP) has been applied to the clinical picture of thrombocytopenia associated with mild to severe bleeding phenomena. Most patients have no anemia, unless from blood loss. The thrombocytopenia has been characterized by an abnormal morphology of the platelets observed on the peripheral blood smear, decreased life span of the platelets, and a bizarre morphology of the megakaryocytes in bone marrow. In addition, the bone marrow often shows megakaryocytic hyperplasia.

As ITP has been observed in past decades, clinicians have appreciated that the platelet deficiency may be self-limited to a few weeks or months. This type of idiopathic disease is usually observed in children and is classified as *acute ITP*. In the adult, the thrombocytopenia generally persists for months or years and has been designated *chronic ITP*. Until the etiology of the thrombocytopenia is clarified, this definition may be used for the idiopathic disease. However, a transitory thrombocytopenia may be related to drug ingestion (see later). In recent years, the association of thrombocytopenia with collagen disorders has been emphasized, especially in systemic lupus erythematosus (SLE).

ACUTE ITP

In general, this designation applies to thrombocytopenia that is associated with purpuric manifestations in children and, as stated, is transitory, lasting no longer than three months [1]. Eighty-five percent of patients are below 8 years of age, and both sexes are affected equally (Fig. 75-1). In the United States, the majority of patients with acute thrombocytopenia are seen in December through May, when bacterial and viral respiratory infections are most common. Two thirds of the patients have had antecedent infectious illness [2]. This relationship has been the basis for proposing an immune mechanism for acute thrombocytopenia through contact of human platelets with a viral or bacterial antigen and its antibody. In many instances, the infection occurs within the two weeks preceding the abrupt onset of purpura. Probably many infections with consequent thrombocytopenia are overlooked, since the diagnosis of thrombocytopenia is usually made only after overt bleeding occurs. Although sporadic cases of thrombocytopenic purpura associated with infectious mononucleosis have been reported, Angle and Alt [3] noted that in four of seven patients without purpura, the platelet count was below normal. Routine survey data probably would show transitory lowering of the blood platelet count in most viremias. Although the relationship of thrombocytopenia to measles has been emphasized, the innocuous character of this illness nowadays has lessened the opportunity for hospital observation and laboratory measurement [2]. A large outbreak of measles in an orphanage, or a similar situation, might be utilized to clarify this problem.

The onset of purpura is sudden in children, and it is rare to observe a slow decline in the platelet count. Transfused isologous† platelets are destroyed rapidly (Fig. 75-2) [4]. The rapid destruction of transfused platelets in these recipients implies (1) that a plasma factor agglutinates, alters, or "coats" the platelet for phagocytic removal, or (2) that the reticuloendothelial system (RES) has an abnormal phagocytic response to the circulating platelet. The evidence of a plasma factor in the chronic form of this disease has suggested that a similar mechanism may be present in the acute type. The thrombocytopenia exists despite adequate

* Some studies in this report were done under a grant from the U.S. Public Health Service Grant No. H-5895 (C1-2), and the John A. Hartford Foundation, Inc. Dr. Gardner is a recipient of the U.S.P.H.S. Research Career Award HE-K-1497.

† *Editor's comment:* Homologous is the more proper term. See footnote [†], page 847.—J. H. V.

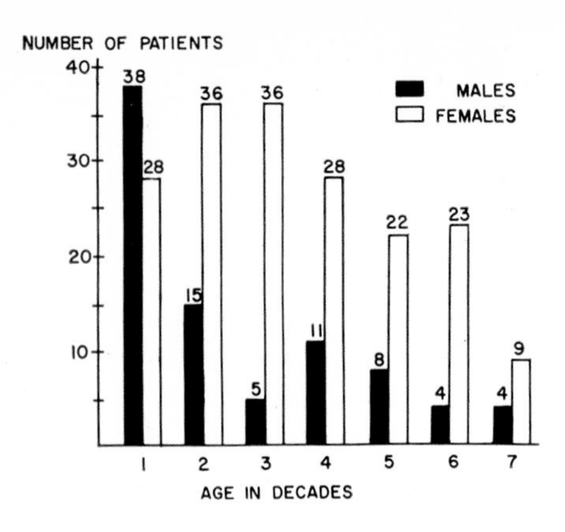

Fig. 75-1. Age and sex of patients with ITP. After age 10, females predominate throughout life. (Modified from Doan *et al.* [12].)

megakaryocytes in the bone marrow, yet there has been conflicting evidence of serological abnormalities (agglutinins or lysins) in the acute type of this disorder. Platelet agglutinins have been described, but the observations have not been reproduced in most laboratories. Most workers, primarily pediatricians, have accepted the concept that the acute disease is associated with an antiplatelet factor that cannot be defined adequately with the techniques available.

An enzyme, acid β-glycerol phosphatase, is found both in platelets and in plasma. During acute thrombocytopenia, the plasma acid phosphatase level is elevated, returning to normal as the platelet count rises (Fig. 75-3) [5]. The plasma level is taken to be a very useful measurement of platelet destruction, and it should be used early for differential diagnosis. It is more helpful than any "antibody test" in establishing evidence of increased platelet destruction. The test has the added advantage that it requires techniques generally available in hospital laboratories and therefore is easily instituted.

Most patients with acute ITP have a benign course whether they are treated or not. Five percent have some cerebral bleeding [2]. For this reason, most children today are treated with corticoids during the period of severe thrombocytopenia (platelets less than 40,000 mm.^{3}). Despite the experience with corticoids in the past decade, however, it is difficult to determine if the course of the illness has been altered. Because of the ability of corticoids to improve capillary integrity nonspecifically, their use seems advisable if there is bleeding. Prednisone is the drug of choice. There is little to be gained from doses above 30 to 45 mg. daily. After one week, the dose should be tapered and finally the drug withdrawn. There is no reason to consider splenectomy during the first three months of the illness unless the platelet count cannot be raised above 40,000 mm.^{3} by corticosteroid therapy. In such patients, one should consider the presence of another disorder (SLE, leukemia, or lymphoma) and carry out careful, appropriate diagnostic procedures. During the past decade, as these children have been followed very

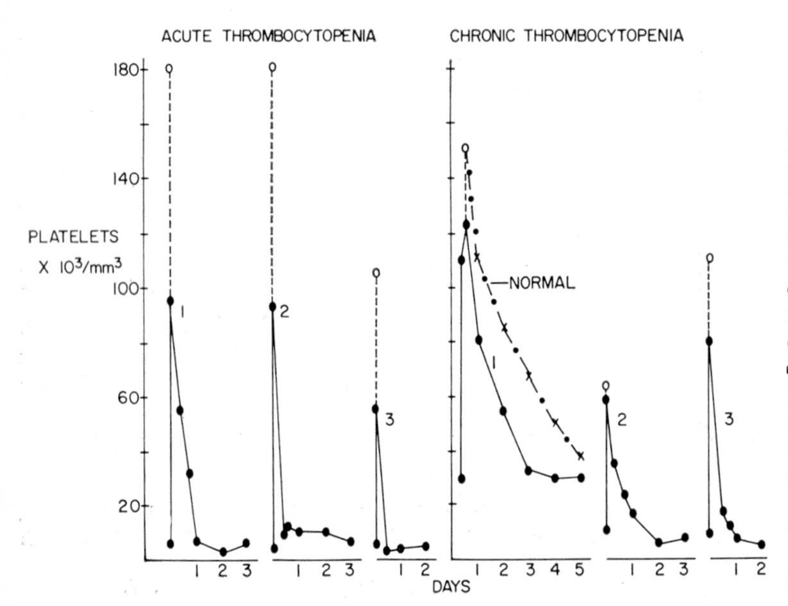

Fig. 75-2. Survival of compatible transfused platelets in patients with acute and chronic ITP. Patient with acute ITP has rapid destruction of platelets. Patient with chronic ITP has a variable response from moderate (*curve 1*) to rapid (*curve 3*) destruction; a normal platelet life span in aplastic anemia is drawn next to *curve 1* for comparison. *Broken lines* indicate calculated platelet level that might be expected within one hour after transfusion. (Redrawn from data of Hirsch and Gardner [4].)

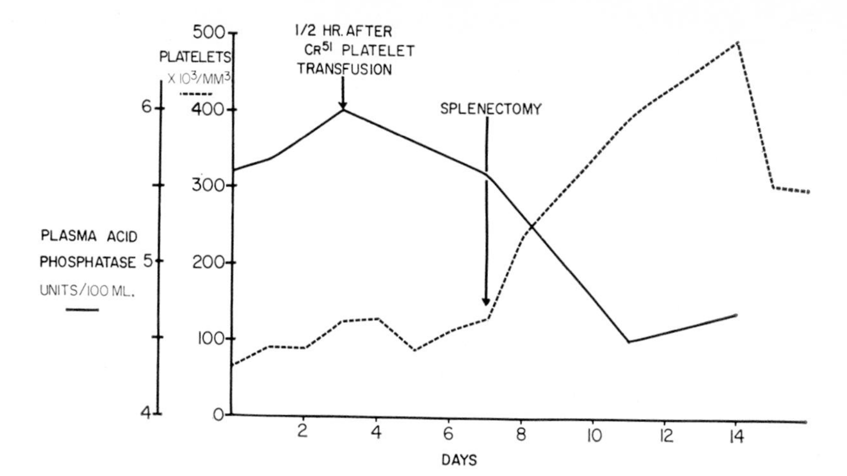

Fig. 75-3. Elevation of plasma acid phosphatase (*solid line*) until ITP is controlled by splenectomy. As platelet count rises, and destruction diminishes, plasma acid phosphatase levels decline. (Modified from Oski *et al.* [5].)

carefully, about 10 percent have progressed to a chronic type of illness that persists into adult life. In these patients, splenectomy is warranted if a spontaneous remission does not occur after a six-month observation period [2].

Since there is no laboratory model for study of ITP, one can only speculate about possible mechanisms to explain idiopathic acute thrombocytopenia. The following concept is presented to relate acute ITP to previous infection. The platelet has been described as a sponge. Indeed, the platelet membrane will bind virus particles, bacteria, soluble antigen-antibody complexes, and endotoxins [6]. Such adsorbed substances may affect the viability of the platelet both by morphological alteration and by metabolic interference. Damaged platelets probably no longer circulate, but are phagocytized rapidly by the RES. We have assumed this to be a physiological method for removal of nonfunctioning platelets. In the presence of viremia, a delay in RES phagocytosis of aggregated proteins or colloids (equated to platelets) has been noted. This was seen with iodinated aggregated albumin in dengue and sandfly fever [7] and with radioactive chromic phosphate in infectious mononucleosis [8]. It is tempting to speculate, therefore, that during viremia, delay in removal of a platelet-virus-antibody complex would allow sufficient platelet membrane changes from the adsorbed complex for an antibody response to altered membrane antigens to occur.

This explanation leans on analogy from certain features of sensitization to Rh antigens. Rh sensitization is initiated in the Rh-negative mother by introduction of Rh-positive red cells from the fetus at the time of first delivery. In a series of studies by Clarke *et al.* [9], the degree of sensitization appeared to be related to the concentration of fetal red cells introduced into the circulation at the time of delivery. If these "foreign" Rh-positive cells are removed immediately by agglutination with an infusion of sera containing incomplete anti-Rh antibody, the Rh-negative recipient will not be immunized. One could say that with the antibody coating, the red cells are quickly removed and the membrane antigen does not come into contact with the maternal antibody-forming cells.* In converse manner, platelets complexed with virus or bacteria may not be phagocytized rapidly because of an impaired RES, and altered platelet membranes could form and act as antigens to elicit an immune response. Although such proposals may be helpful in establishing a working hypothesis for acute ITP, there are no data to support this concept.

CHRONIC ITP

The thrombocytopenia seen in the adult (beyond age 15) is in striking contrast to the acute disease in children. Although one continues to see self-limited episodes that persist for only a few weeks in young adults, most patients have an illness that persists beyond

* *Editor's comment:* Levine (*Hum. Biol.* 30:14, 1958) has marshaled evidence to indicate that ABO incompatibility also will hinder the ability of mothers bearing Rh-positive children to make anti-Rh antibody, presumably through the same mechanism described. —J. H. V.

three months. Once thrombocytopenia has developed, the platelet depression usually continues unless drug therapy or surgery alters the course. A few patients have an unusual episodic course; i.e., severe thrombocytopenia may continue for 1 to 3 months, followed by a spontaneous remission and then recurrence of the thrombocytopenia years later [10]. In many respects, these patients appear to have repeated episodes of the acute type of disease seen in childhood associated commonly with respiratory infections. After any one of the numerous episodes, the patient may continue to have thrombocytopenia for months and thereafter follow a chronic course. One patient in our clinic had a 14-year interval between two severe episodes of thrombocytopenia with purpura and bleeding. Such a long interval is unusual, but remissions for 1 to 3 years are seen occasionally. One may assume that the fundamental derangement is never lost and may be reactivated by such factors as infections and drugs.

In contrast to the equal sex incidence in children, in adults the illness predominates in females, ranging from 65 to 80 percent in various series (Fig. 75-1) [11, 12]. In fact, after age 10, the frequency even of the acute type of ITP in children has a female : male ratio of 3 : 1 [2]. A possible explanation for this ratio is a hormonal influence on the RES. From age 8 to 11, urinary estrogen levels are slowly increasing in girls, usually for 18 months before onset of the menses, and the urinary estrogen excretion follows the adult cyclic pattern [13]. In rodents, estrogens influence the phagocytic activity of the RES [14]. With murine hepatitis, estrogens enhance the mortality from the viremia [15]. Estrogens will also increase the titer of circulating agglutinins in rabbits following immunization with *Escherichia coli,* sheep red cells, and pneumococcus [16, 17]. Data on human beings are, however, quite sparse. In one report [18], two women were studied through the menstrual cycle for variations in type II pneumococcus antibody. The antibody level declined with the estrogen levels after ovulation. The normal heterologous hemolysins for sheep and rabbit red cells are higher in women than in men, with this preponderance declining after age 40 [19]. Thus data from animals and man may suggest that the female has a more active system to respond to (or recognize) a "damaged platelet." Hormonal variations possibly are significant in the prevalence of all "autoimmune" disorders in females.*

The degree of thrombocytopenia is more variable in the chronic than in the acute type of disease. If the platelet level is moderately high (80–100,000 $mm.^3$), the patient will have few if any symptoms. In practice, patients with platelet counts above 100,000 $mm.^3$ do not have a destructive type of thrombocytopenia. However, most patients have platelet counts below 40,000 $mm.^3$. Changes in any patient or group of patients probably reflect variations in the circulating plasma factors that destroy platelets. In the female during the menstrual cycle, there is a physiological undulating rise and fall of the platelets, with a decline at the onset of menses and recovery within 48 hours, followed by mild thrombocytosis at the time of ovulation. A patient with only moderate platelet depression (80,000 $mm.^3$) may well be free from hemorrhagic symptoms until the accentuation of thrombocytopenia at the onset of menses [20]. The only history may then be years of menorrhagia with eventual onset of iron deficiency anemia. All types of therapy may be tried to control the menstrual bleeding before the thrombocytopenia is discovered. The onset of dependent purpura, epistaxis, gingival bleeding, or bleeding at surgery usually prompts the patient to seek further medical care.

In the past 10 years, corticoid therapy has been used with great success to control chronic thrombocytopenia. Usually a program of 15 to 25 mg. of prednisone thrice daily has been satisfactory, with slow decrements of dosage as the platelet count rises. It is of utmost importance not to maintain excessively large doses of prednisone, for its catabolic effect may impair platelet production [21, 22]. Therefore, despite a satisfactory initial elevation of platelets, maintenance of high dosage can cause the count to fall to the pretreatment level [22]. In this instance, the recurrent thrombocytopenia possibly is related to impaired platelet formation from excessive pro-

* *Editor's comment:* This striking predominance in females is indeed worth attention. The meager evidence suggesting that estrogens are responsible for this by enchancing antibody responsiveness in women can, however, be equally balanced by references to estrogen effects on vascular physiology which may make women more susceptible to immunological or other injury. Needless to say, still other postulates could be put forward, including ones that do not focus on estrogens at all.—J. H. V.

tein catabolism induced by corticoids. Low maintenance dosage (10 to 20 mg. of prednisone daily) may be used for four to six weeks. Thereafter, efforts should be made to lower this dosage to see whether the episode is self-limited. If the thrombocytopenia recurs, the drug, at a dosage to maintain a protective platelet level, should be given for periods of three to six months, with the expectation that splenectomy will be performed to avoid the complications of long-term corticoid therapy. Some clinicians have proposed prolonged corticoid therapy for ITP because splenectomy has "unmasked" some cases of SLE (with the symptoms of thrombocytopenia). The onset of systemic symptoms of SLE following surgery has not been frequent enough to suggest a valid correlation. Certainly, the complications of prolonged corticoid therapy, even in small doses of 5 to 15 mg. of prednisone daily, outweigh the risk of splenectomy (0.5 percent mortality). In addition, the variable course of SLE, with spontaneous remissions and exacerbations, is too treacherous to allow a deduction of such a cause-and-effect relationship between splenectomy and activation of the disease.

One further indication for splenectomy is the chance that it affords to establish a positive tissue diagnosis. The percentage of idiopathic cases of thrombocytopenia shrinks as awareness of sarcoidosis, SLE, splenic lipidosis, lymphoma, and leukemia becomes more acute. In our clinic, at least 15 percent of patients undergoing splenectomy for thrombocytopenia yield a positive tissue diagnosis that may be important in prognosis or therapy, or both.

THE PLATELETS IN ITP

Most of our current concepts of ITP are derived from laboratory studies of heterologous platelet antibodies (experimental thrombocytopenia) and the antibody measurements in drug-induced purpura. These observations will be presented briefly as background for the clinical studies suggesting an immune mechanism in ITP.

Experimental Thrombocytopenia. For decades it has been evident that platelet agglutinins and lysins could be produced in animals by immunization with heterologous platelets. Such antiplatelet serum will cause profound thrombocytopenia when injected into the original donor [23]. *In vitro* tests by direct observation of the recipient's platelets, or with antigen-coated (platelet-coated) tanned red cells, show agglutination by the antiplatelet serum. The mixture of antiserum and platelets *in vitro* causes the release of serotonin, amino acids, and histamine from the platelets, implying damage to the platelet membrane [24, 25]. If enough immune antiserum is injected, circulating platelets are removed completely by agglutination and lysis. Normal platelet levels return in four to six days. In the rabbit, the induction of platelet antibodies by injection of heterologous platelets can be inhibited by prolonged administration of corticoids [26].

There is evidence that the spleen participates in the development of the thrombocytopenia. In this respect, immunologically induced thrombocytopenia is similar to the removal of antibody-coated red cells by the spleen. If the recipient animal is splenectomized before injection of the antiserum, the platelet depression is less (Fig. 75-4) [23]. If

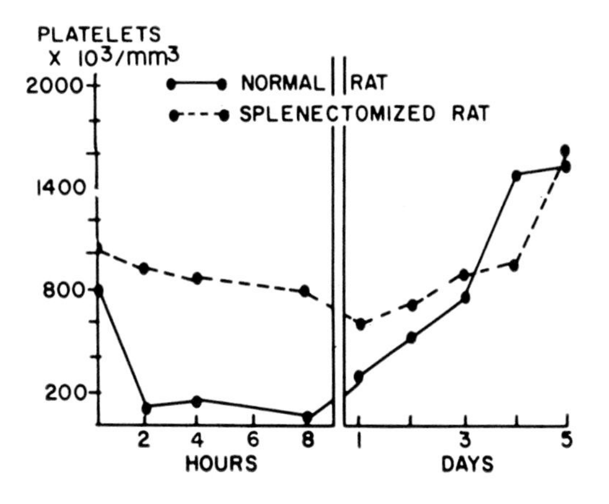

Fig. 75-4. Platelet response in rat following infusion of antirat platelet serum. Serum dosage is adjusted to demonstrate that the splenectomized rat is less susceptible to thrombocytopenia from the immune serum than the paired normal litter mate. (From Harrington *et al.* [41].)

the splenic artery is tied, a similar effect is observed. Harrington *et al.* [23] have published a most convincing demonstration of the splenic sequestration of platelets after injection of antiserum. If parabiotic rats are given injections of platelet antiserum, both will have a fall in platelets. However, if one parabiont is splenectomized and the other is not, the splenectomized animal does not show the thrombocytopenia after injection of antiserum. Corticoids will not prevent the heterologous platelet antibody from uniting with the platelet membrane, but they will delay the removal of these coated platelets from the circulation.

Drug Hypersensitivity. Thrombocytopenia in man which follows drug ingestion has been helpful in clarifying the mechanisms of platelet destruction. Various drugs have been related to purpura. The reader is referred to the current Registry on Blood Dyscrasias by the Council on Drugs of the American Medical Association. Drug reactions with thrombocytopenia are rare. Of the drugs in current use, sulfonamides, chlorothiazide derivatives, chlorpropamide, meprobamate, phenylbutazone, and quinidine are particularly noted; quinidine has been implicated most frequently [27]. Sedormid (allylisopropylacetyl carbamide), a sedative rarely used in this country, has been studied extensively by Ackroyd [28] as a model of drug purpura.

The onset of thrombocytopenia is abrupt. Formerly, small test doses of the drug were given to patients with suspected drug sensitivity after the thrombocytopenia had disappeared. This is not recommended because the sensitive patient may develop fulminating thrombocytopenia, with the possibility of cerebral hemorrhage. When a patient with a history of thrombocytopenia has a problem calling for a drug suspected of having caused purpura, the pharmacological armamentarium available to us today will usually permit substitution with another effective agent, e.g., procaine amide instead of quinidine for cardiac arrhythmias. Only if no other therapeutic approach is available should trial administration of the possible offending drug be considered. Most cases of drug thrombocytopenia can, however, be diagnosed by simple *in vitro* techniques. Addition of saturated solutions of the offending drug to whole blood or platelet-rich plasma usually will impair clot retraction. The drug can be added to such plasma to initiate platelet agglutination, lysis, or complement fixation [29].

Plasma from a sensitized patient can be infused into a normal recipient without change in the recipient's platelet level. Thereafter, injection of the offending drug will initiate a fulminating thrombocytopenia in the recipient (Fig. 75-5) [23]. From this it is presumed that the drug (hapten) combines with circulating proteins to form complexes

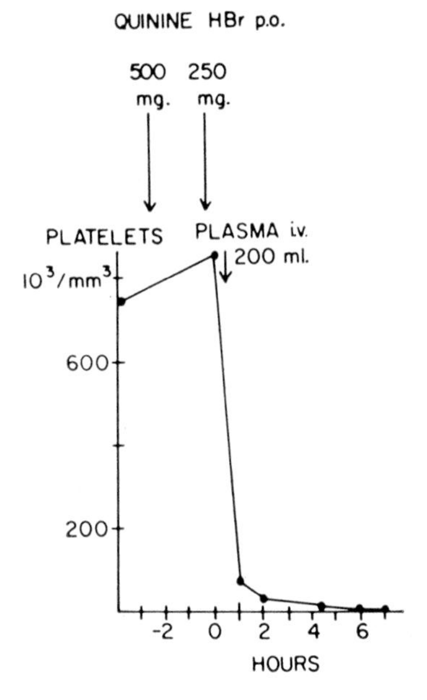

Fig. 75-5. No platelet depression is observed in a normal recipient receiving quinine orally. However, if it is given with plasma from a patient previously sensitized, the recipient has abrupt destruction of circulating platelets. (Figs. 75-5 and 75-10 from Harrington *et al.* [23] in Tocantins, L. M. (Ed.), *Progress in Hematology* [New York: Grune & Stratton, Inc., 1956].)

and that these interact with the platelets. It might be that the drug combines first with platelets to form antigen. However, in test systems the platelet does not exhibit a firm bond with the drug. This unstable interaction may explain in part why drug reactions with thrombocytopenia are rare. Drug-induced antibodies are complement-binding. The studies of Shulman [30] have elucidated this reaction in detail.

After removal of the offending drug, recovery of the peripheral platelet count is delayed by the time necessary for maturation of the megakaryocytes. Direct injury to the megakaryocyte by the drug-antibody complex has been suggested. This is doubtful, and probably the early platelet fragments attached to the megakaryocyte are injured by the drug and the platelet population must be replaced in toto over a 7 to 10 day period.

PLATELET PHYSIOLOGY IN ITP

The experimental induction of heterologous platelet antibodies and the evidence of antibodies in drug purpura initiated studies to explain the platelet destruction in ITP. Reduced peripheral blood platelet levels associated with adequate bone marrow megakaryocyte precursors are the laboratory hallmarks of ITP. With the perfection of nonwettable surfaces, direct transfusion studies were undertaken with silicone-coated syringes. In contrast to the normal platelet life span of five to seven days in aplastic anemia with thrombocytopenia, in ITP there was a variable but rapid destruction of transfused compatible isologous platelets (Fig. 75-2) [4]. The accelerated disappearance of normal donor platelets implied that a lytic or agglutinating factor was present in the plasma or that there was excessive phagocytic activity of the RES, or both. These studies could only be done in the thrombocytopenic recipient, since changes in the circulating platelet level were used for evaluation of platelet survival. It soon was obvious that a spectrum of survival curves existed, varying from abrupt destruction of the transfused platelets in acute ITP to a modest survival of two to four days in chronic ITP. In many respects this is similar to the varying intensities of hemolysis noted in acquired (Coombs-positive) hemolytic anemias.

Multiple transfusions to patients with pancytopenia from bone marrow aplasia soon demonstrated that patients could be immunized to isologous platelet transfusions. Hence, the afore-mentioned shortened isologous platelet survivals in ITP were of uncertain meaning, if previous transfusions had been given to the patient [31]. We have observed isoimmunization of a recipient with rapid destruction of transfused platelets after one previous transfusion. These observations imply that platelets may elicit some type of antibody response. Although efforts to classify platelets into immunological groups have not been satisfactory, some workers believe that blood group substances may be attached to the platelet membrane to cause destruction. The earlier schemes of platelet grouping relied on inadequate methodology and have not yielded reproducible data in different laboratories.

Shulman *et al.* [32] described a type of thrombocytopenia that follows transfusions of mismatched platelet (Pl) groups. Thrombocytopenia occurs after about one week's delay. At this time, the recipient makes an antibody to the antigen of the transfused Pl incompatible platelets which destroys not only the remaining donor platelets but also the recipient's own. The latter appears to occur because Pl antigen can escape from the transfused platelets and adsorb onto the patient's own platelets. The thrombocytopenia is abrupt in onset, and the recovery phase rapid, as in drug purpura. Platelets in whole blood stored in ACD solution at 4° C. for 12 to 24 hours are nonviable and do not remain in the circulation. Nevertheless, delayed thrombocytopenia has been seen after transfusion of stored blood. The mechanism by which nonviable platelets can participate in an antigen-antibody interaction one week after transfusion is obscure. Transfusion of fresh blood provides platelets that could live long enough (7 to 10 days) to act as circulating antigens. There is no evidence of a residual soluble type of circulating platelet debris that could react with the antibody before binding to the recipient's platelets to give thrombocytopenia. However, such a postulate is the best explanation for this type of thrombocytopenia.*

Despite our beginning understanding that human platelets are isoantigenic and may have serological types, these observations have not materially helped us to understand ITP. There has been no correlation of the disease ITP with any pattern of platelet blood group antibody, nor do tests show any pattern of immunization. To study the destruction of platelets, radioisotope techniques for platelet labeling have been developed. A thrombocytopenia below 80,000 mm.^{3} does not allow successful labeling of autologous platelets. The use of sodium phosphate (P^{32}) [33], sodium chromate (Cr^{51}) [34] and diisopropylfluorophosphonate (DFP^{32}) [35] as platelet labels has been studied in many laboratories. Most information has been derived from Cr^{51} labeling of isologous platelets. With such a technique, isologous platelets may be infused in an ITP recipient with ease before and after any specific therapy. In all studies, one must exclude isoimmunization from previous trans-

* *Editor's comment:* It seems reasonable to believe that Pl antigens may adsorb to the recipient's platelets immediately after transfusion and in this way persist in the circulation long enough for the delayed thrombocytopenia to be exhibited. This is my understanding of Shulman's thinking [32].—J. H. V.

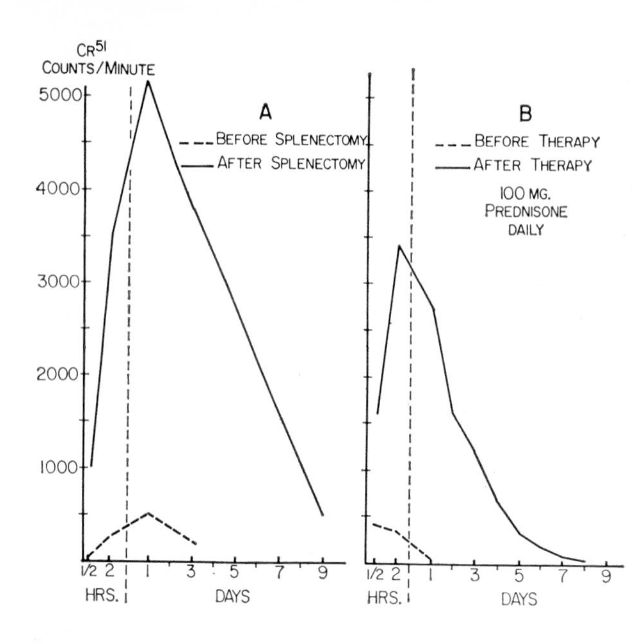

Fig. 75-6. Isologous Cr^{51}-labeled platelet life span in ITP recipients. Life span in untreated patients is quite short and similar to the observations in Figure 75-2. (*A*) Following splenectomy, the Cr^{51} platelet life span is normal. (*B*) During prednisone therapy, the life span is improved and approaches the normal curve. (Modified from Cohen *et al.* [31].)

fusions as an explanation for rapid destruction of the labeled platelets. Radioactive platelet labeling demonstrates the same rapid isologous platelet destruction in ITP as had been noted with direct platelet transfusions (Fig. 75-6) [31]. When the plasma thrombocytolytic factor is of lesser magnitude, as in chronic ITP, the patient will have an opportunity to sequester platelets in the spleen [36]. In some ITP patients given Cr^{51}-labeled platelets before surgery, a high concentration of the injected Cr^{51} has been found in the spleen.

The patient with chronic ITP has elevated plasma concentrations of acid β-glycerol phosphatase, as described in acute ITP. This measurement can be used to follow the changes in platelet destruction with therapy or splenectomy (Fig. 75-3).

Shortly after the demonstration that transfused isologous platelets were destroyed in the recipient with ITP, Harrington *et al.* [37] infused plasma from patients with ITP into normal volunteers. There was a rapid decline in the recipient's platelet count followed by slow recovery over the next 6 to 8 days. These studies demonstrated that a platelet-suppressive factor was present in the plasma in ITP (Fig. 75-7), and this has been fully confirmed [38, 39]. Normal plasma transfusions may induce transitory thrombocytopenia [40], but it is of less than 24 hours' duration and could not be confused with the observations following infusion of ITP plasma. The presence of a Pl agglutinin as described by Shulman could induce a response imitating thrombocytopenia in the recipient. However, such Pl agglutinins have not been observed by Shulman *et al.* [32] in ITP plasma. It is improbable

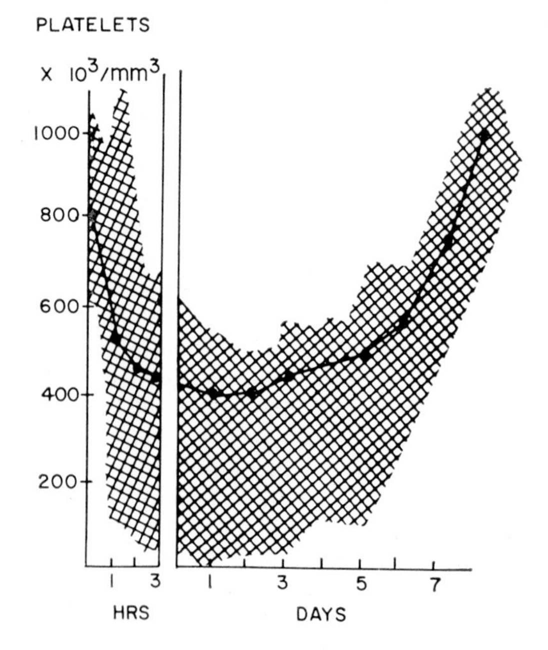

Fig. 75-7. Mean platelet response of eight normal recipients receiving 500 ml. of compatible citrated whole blood from ITP patients. Hatched area is range of response observed. (From Harrington *et al.* [37].)

that previous blood transfusions to the recipient could cause the thrombocytopenia observed after infusion of ITP plasma.* Plasma from ITP patients before and after splenectomy also has shown the thrombocytopenic effect. Patients with normal platelet counts following splenectomy still had a plasma factor capable of reducing platelet levels in normal subjects [23]. This observation implies that the immunological abnormality is not eliminated after splenectomy, but the disease activity is affected because it is related both to the selective sequestering function of the spleen and to the amount of platelet factor (antibody) produced. One could therefore anticipate occasional recurrence of thrombocytopenia months or years after recovery following splenectomy. This is actually observed. In rare instances, hypertrophy of an accessory spleen may explain a recurrence. Localization of splenules by various radioisotope techniques may be helpful in identifying this mechanism. Relapse may be associated with infection, which may well act to restimulate the production of abnormal proteins or to enhance phagocytic function.

The question arises whether the plasma factor resides in part on the platelet, even in the absence of thrombocytopenia. If one wishes to compare with the red cell factors in acquired hemolytic anemia, one might well expect the platelet to be "coated" with a globulin, and this may be demonstrated by the direct antihuman globulin consumption (DAHGC) test discussed later. In the absence of a sequestering spleen, the platelets are not destroyed. Probably the best physiological study of this globulin in man is in the thrombocytopenia existing in the newborn infant of a mother who has had ITP and a resultant normal platelet count following splenectomy. The plasma factor may cross the placental barrier, bind to the infant's platelets, and eventually cause platelet destruction in the intact infant's spleen. Similarly, if the mother has responded to corticoids, the infant will be born with a platelet level similar to the mother's, only to become thrombocytopenic when withdrawn from the maternal supply

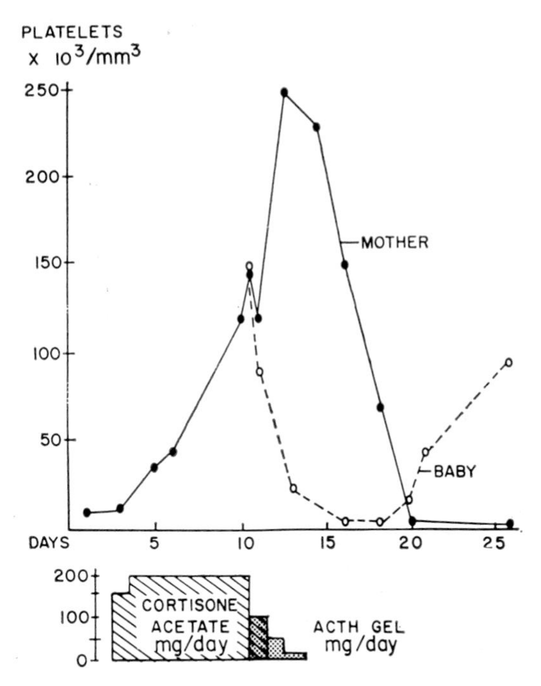

Fig. 75-8. Mother with ITP responds to oral cortisone therapy. At delivery (day 10), mother and infant have similar platelet counts. Withdrawal of steroid now allows plasma thrombocytolytic factor in the infant that has crossed the placenta to destroy platelets. Rapid destruction of platelets in the infant suggests that cortisone had acted primarily to impair reticuloendothelial removal of the platelets. Two years later this mother, after splenectomy, delivered a thrombocytopenic infant, although her platelet count was normal.

of corticoids (Fig. 75-8). In this instance, the corticoids have altered the phagocytosis of the coated platelets, but the plasma factor remained to circulate in the infant.

Since 1951, investigators have reported that platelet agglutinins were present in sera of patients with ITP. Such agglutinins have been demonstrated by a variety of methods, with conflicting results. A few of the results are given in Table 75-1 to emphasize the divergence of results. The initial procedure, popularized by Harrington *et al.* [41], was direct examination for platelet clumps after incubation of a serum platelet suspension. Although these workers did emphasize the frequency of autoagglutination (patients' platelets), most subsequent investigators have used isologous compatible platelets with much less convincing results. Residual thrombin in the serum after clotting will induce viscous meta-

* *Editor's comment:* Harrington has stated (personal communication) that 8 of 17 plasmas positive in passive induction of thrombocytopenia were from ITP patients who had never been transfused and had never been pregnant.—J. H. V.

TABLE 75-1. Platelet Agglutinins in Idiopathic Thrombocytopenic Purpura

Author	Technique	Percent Positive	Total No. of Patients
Harrington *et al.* [41]	Agglutination	74	104
Cohen *et al.* [31]	Agglutination	16	25
Corn and Upshaw [42]	Agglutination	Neg.	25
Tullis [43]	Quantitative agglutination	45	3,000[a]
Dausset *et al.* [44]	DAHGC[b]	50	93
Van de Wiel *et al.* [45]	DAHGC	56	23
Steffen [46]	DAHGC	67	62
Nelken *et al.* [47]	DAHGC	92	12

[a] Author describes this percentage from total number of tests done. Previously, he had listed 56 percent positive tests from 96 cases (including acute and chronic types).
[b] DAHGC = direct antihuman globulin consumption test.

morphosis and eventual clumping of platelets [48]. It should be recalled that prothrombin consumption is reduced in ITP, and the harvested serum has a greater percentage of available prothrombin for autocatalytic conversion to thrombin during the agglutination testing. Trace amounts of thrombin undoubtedly have confused and thwarted accurate evaluation of platelet agglutinations. The DAHGC test also uses the patients' (ITP) platelets. In this test, the absorption by a "coated" platelet reduces the titer of an antihuman γ-globulin serum against Rh(D)-positive red cells coated with anti-D antibody (Fig. 75-9). With all of these tests, some positive results are noted in controls, implying some degree of nonspecificity. Nevertheless the repeated reports of positive results with the DAHGC test in ITP are striking, and they suggest that utilization of autologous platelets in this test may be the only way readily to assess the circulating plasma factor [44]. The autologous platelet in ITP has morphological alterations from normal and may well have a more "sensitized" membrane. Efforts to alter platelets with enzymes (i.e., trypsin) have not, however, increased the platelet membrane reactivity in agglutination tests.

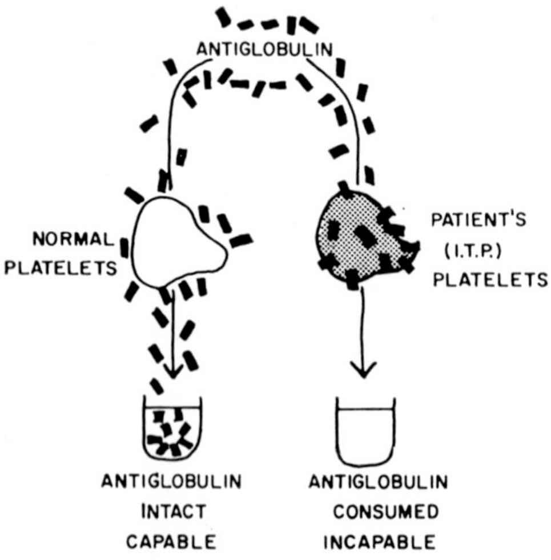

Fig. 75-9. Demonstration of the binding of antihuman globulin serum (AHGS) to ITP platelets. The "coated" platelets remove the AHGS, and it is not capable of agglutinating sensitized anti-D-coated red cells. (From Dausset [61].)

The conflicting findings with platelet agglutination tests have some bearing on the data from drug-induced thrombocytopenia. Shulman [30] emphasized that an intravenous dose of quinidine which would reduce the platelet level in a sensitized recipient was much smaller than the amount predicted from *in vitro* testing. Hence, one can appreciate that thrombocytopenia could develop without platelet factors demonstrable *in vitro*. Although Shulman has used complement fixation to show minute amounts of quinidine antibody, he has never observed such "antibodies" in human ITP. We might conclude that uptake of the plasma factor by platelets may keep the plasma level too low for the usual laboratory procedures to show platelet agglutinins.

The abnormal protein (antibody) in clinical ITP may be related to plasma factors that also coat red cell membranes. Hence one may observe acquired hemolytic anemia concomitant with thrombocytopenia. As noted previously in a few patients with ITP, there may be an associated positive result of the LE cell test or fluorescence test for antibody to nuclear antigens. We are not in a position to state whether these are a common response to a single or multiple antigenic stimuli.* For the most part, the thrombocytopenic plasma factor is usually not associated with the other antibodies, as we are now able to measure them.

Tullis [43] has recently shown that 86 percent of serum samples obtained from ITP patients give positive results in the quantitative platelet agglutination test that he has devised. In this procedure, the substitution of platelets treated with high-energy irradiation increased the positive results from 45 to 88 percent. Like Harrington ten years ago, Tullis and Baudanza [49] have observed patients who demonstrate no serum agglutinins with isologous platelet suspensions but do have positive reactions when autologous platelets are substituted. In another technique, autologous platelets and plasma have been incubated together and elevation of the α-amino nitrogen level noted [50]. The original transfusion studies indicated that the platelet-depressing component in plasma was a globulin. Little further fractionation attempt has been made in *in vitro* studies. Recently, by column chromatography, Tullis [43] defined the platelet agglutinin protein as a 19S globulin.

These observations of positive serum platelet agglutinins have been primarily in chronic ITP. The search for agglutinins in children with acute self-limited ITP has been, for the most part, unsuccessful. Again, the tendency in most laboratories to use isologous platelets in the test for agglutinins could explain the poor yield. Reported results have been more frequently positive with the DAHGC test. Since many patients presumed to have recovered from acute disease may manifest ITP in later years, the criteria for diagnosis of acute disease may not be the same in various clinics.

From the conflicting data it appears that no single procedure has had sufficient reproducibility in more than one laboratory to indicate that platelet agglutinins have been demonstrated satisfactorily *in vitro*. The *in vivo* evidence of a plasma factor can, however, be accepted.

* *Editor's comment:* There is no doubt that the serum factors reactive with red cell antigens in "autoimmune" hemolytic disease and those reactive with the nuclear antigens in SLE are different from each other (Chaps. 66 and 74), and it seems a virtual certainty that thrombocytopenic factors in ITP are different from either.—J. H. V.

RESPONSE TO THERAPY

All forms of adrenal corticoid therapy used have been successful in controlling thrombocytopenia. The platelet count rises over 6 to 12 days with dosages equivalent to 150 to 200 mg. of cortisone. In our clinic, 60 to 70 percent of patients have an initial platelet elevation with corticosteroid therapy. These results are similar to the data of Dameshek [51]. In many instances, the hormone dosage requirement may not allow the patient to be maintained for a prolonged period. In man, steroid therapy may alter the plasma factor described by Harrington *et al.* [23] so that a normal recipient will not manifest a platelet depression following the infusion of plasma from a patient treated with corticoids. This *in vivo* measurement provides the most convincing data to show that the abnormal protein may be effectively obliterated by corticoids in this disease (Fig. 75-10).

Splenectomy has been used in the treatment of ITP with varying degrees of success since 1916. Although the percentage of permanent remissions from splenectomy varies [52–54],

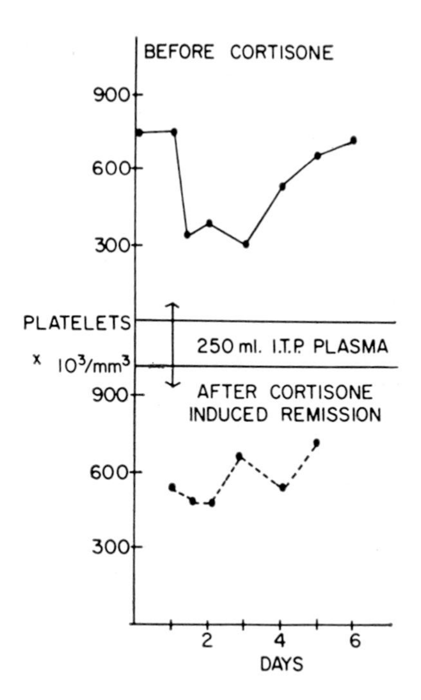

Fig. 75-10. Response in normal recipient to plasma from patient with ITP. The thrombocytolytic factor has disappeared during corticoid therapy, suggesting that production of this factor has been impaired by steroid therapy. (From Harrington *et al.* [23].)

we believe that two thirds of the patients will have a sustained platelet elevation. The successful results have been attributed to removal of a sequestering "filter" for the platelets coated with an abnormal antibody. Some of the Cr^{51}-labeled platelets transfused into a recipient with ITP can be localized in the splenic area by body surface scanning for isotope localization [36]. In our laboratory the results of such scanning have been irregular, possibly related to the type of surface counting probe available. Splenectomy also decreases the reticuloendothelial mass and total antibody (platelet coating protein) synthesis. Techniques for measurement of these variables are unfortunately imprecise. The failure of splenectomy to control thrombocytopenia has been used as evidence of continued extra-splenic antibody formation in adequate titer to coat platelets for removal.

Antimetabolites have been used to suppress antibody response to foreign proteins, especially to limit the response in homotransplantation. Dameshek and Schwartz [55] demonstrated an excellent suppression of hemolysis in acquired hemolytic disease. In some of these patients, transfusion and corticoid therapy have been eliminated. Animal studies by this group suggest that the antimetabolites suppress the proliferation of large lymphocytes (hemocytoblasts) [56]. In our laboratory, we have been encouraged to note that one of these drugs (Imuran; 6-[1-methyl-4-nitro-5-imidazolyl mercaptopurine]) will elevate the platelet count in ITP. The drugs should be used only in the patient who has had no response to splenectomy and requires prolonged corticoid therapy in a dosage that causes a degree of iatrogenic symptoms, such as Cushing's syndrome, that is as harmful as the thrombocytopenia itself. One should not attempt to achieve a normal platelet count with antimetabolites, but rather use the smallest dosage that will maintain the platelet count above the bleeding level (40,000 $mm.^3$). There will be only minor complications of leukopenia and anemia if a minimal drug dosage is maintained. A larger clinical experience is necessary to define the complications of impaired bone marrow function, and the clinician should use antimetabolites with caution. It appears that these drugs have an increasing role in the "splenectomy failure" group of patients.

There must be some reservation about the spontaneous or therapeutic cure rate in ITP. Sixty to 85 percent of patients are improved following splenectomy. At this time, there are no adequate data by which to evaluate long-term therapy with corticoids. In most clinics, requirement for prolonged steroid therapy usually results in splenectomy [53]. Clinical data suggest that the plasma antibody may circulate in variable titers, but sometimes without physiological effect if the spleen is absent. Any stimulus for an anamnestic response may transiently or permanently elevate the antibody protein level to coat the platelet more adequately for destruction [10].

CHRONIC (NONIMMUNE) THROMBOCYTOPENIA

There is a group of patients with chronic thrombocytopenia in whom there is no evidence of immunologically induced platelet destruction. They fall into three categories.

CONGENITAL ABSENCE OF THROMBOPOIETIN

Schulman *et al.* [57] observed a child with chronic thrombocytopenia (40 to 60,000 $mm.^3$) who responded repeatedly to infusions of compatible plasma. Megakaryocytes were present in the bone marrow but were unable to mature. One may predict that other cases of this type will be found. They are attributed to thrombopoietin deficiency.

IMPAIRED PLATELET PRODUCTION

a) Nondestructive ITP. Harrington *et al.* [23] noted that about 20 percent of patients with chronic ITP do not have a thrombocytolytic plasma factor; Cohen *et al.* [31] observed a similar percentage. There is no adequate explanation for this group.

b) Congestive Splenomegaly. Platelet life span in this disorder is close to normal, and the thrombocytopenia must be attributed to decreased platelet production [31].

c) Thrombocytopenia of Pernicious Anemia (PA) and Paroxysmal Nocturnal Hemoglobinuria (PNH). Autologous labeled platelets have a normal life span, implying some bone marrow defect [31]. A nutritional defect with abnormal megakaryocytes may explain the observation in PA, but there are no data to explain thrombocytopenia in PNH.

d) Congenital Cyanotic Vascular Disease [58, 59]. No physiological mechanism has been detected to explain the thrombocytopenia associated primarily with cyanotic congenital heart disease. This type of secondary polycythemia may be associated with platelet counts below 40,000 $mm.^3$. Bone marrow megakaryocytes are in normal number and the degree of thrombocytopenia is not related to the hematocrit elevation. In contrast, thrombocytopenia is not observed in secondary polycythemia of high altitudes or of pulmonary insufficiency.

NONIMMUNE (MECHANICAL) DESTRUCTION OF PLATELETS

Hemangioma. Clinical reports have related thrombocytopenia to destruction of platelets in the cavernous capillary beds, and Cr^{51}-labeled platelets have a shortened life span in these patients. Removal or obliteration of the hemangioma controls the thrombocytopenia. Although seen primarily in infants, this disorder may appear in young adult life.

REFERENCES

1. Hirsch, E. O., and Dameshek, W. Idiopathic thrombocytopenia. *Arch. Intern. Med.* 88:701, 1951.
2. Allen, D. M., and Diamond, L. K. Idiopathic thrombocytopenia purpura in children: A review of its treatment with corticosteroids and splenectomy. Unpublished data, 1963.
3. Angle, R. M., and Alt, H. L. Thrombocytopenic purpura complicating infectious mononucleosis. *Blood* 5:449, 1950.
4. Hirsch, E. O., and Gardner, F. H. The transfusion of human blood platelets. *J. Lab. Clin. Med.* 39:556, 1952.
5. Oski, F. A., Naiman, J. L., and Diamond, L. K. Use of the plasma acid phosphatase value in the differentiation of thrombocytopenic states. *New Eng. J. Med.* 268:1423, 1963.
6. Adelson, E., Rheingold, J. J., and Crosby, W. H. The platelet as a sponge: A review. *Blood* 17:767, 1961.
7. Wagner, H. N., Lio, M., and Hornick, R. B. Studies of the reticuloendothelial system (RES): II. Changes in the phagocytic capacity of the RES in patients with certain infections. *J. Clin. Invest.* 42:427, 1963.
8. Noller, H. G. Changes in the Storage Capacity of the RES during Different Pathological and Pharmacological Conditions. In Halpern, B. N. (Ed.), *Physiopathology of the Reticuloendothelial System.* Springfield, Ill.: Charles C Thomas, Publisher, 1957.
9. Clarke, C. A., Donohoe, W. T. A., McConnell, R. B., Woodrow, J. C., Finn, R., Krevan, J. R., Kulke, W., Lehane, D., and Sheppard, P. M. Further experimental studies of the prevention of Rh haemolytic disease. *Brit. Med. J.* 1:979, 1963.
10. Dameshek, W., Ebbe, S., Greenberg, L., and Baldini, M. Recurrent acute idiopathic thrombocytopenic purpura. *New Eng. J. Med.* 269:647, 1963.
11. Lozner, E. L. The thrombocytopenic purpuras. *Bull. N.Y. Acad. Med.* 30:184, 1954.
12. Doan, C. A., Bouroncle, B. A., and Wiseman, B. K. Idiopathic and secondary thrombocytopenic purpura: Clinical study and evaluation of 381 cases over a period of 28 years. *Ann. Intern. Med.* 53:861, 1960.
13. Heald, F. P., Daugela, M., and Brunschuyler, P. Physiology of adolescence. *New Eng. J. Med.* 268:299, 1963.
14. Nicol, T., and Bilbey, D. L. J. The Effect of Various Steroids on the Phagocytic Activity of the Reticuloendothelial System. In Heller, J. H. (Ed.), *Reticuloendothelial Structure and Function.* New York: Ronald Press Company, 1960.
15. Jones, W. A. and Cohen, R. B. The effect of estrogen on the liver in murine viral hepatitis. *Am. J. Path.* 42:237, 1963.
16. Weinstein, L. The effect of estrogenic hormone and ovariectomy on the normal antibody content of the serum of mature rabbits. *Yale J. Biol. Med.* 11:169, 1939.
17. Von Haam, E., and Rosenfeld, I. Influence of estrone upon formation of heterophile antibodies. *Proc. Soc. Exp. Biol. Med.* 49:710, 1942.
18. Ross, U., and Peizer, L. R. Fluctuations in type 2 pneumococcus antibody during the menstrual cycle. *Proc. Soc. Exp. Biol. Med.* 35:432, 1937.
19. Baumgartner, L. The relationship of age to immunological reactions. *Yale J. Biol. Med.* 6:403, 1934.
20. Pepper, H., Liebowitz, D., and Lindsay, S. Cyclical thrombocytopenic purpura related to the menstrual cycle. *Arch. Path.* 61:1, 1956.
21. Levenson, S. M., and Watkins, D. M. Protein requirements in injury and certain acute and chronic diseases. *Fed. Proc.* 18:1155, 1959.
22. Cohen, P., and Gardner, F. H. The thrombocytopenic effect of sustained high-dosage prednisone therapy in thrombocytopenic purpura. *New Eng. J. Med.* 265:611, 1961.
23. Harrington, W. J., Minnich, V., and Arimura, G. The Autoimmune Thrombocytopenias. In Tocantins, L. M. (Ed.), *Progress in Hematology.* New York: Grune & Stratton, Inc., 1956.
24. Miescher, P. A., and Gorstein, F. Mechanisms

of Immunogenic Platelet Damage. In Johnson, S. A., Monto, R. W., Rebuck, J. W., and Horn, R. C. (Eds.), *Blood Platelets*. Boston: Little, Brown, 1961. P. 671.

25. Nachman, R. L., and Engle, R. L. Amino acid release following platelet antibody interactions. *Fed. Proc.* 22:673, 1963.
26. Suhrland, L. G., Arquilla, E. A., and Weisberger, A. S. The effect of prednisone on circulating antibody formation in animals: Immunized with human platelet antigen. *J. Lab. Clin. Med.* 51:724, 1958.
27. Erslev, A. J., and Wintrobe, M. M. Detection and prevention of drug-induced blood dyscrasias. *J.A.M.A.* 181:114, 1962.
28. Ackroyd, J. F. Platelet agglutinins and lysins in the pathogenesis of thrombocytopenic purpura, with a note on platelet groups. *Brit. Med. Bull.* 11:28, 1955.
29. Weintraub, R. M., Pechet, L., and Alexander, B. Rapid diagnosis of drug-induced thrombocytopenic purpura. *J.A.M.A.* 180:528, 1962.
30. Shulman, R. Immunoreactions involving platelets. *J. Exp. Med.* 107:697, 1958.
31. Cohen, P., Gardner, F. H., and Barnett, G. O. Reclassification of the thrombocytopenias by the Cr^{51} labelling method for measuring platelet life span. *New Eng. J. Med.* 264:1294, 1961.
32. Shulman, N. R., Aster, R. H., Leitner, A., and Hiller, M. C. Immunoreactions involving platelets: V. Post-transfusion purpura due to a complement-fixing antibody against a genetically controlled platelet antigen; A proposed mechanism for thrombocytopenia and its relevance in "autoimmunity." *J. Clin. Invest.* 40:1597, 1961.
33. Adelson, E., Rheingold, J. J., and Crosby, W. H. Studies of platelet survival by tagging *in vivo* with P^{32}. *J. Lab. Clin. Med.* 50:570, 1957.
34. Aas, K. A., and Gardner, F. H. Survival of blood platelets labeled with chromium. *J. Clin. Invest.* 37:1257, 1958.
35. Leeksma, C. H. W., and Cohen, J. A. Determination of life span of human blood platelets using labelled diisopropylfluorophosphonate. *J. Clin. Invest.* 35:964, 1956.
36. Najean, Y., Ardaillou, N., Caen, J., Larrieu, M. J., and Bernard, J. Survival of radiochromium-labelled platelets in thrombocytopenias. *Blood* 22:718, 1963.
37. Harrington, W. J., Minnich, V., Hollingsworth, J. W., and Moore, C. V. Demonstration of a thrombocytopenic factor in the blood of patients with thrombocytopenic purpura. *J. Lab. Clin. Med.* 38:1, 1951.
38. Stefanini, M., and Dameshek, W. *The Hemorrhagic Disorders*. New York: Grune & Stratton, Inc., 1955. P. 96.
39. Kissmeyer-Nielsen, F. Demonstration of a thrombocytopenic and a leukopenic factor in blood of patients with thrombocytopenia and leukopenia. *Acta Haemat.* (Basel) 9:337, 1953.
40. Stefanini, M., and Adelson, E. Studies on platelets: IV. A thrombocytopenic factor in normal human blood, plasma or serum. *Proc. Soc. Exp. Biol. Med.* 79:623, 1952.
41. Harrington, W. J., Sprague, C. D., Minnich, V., Moore, C. V., Aulvin, R. C., and Dubach, R. Immunologic mechanisms in idiopathic and neonatal thrombocytopenic purpura. *Ann. Intern. Med.* 38:433, 1953.
42. Corn, M., and Upshaw, J. D. Evaluation of platelet antibodies in idiopathic thrombocytopenic purpura. *Arch. Intern. Med.* 109:85, 1962.
43. Tullis, J. L. Leukocyte and thrombocyte antibodies: Current concepts of their origin, identity and significance. *J.A.M.A.* 180:136, 1962.
44. Dausset, J., Columbani, J., and Columbani, M. Study of leukopenias and thrombocytopenias by the direct antigloblulin consumption test on leukocytes and/or platelets. *Blood* 18:672, 1961.
45. Van de Wiel, T. W. M., Van de Weil-Dorfmeyer, H., and Van Loghem, J. J. Studies in platelet antibodies in man. *Vox Sang.* 6:641, 1961.
46. Steffen, C. Results obtained with the antiglobulin consumption test and investigations of auto antibody eluates in immunohematology. *J. Lab. Clin. Med.* 55:9, 1960.
47. Nelken, D., Gurevitch, J., and Gilboa-Garber, N. Direct antiglobulin-consumption test for detection of immune antibodies. *Lancet* 1:742, 1961.
48. Jackson, D. P., Schmid, H. J., Zieve, P. D., Levin, J., and Conley, C. L. Nature of a platelet-agglutinating factor in serum of patients with idiopathic thrombocytopenic purpura. *J. Clin. Invest.* 42:383, 1963.
49. Tullis, J. L., and Baudanza, P. Pathophysiology mechanisms in immunologic purpura (in preparation, 1963).
50. Nachman, R. L., and Engle, R. L. New evidence for the presence of a circulating antiplatelet factor in idiopathic thrombocytopenic purpura. *Blood* 22:828, 1963.
51. Dameshek, W. Controversy in idiopathic thrombocytopenic purpura. *J.A.M.A.* 173:1025, 1960.
52. Carpenter, A. F., Wintrobe, M. M., Fuller, E. A., Haut, A., and Cartwright, G. E. Treatment of idiopathic thrombocytopenic purpura. *J.A.M.A.* 171:1911, 1959.
53. Meyers, M. C. Results of treatment in 71 patients with idiopathic thrombocytopenic purpura. *Amer. J. Med. Sci.* 242:295, 1961.
54. Watson-Williams, E. J., Macpherson, A. I. S.,

and Davidson, S. The treatment of idiopathic thrombocytopenic purpura: A review of 93 cases. *Lancet* 2:221, 1958.

55. Dameshek, W., and Schwartz, R. Treatment of Certain "Autoimmune" Diseases with Antimetabolites: A Preliminary Report. *Trans. Ass. Amer. Physicians* 73:113, 1960.
56. Andre, J. A., Schwartz, R. S., Mitus, W. J., and Dameshek, W. The morphologic response of the lymphoid system to homografts: II. The effect of antimetabolites. *Blood* 19:334, 1962.
57. Schulman, I., Pierce, M., Lukens, A., and Currimbhoy, Z. Studies on thrombopoiesis: I. A factor in normal human plasma required for platelet production: Chronic thrombocytopenia due to its deficiency. *Blood* 16:943, 1960.
58. Hartmann, R. C. A hemorrhagic disorder occurring in patients with cyanotic congenital heart disease. *Bull. Hopkins Hosp.* 91:49, 1952.
59. Hultgren, H. N., and Gerbode, F. Physiologic studies in a patient with a pulmonary arteriovenous fistula. *Amer. J. Med.* 17:126, 1954.
60. Blix, S., and Aas, K. Giant hemangioma, thrombocytopenia, fibrinogenopenia, and fibrinolytic activity. *Acta Med. Scand.* 169:63, 1961.
61. Dausset, J. The direct antiglobulin consumption test on platelets and/or leucocytes: experiences in thrombocytopenic purpura, disseminated lupus erythematosus, and panhematocytopenia. *Bull. Amer. Ass. Blood Banks* 13:149, 1960.

76. Thrombotic Thrombocytopenic Purpura

RICHARD F. BAKEMEIER

THROMBOTIC THROMBOCYTOPENIC purpura (TTP) is a clinical syndrome of unknown cause, characterized by thrombocytopenic purpura, hemolytic anemia, transitory and sometimes bizarre neurologic manifestations, variable degrees of renal dysfunction, and fever. One or more of these features may be absent at any given time in the course of the syndrome. In more fulminating cases, all may occur simultaneously. This multisystemic involvement corresponds to the widespread thrombotic occlusion of arterioles and capillaries found at autopsy.

The etiology and pathogenesis of this syndrome remain obscure, and evidence of the participation of immunologic mechanisms is meager. The occurrence of TTP in patients with certain features of systemic lupus erythematosus has been documented, however [1]. Strong allergic histories have been noted in a series of patients with TTP [2], and hypersensitivities to drugs or vaccines have been suggested as possible precipitating factors [3]. For these and other reasons, such as certain similarities of the lesions of TTP with those seen in the generalized Shwartzman phenomenon [4], this syndrome has interested clinical immunologists for many years.

The possibility exists that the clinical syndrome represents an apparently similar response to a heterogeneous group of primary etiological factors or processes. It should be noted that clinical, hematological, and/or histological manifestations indistinguishable from those commonly associated with TTP have been described in patients known to have carcinoma [5], eclampsia [6], and pregnancy without eclampsia [7].

CLINICAL FEATURES

The TTP syndrome has been reported in patients ranging in age from less than 1 year [8] to 69 years [3], with an equal sex distribution. Prodromata may precede the overt syndrome for months to years, and these include recurrent fever, anemia, proteinuria, abnormal bleeding, arthralgias, and hemiparesis. In many reports, patients have had malaise, increased fatigability, headache, dizziness, nausea, and vomiting for variable periods before the often explosive onset of the characteristic syndrome.

Two general clinical forms of TTP have been recognized: an acute, unrelenting illness which terminates fatally in a few days to weeks, and a more prolonged, recurrently relapsing process lasting several months to years.

Virtually all patients with TTP, at some point in the course, have central nervous system manifestations, such as confusion, delirium, stupor, convulsions, coma, or focal neurologic signs. These are often transitory, suggesting the development of collateral blood supply after vascular occlusions have occurred.

The anemia of TTP is characteristic of an extracorpuscular hemolytic process of varying intensity. A striking feature, which should make one suspect the presence of TTP, may be marked anisocytosis and poikilocytosis, with bizarre erythrocytes, including triangular cells, irregularly contracted and crenated cells, termed "schistocytes," and occasional spherocytes. Severe symptoms of vascular occlusion may antedate the appearance of significant anemia by several weeks or more. Icterus, attributable to hemolysis, and perhaps to hepatic involvement as well, has been reported in one fourth of one series of patients with TTP [2].

Thrombocytopenia is a hallmark of TTP. However, the platelet count may vary considerably when the course of the process is prolonged, with levels ranging from normal to less than 10,000 per cu. mm. These variations may occur independently of variations in the anemia.

Renal abnormalities include microscopic hematuria in virtually all cases, with gross hematuria occurring in 35 percent of one large series [2]. Proteinuria and mild to moderate azotemia have occurred in over half the reported cases in which these were mentioned. Hypertension does not commonly occur in TTP, and when present is usually attributable to some antecedent or associated condition.

Moderate lymph node enlargement is occasionally observed in TTP [3]. In less than half the reported cases has the spleen been palpable or found enlarged at autopsy. Mild hepatomegaly may be somewhat more common. Despite the widespread myocardial involvement seen at autopsy, severe cardiac decompensation is uncommon. Congestive heart failure occurred in 6 percent of one series [2]. Tachycardia and variable electrocardiographic changes are often associated with TTP.

LABORATORY DATA

The hemolytic anemia and thrombocytopenia in TTP have been described above. Moderate neutrophilic leukocytosis is common, with pronounced myeloid immaturity in some cases. The bone marrow usually shows reactive normoblastic erythroid hyperplasia and variable myeloid hyperplasia. Megakaryocytes are characteristically abundant in the marrow and often demonstrate poor fragmentation of the cytoplasm into platelets. Characteristic arteriolar thrombotic lesions may be observed in paraffin sections of sternal marrow aspirates.

Blood coagulation studies, when abnormal, have generally reflected features attributable to thrombocytopenia. Fibrinogen levels in published cases have been normal. A possible pathogenic role of enhanced coagulation cannot be excluded from reported cases of TTP.

Serological studies have, in general, not afforded evidence of an "autosensitivity" basis for this syndrome. Results of the antiglobulin (Coombs) test are usually negative, although there are at least seven published exceptions [1]. When positive, the antiglobulin reaction may be of the "anti-non-γ" type [1], suggesting the presence of complement on the erythrocyte [9].

Attempts to demonstrate antiplatelet antibodies have generally been unsuccessful [2, 10]. Transfusion of normal platelets into patients with TTP has been followed by markedly decreased survival, but this does not necessarily implicate an immunological mechanism. The trapping of platelets in the widespread arteriolar and capillary thrombi has been assumed by many to be a reasonable explanation for this decreased platelet survival. Immunofluorescence studies of these thrombi with antiplatelet and antifibrin sera, however, have suggested that the thrombi may be composed primarily of fibrin rather than platelets [11]. These amorphous or granular, acidophilic thrombi, with associated endothelial proliferation, are found most commonly in the arterioles and capillaries of the myocardium, pancreas, brain, renal cortex, and adrenal cortex. There are characteristically aneurysmal dilatations at arteriolar-capillary junctions and an absence of visible inflammatory reaction around the affected vessels [3, 12].

Other serological studies in TTP have included LE cell tests, results of which have generally been negative, when reported, with rare exceptions [13, 14]. Antinuclear factor tests have not often been reported, but a weakly positive result has been seen in one case with a subsequent histological diagnosis of TTP [1], whereas one other case gave an equivocal result and two cases gave negative results [15].

TREATMENT

Therapy in patients who have shown improvement has included corticosteroids, often in massive doses [16], heparin [17], exchange transfusion [18], and splenectomy [16, 19]. Of patients with prolonged survival (up to eight years has been observed), splenectomy had been performed in more than half.* Although the reasons for this apparent ameliorative effect of splenectomy are not understood, this therapeutic measure definitely should be considered, particularly if initial therapy with corticosteroids, transfusions, and possibly small doses of heparin has not resulted in satisfactory improvement.

* The author has personally observed three severe cases in which dramatic and prolonged clinical remissions were temporally associated with splenectomy.

REFERENCES

1. Bakemeier, R. F. Thrombotic thrombocytopenic purpura: A review. *Medicine* (to be published).
2. Adelson, E., Heitzman, E. J., and Fennessey, J. F. Thrombohemolytic thrombocytopenic purpura. *Arch. Intern. Med.* 94:92, 1954.
3. Singer, K. Thrombotic thrombocytopenic purpura. *Advances Intern. Med.* 6:195, 1954.
4. Shwartzman, G., Klemperer, P., and Gerber, I. E. The phenomenon of local tissue activity in bacterial filtrates. *J.A.M.A.* 107:1946, 1936.
5. Brain, M. G., Davie, J. V., and Hourihane, D. O'B. Microangiopathic haemolytic anaemia: The possible role of vascular lesions in pathogenesis. *Brit. J. Haemat.* 8:358, 1962.
6. Seftel, H. C., and Metz, J. Hemolytic anemia, thrombocytopenia, and uremia in eclampsia. *S. Afr. Med. J.* 31:1037, 1957.
7. O'Leary, J. A., and Marchetti, A. A. Thrombotic thrombocytopenic purpura in pregnancy. *Amer. J. Obst. Gynec.* 83:214, 1962.
8. MacWhinney, J. B., Jr., Packer, J. T., Miller, G., and Greendyke, R. M. Thrombotic thrombocytopenic purpura in childhood. *Blood* 19:181, 1962.
9. Leddy, J. P., Hill, R. W., Swisher, S. N., and Vaughan, J. H. Observations on the Immunochemical Nature of Red Cell Autosensitization. In Grabar, P., and Miescher, P. A. (Eds.), *Immunopathology* (3rd International Symposium). New York: Grune & Stratton, Inc., 1963. P. 318.
10. Brittingham, T. E., III, and Chaplin, H., Jr. Attempted passive transfer of thrombotic thrombocytopenic purpura. *Blood* 12:480, 1957.
11. Craig, J. M., and Gitlin, D. The nature of the hyaline thrombi in thrombotic thrombocytopenic purpura. *Amer. J. Path.* 33:251, 1957.
12. Orbison, J. L. Morphology of thrombotic thrombocytopenic purpura with demonstration of aneurysms. *Amer. J. Path.* 28:129, 1952.
13. Laszlo, M. D., Alvarez, A., and Feldman, F. The association of thrombotic thrombocytopenic purpura and disseminated lupus erythematosus: Report of a case. *Ann. Intern. Med.* 42:1308, 1955.
14. Siegel, B. M., Friedman, I. A., Kessler, S., and Schwartz, S. O. Thrombohemolytic thrombocytopenic purpura and lupus erythematosus. *Ann. Intern. Med.* 47:1022, 1957.
15. Barnett, E. V., and Condemi, J. J. Personal communication, 1964.
16. Hill, J. M., and Loeb, E. Massive hormonal therapy and splenectomy in acute thrombotic thrombocytopenic purpura: Report of 3 cases with one 8-year cure. *J.A.M.A.* 173:114, 1960.
17. Bernstock, L., and Hirson, C. Thrombotic thrombocytopenic purpura: Remission on treatment with heparin. *Lancet* 1:28, 1960.
18. Rubenstein, M. A., Kagan, B. M., MacGillviray, M. H., Merliss, R., and Sacks, H. Unusual remission in a case of TTP syndrome following fresh blood exchange transfusions. *Ann. Intern. Med.* 51:1409, 1959.
19. Cahalane, S. F., and Horn, R. C. Thrombotic thrombocytopenic purpura of long duration. *Amer. J. Med.* 27:333, 1959.

77. *Pernicious Anemia and Gastritis*

EUGENE V. BARNETT

GASTRIC ATROPHY OR ATROPHIC gastritis is a consistent feature of Addisonian pernicious anemia (PA). Treatment of PA with liver extracts or vitamin B_{12} results in remission of the anemia and improvement of the combined system disease, but no change occurs in the gastric lesion or achlorhydria. The primary defect in PA is apparently a deficiency of intrinsic factor associated with gastric atrophy and a consequent failure to absorb vitamin B_{12}. Taylor in 1959 and Schwartz in 1960 [1] demonstrated that the serum of untreated PA patients would inhibit the effect of exogenous intrinsic factor in mediating the absorption of vitamin B_{12} in patients with PA. Subsequent work has shown that the γ-globulin fraction of certain PA sera will bind to human intrinsic factor complexed with vitamin B_{12}. Forty percent of PA patients have been shown to have antibody to intrinsic factor [2]. By indirect immunofluorescence staining, Taylor *et al.* [3] found that the sera of 86 percent of their PA patients had γ-globulin that binds to the cytoplasm of the parietal (acid-producing) cells. Similar staining was detected in sera of 11 percent of 100 controls. There was no correlation between the positivity of the test for parietal cell antibody and the presence of antibody to intrinsic factor. They found that, as has been the case with other autoantibodies, the incidence of gastric parietal cell antibodies in normal controls increased with age, the antibodies occurring in 16 percent of their controls over age 60. These antibodies have been shown to react with autologous [4, 5], homologous, heterologous and fetal parietal cells by both complement fixation and immunofluorescence staining. Their specificity has been confirmed by their failure to react with antigens from other tissues, including the pyloric portion of the stomach, where few or no parietal cells are found.

In 1939, Brunschwig *et al.* [5] demonstrated that the intravenous injection of human gastric juice produced acute inhibition of acid secretion in Heidenhain-pouch dogs. In 1962, Hennes *et al.* [6] induced gastric atrophy in dogs by the intradermal injection of autologous, homologous, or heterologous gastric juice in Freund's adjuvant. They detected antibodies reacting with gastric juice and with saline extract of dog stomach mucosa. Histamine-fast achlorhydria was found for up to seven months after the start of the injections. After nine months, the mucosa in most of the experimental dogs had returned to normal. In September, 1963, Sircus *et al.* [7] reported the failure to induce gastric atrophy in dogs by repeated intravenous administration of histamine-stimulated human gastric juice, although Smith *et al.* [8] had earlier reported inducing gastritis by this method. These contradictory reports are reminiscent of the many earlier reports of attempts to produce organ-specific autoimmune disease in animals without the use of adjuvant. The work of Hennes' group [6] does suggest that the stomach may contain organ-specific antigens capable of inducing an immune response when combined in injections with Freund's adjuvant. Such an immune response may result in injury to the stomach.

Not only do PA patients have a high incidence of antibody to intrinsic factor and antibody to parietal cell antigens, but up to 43 percent have antibody to the microsomal antigen of thyroid [1]. Frequently, PA is associated with thyroid disease, and patients with Hashimoto's thyroiditis have a high incidence of antibodies to parietal cells. Roitt [9] has noted an unusually high incidence of antibodies to both thyroid and parietal cells in relatives of PA patients. The association of organ-specific autoantibodies in both PA and thyroiditis has prompted suggestions that these diseases are indeed autoimmune with organ specificity, in contrast with lupus erythematosus which is generally considered an autoimmune disease with no organ specificity. No evidence has been presented, in man or experimental animals, to suggest that the serologic entities themselves cause the disease. Indeed, the high incidence of serological abnormalities detected by tests for thyroid antibodies, intrinsic factor antibody, antinuclear factors, and Wassermann antibody in "normal" old people suggests that increasing tissue breakdown during aging results in increasing autoimmunization, with or without disease secondary to the autoimmunization.

REFERENCES

1. Roitt, I. M., Doniach, D., and Taylor, K. B. Auto Antibodies in Pernicious Anemia. In Gell, P. G. H., and Coombs, R. R. A. (Eds.), *Clinical Aspects of Immunology*. Philadelphia: F. A. Davis Company, 1963. Chap. 36, p. 799.
2. Taylor, K. B. Immune phenomena in pernicious anemia. *Gastroenterology* 45:670, 1963.
3. Taylor, K. B., Riott, I. M., Doniach, D., Couchman, K. G., and Shapland, C. Autoimmune phenomena in pernicious anemia: Gastric antibodies, *Brit. Med. J.* 2:1347, 1962.
4. Irvine, W. J. Gastric antibodies studied by fluorescence microscopy. *Quart. J. Exp. Physiol.* 48:427, 1963
5. Brunschwig, A., Van Prohaska, J., Vlarke, T. H., and Kandel, E. A secretory depressant in gastric juice of patients with pernicious anemia. *J. Clin. Invest.* 18:415, 1939.
6. Hennes, A. R., Sevelius, H., Lewellyn, T., Jowl, W., Woods, A. H., and Wolf, S. Atrophic gastritis in dogs. *Arch. Path.* 73:33, 1962.
7. Sircus, W., Preshaw, R. M., Wynn-Williams, A., and McConnell, R. B. A failure to induce gastric atrophy in dogs by administration of histamine-stimulated gastric juice. *Gastroenterology* 45:384, 1963.
8. Smith, W. O., Joel, W., and Wolf, S. Experimental atrophic gastritis associated with inhibition of parietal cells. *Trans. Ass. Amer. Physicians* 71:306, 1958.
9. Roitt, I. M. Personal communications, 1963.

78. *Diseases of the Liver**

T. B. TOMASI, JR.

ALTHOUGH DESCRIPTIONS OF HEpatic injury associated with immunological reactions in experimental animals and in human allergic reactions have appeared since the early 1900's, it is only recently that immunological mechanisms have been directly implicated in the pathogenesis of certain acute and chronic liver diseases. With the advent of theories of autoimmunization as etiological factors in many human diseases, there has been considerable interest in the possibility that autoimmune phenomena are involved in diseases of the liver. Particular emphasis has been placed on the possibility that some forms of chronic active hepatitis result from persisting damage caused by immunological reactions. This theory was given impetus by the recent descriptions of chronic hepatitis in young women [1–3] thought to be a variant of systemic lupus erythematosus (SLE), referred to as lupoid hepatitis.

It might be expected for several reasons that the liver would be an important organ in immunological reactions. As a highly vascular organ receiving a large part of its blood supply from the portal system it is exposed to a variety of potential antigens absorbed from the gastrointestinal tract. Many of these are detoxified in hepatic cells. The liver contains abundant reticuloendothelial (RE) cells, which are known to be involved in the phagocytosis and metabolism of antigens. There is evidence that certain antigens, such as pneumococcal polysaccharide, may persist for months in hepatic cells [4]. Marked elevations in serum γ-globulins occur in many chronic liver diseases, and recent observations suggest that the liver may, under certain conditions, produce γ-globulin and therefore presumably antibody [5].

In this chapter the participation of the liver in immunological phenomena will be examined primarily from three aspects: (1) the experimental production of liver injury; (2) immunological reactions in the origin and perpetuation of human liver diseases; (3) the origin and significance of the elevation of γ-globulin in liver diseases and the possible role of the liver in the production of antibodies. Excellent recent reviews of these subjects are available [6–9].

EXPERIMENTAL IMMUNOLOGICAL LIVER INJURY

PARTICIPATION OF LIVER IN ALLERGIC REACTIONS FOLLOWING IMMUNIZATION WITH FOREIGN PROTEINS

A number of reports [10–15] indicate that hyperimmunization of animals with foreign proteins leads to the development of focal parenchymal cell necrosis and cellular infiltration in the liver. In certain animals, especially the rabbit, chronic immunization may lead to the development of a fine, nodular overgrowth of connective tissue which, at least superficially, resembles that seen in human cirrhosis [12]. Focal necrosis can also be produced when the antigen is injected directly into the portal vein of an immune animal [16]. It seems likely that the mechanism of liver damage in these cases involves the formation of antigen-antibody complexes in the circulation with subsequent deposition in the hepatic sinusoids. Electron microscopic studies [17, 18] indicate that the liver cell is in direct contact with the blood stream without intervening endothelium or basement membrane, so that the deposited complexes could exert their effect directly on the parenchymal cells. This interpretation of the pathogenesis of the hepatic lesions is also suggested by studies reviewed by Weigle [19] implicating soluble antigen-antibody complexes in several experimental and clinical diseases. The biological activity of

* This research was supported by Grant No. G 19 381 from the National Science Foundation and U.S. Public Health Service Grant No. AM-03986-03S1.

soluble immune complexes is shown not only by their skin toxicity [20] but also by their ability to cause serum sickness and acute nephritis when injected intravenously [21–23]. Steiner [17] has shown that the injection of preformed antigen-antibody complexes into the portal vein produces hepatic cell damage. Ultrastructure studies [17] have shown that, following the injection of complexes, the earliest changes were a swelling of the terminal trabeculae of the Kupffer cells and of the microvilli of the liver cells where they projected into the perisinusoidal space and subsequently the detachment of the swollen microvilli and extrusion into the lumen of the sinusoids. The midzonal necrosis of liver cells produced when a large excess of antigen or soluble antigen-antibody complexes were injected directly into the portal vein was indistinguishable from that produced when insoluble immune aggregates were administered. By use of fluorescent-tagged antigen, precipitates were found in the necrotic areas similar to those described in the lungs and kidneys following the intravenous injection of soluble complexes into the systemic circulation. Whether the liver cell damage is a result of ischemia produced by the precipitates or represents a specific toxicity of the complexes is unresolved. Although the changes in the liver following intravenous injection of immune complexes into the systemic circulation are definite, in general they are less impressive than those in the lung and kidney. The pathogenesis of the lesions in all of these organs is probably similar and results from the toxicity of antigen-antibody complexes.

In acute anaphylactic shock following the intravenous administration of a protein antigen to an immune animal, there is an intravascular precipitation of complexes, particularly in the lung, but such precipitates also occur in the hepatic sinusoids [24]. During anaphylactic shock in several species, especially the dog, there appears to be a constriction of the hepatic vein resulting in a diminished hepatic outflow of blood and centrilobular congestion. The decreased hepatic outflow may result in sufficient diminution in cardiac output to be a significant contributing factor in the etiology of the shock. This is further suggested by the observations that portacaval shunt in dogs prevents the fall in blood pressure in anaphylactic shock [7]. In reports [25, 7, 26] of autopsies on patients dying of anaphylactic shock, the liver has shown congestive changes and lesions similar to those in experimental anaphylaxis. Autopsy studies have been described relatively infrequently on patients with serum sickness. From the available reports [15, 27–29], the most prominent pathological findings are vascular lesions consisting of necrosis and fibrinoid changes together with infiltration of the wall of affected arteries by mononuclear, polymorphonuclear, and eosinophilic cells. The lesions are indistinguishable from those found in cases of periarteritis nodosa of undetermined etiology. In several of the reported cases, the hepatic vasculature has been involved, and infiltration of the portal areas by lymphocytes and eosinophilic leukocytes has been described. In several cases [30–32], hepatomegaly and jaundice following injection of foreign serum were suggested to be hepatic signs of serum sickness. Although it is difficult in these cases to attribute the hepatic findings to a hypersensitivity reaction, it is likely that the hepatic vasculature participates in the generalized Arthus type reaction seen in serum sickness. This is evident from the hepatic vascular lesions and necrosis of parenchymal cells seen in the experimental hypersensitivity lesions produced in animals [29, 33] and also from the common involvement of the liver in human periarteritis nodosa [34].

PRODUCTION OF LIVER LESIONS BY INJECTION OF LIVER HOMOGENATES AND ANTILIVER ANTISERA

There are several reports [6, 35–37] of the injection of homologous liver tissue with Freund's adjuvant into animals with the production of isoantibodies and liver lesions. Despite the production of liver lesions, however, these experiments are inconclusive for the following reasons: (1) Variation in the type of liver damage produced by isoimmunization occurs in different species of animals and within the same species at different ages. Behar and Tal [36] produced massive liver necrosis in young guinea pigs, whereas Jahiel and Koffler [37] were unable to produce similar lesions in the adult guinea pig but a high proportion of animals showed multiple hepatic granulomata. In rabbits, Steiner [6] produced predominantly granulomatous lesions similar to those reported by Jahiel and Koffler, but approximately 25 percent of the animals developed widespread necrotic lesions. In mice, isoimmunization produced predominantly a lesion resembling amyloidosis [38]. Immunization of ducks against killed malaria parasites with adjuvants produced amyloidosis with extensive involvement of the liver [39]. (2) In some normal animals and in animals receiving Freund's adjuvant only, lesions are produced which are similar to those found in the experimental model. For example, the granulomatous lesions of Jahiel and Koffler and the amyloidosis produced in mice and ducks are similar to lesions produced in these animals by adjuvant alone [40, 41]. (3) The administration of homologous liver antigens produces lesions in organs other than the liver, including nephrosis in the rat [42] and demyelination in the central nervous system of guinea pigs [43]. (4) Isoimmunization of guinea pigs with adrenal tissue produced hepatic lesions similar to those produced by liver homogenates [44].

When animals are immunized with heterologous liver homogenates, a variety of antibodies are formed which can be demonstrated by precipitin and complement-fixing techniques [6]. These homogenates contain serum, erythrocytes, blood group substances, and, in some cases, Forssman antigen as well as liver cell proteins. It is not surprising, therefore, that heterologous antisera have been shown to contain antierythrocyte antibodies, Forssman antibodies, and a variety of other nonliver-specific antibodies. There is little question that liver cells contain liver-specific antigens, primarily in the microsomal fraction [45, 46]. Although there is evidence in heterologous antisera of antibody specific for liver [47, 35] which probably represents antibody to the microsomal proteins mentioned above, there are also antibodies which cross-react with other organs such as kidney and blood vessels [48, 49]. The cross-reaction can be shown by using labeled heterologous antisera which bind to a variety of tissues other than liver [50, 51]. Reports have appeared on the administration of heterologous antiliver antiserum in different animals [6, 52–54]. The results of various investigations are inconsistent and confusing. The difficulties in evaluating the significance of these experiments result from: (1) wide differences in the ability to produce hepatic lesions and in their extent; (2) the variation in pathological lesions resulting from injection of the heterologous antiliver antisera; (3) failure in some reports to exclude the possibility of participation of nonliver-specific antibodies, such as antierythrocyte or antiserum protein antibodies, in the pathogenesis of the hepatic damage; (4) failure in some reports to exclude the possibility of direct toxic effect of the injection of a foreign serum; (5) the production of similar lesions following administration of adjuvants alone; (6) the production by antiliver antisera of lesions in organs other than liver; and (7) the hepatotoxicity of antiserum to other tissues, e.g., rabbit antidog muscle serum [55].

It appears, therefore, that although the injection of liver homogenates with Freund's adjuvant or the intravenous administration of heterologous antiliver antisera is capable of producing hepatic lesions, at the present time these experiments contribute little to our understanding of immunological liver injury.

RUNTING SYNDROME AND SECONDARY DISEASE

Perhaps the best experimental demonstration that immunological reactions can lead to liver disease is the runting syndrome and secondary disease [56]. In these conditions, immunologically competent cells are injected into neonatal animals (runting syndrome) or into irradiated adults (secondary disease). The injected cells colonize in the recipient and react immunologically against the foreign tissues of the host. The donor-versus-host immune reaction is mediated by a delayed hypersensitivity mechanism, humoral antibody, or possibly both [57]. Animals with runting syndrome develop hepatomegaly, the livers are infiltrated by lymphoid cells, and focal areas of liver cell necrosis develop. Such lesions resemble those seen in certain forms of chronic hepatitis, particularly lupoid hepatitis. The possibility has been suggested that immunological damage analogous to that occurring in runting syndrome may be involved in the pathogenesis of certain cases of chronic hepatitis [58].

ALEUTIAN MINK DISEASE

This is a naturally occurring disease of mink which is characterized by marked hypergammaglobulinemia and pathological lesions similar to those described in certain human autoimmune diseases. There are extensive perivascular infiltrations of parenchymal organs by lymphocytes and plasma cells particularly in association with necrotizing arteritis. Hepatomegaly occurs, and the lymphocytic infiltration in the liver resembles that seen in some human cases of chronic hepatitis [59]. Recent investigations show that the disease can be transmitted by cell-free filtrates derived from affected tissues [60]. Mink which are homozygous recessive for the Aleutian gene are significantly more susceptible to both the spontaneous and the experimental disease [60]. Steroid therapy reduces the serum protein levels, but the hypergammaglobulinemia returns on cessation of drug therapy.

Aleutian disease of mink is of particular interest to the physician and immunologist because of the possibility that it represents a naturally occurring autoimmune disease in animals. It has been suggested [60] that the filtrable agent, presumably a virus, initiates the disease either by stimulating somatic mutation and the development of forbidden clones or by releasing "self-antigens" from the liver and possibly other organs. The progressive rise of γ-globulin and increasing infiltration of tissues by lymphoid cells presumably results from a continuing autoimmune reaction.*

LIVER DISEASES IN MAN

INFECTIOUS HEPATITIS

The impression that immunological phenomena play a role in the pathogenesis of infectious hepatitis is based primarily on three observations: (1) a high frequency of associated allergic manifestations, including urticaria, angioneurotic edema, rashes, and arthralgia [61, 62]; (2) the occurrence of γ-globulin-producing cells in the liver, as demonstrated by the fluorescent antibody technique [4]; (3) the presence of serum agglutinins. Gajdusek [63] found that the sera of 30 percent of 75 patients with viral hepatitis contained complement-fixing antibodies against aqueous extracts of normal human liver. Similar findings (33 percent of 106 cases) were reported by Mackay and Larkin [64] and by Bjorneboe and Krag [65]. This reaction, however, is not specific for liver, similar titers being found against renal and other tissue antigens. The occurrence of hemagglutinating substances in the sera of patients with acute hepatitis reactive against erythrocytes from a variety of animals suggests the possible occurrence of immunological phenomena accompanying viral hepatitis. Eaton *et al.* [66] described a heterogenic antibody in the serum of patients with acute hepatitis which fixed complement with alcohol-soluble antigens from human liver. This antibody also agglutinated red cells of sheep, horses, rabbits, cows, and rhesus monkeys, but unlike the heterophil antibody of infectious mononucleosis was absorbable by human tissues. Havens and Eichman [67] reported agglutination of chick erythrocytes in approximately 70 percent of patients in the acute phase of viral hepatitis and in 17 percent of those with other acute and chronic diseases, and 7 percent of normals. This antibody differs from that described by Eaton *et al.* in that it does not react with sheep erythrocytes.

Since both the hemagglutinating reactions and the antiliver antibodies are nonspecific and are seen in a number of nonhepatic diseases, their role and that of hypersensitivity in acute hepatitis remains to be determined.

DRUG-INDUCED LIVER DISEASE

In a consideration of the effect of drugs on the liver it is important to distinguish between those drugs such as chloroform which are true hepatotoxins and those such as chlorpromazine which are primarily sensitizing agents. The hepatic disease produced by sensitizing drugs is frequently accompanied by allergic manifestations such as rash, fever, arthralgia, and eosinophilia. The appearance of the lesion cannot be correlated with the dose of drug administered, and the disease occurs only in certain "susceptible" individuals. An unexplained characteristic of drug-induced hepatitis is the inconstancy between exposure to drug and the development of reactions. In some cases, a reaction appears almost immediately following a small dose; in others, only after many months of drug administration, and, on occasion, weeks following the cessation of therapy [68]. Many sensitizing drugs produce primarily canalicular damage (cholestatic hepatitis), although in some cases, both cholestasis and hepatocellular injury occur simultaneously. Because

* *Editor's comment:* Aleutian mink disease has provided a provocative and popular model for students of several of the rheumatic, hypersensitivity, or autosensitivity diseases. No one has yet, however, brought forth evidence that autoantibodies constitute part of the hypergammaglobulinemia of the disease. The most significant feature about the disease, it seems to me, is the apparent role of the genetic constitution of the host in determining susceptibility to the disease.— J. H. V.

of the characteristics mentioned above, several drugs, including arsphenamine, sulfonamides, phenylbutazone, phenobarbital, probenecid, and chlorpromazine, are thought to produce hepatitis by a hypersensitivity mechanism. Although beneficial results have been reported following the administration of corticosteroids [69, 70], the efficacy of these drugs has not been fully established. As pointed out by Klatskin [68], the mode of action of methyltestosterone in producing cholestatic hepatitis may be different from that of chlorpromazine. Methyltestosterone hepatitis is not associated with hypersensitivity phenomena, and there is evidence [71, 72] suggesting hepatotoxicity. Most patients with cholestatic hepatitis recover after a variable course and show no residual hepatic disease. Occasionally, however, progressive and persistent inflammation is associated with the development of a syndrome indistinguishable from primary biliary cirrhosis [73, 74].

Although it seems likely that hypersensitivity mechanisms are involved in drug-induced hepatitis, circulating antibodies and skin sensitivity have not been regularly demonstrated. Failure to find antibodies may be related to defects in the mechanisms of testing, particularly in conjugating the drug to an appropriate carrier.

BILIARY CIRRHOSIS

The clinical features of biliary cirrhosis, also called xanthomatous, cholangiolitic, and Hanot's cirrhosis, have been reviewed elsewhere [75, 76]. Briefly, the disease consists of prolonged jaundice, usually of insidious onset, occurring in middle-aged women with biochemical evidence of biliary obstruction but in whom normal extrahepatic biliary passages are found at laparotomy. Marked elevations of serum lipids and cholesterol are associated with cutaneous xanthomata. In addition to the clinical and biochemical features found in chronic biliary obstruction, there are also manifestations such as steatorrhea and osteoporosis due to malabsorption of fat and fat-soluble vitamins. The course is usually slowly progressive, and eventually cirrhosis develops and the clinical features associated with portal hypertension appear. In only a few cases is a potential initiating factor such as acute cholangiolitic hepatitis or drug administration recognized. Early in the disease, the histological features are those of a pericholangiolar reaction, with little fibrosis or evidence of bile duct proliferation. Ultimately, fibrosis appears in the portal areas and the histological picture is similar to that seen in portal and postnecrotic cirrhosis. The evidence that can be marshaled for the participation of immunological phenomena in the pathogenesis of primary biliary cirrhosis is: (1) infiltration of the liver and occasionally other organs by lymphoid cells [77]; (2) a small but probably significant number of cases which appear to result from the administration of sensitizing drugs [74, 78, 79]; (3) hypergammaglobulinemia appearing early in the course of the disease, sometimes before any clinical evidence of cirrhosis, and the recent description [80] of γ-globulin-producing cells in the livers of patients with primary biliary cirrhosis; and (4) the occurrence of antitissue antibodies.

Mackay [77] reported 2 cases of primary biliary cirrhosis in which there were high titers in the autoimmune complement fixation (AICF) reaction. Serum titers of 1 : 2,048 and 1 : 512 were found against liver antigen. Similar titers were present against kidney antigens. Deicher *et al.* [81] studied 11 patients with primary biliary cirrhosis, 7 of whom showed positive AICF reactions against a variety of human tissue antigens. In the majority of cases, the AICF reactions were positive primarily with cytoplasmic and not with nuclear extracts. Several cases of biliary cirrhosis with positive LE cell reactions, however, were reported by Kunkel [76]. Paronetto *et al.* [82] found that the sera of 4 of 5 patients with primary biliary cirrhosis bound γ-globulin to nuclei of ductule cells as demonstrated by the indirect Coons' fluorescent antibody technique. The nuclear binding was neither species- nor organ-specific and was decreased by steroid therapy; LE preparations were negative in cases with positive binding. The ability to detect nuclear staining by the fluorescent technique in the presence of negative results of LE tests is probably due to the greater sensitivity of the fluorescent technique. Several cases of Sjögren's syndrome with arthritis and antitissue antibody which were associated with biliary cirrhosis have been reported [3].

CHRONIC HEPATITIS AND POSTNECROTIC CIRRHOSIS

Recently there has been increased awareness that some, if not the majority, of the cases of postnecrotic cirrhosis result from a chronic progressive form of hepatitis. Chronic hepatitis or, as it is referred to by Tisdale [83], subacute hepatitis, occurs predominantly in females [84–86] and is characterized by chronic or acute recurrent episodes of liver dysfunction and, in the early stages, by a dense lymphoid infiltration in the liver (Fig. 78-1). In some cases the lymphocytic infiltration is extensive and takes the form of small follicle-like structures resembling the germinal centers of lymph nodes. Cellular destruction is widespread and, in the majority of cases, progressive to a coarse nodular (postnecrotic) cirrhosis.

The etiology of chronic hepatitis is unknown. Some authors believe that most cases of postnecrotic cirrhosis result from the repair of necrotic lesions resulting from a single episode of acute viral hepatitis. Despite the lack of definite episodes of acute viral hepatitis as initiating factors in most patients with chronic hepatitis, many cases have been reported (approximately 25 percent of several series) [87–89] in which there are histories of prior illnesses resembling acute viral hepatitis or in which onset followed blood transfusion or other inoculations. Baggenstoss [90] and Tisdale [83] have reviewed the evidence, obtained largely by serial biopsies, that the earliest lesions closely resemble those seen in acute viral hepatitis. Although in some, if not in the majority, of the cases, acute hepatitis may be an initiating event, the occurrence of continuing hepatic injury and frequently a progressive course suggest a persisting cause. There is no good evidence that persistent low-grade inflammation results from a continuing viral infection.

One of the most widely accepted theories is that of continuing damage resulting from an autoimmune process [9, 80]. Several possible mechanisms for the development of autoimmune disease have been suggested. Initial damage may be caused by the hepatitis virus or a toxin resulting in the release of potentially antigenic material and the formation of antibody locally and perhaps systemically. Interaction of antigen and antibody could then produce the antigen-antibody complexes which result in liver cell damage. Popper [80] found that the serum of patients with chronic liver disease binds to PAS-positive material in the lumen of bile ductules and the cytoplasm of the ductal epithelial cells. He has postulated that the PAS-positive material is antigenic and that locally formed antibody interacts with this material to form cytotoxic antigen-antibody complexes. Mackay and Wood [9] suggested the possibility that an autoimmune destructive reaction results from the appearance of immunologically competent lymphoid cells in the liver. These cells may be responsible not only for the destruction of liver tissue but also for the appearance of hypergammaglobulinemia and a variety of antitissue antibodies which are found in the sera of patients with chronic hepatitis. According to this hypothesis, the continuing immunological activity of the intrahepatic lymphoid cells is responsible for the persistent liver cell de-

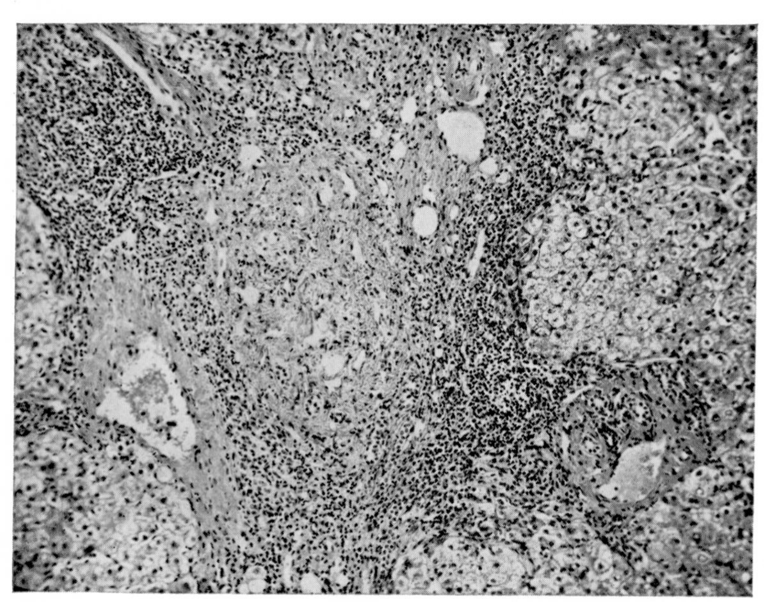

Fig. 78-1. Section of liver from a patient with postnecrotic cirrhosis. An initial illness suggestive of viral hepatitis progressed to chronic hepatitis and eventually cirrhosis. Hepatocellular necrosis, fibrosis, and dense lymphoid infiltration are evident. (Courtesy Dr. Thomas Trainer, University of Vermont College of Medicine.)

struction and eventually the development of coarse nodular cirrhosis. The lymphocytic response could in turn be triggered by virus infection in susceptible individuals or, as Burnet suggested, by a loss of a normal homeostatic mechanism for removing "forbidden clones" which arise as a result of spontaneous somatic mutation. Although the hypotheses of Popper and of Mackay and Burnet are attractive and provide a facile explanation for certain forms of chronic hepatitis, they are not well substantiated by experimental facts and must be regarded as highly speculative. The evidence implicating autoimmunization in chronic hepatitis is discussed later.

PORTAL CIRRHOSIS (LAENNEC'S CIRRHOSIS)

Classically, the liver of patients with portal cirrhosis shows a finely nodular lesion. The pathological differentiation from postnecrotic cirrhosis (coarsely nodular) is, however, not always clear-cut [91]. Whether viral hepatitis leads to portal cirrhosis remains an unsettled question. In a significant number of cases, however, patients with cirrhosis, apparently following an episode of hepatitis, have a finely nodular lesion. In other instances, a coarsely nodular cirrhosis is found in patients having a history most compatible with alcoholic or nutritional cirrhosis. The available evidence indicates that chronic alcoholism and malnutrition are important etiological factors in the pathogenesis of Laennec's cirrhosis [91, 92]. In most cases, the continuing damage can be attributed to the persistence of the injurious factors, and there is little reason to postulate the existence of autoimmune mechanisms to explain the ultimate development of cirrhosis. However, many of the features which suggest autoimmune phenomena in chronic hepatitis and postnecrotic cirrhosis also occur in Laennec's cirrhosis. For example, lymphocytic infiltration, hypergammaglobulinemia, association with other diseases such as ulcerative colitis, and the occurrence of a variety of circulating antibodies are also noted in portal cirrhosis. In general, however, the evidence for autoimmunization is less suggestive in portal cirrhosis than in chronic hepatitis and postnecrotic cirrhosis, since all of the points mentioned above with the possible exception of the hypergammaglobulinemia are not prominent manifestations of portal cirrhosis. Antinuclear and antiliver antibodies occur less commonly in portal cirrhosis than in chronic hepatitis, and as shown by Popper [80] and his co-workers, there is little evidence of γ-globulin production in the liver of patients with portal cirrhosis.

LUPOID HEPATITIS

The term lupoid hepatitis has been used to describe a form of chronic hepatitis usually occurring in young women who manifest, in addition to the symptoms of hepatitis, certain clinical and laboratory features also found in SLE [93, 1, 94, 3]. The clinical features are those of chronic hepatitis, including hepatosplenomegaly, spider angiomata, jaundice, and endocrine disturbances with amenorrhea and infertility. In addition, these patients often manifest some of the stigmata of SLE, most commonly arthralgia and rash but occasionally nephropathy, hemolytic anemia, pleuritis, and rarely other symptoms of SLE. Usually, symptoms suggestive of SLE appear later in the course of the hepatic disease, although Bartholomew *et al.* [93] reported seven cases in which the symptoms of SLE appeared before the liver disease became manifest. Such patients have hypergammaglobulinemia, positive LE cell and, some, positive AICF reactions. Pathological examinations of the livers of patients dying of SLE are frequently unremarkable, and when abnormalities are present, they consist primarily of nonspecific findings such as mild fatty infiltrations, focal necrosis, or, if heart failure has occurred, central congestion of the lobules [95]. In contrast, the histological features in lupoid hepatitis are similar to those of chronic hepatitis and postnecrotic cirrhosis.

The clinical course is variable but is frequently characterized by recurrent episodes of fever and jaundice and progression after a variable period of time to a classic picture of postnecrotic cirrhosis. Death usually occurs from hepatic failure rather than as a consequence of SLE. In our experience, many patients with lupoid hepatitis respond to corticosteroid therapy. In some, the effects are striking, with a rapid fall in serum bilirubin and transaminase levels and improvement in parenchymal cell damage, as seen on liver biopsy. Similar beneficial effects of steroids have been noted by others [96–99]. Once the acute episode has subsided, prednisone in doses of 30 to 40 mg. per day should be continued for at least three to four months before its withdrawal. Transaminase as well as other liver function tests provide good indications of activity and are helpful, along with the clinical symptomatology and liver biopsy, as indicators of disease activity. In some cases, chronic steroid administration is necessary because of increased activity on withdrawal, and in other cases fatal cirrhosis develops rapidly despite steroid therapy. Beneficial results have been obtained in a small number of cases from lymphocytotoxic antimetabolites such as 6-mercaptopurine and 6-thioguanine [9, 100]. Further clinical trials are necessary, however, before any conclusions can be drawn concerning their efficacy, particularly in view of their serious bone marrow suppressive and hepatotoxic potentials.

EVIDENCE OF AUTOIMMUNITY IN CHRONIC AND LUPOID HEPATITIS

REASONS FOR CONSIDERING CHRONIC AND LUPOID HEPATITIS AS AUTOIMMUNE DISEASES

1. *Association with Diseases Thought to Be Caused by Autoimmune Reactions.* As mentioned above, in certain cases of chronic hepatitis there are positive LE reactions and clinical features such as arthralgia and rash resembling SLE. Since the symptoms and also the LE cell tests are not specific for LE, it is not known whether this form of chronic hepatitis is a variant of SLE. Other autoimmune syndromes which have been associated with chronic hepatitis include acquired hemolytic anemias [101], Sjögren's syndrome [102, 3], and Hashimoto's thyroiditis [2].

2. *Infiltration of the Liver by Lymphocytes and Plasma Cells.* The ability of these cells to produce γ-globulin has been demonstrated by Popper [80], using an immunofluorescence technique. It is well known that these cell types are involved in the formation of circulating antibody as well as in delayed type immune reactions. In some cases, the proportion of plasma cells may be very high (approximately 40 percent) [103]. However, plasma cells are not necessary for the development of hepatitis, since it has been described in two cases of agammaglobulinemia associated with a severe plasma cell deficiency [104]. Although the appearance of these cell types is consistent with an autoimmune reaction and their postulated role as autodestructive agents, they could also represent a nonspecific response following contact with an exogenous antigen such as a virus.

3. *Beneficial Effect of Corticosteroids.* This has been noted in many cases of chronic and lupoid hepatitis.

4. *Hypergammaglobulinemia.* This is discussed in detail later, under a separate heading.

5. *Presence of a Variety of Circulating Antibodies.* These include antinuclear and anticytoplasmic factors (antiliver antibodies), antithyroglobulin antibodies, rheumatoid factor, antierythrocyte antibodies, and Wassermann-like antibodies.

The LE cell reaction, which occurs in about 25 percent of the patients with chronic hepatitis, is usually only weakly positive. However, a few instances of strongly positive reactions have been reported [93, 2]. Although the formation of LE cells occurs most frequently in SLE, antinuclear antibodies can also arise in the course of certain diseases, such as miliary tuberculosis [105], which bear little relation to SLE. Moreover, the majority of patients with chronic hepatitis do not have positive LE preparations [1, 106], and liver disease indistinguishable from that seen in so-called lupoid hepatitis may exist for years without the development of positive LE cell reactions. Using the sensitive fluorescent antiglobulin technique, Calabresi and Greenberg [107] found nuclear fluorescence in 10 of 24 alcoholics with cirrhosis and 3 of 8 patients with postnecrotic cirrhosis. Antinuclear factors have also been described in chronic liver disease by Pollak *et al.* [108] and in a miscellaneous group of acute and chronic liver diseases in several other reports [109–111]. In view of the occurrence of these factors in classic portal cirrhosis and a variety of other diseases [110], their presence in the serum of patients with liver disease does not necessarily indicate a close relationship with SLE. More studies are necessary before an understanding of the (immunological?) processes responsible for the formation of antinuclear factors and their role in liver disease can be interpreted. At present, there is insufficient evidence to decide whether the positive LE cell reaction seen in chronic hepatitis represents a "false positive" result or the hepatic disease is a variant of SLE.

The AICF reactions occur between the patient's serum and human tissue homogenates. Mackay and Burnet [2] reported an incidence of positive AICF reactions of 21 percent in chronic hepatitis and 40 percent in lupoid hepatitis, the latter more frequently having the higher titers. Other types of chronic liver disease such as portal and biliary cirrhosis and hemochromatosis have approximately a 12 percent incidence of positive AICF reactions. Similar studies by Hackett *et al.* [112] showed a 35 percent incidence in 78 patients with miscellaneous liver diseases. High titers have also been found in a large variety of human diseases, including macroglobulinemia, SLE, and some cases of biliary cirrhosis [81, 113]. The antigens in the AICF reactions of chronic hepatitis can be derived from a variety of tissues in addition to liver and are of cytoplasmic rather than nuclear origin [114]. By immunofluorescence [109], the cytoplasm of ductule epithelial cells and bile are stained. Asherson and Broberger [115] found that sera from 8 of 28 patients with chronic liver disease reacted with phenol extracts of human liver or colon. These findings are consistent with the carbohydrate nature of the liver antigen proposed by Popper [80]. Despite these findings, however, the chemical nature of the liver antigens responsible for the AICF reactions remains unknown. The reaction of fluorescein-conjugated globulin from certain liver disease sera with sections of the patients' liver obtained by needle biopsy [116] indicates the autologous nature of the antiliver antibodies. In several reported cases [64], the sera failed to react with autologous tissues although it reacted in high titer with isologous tissues. It should be pointed out that the AICF reaction also occurs in low titers in an occasional normal human serum [117]. Duran-Reynals [118] also showed a striking rise in flocculating antihuman tissue antibodies following immunization of rabbits or chickens with a totally unrelated antigen such as a bacterium.

We have recently immunized six rabbits with *Escherichia coli*, using the technique described by Abruzzo and Christian [119]. Immunization resulted in the appearance of a rheumatoid-like factor (Chap. 65) and a rise in titer in the complement fixation reactions against both calf thymus nuclei or human tissue homogenates. The rise in titers of complement-fixing antibodies paralleled the rise in rheumatoid factor titers but was of smaller magnitude. Some normal rabbit sera were found to contain low titers of complement-fixing antibodies against human tissue homogenates. These are probably identical with the so-called natural antibodies of normal rabbit serum described by Kidd and Friedewald [120] and with the flocculating antibodies of Duran-Reynals mentioned above. These findings suggest that the factors responsible for the AICF reactions may be normally present in small amounts and that the elevated titers found in chronic hepatic diseases result from nonspecific stimuli.

There is considerable evidence that the circulating antitissue antibodies are not by themselves directly responsible for the liver disease. Antitissue antibodies have not been clearly shown to be capable of entering intact cells, and there is no good evidence that they produce lesions in solid organs. Most patients with SLE or with other diseases with high titers in the AICF reactions have no demonstrable evidence of liver disease. Positive AICF reactions are seen in a variety of liver diseases, including infectious hepatitis, with apparent complete recovery. Moreover, in most AICF reactions associated with liver disease, the antibody has not been shown to be specific for liver tissue. The report by Dausset and Marchal [121] of a case of cirrhosis having a liver-specific antibody represents an exception. For these reasons, the significance of anticytoplasmic reactions remains uncertain. It seems probable that they represent markers of an abnormal immunological response rather than etiological agents. This is probably also true of the rheumatoid factor which is present, usually in low titer, in approximately 50 percent of patients with acute and chronic liver disease [106, 122].

ORIGIN AND SIGNIFICANCE OF HYPERGAMMAGLOBULINEMIA IN LIVER DISEASE

A characteristic abnormality of the serum proteins in both acute and chronic liver diseases is an elevation of γ-globulin. In acute hepatitis, γ-globulin levels are usually moderately elevated and gradually return to normal as the disease subsides over a period of two to three months [123]. Persistent or increasing hypergammaglobulinemia may indicate the transition from acute to chronic hepatitis [124]. The levels of γ-globulin in chronic liver disease are much higher and may reach values four to five times greater than those of normal serum. Elevations are seen in biliary cirrhosis (both primary and secondary to chronic obstruction) and granulomatous diseases of the liver, such as tuberculosis and sarcoidosis, as well as in chronic hepatitis and Laennec's cirrhosis. In chronic hepatitis, the degree of disease activity roughly correlates with the γ-globulin levels.

FLOCCULATION REACTIONS

These have been reviewed in detail elsewhere [125, 8]. Briefly, two types of mechanisms are involved in flocculation reactions: (1) Certain stabilizing factors which are normally present disappear immediately following an acute parenchymal injury to the liver, and their absence results in a positive cephalin flocculation reaction. In this instance, there is no demonstrable quantitative change in the serum γ-globulin levels. (2) Cephalin flocculation reactions, on the other hand, may depend upon an elevated γ-globulin level. The correlation between positive cephalin flocculation reactions and total serum γ-globulin in various diseases is, however, poor. Franklin [126] found that the cephalin flocculation as well as the thymol turbidity reaction depends primarily on the most basic γ-globulins. In addition, the thymol reaction depends on other promoting and stabilizing factors in the α, β, and the albumin regions [127].

ORIGIN OF GAMMA-GLOBULIN

Miller and Bale [128] have shown that the normal liver does not form γ-globulin. They perfused rat livers with mixtures of amino acids containing C^{14}-labeled lysine and measured the degree of incorporation of the isotope into the plasma protein fractions appearing in the perfusate. All of the protein fractions except γ-globulin were labeled. Popper [80], using the fluorescent antibody technique, also failed to demonstrate γ-globulin-producing cells in normal livers. The livers from patients with portal cirrhosis, biliary cirrhosis, and cardiac cirrhosis showed little evidence of γ-globulin production despite marked elevations of serum γ-globulin levels. Nevertheless, in many cases of chronic hepatitis, γ-globulin could be demonstrated in the cytoplasm of cells lining the sinusoids and also in mononuclear cells in the fibrous septum. The γ-globulin-containing cells were thought to be derived from Kupffer cells. Although confirmation and extension of these interesting studies are necessary, they suggest that at least in some cases of chronic hepatitis, a fraction of the serum γ-globulin is produced in the liver. The antigenic stimuli responsible for the elevation of γ-globulin levels is unknown. Mackay and Wood [9] suggested that although the hepatitis virus may be the initiating factor, the continuing antigenic stimulus is produced by an endogenous autoantigen released by the initial damage.

Havens [129] demonstrated an enhanced capacity of patients with chronic liver disease to produce antibodies to bacterial antigens such as diphtheria and tetanus toxoid. Patients with chronic hepatitis and cirrhosis produced two to three times as much antitoxin as did controls, and the greatest production was in patients with more advanced cirrhosis.

PROPERTIES OF GAMMA-GLOBULIN

Despite suggestions [130, 131] that the electrophoretic elevations in the γ-globulin region represent, at least in part, the release of liver proteins into the circulation, the available evidence does not support this view. Quantitative immunological studies indicate that most of the elevation in the γ-globulin in cirrhosis can be accounted for by an increase in one of the known types of γ-globulin [132]. These experiments, reported in part in Table 78-1, also

TABLE 78-1. Quantitation of Immunoglobulins in Sera of Patients with Portal Cirrhosis

Serum	Total Protein (gm. %)	mg./cc.			Ratio
		γ_2	γ_{1A}	γ_{1M}	γ_2/γ_{1A}
Ya	9.0	19.8	8.92	1.88	2.21
Ru	8.5	24.2	7.02	1.56	3.44
Cl	7.8	17.6	5.0	1.56	3.52
Bo	7.7	19.0	6.20	1.38	3.06
McN	6.7	15.1	6.2	3.2	2.43
He	5.4	17.6	8.04	1.38	2.18
Cirrhosis	aver.	18.9	6.9	1.84	2.81
Normal	aver.	10.0	1.56	1.08	6.4
(18 cases)	range	(8.6–12)	(1.04–2.20)	(0.66–1.88)	

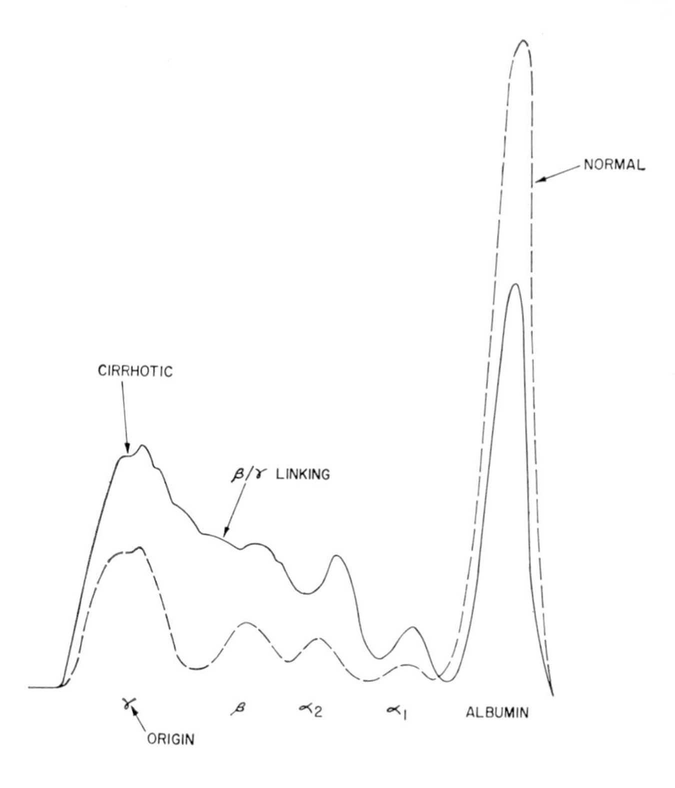

Fig. 78-2. Paper electrophoresis patterns of normal serum and serum of a patient with classic portal cirrhosis. The marked hypergammaglobulinemia and beta-gamma linking of the cirrhotic serum are evident.

show that there is a relatively greater increase in the γ_{1A}-globulin in portal cirrhosis. This is evident from the striking decrease in the γ_2/γ_{1A} ratios in all of the sera studied. It should be noted that except in cases of liver disease associated with high titers of rheumatoid factor, the γ_{1M} fraction is normal or only slightly elevated. The observation that the γ_{1A} fraction is markedly elevated in cirrhosis is consistent with the finding on paper electrophoresis of a diffuse elevation of γ-globulin extending into the β region (Fig. 78-2). This beta-gamma linking eliminates the normal demarcation between the β- and γ-globulins and is a feature regularly observed in the serum of patients with portal cirrhosis. Analysis of the sera of several patients with advanced portal cirrhosis by density gradient ultracentrifugation has indicated that the γ_{1A} globulins are of the 7S size.

Recent observations [132] have shown that unlike Laennec's cirrhosis the ratio of γ_2/γ_{1A} in sera of patients with acute infectious hepatitis and lupoid hepatitis are normal or elevated. The significance of the variations in γ_2/γ_{1A} ratios observed in different types of liver diseases is unknown. It is interesting and perhaps significant that recent studies have shown that γ_{1A} is the predominant type of γ-globulin present in certain external fluids including tears, saliva, nasal and bronchial fluids, and perhaps gastrointestinal fluids and bile as well [133].

REFERENCES

1. Bearn, A. G., Kunkel, H. G., and Slater, R. J. Problem of chronic liver disease in young women. *Amer. J. Med.* 21:3, 1956.
2. Mackay, I. R., and Burnet, F. M. *Autoimmune Diseases.* Springfield, Ill.: Charles C Thomas, Publisher, 1963.
3. Holman, H., and Tomasi, T. B. "Lupoid" hepatitis. *Med. Clin. N. Amer.* 44:633, 1960.
4. Felton, L. D., Prescott, B., Kauffmann, G., and Ottinger, B. Pneumococcal antigenic polysaccharide substances from animal tissues. *J. Immun.* 74:205, 1955.
5. Cohen, S., Ohta, G., Singer, E. J., and Popper, H. Immunocytochemical study of gamma globulin in the liver in hepatitis and postnecrotic cirrhosis. *J. Exp. Med.* 111:285, 1960.
6. Steiner, J. W., *et al.* Experimental immuno-

logical liver injury and the concept of autodestruction: I. *Canad. Med. Ass. J.* 85:1369, 1961; II., *Ibid.*, p. 1425.
7. Goldgraber, M. B., and Kirsner, J. B. Summary of the hypersensitivity state in the liver: A critical review. *Amer. J. Med. Sci.* 241:109, 1961.
8. Osserman, E. F., and Takatsuki, K. The plasma proteins in liver disease. *Med. Clin. N. Amer.* 47:679, 1963.
9. Mackay, I. R., and Wood, I. J. Lupoid hepatitis: A comparison of 22 cases with other types of chronic liver disease. *Quart. J. Med.* 31:485, 1962.
10. Flexner, S. The pathologic changes caused by certain so-called toxalbumins. *Med. News* 65:116, 1894.
11. Wells, H. G. Experimental cirrhosis of the liver in chronic albumose intoxication. *Trans. Chicago Path. Soc.* 5:240, 1901–03.
12. Longcope, W. T. Cirrhosis of the liver produced by chronic protein intoxication. *Trans. Ass. Amer. Physicians* 28:497, 1913.
13. Cornil, L., and Mosinger, M. Sur les réactions hépatiques consécutives à l'injection intra-abdominale répétée de sérum hétérogène. *C. R. Soc. Biol.* (Paris) 121:61, 1936.
14. Choi, C. Y. The local anaphylactic reaction of liver tissue. *Trans. Jap. Path. Soc.* 20:587, 1930.
15. Hawn, C. V., and Janeway, C. A. Histological and serological sequences in experimental hypersensitivity. *J. Exp. Med.* 85:571, 1947.
16. Hartley, G., Jr., and Lushbaugh, C. C. Experimental allergic focal necrosis of the liver. *Amer. J. Path.* 18:323, 1942.
17. Steiner, J. W. Investigations of allergic liver injury: I. Light, fluorescent and electron miscroscopic study of the effects of soluble immune aggregates. *Amer. J. Path.* 38:411, 1961.
18. Korson, R. Personal communication, 1964.
19. Weigle, W. O. Fate and biological action of antigen-antibody complexes. *Advances Immun.* 1:283, 1961.
20. Ishizaka, K., and Campbell, D. H. Biological activity of soluble antigen-antibody complexes: I. Skin reactive properties. *Proc. Soc. Exp. Biol. Med.* 97:635, 1958.
21. Benacerraf, B., Potter, J. L., McCluskey, R. T., and Miller, F. The pathologic effects of intravenously administered soluble antigen-antibody complexes: II. Acute glomerulonephritis in rats. *J. Exp. Med.* 111:195, 1960.
22. McCluskey, R. T., and Benacerraf, B. Localization of colloidal substances in vascular endothelium, a mechanism of tissue damage: II. Experimental serum sickness with acute glomerulonephritis induced passively in mice by antigen-antibody complexes in antigen excess. *Amer. J. Path.* 35:275, 1959.
23. McCluskey, R. T., Benacerraf, B., Potter, J. L., and Miller, F. The pathologic effects of intravenously administered soluble antigen-antibody complexes: I. Passive serum sickness in mice. *J. Exp. Med.* 111:181, 1960.
24. McKinnon, G. E. Role of *in vivo* Antigen-Antibody Precipitation in Hypersensitivity Reactions. In Shaffer, J. H., LoGrippo, G. A., and Chase, M. W. (Eds.), *Mechanisms of Hypersensitivity*. Boston: Little, Brown, 1959.
25. Dean, H. R. The histology of a case of anaphylactic shock occurring in a man. *J. Path. Bact.* 25:304, 1922.
26. Sumner, F. W. Sudden death from anaphylactic shock. *Brit. Med. J.* 1:465, 1923.
27. Clark, E., and Kaplan, B. I. Endocardial, arterial and other mesenchymal alterations associated with serum sickness in man. *Arch. Path.* 24:458, 1937.
28. Longcope, W. T. Serum sickness and analogous reactions with certain drugs, particularly the sulfonamides. *Medicine* 22:251, 1943.
29. Rich, A. R. The role of hypersensitivity in periarteritis nodosa. *Bull. Hopkins Hosp.* 71:123, 1942.
30. Alechinsky, A. Contribution à l'étude des phénomènes hémorragiques. *Ann. Inst. Pasteur* (Paris) 63:41, 1939.
31. Bierry, H., and Mayer, A. Sur l'action du sang rendu hépatotoxique par injections intrapéritonéales de nucléoprotéides du foie. *C. R. Acad. Sci.* (Paris) 138:1639, 1904.
32. Flandin, C., and Valléry-Radot, P. Anaphylaxie sérique ictérigène. *Bull. Soc. Méd. Hôp. Paris.* 45:1072, 1921.
33. Rich, A. R., and Gregory, J. E. The experimental demonstration that periarteritis nodosa is a manifestation of hypersensitivity. *Bull. Hopkins Hosp.* 72:65, 1943.
34. Mowrey, F. H., and Lundberg, E. A. The clinical manifestations of essential polyangiitis (periarteritis nodosa), with emphasis on the hepatic manifestations. *Ann. Intern. Med.* 40:1145, 1954.
35. Vorlaender, K. O. Ueber der Nachweis komplementbindender Auto-antikörper bei Nieren- und Lebererkrankungen. *Z. Ges. Exp. Med.* 118:352, 1952.
36. Behar, A. J., and Tal, C. Experimental liver necrosis produced by the injection of homologous whole liver with adjuvants. *J. Path. Bact.* 77:591, 1959.
37. Jahiel, R. I., and Koffler, D. Hepatic granulomas induced in guinea pigs by Freund's adjuvant with and without homologous liver. *Brit. J. Exp. Path.* 42:338, 1961.
38. Tal, C., and Laufer, A. Amyloidosis in mice following injections with Freund's adjuvant, its components separately and homologous liver-adjuvant mixture. *Brit. J. Exp. Path.* 41:605, 1960.

39. Thomson, K. J., Freund, J., Sommer, H. E., and Walter, A. W. Immunization of duck against malaria by means of killed parasites with or without adjuvants. *Amer. J. Trop. Med.* 27:79, 1947.
40. Waksman, B. H., Pearson, C. M., and Sharp, J. T. Studies of arthritis and other lesions induced in rats by injection of mycobacterial adjuvant. *J. Immun.* 85:403, 1960.
41. Laufer, A., Tal, C., and Behar, A. Effect of adjuvant (Freund's type) and its components on the organs of various animal species: A comparative study. *Brit. J. Exp. Path.* 40:1, 1959.
42. Heymann, W., Hackel, D. B., and Hunter, J. L. P. Autoimmune nephrosis in rats. *Fed. Proc.* 19:195, 1960 (abst.).
43. Tal, C., and Behar, A. J. A demyelinating disease of the brain produced by injection of liver or liver proteolipid. *J. Path. Bact.* 76:483, 1958.
44. Steiner, J. W., Langer, B., Schatz, D. L., and Volpe, R. Experimental immunologic adrenal injury: A response to injections of autologous and homologous adrenal antigens in adjuvant. *J. Exp. Med.* 112:187, 1960.
45. D'Amelio, V., and Perlmann, P. The distribution of soluble antigens in cellular structures of rat liver. *Exp. Cell Res.* 19:383, 1960.
46. Vogt, P. K. The immunology of liver microsomes: I. The properties of the quantitative precipitin system. *Z. Naturforsch.* 15B:213, 1960.
47. Estes, H. R. Effect of anti-rat-liver serum on rats. *Arch. Path.* 47:399, 1949.
48. Bollag, W. Nachweis von organspecifischen Antikörpern. *Experientia* 12:210, 1956.
49. Frank, M., and Bozsoky, S. Versuche zur Hertstellung eines leberspezifischen heterologen Immunserums. *Z. Immunitaetsforsch.* 119: 110, 1960.
50. Korngold, L., and Pressman, D. The *in vitro* purification of tissue localizing antibodies. *J. Immun.* 71:1, 1953.
51. Pressman, D., Sherman, B., and Korngold, L. The zone of localization of antibodies: XIII. The *in vivo* localization of anti-liver-blood-vessel antibodies in the rat. *J. Immun.* 67:493, 1951.
52. Joannovics, G. Ueber das Hepatotoxin. *Wien. Klin. Wschr.* 22:228, 1909.
53. Masugi, M. Ueber das Wesen der spezifischen Veränderungen der Niere und der Leber durch das Nephrotoxin bzw. das Hepatotoxin: Zugleich ein Beitrag zur Pathogenese der Glomerulonephritis und der eklamptischen Lebererkrankung. *Beitr. Path. Anat.* 91:82, 1933.
54. Yokouti, T. Experimentelle Studien über das Hepatotoxin. I. Ueber das aus Leberzellkernen hergestellte Immunserum, mit besonderer Berücksichtigung seiner Beziehungen zum Immunserum aus Leberzellprotoplasma. *Tohoku J. Exp. Med.* 32:198, 1938.
55. Benstz, W., and Meyer-Krahmer, H. G. Zum Mechanismus der "inversen Anaphylaxie" unter Berücksichtigung der Anti-histaminwirkung bei experimenteller allergischer Leberschädigung (Masugi-Hepatitis). *Z. Ges. Exp. Med.* 119:76, 1952.
56. Billingham, R. E. Reactions of grafts against their hosts. *Science* 130:947, 1959.
57. Silverman, M. S., and Chin, P. H. Differences in the rejection of skin transplants and blood cells of donor marrow origin by radiation-induced chimeras. *Ann. N.Y. Acad. Sci.* 99:542, 1962.
58. Mackay, I. R. The problem of persisting destructive disease of the liver. *Gastroenterology* 40:617, 1961.
59. Helmboldt, C. F., and Jungherr, F. L. The pathology of Aleutian disease in mink. *Amer. J. Vet. Res.* 19:212, 1958.
60. Hensen, J. B., Letter, J. R. W., and Wagner, B. M. Experimental hypergammaglobulinemia in mink. *J. Exp. Med.* 165:7, 1962.
61. Mirick, G. S. Infectious Hepatitis In Hoffbauer, F. W. (Ed.), *11th Liver Conference on Liver Injury*. New York: Josiah Macy, Jr. Foundation, 1952.
62. Hawley, W. F., McFarlan, A. M., Steigman, A. J., McMichael, J., and Dible, J. H. Hepatitis and mumps convalescent serum. *Lancet* 1:818, 1944.
63. Gajdusek, D. C. An autoimmune reaction against human tissue antigens in certain acute and chronic diseases: I. Serological investigations. *Arch. Intern. Med.* 101:9, 1958.
64. Mackay, I. R., and Larkin, L. The significance of the presence in human serum of complement fixing antibodies to human tissue antigens. *Aust. Ann. Med.* 7:251, 1958.
65. Bjorneboe, M., and Krag, P. Studies on complement fixation in hepatitis with liver extract as antigen. *Acta Path. Microbiol. Scand.* 24: 352, 1947.
66. Eaton, M. D., Murphy, W. D., and Hanford, V. L. Heterogenetic antibodies in acute hepatitis. *J. Exp. Med.* 79:539, 1944.
67. Havens, W. P., Jr., and Eichman, H. L. Hemagglutination in viral hepatitis. *New Eng. J. Med.* 259:1202, 1958.
68. Klatskin, G. Toxic and Drug-induced Hepatitis. In Schiff, L. (Ed.), *Diseases of the Liver* (2nd ed.). Philadelphia: J. B. Lippincott Company, 1963.
69. Cutts, M. Chlorpromazine hepatitis treated with cortisone. *Ann. Intern. Med.* 46:1160, 1957.
70. Stein, A. A., and Wright, A. Hepatic pathology in jaundice due to chlorpromazine. *J.A.M.A.* 169:1453, 1959.

71. Heaney, R. P., and Whedon, G. D. Impairment of hepatic bromsulphalein clearance by two 17-substituted testosterones. *J. Lab. Clin. Med.* 52:169, 1958.
72. Kory, R. C., Bradley, M. H., Watson, R. N., Callahan, R., and Peters, B. J. A six-month evaluation of an anabolic drug, norethandrolone, in underweight persons: II. Bromsulphalein (BSP) retention and liver function. *Amer. J. Med.* 26:243, 1959.
73. Hanger, F. M., and Gutman, A. B. Post-arsphenamine jaundice apparently due to obstruction of intrahepatic biliary tract. *J.A.M.A.* 115:263, 1940.
74. Myers, J. D., Olson, R. E., Lewis, J. H., and Moran, J. T. Xanthomatous biliary cirrhosis following chlorpromazine, with observations indicating over-production of cholesterol, hyperprothrombinemia, and the development of portal hypertension. *Trans. Ass. Amer. Physicians* 70:243, 1957.
75. Ahrens, E. H., Jr., Payne, M. A., Kunkel, H. G., Eisenmenger, W. J., and Blondheim, S. H. Primary biliary cirrhosis. *Medicine* 29:299, 1950.
76. Kunkel, H. G. Biliary Cirrhosis. Ref. 68.
77. Mackay, I. R. Primary biliary cirrhosis: A case with systemic lesions and circulating anti-tissue antibody. *Lancet* 2:521, 1960.
78. Berger, S. S., and Appelbaum, H. S. Toxic hepatitis due to sulfanilamide: Report of a fatal case with histopathologic findings in the liver. *J. Lab. Clin. Med.* 26:785, 1941.
79. Bevans, M., and Batchelor, W. H. Cholangiolitic cirrhosis with intrahepatic biliary tract obstruction and xanthomatosis. *Amer. J. Med.* 9:133, 1950.
80. Popper, H. Possible Role of Immune Processes in Self Perpetuation of Liver Disease. In Grabar, P., and Miescher, P. (Eds.), *Mechanism of Cell and Tissue Damage Produced by Immune Reactions.* Basel: Benno Schwabe & Co., 1962.
81. Deicher, H. R. G., Holman, H. R., and Kunkel, H. G. Anti-cytoplasmic factors in the sera of patients with systemic lupus erythematosus and certain other diseases. *Arthritis Rheum.* 3:1, 1960.
82. Paronetto, F., Rubin, E., and Popper, H. Local formation of gamma globulin in the diseased liver and its relation to hepatic necrosis. *Lab. Invest.* 11:150, 1962.
83. Tisdale, W. A. Subacute hepatitis. *New Eng. J. Med.* 268:85 and 138, 1963.
84. Alsted, G. Studies on malignant hepatitis. *Amer. J. Med. Sci.* 213:257, 1947.
85. Salvesen, H. A., and Lodoen, O. Clinical studies on malignant hepatitis. *Acta Med. Scand.* 137:305, 1950.
86. Klatskin, G. Subacute hepatic necrosis and postnecrotic cirrhosis due to anicteric infections with hepatitis virus. *Amer. J. Med.* 25: 333, 1958.
87. Patek, A. J. Postnecrotic Cirrhosis. Ref. 68.
88. Ratnoff, O. D., and Patek, A. J., Jr. Postnecrotic cirrhosis of the liver. *J. Chron. Dis.* 1:266, 1955.
89. MacDonald, R. A., and Mallory, G. K. Natural history of postnecrotic cirrhosis: A study of 221 autopsy cases. *Amer. J. Med.* 24:334, 1958.
90. Baggenstoss, A. H. Postnecrotic cirrhosis: Morphology, etiology and pathogenesis. *Progr. Liver Dis.* 1:14, 1961.
91. Patek, A. J., Jr. Portal Cirrhosis (Laennec's Cirrhosis). Ref. 68.
92. Klatskin, G. Alcohol and its relation to liver damage. *Gastroenterology* 41:443, 1961.
93. Bartholomew, L. G., Hagedorn, A. B., Cain, J. C., and Baggenstoss, A. H. Hepatitis and cirrhosis in women with positive clot tests for lupus erythematosus *New Eng. J. Med.* 259: 947, 1958.
94. Joske, R. A., and King, W. E. L. E. cell phenomenon in active chronic viral hepatitis. *Lancet* 2:477, 1955.
95. Larson, D. L. *Systemic Lupus Erythematosus.* Boston: Little, Brown, 1961.
96. Page, A. R., and Good, R. A. Plasma-cell hepatitis, with special attention to steroid therapy. *Amer. J. Dis. Child.* 99:288, 1960.
97. McDonald, W. C., and Bogoch, A. Chronic hepatitis. *Canad. Med. Ass. J.* 84:1105, 1961.
98. Sborov, V. M., Bluemle, L. W., Jr., Neefe, J. R., and Gyorgy, P. Clinical usefulness of ACTH and cortisone in liver disease. *Gastroenterology* 28:745, 1955.
99. Last, P. M. Treatment of active chronic infectious hepatitis with ACTH (corticotropin) and cortisone. *Med. J. Aust.* 44:672, 1957.
100. Goodman, H. C. Current studies on the effect of antimetabolites in nephrosis, other non-neoplastic diseases in experimental animals. *Ann. Intern. Med.* 59:388, 1963.
101. Mackay, I. R., Taft, L. I., and Cowling, D. C. Lupoid hepatitis and the hepatic lesions of systemic lupus erythematosus. *Lancet* 1:65, 1959.
102. Krook, H. Liver cirrhosis in patients with a lupus erythematosus-like syndrome. *Acta Med. Scand.* 169:713, 1961.
103. Kunkel, H. G., and Bearn, A. G. Cirrhosis in Young Females: Its Possible Relation to Infectious Hepatitis. In Hartman, F. W. (Ed.), *Hepatitis Frontiers.* Boston: Little, Brown, 1957.
104. Good, R. A., and Page, A. R. Fatal complications of virus hepatitis in two patients with agammaglobulinemia. *Amer. J. Med.* 29: 804, 1960.

105. Lee, S. L., Michael, S. R., and Vural, I. L. L. E. (lupus erythematosus) cell. *Amer. J. Med.* 10:446, 1951.
106. Holborow, E. J., Asherson, G. L., Johnson, G. D., Barnes, R. D. S., and Carmichael, D. S. Antinuclear factor and other antibodies in blood and liver diseases. *Brit. Med. J.* 1:656, 1963.
107. Calabresi, P., and Greenberg, M. Circulating antinuclear globulins in patients with chronic liver disease. *J. Clin. Invest.* 39:976, 1960.
108. Pollak, V. E., Mandema, E., and Garstenstein, M. Serum antinuclear factor in patients and relatives: Observations in SLE and liver disease. *J. Clin. Invest.* 40:1071, 1961.
109. Paronetto, F., Schaffner, F., and Popper, H. Immunocytochemical reaction of serum of patients with hepatic diseases with hepatic structures. *Proc. Soc. Exp. Biol. Med.* 106:216, 1961.
110. Alexander, W. R. M., Bremner, J. M., and Duthie, J. J. R. Incidence of anti-nuclear factor in human sera. *Ann. Rheum. Dis.* 19:338, 1960.
111. Weir, D. M., Holborow, E. J., and Johnson, G. D. Clinical study of serum antinuclear factor. *Brit. Med. J.* 2:933, 1961.
112. Hackett, E., Beech, M., and Forkes, I. J. Auto-immune complement fixation reaction in 1,014 patients. *Brit. Med. J.*, 2:17, 1960.
113. Mackay, I. R., and Gajdusek, D. C. "Autoimmune" reactions against human tissue antigens in certain acute and chronic diseases. *Arch. Intern. Med.* 101:30, 1958.
114. Asherson, G. L. Antibodies against nuclear and cytoplasmic cell constituents in systemic lupus erythematosus and other diseases. *Brit. J. Exp. Path.* 40:209, 1959.
115. Asherson, G. L., and Broberger, O. Incidence of haemagglutinating and complement-fixing antibodies. *Brit. Med. J.* 1:1429, 1961.
116. Hunter, F. M., Sparks, R. D., and Salzman, R. T. Autoagglutinins in hepatic disease. *Gastroenterology* 39:394, 1960.
117. Gajdusek, D. C. "Autoimmune" reaction against human tissue antigens in certain acute and chronic diseases. *Arch. Intern. Med.* 101:1, 1958.
118. Duran-Reynals, F. Flocculation of tissue extracts by normal and immune sera of fowls and of other animals. *Yale J. Biol. Med.* 12:361, 1940.
119. Abruzzo, J. L., and Christian, C. L. The induction of a rheumatoid factor-like substance in rabbits. *J. Exp. Med.* 114:791, 1961.
120. Kidd, J. G., and Friedewald, W. F. A natural antibody that reacts *in vitro* with a sedimentable constituent of normal tissue cells. *J. Exp. Med.* 76:543 and 557, 1942.
121. Dausset, J., and Marchal, G. Cirrhose hépatique avec une substance sérique antifoie. In Grabar, P., and Miescher, P. (Eds.), *Immunopathology* (1st International Symposium). Basel: Benno Schwabe & Co., 1959.
122. Atwater, E. C., and Jacox, R. F. The latex-fixation test in patients with liver disease. *Ann. Intern. Med.* 58:419, 1963.
123. Havens, W. P., Jr., and Williams, T. L. Changes in the serum proteins in patients with experimentally induced infectious hepatitis. *J. Clin. Invest.* 27:340, 1948.
124. Krugman, S., Ward, R., and Giles, J. P. Natural history of infectious hepatitis. *Amer. J. Med.* 32:717, 1962.
125. Hanger, F. M. Liver function tests. *Med. Clin. N. Amer.* 44:681, 1960.
126. Franklin, E. C. Role of the basic fraction of γ-globulin in the flocculation tests. *Clin. Chim. Acta.* 4:259, 1959.
127. Cohen, P. P., and Thompson, F. L. Mechanism of the thymol turbidity test. *J. Lab. Clin. Med.* 32:475, 1947.
128. Miller, L. L., and Bale, W. F. Synthesis of all plasma protein fractions except gamma globulins by the liver: The use of zone electrophoresis and lysine-E-C^{14} to define the plasma proteins synthesized by the isolated perfused liver. *J. Exp. Med.* 99:125, 1954.
129. Havens, W. P., Jr. Liver disease and antibody formation. *Int. Arch. Allerg.* 14:75, 1959.
130. Berg, G., Roller, E., and Seisle, H. Experimental and clinical investigations of pathogenesis of dysproteinemia in hepatic disease. *Gastroenterology* 95:88, 1961.
131. Gordon, A. H. Detection of liver proteins in circulating blood. *Nature* (London) 189:727, 1961.
132. Tomasi, T. B., Jr. Human γ-Globulins. *Blood.* (In Press.)
133. Tomasi, T. B., Jr., Tan, E. M., Solomon, A., and Prendergast, R. A. Characteristics of an immune system common to certain external secretions. *J. Exp. Med.* 121:101, 1965.

79. *Ulcerative Colitis**

JOSEPH BARNETT KIRSNER

ULCERATIVE COLITIS IS AN ACUTE and chronic inflammatory and ulcerative disease of the colon and rectum, characterized clinically by rectal bleeding, diarrhea, abdominal discomfort, and by numerous complications [1, 2]. The disease occurs at any age from the very young to very old, but is most common in young adults and in children. The sex incidence is approximately equal, females predominating slightly. The incidence is relatively low, but the disease is not uncommon. It occurs in most ethnic groups for whom adequate information is available but appears to be more frequent among persons of Jewish origin. It apparently is found throughout the world. The disease seems uncommon in charity hospitals, but increased awareness and careful observation may reveal more cases in these circumstances. Ulcerative colitis is not infective, epidemic in occurrence or transmissable in the usual sense. Multiple family occurrences are being recognized with increasing frequency [3]. The disease develops at any time of the year; once established, it may recur more often in the fall and winter although exacerbations occur at all seasons. It often affects individuals seemingly in good health, but a history of significant emotional trauma is not unusual. Other initiating circumstances include acute respiratory infections, use of antibiotics, physical fatigue, pregnancy and operations.

THE CLINICAL DISEASE

CLINICAL MANIFESTATIONS

Besides rectal bleeding, diarrhea, and cramping abdominal pain, there are fever, malaise, anorexia, and weight loss. In mild disease, the symptoms may be limited initially to vague abdominal discomfort and slightly increased frequency of bowel movements. In acute severe colitis, the patient is seriously ill, with 20 to 30 watery bloody stools per 24 hours, dehydration, and toxemia. In chronic active ulcerative colitis, the bloody diarrhea approximates 6 to 8 bowel movements daily. Bleeding from the rectum may be the sole symptom initially. Fever, vague abdominal discomfort and weight loss may be the only or principal manifestations, especially in children.

Ulcerative colitis is a chronic disease, continuing in most patients for 5, 10, 20 years and longer [4]. Recurrences are frequent and often unpredictable. The exacerbations commonly are associated, at least chronologically, with upper respiratory and other infections, emotional disturbances, physical fatigue, dietary excesses, use of antibiotics, enemas and cathartics, surgery, and, in women, with the menses. The course varies considerably. The disease may remain mild; intermittent with decreasing severity; intermittent with increasing severity; constantly active without remission; initially severe with eventual recovery; of insidious onset, becoming fulminating; or initially fulminating, terminating fatally.

The physical findings depend on the severity of the colitis. In mild disease, the patient may appear healthy. In severe colitis, there are fever, loss of blood, dehydration and malnutrition, and signs of any of the complications which are listed later. Clubbing of the fingers may be present. The abdomen may or may not be tender diffusely, and often is distended. Rectal examination may disclose perianal irritation, hemorrhoids, and narrowing of the lumen.

DIAGNOSTIC PROCEDURES

Proctosigmoidoscopy reveals, in most patients with active disease, evidence of diffuse inflammation of the rectum and sigmoid, including hyperemia, edema, multiple tiny

* These studies were supported in part by grants (RGAM-02133) from the National Institute of Arthritis and Metabolic Diseases.

hemorrhages and ulcerations, friability of the rectal mucosa, and a sanguinopurulent fecal discharge. In about 5 percent of cases, the examination may reveal only hyperemia and mild granularity of the mucosa, with the disease primarily involving the colon proximal to the sigmoid. In chronic colitis, proctosigmoidoscopy also may disclose "pseudopolypoid" thickening of the mucosa, polyps, "epithelial bridges," the internal orifices of fistulous tracts, narrowing of the bowel lumen, and membranous strictures in the rectum. In healed colitis there may be the smooth gray appearance of an atrophic mucosa. In mild or moderately severe cases, prompt and sustained healing may be followed by apparently complete subsidence of the tissue reaction. Often, improvement in the appearance of the rectal mucosa chronologically lags behind the clinical response.

Roentgen examination facilitates recognition of the disease above the level of the sigmoid. It reveals the extent of involvement as well as the presence of complications, such as stricture and carcinoma. The colon appears to be diseased in at least 90 percent of cases. In 10 percent, almost invariably in patients with mild disease, the colon seems to be normal. In about 50 percent, the entire colon is affected. Involvement of the terminal ileum occurs in a varying proportion (5 to 15 percent). Probably, the earliest roentgenologic findings are a fine marginal serration of the mucosa of the rectum or colon, produced by the ulcerations, and decreased distensibility of the rectal ampulla. Other typical roentgenological changes are decreased to absent haustrations, smoothening, narrowing, and contraction of the colon, and an irregular polypoid appearance of the mucosa. Further findings include stricture and thickening of the colonic wall and an increase in the retrorectal soft tissue space, denoting periproctitis. The so-called "toxic megacolon" is characterized by tremendous distention of the bowel, especially the transverse portion, but it may affect any segment of the colon. The distention is the result of severe inflammation involving all layers of the bowel wall and is associated with a pericolitis.

LABORATORY FINDINGS

These reflect the severity of the colitis. The white blood count usually is normal, except in the presence of complications. The hemoglobin, red cell, and hematocrit values are decreased in proportion to the loss of blood. The sedimentation rate may be elevated, but often is normal. The feces almost invariably contain no identifiable pathogenic bacteria and parasites. Hemolytic coliform organisms are common, and alterations in the usual bacteriological patterns are related to antibacterial therapy. Infrequently, *Salmonella* organisms may be cultured, as secondary invaders; trophozoites and cysts of *Entamoeba histolytica* are noted rarely. The stools contain blood, and occult blood often persists for long periods after subsidence of the clinical symptoms. With prolonged severe diarrhea, the serum sodium and chloride levels may decrease; more often, electrolyte abnormalities are related to the use of ACTH and adrenal corticosteroids. The nitrogen balance is negative during active disease, and hypoproteinemia may be pronounced. After subsidence of the active disease, the serum protein levels return to normal, albeit slowly, and the globulin levels subsequently may exceed normal in patients with and without hepatic disease. Skin reactions are negative for tuberculosis, lymphopathia venereum, histoplasmosis and coccidioidomycosis. There are no known enzymatic defects. The serum alkaline phosphatase level often is increased, particularly in young individuals and in colitis patients with associated pericholangitis of the liver, but in other circumstances as well. Results of the usual chemical tests of hepatic function often are normal, although retention of bromsulphalein is common. Needle biopsy of the liver frequently reveals inflammation or fat in the liver, pericholangitis, or cirrhosis. Malabsorption, secondary to associated inflammation of the small intestine, is indicated by excessive excretion of fat, lowered plasma carotene levels, and decreased urinary excretion of D-xylose after oral administration. The urinary output of 5-hydroxyindole acetic acid is normal. Renal function usually is normal, although it may be impaired by recurrent infection of the urinary tract, especially pyelonephritis. Exfoliative cytologic examination of the colon demonstrates large colonic columnar cells that disappear when the active disease subsides, giant tissue macrophages containing large nuclei, and single cells with increased nuclear cytoplasmic ratios, enlarged hyperchromatic nucleoli and chromatin clumping, resembling neoplastic cells [6]. Touch cytologic preparations of the rectosigmoidal mucosa may disclose neutrophilic and eosinophilic granulocytes as well as lymphocytes and plasma cells.

COMPLICATIONS

Practically every organ and system in the body may be involved. In the colon, complications may include massive hemorrhage, toxic megacolon, strictures, pseudopolyps, carcinoma, abscesses, or fistulae. Electrolyte depletion and malabsorption usually depend on involvement of the small intestine. Systemic complications include malnutrition with anemia, hypoproteinemia, stomatitis, and stomal ulcerations. Iritis, iridocyclitis, erythema nodosum, and pyoderma gangrenosum occur in perhaps 5 percent of cases. These complications may represent phenomena of hypersensitivity or may be related to other unknown mechanisms, as may the arthritis [5], tenosynovitis, peritendinitis, spondylitis, and amyloidosis which may develop. Hypercoagulability of the blood and vascular thromboses have been reported. Pericholangitis and fatty infiltration and cirrhosis of the liver occur frequently. Degenerative and inflammatory changes in the pancreas and glomerulonephritis have been described. Retardation of growth in children, myocarditis, nephrolithiasis, drug sensitivities, peripheral neuritis, narcotic addiction, and serious emotional difficulties are other problems. Thus, although the initial and predominant manifestations of ulcerative colitis are in the colon, in its totality it is a systemic disease.

PATHOLOGY

Ulcerative colitis begins in the mucosa and submucosa of the colon and may persist there, although extension to the muscular and serosal layers is common. The anatomical changes vary with the severity and stage of the disease and with the presence or absence of complications [7, 8]. The external appearance of the colon, characterized by increased vascular markings and hyperemia, usually does not reflect completely the severity of the colitis as observed internally. In the acute form, the mucosal surface is congested, with numerous hemorrhages and erosions. The histological features include vascular congestion, edema, hemorrhage, and superficial ulceration. Polymorphonuclear leukocytes in the crypts of Lieberkühn predominate, but the cellular infiltration includes lymphocytes, plasma cells, and eosinophils. Vascular lesions, including thromboses, endarteritis or perivasculitis, are uncommon.

In the subacute form, the mucosal surface contains ulcerations and "pseudopolyps," including mucosal remnants, areas of granulation tissue with or without an overlying layer of colonic epithelium, and adenomatous polyps. The number of goblet cells is decreased. The crypts are few in number and are arranged abnormally. The highly vascular granulation tissue, infiltrated by lymphocytes, plasma cells, and eosinophils, is a prominent feature. In chronic ulcerative colitis, the wall of the colon may be thickened as a result of inflammation and edema, muscle hypertrophy, infiltration by fat, and the deposition of fibrous tissue. Usually, the colon is contracted and narrowed. The mucosa may present a hyperplastic appearance as a result of the severe inflammation. The histological features include vascular engorgement, cellular infiltration, and occasional crypt abscesses. The submucosa is thickened and fibrotic and contains dense cellular infiltrates, aggregates of lymphocytes, and variable amounts of fat.

The periodic acid–Schiff stain reveals less of the basement membranes of the epithelial cells and, with toluidine blue, metachromatic staining of the ground substance of the connective tissue. These changes disappear with subsidence of active disease. Other histochemical studies may demonstrate alterations in the normal disposition of enzymatic constituents of colon epithelial cells, such as DPN diaphorase, succinic dehydrogenase, and alkaline phosphatase. The significance of these findings is not known.

In fulminating cases, the ulcerations are extensive, and the bowel wall is thinned. There may be necrosis of blood vessels, fragmentation of the muscle layers, and disintegration of the bowel wall, with sloughing of large portions of muscosa and submucosa.

Injury and healing in the bowel proceed concurrently, so that different areas simultaneously may manifest all stages of reaction from acute inflammation to epithelial regeneration. In areas of colon adjacent to obviously diseased bowel, but appearing normal grossly, careful study may disclose focal infiltrates of polymorphonuclear leukocytes in crypts, tiny erosions and ulcerations, mild capillary dilatation, and infiltration of the lamina propria by lymphocytes and plasma cells. Epithelial regeneration occurs by the growth of a single layer of flat cuboidal cells, emerging from surviving crypts and extending over the denuded surface. Complete restitution to normal with mucosal differentiation is uncommon. Residual evidence of colitis includes an atrophic mucosa with flattened epithelium, fewer and abnormally arranged crypts of Lieberkühn, congestion, round cell infiltration of the lamina propria, granulomata with or without giant cells, and the presence of fibrous tissue and fat. The granulomata may represent "granulomatous" disease of the colon, reaction to foreign material, or a hypersensitivity reaction [9]. An apparently increased number of autonomic nerve ganglia has been observed in the wall of the colon, but their significance remains to be determined.

In proctitis, the tissue reaction, as observed at proctosigmoidoscopy, appears to be limited to the rectum. Regional or segmental colitis, as visualized by x-rays, involves portions of the bowel proximal to the rectum. Ileocolitis affects chiefly the distal portion of the small intestine, the cecum, ascending colon, and the proximal portion of the transverse colon. The histological appearance may be that of a "granulomatous" process, resembling or identical with regional enteritis, an inflammatory ulcerative process comparable to ulcerative colitis, or both.

TREATMENT

In the absence of knowledge as to the specific cause of ulcerative colitis, treatment is symptomatic, comprehensive and prolonged [10]. The objectives are physical and emotional rest, correction of nutritional deficits, control of infection, restoration of normal bowel function, and the management and prevention of complications in order to return the patient to an effective life.

Medical Therapy. A bland, nutritious diet, bed rest, especially during the acute illness, and administration of sedatives, antispasmodics in judicious amounts, and, temporarily, codeine or deodorized tincture of opium form the basis of medical therapy. Supportive measures include transfusions of blood, plasma, and albumin and the intravenous administration of electrolytes, glucose, and fluids. Antibacterial medication consists chiefly of sulfonamides, furazolidone (Furoxone), occasionally penicillin and streptomycin intramuscularly, tetracycline, chloramphenicol or paramomycin, to control existing secondary infection and perhaps to eliminate unidentified pathogenic bacteria.

Corticotropin (ACTH) and adrenal corticosteroids do not cure ulcerative colitis, and their influence on the long-term course of the disease remains to be determined. However, administered carefully, in sufficiently large amounts, they are useful adjuncts, initiating and enhancing recovery. They are indicated chiefly in severe cases unresponsive to comprehensive treatment in the hospital, in fulminating disease, and in the presence of arthritis, erythema nodosum, pyoderma gangrenosum, and iritis. They are contraindicated in the presence of perforation of the bowel, peritonitis, and abscess formation. Hemorrhage, or pericolitis, may respond dramatically to these drugs. Formation of pseudopolyps is not a contraindication, because a sustained favorable response may decrease the hyperplastic inflammatory reaction. As in other disorders, the use of ACTH and adrenal steroids may be accompanied by complications and undesirable effects; however, these can be controlled by careful observation of the patient. They usually are administered intramuscularly, and occasionally intravenously. In patients with disease limited to the rectum and sigmoid, steroids also may be given as retention enemas. Initial courses of such therapy usually are more effective than repeated courses. The steroids often are remarkably helpful in controlling severe ulcerative colitis. The mechanism of the beneficial effect is not known. It may involve suppression of an antigen-antibody interaction or nonspecific inhibition of the tissue response to inflammation.

Management also involves careful attention to the commonly observed emotional difficulties either by formal psychotherapy in conjunction with medical treatment or as supportive psychotherapy by the informed attending physician. The favorable response may reflect control of associated physiological disturbances triggered by emotional stimuli and not necessarily the elimination of etiological psychogenic mechanisms.

Surgical Treatment. Sustained, comprehensive medical management controls ulcerative colitis in 75 to 80 percent of patients. Surgical treatment is necessary in perhaps 15 or 20 percent for the following reasons: (1)

failure of medical treatment; (2) acute fulminating colitis not responding promptly to intensive therapy; and (3) uncontrollable hemorrhage, obstruction, carcinoma, extensive perianal and perineal fistula formation, and significant retardation of growth in children.

The operative procedure of choice is total colectomy and ileostomy. Partial resection of the colon may be considered for segmental colitis; abdominoperineal resection for removal of a severely diseased rectum; and subtotal colectomy, with anastomosis of the ileum to the rectum, may be considered in the occasional patient with an apparently normal rectum. Limited surgical procedures may be indicated for the management of painful hemorrhoids and perianal abscesses. Colectomy and the establishment of an ileostomy do not necessarily eliminate all problems. Ileostomy complications include bleeding, prolapse, retraction, fistula formation, perforation, stenosis, volvulus, peristomal ulceration, ulcerative enteritis with electrolyte and fluid depletion, and emotional difficulty in adjusting to the ileostomy appliance. However, the frequency and the severity of these problems are diminishing with improvements in surgical technique and in the care of the patient.

PROGNOSIS

Since ulcerative colitis tends to be a chronic, recurrent disease with many complications, the outlook for return to complete health is uncertain, although many patients are able to live normal lives. Fatalities are most common during the initial one or two years of illness. The important causes of death are perforation of the bowel and peritonitis, massive hemorrhage, carcinoma of the colon, and the problems associated with surgery, often undertaken in critical circumstances. Associated factors include electrolyte depletion, malnutrition, and vascular thromboses. In individual cases, other causes of death include hepatic disease, hepatorenal insufficiency, acute pancreatitis, and cardiovascular disease. Improved methods of controlling infection and restoring nutrition, advances in general medical care, and increased surgical skill have combined to reduce the mortality to approximately 5 percent and to diminish the invalidism of many patients. Initial observation does not always accurately reflect the subsequent course. At times, the most severely ill individual may undergo a remarkable improvement during medical treatment. The associated circumstances usually are as obscure as those surrounding the onset of the disease. The improvement may be characterized radiologically by the striking reappearance of haustrations and by increase in the length and caliber of the colon [11].

ETIOLOGICAL CONSIDERATIONS

The cause of ulcerative colitis is not known, and the possibility exists that a heterogeneous group of diseases may be involved. The many theories include bacterial (aerobic, anaerobic) and viral infections, the action of bacterial (gram-negative) endotoxins or fungi, the destructive effect of proteolytic enzymes on the bowel wall, allergy to food and pollens, abnormalities in the lymphatic and vascular circulation to the colon, including ischemia of the bowel, "abnormalities" in the connective tissue of the colon, defective regeneration of the colonic epithelium, obscure nutritional and metabolic disorders, and overactivity of the parasympathetic nervous system, related indirectly or directly to emotional disturbances [12, 13]. Although clinical evidence appears to support some of these concepts, especially those emphasizing infection and psychogenic mechanisms, the details of pathogenesis are obscure and conclusive evidence is lacking. Interest in possible contributing factors recently has been directed to fibrinolytic mechanisms, subtle vascular injury, and to a genetically determined individual vulnerability.

Efforts to reproduce ulcerative colitis in the experimental animal remain unsuccessful [14]. Abnormalities in the colon have been induced by deficiencies of vitamin A, folic acid, pyridoxine, and proteolytic enzymes including lysozyme; the administration of broad-spectrum antibiotics, analogues of folic acid, histamine, and histamine-releasers; application of Shiga toxin to colon explants; administration of *Staphylococcus* toxin; repeated injection of cholinergic drugs; and by experimentally designed "self-stimulation" of the brain in monkeys. The lesions produced are acute, superficial, and transient, disappearing with discontinuance of the noxious influence, and the experimental lesions do not resemble ulcerative colitis.

IMMUNOLOGICAL CONSIDERATIONS

The gastrointestinal tract is well endowed biologically to participate in and to generate immunological reactions [15]. Anatomically, the alimentary canal, especially the small intestine and colon, is rich in lymphoid tissue, lymphocytes, and plasma cells, potential sources of antibody. Mast cells are common throughout the digestive tract, including the colon, and are more numerous in the colon of ulcerative colitis; their products—heparin, histamine, and capillary permeability factor—have been implicated in hypersensitivity reactions. Immunologically, abundant sources of antigen are present in the digestive tract. Immunological responses to ingested antigens have been demonstrated in animals, as well as local antibody formation within the alimentary canal.*

FOOD AND POLLEN ALLERGY

Allergic reactions to foods such as milk, eggs, cheese, and wheat and to pollens and other inhalants have been implicated in the onset and recurrences of ulcerative colitis on the basis of amelioration of symptoms upon withdrawal of the allergen and recurrence following its reintroduction. However, intensification or renewal of symptoms is noted with foods on the basis of mechanical or chemical stimulation of bowel activity, and milk has been implicated in the abdominal distress of irritable colon and diverticulitis without involving immunological disorders. Hemagglutinins to proteins in cow's milk (casein, β-lactoglobulin) have been observed in patients with ulcerative colitis without a direct relationship between the titers and the activity of the disease. Since similar hemagglutinins are demonstrable in normal individuals, in children with celiac disease, chronic respiratory illnesses, and other disorders [16], the immunological significance of this observation in relation to ulcerative colitis seems questionable. The circulating antibodies to jack-bean urease similarly are difficult to evaluate. The local reaction to injections of powdered extracts of wheat, eggs, and milk into the rectal mucosa of patients with ulcerative colitis likewise does not provide an adequate explanation for the origin of the disease; the colitis mucosa also is hyperresponsive to mechanical and other stimuli [17].

CLINICAL OBSERVATIONS SUGGESTING AN IMMUNE PROCESS

The possible implication of an immunological mechanism in the pathogenesis and course of ulcerative colitis is suggested by numerous considerations [17, 18]. Hypergammaglobulinemia may be seen with the presence of autoreactive antibodies. Clinically, the frequency of the disease among young adults and children, the common personal or family history of hay fever and asthma, the multiple family occurrences of the disease, and the very occasional association of ulcerative colitis with disorders ascribed to hypersensitivity mechanisms, including arthritis, iritis, rheumatic fever, Hashimoto's disease, autoimmune hemolytic anemia, erythema nodosum, periarteritis nodosa, scleroderma, systemic lupus erythematosus (SLE), and allergic granulomatous angiitis may be listed. Lupoid hepatitis and chronic cholangitis may be seen in occasional patients. Chronic hepatic disease among young men and women may at times precede the colitis and has been linked with hypersensitivity mechanisms. The multiplicity of "disorders of connective tissue" in the occasional colitis patient suggests a systemic tissue vulnerability, possibly of immunological origin, as in a young woman with scleroderma, arthritis, febrile episodes resembling SLE and ulcerative colitis, or in a young man who successively developed rheumatic fever and heart disease, recurrent streptococcal pharyngitis, pneumonitis, ulcerative colitis, hyperglobulinemia, hepatitis, and hemolytic anemia [1, 12]. The occasional onset of ulcerative colitis in only one of many individuals simultaneously ill with an acute enteric infection may connote an individual vulnerability, perhaps genetically conditioned.

HISTOLOGICAL OBSERVATIONS SUGGESTING AN IMMUNE PROCESS

Histologically, the infiltration of the lamina propria of the colon by lymphocytes, plasma

* *Editor's comment:* It is remarkable that, despite all these factors that would seem to favor the development of hypersensitivity in the gut, relatively little of it actually occurs. Chase (*Proc. Soc. Exp. Biol. Med.* 61:257, 1946) pointed out that a potent contact sensitizer such as dinitrochlorobenzene is incapable of sensitizing animals that have been exposed to the chemical by prior feeding. The digestive tract holds some secrets from us, but Battisto and Miller are pursuing them (*Proc. Soc. Exp. Biol. Med.* 111:111, 1962).—J. H. V.

cells, and eosinophils, in addition to polymorphonuclear cells, and the disorganization of the ground substance of the connective tissue and loss of the basement membranes of the epithelial cells of the colon, although not diagnostic of immune responses, have been described in tissue reactions of known hypersensitivity origin. The granulomata and giant cells in the resected colon of some patients with ulcerative colitis also have been ascribed to immune mechanisms, but they also may reflect a "regional enteritis" of the colon. Anatomical findings of related interest include the intense necrosis that denudes the mucosa and submucosa in severe colitis and the absence of enlargement of regional lymph nodes, which contrasts with the findings usually associated with suppurative diseases of the colon.

EXPERIMENTAL HYPERSENSITIVITY REACTIONS OF THE COLON

Passive local sensitization has been accomplished in the ileum, cecum, colon, and rectum; and the Arthus and Auer reactions, as well as the Shwartzman phenomenon, have been induced in the rabbit colon [15]. In experimental systemic tuberculin reactions, presumably involving a delayed hypersensitivity response, hemorrhagic involvement of the intestine has been described [19].

The Shwartzman reaction, though nonspecific immunologically, histologically resembles the Arthus response [20, 21]. The phenomenon in the colon, as initiated with filtrates of *Serratia marcescens,* is characterized by hemorrhage, vascular thromboses, and tissue necrosis. The cellular reaction, initially polymorphonuclear in type, includes lymphocytes, plasma cells, and mononuclear cells with granulomata and giant cells appearing one to several weeks later. Similar responses in the colon can be elicited with *Escherichia coli* lipopolysaccharide and other gram-negative bacterial endotoxins, abetted by vasoconstriction with epinephrine or norepinephrine. In two patients with ulcerative colitis, the histological appearance of the colon and the kidneys was comparable to that of the Shwartzman reaction. A similar relationship has been suggested in a case of fatal diarrhea attributed to *E. coli* 0-111 B_4 in a woman with ulcerative colitis and gangrenous skin lesions, and in the dermatological complication, pyoderma gangrenosum.

The Arthus reaction may be induced by the injection of specific antigen (e.g., crystalline egg albumin) into the colon of rabbits previously sensitized to the antigen [22]. The histological findings include: cellular infiltration at the bases of the crypts and hemorrhage and necrosis of the muscularis propria; vascular thromboses and, occasionally, perivascular accumulations of eosinophils, associated with hyaline degeneration and necrosis of blood vessels; and, subsequently, the formation of granulomata.

The Auer phenomenon is based on a sequence of systemic sensitization and localization of specific antibody and reinjected antigen in the colon (facilitated by prior exposure of the bowel to a mild irritant which increases local capillary permeability). The union of specific antigen and antibody locally produces a cytotoxic reaction [23, 24]. The response in the colon is characterized grossly by hemorrhage and superficial ulcerations. The histological features include vascular congestion, edema, infiltration by polymorphonuclear leukocytes, lymphocytes, plasma cells, monocytes, and eosinophils, occasional perivascular infiltrates, and dilatation of lymphatics and blood vessels. Concentration of specific antigen and antibody, respectively, in the tissue reaction can be demonstrated immunohistochemically [25]. The antigen often is visible in perivascular areas of edematous submucosa, especially in areas of cellular infiltration adjacent to dilated blood vessels and lymphatics, by fluorescence techniques. Antigen also is seen among glands of the reactive mucosa, occasionally attached to mononuclear cells of the inflammatory exudate. The increased tissue globulins (presumably antibody) are localized in the same areas as the specific antigen.

These experimental immune reactions in the colon do not reproduce human ulcerative colitis, and their occurrence does not necessarily relate the disease to an Arthus, Auer, or Shwartzman phenomenon. The significance of their occurrence consists in establishing the capacity of the colon to participate in hypersensitivity reactions.

AUTOIMMUNE POSSIBILITIES

A priori, no obvious explanation exists for the development of autoantigenicity in the normal colon of man. According to current concepts, autoimmune reactions might develop in ulcerative colitis: (1) without alteration in the biological characteristics of colon tissue, by an acquired abnormality or excessive response of the antibody-producing cells; (2) as a consequence of genetically induced defects in immunological homeostasis, facilitating increased responsiveness to multiple immunological stimuli, as has been postulated in SLE, or (3) from the "spilling" into the circulation of tissue antigens ordinarily inaccessible to the sites of antibody formation and hence stimulation by antigens to which immunological tolerance may never have been established. There is no conclusive evidence of the operation of any one of these mechanisms in ulcerative colitis; other possibilities may exist. Antigenicity of colon tissue would seem more likely to result from a change in its structure, perhaps by an antecedent unrecognized bacterial or viral infection or by unidentified metabolic, physical, chemical, or enzymatic influences.

DIRECT IMMUNOLOGICAL OBSERVATIONS

The presence of a circulating globulin with affinity for leukocyte nuclei has been interpreted as reflecting an altered immunological state in ulcerative colitis; and the finding of similar antinuclear factors in the sera of relatives of patients with ulcerative colitis has suggested a genetic component in the presumed immunological vulnerability to the disease. Antinuclear globulins also have been noted in the sera of patients with regional enteritis. However, the precise immunological significance of antinuclear factors awaits clarification, and the presence of antithyroid and rheumatoid factors in the blood relatives of colitis patients raises the possibility of nonspecific phenomena. Normal levels of serum complement have been reported, and negative complement fixation against normal fetal colon and ulcerative colitis colon has been interpreted to mean that complement plays no important role in the pathogenesis of the disease.

Hemagglutinins, presumably antibodies, to antigenic constituents in normal colon and ulcerative colitis colon are demonstrable in the sera of many patients with ulcerative colitis. Broberger and Perlmann [26] employed a phenolic extract of human fetal colon obtained at autopsy. Sheep cells coated with this extract gave hemagglutination reactions with sera from 28 of 30 children with ulcerative colitis; positive results (lower titers) were obtained in a smaller proportion of adult patients. The reaction could be inhibited by prior absorption of the colitis serum with extracts of colon and also with extracts of liver or kidney. Colon antigens also were obtained from sterile juvenile and adult colon by extraction with phenol and water at 65° C. Broberger and Perlmann also demonstrated colon antibodies in microsomal fractions of extracts of regional colonic lymph nodes from 2 children with ulcerative colitis, but not in extracts from ileal lymph nodes from the same patients.

Bregman and Kirsner [27], utilizing sterile saline extracts of mucosal scrapings from the colon in ulcerative colitis or of colon from patients with other diseases of the bowel (carcinoma, polyps) and tanned human erythrocytes coated with these extracts, also observed positive hemagglutination reactions with the sera from many patients with ulcerative colitis. Positive reactions were noted very occasionally with sera from patients with abnormal serum proteins, e.g., SLE, hepatic and hematological diseases, or rheumatoid arthritis, but not with sera of normal individuals. Nonspecific reactions occurred with extracts of whole colon. The anticolon mucosa hemagglutinin titers were low and were not correlated consistently with the severity of the disease, the presence of systemic complication, or with the use of corticotropin or adrenal corticosteroids in therapy. These hemagglutination reactions also could be eliminated by prior absorption of the colitis serum with saline extracts of normal colon or colitis colon mucosa, but not with extracts of other human organs.

In gel diffusion experiments, Broberger and Perlmann reported positive reactions with 22 of 30 colitis sera when tested with phenol-water extracts of fetal colon; 4 sera also gave precipitates with extracts from liver and 6 sera with extracts from kidney. Immunoelectrophoresis of the patients' sera revealed that the precipitation reactions were due to γ-globulins. Similar results were obtained with saline extracts of lymphatic glands, apparently containing colon antibody. Bregman and Kirsner also noted positive agar gel precipitations between ulcerative colitis serum and saline extracts of ulcerative colitis colon mucosa, and of colon obtained from premature infants, but because of the low concentrations of colon precipitins, positive results were less frequent than in the hemagglutination tests. Positive reactions were not observed when normal human serum was utilized.

Immunological studies in ulcerative colitis utilizing extracts of adult colon are of limited value because of the possible involvement of bacterial antigens in the reactions. The absence of viable bacteria in aerobic and anaerobic cultures of the adult colon tissue extracts employed, and the preparation of satisfactory colon antigens from colons of premature infants presumably uncontaminated by microorganisms, suggest no direct role for bacteria in the positive reactions. Absorption of colitis sera with several bacterial suspensions (*Spherophorus necrophorus, Proteus vulgaris, E. coli*) did not alter the positive reactions, and hemagglutination tests with extracts of these bacteria and ulcerative colitis sera were negative. Broberger and Perlmann also found no cross-reactivity between their colon antigen and its antibodies, on one hand, and a number of bacterial lipopolysaccharides, on the other.

Other investigators have utilized phenol-water extracts of human fetal colon mucosa, colon from patients with ulcerative colitis or colonic carcinoma, saline extracts of whole normal colon obtained at autopsy, and resected ulcerative colitis colon from adults or from children with colitis dying of other causes. Negative results have been reported with the hemagglutination, collodion particle, agar gel precipitation, and complement fixation techniques [17]. The divergent findings presumably reflect technical problems inherent in the methodology.

IMMUNOFLUORESCENCE STUDIES

In 3 of 10 children with ulcerative colitis studied by Broberger and Perlmann [28], positive hemagglutinations correlated with immunofluorescent staining of the cytoplasm of normal colon mucosal epithelial cells by conjugated serum or γ-globulin. Fluoresceinated serum prepared from patients with rheumatoid arthritis also stained sections of human colon, but localization of the stainable antigens apparently differed from that noted with ulcerative colitis sera, and differences also were demonstrated by absorption and cross-inhibition experiments. Six of 15 colitis sera reacted positively, with staining of the cytoplasm, when tested by the indirect immunofluorescence method utilizing conjugates of sheep antihuman γ-globulin.

Koffler *et al.* [29], using the indirect immunofluorescence technique, demonstrated in the sera of 6 of 31 patients with ulcerative colitis a γ-globulin factor binding with cytoplasm of the epithelial cells in normal adult human colon after pretreatment with ulcerative colitis sera and then exposure to fluoresceinated rabbit antihuman γ-globulin. Autoantibodies were found in the sera of 3 of 4 patients from whom tissues for testing were available. Hepatic bile ductules and ileum contained an antigen reacting similarly to the polysaccharide antigen of the colonic mucosa, and a similar polysaccharide antigen was observed to react with serum globulins of patients with hepatic disease. The failure to demonstrate similar antibodies in granulomatous disease of the ileum and colon indicated that acute and chronic inflammation per se did not account for the reaction. The presence of a similar antigen in fetal colon suggested that bacteria did not provide a significant part of the antigenic substrate. In addition, occasional small foci of γ-globulin-containing plasma cells were distributed in the mucosa and submucosa. These cells were particularly abundant in tissue sections of active ulcerative colitis and regional ileitis. The demonstration of complement (β_{1C}-globulin), in association with fibrinogen and γ-globulin, in the inflammatory cells in 2 of 12 ulcerative colitis tissues and in 3 of 10 regional enteritis tissues was interpreted as evidence of local, potentially cytotoxic antigen-antibody complexes. Klavins [30] by a similar indirect immunofluorescence method utilizing horse antihuman γ-globulin, also demonstrated cytoplasmic staining of the colonic mucosal cells in 4 of 11 patients with ulcerative colitis. Fluorescence also was observed in occasional round cells in the lamina propria.

Other investigators have reported negative results with the indirect immunofluorescence technique, utilizing the sera of adult patients with ulcerative colitis and sections of freshly frozen human colonic mucosa. Recent direct and indirect fluorescence antibody studies in our laboratory, involving careful control of the fluorescein : protein ratio and related technical modifications, have failed to demonstrate the specificity of the fluorescence observed occasionally in colonic epithelial cell cytoplasm. Fluorescence commonly is limited to the cellular infiltrate of the lamina propria and submucosa [31]. Some green fluorescence is associated with leukocytes and eosinophil granules; and there also appears to be fluorescence associated with the cytoplasm and immediately adjacent areas of lymphocytes and plasma cells. The significance of these observations is being studied further. Since some of this cellular fluorescence pattern is not obtained with conjugated globulins from normal individuals, and since the amount and degree of the pericellular fluorescence are less in tissues from normal individuals than in tissues from patients with ulcerative colitis, the possibility arises that the fluorescence represents either antigen or antigen-antibody complexes in the process of phagocytosis. Antigen-antibody complexes also have been shown to be chemotactic for polymorphonuclear leukocytes as well as eosinophils. We also have obtained immunofluorescent evidence to support the interpretation of increased numbers of antibody-producing cells in ulcerative colitis tissue.

COLON ANTIGENS

Several types of colon extracts have been employed in immunological studies of ulcerative colitis. Broberger and Perlmann utilized an extract of normal human fetal colon with phenol-water at 65° C., containing mostly lipopolysaccharides. In extracts of colon mucosa prepared with slightly acid saline, modified Krebs buffer, or phosphate buffer, Bregman and Kirsner demonstrated apparently similar antigenic components containing proteins, lipoproteins, free amino acids, and some polysaccharide. An antigen chemically associated with an acid mucopolysaccharide, specific for gastrointestinal mucosa but common to all parts of the digestive tract, has been demonstrated by the injection into rabbits of microsomal material prepared from normal human colon mucosal scrapings. Similar antigenic material also has been demonstrated in the intestines of sheep, cattle, dogs, and rats, but not of rodents. Immunofluorescence studies revealed the antigen in the goblet cells of the small intestine and epithelial cells of the colon. The many substances with varying antigenic activities extracted from colon tissue reflect the complexity of the potential immunological systems of the colon [17]. More precise definition of the immunological reactivity of colon mucosa probably will necessitate study of individual constituents of colon tissue, such as may be obtained from the epithelial cells, separated individually or in clones, and grown in tissue culture. Such a method would perhaps obviate the technological problem presented by the intestinal bacterial flora.

SIGNIFICANCE OF CIRCULATING COLON ANTIBODIES

The presence of circulating antibodies to constituents of colon mucosa (saline-extractable and phenol water-extractable cytoplasmic constituents) in patients with ulcerative colitis does not necessarily establish an etiological role for the antibodies [32]. Even if the cytotoxicity of the antibodies to colon mucosa were established by *in vitro* tests, this would not necessarily establish a primary injurious effect *in vivo* on normal colon tissues. Broberger and Perlmann [33, 34] observed no demonstrable cytotoxic effects, as estimated by the release of organically bound P^{32} or C^{14} into the medium from prelabeled colon cells on exposure of fetal colon cells to fresh colitis serum, with or without the addition of normal human serum. However, exposure of cultures of colonic cells to circulating white blood cells, predominantly lymphocytes, from colitis patients apparently produced cell damage more often than did exposure to white blood cells from healthy individuals (75 vs. 40 percent). Most of the specifically released isotope was found in the phospholipid and acid-soluble fractions, suggesting that lymphoid cells can disturb the structural integrity of the surface of the epithelial cells to which they had acquired sensitivity. The reaction required complement and was inhibited by pretreatment of the colitis leukocytes with the same colon antigen as was employed in the hemagglutination test. No specific cytotoxic effect was conferred by colitis serum on normal leukocytes. The significance of this observation awaits further study in view of the need for control observations with leukocytes from patients with rheumatoid arthritis, SLE, regional enteritis, cirrhosis of the liver, and hematological disorders. The observation nevertheless focuses attention on the possible role of "hypersensitive" cells in the tissue reaction of ulcerative colitis.

ATTEMPTS TO PRODUCE "IMMUNE COLITIS" EXPERIMENTALLY

The unequivocal production of an "immune ulcerative colitis" with animal antisera to colon tissue has not been accomplished [17, 18]. Negative results have been obtained with rabbit antisera to normal dog and rabbit colon, to dog colon previously altered by systemic injections of methacholine, to normal and chemically irritated guinea pig colon, and to rat colon mixed with Freund's complete adjuvant or with sodium alginate; or by the injection of extracts of gastrointestinal tissues. Hemorrhages and ulcerations were noted in the colon of guinea pigs given rabbit antisera to guinea pig colon, after prior rectal instillation of dilute formalin. However, similar changes appeared occasionally in the small intestine and in control animals given injections of antikidney serum or nonimmune serum. In another study, antiserum to dog colon prepared by the injection of saline extracts of sterilized, homogenized colon mucosa into rabbits and ducks was injected into dogs after partial colectomy, done in the hope of intensifying the anticipated antigen-antibody interaction in the colon. However, the tissue changes seemed relatively mild and apparently did not include the presence of plasma cells, eosinophils, or perivascular infiltrates. A similar experiment involved the administration of antidog colon serum produced in response to injection into rabbits of extracts of dog colon and Freund's adjuvant. Since Freund's adjuvant apparently alters the antibody response, and since the injection of Freund's adjuvant alone may produce pathological changes in tissues, the observations are difficult to evaluate. The experiments have failed to provide conclusive evidence of the presence of antibodies specific for the colonic epithelium in the antisera or of their exclusive localization in the exact sites of the tissue reaction. Studies involving the injection of heterologous antisera require elaborate controls, including the injection of normal animal serum, absorbed anticolon antiserum, antiserum to colonic epithelium from other species, antiserum to homologous organs or tissues, and Freund's adjuvant alone. The production of significant lesions in the residual colon of an animal given injections of an antiserum to its own colon, absorbed with homologous tissue to remove species-specific reactants, if it were readily reproducible and correlated with immunohistochemical localization of both specific antigen and antibody, would constitute valid evidence of the experimental production of an autoimmune reaction in the colon. This has not been achieved.

The resemblance of the homograft reaction to other cell-bound hypersensitivity phenomena provides another interesting approach to the study of immune phenomena involving the bowel [17]. The runting syndrome complicating the transplantation of immunologically competent cells in the mouse is characterized by the occurrence of diarrhea and inflammatory and degenerative changes in the small bowel in addition to hemolytic anemia, leukopenia, thrombocytopenia, splenomegaly, weight loss, and alopecia. Noteworthy findings in the ileum include atrophy, clubbing and bridging of villi, and an appearance suggestive of colitis mucosa. A possible immunological basis for the intestinal lesions is under investigation.

EVALUATION OF AVAILABLE IMMUNOLOGIC INFORMATION

The evidence clearly demonstrates the capacity of the colon to participate in local immunological reactions. The combination of specific exogenous antigen and antibody within the bowel produces an inflammatory tissue reaction, recognizable morphologically and identifiable immunohistochemically. However, the lesions do not resemble ulcerative colitis. Truly ulcerative colitis has not been produced by immunological approaches or, indeed, by other techniques. The clinical and laboratory information suggesting the participation of immune phenomena in ulcerative colitis is nevertheless persuasive. Hemagglutination and precipitin tests, less often immunoelectrophoresis and other immunological methods, appear to indicate a spectrum of circulating reactants, presumably antibodies, directed against components of colonic epithelium in the serum of many patients with ulcerative colitis. The antibodies are present in low concentration, and their titers do not parallel closely the severity of the disease. Most studies have been with homologous colon tissue, since this material is most readily available. Autologous antibodies also have been demonstrated with colon tissue and serum from the same patient. There is no conclusive evidence that the demonstrated colon antibodies are of primary importance in the pathogenesis of ulcerative colitis. They may represent a secondary immunological response to existing nonimmunological cellular injury of the colon. An immune process developing secondarily may nevertheless contribute to the tissue reaction of ulcerative colitis and to its chronicity. The localization of antibody globulin in colitis colon likewise does not necessarily establish its participation in the pathogenesis of ulcerative colitis, since the attachment of globulin to colon tissue may occur not only by binding to specific antigen but also nonspecifically. The possible involvement of an immune process mediated by cell-bound antigen-antibody complexes, as in delayed hypersensitivity reactions, is suggested by the studies on the effect of "hypersensitive" lymphocytes upon colon tissue *in vitro*.

Available data are still insufficient to answer several fundamental questions about immune phenomena in ulcerative colitis: Is the normal colon in man autoantigenic? Is colon antigenicity induced by the incorporation of bacteria or their metabolic products or constituents into colon tissues? Pertinent further studies might include the identification of specific colon antigens and antibodies, possibly by utilizing clones of colonic epithelial cells, study of the role of "hypersensitive" cells (lymphocytes, plasma cells, mononuclear cells) in the tissue reaction; biochemical studies of normal and diseased colon tissues, and further attempts at experimental reproduction of the disease by immunological techniques, guided by stringent criteria for the evaluation of immunological phenomena. In the investigation of an autoimmune basis for ulcerative colitis, certain criteria, adapted by us from Witebsky [35] and others, may be useful guides: (1) the direct demonstration of circulating colon antibodies or perhaps antigen-antibody complexes that are active at body temperature, at the onset or early stage of the disease; (2) identification of the specific antigen or antigens in normal or diseased colon; (3) production of antibodies against the same antigen in experimental animals; (4) production of pathological changes, similar to those of the human disease, in the colon of actively sensitized animals given injections of antiserum against the specific colon antigen, or perhaps antigen-antibody complexes; (5) demonstration of absence of similar changes with antisera against species-specific tissue constituents other than from colon; (6) demonstration of autoantigen, autoantibody, and perhaps antigen-antibody complexes in ulcerative colitis colon tissue; (7) possibly, transfer of the disease by the use of immunologically competent cells, and perhaps (8) effective treatment of ulcerative colitis with compounds suppressing or eliminating immune phenomena or the specific antigen-antibody interaction. Although available evidence is inadequate to establish an immune or autoimmune mechanism for ulcerative colitis, it is sufficient to justify continued investigation of the problem.

REFERENCES

1. Kirsner, J. B. Ulcerative colitis: Observations on its etiology, course, and management. *Postgrad. Med.* 22:132, 1957.
2. Kirsner, J. B. Ulcerative colitis: Certain clinical aspects and problems. *Gastroenterology* 40:287, 1961.
3. Kirsner, J. B., and Spencer, J. A. Family occurrences of ulcerative colitis, regional enteritis and ileocolitis. *Ann. Intern. Med.* 59:133, 1963.
4. Kirsner, J. B., Palmer, W. L., Maimon, S. N., and Ricketts, W. E. Clinical course of chronic non-specific ulcerative colitis. *J.A.M.A.* 137: 922, 1948.
5. McEwen, C., Lingg, C., Kirsner, J. B., and Spencer, J. A. Arthritis accompanying ulcerative colitis. *Amer. J. Med.* 33:923, 1962.
6. Galambos, J. T., Massey, B. W., Klayman, M. I., and Kirsner, J. B. Exfoliative cytology in chronic ulcerative colitis. *Cancer* 9:152, 1956.
7. Goldgraber, M. B., Kirsner, J. B., and Palmer, W. L. The histopathology of chronic ulcerative colitis and its pathogenetic implications. *Gastroenterology* 38:596, 1960.
8. Warren, S., and Sommers, S. C. Pathogenesis of ulcerative colitis. *Amer. J. Path.* 25:657, 1949.
9. Goldgraber, M. B., and Kirsner, J. B. Granulomatous lesions—an expression of a hypersensitive state. *Arch. Path.* 66:618, 1958.
10. Kirsner, J. B., Bicks, R. O., and Palmer, W. L. The treatment of ulcerative colitis. *Arch. Intern. Med.* 99:642, 1957.
11. Kirsner, J. B., Palmer, W. L., and Klotz, A. P. Reversibility in ulcerative colitis: Clinical and roentgenologic observations. *Radiology* 57:1, 1951.
12. Kirsner, J. B., and Palmer, W. L. Ulcerative colitis: Considerations of its etiology and treatment. *J.A.M.A.* 155:341, 1954.

13. Kirsner, J. B., *et al.* Symposium on "New Frontiers in Ulcerative Colitis." *Gastroenterology* 40(2):286, 1961.
14. Kirsner, J. B. Experimental colitis with particular reference to hypersensitivity reactions in the colon. *Gastroenterology* 40(2):307, 1961.
15. Kirsner, J. B., and Goldgraber, M. B. Hypersensitivity, autoimmunity and the digestive tract. *Gastroenterology* 38:536, 1950.
16. Peterson, R. D. A., and Good, R. A. Antibodies to cow's milk proteins—their presence and significance. *Pediatrics* 31:209, 1963.
17. Kirsner, J. B., Bregman, E., Kraft, S. C., and Reilly, R. W. Immune Reactions of the Intestines with Reference to Ulcerative Colitis. In Gamble, J. R., and Wilbur, D. L. (Eds.), *Current Concepts of Clinical Gastroenterology.* Boston: Little, Brown, 1965.
18. Kirsner, J. B. Immunologic considerations in ulcerative colitis. *Surg. Clin. N. Amer.* 42:1115, 1962.
19. Crowle, A. J. *Delayed Hypersensitivity in Health and Disease.* Springfield, Ill.: Charles C Thomas, Publisher, 1962.
20. Goldgraber, M. B., and Kirsner, J. B. The Shwartzman phenomenon in the colon of rabbits: A serial histological study. *Arch. Path.* 68:539, 1959.
21. Patterson, M., Terrell, J. C., II, Waldron, R. L., and O'Bryan, B. C. The Shwartzman phenomenon in the colon of rabbits: The effects of epinephrine, norepinephrine, and mecholyl *Amer. J. Dig. Dis.* 8:213, 1963.
22. Goldgraber, M. B., and Kirsner, J. B. The Arthus phenomenon in the colon of rabbits. *Arch. Path.* 68:556, 1959.
23. Kirsner, J. B., and Elchlepp, J. The production of an experimental ulcerative "colitis" in rabbits. *Trans. Assoc. Amer. Physicians* 102: 102, 1957.
24. Callahan, W. S., Goldman, R. G., and Vial, A. B. The Auer phenomenon in colon-sensitized mice. *J. Surg. Res.* 3:395, 1963.
25. Kraft, S. C., Fitch, F. W., and Kirsner, J. B. Histologic and immunohistochemical features of the Auer colitis in rabbits. *Amer. J. Path.* 43:913, 1963.
26. Broberger, O., and Perlmann, P. Autoantibodies in human ulcerative colitis. *J. Exp. Med.* 110:657, 1959.
27. Bregman, E., and Kirsner, J. B. Immunologic studies in ulcerative colitis (to be published)
28. Broberger, O., and Perlmann, P. Demonstration of an epithelial antigen in colon of man by fluorescent antibodies from children with ulcerative colitis. *J. Exp. Med.* 115:13, 1962.
29. Koffler, D., Minkowitz, S., Rothman, W., and Garloch, J. Immunocytochemical studies of ulcerative colitis and regional enteritis. *Amer. J. Path.* 41:733, 1962.
30. Klavins, J. V. Cytoplasm of colonic mucosal cells as site of antigen in ulcerative colitis. *J.A.M.A.* 183:547, 1963.
31. Kraft, S. C., and Kirsner, J. B. Immunohistochemical studies in ulcerative colitis. *Gastroenterology* 46:329, 1964.
32. Kraft, S. C., Bregman, E., and Kirsner, J. B. Criteria for evaluating autoimmune phenomena in gastrointestinal disease. *Gastroenterology* 43:337, 1962.
33. (*a*) Broberger, O., and Perlmann, P. *In vitro* studies of ulcerative colitis: I. Reactions of patients' serum with human fetal colon cells in tissue culture. *J. Exp. Med.* 117:705, 1963. (*b*) Perlmann, P., and Broberger, O. II. Cytotoxic actions of white blood cells from patients on human fetal colon cells. *Ibid.*, p. 717.
34. Perlmann, P., and Broberger, O. The Possible Role of Immune Mechanisms in Tissue Damage in Ulcerative Colitis. In P. Grabar and P. Miescher (Eds.), *Mechanism of Cell and Tissue Damage Produced by Immune Reactions.* Basel: Benno Schwabe & Co. 1962. P. 288.
35. Witebsky, E. The question of self-recognition by the host and problems of autoantibodies and their specificity. *Cancer Res.* 21:1216, 1961.

80. *Adrenalitis; Aspermatogenesis, Orchitis, and Infertility*

EUGENE V. BARNETT AND JOHN P. LEDDY

ADRENALITIS

In 1958, Colover and Glynn [1] reported round cell invasion of the adrenal cortex and adrenal necrosis in guinea pigs following immunization with homologous adrenal in Freund's complete adjuvant. In 1960, Steiner *et al.* [2] reported similar results in guinea pigs, but in rabbits immunized with homologous adrenal in adjuvants, they obtained no adrenal damage. In 1962, Witebsky and Milgrom [3] obtained antibody in hemiadrenalectomized rabbits after immunization with autologous adrenal in Freund's adjuvant. They also obtained complement-fixing antibodies in guinea pigs directed against guinea pig adrenal following immunization with homologous adrenal in Freund's adjuvant, but they were unable to confirm the earlier reports of induction of adrenalitis. In the same year, Barnett *et al.* [4] found that rabbits immunized with homologous and heterologous adrenal homogenates in complete adjuvant responded with autoantibody primarily directed against adrenal. The antibody was detected in complement fixation tests and was shown to react with cytoplasm of adrenal cortex and with ovarian and testicular cells, as detected by the immunofluorescence test. Histological evidence of adrenalitis was present only in those rabbits immunized with heterologous adrenals.* Guinea pigs immunized with heterologous adrenal homogenate developed more extensive adrenal infiltrates than did guinea pigs immunized with homologous adrenal. Antibody from guinea pigs immunized with heterologous adrenals reacted with autologous as well as heterologous adrenals. Skin tests with homologous adrenal revealed no evidence of delayed type hypersensitivity in either the guinea pig or the rabbit. There have been no reports of passive transfer experiments in animals that would incriminate the serological entities in the induction of adrenalitis.

Adrenal insufficiency in man, described by Addison in 1855, is characterized by asthenia, weight loss, pigmentation of the skin and mucous membranes, and gastrointestinal disorders. It is almost invariably associated with complete destruction of both adrenal glands. In 1957, Anderson *et al.* [5] detected complement-fixing antibodies with adrenal and thyroid extract in 2 of 10 patients with Addison's disease. They detected no complement-fixing antibody to adrenals in 2 cases of Simmond's disease, 12 cases of thyrotoxicosis, 17 cases of Hashimoto's disease, or in 54 controls. In 1962, Mead [6] reported on a patient with a histological diagnosis of Hashimoto's thyroiditis and adrenocortical insufficiency. The patient's serum was shown to contain complement-fixing antibody reactive with crude adrenal and thyroid extracts but not with extracts of kidney, pancreas, or liver. Blizzard *et al.* [7], using an indirect immunofluorescence technique, detected antibodies to adrenal in 16 of 30 patients with Addison's disease. They also detected adrenal antibodies in 4 of 18 patients with idiopathic hypoparathyroidism. Four of their patients with Addison's disease and detectable adrenal antibodies also had idiopathic hypoparathyroidism. Other reports of coexistent adrenal and parathyroid insufficiency with autoantibodies have added pernicious anemia and superficial moniliasis to the symptom complex [8]. Gass [9] pointed out the association of keratoconjunctivitis with superficial moniliasis, idiopathic hypoparathyroidism, and Addison's disease, but he made no antibody studies. Blizzard *et al.* [7] detected no adrenal anti-

* *Editor's comment:* It must be noted that the inflammation was highly focal, sparing the vast majority of the cortex.—J. H. V.

bodies in 15 patients with viralizing adrenal hyperplasia or Cushing's syndrome. Seven Addisonian patients with adrenal antibodies also had thyroid antibodies, an association pointed out previously by both Anderson and Mead. The Addison's disease was idiopathic in all (see also Ref. 8). Anderson suggested that adrenal atrophy, with or without round cell invasion, might have an autoimmune etiology. Irvine's data [10] suggest that adrenal insufficiency due to tuberculosis is not associated with adrenal antibodies. There have been no reports in man, however, correlating the histopathology of the adrenal with the presence of adrenal antibodies.

ASPERMATOGENESIS, ORCHITIS, AND INFERTILITY

Immunization of guinea pigs (or rats) with homologous or autologous testis or spermatozoa incorporated in Freund's complete adjuvant is capable of inducing progressive degeneration of the germinal cells of the seminiferous tubules, culminating in aspermatogenesis [11–15]. The earliest degenerative changes appear 8 to 14 days after immunization. In most studies [12–14], testicular inflammation is described as conspicuously sparse or absent, suggesting that the germinal cell damage is not secondary to an inflammatory reaction. Waksman [15], however, has particularly emphasized focal perivenous accumulations of lymphocytes and histiocytes in the epididymis, rete testis, and seminiferous tubules and on this basis has argued for mediation of the lesion by inflammatory cells. In Waksman's study, none of the affected animals exhibited "clinical" signs of testicular inflammation.

Complement-fixing, immobilizing, and skin-sensitizing antibodies against sperm or testis have regularly been demonstrated in the sera of affected animals [12–14, 16]. The appearance and titer of these antibodies, however, did not correlate consistently with the severity and progress of the testicular lesions. Attempts to transfer the disorder to normal animals with homologous serum containing antibodies have uniformly failed. Positive delayed-type skin reactions to testicular extracts or sperm are regularly, but not invariably [14], apparent shortly before and during the development of the histological changes. Accordingly, the pathological process has been regarded by some workers [12, 15] as one mediated by the delayed or "cellular" mechanism of autoimmunity. This view has been challenged [14], however, particularly on the grounds that "cellular" immunity ought to show the appropriate cellular response. Attempts to transfer the process to normal animals with the lymphoid cells of affected animals have not been reported.

As with most experimental inductions of autoimmunity, the use of mycobacteria in the immunizations has generally been essential for the production of tissue lesions (and of delayed hypersensitivity). Immunization in *incomplete* adjuvant leads to antibody formation without tissue damage [12–14]; indeed, such circulating antibodies were found to protect against subsequent induction of testicular lesions by immunization in *complete* adjuvant [14].* Because of the seemingly "unphysiological" nature of adjuvants, it is of considerable theoretical interest that similar, although milder, germinal cell degeneration has been produced in guinea pigs by repeated intradermal injections of minute quantities of testicular homogenate alone [17]. The critical antigen(s) capable of inducing aspermatogenesis is apparently shared to some extent by brain, but not by other organs or by heterologous sperm [12–14]. The process thus appears to possess a high degree of organ and species specificity. Some progress has been made in localizing and characterizing the inducing antigen(s) [12, 18, 19]. Without further immunization, gradual recovery has been observed in some animals followed a year or more [14].

Spermatogenesis is known to be sensitive to a variety of chemical or physical stresses, e.g., regional injection of adjuvant alone [12], subcutaneous turpentine abscess [15], and intercurrent infection [15]. As Bishop *et al.* [16] pointed out, unraveling of the mechanism responsible for this experimental disease demands a clear separation of such nonspecific factors from specific (immunological) responses.

The relevance of the foregoing experimental findings to human disease is still unclear. Since the observations of Landsteiner, Metchnikoff, and Metalnikoff at the turn of the century, spermatozoa have been known to be

* For another example of the protective effect of circulating antibody, see Chapter 71.

autoantigenic without adjuvants, suggesting that sperm may carry "cloistered" antigens to which immunological tolerance is poorly developed. In clinical studies, agglutinins against homologous sperm have been described in the sera or seminal plasma of 3 of 150 [20] and 67 of 2,015 [21] infertile men, some of whom had aspermia or oligospermia. In the latter series, one third of the "positive" patients exhibited autoagglutination of living sperm in their semen. Sperm agglutinins were not found in the sera of 416 fertile men [21]. In some cases, the agglutinins were eluted from agglutinated sperm and their activity demonstrated against homologous or autologous sperm [21]. Red cells, leukocytes, and platelets were not agglutinated. Several writers considered that such sperm agglutinins might arise after escape of sperm or related testicular antigens into the circulation consequent upon obstruction of seminal ducts, infection, local surgery, or other trauma. Seventeen patients with sperm agglutinins underwent testicular biopsy; 15 specimens were normal [21], emphasizing that in man, as in experimental animals, antibodies to sperm do not necessarily lead to testicular pathology. In patients with histologically normal seminiferous tubules and, therefore, presumably some capacity to produce sperm, the presence of sperm agglutinins in their seminal plasma might well be conceived to prejudice the individual's fertility, particularly since agglutinated sperm may be unable to penetrate cervical mucus [20, 21]. The available serological evidence, however, suggests "autoimmune" mechanisms in only a minority of cases of male infertility.

The clinical problem of idiopathic germinal cell aplasia [22], on the other hand, clearly deserves further study, as Waksman [15] has pointed out. Occasional patients with "nonspecific" granulomatous orchitis have been reported to have sperm agglutinins in their serum [23]. Certain features of mumps orchitis have focused the attention of immunologists on the problem: (1) difficulties in isolating virus from inflamed testis, (2) the characteristic delay between the parotitis and the onset of orchitis, and (3) certain histological similarities to the adjuvant model in animals [15]. Serological evidence of autoimmunization in mumps orchitis has been scant, however.

Finally, turning to isoimmunity, the idea that certain women may fail to conceive because of antibodies to their husband's sperm has been lent uneven support by animal experiments. Furthermore, it is not corroborated by convincing evidence in human subjects. Serum agglutinins against standard donor sperm have been reported in a small percentage of infertile women [24], but a sufficient number of positive reactions were encountered in fertile control women to make interpretation difficult. In this connection, the association of blood group A and B substances with human spermatozoa [25, 26], whether an intrinsic property or acquired by adsorption from seminal fluid, may deserve consideration.

REFERENCES

1. Colover, J., and Glynn, L. E. Experimental iso-immune adrenalitis. *J. Immun.* 2:172, 1958.
2. Steiner, J. W., Langer, B., Schatz, D. L., and Volpe, R. Experimental immunologic adrenal injury: A response to injections of autologous and homologous adrenal antigens in adjuvant. *J. Exp. Med.* 112:187, 1960.
3. Witebsky, E., and Milgrom, F. Immunological studies on adrenal glands: II. Immunization with adrenals of the same species. *J. Immun.* 5:67, 1962.
4. Barnett, E. V., Dumonde, D. C., and Glynn, L. E. Induction of autoimmunity to adrenal gland, *J. Immun.* 6:382, 1963.
5. Anderson, J. R., Goudie, R. B., Gray, K. G., and Timbury, G. C. Auto antibodies in Addison's disease. *Lancet* 1:1123, 1957.
6. Mead, R. K. Autoimmune Addison's disease: Report of a possible case. *New Eng. J. Med.* 266:583, 1962.
7. Blizzard, R. M., Chandler, R. W., Kyle, M. A., and Hung, W. Adrenal antibodies in Addison's disease. *Lancet* 2:901, 1962.
8. Hung, W., Migeon, C. J., and Parrott, R. H. A possible autoimmune basis for Addison's disease in three siblings, one with idiopathic hypoparathyroidism, pernicious anemia and superficial moniliasis. *New Eng. J. Med.* 269: 658, 1963.
9. Gass, J. D. M. The syndrome of keratoconjunctivitis, superficial moniliasis, idiopathic hypoparathyroidism and Addison's disease. *Amer. J. Ophthal.* 54:660, 1962.
10. Irvine, W. J. A clinical and immunological study of adrenal insufficiency. *J. Endocr.* 26: 32, 1963.

11. Voisin, G., DeLaunay, A., and Barber, M. Sur les lésions testiculaires provoquées chez le cobaye par iso- et auto-sensibilisation. *Ann. Inst. Pasteur* (Paris) 81:48, 1951; Sur les lésions testiculaires observées chez des animaux soumis à des injections de substances adjuvantes seules ou mélangées avec des extraits de tissus homologues. *Ibid.* 89:307, 1955.
12. Freund, J., Lipton, M. M., and Thompson, G. E. Aspermatogenesis in the guinea pig induced by testicular tissue and adjuvants. *J. Exp. Med.* 97:711, 1953; Impairment of spermatogenesis in rat after cutaneous injection of testicular suspension with complete adjuvants. *Proc. Soc. Exp. Biol. Med.* 87:408, 1954; Aspermatogenesis, anaphylaxis and cutaneous sensitization induced in the guinea pig by homologous testicular extract. *J. Exp. Med.* 101:591, 1955.
13. Katsh, S., and Bishop, D. W. The effects of homologous testicular and brain and heterologous testicular homogenates combined with adjuvant upon the testes of guinea pigs. *J. Embryol. Exp. Morph.* 6:94, 1958.
14. Brown, P. C., Glynn, L. E., and Holborow, E. J. The pathogenesis of experimental allergic orchitis in guinea pigs. *J. Path. Bact.* 86:505, 1963.
15. Waksman, B. H. A histologic study of the auto-allergic testis lesion in the guinea pig. *J. Exp. Med.* 109:311, 1959.
16. Bishop, D. W., Narbaitz, R., and Lessof, M. Induced aspermatogenesis in adult guinea pigs injected with testicular antigen and adjuvant in neonatal stages. *Devel. Biol.* 3:444, 1961.
17. Bishop, D. W. Aspermatogenesis induced by testicular antigen uncombined with adjuvant. *Proc. Soc. Exp. Biol. Med.* 107:116, 1961.
18. Katsh, S. Localization and identification of antispermatogenic factor in guinea pig testicles. *Int. Arch. Allerg.* 16:241, 1960.
19. Katsh, S., and Katsh, G. F. Antigenicity of spermatozoa. *Fertil. Steril.* 12:522, 1961.
20. Wilson, L. Sperm agglutinins in human semen and blood. *Proc. Soc. Exp. Biol. Med.* 85:652, 1954; Sperm agglutination due to antibodies: A new cause of sterility. *Fertil. Steril.* 7:262, 1956.
21. Rumpke, P., and Hellings, G. Autoantibodies against spermatozoa in sterile men. *Amer. J. Clin. Path.* 32:357, 1959.
22. Howard, R. P., Sniffen, R. C., Simmons, F. A., and Albright, F. Testicular deficiency: A clinical and pathologic study. *J. Clin. Endocr.* 10:121, 1950.
23. Cruickshank, B., and Stuart-Smith, D. Orchitis associated with sperm-agglutinating antibodies. *Lancet* 1:708, 1959.
24. Nakabayashi, N. T., Tyler, E. T., and Tyler, A. Immunologic aspects of human sterility. *Fertil. Steril.* 12:544, 1961.
25. Landsteiner, K., and Levine, P. On group specific substances in human spermatozoa. *J. Immun.* 12:415, 1926.
26. Gulbring, B. Investigation on the occurrence of blood group antigens in spermatozoa from man, and serological demonstration of the segregation of characters. *Acta Med. Scand.* 159:169, 1957.

81. *Myasthenia Gravis**

KERMIT E. OSSERMAN AND ARTHUR J. L. STRAUSS

MYASTHENIA GRAVIS IS A DISORDER characterized by fatigability and abnormally rapid exhaustion, with loss of strength in the muscles under voluntary control. There is a return of strength, at least in part, after a period of rest [1]. The etiology is still unknown. In the past twenty-five years, clinical, pharmacological, and experimental neurophysiological evidence has established the essential defects in neuromuscular transmission in myasthenia gravis [2, 3].

The precise nature of biochemical or morphological defect remains to be clarified, although altered responsiveness of myasthenic patients to anticholinesterase medications and curare is well established. The neuromuscular defect is now postulated to be one of three: (1) diminished acetylcholine production; (2) increased cholinesterase activity at the motor endplate; and (3) a dual mechanism with alteration of endplate properties [1]. Most studies indicate that the functional defect at the neuromuscular junction is postsynaptic [2, 3]. There is some indication that there may also be a presynaptic derangement, suggested by the experiments of Desmedt [4] using a hemicholinium base. His observation indicates that inhibition of acetylcholine release from presynaptic sites recapitulates the electrophysiological events seen in myasthenia gravis more satisfactorily than does curare. Dahlbäck *et al.* [5] suggest that, in the skeletal muscles not clinically involved, acetylcholine synthesis or release may be impaired in the presynaptic region and thereby precede any changes in the motor endplate. Anatomical changes have been described in terminal motor neuroarborizations and in motor endplates of myasthenic muscle [6, 7]. Electron microscope studies of the neuromuscular apparatus are of a preliminary nature, and no certain inference can be drawn from them in favor of either a pre- or a postsynaptic change [8, 9].

Since 1956, observations have been reported concerning immunological abnormalities associated with the disease. A few authors have hypothesized an autoimmune etiology or pathogenesis, based on the character and progression of clinical symptomatology and changes in serum hemolytic complement activity which correlate with remission and exacerbations of this syndrome [10, 43]. More recently, Burnet [13] and others have commented on the well-known association of thymic hyperplasia or thymoma with myasthenia gravis. They have suggested an immunopathological function of the thymus. The subject is reviewed by Miller *et al.* [14]. Functional connections, if indeed there are such, between a neuromuscular defect, immune concomitants, and thymic pathology in myasthenia gravis are not known. A review of these three areas of interest, together with an introductory description of clinical manifestations of the disease, can serve to delineate gaps in our understanding and suggest a direction and form for future research into the etiology and pathogenesis of this condition.

CLINICAL ASPECTS

The first clinical description of myasthenia gravis is attributed to Sir Thomas Willis [15] who, in 1672, recognized the chief symptoms of asthenia of voluntary muscle with recovery after rest. It was over two hundred years before this syndrome was again referred to in the medical literature. In 1877, Samuel Wilks [16], an English physician at Guy's Hospital, London, reported a case with symptoms suggestive of myasthenia gravis. Autopsy revealed a medulla oblongata "quite healthy to the naked eye and the microscope discovered no manifest change in the tissue." Jolly [17], in 1895, was first to use the name "myasthenia

* This publication conforms to the regulations of the U.S. Department of Health, Education and Welfare and the U.S. Public Health Service governing *nonofficial* publications by their employees.

gravis pseudo-paralytica" to describe this syndrome and noted in his first two patients that when muscles were stimulated repeatedly by faradic current, the reaction of asthenia was promptly demonstrated by a recorded tracing. This is the so-called myasthenic reaction or Jolly test that led the way, in part, to further electrophysiological study of neuromuscular junction function. In 1901, Laquer and Weigert [18] reported the first case of thymoma in a myasthenic patient. Currently, involvement of the thymus is reported to be frequent, either as hyperplasia (65 percent) or as thymoma (15 percent) [19, 20].

Any striated muscular group may be affected. Usually, symptoms are multiple: ptosis, diplopia, myasthenic facies, dysarthria, difficulty in chewing, dysphagia, weakness of neck and jaw muscles, respiratory weakness, and weakness of extremities, including a waddling gait. Not all of these need be present in a given patient; in fact, there may be only one symptom. In a study of more than 650 myasthenics, one is impressed by several forms of the clinical syndrome. The classification given below, based on many variables such as sex, age of onset, localization or spread of symptomatology, and prognosis, has been helpful to us in assessing the effects of treatment [1], but it is recognized that certain of the groups may overlap or evolve one into another.

Clinical Classification [1]

Pediatric

Neonatal: Transient neonatal myasthenia occurs in infants born of myasthenic mothers. It is characterized by masklike facies, inability to cry or suck, extremity weakness, absence of Moro's reflex and brisk response to administration of anticholinesterase drugs. Permanent and complete remission always occurs no later than the sixth week of life and may occur as early as the third day. The etiological factor is possibly some substance transported across the placenta from mother to child.

Juvenile: Unlike those of the neonatal type, these children are born of *non*myasthenic mothers and have a permanent form of the disease. The condition may be present at birth or appear at any time to the age of puberty. There may be more than one myasthenia patient in a family: sisters, brothers, and cousins have been reported. Ophthalmoplegia, complete or partial, with severe bilateral ptosis, relatively unrelieved by drug therapy, is characteristic.

Adult

Group I: This is a localized nonprogressive form with perhaps only one eye affected. Occasional patients are resistant to drug therapy. Prognosis is excellent.

Group II: This is generalized myasthenia of gradual onset involving more than one group of striated muscles, both bulbar and skeletal. It may remain static for long periods. Spontaneous remission or exacerbation may occur early or late. Symptoms are usually amenable to drug treatment, and prognosis is fairly good.

Group III: There is acute fulminating onset of generalized myasthenia gravis with severe bulbar manifestations. Usually the respiratory system is involved early and myasthenic crisis may develop. These patients do not respond well to drug treatment, and prognosis is very poor.

Group IV: Late, severe myasthenia may develop in patients who have had at least *two or more years* of a clinical course typical of group I or II. Prognosis is poor.

Group V: This is a descriptive category characterized by muscle atrophy. Most patients start in group II, but as early as *six months* after onset begin to show atrophy, which is not caused by disuse of their muscles. Prognosis and mortality depend on other features noted in these patients.

Table 81-1 shows the experience in a large metropolitan hospital, with data given according to our classification.

TABLE 81-1. Classification of 650 Patients[a] Seen at Mount Sinai Hospital, New York, to August, 1963

Classification	No. of Patients	%
Neonatal	12	1.8
Juvenile	63	9.7
Group I	141	21.7
II	260	40.0
III	87	13.4
IV	56	8.6
V	31	4.8
	650	100.0

[a] Males, 251; females, 399.

In the series analyzed by Schwab and Leland [21] myasthenia gravis developed in 62 percent of 202 females before age 31, but in only 27 percent of 167 males before age 30. For the females, the mode 21 percent onset age was 21 to 25 years, whereas for the males, the mode 30 percent onset was 61 years and over. Observations at The Mount Sinai Hospital, New

York, and elsewhere are in essential agreement with those of Schwab and Leland. Myasthenia gravis may occur from birth to the ninth decade of life.

DIAGNOSIS

A high degree of suspicion of myasthenia gravis is most important in the differential diagnosis of weakness. Information regarding variability of symptoms in relation to rest, activity, and the time of day is important. Physical examination may show no abnormality except localizing symptoms. It should include repetitive use of muscle groups to permit evaluation of the influence of fatigue. There are no sensory defects or reflex changes.

Responses to chemical agents have been the major accepted criteria for diagnosis. Two types of drugs are used: stimulants and depressants. Muscle weakness should respond to stimulant or reparative drugs such as edrophonium chloride (Tensilon). Two mg. should be administered intravenously, with the needle left in the vein. If there is no response, an additional 8 mg. is injected. Alternatively, 1.5 mg. of neostigmine (Prostigmin) can be given subcutaneously or 0.5 mg. intravenously, provided such testing is adequately controlled by placebo administration before the test. Onset of action of edrophonium is in 30 to 45 seconds and its duration of action 2 to 5 minutes. Onset of action of neostigmine is in 10 minutes when given subcutaneously and 1 to 2 minutes when given intravenously; duration of action is at least 1 hour. In the myasthenic, there should be an increase of muscle strength with minimal fasciculations or muscarinic side reactions.

There are two depressant or provocative drugs: curare and quinine. Use of quinine has been discontinued because there is no antidote to counteract its paralyzing action. D-Tubocurarine in dosage of 0.6 mg. per 40 lb. of body weight is diluted to 10 ml., and increments of 1, 2, 3, and 4 ml. are given every 2 minutes intravenously. Onset of action is usually within 1 minute, and duration of action is 30 minutes. The myasthenic's increased sensitivity to this drug elicits subclinical muscular weakness, which can be confirmed by ergograms or electromyography. Provocative tests are to be used only in the hospital, with proper stand-by equipment for ventilatory assistance. Mechanical and electrical tests are rarely required to establish diagnosis, but can be helpful at times.

Wide variability in age of onset of myasthenia gravis, periods of remission, constant localization of symptoms in certain areas, production of symptoms from muscle weakness without recognition of the weakness, and atypical response to medication may all confuse the examiner [22]. For example, periods of remission in myasthenia gravis may simulate those of multiple sclerosis. Isolated bulbar symptoms may suggest bulbar poliomyelitis, amyotrophic lateral sclerosis, pseudobulbar palsy, encephalitis, or multiple sclerosis. Isolated ocular symptoms are like those found in cranial neuropathies seen with diabetes, diphtheria, syphilis, certain intracranial neoplasms, and the so-called Guillain-Barré syndrome. Weakness limited to the limbs and trunk may simulate muscular dystrophy, motor neuropathies, or myotonia congenita. Almost any myasthenic symptom unaccompanied by demonstrable muscular weakness may be seen in psychoneurosis in which conversion symptoms, especially neurasthenia, may be the main feature.

Eaton and Lambert [23] have described electromyographic evidence of neuromuscular defects in amyotrophic lateral sclerosis, syringomyelia, and bronchogenic carcinoma of the oat cell type. Pharmacological response in some of these patients to edrophonium and other anticholinesterase agents resembles that seen in the true myasthenic's electromyographic recordings. Clinical symptomatology in these patients generally is distinct from that associated with classic myasthenia gravis, and they do not respond to anticholinesterase drugs as dramatically as does the true myasthenic. Other myopathies [24, 25] may sometimes be confusing. Hyperthyroid myopathy has not, in our experience, responded to edrophonium or neostigmine.

THERAPY

Jolly [17] pointed out similarities in the weakness in myasthenia gravis to that which can be induced by curare poisoning. It was 50 or more years before Mary Walker utilized this observation to administer to a patient the antidote to curare, namely, physostigmine, with a dramatic response [26]. Curare sensitivity is, however, only superficially similar in that, in curare poisoning, all voluntary muscles are involved, and there are more precise neurophysiological differences. An analogue of physostigmine, neostigmine, was soon used, first in a diagnostic test and later in tablet form for therapy [27]. Many anticholinesterases (nerve gas poisons) became available after the end of the Second World War.

Double-bond phosphorus drugs, although effective, are no longer used because of severe toxic reactions. In the mid-1950's, new quaternary ammonium anticholinesterases became available—pyridostigmine bromide (Mestinon) [28] and ambenonium chloride (Mytelase) [29]. Edrophonium has proved to have great advantage for a rapid diagnostic test [30] and also as a means of management of drug dosage [31], but it has no other value in a treatment. Now available for treatment are three quaternary ammonium compounds—neostigmine, pyridostigmine and ambenonium (Table 81-2).

Pyridostigmine is the drug of choice with which to begin treatment in the newly discovered myasthenic. This drug has the advantage of causing minimal muscarinic side reactions and therefore a more suitable therapeutic index. It tends to relieve bulbar symptoms better than neostigmine and has a slightly longer duration of action. Ambenonium is the second drug of choice. It, too, has minimal muscarinic side effects. Its earliest sign of cholinergic toxicity is headache and muscle fasciculations. One disadvantage of ambenonium is the absence of the blood-brain barrier to this agent present with neostigmine and pyridostigmine. Cholinergic toxicity may approach without the usual muscarinic early warning symptoms such as sweating, salivation, lacrimation, epigastric distress, and diarrhea that are associated with other anticholinesterase medications. Pyridostigmine in the Timespan preparation has its greatest value in nighttime usage, permitting the patient a full night's sleep without awakening for additional medication.

Many drugs have been advocated for adjuvant medication. Some are still widely employed, such as ephedrine sulfate, 25 mg., and potassium liquid supplement, approximately 30 mEq., each three times a day after meals. These adjuvants are utilized when specific anticholinesterase drugs do not afford adequate clinical response. *At best, no drug produces more than 90 percent return to normal muscle function unless the patient is fortunate enough to experience complete remission of his disease.*

It is now generally accepted that anticholinesterase drugs, when given in excess, can create muscle weakness similar to the weakness of the disease itself [1]. Two mg. of edrophonium chloride injected intravenously 1 hour after an oral dose of any quaternary ammonium salt will indicate within 30 to 60 seconds whether the antecedent oral dose was adequate, too little, or too much. If the dose was insufficient, there is pronounced improvement of muscle strength without fasciculations or muscarinic side reactions. If the dose was excessive, the patient will have increasing myasthenic symptoms, muscarinic side reactions, and muscle fasciculations. Atropine, 0.04 mg., or other belladonna derivatives can alleviate the muscarinic side effects.

With severe overdosage, cholinergic crisis may ensue [32], the respiratory muscles become involved, and breathing may stop. It

TABLE 81-2. Equivalents Used in Transferring Patients from One Drug to Another

Drug	Route		
	I. V. (mg.)	I. M. (mg.)	Oral (mg.)
Neostigmine			
Bromide	—	--	15
Methylsulfate	0.5	1.5	—
Pyridostigmine			
Bromide	2.0	2.0	60 (regular)
Bromide	2.0	2.0	180 (Timespan)
Ambenonium chloride	—	—	6

SOURCE: Osserman [1].

has been advocated that, in addition to atropine, para-amino aldoxime (PAM) will correct the cholinergic crisis [33, 34]. In the experience of The Mount Sinai Hospital Myasthenia Gravis Clinic, PAM is most effective if crisis has been caused by overdosage of alkyl phosphates. Early tracheotomy with ventilatory assistance is often necessary, whether the crisis be due to the drug treatment (cholinergic) or to the disease itself (myasthenic) [34].

The often-noted occurrence of thymic pathology in myasthenia gravis patients has led to consideration of thymectomy in treatment. In the 1930's, with progress in anesthesia for thoracotomy, Blalock performed the first thymectomy on a myasthenic patient, followed by clinical remission [35]. This led to frequent use of this procedure in many centers. After 15 years, however, there was no consensus as to the merits of thymectomy. Schwab and Leland [21], in a retrospective study at Massachusetts General Hospital, outlined their idea of the indications for thymectomy: (1) young females under 30 years of age, (2) hyperplasia of thymus without thymoma, and (3) operation within five years of onset of myasthenia.

The Mayo Clinic, in 1954, using the above criteria, reported results similar to those of the Massachusetts General Hospital [2]. In more recent years it has been felt that there is no usefulness in sex differentiation for the selection of patients with myasthenia gravis for thymectomy [36]. Keynes [37], in Great Britain, has advocated early thymectomy, almost at the onset of the disease. In the United States, we have not yet approached this attitude. Unfortunately, there are no real controls in any of the reported thymectomy series, since there has been no attempt to match patients with controls before the decision to operate; controls have been those who refused to have surgery.

An unequivocal indication for thymectomy in myasthenia gravis is the presence of thymoma. This is a potentially malignant tumor, despite the fact that it does not appear to be anaplastic histologically and does not metastasize to distant sites. It spreads by contiguity and may involve any of the organs within the thorax [36]. At the Mayo Clinic, 25 percent of the myasthenic patients with thymoma have had symptoms ameliorated by operation [38]. This is in contrast to the 60 to 70 percent improvement reported by Keynes and by Schwab and Leland from thymectomy for hyperplasia alone.

ETIOLOGY AND PATHOGENESIS

Certain clinical observations are apparent which are not explicable *solely* on the basis of the well-established concept of a neuromuscular transmission defect in myasthenia gravis: the unanswered question as to why certain muscle groups seem to be involved in some patients and not in others; the spotty distribution of symptoms; the waxing and waning of symptomatology; and the occurrence of transient, bizarre neurological findings unexplainable by lesions in the central nervous system. Harvey and Johns [39] have stated: "With increasing severity of disease there is a progressive degree of basal weakness at rest and progressive limitation in the ability of the anticholinesterase drugs to improve strength. Such observations indicate that these measures do not correct the basic defect in myasthenia gravis. . . ." Exacerbation of the disease is often seen with intercurrent infections, psychic stress, and onset of menses. Administration of adrenocorticotrophic hormone (ACTH), in early clinical trials, frequently caused exacerbation and even death in patients with generalized and severe forms of the disorder. Pregnancy in the majority of female patients tends to influence the course of the myasthenia, either improving it or making it worse.

CIRCULATING FACTORS

Historically, Walker [40] observed that ptosis could be induced in a myasthenic patient by releasing blood in an extremity which had been occluded by a tourniquet during a period of exercise. Appearance of transient neonatal myasthenia in about 20 percent of infants born of myasthenic mothers possibly points to the placental transfer of a neuromuscular inhibitor [1]. These clinical observations have suggested a possible investigative approach to the etiology and pathogenesis of myasthenia gravis: the neurophysiological effect of serum or plasma from patients *in vitro* and *in vivo*. Exchange transfusions between normal individuals and myasthenics have been attempted without relief of symptomatology in the myasthenic and, conversely, without the production of myasthenia gravis in the normal recipient. An extensive review [41] of published reports of other experimental attempts to assay for such a factor or factors suggests that the results must be deemed inconclusive; a possible exception is an unconfirmed report of Windsor [42] which appeared after this review. Nastuk *et al.* [10, 41] called attention to the fact, however, that a heat-labile serum factor in myasthenia gravis had cytolytical activity for frog sartorius muscle.

AUTOIMMUNE HYPOTHESIS

Nastuk *et al.* [10] in the United States and Simpson [43] in Great Britain simultaneously suggested that autoimmunity may play a role in myasthenia gravis. The views of Nastuk *et al.* were predicated on their neurophysiological experience in myasthenia, their observation of fluctuations in serum complement activity during remissions and exacerbations of the disease, and the finding of a muscle-binding, complement-fixing reactivity of serum globulins from some patients with myasthenia gravis [11]. Simpson based his theoretical formulation primarily on his evaluation of symptoms, signs, and pathophysiological and neuroanatomical findings in 440 patients with myasthenia gravis. The possible properties of a hypothetical inhibitor of neuromuscular transmission in this disease were considered. Simpson was careful to point out that "this [hypothesis] will probably require modification in detail but [it] has the double merit of incorporating all the clinical phenomena without exception and of suggesting completely new lines of inquiry."

While evaluating techniques for the detection of a serum-borne inhibitor of neuromuscular transmission, Nastuk *et al.* [10, 41] observed that some myasthenic sera produced cytolysis of surface fibers of teased frog sartorius muscle. The assay involved measurement of changes in muscle tension of an indirectly stimulated frog sartorius-sciatic nerve preparation immersed in diluted serum (up to 72 percent serum). Serum samples from a few myasthenic patients caused a reduction in muscle tension, and this result appeared to parallel the cytolytic activity of these sera. Sarcolemma appeared to be disrupted, fibers grew cloudy, and striational pattern, when viewed under a light microscope, was obscured. It was subsequently determined that heating of these sera to 56° C. for one hour obliterated cytolytic activity; activity could be restored to a heated sample by the addition of fresh normal serum which in itself did not possess cytolytic activity. A more extensive study showed that 44 percent of myasthenic sera and 22 percent of normal sera possessed cytolytic activity for frog sartorius muscle [10]. The relative strengths of active sera found in each group were not determined. These findings, whether significant or not in elucidating the pathogenic processes in myasthenia gravis, had heuristic value in prompting a study of hemolytic complement activity in the sera of myasthenic patients during the course of their disease [10].

Serum complement (C′) activity was determined on serial or solitary samples of serum from 68 patients with myasthenia gravis and on 32 samples from 13 normal individuals. In the normal group of samples, C′ activities showed a standard deviation from the mean of ±2 percent and maximal deviation from the mean of 19 percent.

In 46 cases of myasthenia gravis, from 2 to 14 serial C′ determinations were carried out over a timespan of 1 week to 44 months. In 22 cases, single C′ determinations were made. Serum C′ activities determined for these patients were distributed over a wide range, frequently well below or above the extremes of the control series (Fig. 81-1).

Nastuk *et al.* [10] were able, furthermore, to develop correlations between clinical course of disease and serum C′ activity in 46 of the 68 patients. Evidence of exacerbation was seen in 15 patients. Among these, the sera of 11 showed C′ activities below the normal range, 1 in the normal range, and 3 above normal. Evidence of disease remission was seen in 21 of the 46 patients. This was accompanied in 11 cases by a rise in C′ activity, which reached the supernormal range, and in 4 by no change or a drop in C′ activity. In 14 cases, there was no notable variation in disease activity over the course of the study. In 6 of these, C′ reactivities remained within the normal range and showed little variation. But in 8 cases, C′ activities were aberrant. Three patients were pregnant women, each of whom gave birth to an infant exhibiting transitory neonatal myasthenia gravis. Two of the 3 had low C′ activities, and 1, supernormal activities. The 5 other patients displayed varied

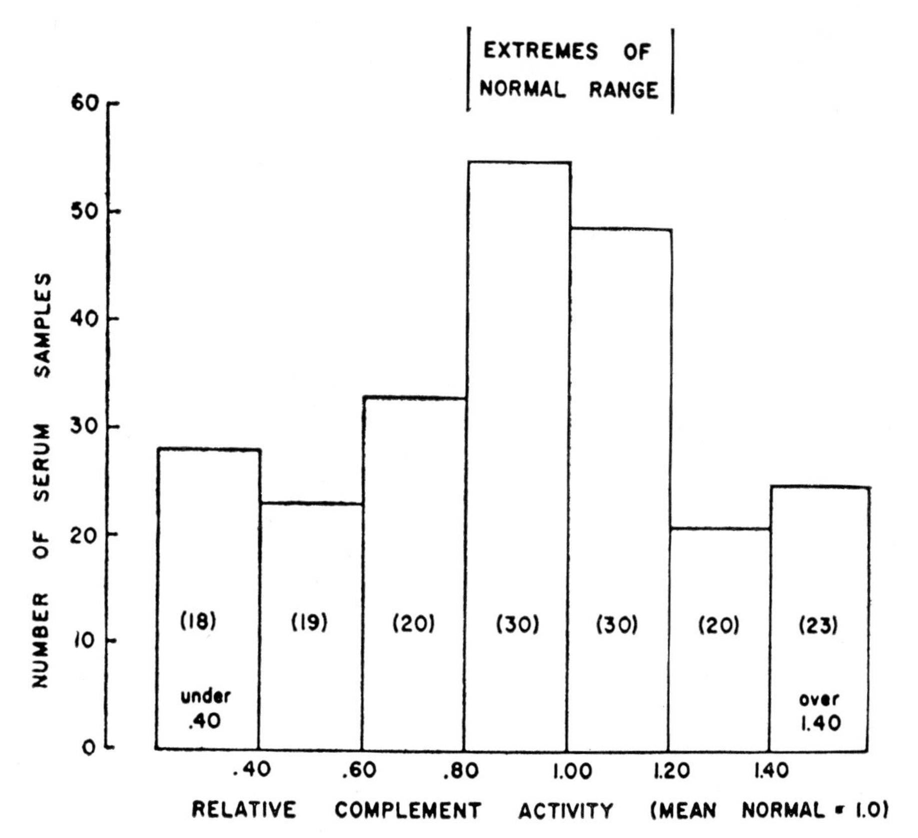

Fig. 81-1. Distribution of C′ activities in serum samples from 68 patients with myasthenia gravis. Numerals in parentheses give number of patients contributing serum samples whose C′ activities fell in the range indicated. (From Nastuk *et al.* [10], courtesy *Proc. Soc. Exp. Biol. Med.;* and Viets, H. R. (Ed.), *Second International Symposium on Myasthenia Gravis,* 1961, courtesy Charles C Thomas, Publisher, Springfield, Ill.)

trends, 1 exhibiting fairly constant but subnormal C′ activities, another varying between subnormal and normal range, another showing a marked drop into the low subnormal range during the observation period, and another a rise from a high normal to a supernormal range. In the remaining patient, C′ activities were continually in the supernormal range. Administration of anticholinesterase medications did not appear to be involved in the variation in serum C′ activity.

Nastuk *et al.* [10] emphasized that fluctuations in C′ could come about by several means; but a possible one was consumption of complement components in an autoimmune reaction between an immune serum globulin and one or more constituents of the terminal motor neuronal apparatus or skeletal muscle. Several preliminary attempts were made to detect such antibody. Agar diffusion, tanned red cell agglutination [10], and other techniques were unsuccessful [43]. In immunofluorescence, however, the globulins from pooled myasthenia gravis sera were shown by Strauss, *et al.* to stain brilliantly the alternate striations in normal or myasthenic skeletal muscle and rat skeletal muscle [11] (Fig. 81-2, *A*). Similar sections treated in the same manner with fluorescein-conjugated pool of normal human serum globulin did not stain skeletal muscle sections (Fig. 81-2, *B*). Sections of auricular appendage myocardium failed to stain, as did sections of myometrium and thymic tissue from myasthenic patients. Prior treatment of skeletal muscle sections with unconjugated myasthenic serum globulin substantially inhibited fluorescence from fluorescein-conjugated myasthenic globulin subsequently applied. Unconjugated normal serum globulins did not produce inhibition.

In view of this apparent demonstration of a muscle-binding globulin in the myasthenic globulin pool, and because of the observations of Nastuk *et al.* [10], immunohistological dem-

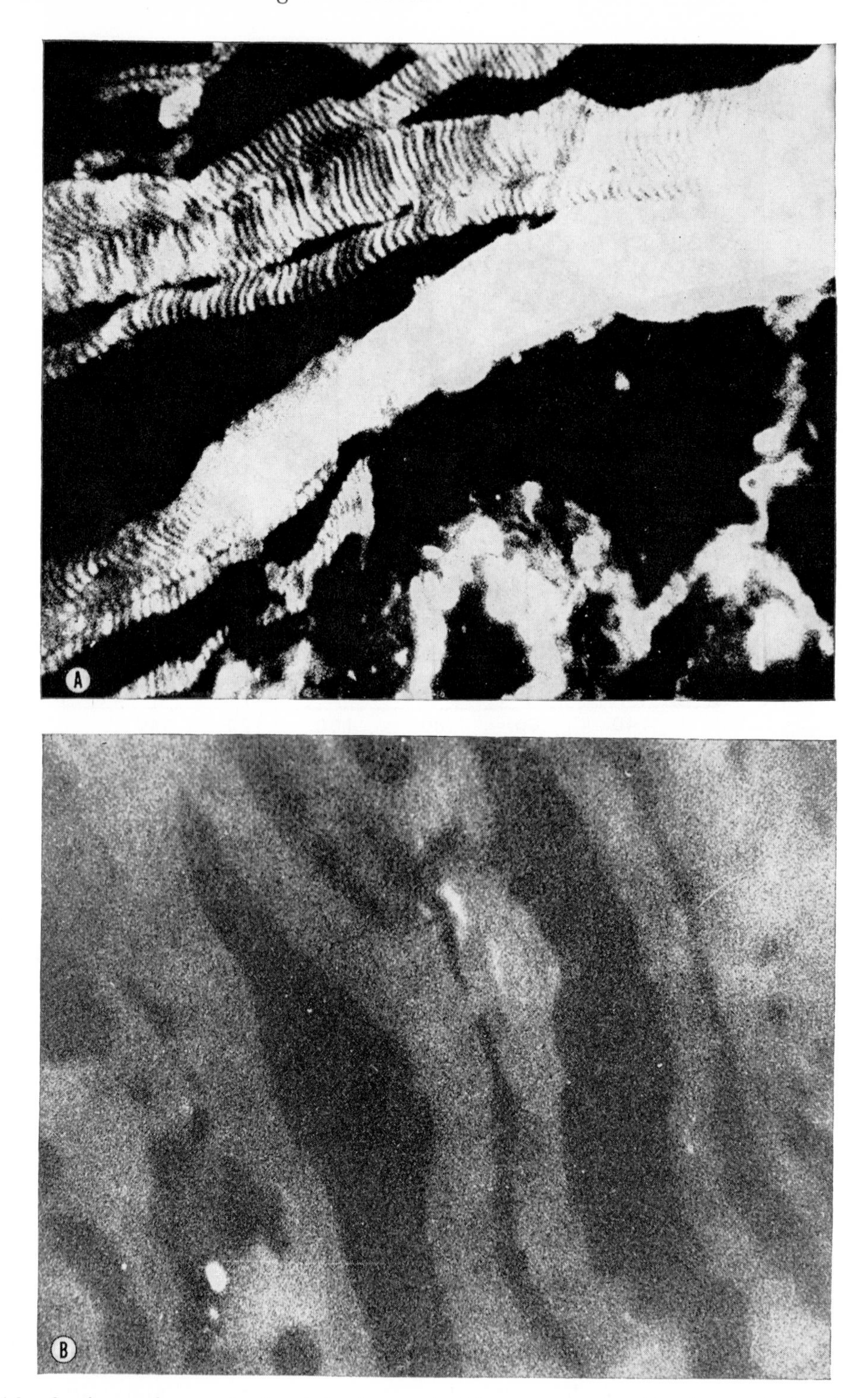

Fig. 81-2. Sections of myasthenic skeletal muscle biopsy stained with fluorescein-isothiocyanate-conjugated serum globulins from: (*A*) a pool of 10 myasthenia sera, and (*B*) a pool of 12 sera from healthy human subjects. In *A,* note alternate fluorescent striations; haziness of fluorescence in mid-diagonal fiber is due, in part, to its being out of critical focus; wavy fluorescence in lower middle field represents autofluorescence of tunica elastica of an arterial vessel. (×1,200, before 50% reduction.) (Prepared by Dr. K. C. Hsu with A. J. L. S.; courtesy of *Proc. Soc. Exp. Biol. Med.*)

onstration of complement fixation to muscle treated with myasthenic serum globulin was attempted [11]. Sections of skeletal muscle were treated successively with (1) unconjugated, undiluted whole myasthenic sera or serum globulins, (2) guinea pig serum as a source of complement, and (3) fluorescein-conjugated rabbit antiguinea pig complement. As with the direct procedure, fluorescence was noted in alternate skeletal muscle striations. Sera were deliberately selected for study from 10 patients with generalized progressive, or exacerbating, disease who also had evidence of thymic pathology and who had had the disease for less than three years. Eight fixed complement by the immunohistochemical criterion. None of 11 normal sera similarly studied fixed complement. Serum from 1 patient with paroxysmal myoglobinuria also fixed complement in alternate striations, while the serum from 1 patient with acute dermatomyositis appeared to fix complement to sarcolemma. Later, 100 randomly selected myasthenic sera were examined, together with an equal number of normal controls. Thirty-five of the 100 myasthenic sera fixed complement [44], all to alternate skeletal muscle striations. None of the normal samples fixed complement.

Beutner *et al.* [12] and Feltkamp *et al.* [45] have studied reactivity of myasthenic sera for alternate skeletal muscle striations by means of an indirect immunofluorescence technique for detection of γ-globulin binding: successive application of the patient's serum in varying dilutions [12], or undiluted [45], and then fluorescein-conjugated antihuman γ-globulins to skeletal muscle sections. This technique is far less cumbersome than either direct conjugation of the patients' sera or the complement-staining technique, particularly when large numbers of sera are to be examined. In subsequent experience with the indirect technique we noted binding of normal serum γ-globulin to skeletal muscle in many instances. This reactivity is less intense than that seen with positive myasthenic sera; it is diluted out at titers from 1 : 10 to 1 : 30 and is noncomplement fixing.* We have titered muscle-binding activity of many myasthenic sera by the indirect technique to 1 : 1,920, 1 : 3,840, or more, and to 1 : 256,000 in one instance. Minimal binding by undiluted normal sera, noted by us, appears to support the findings of Feltkamp *et al.* [45], and Nastuk and Kessler [45a] that some individual normal human globulin samples, *undiluted* and *directly* conjugated with fluorescein isothiocyanate, also adhered to skeletal muscle striations.†

The precise morphological localization of binding by myasthenic serum globulins to skeletal muscle striations has been studied [46]. Comparison of dark-field fluorescence, positive phase contrast, and polarized light photomicrographs of identical fields indicated that fluorescence was localized to the lateral portions of the A-band (Fig. 81-3, *A–C*). Dr. W. K. Engel of the National Institute of Neurological Diseases and Blindness subsequently examined some of our preparations and sometimes noted fluorescence within the Z-line; this observation was also made by Nastuk and Kessler [45a] (Fig. 81-3, *D* and *E*). Lateral portions of skeletal muscle A-bands have been characterized [47] by a concurrence of myosin and actin filaments with connecting cross bridges. These regions are rich in myosin adenosinetriphosphatase activity [48]. The characterization of the Z-line is less certain. Grob and Namba [49] and Lang and Shulman [50] have reported attempts to characterize muscle antigens which react with myasthenic sera. What relation their preparations bear to the morphologically localized reactants that are demonstrated by immunofluorescence techniques does not seem to be clear.

In the study by Beutner *et al.* [12], 10 myasthenic sera and suitable controls were examined for reactivity with skeletal muscle and cardiac muscle by the direct, indirect, and complement-staining immunofluorescence techniques. Two of the 10 sera (from patients with thymoma) displayed strong reactivity for

* Normal sera, as noted earlier, were not reactive, even when studied undiluted with the complement-staining immunofluorescence technique.

† *Editor's comment:* This capacity of undiluted normal serum to stain cross-striations in indirect immunofluorescence has been the source of much confusion. Neither the specificity of the normal serum reaction nor what class of immunoglobulin mediates it has been adequately worked out. It seems possible that the difference between normal serum and serum of myasthenia gravis is quantitative rather than qualitative. It seems to me that this area deserves more investigative attention.—J. H. V.

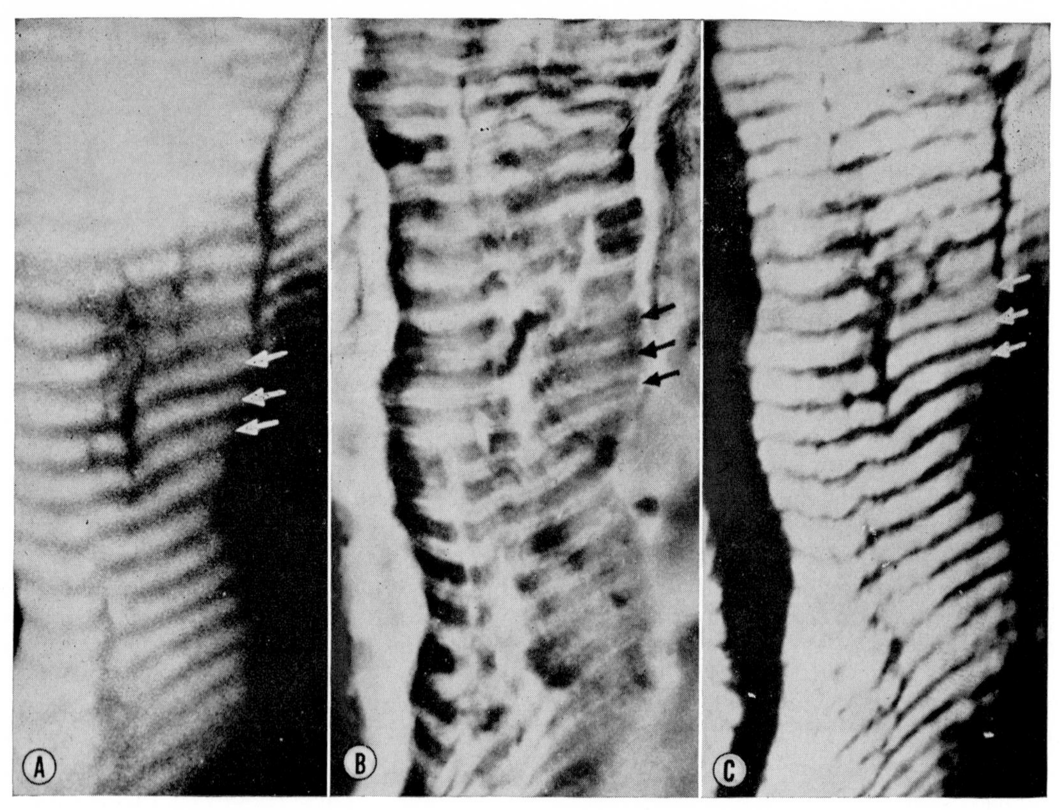

Fig. 81-3. (*A*) immunofluorescence, (*B*) positive phase contrast, and (*C*) polarized light views of an identical section from myasthenic skeletal muscle biopsy treated with fluorescein-isothiocyanate-conjugated myasthenic serum globulins. Arrows in each point to identical A-band regions. Resolution of immunofluorescence photomicrograph (*A*) is insufficient to reveal nonfluorescent central portions of A-bands (H-zones); see *D* for this detail. (×2,400, before 40% reduction.) (Prepared by Dr. A. Deitch with A. J. L. S.) (*D*) Immunofluorescence and (*E*) positive phase contrast views of rabbit skeletal muscle myofibrils stained with fluorescein-isothiocyanate-conjugated myasthenic serum globulins, illustrating localization of the globulins in lateral portions of the wide muscle A-bands and in narrow Z-lines. (×1,200) (Courtesy Drs. H. Kessler and W. L. Nastuk.)

alternate striations in skeletal muscle by all three procedures, whereas the remaining 8 showed either low, questionable, or no reactivity. Among 32 control sera, 3 gave questionable reactions (2 were from patients with muscular dystrophy). Beutner *et al.* demonstrated reactivity between a patient's serum and muscle *in vitro* and cited this as evidence of the autoantibody nature of the globulin;* they also confirmed that this reactivity of myasthenic serum was attributable to the γ-globulins. They further distinguished two types of serum reactivity for muscle tissue: complement-fixing reactivity exclusive for skeletal muscle (S), and noncomplement-fixing serum reactivity for both skeletal muscle and heart muscle (SH). Selective absorption of the noncomplement-fixing reactivity (SH) with a saline-insoluble fraction of heart muscle could be accomplished, leaving complement-fixing reactivity for skeletal muscle (S) [51, 51a]. Both serum reactivities could be demonstrated with dog, rat, duck, turtle, and frog muscle, as well as with human and monkey muscle. Beutner *et al.* [51] also described *in vivo* localized γ-globulins in biopsies of clinically affected muscle.

A tanned cell hemagglutination test for the demonstration of antimuscle activity in myasthenic serums has been reported by Djanian *et al.* [52]. It was their impression that the major activity demonstrated by this technique

* Although Strauss *et al.* [11] studied autologous skeletal muscle and serum, they made no explicit claim that the reactions observed were of an autoimmune nature.

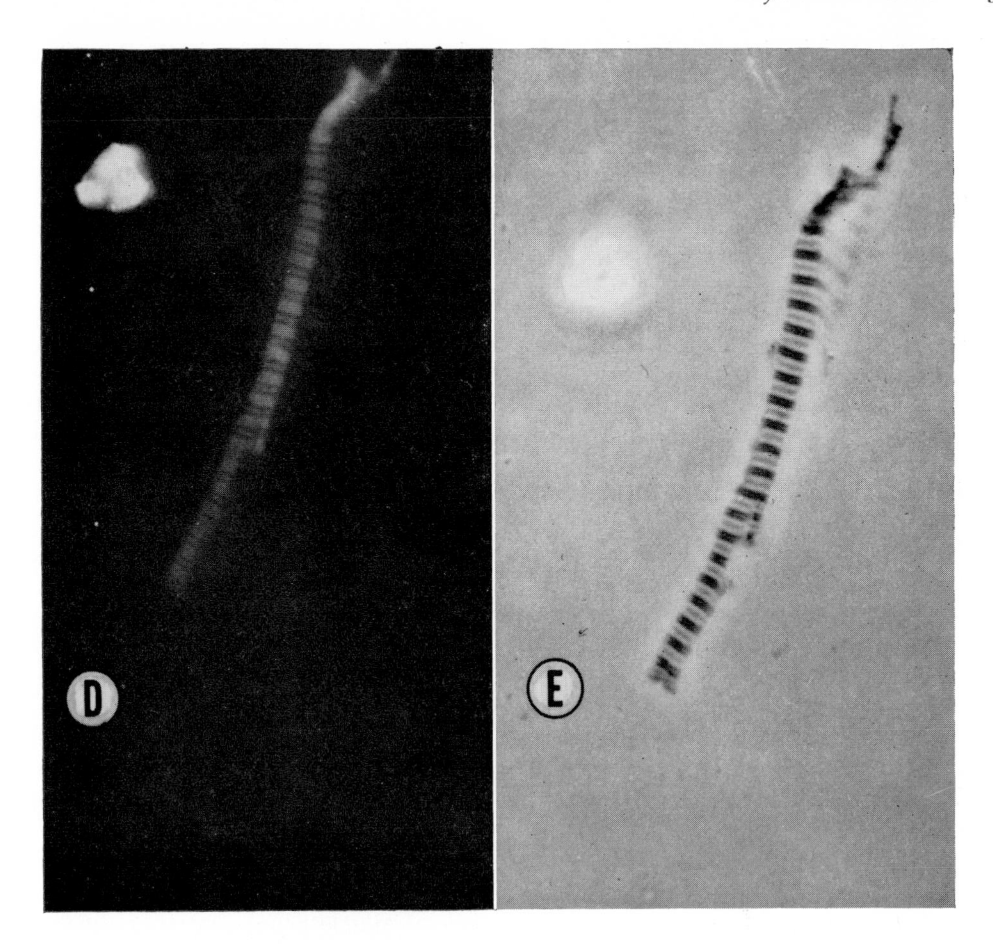

corresponds to the SH antibody-antigen system described by Beutner *et al.* [12, 51].

Hess *et al.* [53] have reported evidence of the binding of fluorescein-conjugated serum γ-globulins from a patient with myasthenia gravis to the sarcolemmal region of isologous skeletal muscle. There was no reaction between fluorescein-conjugated normal γ-globulins and myasthenic muscle. In one patient, in whom studies were performed at one-year intervals, the staining reaction was reported to have been much more intense at the time of exacerbation of the disease.

Feltkamp *et al.* [45] have studied γ-globulin binding to rat diaphragm skeletal muscle. The *undiluted* sera of 111 patients with myasthenia gravis were examined. In 20, prominent fluorescent staining of cross-striations was seen. In 15, the staining was less striking. Three sera produced striking fluorescence of the sarcolemmal region; 4 did so less intensely. Two myasthenic sera produced a so-called "zebra" pattern, with only approximately one-half the muscle fibers in longitudinal sections showing fluorescence. Sera from 20 normal individuals showed no fluorescence.*

Antinuclear reactivity in myasthenic sera, demonstrated by indirect immunofluorescence, was first reported in 6 of 16 patients by White and Marshall [54], by Beutner *et al.* [12] in several of 10 patients, subsequently in 15 of 44 patients by Sturgill *et al.* [55], and in 15 of 111 patients by Feltkamp *et al.* [45]. The possible relationship to antinuclear factors seen in sera from patients with systemic lupus erythematosus, Sjögren's syndrome, and rheumatoid arthritis has not been determined. Sturgill *et al.* [55] have shown, however, that 9 of the 15 myasthenic sera with antinuclear reactivity also reacted with thermally denatured desoxyribonucleic acid on bentonite particles, as did 23 of 35 lupus sera tested.

* Van der Geld (Feltkamp's coauthor) contends that minimal binding produced by undiluted normal sera in the indirect immunofluorescence technique can be eliminated by extensive washing of sections with buffer heated to 37° C. Binding of myasthenic serum reactivity is unaffected by the procedure.

Antinuclear reactivity in myasthenic sera has rarely been found by Strauss *et al.* [56] to exceed a titer of 1 : 30 or 1 : 60, whereas titers of 1 : 240, 1 : 480, 1 : 960, and 1 : 1920 are quite common in systemic lupus erythematosus sera. In one instance, we have observed a sustained titer of antinuclear reactivity of 1 : 240 in a female patient with myasthenia gravis, before and for one year after thymectomy. Interestingly, this patient's serum never, during our study, demonstrated reactivity with skeletal muscle striations. In another patient with thymoma and antimuscle activity in a titer of 1 : 960, we have demonstrated antinuclear reactivity in a titer of 1 : 480; this patient is also reported to have antibody to thyroid protein [56a].

Grob and Namba [49] have described complement-fixing reactivity in sera from 29 of 51 myasthenic patients for a ribonucleoprotein-rich fraction of skeletal muscle precipitated by D-tubocurarine or 1.2 to 2.4 M ammonium sulfate. This reactivity was not encountered with 201 sera from various patients without myasthenia gravis, nor with 75 normal controls. Some reactivity occurred, however, with 1 of 3 sera from patients with muscular dystrophy, 2 of 3 with polyarteritis, 1 of 3 with myositis, 1 of 4 with scleroderma, 1 of 9 with systemic lupus erythematosus, and 2 of 3 with ulcerative colitis. The reactive material in positive myasthenic sera was shown to be in the 7S γ-globulins. These investigators believe that the appearance of this reactivity in myasthenia gravis was probably secondary to degenerative changes in muscle rather than the cause of impaired muscle function, because it had also occurred in sera from patients with other diseases involving skeletal muscle and smooth muscle.

Van der Geld *et al.* [57, 58] have employed the anti-γ-globulin consumption test (AGCT) to study reactivities of myasthenia gravis sera for skeletal muscle and thymus. In this procedure, binding of γ-globulins by the tissues is detected by a reduction of the amount of *anti*-human γ-globulin in a horse or rabbit immune serum after the immune serum is exposed to the tissue. The antigens used for the test were lyophilized human skeletal muscle, heart muscle, thymus, thyroid, pancreas, and kidney. The result was positive with the sera from 38 patients with myasthenia gravis, and negative in 60. Reactions were seen only with muscle or, in 2 cases, with thymus as well. Cross-absorption experiments established two types of reactivities, one with both skeletal muscle and thymus, and the other with skeletal muscle only. Eight of the myasthenic patients had associated thymomas; all 8 had serum reactivity against skeletal muscle.

The same sera were studied by indirect immunofluorescence against rat skeletal muscle. Forty-five were positive, 27 of which had also been positive in the AGCT. In the same series, antithyroid reactivity was demonstrable in 36 or 111 sera, antinuclear reactivity in 11, and rheumatoid factor in 5. Ten percent of the patients with myasthenia gravis also had thyroid lesions, type(s) unspecified. Five had rheumatoid arthritis. These investigators concluded that: "1. Patients whose myasthenia was associated with a thymoma had a higher incidence of anti-muscle antibodies, and their clinical condition was more severe. 2. Patients with ocular myasthenia only had a lower incidence of anti-muscle antibodies. 3. Anti-muscle and anti-thymus antibodies were demonstrable."

Nastuk and Kessler [45a] studied the reactivity of myasthenic serum globulins for skeletal muscle before and after thymectomy. A fall in muscle-binding activity was noted with some patients after thymectomy. This took place over many months. Similar findings have been noted by van der Geld and Oosterhuis [57] and by Osserman and Weiner [59]. Unfortunately, possible "natural" fluctuations in muscle-binding activity have not been wholly excluded in these studies, neither by a serial study before thymectomy nor in a serial study of nonthymectomized myasthenic patients.

Hess *et al.* [53] noted binding of myasthenic serum γ-globulins to sections removed from a myasthenic patient's thymoma. The binding occurred with cytoplasm of cells in scattered areas of a lymphoepithelioma [59a].

Van der Geld *et al.* [60] have described reactivity of myasthenic sera, by indirect immunofluorescence, for cytoplasm of scattered groups of large (epithelial?) cells in bovine thymus. Van der Geld and Strauss have also observed the same serum reactivity with similar-appearing cells of fetal human thymus.* It has been noted only in sera which also display reactivity for skeletal muscle; it has occurred in sera from virtually all patients with associated thymoma (Fig. 81-4, *A* and *B*).

SPECIFICITY STUDIES

Strauss, van der Geld *et al.* [56] have randomly examined in coded fashion the sera from 1,139 individuals with assorted diseases and healthy controls, by indirect immunofluorescence technique, for reactivity against skeletal muscle and thymus. The series included sera of 129 healthy individuals, 336 myasthenia gravis patients, and 674 patients with inflammatory myopathies, endocrinopathic myopathies, carcinomatous myopathies, muscular dystrophies, heredofamilial neuromuscular disorders, demyelinating diseases, systemic lupus erythematosus, rheumatoid arthritis, dermatomyositis, scleroderma, Sjögren's syndrome, Hashimoto's thyroiditis, and thymomas unassociated with myasthenia gravis. Muscle-binding reactivity in titers of 1 : 60 through 1 : 1,920 or greater were encountered only in sera from 99 patients with myasthenia gravis (about 30 percent), in serum from one healthy individual, and from one patient with thymoma and an associated aregenerative anemia. Many

* Strauss *et al.* [56] have recently examined surgically removed thymomas and thymic hyperplasias from myasthenic patients. Interestingly, thymic epithelial cells, though present on hematoxylin-eosin preparations, have *not* reacted by immunofluorescence with the regularity encountered with calf thymus and human fetal material. Does this reflect an antigenic change in the abnormal organ?

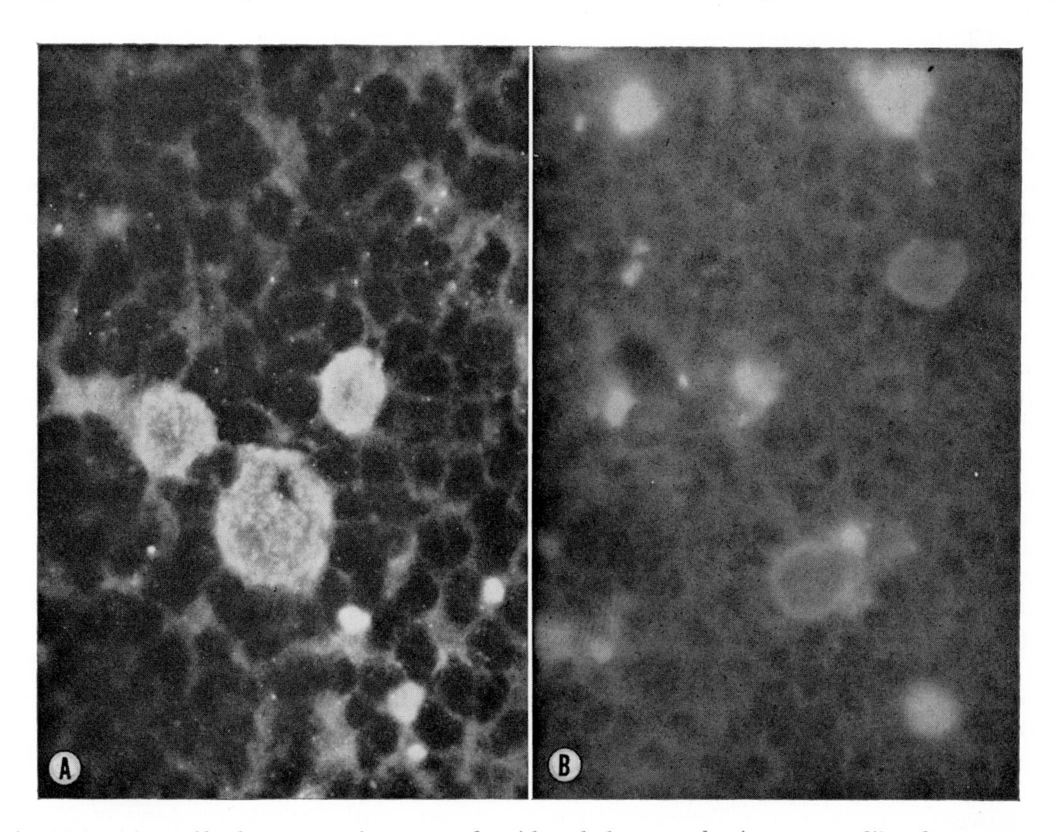

Fig. 81-4. (*A*) Calf thymus section treated with whole *myasthenic* serum, diluted 1 : 60, and fluorescein-isothiocyanate-conjugated rabbit antihuman γ-globulin (specific). Apple-green fluorescence is confined to the cytoplasm of the three large (epithelial?) cells in center of field. Smaller fluorescent areas are white, blue-white, or pale yellow and represent autofluorescent granules in other cell types. (*B*) Calf thymus section successively treated with whole *normal* serum, diluted 1 : 60, and fluorescein-conjugated-rabbit antihuman γ-globulin (specific). Two large (epithelial?) cells, devoid of immunofluorescence, are seen to right of center. White and blue-white granules, of autofluorescent character, are seen in other, small cell types. (× 1,000, before 40% reduction.) (Prepared by Dr. H. van der Geld with A. J. L. S.)

normal and disease control sera manifested reactivity of low intensity for skeletal muscle striations in titers up to 1 : 30.* This was no more common in the disease control group than in the normal control group. Reactivity for skeletal muscle striations in myasthenia gravis sera was universally associated with reactivity for large thymic cells. Reactivity for thymic cells has been observed only in myasthenia gravis sera and only in those showing reactivity with skeletal muscle striations. Sera from 19 of 20 patients with myasthenia gravis and thymoma were reactive. As van der Geld *et al.* [60] reported, reactivity for both skeletal muscle and thymus could be absorbed with sediments or lyophilized powders of striated muscle but not with similar preparations from other tissues. This has been confirmed with randomly selected positive sera in our larger series [56] and suggests the presence of antigenic determinants common to striated muscle and thymus.

CLINICAL CORRELATIONS

Osserman and Weiner [59] recently reevaluated the criteria used by Strauss *et al.* [11] in 1960 for selection of myasthenic sera for potential immune reactivity against skeletal muscle. They studied coded randomized sera of 256 myasthenic patients, using the indirect immunofluorescence technique for γ-globulin binding.† Laboratory findings were subsequently correlated with (1) duration of disease, (2) progression and severity of disease, and (3) association with thymic pathology. Two thirds of the patients with disease for two years or less had reactive sera. Reactivity reached its peak incidence in patients with disease of two years' duration and showed a marked drop after five years' duration of illness. The over-all percentage of patients whose sera were reactive at a single point in time was 30, whereas in patients classed as group III and IV (described earlier), percentages of reactive sera were 68 and 45, respectively. Reactivity for skeletal muscle striations was three times as high in individuals whose symptoms were exacerbating, especially in those who had experienced myasthenic crisis. Sera from all twelve patients who were subsequently shown to have thymomas were reactive.

INTERPRETATIONS

We have dealt with reactivities of myasthenic sera in some detail because they provide the bulk of experimental evidence on which an autoimmune hypothesis for myasthenia gravis is based. None of the data can, however, be taken to indicate that any of these immune concomitants participate primarily or secondarily in production of muscle damage, impaired neuromuscular transmission, or clinical symptoms. The fact that antibodies to muscle occur in only one third of patients with myasthenia gravis who are randomly studied at one point in time might be taken as meaning that such reactivity is an incidental rather than a causative or functionally related factor. A single negative serum sample from a patient may, however, indicate very little retrospectively or prospectively about antibody in that patient. Osserman and Weiner [61] restudied 118 of the 256 myasthenic patients previously described [59] over an average period of one year. Twenty-seven (23 percent) of this group showed changes in immunofluorescence reactivity for skeletal muscle striations during the period of study. Changes were of two major types: (1) from positive to negative, and (2) from negative to positive. Several individuals showed further changes in that their sera showed more than one reversal during the study.

The virtually universal occurrence of antimuscle antibodies in sera of patients with myasthenia gravis having associated thymomas and the concurrence and probable cross-reactivity of antimuscle and antithymus factors in myasthenia gravis sera may provide the first clues to a possible functional relationship between this disease and thymic pathology.

Thymic pathology, in the form of "hyperplasia" with germinal follicle formation or a lymphoepithelioma-thymoma, is found in about 80 percent of patients with myasthenia gravis. "Hyperplasia" is roughly four to five times more common than thymoma. Specific facts regarding incidence and histopathology have been reviewed by Castleman [62] and others. Marshall and White [63, 64] have shown that injections of antigens into the

* Normal and disease control sera, when studied undiluted and in dilutions through 1 : 30, produced diffuse fluorescence of thymic tissue. No discrete reactivity in thymic epithelial cells could be detected under these conditions. We believe that the reactivity demonstrable in low titer against skeletal muscle when present in a nonmyasthenic serum is *not* associated with reactivity against thymic epithelial cells.

† Examined at a serum dilution of 1 : 60.

thymus of the guinea pig induced the formation of germinal centers, plasma cells, and antibody in that organ. The histology was reminiscent of that encountered with thymic "hyperplasia" associated with myasthenia gravis. Parenteral administration of the same antigens failed to induce these changes in the thymus. Marshall and White [63] suggested that a hemothymic barrier may exist under normal physiological conditions to prevent the antigenic stimulation of otherwise immunologically competent thymic cells and that germinal follicle formation in the thymus associated with myasthenia gravis may be the result of an intrinsic immunological disturbance in the thymus. Epithelial cells in thymoma associated with myasthenia gravis undergo neoplasia; the nature of any antigenic changes which might accompany this transformation is unknown. White and Marshall [54] have also demonstrated γ-globulin in cell sites within the medullae of myasthenic thymic "hyperplasias"; these sites appear, from published account, to correspond to germinal follicles. These observations, and those of van der Geld *et al.* [60] which strongly suggest cross-reactive antigenic determinants in skeletal muscle and thymus, indicate the need for tentative refinements and modification of the autoimmune hypothesis proposed by Nastuk *et al.* [10] and Simpson [43].* The hypothesis, with such changes, should accord the thymus some functional or pathogenic role in myasthenia gravis based on an immunological response perhaps intrinsic to the thymus. On the other hand, it may be that thymus and striated muscle, because of common and unique antigenic features, are subject to similar or identical pathogenic influences. These may be capable of producing disease in two otherwise unrelated tissues; the occurrence of cross-reacting antibodies may merely be nonfunctional indicators of this. Although the autoimmune hypothesis is still highly speculative, it offers promise for continued investigation.

REFERENCES

1. Osserman, K. E. *Myasthenia Gravis.* New York: Grune & Stratton, Inc., 1958.
2. Viets, H. R., and Gammon, G. (Eds.) First International Symposium on Myasthenia Gravis. *Amer. J. Med.* 19:655–742, 1955.
3. Viets, H. R. (Ed.) *Second International Symposium on Myasthenia Gravis.* Springfield, Ill.: Charles C Thomas, Publisher, 1961.
4. Desmedt, J. E. Myasthenic-like features of neuromuscular transmission after administration of an inhibitor of acetylcholine synthesis. *Nature* (London) 182:1674, 1958.
5. Dahlbäck, O., Elmqvist, D., Johns, T. R., Radner, S., and Thesleff, S. An electrophysiologic study of the neuromuscular junction in myasthenia gravis. *J. Physiol.* 156:336, 1961.
6. Coërs, C., and Desmedt, J. E. Improved method of obtaining biopsies of neuromuscular junction in man: Oscillographic delimitation of end-plate on exposed muscle. *Neurology* (Minneap.) 9:238, 1959.
7. MacDermot, V. The changes in the motor end-plate in myasthenia gravis. *Brain* 83:24, 1960.
8. Bickerstaff, E. R., and Woolf, A. L. The intramuscular nerve endings in myasthenia gravis. *Ibid.,* p. 10.
9. Zacks, S. R., Bauer, W. C., and Blumberg, J. M. The fine structure of the myasthenic neuromuscular junction. *J. Neuropath. Exp. Neurol.* 21:335, 1962.
10. Nastuk, W. L., Plescia, O. J., and Osserman,

* Additional information about the immunological aspects of myasthenia gravis is accumulating rapidly. Since the writing of this chapter, Adner *et al.* (*New Eng. J. Med.* 271:1327, 1964) reported that myasthenia gravis patients as a group are less susceptible than a group of controls to cutaneous sensitization with 1-chloro-2,4 dinitrobenzene (DNCB). In a recent Conference on Myasthenia Gravis (*Ann. N.Y. Acad. Sci.* 1965), several authors discussed the nature of immune globulins which develop during the course of this disease, and of related diseases. Strauss *et al.* found circulating antibodies against skeletal muscle and thymus in 10 of 33 nonmyasthenic individuals with thymomas, or histories of thymomas. Titers were in the same range as titers in the serum of myasthenia gravis patients. Sera from 200 patients with other neoplasms, on the other hand, did not contain antibodies. Douglas, Gottlieb, and co-workers examined the fine structural details of the binding of globulin to muscle with direct and indirect ferritin-immunoelectronmicroscopic techniques: ferritin conjugated gamma globulin localized in the H-Zone of the A-Band excluding the bare area [45a, 46]. McFarlin *et al.* were unable to demonstrate localization of fluorescent myasthenic serum γ-globulins in those neuromuscular junctions which could be identified by enzymatic staining. Weiner and Osserman established that the highest incidence of positive immunofluorescence to muscle and thymus occurs within the first year of the disease, in blood samples of patients obtained shortly after its onset.

K. E. Changes in serum complement activity in patients with myasthenia gravis. *Proc. Soc. Exp. Biol. Med.* 105:177, 1960.

11. Strauss, A. J. L., Seegal, B. C., Hsu, K. C., Burkholder, P. M., Nastuk, W. L., and Osserman, K. E. Immunofluorescence demonstration of a muscle binding, complement-fixing serum globulin fraction in myasthenia gravis. *Ibid.,* p. 184.
12. Beutner, E. H., Witebsky, E., Ricken, D., and Adler, R. H. Studies on autoantibodies in myasthenia gravis. *J.A.M.A.* 182:46, 1962.
13. Burnet, F. M. The new approach to immunology. *New Eng. J. Med.* 264:24, 1961.
14. Miller, J. F. A. P., Marshall, A. H. E., and White, R. G. The Immunological Significance of the Thymus. In Taliaferro, W. H. and Humphrey, J. H., (Eds.), *Advances in Immunology,* Vol. 2. New York: Academic Press, Inc., 1962.
15. Willis, T. *Two Discourses Concerning the Soul of Brutes* (tr. by S. Pordage). London: 1683.
16. Wilks, S. On cerebritis, hysteria and bulbar paralysis, as illustrative of arrest of function of the cerebrospinal centres. *Guy's Hosp. Rep.* 22:7, 1877.
17. Jolly, F. Ueber Myasthenia gravis pseudoparalytica. *Berl. Klin. Wschr.* 32:1, 1895.
18. Laquer, L., and Weigert, C. Beiträge zur Lehre von der Erb'schen Krankheit (Myasthenia Gravis). *Neurol. Zbl.* 20:594, 1901.
19. Castleman, B., and Norris, E. H. Pathology of the thymus in myasthenia gravis. *Medicine* 28:27, 1949.
20. Genkins, G., Mendelow, H., Sobel, H. J., and Osserman, K. E. Myasthenia Gravis: Analysis of Thirty-One Consecutive Post-Mortem Examinations. Ref. 3.
21. Schwab, R. S., and Leland, C. Sex and age in myasthenia gravis as critical factors in incidence and remission. *J.A.M.A.* 153:1270, 1953.
22. Osserman, K. E., and Genkins, G. Studies in myasthenia gravis. *New York J. Med.* 61:2076, 1961.
23. Eaton, L. M., and Lambert, E. H. Electromyography and electric stimulation of motor unit. *J.A.M.A.* 163:1117, 1957.
24. Rowland, L. P., and Eskenazi, A. N. Myasthenia gravis with features resembling muscular dystrophy. *Neurology* 6:667, 1956.
25. Osserman, K. E., and Silver, S. The Differential Diagnosis of Myopathy as Seen in Hyperthyroidism and Myasthenia Gravis. In Pitt-Rivers, R. (Ed.), *Fourth International Goitre Conference.* London: Pergamon Press, 1960.
26. Walker, M. B. Case showing effect of prostigmin on myasthenia gravis. *Proc. Roy. Soc. Med.* 28:759, 1935.
27. Viets, H. R., and Schwab, R. S. Prostigmin in the diagnosis of myasthenia gravis. *New Eng. J. Med.* 213:1280, 1935.
28. Osserman, K. E. Progress report on Mestinon bromide (pyridostigmine bromide). *Amer. J. Med.* 19:737, 1955.
29. Schwab, R. S. WIN-8077 in the treatment of sixty myasthenia gravis patients: A twelve-month report. *Ibid.,* p. 734.
30. Osserman, K. E., and Kaplan, L. I. Rapid diagnostic test for myasthenia gravis: Increased muscle strength without fasciculations after intravenous administration of edrophonium (Tensilon) chloride. *J.A.M.A.* 150:265, 1952.
31. Osserman, K. E., Kaplan, L. I., and Besson, G. Studies in myasthenia gravis: Edrophonium chloride (Tensilon) test as a new approach to management. *J. Mount Sinai Hosp. N.Y.* 20: 165, 1953.
32. Osserman, K. E., and Kaplan, L. I. Studies in myasthenia gravis: Use of edrophonium chloride (Tensilon) in differentiating myasthenic from cholinergic weakness. *Arch. Neurol. & Psych.* (Chicago) 70:385, 1953.
33. Grob, D., and Johns, R. Use of Oximes in the treatment of intoxication by anticholinesterase compounds in patients with myasthenia gravis. *Amer. J. Med.* 24:512, 1958.
34. Osserman, K. E., and Genkins, G. Studies in myasthenia gravis: Reduction in mortality rate after crisis. *J.A.M.A.* 183:97, 1963.
35. Blalock, A., Mason, M. F., Morgan, H. J., and Riven, S. S. Myasthenia gravis and tumors of the thymic region. *Ann. Surg.* 110:544, 1939.
36. Genkins, G., Kreel, I., Jacobson, E., Osserman, K. E., and Baronofsky, I. D. Studies in myasthenia gravis: Technical care of thymectomy patient. *Bull. N.Y. Acad. Med.* 36:826, 1960.
37. Keynes, G. Surgery of the thymus gland: Second (and third) thoughts. *Lancet* 1:1197, 1954.
38. Bernatz, P. E., Harrison, E. G., and Clagett, O. T. Thymoma: A clinicopathologic study. *J. Thorac. Cardiov. Surg.* 42:424, 1961.
39. Harvey, A. M., and Johns, R. J. Myasthenia gravis and the thymus. *Amer. J. Med.* 32:1, 1962.
40. Walker, M. B. Myasthenia gravis: A case in which fatigue of forearm muscles could induce paralysis of the extra-ocular muscles. *Proc. Roy. Soc. Med.* 31:722, 1938.
41. Nastuk, W. L., Strauss, A. J. L., and Osserman, K. E. Search for a neuromuscular blocking agent in the blood of patients with myasthenia gravis. *Amer. J. Med.* 26:394, 1959.

42. Windsor, C. E. Preliminary Report on the Effect of the Serum of Myasthenia Gravis Patients on the Neuromuscular Transmission of the Intact Frog. Ref. 3.
43. Simpson, J. A. Myasthenia gravis: A new hypothesis. *Scot. Med. J.* 5:419, 1960.
44. Strauss, A. J. L. Autoimmune response in myasthenia gravis. *Lancet* 2:351, 1962.
45. Feltkamp, T. E. W., van der Geld, H., and Oosterhuis, H. J. G. H. Studies on sera from cases of myasthenia gravis, using the fluorescent antibody technique. *Vox Sang.* 8:317, 1963.
45a. Nastuk, W. L., Kessler, H. J., Grynbaum, A., Smith, M., and Herman, Jr., C. Effect of thymectomy on circulating anti-muscle antibodies, serum complement activity and the clinical status of patients with myasthenia gravis. To be published.
46. Strauss, A., Deitch, A., and Hsu, K. Further observations on the localization of a muscle binding, complement fixing serum globulin fraction in myasthenia gravis. *Fed. Proc.* 20:38, 1961.
47. Huxley, H. E., and Hanson, J. The Molecular Basis of Contraction in Cross Striated Muscles. In Bourne, G. H., (Ed.), *Structure and Function of Muscle;* Vol. I., *Structure.* New York: Academic Press, Inc., 1960.
48. Engel, W. K. The essentiality of histo- and cytochemical studies of skeletal muscle in the investigation of neuromuscular disease. *Neurology* (Minneap.) 12:778, 1962.
49. Grob, D., and Namba, T. Complement fixation by muscle nucleoprotein and serum of patients with myasthenia gravis and other diseases. *J. Clin. Invest.* 42:940, 1963.
50. Lang, R., and Shulman, S. Precipitation analysis of muscle antibodies in human serum. *Fed. Proc.* 23:342, 1964.
51. Beutner, E. H., Witebsky, E., and Leff, I. Autoimmune responses in myasthenia gravis: Observations on S and SH antigens, on species specificity and on *in vivo* reactions. *Fed. Proc.* 22:217, 1963.
51a. Beutner, E. H., Witebsky, E., and Djanian, A. Y. Serologic studies of myasthenia gravis. *Ann. N.Y. Acad. Sci.,* 1965.
52. Djanian, A. Y., Beutner, E. H., and Witebsky, E. Tanned-cell hemagglutination test for detection of antibodies in sera of patients with myasthenia gravis. *J. Lab. Clin. Med.* 63:60, 1964.
53. Hess, J. W., Stecker, S., Gordon, S., and Wolf, P. L. Evidence for the binding of fluorescein-tagged gamma globulin to muscle in myasthenia gravis. *Clin. Res.* 10:294, 1962.
54. White, R. G., and Marshall, A. H. E. The autoimmune response in myasthenia gravis. *Lancet* 2:120, 1962.
55. Sturgill, B. C., Carpenter, R. R., Strauss, A. J. L., and Goodman, H. C. Antibodies in systemic lupus erythematosus and myasthenia gravis which react with thermally denatured DNA-coated bentonite. *Proc. Soc. Exp. Biol. Med.* 115:246, 1964.
56. Strauss, A. J. L., van der Geld, H. W. R., Kemp, P. G., Jr., Exum, E. D., and Goodman, H. C. Immunological concomitants of myasthenia gravis. *Ann. N.Y. Acad. Sci.,* 1965 (in press); see also *Fed. Proc.* 23:341 and 342, 1964.
56a. Rowland, L. P. Personal communication, 1964.
57. Van der Geld, H., and Oosterhuis, H. J. G. H. Muscle and thymus antibodies in myasthenia gravis. *Vox Sang.* 8:196, 1963.
58. Van der Geld, H., Feltkamp, T. E. W., van Loghem, J. J., Oosterhuis, H. J. G. H., and Biemond, A. Multiple antibody production in myasthenia gravis. *Lancet* 2:373, 1963.
59. Osserman, K. E., and Weiner, L. B. Studies in myasthenia gravis: fluorescent tagging of muscle striation with antibody from serums of 256 myasthenic patients. *Ann. N.Y. Acad. Sci.,* 1965 (in press).
59a. Hess, J. W. Personal communication, 1964.
60. Van der Geld, H., Feltkamp, T. E. W., and Oosterhuis, H. J. G. H. Reactivity of myasthenia gravis serum γ-globulin with skeletal muscle and thymus demonstrated by immunofluorescence. *Proc. Soc. Exp. Biol. Med.* 115: 782, 1964.
61. Osserman, K. E., and Weiner, L. B. Studies in myasthenia gravis: Changes in muscle binding reactivity in patient serums, as demonstrated by immunofluorescence, and correlated with clinical course (to be published).
62. Castleman, B. Tumors of the Thymus Gland. *Atlas of Tumor Pathology,* Sect. V, Fasc. 19. Washington, D.C.: American Registry of Pathology, Armed Forces Institute of Pathology, 1955.
63. Marshall, A. H. E., and White, R. G. Experimental thymic lesions resembling those of myasthenia gravis. *Lancet* 1:1030, 1961.
64. Marshall, A. H. E., and White, R. G. The Immunological reactivity of the thymus. *Brit. J. Exp. Path.* 42: 379, 1961.

Index

p 27 – antigen sRNA complex
? antibodies develop through incorporation of foreign protein into host mRNA ? specifying antibody